Southern Medicine and Surgery

(Volume CVI)

Editor

James M. Northington

Alpha Editions

This edition published in 2020

ISBN : 9789354047800

Design and Setting By
Alpha Editions
www.alphaedis.com
email - alphaedis@gmail.com

As per information held with us this book is in Public Domain.
This book is a reproduction of an important historical work. Alpha Editions uses the best technology to reproduce historical work in the same manner it was first published to preserve its original nature. Any marks or number seen are left intentionally to preserve its true form.

SOUTHERN MEDICINE & SURGERY

•

Official Organ
of the
TRI-STATE MEDICAL ASSOCIATION
of the
CAROLINAS AND VIRGINIA

JAMES M. NORTHINGTON, M. D., *Editor*

VOLUME CVI

Published by
Charlotte Medical Press
Charlotte, N. C.

THE JOURNAL OF SOUTHERN MEDICINE AND SURGERY

306 North Tryon Street, Charlotte, N. C.

The Journal assumes no responsibility for the authenticity of opinion or statements made by authors or in communications submitted to this Journal for publication.

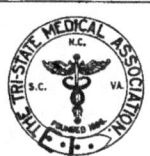

JAMES M. NORTHINGTON, M. D., Editor

VOL. CVI   JANUARY, 1944   No. 1

Clinical Effects of Suspensions of Estrone and Stilbestrol*

Herbert S. Kupperman, Ph.D., and Robert B. Greenblatt, M.D.**
Augusta, Georgia

IT HAS BEEN THE AIM of clinical endocrinologists to find a proper vehicle for hormone medication which would allow for slow and continuous release of the active principle to the organism in much the same manner that endogenous hormone is secreted into the blood stream from the glands of internal secretion. While it is true that the pellet method of hormone administration has been shown to fairly closely fill these requirements, it still has some major disadvantages such as expense, difficulty of manufacture of sterile pellets, and the procedure of implantation which, in itself, is not without some discomfort. On the other hand parenteral administration of aqueous suspensions or ester suspensions of gonadal hormones, although not having the physiological effect of implanted pellets, nevertheless have a relatively prolonged action, while the mode of administration entails little discomfort.[1] Esterification of the steroid hormones particularly by the higher fatty acids results in some loss of actual activity.[2] However, this is more than compensated for since the esterified preparation has a prolonged action in comparison to the unconjugated compound through the slow absorption of the hormone from the site of injection. Administration of aqueous estrone simulates pellet implanted estrogens in action since by the injection of these suspensions minute amounts of estrogens are implanted subcutaneously or intramuscularly. This process likewise insures a slow absorption of the hormone with a relative prolonged effect. The following report presents some of the results in the clinical investigation of two such preparations, stilbestrol dipalmitate suspended in sesame oil and aqueous estrone, and is only preliminary in scope.*

Clinical studies were done on a total of twenty-two patients. Sixteen had typical menopausal symptoms, four complained of dysmenorrhea of long duration, and two suffered from senile vaginitis. In all cases therapy consisted of single doses of 5 mg. of stilbestrol dipalmitate or aqueous estrone administered at weekly intervals. In only two cases untoward side reactions of nausea were noted. This developed in one patient receiving aqueous estrone and another treated with stilbestrol dipalmitate.

All the patients with a menopausal syndrome so treated obtained general symptomatic relief after one injection of the hormone. The predominant complaint of hot flashes in this group of patients was effectively controlled. Paresthesia (formication), present in about 75 per cent of the patients, was also alleviated by this hormone therapy. In two patients whose major complaint was menopau-

---

*The stilbestrol dipalmitate and aqueous estrone were supplied by Abbott Laboratories, North Chicago, Illinois.

*From Department of Experimental Medicine, University of Georgia School of Medicine, Augusta.
**Present address: Surgeon, Reserve Corps, U. S. P. H. Service, Southeastern Medical Center, Oatland Island, Savannah.

sal headaches, stilbestrol dipalmitate therapy produced complete relief in one and partial alleviation in the other.

Vaginal smears were made before and after therapy. Both forms of estrogens brought about complete maturation of the vaginal epithelium in those patients who exhibited an atrophic or castrate smear on examination. An indication of the high estrogenic potency of these hormone preparations and of their prolonged effect may be noted from the fact that after a single injection of either hormone maturation of the castrate vaginal epithelium frequently occurred, with maintenance of this state for one to two weeks.

Four patients in the menopausal series complained of concomitant arthralgia. Of these one received complete relief, one partial, and no alleviation of pain was noted in the remaining two.

The two patients treated for senile vaginitis received complete relief after one injection of 5 mg. of stilbestrol dipalmitate. Complete restoration of the atrophic vaginal epithelium followed the initial injection and was accompanied by symptomatic relief. Recurrence of vaginal irritation was prevented by weekly or biweekly injections of 5 mg. of stilbestrol dipalmitate.

In the treatment of patients with dysmenorrhea we have found that many cases have responded favorably to large doses of estrogen administered at least one week prior to expected onset of menses. We have tried this same regimen in cases of severe dysmenorrhea of long duration, using 5 mg. of stilbestrol dipalmitate for the therapeutic dose. In all four patients complete relief was obtained after one injection of the hormone when given one week to ten days before the expected menstrual period. One case in particular is worthy of note: This patient—a colored girl, 17 years of age—for the past few years suffered intense pain with each menstrual period, which completely incapacitated her for several days. She had so despaired of further unfruitful treatment that she had requested hysterectomy if relief could not be obtained from the dipalmitate therapy. A single injection of 5 mg. of stilbestrol dipalmitate was given seven to ten days before the expected menstrual period for three successive months. The patient obtained complete relief from her painful menstruation. In addition, it may be said that in this case the treatment has resulted in more than a temporary alleviation of the dysmenorrhea since the patient has experienced normal periods for the past six months.

Although our series of patients is too small to make any statistical comparison of the effectiveness of stilbestrol dipalmitate and aqueous estrone with other parenteral estrogens, some general conclusions may be stated. Suspensions of aqeous estrone and stilbestrol dipalmitate are found to be effective estrogens in controlling the symptoms of the climacteric, senile vaginitis, and dysmenorrhea. Invariably 5 mg. of either substance, when given in one injection, was of sufficient strength to alleviate the major complaint and had such a prolonged action that one injection sufficed for at least one to two weeks. The only toxic phenomenon produced by the drug was nausea and this was found to present in only two of the twenty-two patients (9.0%). The degree of nausea or gastro-intestinal disturbance observed by us compares favorably with that reported in an earlier paper on stilbestrol dipalmitate.[3]

SUMMARY

Suspensions of crystalline estrone in water and stilbestrol dipalmitate in sesame oil were injected in doses of 5 mg. each into a series of patients complaining of menopausal symptoms, senile vaginitis, or dysmenorrhea. The vasomotor and autonomic complaints of the menopausal patient were temporarily but effectively controlled and dissipated by a single weekly injection of these substances. Restoration of the atrophic vaginal epithelium in the climacteric individual was brought about by this mode of therapy. Senile vaginitis observed in two patients was alleviated by a single injection of stilbestrol dipalmitate and the mature "estrus" phase of the vaginal epithelium was maintained by weekly injections of the estrogenic substance. Four cases of dysmenorrhea were effectively treated by administering a single dose of 5 mg. of stilbestrol dipalmitate seven to ten days prior to the expected menstrual period. This method of treatment has proved to be a satisfactory regimen for the control of dysmenorrhea and in certian instances has led to a permanent alleviation of the syndrome. Nausea, the only untoward reaction that was noted, was experienced by only two of the twenty-two patients treated with these preparations.

Aqueous estrone and stilbestrol palmitate are worthy additions to our hormonal armamentarium.

References

1. FREED, S. C., and GREENHILL, J. P.: Therapeutic Use of Estrone Suspensions. *J. Clin. End.*, 1, 983; 1941.
2. DODDS, E. C., GOLBERG, L., LAWSON, W., and ROBINSON, SIR ROBERT: Synthetic estrogenic compounds related to stilbene and diphenylethane. *Proc. Roy Soc. London*, S. B. 127, 140; 1939.
3. FREED, S. C., EISIN, W. M., and GREENHILL, J. P.: Therapeutic efficiency of diethylstilbestrol esters. *J. A. M. A.*, 119, 1412; 1942.

SMALLPOX.—For the month of July 738 cases were reported in Turkey. It is of interest to reflect that it was in Turkey Lady Mary Wortley Montague learned of *inoculation* against smallpox, had her little son so treated and took the information home to England. 80 years before Jenner announced his discovery of the protective value of *vaccination*.

Differential Diagnostic Implications From the Complaints of Patients With Cardiovascular Disease*

T. S. USSERY, M.D., Statesville, North Carolina
Henry F. Long Hospital

THE MOST striking and most important of the acute manifestations in a cardiac case is cardiac pain proper, and angina pectoris is the most important cardiac pain. Since the days of pseudo angina terminology there has been a distinction between the nervous and organic forms of heart disease, whose differentiation is of the greatest importance. Genetically, these forms are also extremely different. In the nervous form a moderate spasm occurs in the coronary vessels without the change pathologic in the vessels. It is different in genuine angina pectoris; to be sure, spasms occur here but only in changed vessels. Marked changes in the nutrition of the heart muscles are likely to occur; as a result of over-working of the heart muscles, a blood vessel can become thrombosed and then a grave condition develops, coronary thrombosis or occlusion.

The nervous form found in young persons, more frequent in the young physically and mentally unstable woman, unhappily married.

Genuine angina pectoris appears at a later age (45 to 60), is in most cases independent of psychgenic factors and depends strongly upon physical exertion. Between the attacks the patients do not impress one as being ill or nervous. In the nervous forms, no pains are experienced at night and no attacks occur.

Of great significance in the differential diagnosis are previous diseases. In these cases the heart and vessels are usually normal. In true angina pectoris the vessels of the heart show organic changes by the ecg. tracings. In the functional type no pathologic changes can be demonstrated. The accounts of the patient in the nervous forms are usually dramatic: "I was sure death had struck me," or "I was sure I was dying." These cases as a rule have a rapid heart rate. In organic diseases the pain is as of a dagger piercing the chest or of a claw gripping the heart hard; with radiation of the pain to the left shoulder and arm, rarely to the right shoulder and arm and into the neck and back, or to either or both angles of the jaw. In a very short time the patient can perform considerable work. In contrast, a heart after a real attack of angina is not capable of carrying on its work in a normal way.

Most reliable for the recognition of the severity of the attack are the duration and severity of the pain with transition into a status anginosus—an occlusion with cardiac infarct. White, Christian and Roberts agree that an attack of real angina, lasting longer than 30 to 40 minutes, not relieved by the nitrites, should be considered coronary occlusion until proven otherwise.

Cardiac oppression must be differentiated from attacks of angina pectoris. Its intensity is much less, the duration of the complaint is often prolonged, and there is a sensation of anxiety. Patients frequently report that it is not a real pain that tortures them. This uneasy sensation in the precordial region is frequently found in old individuals with coronary sclerosis, in all forms of hypertension and kidney affections, also improperly functioning hearts. The ecg. is helpful in making a correct diagnosis.

A wholly different form of cardiac pain in the aortic region is the so-called aortalgia, especially in the syphilitic or aortic type. These pains are overwhelming and often of considerable duration, felt over the upper part of the sternum, and not over the entire heart. The differentiation is made solely by röntgenologic evidence of dilatation of the arch of the aorta and a history of syphilis.

Other pains in the cardiac region, as those caused by acute pericarditis, are more commonly localized in the upper part of the heart. Demonstration of a pericardial rub and a high white and pmn. count are of great importance.

A common complaint in a cardiac case, real or functional, is shortness of breath, dyspnea, especially with diseases of the pleura and mediastinal disturbances, such as mediastinal tumors, either benign or malignant. When these diseases can be excluded and there is definite evidence of cardiac changes, dyspnea has a considerable significance in differential diagnosis. Shortness of breath often occurs in organic heart disease during rest. The attacks are short but may be frequent. Cerebral dyspnea occurs especially at night, when the blood supply to the vasomotor center is insufficient, and cardiac asthma is not at all simple to differentiate in these cases. Dyspnea may be caused by restriction of the function of the lungs. Hypostasis and

*Presented to Ninth (N. C.) District Medical Society meeting at Statesville, September 30th.

bronchopneumonia or stasis may develop in the lungs and result in pulmonary edema. Often in the aged an effusion occurs in the right pleural cavity. I have seen two such cases in the Walter Reed Hospital and all of these cases lead to dyspnea. Some cardiac patients complain of pressure in the stomach and loss of appetite as the first sign, and these symptoms may be considered by the patient and physician as independent gastric signs, until the disappearance of the symptoms after cardiac therapy.

Paralleling processes in the blood vessels of the brain are frequent in the syphilitic and the arteriosclerotic. These bring about slight or profuse hemorrhages, especially in all types of hypertension. Similar disturbances may be caused by a poor blood supply to the brain of the cardiac patients. Thus, one sees Cheyne-Stokes breathing, irrational states, and disorientation—always giving a bad prognosis. These patients must be closely guarded.

Hepatic congestion occurs but is easily recognized. With the exception of infarct, splenic lesions seldom cause discomfort in cardiac conditions.

Renal congestion does not cause pain, but produces congestive urine. Its quantity is small, the decrease paralleling the cardiac insufficiency. The urine is highly colored, of high specific gravity, often contains much albumin and many casts, and in many cases there is erroneous assumption that, apart from the cardiac insufficiency there is an independent kidney affection. As improvement goes on urinary secretion increases and the pathological elements disappear.

Differentiation of a real kidney condition can be today easily made through blood chemistry examinations. Often in the aged, it is necessary to observe the quantity of residual urine, and the chemical constitution of the blood over a period of several days, even weeks, before one can definitely diagnose real kidney pathology.

MEDICAL ETHICS IN ANCIENT CHINA
(T'ao Lee, Peiping, in *Chinese Med. Jl.*, April-June)

Sun Ssu-miao (581-673 A. D.), the father of medicine in China, discusses the duties of a physician to his patients and to the public.

"Medicine is an art which is difficult to master. A foolish fellow, after reading medical formularies for three years, will believe that all diseases can be cured. But, after practicing for another three years, he will realize that most formulae are not effective. A physician should, therefore, be a scholar, mastering all the medical literature and working carefully and tirelessly.

A doctor, when treating a patient, should make himself quiet and determined. He should have bowels of mercy on the sick and pledge himself to relieve suffering among all classes. He should look upon the misery of the patient as if it were his own and be anxious to relieve the distress, disregarding his own inconveniences. Even foul cases, such as ulcer, abscess, diarrhoea, etc., should be treated without the slightest antipathy. One who follows this principle is a great doctor, otherwise, he is a great thief.

It is a great mistake to boast of himself and slander other physicians.

He should not prescribe dear and rare drugs just because the patient is rich or of high rank, nor is it honest and just to do so for boasting.

Lao Tze said: "Open acts of kindness will be regarded by man while secret acts of evil will be punished by God."

A NEW SULFA COMPOUND, DESOXYEPHEDRONIUM SULFATHIAZOLE, FOR THE TREATMENT OF SINUSITIS
(W. F. Hamilton *et al.*, Los Angeles, in *The Laryngoscope*, Aug.)

A new group of sulfa compounds was discovered as a result of work on stabilization of aqueous solutions of salts of the sulfa drugs, and incorporation of vasoconstrictors, to give the optimum shrinkage, drainage and ventilation, without the after-effects so commonly experienced with use of the usual vasoconstrictors—sneezing, tachycardia and nervousness.

In acute sinusitis the treatment included spraying the nasal membranes with 1 per cent solution of cocaine, followed by insertion of tampons medicated with 20 minims of D.O.E. Sulfa, shrinking the congested mucous membrane just short of that noticed with the use of adrenalin, yet without blanching, sneezing or subsequent swelling.

For home treatment patients were instructed to use spray or drops often enough to keep the nose open, beginning at five-minute intervals, usually two or three times, until the deeper tissues in the nose were reached.

Chronic sinusitis was treated by irrigating the affected sinuses and following with the instillation of the solution into the sinuses, and the use of spray or drops at home.

Acute pharyngitis and laryngitis, too, were treated by spraying the nose and throat and, in office treatments, also the larynx and upper trachea.

Acute suppurative otitis media was treated by myringotomy and medicated tampons in office treatment, and by drops in the ear and nose and in the epipharynx by the patient at home.

VALUE OF PROCTOSCOPY IN THE DIAGNOSIS OF AMEBIASIS
(R. J. Jackman & W. L. Cooper, Rochester, Minn., in *Jl. Dig. Dis.*, Oct.)

A study of 115 consecutive patients who had amebic dysentery was made for evaluating proctoscopy in the diagnosis of the condition.

Ulceration of the lower part of the bowel, suggestive of amebiasis as determined by proctoscopy, was found in 20.8% of the cases.

Biopsy and scrapings from the ulcers at the time of proctoscopy afforded the diagnosis in two cases in which repeated examinations of stools had given negative results.

In comparison with the other infectious types of diarrhea, anal abscess and anal fistula were not common complications.

The occasional coëxistence of a carcinoma or other tumefactive lesion with amebic dysentery is sufficient frequent to warrant proctoscopy in every case in which amebic dysentery is suspected.

"IN ONE large Eastern city the names of the two leading abortionists are more widely known than that of the local Methodist bishop or the baseball manager," says Associate Professor of Obstetrics Guttmacher, of Johns Hopkins, in the *West. Va. Med. Jl.*

INTESTINAL PARASITES have been demonstrated by giving the patient a specially prepared meal and showing by x-ray examination that the worms have ingested some of the opaque material.—*Donaldson.*

Diagnosis and Treatment of Primary Atypical Pneumonia*

VERNON D. OFFUTT, M.D., Kinston, North Carolina

RECENTLY the widespread occurrence in this country of an epidemic form of nonbacterial pneumonia, described variously as acute influenzal pneumonitis, desseminated focal pneumonia and viral pneumonia, has renewed our interest in this respiratory disease.

The essential clinical characteristics of primary atypical pneumonia have been described in a number of publications over the past nine years. Allen, in 1935, analyzed and reported on 50 cases at Fort Sam Houston, which conformed essentially to those seen recently. He used the term acute pneumonitis to designate a form of respiratory infection characterized by a benign course, few physical signs and x-ray evidence of a localized inflammatory process in the lungs.

In 1938, Reimann reported on eight cases occurring in Philadelphia and made studies to determine the etiological agent. These were all negative for the influenza virus A and B, as well as for psittacosis virus, which is known to produce similar pulmonary lesions. A filterable infectious agent was recovered from the nasopharynx of one and from the blood of another, but evidence that it was actually the cause of the disease was incomplete. Reimann was therefore led to regard it as a separate disease entity pending further study. According to British investigators the probability of obtaining the virus diminishes rapidly after the third day and they also suggest that when the virus attacks the lungs there is less of it in the upper respiratory tract.

Examinations of the sputum in all our cases but one showed the usual nasopharyngeal and upper bronchial flora such as streptococcus viridans, staphylococci, diphtheroids, gram-negative bacilli and occasionally pneumococci of the higher types. In the one case which showed tubercle bacilli, tuberculous disease coëxisted.

CLINICAL FEATURES

Reports of this disease indicate that there is a wide variation in the intensity of the symptoms and a great diversity of signs—from the most severe cases with encephalitis to the milder respiratory cases—which would suggest that no single etiologic factor is in all instances responsible for the disease.

The essential features of our cases were as follows:

1. Variable upper respiratory symptoms and signs.
2. Repeated chills and fever.
3. Profuse sweating.
4. Non-productive cough.
5. Lacks of physical signs first 3 to 5 days.
6. Normal leucocyte count and differential.
7. Normal sedimentation rate.
8. Non-specific sputum.
9. Non-response to sulfonamides.
10. X-ray evidence.

The discrepancy between the physical and the x-ray signs is marked, and neither are always characteristic. Diffuse soft mottling fanning out from the hilum and fading into normal lung is the rule, not as dense as in lobar pneumonia and may show involvement of one or all lobes simultaneously or successively. The lesion may advance in one portion of lung while regressing at the original site. Resolution as shown by x-rays generally lags considerably behind clinical improvement.

TREATMENT

The treatment of the disease has been entirely symptomatic and quite unsatisfactory. Adequate fluid intake, codeine sufficient to control cough and medicated steam inhalations appear to have some effect in loosening secretions. The sulfonamides if used at all are given in the first days as a diagnostic and therapeutic test. If there is no response in 36 to 48 hours, certainly after the diagnosis is established, drugs of this class are discontinued. There is evidence that they may do harm if their use is continued, or even used at all.

Due to this unsatisfactory state of treatment and because of the prolonged period of fatigue which disables some victims for as long as four to six weeks we have endeavored to find more effective means of treatment. Although the results of x-ray therapy of lobar pneumonia are well known there is little information available on treatment of atypical pneumonia. Oppenheimer[1] has reported on a series of 56 cases, in none of which had there been favorable response to medical treatment, and failure to respond to sulfonamide therapy was considered diagnostic of this atypical form of pneumonia. Forty-five were termed cured in three to five days. The remainder were of over 14 days duration. Answers to inquiries made of several institutions are that x-ray treatment has not been

---
*Presented to the 1943 (Dec.) meeting of the Seaboard Medical Assoc. held at Richmond.

used so far in treatment of the viral pneumonias.

Accordingly, we made a point to treat all cases of primary atypical pneumonia with x-ray therapy since September and we have thus handled twelve cases to this writing. Our cases received 100-r. doses, daily or every other day, depending on severity and response, alternating front and back or alternating sides if both lungs were involved. None received more than the fourth dose and the majority had three. The temperature began to decline after the first treatment and usually after the second or third dose responded by rapid lysis. One case which was referred after ten days treatment for an associated sinus infection responded equally well after the second treatment.

With surprising uniformity fever and symptoms subsided and after one or two treatments most of the patients spent their first comfortable night after days of harassing cough and great discomfort. With but one exception all cases were fever-free and discharged from the hospital in one week or less. The one exceptional case was complicated by severe diabetes and in this case there developed a sterile effusion after treatment which was later absorbed and a normal recovery was made. No unfavorable reactions occurred in our cases with this therapy. In the presence of leukopenia no further decrease in white cells was observed.

Our investigation is continuing. However, with the cases thus far handled it is our opinion that röntgen therapy is the most effective mode of treatment for control of the cough and fever, and that it greatly hastens convalescence.

REFERENCES

ALLEN, W. H.: Acute Pneumonitis. *Ann. Int. Med.*, 10: 441; 1936.
REIMANN, H. A.: An Acute Infection of Respiratory Tract With Atypical Pneumonia. *Jour. A. M. A.*, 111: 2377; 1938.
MACLEOD, C. M.: Primary Atypical Pneumonia. *Med. Clinics of N. America*, May, 1943.
OPPENHEIMER, A.: Röntgen Therapy of Virus Pneumonia. *Amer. Jour. of Roentgenology*, 49: No. 5.
—Kinston Clinic

MEDICAL AND SURGICAL RELIEF COMMITTEE
OF AMERICA
(420 Lexington Avenue, New York City)

This committee appeals to every doctor for help:
Dear Doctor:
There is a critical need for medical and surgical supplies that may lie hidden and forgotten in your office: discarded or tarnished instruments . . . surplus drugs . . . vitamins . . . infant foods. Collected, packaged, sent to the Medical and Surgical Relief Committee, they can play a vital role in its program of medical relief for the armed and civilian forces of the United Nations.
The work of warzone hospitals and welfare agencies is too often crippled by the lack of medical supplies. Community nurseries in this country, refugee camps abroad cry out for vitamins and baby foods for their ill-nourished charges.

This committee has supplied over 900 sub-hunting and patrolling ships of the Navy with emergency medical kits; equipped battle-dressing stations on warships. The Fighting French in North Africa; the Royal Norwegians in Canada and Iceland; the West Indies; South and Central Africa; China; India; Great Britain; Yugoslavia; Greece; Syria; Russia and Alaska call on us.

To meet the demands that pour in the committee needs all types of instruments, especially clamps, scalpels, forceps and all kinds of drugs from iodine to sulfa products. By contributing what you can spare, you will help speed another shipment of sorely-needed medical aid.

(Signed) Joseph Peter Hoguet, M.D.,
Medical Director.

CRITICAL EVALUATION OF SKIN TESTS IN ALLERGY DIAGNOSIS
(Louis Tuft, in *Jl. Allergy*, July)

Skin testing could be made more accurate diagnostically by: 1) Better preparation and standardization of the allergens used for testing; 2) standardization of the technic of application; 3) report of reactions as simply positive, negative or doubtful (with possible explanatory detail); 4) more accurate differentiation between clinical and non-clinical positive reactions; 5) better standardization of the inhalants used for nasal application; 6) elimination of many substances known to be of little or no allergic importance; 7) additional research to isolate active excitants and to determine their nature and their antigenic relationships.

CHLOROFORMED IN BATTLE-WAGONS
(*Squibb Memoranda*)

Severely injured tankmen, who cannot be removed from their "battle-wagons" without the danger of further shock, are anesthetized before their rescue is attempted through the narrow aperture leading from the tank. In this work a cloth mesh chloroform ampul, now being produced by Squibb, is in wide use on battlefields where tanks comprise the spearhead of attack. Chloroform can be used here because it is not explosive and therefore does not add to the fire hazard. It is also easy for a non-medical person to administer chloroform, and under combat conditions the emergency may call for such administration.

IT WOULD APPEAR unlikely that heredity is of primary importance in the etiology of hypertension.—Feldt, R. H., & Wenstrand, D. E. W., in *Amer. Jl. Med Sci.*, Jan.

SHOULD VITAMIN D BE GIVEN ONLY TO INFANTS?

Vitamin D has been so successful in preventing rickets during infancy that there has been little emphasis on continuing its use after the second year.

A careful study* reveals a high incidence of rickets in children 2 to 14 years old. Postmortem examination of 230 children of this age group showed the total prevalence of rickets to be 46.5%.

Rachitic changes were found as late as the fourteenth year, and the incidence was higher among children dying from acute disease than in those dying of chronic disease.

The authors doubt if the slight degrees of rickets found in many of the children interfere with health and development, but "our studies afford reason to prolong administration of vitamin D to the fourteenth year, and especially indicate the necessity to suspect and to take the necessary measures to guard against rickets in sick children."

*R. H. Follis, D. Jackson, M. M. Eliot and E. A. Park: Prevalence of rickets in children between two and fourteen years of age. *Am. J. Dis. Child.*, 66:11, July, 1943.

DEPARTMENTS

HUMAN BEHAVIOUR

JAMES K. HALL, M.D., *Editor*, Richmond, Va.

PROHIBITION RESURGENT?

IS THERE ANY BASIS for the hope of the prohibitionist that man will ever develop the willingness to deny himself the cup; or that he will ever permit another to say to him authoritatively: thou shalt not drink alcohol?

After the captains and the kings have departed from the field of battle, after the killed have been counted; the wounded ministered to; the prisoners segregated and demilitarized, a general inventory is made of losses and of gains. There is a stacking of arms. At the assembled peace conference an infinite amount of solemn and futile lying is indulged in. Deep breaths are taken; the weary, battered soldiers rest and recuperate, and eventually they are restored to the capacity to fight again. And a youthful group of warriors may have grown up to join them. Another war is loosed, and that which had been done again and again is that which is done once more. But the soldier makes war upon another; upon his country's and his own enemy; the bibulous alcoholic makes war against himself.

Suicide, the voluntary killing of self, is generally thought to be the act of a mentally disordered individual; and suicide is usually looked upon, too, as the sudden, impulsive taking of one's own life. But neither assumption may be valid. An individual may be slowly, inexorably and certainly engaged in robbing himself of his own life, without being aware of it. He may be carrying the sword from which he will perish without even knowing that he has taken up a sword. Any physician can name you a number of persons who are slowly but certainly killing themselves. But neither the individuals nor their neighbours may be aware of it.

For a number of years the government of the United States, the government of many of the states and the government of many municipalities and of other political subdivisions have been busily engaged in selling alcoholic beverages to the citizenship. The alcohol so sold is a universal poison. Neither animal nor plant life can survive immersion in alcohol or saturation with alcohol. He who alcoholizes is as certain to die as he who sins.

The toxicity of beverage alcohol is wholly unaffected by the legality or the illegality of the use of the alcohol. Living tissue knows no difference between bootleg alcohol and government-sold alcohol.

The thoughtful and honest citizen is unable to understand how his own government can allow itself to engage in selling poisonous drinks, not labeled as poisonous, to the citizens who support the government. The individual who answers for his crime by the payment of an enforced contribution to a public treasury is left civically stigmatized, however small the fine may have been. The government of the people, our very own democratic government, that dispenses for commercial gain to the individual citizen a poisonous drink, is undeniably causing nation-wide destruction of life. No public treasury made plethoric by the inflow of revenue from such sources can offer compensation to the civic structure adequate to the damage done.

Prohibition, long thought to be dead, is slowly resurging. Eventually the voter will be regaled but sometimes shocked by the loud outcry of the lawmaker for prohibition who only yesterday was delivering phillipics against all legislation that would tend to lessen bibulosity.

He who expressed doubt that beverage alcohol rides high amongst those who travel on the Chariot of Death are either uninformed or unveracious.

Does one hear the question: would you have the bootlegger once again? And one makes answer: yea, it is better that reprehensible conduct be fathered by the reprobate than by the State.

ORTHOPEDIC SURGERY

JOHN T. SAUNDERS, M.D., *Editor*, Asheville, N. C.

THE LOW-BACK PROBLEM

LOW-BACK PAIN with sciatic nerve symptoms continues to be the outstanding problem in orthopedic surgery. There is a sustained interest in lesions of the intervertebral discs and their relation to these symptoms. The trend is toward less frequent use of contrast mediums for visualization of protruding discs, or even toward relying solely upon a careful evaluation of symptoms and a thorough neurologic examination.

Much discussion continues in recent literature concerning the relation of fusion operations and disc removal with a definite trend toward a combination of both procedures. Recent studies show approximately twenty-five per cent more recoveries following this combination than from laminectomy alone.

My opinion is that a protruding or ruptured intervertebral disc is secondary to mechanical instability of the area involved following developmental variations, trauma, postural changes, wear and tear, or arthritic change. These changes are frequently seen at the lumbo-sacral region and less frequently in the cervical, dorso-lumbar or mid dorsal spine. At the lumbo-sacral junction instability is frequently seen, especially an increased range of motion of the fifth lumbar vertebra on the sacrum associated with asymmetric lateral articulations and narrowing of this interspace. An exaggerated angle of weight thrust here, a narrow disc and a posterior rotation of the pelvis are the chief factors causing pain.

All intervertebral discs are subject to physiologic aging—similar to involution processes of the discs of the sacrum. Disc changes at the lumbo-sacral junction frequently follow chronic strain resulting from mechanical factors at this unstable region. Sciatic nerve pain from disc protrusion is present in perhaps four per cent of patients with low back symptoms seen in an active practice. It must be remembered that synovitis of the lateral articulations at the lumbo-sacral level is adjacent to the lumbo-sacral nerve plexus, and pain may be referred along the sciatic nerve. Neurologic examinations show changes often more consistent with a plexus distribution than with a nerve-root distribution.

It is clinically well known that many patients with definite symptoms referrable to disc protrusion recover spontaneously, and for this reason a plea is hereby made for adequate conservative treatment before surgery is advised.

GYNECOLOGY

CANCER, ESPECIALLY GYNECOLOGICAL CANCER

ROBERT THRIFT FERGUSON, M.D., *Editor,* Charlotte, N. C.

AT ONE TIME it was thought that the nature of a malignant cell could be demonstrated by the abnormalities which might be seen under a high-power lens of a microscope; and, although it is true that certain abnormalities are frequently present in the anatomy of a malignant cell, yet no one abnormality is always present, and, indeed, any of the histological abnormalities seen in a malignant cell may be found under certain conditions in non-malignant cells. It is now realized that the physiology of a tumor cell is more important than its structure. There is an increasing amount of evidence that in some cells the abnormality of the physiology can be rectified. This is a new point of view to some of us and is one that should be kept in mind.

These important points serve as an introduction to a discussion[1] which must be of great interest to us all.

It is true that a greater percentage of multiparae suffer from carcinoma of the cervix than nulliparae, but Donaldson regards it as very questionable whether trauma has anything to do with this. It is true that carcinoma of the body of the uterus occurs more frequently in nulliparae but the cause is not known.

Before the war the British Empire Cancer Campaign organized lectures to lay audiences and over 1200 such lectures were given. At first very considerable opposition was raised on the grounds that such lectures would turn the population into neurasthenics. Donaldson is convinced from the numerous letters received from people who attended these lectures that the opposite is true, that as soon as people are able to talk freely about cancer in the same way that they talk about other diseases it will be possible to do away with the fear and ignorance which are so largely responsible for the late diagnosis of cancer, that it is essential that many more lectures to the public be given after the war. But how can the individual gynecologist help? We all have many patients suffering from cancerphobia. The patient should be told of the early symptoms of the more common types of cancer, care being taken to emphasize that other diseases may cause these symptoms, but that in any case they should be investigated; for instance, lumps in the breast, vaginal haemorrhage, or haemorrhoids. These persons should be encouraged to visit a doctor once a year and to explain that they are anxious to have an overhaul.

Cancer should be regarded as an acute disease. A five-years' survival rate gives an idea of the effect of treatment; but, in order to use this method for comparing the efficiency of different techniques, it is necessary to have at the start the same biological and other conditions present in the two series of cases. This difficulty is one of the factors that in the past has caused such heated arguments on the respective merits of surgery and radiotherapy in carcinoma of the cervix.

A great deal can be done by keeping accurate records. It is essential to have a stenographer in the operating theatre with a form containing multiple headings. The stenographer calls out the headings and the operator dictates the note.

Another criterion makes it possible within a few weeks of the start of treatment to assess the effect on the primary growth. This method consists in counting the entire cell population of an area of tissue taken from the growing edge before and after irradiation, and then determining the number of cells in each of four categories—dividing, degenerating, rest and differentiating cells.

Capacity for differentiation varies for different tumours and also among different cells of the same tumour. One must search for an optimum dose of irradiation which will encourage differentiation. *It is possible that a large dose may have the opposite effect.*

For the pain in advanced cases of cancer, there

---
1. Malcolm Donaldson, in *Proc. Royal Soc. of Med.* (Eng.), Nov.

is a tendency to be content with ordering morphine and to leave it at that. Need is seen for a committee or group of workers to devoting their whole time and energy to finding a method for the abolition of pain.

The Cancer Act of 1939, it is believed, will prove to be one of the very greatest benefits in helping to solve the cancer problem. The Act compels certain of the local authorities to submit plans to the Ministry of Health that will provide efficient diagnosis and treatment for cancer patients within their area. It does not require each local authority to have a separate plan; on the contrary powers are provided to compel them, where desirable, to set up joint plans. The Act also compels localauthorities to consult with the voluntary hospitals and other medical bodies within their boundary. Since most of the treatment of cancer is carried out in the voluntary hospitals, the Act provides a golden opportunity for the hospitals to get together and draw up programs and provide a first-class cancer organization, diagnostic and consultative centers, treatment after consultation between the surgeon and radiotherapist, efficient follow-up departments, statistical departments for the whole area as well as for the individual hospitals, and educational lectures to the public. Such an organization will provide not only for more efficient routine treatment than is obtained at present by most patients, but an ever-increasing opportunity for planned research.

This English teacher of gynecology gives us an excellent outline for the discovery, examination and treatment of cancer. I would urge especial attention to hemorrhages occurring during the menopause. Trauma should not be given too much consideration in regard to etiology, for we all see too many cases in maiden ladies who have had no trauma.

It has been decided that five years is too short a time for evaluating the treatment in any form of cancer, for it has been found that at the end of a ten-year period most of these patients have expired. Education has done more than any other one thing to bring the subject before the public and I advocate this very strongly from every standpoint possible.

GENERAL PRACTICE

JAMES L. HAMNER, M.D., *Editor*, Mannboro, Va.

THE TREATMENT OF CARDIOVASCULAR EMERGENCIES IN THE HOME

THE INITIAL TREATMENT in cardiac emergencies is usually required to be given in the home. A Wisconsin teacher[1] who has confidence in his teach-

1. F. D. Murphy, Milwaukee, in *Wisc. Med. Jl.*, Aug.

ing writes helpfully on the subject.

Angina pectoris. Over 40 years of age, pain comes following exercise, emotional disturbances, or a heavy meal. Pain is under the sternum, radiates to the neck and down the shoulder into the arms; patient is very apprehensive. The spell lasts from 5-10 minutes and then passes away. Relief is obtained from nitroglycerin. Pain continuing for more than 5 to 10 minutes, with evidence of cardiac embarrassment, the chances are that the condition is coronary thrombosis.

Treatment nitroglycerin 1/100 grain under the tongue or the contents of an amyl nitrite ampule, subsequent regulation of the patient's life accomplished by limiting the quantity and quality of work, and avoiding the things that the patient knows will precipitate an attack. For the hypertension, xanthine drugs, sedatives and regulation of the diet and work are as helpful in the one condition as in the other. Rigid prohibition of tobacco is necessary in both.

Coronary thrombosis, too, comes on in people over 40, but the attack usually occurs independently of exercise, emotional disturbances, and heavy meals, may come on while asleep. As the minutes wear on, the pain takes a tighter grip and is not relieved by simple remedies. The blood pressure falls; the pulse becomes rapid and irregular, occasionally remains normal. Slight pulmonary edema is manifested by crepitant rales in the bases of both lungs, cyanosis, clammy perspiration, exhaustion. Pain may not be in chest but in upper abdomen, and nausea and vomiting are common. Ailments always to be considered when pain is in the chest, are spontaneous pneumothorax, pulmonary embolism, massive collapse of the lung and acute disease of the upper abdominal viscera. Emergency treatment of coronary thrombosis—clear the room of all the curious, place the patient in a semireclining position or in position most comfortable, 1/3 grain of pantopon intramuscularly, or ¼ grain of morphine hypodermically, or, probably best of all, ½ grain of papaverine intravenously. Give 7½ to 15 grains of caffeine sodium benzoate subcutaneously every few hours to counteract shock. Coramine is sometimes a lifesaver, given intravenously. Oxygen is the sovereign remedy.

An intravenous injection of 8 grains of aminophylline with 50 c.c. of 50 per cent glucose solution has often been followed with relief of the pain, of the shock syndrome and of pulmonary edema.

Digitalis is contraindicated, as is epinephrine.

Paroxysmal tachycardia starts abruptly and ends so, usually occurs in nervous individuals without heart disease, may be associated with heart disease. Appraise on the condition of the heart muscle.

Pressure over the carotid sinus for 1 or 2 min. in the upper part of the neck or ice-pack on the precordial area may be effective. Most effective is 10 to 15 grains of quinidine sulphate given at once, then 5 grains once or twice a day, and finally a few grains once a day to protect from subsequent attacks.

Paroxysmal auricular fibrillation and flutter with a very rapid ventricular beat can usually be recognized without difficulty. It is often allied with genuine heart disease. Give digitalis 3 or 4 grains of the powdered leaf a day. Phenobarbital is helpful. If digitalis does not alleviate the condition speedily, quinidine sulphate 5 grains 3 or 4 times a day. Quinidine must be used with great care in fibrillation that has been present for a number of weeks or months, but it is the drug of choice when fibrillation is an acute emergency.

Extrasystoles are more of a nuisance than a disease, may interfere with sleep. Fatigue, liquor, tea, coffee and tobacco are the main causes.

Left ventricular failure requires absolute rest in bed for a number of weeks. Greater relief is given by sitting up in bed than by lying flat. Oxygen for cyanosis or dyspnea. It is wise to give it in any case of heart failure; in most cases 1/4 grain morphine. Fifty to 100 cc. of 50 per cent glucose with 7 grains of aminophylline intravenously augments the pulmonary circulation and relieves dyspnea. Digitalis 1 1/2 gr. is usually indicated; for rapid digitalization, 1/100 grain of strophanthin at once and repeated in six hours, providing no digitalis has been given previously. The fluid should be limited to 1,200 to 1,500 c.c. a day and the salt in the diet kept low. Mercupurin, 1 c.c., in the forenoon for a few days (edema need not be present) often relieves the dyspnea as well as the edema. Occasionally 1/2 grain of codeine phosphate or codeine sulfate with ammonium chloride in a proper vehicle three or four times a day relieves cough. When an acute attack of paroxysmal dyspnea sets in, aminophylline intravenously generally relieves. If not, give 1/3 grain of pantopon. Paroxysmal dyspnea at night may be prevented by giving 3 grains of aminophylline by mouth before going to sleep. The diet must be simple, distention of the abdomen kept at a minimum.

These principles prevail also in *right heart failure*, but venous congestion may be so great that nothing short of a venesection of one pint or more of blood will relieve, repeated once or twice within a period of a week if necessary for the relief of symptoms. Fluid often is present in the chest cavity and requires thoracentesis. Fluid in the abdominal sac requires tapping. In right ventricular failure the symptoms are much more responsive to diuretics of the mercury group than those of left failure.

Rest. A proper way of living may be more important than medicine. One of the best therapeutic aids is to add a word of encouragement to the patient.

In heart failure, auricular fibrillation or coronary obstruction, embolic phenomena are likely to occur. Thrombi may form on the walls of auricle or ventricle. Pieces of the thrombotic mass may break off and lodge in the extremities, brain, spleen, lung or kidney. The outlook depends on the size of the embolus and the organ in which it lodges. Specific treatment consists of the injection of 1 grain of papaverine hydrochloride intravenously and 1 ampule of metrazol subcutaneously. Other measures are purely symptomatic.

* * * * *

THE PROGNOSIS OF ANGINA PECTORIS

A FOLLOW-UP STUDY was made[1] in 1943 of 497 cases of angina pectoris that were first observed from 1920 to 1930, and a few observations added on a supplementary series of 75 cases with angina pectoris decubitus.

Of the 497 patients with angina pectoris 445 are dead and 52 are still living. The average duration to death of the 445 was 7.9 years, while the average from onset of the disease in the living is 18.4 years. The average duration to date for the combined dead and living is 9.0 years, which will increase when all the present survivors succumb—a duration of life about double that at present widely regarded as the expectation of life after angina pectoris first appears.

Seventy-six per cent of the deaths were due to cardiac causes one-fifth of the entire group and normal cardiac examinations, blood pressures and ecgs. at the time of the first examination, and these patients as a rule lived longer.

Angina pectoris decubitus was found in 103 of the 497 cases. There were no significant differences in the average duration of the disease to death or in the living between this group and that of the group as a whole. In 75 additional cases of angina pectoris decubitus, life averaged 2.8 years in 47 cases followed to death. However, the average duration of the precedent angina of effort brought the overall average duration of life close to that of the larger group. Gross myocardial infarction recognizable clinically followed angina pectoris decubitus within 24 hours in 22 of the 75 cases, and within a period of three months in 19 more. The follow-up study of these groups will further affect the prognosis.

The coronary artery damage may be permanent and therefore chronic, but its effect on the heart itself is the important point; thus coronary artery disease and coronary heart disease must be clearly differentiated. Special care over the periods of the

---

1. Paul D. White *et al.*, Boston, in *Jl. A. M. A.*, Nov. 27th.

acute and subacute phase of coronary heart disease, replacing the old fatalistic point of view, is disclosed to be the most important part of the treatment of coronary heart disease, at times lost to view in the course of the introduction of new therapeutic measures.

THERAPEUTICS

J. F. NASH, M.D., *Editor*, Saint Pauls, N. C.

NEUROLOGICAL TREATMENT IN GENERAL PRACTICE

THE NEED FOR CONSERVATION of time and energy has prompted the listing[1] a few neurological conditions with recent treatment trends.

Syphilis of the Central Nervous System: Any case under treatment which develops a positive serological reaction after once having a negative test, or a case that shows a Wassermann-fast reaction, should have a spinal fluid examination—cell count, protein, colloidal gold curve, and quanitative Kahn. Other diagnostic leads are urinary incontinence, migratory or radiating pains, transitory visual disturbances, diplopia and changes in personality.

The arch stone of neurosyphilis treatment is fever therapy supported by arsenicals as tryparsmide or mepharsen, heavy metals as bismuth, and arsphenamine for systemic syphilis. In the middle-age patient a course of heavy metal and arsenicals should precede fever therapy. Mechanical fever is the first choice, as that produced by the inductotherm or the hypertherm cabinets. An excellent method of fever production is the triple typhoid vaccine infusion, by drip method in normal saline.

Apoplexy: When the onset of unconsciousness, hemiplegia and aphasia is slow with prodromes lasting several hours, the pathological condition is very apt to be cerebral thrombosis rather than hemorrhage or embolism. For the latter conditions treatment is very discouraging indeed. For cerebral thrombosis rational treatment is often of benefit. The head should be lowered and feet elevated, body warmth maintained, with frequent change of position to avoid pulmonary hypostasis. If seen early, normal saline 400-500 c.c. given intravenously with 10 c.c. of heparin, 20-25 drops per minute, and repeated every one hour, as the anticoagulant effect of the heparin passes away after one hour. Circulation is maintained by heat, small amount of wine or whisky, every two or three hours, nicotinic acid 50 mg. t.i.d. before meals. Small meals. Care of the contracture deformities require heat, massage, active and passive movements of joints, and part-time wearing of splints.

most useful in the control of grand mal convulsions

---
1. H. R. Carter, Denver, in *Rocky Mountain Med. Jl.*, Nov.

Epilepsy: Phenytoin sodium (dilantin sodium) is where phenobarbital is ineffective. As we digitalize hearts so must we "dilantinize" brains. The minor toxic symptoms are transitory and should not deter us from giving ample dosage, up to nine grains daily, dosage being maintained just below the toxic level.

Petit Mal: Bromide treatment is effective in some cases. Phenytoin is not as effective as phenobarbital, and even when the latter is given, there may be only a reduction in number of seizures. Epileptic children tolerate much larger dosages than non-epileptic—1½ to 10 grains in 24 hours. Drowsiness can be counteracted by small doses of amphetamine sulfate in the morning. Any treatment program should be continued for several *years* after the patient is symptom-free.

Status Epilepticus: First to be tried should be sodium amytal 7½ to 15 grains intravenously, secondly avertin anesthesia. Later 2 c.c. of magnesium sulfate, 20% solution intravenously, together with spinal drainage. Morphine sulfate may be used when other remedies are not at hand .

Alcoholic Intoxication: Deep coma, dilated pupils, irregular pulse indicate two to three c.c. of metrazol, 10% solution, given slowly. Supportive treatment is given in the form of high carbohydrate intake as sweetened fruit juices, later solid carbohydrate foods. Fluids by mouth and per rectum, and with vomiting, parenteral normal saline with 5% glucose, and sodium chloride (enteric coated tablets or capsules) 2 grains every four hours. Thiamin chloride or B complex intravenously. Vitamins A and C are added to the fluid intake. Paraldehyde is of value in controlling the restlessness—8 to 24 c.c., can be given by rectum or by mouth.

Meningococcus Meningitis: Spinal fluid is drawn under avertin or pentathol sodium anesthesia. The examination of a Gram-stained smear and culture of the organism will confirm the clinical diagnosis. It is but a complication of meningococcus septicemia. Sulfadiazine, 4-6 grams by mouth and a quarter of the dosage every four hours for 10 days; may be given intravenously. A concentrattion of 15 mg. per 100 c.c. of blood should be maintained. The drug should not be discontinued too early even though the patient is largely symptom-free. Restlessness is best controlled by paraldehyde and moderate dosages of barbiturates.

Pneumococcus Meningitis: Requires in addition to sulfonamide therapy the specific rabbit antipneumococcic serum started four to eight hours after the sulfonamide—one million units, repeated as needed. Chemotherapy should be continued one week after sterile spinal fluid cultures are obtained. Blood transfusion and 5% glucose in normal saline may be required.

Influenzal Meningitis: Mortality 90% in children under two years of age, when the type B bacillus is found in the spinal fluid. Sulfadiazine, 0.1 grain per kilogram body weight, should be given intravenously by continuous drip. Later 0.1 gram per kilogram body weight, in 40 c.c. of normal saline intravenously q. 4 h. Type B globulin-refined rabbit serum is administered by continuous intravenous drip. Ringer's solution given intravenously by drip, taking two hours for 200-300 c.c. Serum may be stopped when a 1-10 dilution of patient's serum shows a capsular swelling of the influenza bacillus.

Migraine: Ergotamine tartrate 0.25 mg. intravenously, followed by 0.5 mg. subcutaneously after two hours—6-10 mgms. within 24 hours—is effective in the majority of cases. Amphetamine sulfate 3-20 mg. intravenously until an elevation of systolic pressure of 20-40 mm.; then 10-40 mg. of amphetamine sulfate by mouth at the onset of the next attack. One hundred per cent oxygen continued for two hours gives relief in many cases.

Herpes Zoster: Early treatment consists of x-radiation to the area over the dorsal roots and ganglia involved. To the areas of vesicular pain a powder of menthol 3.0 gram, starch 15.0 grams and zinc oxide 90.0 grams. Intense pain alleviated by cocaine alkaloid one per cent in lanolin.

OPHTHALMOLOGY

HERBERT C. NEBLETT, M.D., *Editor*, Charlotte, N. C.

BILATERAL CATARACT FROM ELECTRICAL SHOCK? CASE REPORT

WHETHER or not a cataract of the crystalline lens is of traumatic origin cannot be proven with the knowledge now at hand unless the status of the eyes was known immediately prior to an alleged injury, and this fact augmented by the history and evidence of an injury which produced a clouding of the lens while the case was under the care of an oculist. The history and evidence of an injury alone to a patient who had cataract at the time the case was presented for the first treatment of the injury is not proof that a cataract did not previously exist or was the result of the immediate trauma. The circumstances attending such a case may be considered strong evidence in support of the causative factor but medico-legal proof to sustain such a contention is wanting. Without an exact knowledge of all the foregoing facts in his record of the case no oculist should venture to prove before a court the existence of a traumatic cataract. It has been argued that a cataract of traumatic origin presents a definite pattern from which a probable diagnosis can be made. This has no basis of fact since trauma may cause any type of opacity in the human lens as to shape, size, density, color and area. The same may be said of any of the other (non-traumatic) types of cataract of which there are many.

Cataract of electrical origin, whether by commercial voltage or by lightning stroke, is not common. If a person is shocked by either of the foregoing agencies the following noteworthy facts are of interest for careful consideration by the oculist who treats or reviews the eyes in such a case. The initial changes in the lens, when present, are seen as numerous dust-like opacities beneath the anterior capsule. The absence of progression of these opacities is characteristic; they are usually partial, rarely complete; bilateral involvement is uncommon; foveal degeneration may be an early manifestation; optic atrophy may begin early and become complete within 6 to 12 weeks. These latter two conditions either alone or jointly may be present with or without any changes in the lens. If neither the retinal nor optic nerve elements are too severely damaged and the cataract is the main or only bar to vision there is no contraindication for extraction of the lens. Equally as good or better visual results are obtained after extraction than in the average type of senile cataract for reasons which are obvious when dealing with the aged. Early examination of the eyes of such patients is of great importance, and with the slit-lamp if possible, and a review 3 or 4 months later should be suggested in the oculist's report, especially in cases where liability exists. Dust-like opacities may occur in the lens within a few days to several months after electrical shock and may be partially or completely absorbed or remain stationary.

The production of opacities in the human lens from electrical shock is based upon the following theories: The power of an electric discharge to kill living cells without the development of heat, to concussion of the lens, to the intense iridociliary hyperemia present which causes osmotic interchanges between the vitreous and the lens, the production of a subepithelial albumic degeneration of the epithelium, followed by penetration of the aqueous, changing the aqueous so that it is unfit for osmosis.

Case Report

An electrical lineman, 30, of powerful build and in excellent physical condition was rendered partly unconscious for 4 or 5 days the result of 11,000 volts of electricity passing through his body, from his forehead coming in contact with a high-voltage wire while he was working on a pole 30 feet above the ground. He did not fall from the pole, his body being suspended by his emergency belt. There was a large third-degree burn of two-thirds of the forehead, with a deep depression in the frontal bone above the left supraorbital arch; two toes on the left foot burned off and a third-degree burn of the right foot. The accident occurred on May 14th, 1942. He was first seen by me on the following August 24th, having been referred because of progressive dimness of vision of the right eye for 3 or 4 weeks. On examination there was no evidence of injury or disease of the lids and their adnexa or of the globes externally. Uncorrected vision right eye was 20/40, left 20/30. With minus 0.75 sphere each eye, vision right 20/30, left 20/20. The fundi and optic nerves showed no pathological changes. With the ophthalmoscope and slit lamp the anterior surface of the right lens was seen to be studded with fine dust-like opacities, the left lens presented an occasional similar type of opacity. The field of vision and color sense of each eye was normal.

No previous record of this man's vision could be obtained although he claimed to have had excellent vision in each eye up to the time as stated prior to my examination. Family history for cataracts was negative.

Diagnosis: Electrical shock cataract in each eye, the greater involvement in the right?

On the basis of this diagnosis being probable request was made in my report to have the man return in three months. This was done on December 29th. At this examination vision r. eye 20/100, l. 20/70 from progressive generalized cloudiness of the lenses. There were no pathological changes in the fundi.

At final review of the case June 28th, 1943, vision in each eye was ability to count fingers at three feet. The opaque lenses presented an interesting and identical pattern. Viewed with the ophthalmoscope the opacity looked like hammered brass and in the vertical diameter of the anterior capsule just above the horizontal was a whitish-gray oval opacity 3 millimeters in its longest diameter which gave the appearance of being suspended by four whitish-gray lines running to the periphery of the lens at 12, 3, 6 and 9 o'clock positions. Viewed with the slit lamp and with a loupe and condenser the cataract gave the appearance of hammered silver and the whitish-gray body in the anterior capsule as above described.

Cataract extraction on the right eye was advised and accomplished by the intracapsular method with a small iridectomy on July 15th, 1943. Convalescence was uneventful. The extracted lens was a firm solid mass similar to a senile cataract. The small grayish-white opacity did not come away with the lens but fell downward and to the nasal side of the pupillary area and was allowed to remain. At the present writing its shape, size and color has not changed and its presence does not cause any untoward effect. Two of its suspension lines, at 9 and 12 o'clock position, were broken at the time of the extraction allowing it to drift nasally.

On Sept. 29th, extraction of the left lens was successfully accomplished via the same method and with a similar result, with the exception that the grayish-white mass came away with the anterior capsule of the lens. It was of moderate consistency, thin and flat and very loosely attached to the capsule with its faint suspensory lines radiating across the anterior capsule in the positions as before mentioned. From the findings described concerning these suspensory lines and their behavior during the extractions their terminal attachment must have been at some point beneath the body of the iris. How this interesting anomaly became a part of, though practically separated as it was from, the cataractous lenses is unknown. It was not seen during the early stages of either cataract, having been found 10 months after my first examination. It may be surmised that it and its suspensory lines were a terminal product of the intense iridociliary hyperemia produced at the moment of the electrical stroke, or the result of a severe electrolytic reaction in the apex of the anterior capsule or both.

At final examination and refraction on December 18th no pathological changes were to be found in the media or fundi. There was found, however, a left hyperphoria of 5 to 6 prism diopters cataract bifocals were prescribed with a prism of 5 diopters, divided equally between the two eyes, correcting vision to 20/20, Jaeger 1 each eye.

Prescription: O. D. + 10.00 s. with + 3.00 cyl. ax. 90 with 2.5 P. D. base up; O. S. + 10.00 s. with + 3.00 cyl. ax. 90 with 2.5 P. D. base down, + 2.50 s. addition each eye for reading.

Summary: Affirmative data—This is not a proven case of electrical shock cataract but the findings presented are so strongly circumstantial as to make the etiological factor almost a certainty. The initial lesions in the lenses were of a pattern often found in electrical stroke cases.

Negative data—The opacities in the lenses did not tend to absorb or remain stationary, but rapidly progressed, involved the entire structure of the lens, and were bilateral. There were no foveal or optic nerve changes which are often a complication or sequela of electrical stroke, with or without cataract. No report can be found of a similar opacity suspended in front of the lens in such a case as herewith described.

REFERENCES
FUCHS: *Ophthalmology*, Duane 8th Edt.
WURDEMANN: *Injuries of the Eye*, 2nd Edt.
RAE: *Neuro-Ophth.* 1st Edt.
DUKE-ELDER: *Text-Book of Ophth.*

INSURANCE MEDICINE
H. F. STARR, M.D., *Editor*, Greensboro, N. C.

THE APPLICANT FOR LIFE INSURANCE

FOR EACH SALE there must be a buyer. Persuasive selling efforts of the agent notwithstanding, the applicant for life insurance is a buyer. He may have been slow to reach a decision and sales ingenuity and persistence may have been required to convert him, yet at the time of application he wants the protection afforded by insurance and his psychological reaction is that of a purchaser. It is important for the medical examiner to realize this and to take the mental attitude of the applicant into account during the examination and in weighing the evidence.

Life insurance was not always bought and sold to the insured as protection. There was a time when it was bought and sold as a speculation, pure and simple. Lloyds and the merchants of the Royal Exchange charged 25 per cent against the return of George II when he fought at Dettingen. Premiums were quoted on the lives of Warren Hastings, Sir Robert Walpole, Admiral Byng, and others, including prisoners who might be executed.*[1]

The beneficiary was the purchaser and the in-

*[1]. Dingman: Insurability, Prognosis and Selection. The Spectator Company, 1927.

sured was not necessarily aware of the transaction. The evils of such procedures are self-evident. As one commentator remarked in 1768, "This inhuman sport affected the minds of men depressed by long sickness; for when such persons, casting an eye over a newspaper for amusement, saw their lives had been insured in the Alley at 90 per cent, they despaired of all hopes and thus their dissolution was hastened." Of this vicious practice John Francis said in 1853: "A pecuniary interest in the death of anyone is fearful odds against benevolent feeling; and it was hardly to be expected that men should throw what influence they possessed into the scale of mercy. The power of opening merely speculative policies on private persons was also demoralizing, and perhaps dangerous to life itself. It was not possible—it was not in human nature— to have money depending on the existence of the inmate of your home without watching him with feelings which the good man would tremble to analyze, and even the bad man would fear to avow."

By an act of Parliament, in 1774, it was declared that no policy should be granted without the name of the beneficiary being properly inserted and that no greater sum should be recovered than the amount of interest of the beneficiary. This principle still stands and is routinely followed in the selection of risks.

Now the applicant buys insurance on his own life to enable him to meet his responsibilities to his family, business associates, creditors or dependents—a motive highly commendable. But the examiner must remember that the applicant tries to present himself in the most favorable light. He may insist, and with a degree of sincerity, that he really does not want the insurance. Yet when he presents himself for the examination he subconsciously senses that his soundness is being questioned and proceeds on the basis that he owes it to himself to make the best showing possible. His tendency nearly always is to minimize or even forget unfavorable factors. Some go so far as to lie outright and to commit fraud. The life insurance policy is nothing more nor less than an agreement that one party will do a certain thing in view of a certain consideration. As with all contracts, the agreement is based upon a common understanding or meeting of the minds of the two parties. If the applicant is guilty of material concealments, reservations or falsifications, the contract becomes jeopardized, for under such conditions there can be no common ground for a meeting of minds, a condition to which both parties are legally entitled when entering into a contract. The applicant should see that correct answers are recorded and should not attempt to relieve his conscience by trying to shift his responsibility to the agent or examiner who may be unfamiliar with the facts or careless in making the report.

The power of selection exercised by the applicant is fully appreciated by the underwriter. The applicant knows more about his own health and physical condition than the company will ever learn. His is the decision as to whether he will apply for insurance, and with experience and information he is in a position to act to his own advantage. He determines the amount he will buy and the plan, and after the policy is issued he may continue it or lapse it as he chooses. The applicant has the opportunity to prove his insurability at any time to any company, but any decision the company makes is to a certain degree final as far as the obligation of the company is concerned.

The effectiveness of self selection is amply demonstrated by the fact that those who buy annuities, thereby receiving regular payments for life, live longer than those who buy life insurance payable at death. Purchasers of endowment insurance expect to live to collect the face amount and the death rate among them is better than among those who purchase term or ordinary life policies. Many insurance figures have been compiled which show that without apparent design, the coverage most profitable to the purchaser is consistently chosen. After the applicant has become a policyholder he continues self-selection against the company in determining whether to continue the policy or lapse it.

A realization of the very great power of self-selection exercised by the applicant is important to medical examiners for life insurance. Consideration of the factors involved makes it clear why the history obtained from the applicant for insurance is entirely different from the history given when he consults a physician concerning his health. The successful medical examiner bears this in mind and uses a suitable technique to get the history from the applicant which is different from that used at the bedside. He realizes, too, that the statements of the applicant must be analyzed and regarded in a somewhat different light than if they came from a patient seeking medical advice.

OBSTETRICS
HENRY J. LANGSTON, M.D., *Editor*, Danville, Va.

BICORNATE UTERUS WITH PREGNANCY IN EACH HORN

THE TWO MULLERIAN DUCTS fuse from below upward to form the vaginal tract and the uterus. Anomalies of the female genital system are due in most cases to failure of fusion at any location throughout the extent of the two canals and in the remainder to the rudimentary development of one duct. In some animals the ducts normally do not fuse and two tubular uteri are present.

Usually menstruation occurs from the two uteri simultaneously; however, it may come from one horn at a time. Pregnancy may occur in one or both horns. Menstruation occurs from the empty horn during the pregnancy. In one instance twins were found in one horn. In case each horn contains an ovum, superfetation may occur. Several such cases have been reported.

In the ordinary course of pregnancy in one horn the nonpregnant horn forms a decidual membrane typical of that found in an ectopic pregnancy. This decidua may be expelled without disturbing the pregnancy of the other horn, or the course may be that of an abortion. Foreknowledge of an anomalous development of the uterine tract will cause the surgeon to proceed with extreme caution during the curettage.

It is unusual for gestation in a bicornate uterus to continue uneventfully to term.

Braze[1] reports an instructive case:

On Jan. 20th, 1941, a white woman, 24, in active labor, was referred to me. The menstrual history was normal, profuse. One year previously she had had a delivery in the home; membranes ruptured spontaneously prior to onset, severe dystocia for 12 days.

Examination: Broad abdomen, two sets of fetal heart tones—140 per minute on the right, 135 on the left. Both fetal heads were palpable and the diagnosis of twins was readily made. A depression between the two fetuses aroused suspicion of bicornate uterus. The two fetal heads were above the pelvic inlet. Both presenting, one on each side of the pelvis. The fetal spines were directed laterally and the small parts toward the maternal spine, no developmental anomalies of the fetuses or of the maternal pelvis.

At 10 a. m., spontaneously, a viable boy was born, wt. 5 lbs. 12½ oz. The placenta was delivered intact at 10:12 a. m. from the right horn, but despite firm contraction of this horn, profuse hemorrhage continued. At 10:19 a. m. a living girl, wt. 6 lbs. 9 oz., was delivered by manual pressure over the left fundus and its placenta followed intact in six minutes. The left horn remained atonic but with continued gentle massage and the administration of pitocin and ergotamine tartrate eventually contracted nicely. There were no lacerations. Profuse hemorrhage again occurred at 1 p. m., but responded well to treatment.

The mother's hemoglobin was 38 per cent and red blood corpuscles 2,910,000. She was given a transfusion of 550 c.c. of whole citrated blood. The puerperium was otherwise uneventful.

---
1. Maj. Alexander Braze, M. C., U. S. A., in *Jl. A. M. A.*, Oct. 23rd.

UROLOGY

RAYMOND THOMPSON, M.D., *Editor*, Charlotte, N. C.

SULFONAMIDE-RESISTANT GONOCOCCIC INFECTIONS

"SULFONAMIDE RESISTANCE is an important factor in the therapy of gonorrhea and constitutes a formidable barrier in the present campaign for the complete eradication of this disease."[1]

Thirty per cent of cases of gonorrheal urethritis show some degree of resistance such as persistence of symptoms with positive cultures, or persistence of positive cultures in asymptomatic carriers. The strain of gonococcus is probably responsible for the resistance, rather than the constitution of the host. It is also reported that certain species of bacteria can protect susceptible bacteria from the action of the drug in mixed culture.

A recent laboratory method for differentiating the sulfonamide resistant from the sulfonamide responsive strains has been reported by Goodale *et al.*, who primarily aimed at correlating clinical and in vitro response to sulfonamides. In cases of untreated acute gonorrheal urethritis, we are told, the test may be completed in less than twenty-four hours.

These investigators have drawn up tables comparing their new methods, which they regard as furnishing only presumptive evidence, with the original method. The comparison is gratifying as to reliability, and it is suggested that the method could be used routinely as a guide to therapy, for it permits an accurate prognosis of the results of sulfonamide therapy, and could be used for selecting any limited few cases to be treated with penicillin.

No relationship was found between the speed of cure with sulfonamides and the time after onset of symptoms at which sulfonamide therapy was started; sulfathiazole, sulfadiazine and sulfamerazine all appear to be in hibitory; but, weight for weight, it was concluded that sulfathiazole is several times as powerful as either of the other two.

The test is of value "in focusing attention on patients who become asymptomatic carriers." These are the patients who are not only more likely to infect others, but who spread strains of the resistant types.

---
1. Laboratory Identification of Sulfonamide Resistant Gonococcic Infections. Walter T. Goodale, R. Gordon Gould, Louis Schwab and Virginia G. Winter. *J. A. M. A.*, October 30th, 1943.

No UNTOWARD reactions were noted in any instance when 35 administrations of plasma prepared from patients with active malaria were made. The type of preservation used had no obvious effect on the results obtained.

SURGERY

GEO. H. BUNCH, M.D., *Editor*, Columbia, S. C.

SODIUM CHLORIDE POISONING

FOR A DECADE Coller of the University of Michigan has strongly advocated the intravenous administration of normal salt solution in large amounts to patients who are dehydrated or in shock following operation. Giving five or six liters a day was recommended for adults. Salt solution was considered somewhat of a harmless panacea and if the patient did not do well it was because not enough solution had been given, and more was administered. It was believed that the patient could eliminate salt solution even in large amounts readily and without deleterious effect.

Coming from such an authority the wisdom of the practice has been accepted without question by surgeons generally over the nation so that the administration of salt solution parorally is almost a universal practice after severe operations. It had long been observed that overdosage of sodium chloride in the average individual caused edema; and patients to whom salt was being continuously given should be watched for this, and when edema appeared glucose in distilled water was given instead of salt solution. Edema from retention of sodium chloride in the tissues was not considered dangerous and could be readily relieved by giving glucose.

In a paper read before the Southern Surgical Association (Dec., 1943) and not yet published, Doctor Coller has the courage to frankly admit that he has been in error and that the administration of salt solution in susceptible patients is not without danger and may cause death. He says that many of the postoperative patients who sink into progressively deepening coma with or without high fever and with or without anuria, are, in his opinion, suffering from acute sodium chloride poisoning. He is convinced that patients with an idiosyncrasy may succumb from the administration of even a single liter of normal salt solution. He thinks that water should be given parorally as glucose solution without any sodium chloride content for the first postoperative day or until the urinary output has again risen to normal. When a patient complains of thirst water should be given orally, unless certainly contraindicated; otherwise intravenously as glucose solution, never as normal salt solution.

It is of interest to note that Dr. Coller no longer relies upon blood chemistry findings in giving salt solution. That the indications for the administration of water or of salt have been found to be essentially clinical should be a peculiar satisfaction to those of us who have, over the years, had to work without having the advantage of adequate laboratory facilities.

This sketchy outline of Coller's paper is given at this time from memory that our readers may be warned of the danger of the routine and the indiscriminate administration of sodium chloride solution postoperatively.

DENTISTRY

J. H. GUION, D.D.S., *Editor*, Charlotte, N. C.

THE FATE OF BACTERIA SEALED IN DENTAL CAVITIES

THERE HAS ALWAYS been much speculation as to what happens to the bacteria sealed in the dental cavities under filling materials. From this speculation controversy has arisen over the need of cavity sterilization, the employment of germicidal filling materials, and the importance of removing every trace of carious dentin even to the point of pulpal exposure. If the bacteria die shortly after filling without the employment of any germicidal agent then these problems lose importance and technical procedures can be greatly simplified.

It is generally accepted that bacteria penetrate the dentinal tubules beyond the limits of the softened, carious lesion. The known sterilizing and germicidal agents on hand probably are effective on the surface of the lesion but their penetrating action into the tubules is doubtful.

Millions of teeth have been filled and in the great majority of cases there has been no noticeable recurrence of decay *under* the filling and local symptoms of pulpal difficulties have been few. But if pathogenic bacteria can grow and multiply in dentinal tubules for any length of time could they not in some cases enter the pulp and the general circulation, or could their toxins not be the cause of some of the unexplained cases of sensitive teeth and even systemic intoxication?

If there is any basis to the popular theory of focal infection we should be aware of the fate of the bacteria sealed in dental cavities so that our tratment may be on a rational basis.

A careful study has been made[1] recently, the result of which cannot fail to interest thoughtful physicians and dentists alike.

In this study only molar teeth with occlusal cavities were used. No antiseptics were used in the tooth cavity. Control cultures were made to determine contamination of the operating tray just before inoculating the media with specimens from the cavity. All tests were made of teeth in situ.

A rubber dam was applied to isolate the tooth;

---
1. F. B. Besic, Chicago, in *Jl. Dental Research*, Oct.

the field was dried and all areas inspected for leaks in the dam; the whole field was painted with 7 per cent tincture of iodine (cavity in tooth not touched with antiseptics); the iodine was allowed to dry and then washed off with 70 per cent alcohol. All instruments, materials, and the tray were sterilized.

All undermined enamel was chipped away and all decay at the dentino-enamel junction was completely removed, but a small amount of decayed dentin was allowed to remain in the base of the cavity in all but a few cases.

Sterile normal saline was carried to the cavity with a sterile cotton pellet and agitated in the open cavity, then dropped into a culture tube or streaked over a culture plate. Also small bits of decayed material were dropped in the media. The cavity was wiped dry with cotton pellets. A portion of a dry pellet was left in the cavity and covered first with sterile baseplate gutta percha packed down tightly, and that in turn covered by oxyphosphate of zinc cement.

The tooth was left in this condition for two weeks and was then reopened and recultured. A third culture was made in two more weeks and successive cultures at various intervals for a period as long as 18 mos. in certain cases.

In the 10 cases studied in detail streptococci were present in eight; lactobacilli in five, staphylococci in two. Lactobacilli in all cases died out at some time between two and 10 months. Staphylococci remained for at least one year in one case and in the other could not be followed up. Streptococci in one-third of the cases remained after being sealed for more than a year.

One of the three cases that still remained positive after $1\frac{1}{2}$ years had all clinical traces of decay removed. In no case was there any gross indication of progress of decay.

Conclusions arrived at were:

Apparently an effective, penetrating sterilizing agent may be necessary in deep decayed lesions near the pulp—*not* to stop the carious process from progressing, because it ceases automatically upon filling of the cavity; *but* to destroy the possible surviving organisms and eradicate a possible focus of bacterial growth that *may possibly* injure the dental pulp or tissues elsewhere in the body through focal infection.

PEDIATRICS

CONVULSIONS IN CHILDHOOD

CONVULSIONS remain one of the commonest of the alarming symptoms shown by infants and young children. Specific authoritative information as to what to do and what not to do[1] should be kept in the front of our stores of knowledge.

Do not put the child in a hot bath, and do not give morphine. Morphine will depress the respiratory center, contract the pupils, inhibit peristalsis, and mask the symptoms. The child will usually have a fever, in which case a tepid or cool sponge or pack and a cool enema to reduce the temperature. This should be followed by antipyretics to keep the temperature down.

If there is no fever, or if the convulsion persists, the most effective and the simplest treatment is to administer vinyl ether or chloroform by the open drop method. The danger of these drugs is nothing compared to the injurious effects of a continued convulsion. If chloroform or vinyl ether is not available, sodium phenobarbital by hypo. Magnesium sulphate is effective in a saturated (50%) solution by mouth or in a retention enema, $\frac{1}{2}$ to 1 ounce q. 4 h. For quick action this drug may be given intramuscularly or intravenously in sterile solution. Two to 8 c.c. of 50% solution may be injected deep into the muscles q. 4 h. Two to 5 c.c. of 25% solution may be given intravenously by slow injection.

Immediate Treatment
1. Protect against injury; no opiates.
2. Reduce fever.
3. Chloroform or vinyl ether anesthesia.
4. Magnesium sulfate, q. 6 h.
   60 to 180 c.c. of 50 to 25% solution by mouth or rectum, or 5 to 20 c.c. of 25% sterile solution intramuscularly, or 2 to 10 c.c. of 20 to 10% sterile solution intravenously *slowly*.
5. Calcium gluconate by mouth or intramuscularly.
6. Calcium chloride by mouth for tetany.
7. Tribromethanol by rectum for tetanus.
8. Phenobarbital sodium subcutaneously.
9. Chloral by rectum.
10. Absolute rest and quiet for days after.

Important in an acute generalized convulsion is a realization of the injury which the convulsion often causes the brain. Therefore it is essential to keep every patient who has had a convulsion at absolute rest for several days thereafter.

For *epilepsy* the ketogenic diet remains the most effective treatment available. It is the only treatment which has any effect on petit mal epilepsy. Phenobarbital remains the drug of choice in those cases in which the ketogenic diet is not practicable or in which the results have been unsatisfactory.

* * * * *

TECHNIC OF INTRAVENOUS INJECTION IN INFANTS

GIVING A TRANSFUSION to an infant is not difficult, if the best method and apparatus is used for the successful insertion of a needle into a vein and maintaining it there.[1] Two technics are available, the less certain method of penetration of the skin and vein with a sharp needle and the more reliable method of exposure of the vein by dissection and

---
[1] M. G. Peterman, Milwaukee, in *Ill. Med. Jl.*, Nov.

[1] M. L. Scivek, Chicago, in *Ill. Med. Jl.*, Nov.

entering with a blunt needle. The sharp method appears to be the simpler of the two, but in actual practice it is the more difficult and carries a higher percentage of failure.

The best method exposes the vein by dissection and then threads it with a blunt needle. The vein most commonly used is the small saphenous just anterior to the internal malleolus. Unless this vein can be demonstrated by sight or feel no vein will be found on dissection, since it is not always present.

The ankle is restrained by taping the foot in external rotation to a padded splint with 1-in. adhesive tape, applied to the underside of the splint at the heel side, passed up and over the heel over the foot and toes and down and around the underside of the splint around once more to the heel side, over the instep and down and around to be secured on the underside of the splint. The assistant seated alongside of the baby holds the splint down on the table.

The site of operation is prepared with iodine and alcohol. The adhesive tape immediately adjacent is also liberally sponged with the solution. With the vein's position known, a local anesthetic is injected directly over the center of the vein. The wheal raised obliterates the vein, but the needle mark then acts as a marker, accurately locating the underlying vein.

Two towels are used as sterile drapes. A sharp knife is used to make a ¼- to ½-in. incision transverse to the vein. The wound is spread with a forceps and the vein is scooped up with an iris forceps. A piece of catgut is passed under the vein to lift it out of the wound. A small opening is cut in the vein wall with the sharp pointed iris scissors after fat and adventitia have been cleaned from it. Through this opening a blunt No. 22 needle is made to slip into the vein. To secure the needle in position and prevent its being pulled out, a forceps with a notched tip is clamped on the needle catching the vein and needle in its jaws.

At completion, the vein is not tied off and no sutures are used to close the incision. A tight pressure bandage controls bleeding and approximates skin edges giving eventually a small scar.

If continuous intravenous fluids are to be given, the needle is tied into place with a dermal ligature and the needle and cannula are taped securely to the skin of the ankle.

This common-sense article should help a lot. Without its encouragement we would be apt to feel ashamed to cut down on a vein in order to make an intravenous injection so often needed by a baby or child.

THE TUBERCULOSIS DEATH RATE has been reduced *three-fourths* in the past 40 years.

THE SIGNIFICANCE OF THE WIDAL REACTION IN ENTERIC DISEASES OF CHILDREN

IT IS IMPORTANT to know, even in this day of little typhoid, that the diagnosis of typhoid or paratyphoid fever on the basis of a positive Widal test is not justifiable, that such a positive test may be the result of an infection with another member of the Salmonella group.[1] The stools may contain *Salmonella eastbourne* or *Salmonella enteritidis*.

Salmonella includes the organisms commonly associated with food poisoning as well as the typhoid, paratyphoid A, and paratyphoid B bacilli. The only pathogenic organisms commonly associated with the enteric tract not covered by this definition are the bacillary dysentery group.

Very enlightening is a discussion of the two typhoid bacillus antigens, known as O and H. The O antigen is obtained from the body of the bacillus, the H antigen from the flagella. Organisms in the Salmonella group are motile and have flagella, they all have O and H antigens.

When the clinician makes a diagnosis of paratyphoid fever on the basis of suspicious clinical symptoms, a leucopenia, and agglutination by the patient's serum, of paratyphoid A or B organisms, he is on even more uncertain ground than in making a diagnosis of typhoid fever, since most laboratories do not report agglutinations with the O and H antigens of paratyphoid A and B as they do with typhoid. In one case a diagnosis of paratyphoid B fever was made on the basis of a Widal test which was positive for paratyphoid B in a high dilution.

The question may be raised as to what difference it makes whether the causative organism of the infection be typhoid or paratyphoid B or *S. typhi murium*. Typhoid and paratyphoid fevers have higher mortalities than the fevers caused by the other Salmonella organisms. Carriers of typhoid and paratyphoid occur in from 5 to 10 per cent of all cases, and are a chronic and a continuous danger to the community. Infections with the other Salmonella organisms are usually short-lived, and chronic carriers of the organism are uncommon.

1. Morris Greenberg, New York, in *Jl. of Pediatrics*, Aug.)

INTERNAL MEDICINE

GEORGE R. WILKINSON, M.D., *Editor*, Greenville, S. C.

DYSENTERY AND ITS TREATMENT

FREQUENTLY the amoebae and the bacilli are associated and cause mixed dysentery, which is found in India as frequently as either amoebic or bacillary dysentery alone.[1] This Calcutta physician

1. Frank McCay, Calcutta, India, in The *Practitioner* (Lond.), Sept.)

goes on to give his experience with dysentery.

To establish the correct diagnosis, the exudate from a freshly passed stool must be examined under the microscope. A culture can be made at the same time to confirm the smear findings. If the stool is more than four hours old it is not worth investigation. Free forms of Entamoeba histolytica encyst quickly on cooling or drying, and Charcot-Leyden crystals are no longer considered pathognomonic of amoebic dysentery.

In Flexner epidemics—usually waterborne—the proportion of bacillary cases will rise steeply, and the number of mixed dysentery cases will also increase as people with amoebiasis go down with bacillary infection and conditions thus become suitable for their own resting amoebae to get active.

In India it has often been found that by insisting on bearers washing their hands with a soap and water before serving meals the incidence of intestinal infection in the household has been decreased. Filtering drinking water through a Berkefeld or Chamberland filter also reduces the amount of bowel disease, and has the added advantage of allowing any bacteriophage present in the water to pass through.

Most patients with acute dysentery suffer from the onset and have 20 stools in the 24 hours, colic and griping, tenesmus. The ulcers of bacillary dysentery tend to form at the lower end of the large gut so blood appears earlier in this condition than in amoebic dysentery in which the ulcers often appear first in the region of the caecum.

The usual treatment by purging with magnesium sulphate is completely wrong. A good mixture is:

Tincture of opium .... 10 minims
Tincture of belladonna .... 5 minims
Peppermint water............to ½ ounce

Three or four such doses a day in the acute stage give freedom from tenesmus and yet let him have an occasional fluid stool. In collapsed patients saline by vein is indicated.

Dysentery in babies is a dangerous condition. Most practitioners have learned by experience the value of chlorodyne.

All patients with dysentery, while temp. is above normal, should be kept strictly in bed and have fluid feeds only—milk, soup and sugar drinks with malt, and flavoured to taste ad lib.—with perhaps one small diluted peg of whiskey in the evening to those used to it. A total fluid intake of at least 1 gallon daily should be insisted upon. When the temp. comes down to normal milk puddings, jellies, ice cream, egg flips and glucose sweets can be added, and, when the stool first appears to be free microscopically from blood and mucus, soft eggs, poached, scrambled or lightly boiled, and strained porridge. Later soft fish, then boiled chicken and then other meat can be taken. A little mucus and blood with a single stool two or three days after normal motions have started does not necessarily mean a relapse.

A patient with either sort of dysentery should not be allowed to go back to normal life until a negative microscopic and cultural report on a purged stool has been obtained.

The writer has never seen serum do any good.

The writer has had excellent results with Shillong bacteriaphage, three or four 2 c.c. double ampoules daily, ½ hr. a. c., until the stools have been normal for two days, then one ampule in the morning on an empty stomach for the next week helps to destroy any dysentery bacilli that may still persist. In the average early case the fever disappears in 24 to 48 hours and the patient is passing normal stools by the third to the fifth day. In really early cases the response is even more dramatic, and the whole attack of bacillary dysentery is a matter of hours.

Emetine is specific for *amoebic* dysentery, intramuscularly in doses of 1 grain of the bihydrochloride. A course of six injections is usually sufficient, a second course must be given if the liver is still enlarged or the stool pathological. In acute amoebic cases with fever, the patient should be put to bed and the injections given every day. A varying amount of typhlitis often results. Bed is not necessary in mild or convalescent cases but the condition of the heart must be known and no exercise taken. Some people residing in the tropics receive an annual course of emetine with definite benefit.

Intestinal disinfectant drugs which may be useful after emetine or 'phage have coped with the acute infection are stovarsol, carbarsone, yatren, kaolin and enterovioform. They can never take the place of emetine for amoebic dysentery, or of 'phage for bacillary.

A course of atebrin—now mepacrine—has been shown to be specific for *Giardia lamblia* infestation.

Recently McCay has given sulfaguanadine in bacillary dysentery, with promising results. He thinks it would be a great pity for bacteriaphage to be superseded by the sulfa drug.

Two Chunking physicians[2] think highly of the sulfonamides' value in bacillary dysentery.

On the pediatrics service of the Central Hospital in Chunking, between November, 1941, and January, 1943, 57 cases of bacillary dysentery have been admitted. Five cases are excluded from the present series since these patients died within 24 hours of admission. Another six cases were chronic infections, and in these cases chemotherapy was not given until 30 days after onset. The remaining

2. K. T. Chen & L. L. Tael, Chunking, in *Chinese Med. Jl.,* April-June.

46 cases are acute, though in several instances specific therapy was not begun until the second or the third week of the illness. The results are fairly good in the chronic cases as well, so they are included ,making a total of 52 cases. Sulfathiazole was used in the first two cases only. The price was prohibitive for general use. Sulfanilyl guanidine was even more difficult to get. Sulfanilamide was then tried and the results were so excellent that from that time on, in every case in which a clinical diagnosis of bacillary dysentery was made, sulfanilamide was given without delay.

Usually only the severely infected or acutely ill cases are admitted.

The treatment before chemotherapy came into use consisted of general and symptomatic measures only. Specific polyvalent serum has not given the good results expected and has fallen into disuse.

The daily dose of the sulfonamide is 100-150 mgm. to every kilogram. The initial dose a third or a quarter of the total 24-hour dose is followed by the total 24-hour dose, divided into six equal parts and given at 4-hour intervals. Sodium bicarbonate is always given with sulfanilamide.

There were four deaths in the entire series. One case was not benefited by the treatment.

CLINICAL CHEMISTRY and MICROSCOPY

J. M. FEDER, M.D., and EVELYN TRIBBLE, M.T., Editors,
Anderson, S. C.

HISTOPLASMOSIS OF DARLING

A Brief Review of Available Literature

SEVERAL YEARS AGO our group accurately diagnosed three cases of Actinomycosis within as many months. Two of these were obscure and at that time, commenting before our County Medical Society, this writer remarked that these men made the diagnosis because they were thinking about Actinomycosis.

By the same token, other unusual disease conditions often escape detection because the clinicians and laboratory personnel do not bear them in mind It is true that Histoplasmosis is relatively rare but equally true that progressively more and more cases are being reported.

Etiological Factor—A fungus, *Histoplasma capsulatum*. Yeast-like form appears in blood and endothelial cells, when grown outside of the body mycelial threads become evident.

Blood Cultures—Organisms can be grown on ordinary media at the usual body temperature. Growth occurs best when the medium is adjusted to a pH of 6.5. The colonies appear as cotton balls.

Appearance of the Fungus in Tissue Sections— The parasitic bodies have been found in the endothelial cells in nearly every region of the body. They appear as numerous intracellular bodies encapsulated, hyperchromatic and bearing a distinct resemblance to the protozoal organisms of Leishman and Donovan. The wall is described as thicker than the ectoplasmic membrane of these and the Darling organisms appear larger and lack the bipolar staining so common to the protozoa.

Historical—In 1905 Sir Patrick Manson made the statement that kala-azar or some analogous disease might be found in America. Spurred on by this, Dr. S. T. Darling, Pathologist to the Ancon Hospital, Panama Canal Zone, made a special postmortem study for the presence of the Leishman-Donovan bodies in all patients dying in the hospital who had splenomegaly. He found three cases in which organisms were demonstrated that closely resembled those described by Leishman and Donovan and described them as "small or oval microorganisms 1 to 4 microns in diameter and possessing a polymorphous chromatin nucleus, basophilic cytoplasm and achromatic spaces, all enclosed within an achromatic, refractile capsule."

Clinical Manifestations—The disease apparently attacks all age groups but one might judge from the case histories reviewed that it is more prevalent in infancy and childhood. Both sexes appear to be equally susceptible and no organ in the body seems to be immune. From the evidence presented it would appear that we should be especially on guard when vague gastrointestinal symptoms make their appearance.

Synopsis of the clinical findings: A chronic febrile disease characterized by loss of weight, weakness, splenomegaly and more or less generalized enlargement of the lymph-nodes. It is quite possible that in the presence of this latter manifestation, an aspiration biopsy undertaken under the strictest bacteriological antiseptic conditions might provide a diagnostic culture.

Special caution is urged by some writers regarding the presence in some of the tissues of giant cells and areas of endothelial proliferation suggestive of tuberculosis. Perhaps all of us have had these cases in which every effort to demonstrate the tubercle bacillus met with failure. Possibly we weren't thinking about going down with the oil immersion and diligently seeking for the intracellular body of Darling.

Treatment — Antimony compounds, the arsenicals and bismuth have been tried with scant success. The disease terminated fatally in all of the cases reviewed.

Summary—This presentation is made to focus attention upon the fact that the disease is widely distributed throughout the world. Cases have been reported in which the diagnosis was made from blood smears, usually using the thick preparations commonly employed for concentration of the malaria parasites, the search being aided by the dehemoglobinization commonly employed in connection with the staining of these films.

The accrued bibliography is quite extensive, and to those interested in further details of this interesting entity it is suggested that the comprehensive package library of the American Medical Association be obtained. Due credit is given that source for some of the details contained in this commentary.

DERMATOLOGY

J. LAMAR CALLAWAY, M.D., *Editor*, Durham, N. C.

DERMATOPHYTID

VESICULAR ERUPTIONS of the hands may be a dermatophytosis, a dermatophytid, a contact dermatitis, a neurodermatitis, a drug eruption—most commonly, probably, a dermatophytid.

Dermatophytids are secondary "allergic" fungus eruptions which occur in specifically sensitized individuals as a result of the hematogenous spread of the fungi or of their allergenic toxic products by the blood stream from the primary fungus focus to a distant site. There are certain criteria which must be present to establish without question the diagnosis of an "id" eruption.

1. Pathogenic fungi must be demonstrated in the primary focus.
2. Fungi cannot be demonstrated in the secondary site.
3. A positive trichophytin test is always given.
4. The "id" eruption may be precipitated by irritation of the primary focus by trauma or over-treatment or it may result from spontaneous changes.
5. A positive blood culture may be obtained at the time of the hematogenous spread.
6. Spontaneous disappearance of the secondary eruption should occur as soon as the primary focus is eliminated unless other sensitivity is present.

The fingers and the hands are the commonest sites of the "id" eruption although the feet, legs and body generally are sometimes affected. Pustular bacterids or actual dissemination of the fungus itself with a true dermatophytosis may simulate the dermatophytids unless a careful study is carried out. In a like manner, contact dermatitis and drug eruptions may also simulate the dermatophytids.

The commonest manifestation of dermatophytid is the pompholyx type of vesicles along the sides of the fingers or groups of vesicular lesions appearing over the fingers and hands, or on occasion over any or all parts of the body. The vesicles are tense, edematous, and filled with a clear to cloudy sticky fluid. The vesicles are deep, are somewhat painful, and frequently itch intensely. Secondary infection, lymphangitis and lymphadenitis often develop and after the acute phase is over, the vesicles subside, leaving scaling eczematoid patches.

Treatment is directed principally to the primary focus since it is the exciting agent but treatment must be conservative or an exacerbation of the "id" eruption may occur, and treatment consists usually in using simple compresses, 1 per cent gentian violet solution, and other forms of mild treatment. The secondary of "id" eruption is likewise treated with warm wet compresses such as boric acid solution, avoidance of soap and water, and soothing cremes, or a calamine lotion. Efforts must be made to avoid secondary infection and in some instances calcium gluconate intramuscularly, whole b'ood injections, or röntgen therapy may be necessary to complete the involution. Desensitization by autogenous vaccine or by stock vaccine if attempted must be done with extreme caution.

SEX AND THE GORILLA
Sexology, Nov.

Dr. Adolph H. Schultz, Department of Anatomy, of the Laboratory of Physical Anthropology at Johns Hopkins Medical School, was kind enough to furnish us the following information:

"The size of the external genitalia differs greatly in the different types of apes. The gorilla is characterized by exceptionally small testicles and a very short male organ in its flaccid state. These small structures are entirely hidden in the dense coat of hair covering the pelvic region of the gorilla. Since gorillas of more than infantile age are too powerful and untrustworthy to be handled, it is in most cases impossible to examine their genitalia by palpation. Most people have concluded erroneously that a gorilla is a female after having failed to notice any sign of male genitalia. I have never heard of the reversed error, *i.e.*, that a female gorilla was mistaken for a male. An examination of the bodies of dead gorillas, of which I have seen a good many, leaves, of course, no doubt regarding their sex."

DIABETIC IDENTIFICATION TAGS

At the suggestion of the Medical Division of the U. S. Office of Civilian Defense, to prevent dangerous delay in diagnosis and to insure proper treatment during unconsciousness or coma, Eli Lilly and Company, Indianapolis 6, Indiana, in cooperation with the American Diabetes Association, will provide metallic identification tags to be worn by diabetic patients or carried in the pocket. The inscription read "Diabetic; If Ill Call Physician." No advertising of any sort appears on the tags, which will be supplied to the medical profession on request.

LAST YEAR 28,000 soldiers developed jaundice following inoculations against yellow fever. The army switched to another type of anti-yellow fever vaccine which does not contain human blood serum. So far as known this new vaccine has not produced jaundice.—*Victor News*, Oct.

SURGICAL OBSERVATIONS
OF THE STAFF
DAVIS HOSPITAL
Statesville

SPINAL ANESTHESIA AND THE REDUCTION OF MORTALITY IN SURGERY

THE CONTINUED improvement in the method of administering spinal anesthesia and in the drug used has had a great influence in the reduction of mortality in surgery. It has, also, made operations simpler, easier and less distressing.

The almost perfect relaxation which is obtained by spinal anesthesia enables the surgeon to do abdominal work with the greatest possible speed consistent with the maximum safety.

Most patients react from spinal anesthesia feeling so much better than they expected as to have a powerful influence for the best, in great contrast to the depression so common after general anesthesia, with its nausea, vomiting and the general distress.

During the present war spinal anesthesia has been the means of saving an untold number of lives which would have been lost had it been necessary to give some general anesthesia. For the wounded brought to the hospital in the advance sector needing prompt surgery below the diaphragm the spinal anesthetic's immediate action is a boon.

Personal communications from those who are using spinal anesthesia routinely in treatment of wounds of all kinds below the diaphragm, both abdominal and of the extremities, are practically unanimous in its praise.

There was a time when misinformed and irresponsible individuals claimed that spinal anesthesia caused backache, nervousness, weakness of the back and various other complications, but now most of those who once opposed it are to be found its strongest advocates.

* * * * *

TREATMENT OF FRACTURES OF THE NECK OF THE FEMUR

THESE FRACTURES, particularly those within the capsule, even in the aged, have been much more satisfactorily treated since the advent of the Smith-Peterson nail. The operation occasions little shock, a great consideration in these very poor risks. A day or so's observation *after* the occurrence of the fracture finding the patient's condition fairly good, one is warranted in attempting to do an internal fixation in the expectation that end results will justify the procedure.

In another type of fracture, the intertrochanteric, we often have extensive bone comminution. When such a condition occurs in the feeble aged, the outlook is bad. To put patients of this type in a plaster, splint or extension is to get poor results. Patients not able to stand the confinement are not so likely to survive.

In a large number of cases through the years we have found by using the Smith-Peterson nail and an angle bar we have been able to maintain the fragments in position so that healing took place even in the very aged who would ordinarily be considered hopeless risks. We feel that almost every patient, even though he might be considered a doubtful surgical risk, should be treated in this way.

Recently we have had two patients, one man and one woman, each nearly ninety-five years of age, on whom this treatment was used, and both recovered.

Years ago when we first began to use this treatment we felt that perhaps the use of so much metal in patients of this age might cause trouble. However, in no case has the tissue reaction been such as to cause trouble even in the very aged.

The treatment given aged patients with a fracture of the femur immediately after and, also, postoperatively, must be judiciously chosen! All the sources of complications should be eliminated if possible, the patient's strength built up in every way possible, and when necessary blood transfusions should be given.

The anesthesia should give most relaxation, most freedom from pain, and least ill after-effects. We usually find a very low spinal anesthesia the best for accurate and rapid reduction of the fracture under fluoroscopic and x-ray control and the carrying out of the operative procedure on the x-ray table where every necessary facility is available.

The Engle and May method of localization is used with a great deal of satisfaction. We have, also, devised a simplified method of localization which we have found very useful.

Without accurate localization it is impossible to insert the Smith-Peterson nail properly. This operation can only be done properly where there are available a good x-ray department and trained and experienced nurses and doctors.

In simple intracapsular fractures of the neck of the femur patients may be gotten up in twenty-four hours after the operation. Usually we keep them in bed a little longer. Comminuted fractures should have several days in bed—usually until the wound sutures have come out, then in a wheel chair. Fixation of the fragments prevents pain. Getting the patient up restores cheerfulness and promotes healing.

Just the thought of a possible life of invalidism, together with the severe pain that naturally comes in the average fracture not treated in this way, are enough to terrorize any patient, and the resulting depression may be sufficient to tip the scale against a possible recovery. Treated by internal fixation, most of these patients do very well and where there is a failure it is usually due to some cause beyond human control.

Our results at Davis Hospital have been so uniformly satisfactory that we feel that every patient where there is the least possible change of recovery should have the benefit of the doubt and that this method of treatment should be used.

* * * * *

A Letter

To the Medical Profession:

At a recent meeting of the Hurst Turner Post of the American Legion in Statesville, N. C., Mr. Paul G. Noell, Assistant State Service Officer, of Fayetteville, and our local Service Officer, Mr. Oscar R. Mills, of Statesville, requested me to communicate with the medical journals of the state regarding every examination and treatment of an ex-service man or woman, ill or having any disability of any kind, following his or her discharge from the Army or other of the Armed Forces.

Because of the fact that a careful written record of this history, examination and findings must be made, it is important that every such patient have a complete and accurate record of both the history of the trouble and of the findings at the time of the examination.

In order that this record may be as complete and accurate as possible, I would suggest that in all cases, except in cases of emergency, the patient be asked to sit down and write out in his own words a detailed statement of the trouble of which he or she is complaining, in consecutive order if possible; that the physician go over this statement with the patient, correcting, revising and adding to as may be found necessary; and that the examination be complete and thorough and all the findings minutely recorded.

The patient's statement, as nearly as practicable in his own words, plus a record of a complete and thorough examination of all the findings, will be competent medical evidence later on in case the patient should apply for any benefits to which ex-service men and women are entitled. Date of the examination and details of the findings should be accurately recorded, no matter how trivial the case may seem and no matter what the diagnosis.

By keeping this in mind every doctor in North Carolina can do much to protect the interests of ex-service men and women who come to him for examination and treatment, likewise to protect the interests of the Country by eliminating unjust and unwarranted claims to benefits.

Yours for greatest usefulness,

JAMES W. DAVIS,
Statesville.

DR. ROBERT WILSON RESIGNS

(*The Recorder* of Columbia (S. C.) Medical Society.)

Dr. Robert Wilson has tendered his resignation as Dean of the Medical College of the State of South Carolina and as Professor of Medicine in that college, to the Board of Trustees. The board accepted it with regret. Dr. Wilson was elected Dean Emeritus and Professor Emeritus of Medicine and will continue his association with the Medical College as special lecturer in Medical History. Dr. Wilson has been connected with the Medical College throughout his medical career, having served on the staff for the last fifty-two years and he has also served as Dean and Professor of Medicine for the last thirty-six years. He was, at the time of his resignation, the oldest dean of a Medical College in the United States. He was likewise the oldest active Professor of Medicine. No one has had a greater influence on Medical Education throughout the South than Dr. Wilson.

Dr. Wilson is largely responsible for the transformation of the Medical College in Charleston into a State institution, which occurred in 1913, and also for its continued growth and progress. The Medical College of the State of South Carolina has been brought from a reasonably small, privately-owned institution to a college with acceptable standards; standards that have been maintained since the beginning of ratings and inspections. Dr. Wilson's accomplishments have been recognized by other institutions, as he is the recipient of numerous honorary degrees. He has also maintained a high level of efficiency in the practice of medicine and in medical organization, both State and nation. He has held many high offices of honor and trust in both.

The Board of Trustees have unanimously elected Dr. Kenneth M. Lynch, who has been for a number of years Vice-dean and Professor of Pathology, to fill the office of dean. Dean Lynch took office at the end of this last academic year. He will continue as head of the Department of Pathology, in addition to his executive duties connected with his new administrative office.

Dr. Wm. H. Kelley has been chosen to head the Department of Medicine and to fill the chair of Professor of Medicine. Professor Kelley has been connected with the college for the past few years.

Following is a brief biography of Dr. Wilson:

Robert Wilson, M.D., Charleston, S. C. Physician. Born Statesburg, S. C., Aug. 23rd, 1867. Son of Robert Wilson, M.D., D.D., and Nana (Shand) Wilson.

Education: College of Charleston, 3 years; S. C. College 1887, A.B.; Medical College of S. C., 1892, M.D.; University of the South, D.C.L., 1926; LL.D., College of Charleston, 1922. Fraternity:

To Page 26

SOUTHERN MEDICINE & SURGERY

Official Organ

JAMES M. NORTHINGTON, M.D., *Editor*

Department Editors

Human Behavior
JAMES K. HALL, M.D. .... Richmond, Va.

Orthopedic Surgery
JOHN T. SAUNDERS, M.D. .... Asheville, N. C.

Urology
RAYMOND THOMPSON, M.D. .... Charlotte, N. C.

Surgery
GEO. H. BUNCH, M.D. .... Columbia, S. C.

Obstetrics
HENRY J. LANGSTON, M.D. .... Danville, Va.

Gynecology
CHAS. R. ROBINS, M.D. .... Richmond, Va.
ROBERT T. FERGUSON, M.D. .... Charlotte, N. C.

General Practice
J. L. HAMMER, M.D. .... Mannboro, Va.

Clinical Chemistry and Microscopy
J. M. FEDER, M.D.,
EVELYN TREBBLE, M. T. } .... Anderson, S. C.

Hospitals
R. B. DAVIS, M.D. .... Greensboro, N. C.

Cardiology
CLYDE M. GILMORE, A.B., M.D. .... Greensboro, N. C.

Public Health
N. THOS. ENNETT, M.D. .... Greenville, N. C.

Radiology
R. H. LAFFERTY, M.D., and Associates .... Charlotte, N. C.

Therapeutics
J. F. NASH, M.D. .... Saint Pauls, N. C.

Tuberculosis
JOHN DONNELLY, M.D. .... Charlotte, N. C.

Dentistry
J. H. GUION, D.D.S. .... Charlotte, N. C.

Internal Medicine
GEORGE R. WILKINSON, M.D. .... Greenville, S. C.

Ophthalmology
HERBERT C. NEBLETT, M.D. .... Charlotte, N. C.

Rhino-Oto-Laryngology
CLAY W. EVATT, M.D. .... Charleston, S. C.

Proctology
RUSSELL VON L. BUXTON, M.D. .... Newport News, Va.

Insurance Medicine
H. F. STARR, M.D. .... Greensboro, N. C.

Dermatology
J. LAMAR CALLAWAY, M.D. .... Durham, N. C.

Pediatrics

Offerings for the pages of this Journal are requested and given careful consideration in each case. Manuscripts not found suitable for our use will not be returned unless author encloses postage.

As is true of most Medical Journals, all costs of cuts, etc., for illustrating an article must be borne by the author.

TWO NEW DEPARTMENT EDITORS

THE JOURNAL is happy to announce for the New Year accessions of strength. With this issue Dr. John T. Saunders begins the conduct of the Department of Orthopedic Surgery, Dr. Robert Thrift Ferguson the conduct of the Department of Gynecology.

Every reader will look forward to each issue carrying authoritative presentations on some problem of these important divisions of our art.

Dr. Saunders is the head of a renowned orthopedic group in a city of especially accomplished physicians and surgeons. Dr. Ferguson, the first (and I believe the only) surgeon in this Section to devote his talents to gynecology exclusively, has, by the quality of his work, made his name known to doctors far and wide.

The editor has no hesitancy in promising that both the Department of Orthopedics and the Department of Gynecology will keep those who rely on them for information in these fields fully abreast of the times, for there will be served to them the latest of sound developments, the soundness attested by their having passed thoroughly informed, critical judgment.

* * * * *

THE RECORD OF REJECTIONS FOR THE ARMED SERVICES NO REFLECTION ON DOCTORS OF MEDICINE

IN THE WAR now going on, as in and after World War I (and perhaps all other wars) the numbers of young men, from "the cream of our population," rejected for the Army, Navy and Marine Service, is argued by those with more zeal than discretion as evidence of the lack of competence of doctors of medicine.

Let's look at the factual statement of the causes for these rejections.

The ten leading causes of rejection among white 18- and 19-year-old Selective Service registrants are, in decreasing order of occurrence, eye defects, mental disease; musculoskeletal, cardiovascular and ear defects; hernia; neurologic defects, educational deficiencies, underweight, and mental deficiency. For 18- and 19-year-old Negroes the ten leading causes of rejection are educational deficiency, syphilis; cardiovascular and mental disease, musculoskeletal abnormalities, hernia, eye and neurologic defects and diseases, mental deficiency and tuberculosis. Half of the rejections of Negro youths resulted from educational deficiency or from syphilis.

Will those with an itch for writing in defamation of their betters tell us and the rest of the people just which of these conditions is due to lack of attainable knowledge or of care on the part of doctors?

Not one of the ten leading causes for rejection of whites is to any considerable degree preventable. Eye defects, first in the list, are purely developmental; moreover, in only an extremely small percentage of cases, do they constitute a disability in civilian life to the making of a livelihood or the living of a long, happy and useful life.

No candid and half-intelligent person can read into this official statement any indictment of the medical profession.

Only one of the causes for rejection named, and that not as to whites at all and only tenth as to Negroes, may be reasonably said to be preventable—and the medical profession has, within the present century, and despite the apathy and active opposition of the general population, reduced the death-rate from tuberculosis by about 80 per cent!

* * * * *

A NEW THING UNDER THE SUN
GENERAL PRACTITIONER TO BE PAID SAME AS SPECIALIST

From a letter from Dr. Geo. M. Cooper, Assistant State Health Officer of North Carolina:

I am enclosing a copy of the revised fee schedule setting up a new scale of fees for payment to physicians for obstetric and pediatric care for the wives and babies of men in certain of the armed services. We have worked for several months to make this upward revisal in behalf of the general practitioners and have only recently been able to smooth out all the difficulties and to be able to make these changes effective for new cases authorized on and after January 1st, 1944.

1. The new schedule brings up the pay to all the general practitioners in the State participating in this service, making payments to all physicians on the same level. It increases the total that may be received for one of these obstetric cases of a maximum of $45.00. It is contemplated that this service will include a good quality of prenatal care, delivery service and careful postpartum examination from four to six weeks after the birth of the baby.

2. These changes make it possible for us to pay for prenatal visits after authorization at the rate of $2.00 per examination up to a maximum of $10.00. Heretofore we were only permitted to make payment if the minimum of visits or examinations made at the usual time totaled five. If a man now makes, for instance, four careful prenatal examinations he may receive $35.00 base pay, plus the $8.00 for the prenatal care given, making a total of $43.00 in such a case. The former arrangement has been a source of considerable dissatisfaction to physicians and we have made every effort to have it eliminated, working ever since March to do so. We have been successful and we hope that the physicians will find it satisfactory from now on.

There is one rigid requirement applicable in consideration of these higher fees, and that is that a careful postpartum examination should be made and included in the final brief, simplified report which is required. If such an examination and its reported results is not properly recorded, $5.00 will be deducted from the total pay, which would mean that the physician would get $40.00 instead of $45.00 for the otherwise complete case.

I should like to emphasize that the whole program is a voluntary arrangement and has already a two-fold purpose, and that is, in view of the shortage of physicians throughout the country in civilian practice, efforts had to be made to procure medical attention for the wives of these men serving in every part of the world; and second, to provide at least some compensation to physicians called upon to render competent medical service for these young women and children.

Dr. Cooper has always stood up for the general practitioner. He has been one himself. Throughout his many years of invaluable service to his people as Public Health Officer, he has never infringed on the rights of the private practitioner of medicine and he has shown a special concern and deep respect for the foundation stone of medicine—the family doctor.

Today I wrought a miracle. I bought of a Jew and sold to a Scot—and made a good profit.

But my miracle was but a minor one, as compared to Dr. Cooper's miracle of getting the same pay for a general practitioner for a certain kind of work as is paid to a specialist.

Hats off to Cooper.

* * * * *

HOW YOU MAY SAVE ON FIRE INSURANCE COSTS

Some weeks ago an editorial in the *Chapel Hill Weekly* had this to say:

Virginia has a system, established by law 15 years ago, for regulating fire insurance rates. North Carolina has no such system.

In both states, cities are classified first class, second class, etc., according to the quality of fire protection. In first class cities the brick dwelling rate (per $100) in Virginia is 16 cents, in North Carolina 18 cents; the frame dwelling rate in Virginia is 22 cents, in North Carolina 34 cents (54% higher). In fourth class cities the brick dwelling rate in Virginia is 22 cents, in North Carolina 40 cents (82% higher); the frame dwelling rate is 26 cents in Virginia, in North Carolina 63 cents (142% higher).

The reports from the Virginia Corporation Commission show that the companies doing business in that state have been fairly treated and have been able to make a fair profit. The commission has ordered seven rate reductions since the regulation law went into effect. The estimate of a saving of $21,500,000 to policyholders in 15 years is given by a member of the commission.

Until seven or eight years ago my fixed idea had been that fire insurance rates in North Carolina were established by law and, knowing that the State made certain requirements of insurance companies seeking licensure, my practice, based on this idea, was to purchase this insurance from whatever likeable agent happened to be handy.

My disillusionment came when riding with a friend. Happening to pass the scene of a recent house-burning, he mentioned that his insurance cost him only 60 per cent of the ordinary rate. A ten, a five, or even a "one per cent, 10 days," discount interests me—the teaching of a father that "a merchant who doesn't discount his bills is already bankrupt."

The upshot of the matter was that, as my insurance contracts then in force expired, new policies were bought from the company from which my friend and informant was purchasing insurance.

As a matter of course, the hoary lie, "You get what you pay for," was tried out on me, and "you don't want cheap insurance."

This irrefutable answer was given to the intimation that the "cheap insurance" did not afford as ample protection as that offered by the dear: On a substantial property, I owed the Prudential Life Insurance Company a considerable sum. A large part of the security consisted of a fire insurance policy. The Prudential had no interest in any fire insurance company beyond the certainty that, in case of destruction by fire of property on which the Prudential had lent money, the amount of the policy would be paid. The Prudential accepted without question the "cheap" policy purchased of the Mutual Company.

Here is a ready way for "preferred risks"—and most doctors are so rated—saving nearly half on their fire insurance, whether or not North Carolina follow Virginia's lead in this regard.

URTICARIA AND ANGIONEUROTIC EDEMA

MANY PATIENTS with chronic urticaria and angioneurotic edema are sensitive to coal tar products.[1] Most analgesic and soporific drugs and some cathartics are coal-tar derivatives. In addition, artificial colors and flavors are widely used in tooth pastes, mouth washes, candies, soft drinks, chewing gum, condiments, various liquid medicines and in the coating pills.

A practical plan of procedure is worked out:

The first thing to do is to free the patient of all ingested coal-tar contacts for at least two weeks. Over half of the cases will lose their symptoms and will remain free. The rigid restrictions may then be relaxed and various food sources of coal tars allowed from time to time until symptoms recur following the addition of some type of product or

[1] M. B. Coen, Cleveland, in Ohio State Med. Jl., Dec.

until the diet is unrestricted. The causative factors in most cases will then be demonstrated to be the cold, cough or purgative remedy which has been used.

During the time required for these experiments it is necessary to relieve the patient of the distressing symptoms. Epinephrine and ephedrine are the medicines of choice as in other allergic conditions. Ephedrine is usually prescribed in combination with some barbiturate. Sodium bromide is the hypnotic of choice. It may be combined with ephedrine.

```
Ephedrine Hydrochloride or Sulfate......gr. viii
Sodium Bromide ...................................dr. iiss
Syrup ...................................................fl. oz. i
Distilled water ....................................fl. oz. iv
    Sig.: 1 teaspoonful every 4 hours.
```

Relief in more than half of the cases of hives will be afforded by these measures. One-half of the remainder can be relieved by immunization with a histamine conjugate together with attention to the general needs of the patient.

From Page 23

Sigma Alpha Epsilon. Instructor in bacteriology, 1889-1900. Adjunct Professor 1901-03, Professor of Medicine since 1904; Dean since 1908. Medical College of S. C. Chairman State Board of Health, 1907-31; Fellow American College of Physicians; Member A.M.A., Southern Medical Association (president 1915-16); S. C. Medical Association (president 1904-05); National Association Study and Prevention of Tuberculosis; American Climatological and Clinical Association; Tri-State Medical Association of Carolinas and Virginia (president 1927-28). Mason. He is an Episcopalian.

WATTS HOSPITAL SYMPOSIUM
FEBRUARY 16TH-17TH

A two-day Medical Symposium, sponsored by the Staff of Watts Hospital, will be presented at the Washington Duke Hotel, Durham, North Carolina, Wednesday and Thursday, February 16th and 17th, 1944. The following physicians and surgeons will participate in the program:

1) Brig. General Hugh J. Morgan, Washington, D. C.
2) Brig. General James S. Simmons, Washington, D. C.
3) Lt. Col. Baldwin Lucke, Washington, D. C.
4) Lt. Col. Thomas Fitz-Hugh, Jr., Philadelphia, Pa.
5) Dr. Wiley D. Forbus, Professor of Pathology, Duke University Hospital, Durham, North Carolina.
6) Dr. Howard H. Bradshaw, Professor of Surgery, Bowman Gray School of Medicine, Wake Forest College, Winston-Salem, North Carolina.
7) Dr. Kenneth E. Appel, Assistant Professor of psychiatry, University of Pennsylvania, Philadelphia, Pa.
8) Dr. Tinsley Harrison, Professor of Medicine, Bowman Gray School of Medicine, Wake Forest College, Winston-Salem, North Carolina.
9) Dr. Oscar Hansen-Pruss, Associate Professor of Medicine, Duke University Hospital, Durham, North Carolina.

All members of the medical profession are cordially invited to attend. For hotel reservations communicate with the Manager, Washington Duke Hotel, Durham, N. C.

THE TRI-STATE PROGRAM

A SUPERB PROGRAM has been arranged from the offerings of surgeons and physicians who are never too busy or too well satisfied to take part in a first-class medical meeting.

Among the subjects to be discussed are:
Medico-Legal Aspects of Coronary Thrombosis
Prefrontal Lobotomy
The Politico-Economic Situation in Reference to Medicine
Pituitary Disturbances
Asthma
Everyday Problems in Allergy and Endocrinology
Prevention of Postoperative Cystocele
Rapid Treatment of Syphilis
Surgery of the Heart
Treatment of Burns
The Physician as Teacher
Pellagra *sine* Pellagra
Research in Antisepsis
Treatment of Neuro-psychiatric Patients in a General Hospital
Preventive and Early Treatment of Hypertrophy of the Prostate
Hold the Line
Foot Problems
Our neglect of the Deaf Patient

Among the speakers will be:
Dr. J Morrison Hutcheson, Richmond
Drs. James W. Watts, and Walter Freeman, Washington
Dr. H. F. Starr, Greensboro
Dr. Beverley R. Tucker, Richmond
Dr. J. G. Lyerly, Jacksonville
Dr. V. K. Hart, Charlotte
Dr. J. M. Feder, Anderson
Dr. G. H. Bunch, Columbia
Dr. Carl V. Reynolds, Raleigh
Drs. J. Lamar Callaway and R. O. Noojin, Duke University
Dr. Clay W. Evatt, Charleston
Dr. D. L. Maguire, Jr., Charleston
Dr. Wm. H. Prioleau, Charleston
Dr. Raymond Thompson, Charlotte
Dr. Karl Schaffle, Asheville
Dr. Ernest L. Copley, Richmond
Dr. John Stuart Gaul, Charlotte
Dr. William A. Johns, Richmond (now in the Army, stationed at New Orleans)
Dr. Thomas C. Bost, Charlotte
Dr. Archie A. Barron, Charlotte
Dr. Edward J. Williams, Monroe

Additions will be made.

A good attendance is assured from all over our territory. Be making your reservations. The Charlotte Hotel is headquarters, and the management promises that everything will be done for your comfort, and where the management leaves off the local medical profession will take on.

NEWS

CATAWBA VALLEY MEDICAL SOCIETY

At its December meeting the society elected the following officers:

Dr. J. S. Lewis, Hickory, president (succeeding Dr. C. R. Hedrick, Lenoir); Dr. Yates S. Palmer, Valdese, vice-president; Dr. L. A. Crowell, Jr., Lincolnton (re-elected), secretary-treasurer.

Dr. J. R. Saunders, superintendent of the State Hospital, and Dr. Palmer presented a paper on The Treatment of Hip Fractures of the Insane.

Other papers included Common Mistakes in Obstetrics by Dr. J. S. Lewis, Hickory, the new president; and Hyperinsulinism and Hyperglycemia by Dr. G. L. Donnelly of Valdese.

A number of case reports were presented to conclude the technical program.

RICHLAND COUNTY, S. C. (COLUMBIA) MEDICAL SOCIETY

Dr. Hugh E. Wyman is president; Dr. C. Gordon Spivey, vice-president; Dr. William A. Hart, treasurer; Dr. Chapman J. Milling, all of Columbia, for 1944. Delegates to the State Convention are Drs. James E. Boone, Kirby D. Shealy, L. E. Madden, A. F. Burnside and D. F. Adcock; with holdovers from last year, Drs. Benj. Rubinowitz and E. W. Masters.

Publishing Committee for The Recorder: Drs. Wm. Weston, Sr., N. B. Heyward, K. D. Shealy, D. F. Adcock and T. A. Pitts. The new president and secretary of the society ex-officio members.

NEW OFFICERS EDGECOMBE-NASH MEDICAL SOCIETY

Dr. J. Allen Whitaker, city health officer of Rocky Mount, was elected president of the Edgecombe-Nash Medical Society at the December meeting.

Other officers named were Dr. M. L. Stone, vice-president; Dr. Samuel H. Justa, secretary-treasurer; Dr. N. P. Battle, delegate to the state society; Dr. C. W. Bailey, alternate delegate, all of Rocky Mount. Members elected to the board of censors were Dr. Margaret Battle, of Rocky Mount; Dr. J. R. Vann, of Spring Hope, and Dr. J. G. Raby, of Tarboro.

SEABOARD MEDICAL ASSOCIATION NEW OFFICERS

At its recent meeting at Richmond this association of Virginia and North Carolina doctors east of the Atlantic Coast Line Railroad elected—

President—Dr. M. A. Pittman, Wilson, N. C.
First Vice-President—Dr. Ivan Steele, Winslow, Va.
Second Vice-President—Dr. G. G. Dixon, Ayden, N. C.
Third Vice-President—Dr. R. H. Wright, Phoebus, Va.
Fourth Vice-President—Dr. H. A. Ward, Hertford, N. C.
Secretary-Treasurer (re-elected) — Dr. Clarence Porter Jones, Newport News, Va.

The STAFF OF THE PROVIDENCE HOSPITAL, Columbia, S. C., elected officers at the regular December meeting: Dr. F. E. Zemp, Chief; Dr. George H. Bunch, Vice-Chief; and Dr. Ben Miller, Secretary. The Staff Committee is Dr. W. J. Bristow, Dr. H. E. Wyman and Dr. L. W. Pitts.

UNIVERSITY OF VIRGINIA

On November 12th, 1943, the Virginia Alpha Chapter of Alpha Omega Alpha presented Major-General David N. W. Grant, Flight Surgeon of the Army Air Force, as the speaker for their annual initiation program. His subject was "Problems in Aviation Medicine."

Dr. Herbert C. Clark of the Gorgas Memorial Institute, representing the National Research Council, gave two lectures to our student body and staff on November 19th, 1943. The subjects for these lectures were: "The Age Level for the Peak of Acquired Immunity to Malaria" and "The Distribution and Complication of Amœbic Lesions."

Dr. Robert V. Funsten attended a meeting of Orthopedic Specialists in Dallas, Texas, November 12th through 14th, to study treatments of poliomyelitis.

On November 22nd, Dr. Fred W. Stewart, Pathologist of Memorial Hospital for the Treatment of Cancer and Allied Diseases, gave the Phi Beta Pi lecture on "The Relation of Trauma to Malignant Tumors."

On November 25th, Dr. C. J. Frankel gave a lecture on "Functional Backache"; and on November 26th, Drs. W. E. Bray and T. S. Englar lectured on "Dysenteries" at Fort Belvoir, Virginia.

On December 2nd, Dr. Robert V. Funsten gave a lecture on "Fractures," and Dr. David C. Wilson one on "Psychoneurosis, Maladjustment, Neuropsychiatry" on December 16th at the U. S. Naval Hospital and Naval Academy Dispensary, Annapolis, Maryland.

DUKE

Efforts to render blood of animals suitable for human transfusions are being made by Professors Frank W. Putnam and Hans Neurath. In a paper read to the American Chemical Society recently, it was pointed out that protein molecules have a coiled structure which can be loosened or tightened by suitable manipulation with certain organic substances such as urea to modify their chemical nature and hence their disease-curing effects.

It has been discovered by Drs. Neurath and Putnam, in experiments on animals, that various proteins, including blood serums, lose their shock-causing properties after such treatment.

Investigation has shown that synthetic soaps are most effective in modifying the chemical nature of these proteins. Experiments are under way to learn whether they may serve as a means of treating blood proteins to avoid the serum-sickness that is always a risk in immunizing sensitive persons against certain diseases.

These experiments, conducted in laboratories at Duke, are part of the more general problem of investigating factors which cause proteins to produce antibodies when injected into human beings for therapeutic purposes.

RETIREMENT OF DR. CATHCART AND DR. VAN DE ERVE

The Board of Trustees of the Medical College of the State of South Carolina have announced the retirement of Dr. Robert S. Cathcart, head of the department of surgery, and Dr. John van de Erve, head of the department of physiology.

DR. HERBERT S. WELLS and Mr. John J. Thompson of the Bowman Gray School of Medicine, Winston-Salem, N. C., have devised a portable apparatus for estimating the peripheral blood flow. The apparatus is described in the issue for December of the *Journal of Laboratory & Clinical Medicine*.

DR. GEORGE B. ARNOLD, for several years superintendent of the State Colony for Epileptics and Feeble-minded, at the Colony near Lynchburg, has resigned, effective January 1st, 1944. He will be succeeded by DR. A. D. HUTTON, for several years a member of the medical staff of the Southwestern State Hospital at Marion, Virginia.

MARRIED

Dr. Otho B. Ross, Jr., of Charlotte, and Miss Dorothy Maude Lowe were married in Miami on December 22nd.

Dr. Henry Lee Howard, Medical Corps, United States Navy, of Savannah, and Miss Julia Thornton Booker, of Chapel Hill, North Carolina, were married on December 16th.

Lt. Joseph Shelton Bower, Medical Corps, U. S. Navy, of Salem, and Miss Marietta Bagley McGhee, of Lynchburg, were married on December 18th.

Dr. Marion Bailey Murdock, of New York, and Miss Katherine Clay Mallory, of Richmond, were married on December 21st.

Dr. Orin Watts Booth and Miss Elizabeth Amanda Mack, both of Durham, were married on December 18th.

Dr. Edgar Newman Weaver, of Orange, and Miss Evelyn Dabney Richards, of Roanoke, were married on December 20th.

Dr. James Edward McGee, Jr., of Roanoke Rapids, North Carolina, and Miss Jane Katherine Liesfield, of Richmond, were married on December 20th.

Dr. Maston L. Gray, of Huntington, West Virginia, and Miss Roberta C. Shaw, of Beaufort, North Carolina, were married on December 19th.

Dr. Marion Bailey Murdock, of New York, and Miss Catherine Clay Mallory, of Richmond, Virginia, were married on December 21st.

Mrs. Mary Slaughter Kidd, of Lynchburg, was married to Dr. S. G. Miller, of Covington, Virginia, November 6th, in Oak Grove Baptist Church, Petersburg Pike. The couple will live at Covington.

DIED

Dr. Lee Cohen, 69-year-old pioneer in the field of plastic surgery, died Dec. 31st at the Johns Hopkins Hospital following a lengthy illness.

He was one of the first surgeons in America to do plastic surgery on the nose, and designed a number of instruments for use in plastic operations, and was the author of many scientific papers on the subject. He was an attending surgeon at the Sinai Hospital and the Baltimore Eye, Ear and Throat Hospital.

A native of Halifax, N. C., Dr. Cohen was graduated from the University of North Carolina and the University of Maryland School of Medicine, where he completed his work in 1895.

During World War I he was in charge of oral plastic surgery at General Army Hospital No. 11, Cape May, N. J.

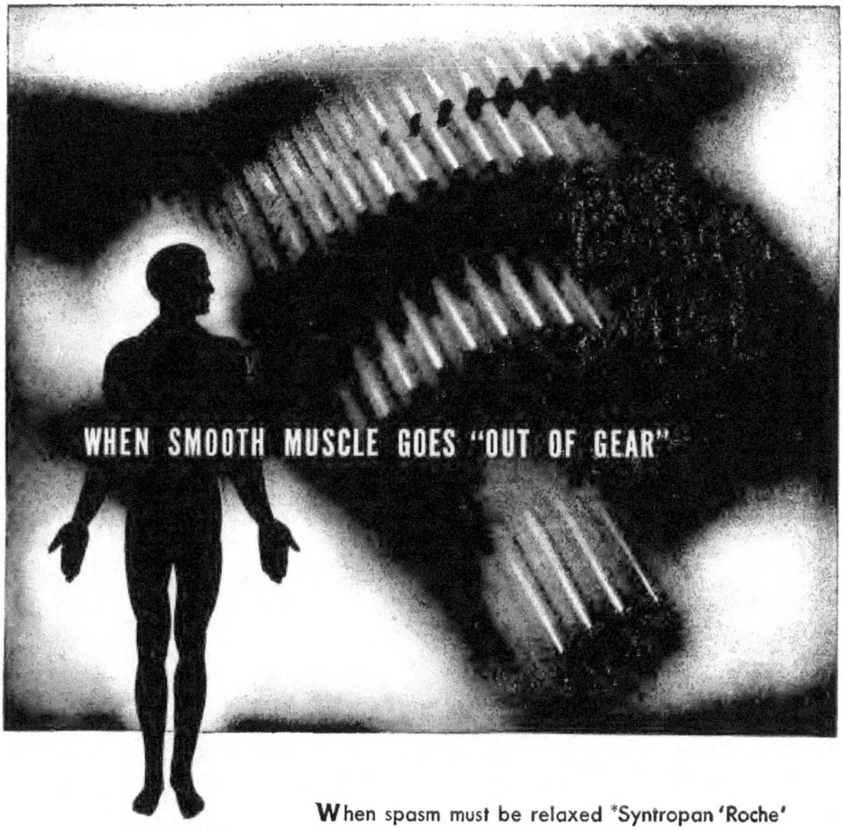

WHEN SMOOTH MUSCLE GOES "OUT OF GEAR"

When spasm must be relaxed *Syntropan 'Roche' is a dependable and effective means of restoring normal tone and activity. **INDICATIONS:** Syntropan 'Roche' is indicated in pylorospasm, cardiospasm, intestinal colic, spastic constipation, gastric spasm, spasms due to peptic ulcer, megacolon, and tenesmus. **DOSAGE:** One tablet (50 mg) three or four times a day, or as required. By subcutaneous or intramuscular injection, one ampul t. i. d., or as required. HOFFMANN-LA ROCHE, INC., NUTLEY, NEW JERSEY

*Phosphate of dl-tropic acid ester of 3-diethylamino-2, 2-dimethyl-l-propanol.

SYNTROPAN 'ROCHE'
NON-NARCOTIC ANTISPASMODIC
"FIGHT INFANTILE PARALYSIS • JANUARY 14th—31st"

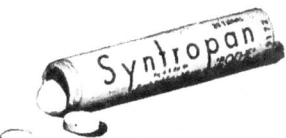

Dr. William I. Wooten, 49, Chief Surgeon of the Pitt County Hospital, Greenville, N. C., and member of the N. C. General Assembly, died suddenly of a heart attack at his home December 12th.

Dr. Charles H. May, 82, ophthalmologist and author of "The Manual of Diseases of the Eye," the most popular text on this subject ever written, died at his New York home December 8th.

Dr. Charles Lloyd Moore, 68, retired, died December 8th at his home at Charlottesville, Va. He was a native of Richmond, was educated at Virginia Military Institute and the Medical Colege of Virginia.

He practiced for many years in West Virginia. During World War I, he served as captain in the Medical Corps with the Seventy-ninth Division, winning special recognition for his work with the wounded at Montfaucon.

Dr. Michael Saliba died at the home of his brother in Savannah, Georgia, on January 5th. He was sixty-eight years of age and for many years he had practiced as a specialist in eye, ear, nose and throat diseases in Wilson, North Carolina.

Dr. George Adams Smith died at the home of a daughter in Fremont on January 7th. He was born in 1859, was graduated from the Louisville Medical College in 1887, and for many years he had practiced in Black Creek, North Carolina.

AN EFFECTIVE, CHEAP TREATMENT FOR PEDICULOSIS CAPITIS

(W. A. Davis, New York, in Jl. A. M. A., Nov. 27th)

The formula used was phenyl cellosolve 40%, ethanol 30%, water 25%, methyl salicylate 5%. The nurses were asked to apply the lotion to the head so that the hair was thoroughly wet and cautioned to keep the fluid out of the eyes and mouths of the children. No further treatment was used. No live lice were ever found after a single treatment. No irritation was observed except a brief mild tingling if the lotion was rubbed into the scalp.

Advantages are ease of application, rapidity of action, freedom from irritant action and efficiency against both insects and eggs. The cost was 1c per treatment. The lotions produced a moderate burning if applied to such tender areas as the eyes, mouth or perineum. The collosolve left the hair in a few days. The treatment proved satisfactory for the treatment of pediculosis capitis and is recommended for general use.

NEW VITAMIN-MINERAL PRODUCT

Hoffman-La Roche, Inc., of Nutley, New Jersey, recently announced to the medical profession a new multivitamin-mineral preparation called *Vitaminets*. This is not "just another" multivitamin combination. *Vitaminets* are palatable tablets of superior merit containing 9 *vitamins and 5 minerals*—vitamins A, B_1, B_2, B_6, C, D and E, calcium pantothenate, niacinamide, iron, calcium, phosphorus, manganese and magnesium. *Vitaminets* have a pleasant licorice flavor and, if desired, they may be chewed and swallowed like any other food. Like all Roche products, *Vitaminets* will be marketed only through professional channels and will never be advertised to the laity. *Vitaminets* are available in bottles of 30 and 100 tablets. A descriptive *Vitaminets* booklet will be furnished upon the request of the physician.

TOLERANCE TO DRIED THYROID does not develop in the myxedematous patient even after years of medication.

BOOKS

ESSENTIALS OF SYPHILOLOGY, by RUDOLPH H. KAMPMEIER, M.D., Associate Professor of Medicine, Vanderbilt University, in Charge Syphilis Clinic, Vanderbilt University Hospital. With chapters by ALVIN E. KELLER, M.D., and J. CYRIL PETERSON, M.D. 516 pages; 87 illustrations. *J. B. Lippincott Company*, Philadelphia. $5.00.

The author's objectives are stated as—

To present the concept of syphilis as a systemic disease presenting problems for every type of specialist, and therefore a disease of peculiar interest to the general practitioner.

To promote better habits in history taking and physical examination.

To emphasize that in acute syphilis, a clinical diagnosis alone is not justifiable.

To develop a critical evaluation of serodiagnosis.

To raise the index of suspicion as to the role syphilis plays in chronic disease years after the infection was acquired.

To stimulate better antisyphilitic treatment.

The records of 6,259 cases are used in this practical book as examples to illustrate points in diagnosis, prognosis and treatment.

The author does his part toward attaining his objectives. If readers will study well his book and follow its direction the result will be all that author, doctor and patient can reasonably desire in the lessening of incidence and ravages of syphilis.

The book sets forth, not only what is desirable to do, but what has been done on a small scale, and can be done on a large scale.

PATHOLOGY AND THERAPY OF RHEUMATIC FEVER, by LEOPOLD LICHTWITZ, M. D., Lately Chief of Medical Division, Montefiore Hospital, New York, and Clinical Professor of Medicine, Columbia University. Foreword by WILLIAM J. MALONEY, M.D., LL.D., F.R.S. (Edin.), Consulting Neurologist, City Hospital, New York. Edited by MAJOR WILLIAM CHESTER, M.C. 225 pages; 69 illustrations. *Grune & Stratton, Inc.*, 381 Fourth Avenue, New York 16, N. Y. $4.75.

Reading of this book cannot fail to impress on one the importance of rheumatism as a crippler and a killer. Constant alertness as to early diagnosis is urged, and adequate management over a longenouhg time to reduce permanent impairment to a minimum. The various therapeutic measures are evaluated, individualized, and described in detail.

Contents

1. Definition.
2. Incidence and Influence of Personal Factors.
3. General Pathology.
4. Systemic Phenomena.
5. Rheumatic Heart Disease.
6. Rheumatic Vascular Disease.
7. Arthritis.
8. Myositis.
9. Manifestations in the Skin.

HE ORDERS THE JUMP... BUT HE'S FIRST TO LEAP

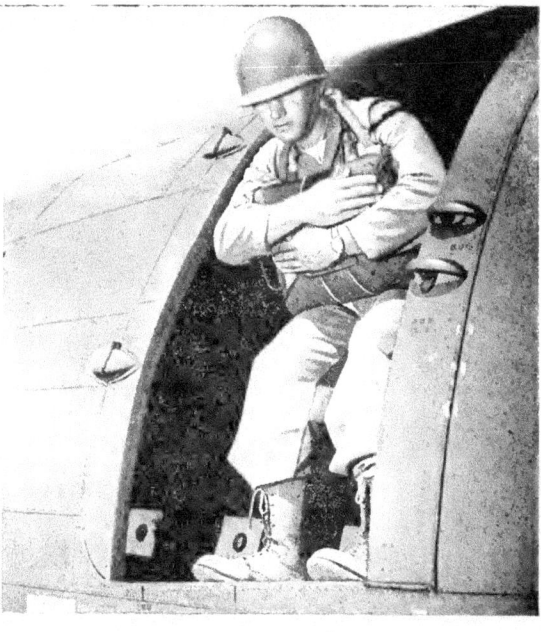

"*Ready!*" the pilot warns...Five tense minutes to go ... the men "hook up" for the last brief check... then the paradoctor's command: "*Stand to the door!*" But it is he who leads them off ... first overside ... first to face the unknown perils that lie below.

Courageous as he is versatile, the war doctor fulfills long, tough missions without thought of rest. When it's time to relax, he keenly appreciates the pleasure of a good smoke ... Camel most likely, the favorite of the armed forces*... for sheer mildness, friendly taste.

Make it *your* pleasure to remember those you know in the services. Send them cartons of Camels ... often!

1st in the Service

*With men in the Army, Navy, Marine Corps, and Coast Guard, the favorite cigarette is Camel. (Based on actual sales records.)

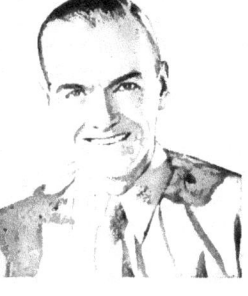

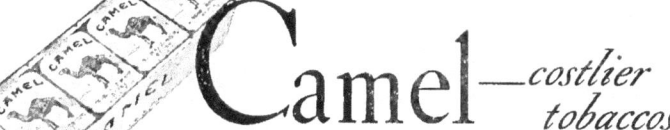

Camel —*costlier tobaccos*

New reprint available on cigarette research—Archives of Otolaryngology, March, 1943, pp. 404-410. Camel Cigarettes, Medical Relations Division, One Pershing Square, New York 17, N. Y.

10. Manifestations in the Nervous System.
11. Manifestations in Other Organs and Areas.
12. Differential Diagnosis and Prognosis.
13. Therapy (Prevention of bacterial invasion. General therapy. Antirheumatic drugs. Fever therapy. Serum; vaccine. Therapy by skin irritation. Sulphur; gold salts. Therapy in carditis. Therapy of Sydenham's chorea. Treatment of Hyperpyrexia).

THE YOUNGEST OF THE FAMILY, HIS CARE AND TRAINING, by JOSEPH GARLAND, M.D., Physician to Children's Medical Department, Massachusetts General Hospital. Revised Edition. *Howard University Press*, Cambridge, Mass. $2.00.

A guide to mother and nurse, remarkably free from fads and extremes, firmly based on sound knowledge and sweet reasonableness. Every pregnant woman, however many children she may have borne already, should have a copy for her study during the pregnancy and afterward; and few physicians who have the care of pregnancy, infancy and childhood—obstetricians, pediatricians, or general practitioners—could make a more profitable investment.

THE 1943 YEAR BOOK OF INDUSTRIAL AND ORTHOPEDIC SURGERY. Edited by CHARLES F. PAINTER, M.D., Orthopedic Surgeon to Massachusetts Women's Hospital and Beth Israel Hospital, Boston. *The Year Book Publishers*, 304 S. Dearborn St., Chicago. $5.00.

The editor deplores the propensity of doctors to lend enthusiastic support to new methods of treatment before their efficacy has been demonstrated. This volume consistently shows throughout that the editor has the wisdom to prove all things and hold fast to that which is good.

Hemohistoblast
Erythrocyte
Proerythroblast
Reticulated
Erythrocyte

(Tablets)
FERRO-SEALS
(B Complex)

Meets the greatly increased iron requirements of pregnancy and lactation.
Samples and literature from

BISHOP LABS., 80 Greenwich St., New York, N. Y.

ASAC

15% by volume Alcohol
Each fl. oz. contains:
Sodium Salicylate, U. S. P. Powder........ 40 grains
Sodium Bromide, U. S. P. Granular........ 20 grains
Caffeine, U. S. P. .... 4 grains

ANALGESIC, ANTIPYRETIC
AND SEDATIVE.

Average Dosage
Two to four teaspoonfuls in one to three ounces of water as prescribed by the physician

How Supplied
In Pints, Five Pints and Gallons to Physicians and Druggists.

Burwell & Dunn ompany

Manufacturing   *Pharmacists*
Established   *in 1887*
CHARLOTTE, N. C.

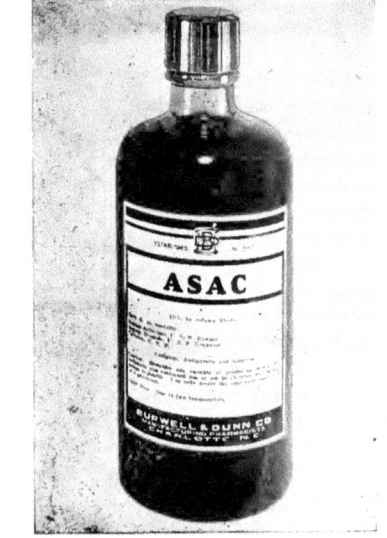

HEALTH EDUCATION ON THE INDUSTRIAL FRONT. The 1942 Health Education Conference of the New York Academy of Medicine. Pages x + 63. *Columbia University Press*, Morningside Heights, New York. $1.25.

These papers deal with the opportunities and obligations that exist for health educators and others in the industrial health field in such matters as nutrition promotion, control of physical illness, restriction of mental disabilities, and limitation of accidents.   *Contents*

Introduction, by Iago Galdston, M.D.

Introductory Comments, by Donald B. Armstrong, M.D.

The Wartime Intensive Industrialization of the Community and Its Health Implications, by Cassius Watson, M.D.

Food and Nutrition in the Home and in the Work Place, by Otto A. Bessey, Ph.D.

Disease and Handicap Detection and Control in Industry, by Leonard Greenburg, M.D.

Mental Problems and Morale in Industry, by Lydia G. Giberson, M.D.

Educational Methods and Control of Accidents in Industry, by Harold R. Bixler.

FUNDAMENTALIST, EVIDENTLY

From an exchange:

"The Reverend Mr. Jacob *Gartenhaus* will bring the message at the evening service Sunday evening at the First Presbyterian Church."

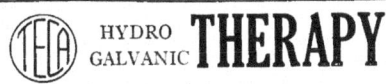

HYDRO GALVANIC **THERAPY**

FULL BATH TREATMENTS
in any available bath tub
TANK TREATMENTS
IONTOPHORESIS

— FOR HOSPITAL AND OFFICE USE —

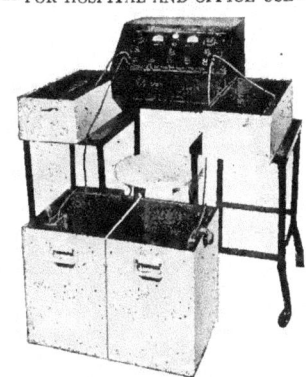

For full information and literature write to

TECA CORPORATION
220 WEST 42nd STREET   NEW YORK 18, N. Y.

FOR
FULLY EFFECTIVE THEORY
B COMPLEX
derived from
RICE BRAN CONCENTRATE

"BEFACLIN*" Rice Bran Concentrate is a natural source of all known B factors observed but not yet positively identified.

Deficiencies in the B vitamins usually occur together.

No single B vitamin, such as Thiamine, will control the deficiencies adequately.

High Thiamine content of so-called B complex preparations is not necessarily a true index of therapeutic value, since all the various B factors must be supplied in properly balanced amounts (1).

"BEFACLIN"—Tablets and Elixir supply the whole Vitamin B Complex.

(1) L. B. Pett, J. A. McKirdy and M. M. Cantor, Canadian Medical Journal, 46:413, 1942.

*"BEFACLIN" is a trademark of Tablerock Laboratories.

TABLEROCK LABORATORIES
GREENVILLE, SOUTH CAROLINA, U. S. A.

SURGERY

R. S. ANDERSON, M.D.

GENERAL SURGERY

144 Coast Line Street   Rocky Mount

R. B. DAVIS, M. D., M. M. S., F. A. C. P.
*GENERAL SURGERY
AND
RADIUM THERAPY*
Hours by Appointment
Piedmont-Memorial Hosp.   Greensboro

(*Now in the Country's Service*)
WILLIAM FRANCIS MARTIN, M.D.
GENERAL SURGERY
Professional Bldg.   Charlotte

OBSTETRICS & GYNECOLOGY

IVAN M. PROCTER, M.D.

OBSTETRICS & GYNECOLOGY

133 Fayetteville Street   Raleigh

SPECIAL NOTICES

TWO LABORATORY TECHNICIANS, being graduated from a High-class Hospital Laboratory, services available January 1st, 1944. Address TECHNICIAN, care *Southern Medicine & Surgery*.

TO THE BUSY DOCTOR WHO WANTS TO PASS HIS EXPERIENCE ON TO OTHERS

You have probably been postponing writing that original contribution. You can do it, and save your time and effort by employing an expert literary assistant to prepare the address, article or book under your direction or relieve you of the details of looking up references, translating, indexing, typing, and the complete preparation of your manuscript.

Address: *WRITING AIDE*, care *Southern Medicine & Surgery*.

THE JOURNAL OF
SOUTHERN MEDICINE AND SURGERY

506 North Tryon Street, Charlotte, N. C.

The Journal assumes no responsibility for the authenticity of opinion or statements made by authors or in communications submitted to this journal for publication.

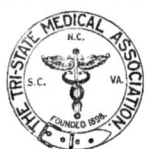

JAMES M. NORTHINGTON, M.D., Editor

VOL. CVI   FEBRUARY, 1944   No. 2

— HELP —

R. M. YERGASON, M.D., F.A.C.S., Hartford, Connecticut

IT IS EASY TO ACCEPT catch phrases at face value, without analysis, and to travel along under the banner of some slogan the implications of which may be broader than we realize.

We hear and we read a great deal about "Postwar Planning" (which has just drawn its first breath), and the importance of the Social Sciences (which, as sciences, are in their swaddling clothes). We are told that psychology and psychiatry must be applied when these subjects (outside of laboratory psychology) are just beginning to become scientific. With these imperfect tools nevertheless we must be dextrous in this production process of postwar planning if we hope to turn out the logical product, social security.

The expression "Social Security" is commonly understood, in a very restricted sense, to refer to compulsory savings for the benefit of old age. It is unfortunate that the term should have been given this limited usage, for its implications are extremely broad. In fact, on a world basis, "Social Security" expresses the very essence and fundamental purpose of our war effort. It is Social Security for all nations and all individuals which we desire and, upon this rock, all purposeful postwar planning must be built.

In *Postwar Planning for World Social Security* we are dealing, probably, with a googol of variables of the form $y = f(x)$, so that most of us are completely bemazed by our first look at this hopeless entanglement of differentials. How clarifying it would be if we could but get together and search out the postulates implied in this expression "Social Security."

To accomplish this, it would seem that the basic principles might be derived through the use of the following:

BASIC SCHEME OF SOCIAL SECURITY

1. Special study of individual *personality* so that, if not a definite referent (designatum), a limited system of references (denotata) will be understood to be implied by this word. (Anatomical consideration of the *cell* of the superorganism.)
(Psychology should function here)

2. Studies of the reactions of individuals to the impingement upon them of environmental factors. (Physiological and pathological consideration of the *cell* of the superorganism.)
(Psychiatry should function here)

3. Studies of the mechanics of local classes and groups of individuals (home, school, church ....) (Anatomical consideration of the *tissues* of the superorganism.)
(Local Social Services should function here)

4. Studies of the interaction of local groups. (Physiological and pathological consideration of the *tissues* of the superorganism.)
(Municipal Social Services should function here)

5. Studies of the Statewide classes and groups of which local ones are a part. (Anatomy, physiology and pathology of the *organs* of the superorganism.)
(State organizations should function here)

6. Studies of the National classes and groups of which local ones are a part. (Anatomy, physiology and pathology of the *systems* of the superorganism.)
(National Social Services should function here)

7. Studies of the mechanics (by the national government) of *Democracy* so that, if not a definite referent (designatum), a limited system of references (denotata) will be understood to be implied by this word. (Anatomical consideration of the *superorganism*.)

(National Representatives should function here)

8. Studies of the reactions of democracy to the impingement of other systems of government (its environmental factors), (presupposing knowledge of their anatomy, etc.) (Physiological and Pathological consideration of the *superorganism*.)

(National Senators and or Supreme Court should function here)

Walter Pitkins says, "Were we all to withhold speech except when we knew exactly what we were talking about, what deathly silence would enshroud this world of born gabblers."* Hence the temerity of a specialist in human body mechanics in this attempt to place on paper some principles which seem to him basic in the hope that, others doing likewise, a clearer vision of the best process for postwar planning may appear.

Addendum: Surveying this schema brings the suggestion of a new specialty, that of Superpsychiatrist, to which might aspire Doctors of Philosophy who have majored in diplomatic subjects upon an early background of deep interest in anthropology.

*A short Introduction to the History of Human Stupidity. Walter B. Pitkin. Simon and Schuster, 1932.

MORE ABOUT RESISTANT GONORRHEA
(E. N. Cook et al., in *Proc. Staff Meetings Mayo Clinic*)

In May, the use of penicillin in sulfonamide-resistant gonorrheal infection was reported. We have now used penicillin in an additional group of 14 cases—3 in women—with equally effective results. All patients had failed to respond to sulfonamide therapy except one.

Penicillin was administered in this group of cases by means of the intravenous drip method. This technic has proved entirely satisfactory and does not require repeated injections at short intervals. Half of the daily dose dissolved in 1 liter of physiologic saline solution was attached to the intravenous apparatus morning and evening, and the material administered at a rate of 30 or 40 drops per minute. Since repeated intravenous or intramuscular injections require frequent visits to each patient throughout the 24 hours, the intravenous method, in addition to the lack of the necessity for repeated injections and discomfort to the patient, conserves the time of the medical personnel.

The intramuscular administration of 10,000 to 20,000 units of penicillin in 5 or 10 c.c. of physiologic saline solutions, at intervals of three to four hours is equally satisfactory.

One of the three women had had the disease for 8½ months; she had, in addition to the pelvic inflammatory disease, a gonorrheal proctitis. It appears that the results in the treatment of women suffering from gonorrhea are comparable to those reported for men.

Since this material was presented Mahoney and others have reported ressults of treatment in 75 cases of sulfonamide-resistant gonorrhea, with success in 74.

POLIOMYELITIS AT ELEVEN DAYS
(Jour. Am. Med. Assn., Jan 29th)

The case of an infant which began to show signs of infantile paralysis in its eleventh day of life and of its mother, who apparently had the disease at the time the child was born and who died from it on the fourth day after delivery, was discovered in the course of a survey of epidemics made for The National Foundation for Infantile Paralysis.

The authors point out that though it is not possible to determine the source of the infant's infection, "it appears to us that the available evidence would suggest that infection occurred at time of birth or shortly thereafter."

The age of susceptibility to infantile paralysis has been of great interest to students of the disease. During pregnancy there is apparently a failure of infection of the child in the womb when the mother has infantile paralysis. Cases occur infrequently in infants under 6 months of age, and several investigators have reported that infants usually show antibodies if the mother has neutralizing antibodies in her blood and that these appear to persist several months after birth.

On the day of birth the child was admitted to the nursery in good condition. At 9 a. m., the child was placed in bed beside the mother for 10 min., the only contact between the mother and the child subsequent to delivery. On the 11th day of life the child became listless, cried seldom and at times was slightly cyanotic, showing some throat congestion. Two days later there was weakness in both lower extremities. . . . A spinal puncture resulted in a diagnosis of infantile paralysis.

The last report on the child on 63d day of life, there was complete paralysis of the right lower extremity except for slight motion of the toes.

PRESCRIPTIONS
(From the *New York Physician*)

For the cold sterilization of metallic instruments:
Sodium Borate	20 Gm.
Solution of Formaldehyde	300 c.c.
Methanol qs.	1000 c.c.

M. et ft. sol. et filtra

A palatable way of prescribing Aspirin for child:
Acid Acetylsal.	3.2
Alcoholis	15.0
Pulv. tragac.	0.2
Syr. rub. id.	45.0
Aquae, qs ad	90.0

M. et Sig.: Teaspoonful p. r. n.

For Coughs:
Papaver. Hydrochlor.	0.4 Gm.
Codein. Sulf.	0.4 Gm.
Elix. Terpin. Hyd. q.s. ad	90.0 c.c.

Sig.: One teaspoonful every 2 or 3 hours.

Ammon. Chlorid	10 Gm.
Elix. Glycyrrh.	60 c.c.
Syr. Acac. qs.	120 c.c.

Sig.: Teaspoonful in half a glass of water q. 2 h.

For Neuralgia:
Phenobarb.	.75 Gm.
Aminopyrin	7.5 Gm.
Liq. Amaranth.	25 c.c.
Elix. Iso-Alc. N.F. q.s.	90.0 c.c.

M. et ft. sol.

Sig.: Teaspoonful in water q. 3 h. to relieve pain and restlessness.

The Relationship of Tonsillectomy and Adiposo-Genital Dystrophy

Max. A. Goldzieher, M.D., New York City

REMOVAL of tonsils and adenoids, as a rule, scarcely affects the otherwise normal child, notwithstanding the occasional claims that retarded growth and development in previously underweight children favorably respond to the pharyngeal surgical procedure. The systemic after-effects of the operation are not striking, according to good authority (Selkirk and Mitchell, Zubkus), and large statistics. Nevertheless, cases have been observed in which abnormal gain in weight, or even the classical manifestations of Fröhlich's adiposo-genital dystrophy, followed in the wake of tonsillectomy. The number of these cases is not large compared to the huge figures comprised in statistics of tonsillectomy. Hence, it is understandable that these rare sequelae of the operation have attracted but little attention on the part of rhinolaryngologists. Pediatricians and particularly endocrinologists who are afforded the opportunity to observe a more select material—*i.e.*, cases of obesity in childhood—have become aware of the fact that the onset of pathologic obesity is sudden in a not negligible percentage of cases upon removal of tonsils and adenoids.

We have called attention to this remarkable coincidence in earlier publications and feel that it cannot be complacently accepted or explained by the hypothesis that removal of oversize tonsils and adenoids, in clearing nasal passages, increases the appetite and vigor of these children or decreases their susceptibility to respiratory infections, as a consequence of which nutrition and growth are improved. It may be reasonably assumed that tonsillectomy on a previously undernourished child might be followed by gratifying growth, provided the response to the operation is self-limited and leads to the attainment of weight average for the age group. The explanation is obviously untenable in case the postoperative gain in weight continues to pathologic proportions. Such obesity may develop in children who were not underweight or in ill health before the operation; the previously normal, healthy child first showing signs of a pathological condition after the operation. In addition to the abnormal weight, the pathologic character of these changes is shown by the peculiar distribution of the fat deposits—above the hips of the girdle or rubber-tire type, or of the abdomen, producing a pendulous apron, while additional bulges appear on the flexor surface of the thigh and extensor surface of the upper arm. These specific deposits are conspicuous regardless of the degree of general obesity.

Peculiarities of fat distribution, the diagnostic significance of which was highly rated by earlier empiricists, find little favor in the eyes of modern students of nutrition, who believe that obesity merely represents the result of excessive food intake; it is assumed to be the result of conditioning by environmental influences or the reaction to emotional disturbances. The reluctance of the nutritional school to consider possible endocrine factors is so great that they are unwilling to recognize even those hormonal influences which are known to govern, or at least influence appetite, partly by regulation of the blood sugar and partly by mediation of the effects of the autonomic nervous system upon the gastro-intestinal tract. The arguments presented in favor of the purely nutritional theory of obesity are outweighed, in our opinion, by evidence to the contrary; yet, assuming that the theory is correct, overindulgence in food and an intake of calories in excess of expenditure might perhaps account for a gain in weight, but hardly for the singular features of fat distribution which vary so characteristically in the individual types of endocrine disorder. Thus, the trunk-obesity of the hypothyroid is in striking contrast to the fat distribution of Fröhlich's adiposo-genital dystrophy which, on the other hand, is identical with that of women of childbearing age whose obesity develops coincidentally to menstrual disorders or upon the onset of the menopause. Obesity of similar type is also noted postpartum, in case of massive puerperal blood loss, the significance of which becomes evident only when the girdle-type obesity gradually changes into emaciation such as characterizes the later stage of Simmonds' disease. Such cases, as supported by animal experimentation, prove conclusively that girdle-type obesity is intimately connected with disease of the pituitary gland. Pathognomonic fat deposits, the distribution of which characteristically differs from that of the thyroid or pituitary type, are also noted in the hypogonad, following castration, or in case of overactivity of the adrenal cortex.

It was necessary to discuss the diagnostic significance of abnormal fat distribution in order to point out that the obesity which is observed subsequent to tonsillectomy is of a specific type and bears the characteristics of pituitary disease. The sudden accumulation of fat is usually accompanied by abnormalities of skeletal growth and genital development. The combination of retarded growth, subnormal genital development, and obesity constitutes the classical syndrome of Fröhlich's adiposo-genital dystrophy. This classical picture, however, is not present in every case, for girdle-type obesity may develop without significant retardation of longitudinal growth; and, though less often, without deficient development of the genital organs. Normal growth and genital development do not contradict the view that abnormal fat deposits indicate an abnormal function of the pituitary gland, for the anterior lobe of the pituitary is an organ of manifold activities, liable to show evidence of dissociation in the sense that one or several of the functions remain unaffected while others are more or less impaired or distorted. The pituitary gland may be capable of promoting normal growth, yet at the same time fail to produce enough gonadotropins to assure normal genital development; or, the direct or indirect effects of the pituitary on intermediary metabolism may become disturbed to an extent which entails accumulation of abnormal fat deposits without interfering with other secretory activities.

The girdle-type obesity and the associated changes of growth and development, observed after tonsillectomy, simulate Fröhlich's disease also in respect to those metabolic peculiarities which we have described as the "pituitary metabolic pattern." The individual deviation from normal values may not seem important or specific, yet they fit into a definite pattern the combination of which points to a metabolic trend of considerable diagnostic significance. These changes consist of:

1. decreased basal metabolism
2. absence or decrease of the specific dynamic action of proteins
3. low fasting blood sugar
4. flat sugar tolerance curve with a delayed hypoglycemic dip
5. increased uric acid
6. increased cholesterol
7. high normal or increased chloride and sodium values.

A relative lymphocytosis is invariably and a slight eosinophilia frequently present.

If the obesity develops at an early age, examination of cranial röntgenograms contributes important information, for the pneumatization of the cranium is found to be deficient; e.g., the frontal sinus and mastoid cells are small or altogether undeveloped, while the cranial vault remains thin and the diploë extremely scanty. These findings cannot be expected in case the pituitary condition starts later, at an age when cranial pneumatization is well advanced.

In cases of adiposo-genital dystrophy in which the symptoms set in immediately upon, or shortly after the performance of pharyngeal surgery, careful investigation reveals the metabolic and radiologic findings of ordinary cases of Fröhlich's syndrome which have developed without any relationship to the removal of tonsils and adenoids.

If the pituitary pathogenesis of Fröhlich's syndrome is accepted—and this applies to both ordinary and post-tonsillectomy cases—the pathogenetic relationship of pharyngeal surgery to the development of pituitary disease will warrant the attitude that this coincidence is merely fortuitous, for Fröhlich's syndrome might have developed irrespective of the surgical performance. It is the purpose of the present paper to call attention to certain anatomical features which are apt to bridge the gap between the post-tonsillectomy incidence of Fröhlich's syndrome and its relationship to the pituitary gland. The connecting link is found in the adenoids which as a rule are removed along with the tonsils. These hyperplastic portions of the pharyngeal lymphatic tissue, however, are located in close proximity to the pharyngeal pituitary and to other residues of the fetal pituitary anlage.

The anterior lobe of the pituitary in the embryo develops from the pharyngeal bursa in the form of a small recess known as Rathke's pouch, which remains connected with the original pharyngeal site by means of a narrow stalk which, imbedded in the body of the sphenoid bone, produces the cranio-pharyngeal canal. This structure disappears later on in most cases, yet grossly demonstrable residues are met with in 10 per cent of all autopsies (Erdheim, Pende). The persistent craniopharyngeal canal leads distally to the original site of the pharyngeal bursa and cranially to the sella turcica; its presence may be, but is not always, shown by an opening in the floor of the sella (Le Double). In a review of 72 cases of persistent cranio-pharyngeal duct, Haberfeld pointed out that an open duct is more frequent in the abnormally developed cranium or with other malformations. It is particularly common in the author's experience in association with eunuchoidism. The patent duct is filled with connective tissue and carries small blood vessels and lymphatics; it often contains residues of the pituitary anlage, such as more or less differentiated cells of anterior-lobe-type as well as epithelial structures of epidermal character, akin to those of cranio-pharyngiomas or adamantinomas of the cranium. The presence of glandular elements within the duct is significant in those cases in which they give rise to the growth of hyperplastic or neoplastic nodules within the sphenoidal bone; such changes have been met with in paradoxical cases of hyperpituitarism, or even in acromegaly in which the pituitary gland was not enlarged nor the sella turcica distended. The distal end of the cranio-pharyngeal canal is the site of the pharyngeal pituitary; the cells of this rudimentary structure ordinarily do not possess secretory activity, at least in so far as morphological criteria may be accepted as conclusive. It cannot be denied, however, that the pharyngeal pituitary may become involved in hyperplastic, or even neoplastic, processes in the course of which the cells may assume secretory function.

The cranio-pharyngeal canal is either patent throughout and terminates in an opening at the bottom of the sella as a small funnel-shaped recess, or the cranial portion of the canal is closed so that the lumen of the duct is retained only in its more distal portion. Nevertheless, it is an open question whether the lymphatic connection between the pharyngeal bursa and the sella turcica also obliterates, even though gross anatomical inspection or röntgenological examination does not reveal a lumen.

The incidence of open cranio-pharyngeal canal is estimated at 10 per cent by anatomists. The author has reviewed a large number of cranial röntgenograms and noted peculiarities in the structure of the sphenoid bone suggestive of a persistent cranio-pharyngeal canal in roughly the same percentage. The röntgenogram may show the funnel-shaped opening at the bottom of the sella turcica which tapers off as a narrow duct in the direction of the pharynx. A typical illustration of this type was reproduced in previous publications. In other cases, the remnants of the canal are indicated by two parallel lines which cut through the body of the sphenoid bone and point upwards to the bottom of the sella and downwards toward the pharynx.

The problem of the postoperative incidence of adiposo-genital dystrophy is not yet solved by demonstration of an anatomical connection between the sella turcica and the site of pharyngeal surgery; this is but the first step of a rational approach to a puzzling question which the following hypothesis might answer:

Removal of the adenoids is likely to traumatize or actually destroy the pharyngeal pituitary and abolish whatever function this rudimentary organ possesses. The probability of function could be assumed in case the pituitary gland proper is defective, either as the result of malformation or of impairment in early childhood as a consequence of which a compensatory process of the pituitary cells in the pharyngeal region sets in, in the form of differentiation and hyperplasia. It can be assumed, moreover, that the abundant lymphatic network of the pharynx is opened up by the surgical trauma so that infection may find its way and ascend through the lymphatics of the craniopharyngeal canal up to the sella turcica. The spread of a low-grade infection through the lymphatics may produce morphologic changes of the anterior lobe. No anatomical data are available to show that pyogenic infections reach the pituitary through the cranio-pharyngeal canal and cause purulent inflammation. On the other hand, interstitial fibrosis of the anterior lobe is not infrequently observed without any demonstrable path of infection.

The interstitial changes are associated, as a rule, with more or less atrophy of the glandular parenchyma. It is not an unwarranted assumption that such otherwise unexplained fibrosis of the pituitary constitutes the terminal stage of an inflammatory process which developed following the lymphatic spread of a non-pyogenic infection.

The pathogenic role of pharyngeal surgery in Fröhlich's syndrome might be more readily acceptable but for the prevalent belief that the syndrome is essentially the product of neoplastic changes within or above the pituitary gland. A careful review of the literature shows, as pointed out in previous publications, that this belief is not valid, for neoplastic lesions are responsible for only a fraction of all cases of Fröhlich's disease; whereas the autopsy findings more often show inflammatory, hemorrhagic, sclerotic or atrophic changes of the anterior lobe. Lesions of this type would include also those which develop as a consequence of pharyngeal surgery.

In order to bear out clinical observations, made more or less casually in the course of time, and in order to substantiate the validity of the preceding discussion, we selected from our files 150 consecutive cases of adiposo-genital dystrophy. In fourteen (9.3%) of these cases, the symptoms of the disease set in within a short time after the removal of tonsils and adenoids. This group of 14 cases includes 12 cases of altogether typical Fröhlich's syndrome — obesity, abnormal fat distribution, slightly retarded longitudinal growth and subnormal genital development. The height of the other two of the children was normal for their age, though all other symptoms were typical.

Suitable cranial röntgenograms were available in ten cases. The cranio-pharyngeal canal was well outlined, all the way up to the bottom of the sella in two cases; the radiologic findings were indicative of residues of the canal within the body of the sphenoid bone in four others, but not in the remaining cases. The complete or partial persistence of the cranio-pharyngeal canal in six of 10 cases is rather high if compared with the incidence of similar x-ray findings which, in our general material approached 10 per cent, but was not more than 2 per cent in the main group of adiposo-genital dystrophy.

SUMMARY

Attention is called to the relatively frequent development of adiposity of the Fröhlich type following removal of tonsils and adenoids. The peculiar fat distribution, retarded genital development and characteristic metabolic pattern proves that the symptoms of these patients are of the same order and pathogenesis as those of ordinary cases of Fröhlich's syndrome.

The pathogenetic role of the pituitary in Fröhlich's syndrome calls for consideration of a possible connection between pharyngeal surgery and subsequent pituitary disease. Anatomical and radiologic evidence offers a clue in the form of the occasional persistence of the cranio-pharyngeal canal.

X-ray findings suggestive of this developmental anomaly were obtained in six of 10 cases of postoperative Fröhlich's syndrome.

The hypothesis is advanced that the removal of the adenoids may be responsible in one of two ways:

1. By destruction of the pharyngeal pituitary, the compensatory hyperplasia and associated secretory activity of which was replacing the function of a congenitally deficient pituitary gland.

2. By injury to the region of the pharyngeal pituitary the cranio-pharyngeal canal or its lymphatics are opened up for an ascending infection of non-suppurative character. Such infection might cause interstitial fibrosis of the anterior lobe and subsequent functional deficiency, responsible for the manifestation of Fröhlich's syndrome.

REFERENCES

ERDHEIM, J.: *Beitr. Path. Anat.*, 46-233, 1909.
GOLDZIEHER, M. A.: *The Endocrine Glands*. D. Appleton Century Co., New York, 1939.
GOLDZIEHER, M. A.: *Penn. Med. Jl.*, April, 1942.
HABERFELD, W.: *Frankf. Ztsch. Path.*, 4:96, 1910.
LE DOUBLE, A. F.: Variations de l'os du crane de l'homme, Paris, 1903.
PENDE, N.: *Beitr. Path. Anat.*, 43:437, 1910.
SELKIRK, K. T., and MITCHELL, A. G.: *Am. J. Dis Child.*, 42:9, 1931.
ZUBKUS, J.: *Monats. f. Ohrenheilk.*, 71:1359, 1937.

MAGNESIUM SULFATE IN PAROXYSMAL TACHYCARDIA
(L. J. Boyd & D. A. Scherf, New York City, in *Modern Med.*, Dec.)

In eight out of eight attacks of paroxysmal tachycardia, 20 cc. of a 20% solution of magnesium sulfate injected intravenously was beneficial. A 10% solution, however, was beneficial in only three out of eight attacks. Disturbances of conduction and ventricular extrasystoles appeared for a short time after the injection. The rate of the paroxysmal tachycardia often diminished before the attack disappeared.

DEPARTMENTS

GYNECOLOGY

ROBERT THRIFT FERGUSON, M.D., *Editor*, Charlotte, N. C.

INJUDICIOUS HORMONAL THERAPY IN GYNECOLOGIC DISORDERS

AN INSTRUCTIVE ARTICLE by Dr. John A. Hepp in the *Pennsylvania Medical Journal* relative to the management of the menopause is discussed editorially in the same issue for restatement and emphasis.

The unwarranted and injudicious use of hormonal therapy is a subject well worthy of our consideration. Attention is properly directed by Dr. Hepp to the fact that many women experience little or no difficulty during the menopausal epoch. A goodly number who do complain of disagreeable symptoms are made fairly comfortable by an explanation of the physiologic changes responsible for their annoyance, plus the reassurance of a negative pelvic examination. A minority require sedation or estrogenic therapy. Too often the menopausal patient is led to believe that courses of "injections," continued over a long period of time, are essential to health and serenity. She may even be prompted to expect terrible experiences with the advent of the "change of life." "These suggestions come not only from her intimates but sometimes from her medical adviser as well."

The use of a potent endocrine product, under whatever trade name, natural or synthetic, should be based on a sound knowledge of its action. "Honesty of purpose and fineness of judgment are essential if good instead of harm is to result from its employment."

The quoted author has pointed out that restrictions are necessary in the use of estrogenic substances, of which diethylstilbestrol is an example, with respect both to indications and dosage. Uterine bleeding may result from excessive and continued dosage with these estrogenic substances, primarily designed to combat the vasomotor phenomena incident to the menopause. In many cases confusion must arise as whether this is due to organic pelvic disease, especially fundal carcinoma, or to the injudicious therapy. Only a diagnostic curettage can solve the problem thus created. Also there is a possibility of a carcinogenic effect on the genitalia or breast, postmenopausal, particularly in cases giving a familial history of genital or mammary cancer, and entirely apart from preëxisting cancer.

Patients are observed who, for indefinite periods of time, have been receiving preparations to control irregular or prolonged bleeding from the uterovaginal tract, without ever having had a pelvic examination. Thus in many instances, organic pelvic disease has been overlooked and, tragically, cancer has often been found to be the cause of the abnormal hemorrhage. Where the cause is found to be a benign lesion, the situation may not yet be beyond effective control; in those cases due to cancer the outlook is often hopeless because of the delay.

It is proper to treat the functional bleeding of adolescence and the early reproductive period with hormonal therapy, including thyroid extract, and along with adequate general measures, provided that a careful examination has been made and that logical consideration has been given to the reasons for using this or that hormonal preparation. Furthermore, the possibility that such therapy may disturb the delicate endocrine balance should always be borne in mind. To be on the safe side, however, a bimanual pelvic examination should never be omitted in the married patient nor a bimanual rectal examination in the virginal woman. Otherwise organic disease is bound to be overlooked in a fair proportion of cases.

In case of abnormal bleeding in the late reproductive, menopausal, or postmenopausal periods, there is little justification for prolonged and experimental hormonal therapy. Effective radiologic and surgical measures are available in such cases, not only for the relief of organic pelvic disease but for the correction of functional bleeding—measures which are surer and less time-consuming by far than prolonged and indecisive hormonal therapy.

It seems that we, as a people, find it next to impossible to appraise a new and useful thing temperately and judiciously. We overvalue and so expect too much. Then, when our ill-founded hopes are not realized, we swing to the other extreme of undervaluation.

The editorial analysis and comment on this article and the article itself are timely. We will do well to take to heart the lessons they teach.

I agree fully with every word written by Dr. Hepp, and can only emphasize the fact that hormones are probably more injudiciously given than any other drug on the market at this time unless it be the wild-cat giving of vitamins.

The effect of certain estrogenic substances during the normal or artificial menopause in many instances is truly remarkable, but I find many patients being given them with no justification.

Also progesteronic substances given in abnormal types of bleeding due to lack of this particular hormone frequently work like a charm.

It is easy to become over-enthusiastic when a new drug is put on the market and the mail is full of descriptive literature, and your office besieged with plausible salesmen.

DERMATOLOGY

J. LAMAR CALLAWAY, M.D., *Editor*, Durham, N. C.

DERMATOLOGY—CUTANEOUS MEDICINE

THAT Dermatology in reality should be designated Cutaneous Medicine is rapidly becoming recognized as the purely morphologic conception of diseases affecting the skin disappears. No longer do dermatologists examine only affected areas and because of certain structural morphologic characteristics of certain configuration and distribution assign a specific diagnosis. It is true that morphology, distribution and configuration play a role in arriving at a diagnosis, but a carefully taken history with a complete and careful physical examination and indicated laboratory studies are much more important.

Many of the common dermatoses merely mirror the systemic disease underlying the cutaneous manifestations. Erythema nodosum, urticaria, acute desseminated lupus erythematosus, and xanthomata are a limited number of systemic diseases producing associated skin lesions. Infiltrations in the skin which may at first sight seem nothing more than a localized neurodermatitis or some form of eczema may on complete investigation turn out to be a serious lymphoblastoma. A localized small translucent nodule may be the only manifestation of generalized sarcoidosis which is diagnosed by x-ray studies and biopsy of adjacent lymph nodes. Velvety pigmentation in the axillae constituting a clinical diagnosis of acanthosis nigricans may mirror a case of abdominal cancer. Not only do dozens of simliar conditions come to one's mind but in many instances a complete physical examination unearths a problem which may be serious and completely unrelated to the cutaneous disease in question.

The necessity for a complete evaluation of all cases which present even localized skin lesions is graphically demonstrated by the following case which was recently seen in my practice.

A prominent lawyer was admitted to Duke Hospital for diagnosis and treatment of a chronic eczematoid dermatitis of both hands which had existed for several months. On casual examination the dermatitis appeared to be primarily a contact eczematoid eruption associated in some way with his occupation. However, skin tests with contact substances (patch tests) had failed to disclose the causative agent, and all types of local treatment including x-ray therapy had failed to affect a cure. While in the hospital numerous foci of infection were removed and with minimal local therapy a complete cure of the dermatosis was affected which did not recur when he returned to his occupation.

More important, however, during the physical evaluation a rectal examination by the house officer disclosed a small nodule to be present in the prostate. Urological consultation confirmed the suspicion of early cancer, biopsy revealed an early carcinoma and the entire encapsulated tumor was excised in situ. It is believed that a permanent cure was thereby obtained.

This is but one example, albeit an important one, in which a complete physical examination resulted in the diagnosis and cure of a serious systemic disease completely unrelated to the localized and much less serious cutaneous manifestation for which the patient sought relief.

A plea for a complete physical examination with accessory laboratory studies should not be necessary. It is obligatory to the adequate evaluation, diagnosis and management of any dermatosis no matter how trivial.

SURGERY

GEO. H. BUNCH, M.D., *Editor*, Columbia, S. C.

BACKACHE FROM RUPTURED INTERVERTEBRAL DISKS

IN THE JANUARY ISSUE of this Journal, Saunders has an interesting and a timely editorial on the low-back problem. This, although as old as mankind, has assumed a new and a greater interest since the discovery of the protruding lumbar disk as a possible cause. Over the years backache has generally been attributed in women to uterine displacement or to some other gynecologic condition, and in men to infection of the prostate. Women have had corrective operations and men prostatic massage by the urologist. The discovery of sacroiliac subluxation by the orthopedic surgeon has automatically thrown much of the backache problem into his lap. Now, since the advent of the intervertebral disk as a cause, so many of these cases are being operated upon by the neurosurgeon that a rather heated controversy on the diagnosis and the indications for operation upon these patients has arisen between the two competing groups.

Dandy,[1] professor of neurosurgery at Johns Hopkins, from a series of over 500 cases, concludes that ruptured lumbar disks are now among the most common lesions coming to surgery; that their diagnosis and localization are simple, almost absolutely certain, and a cure is practically assured, and almost without risk. The diagnosis can now be made solely upon the history of low-back pain, plus sciatica down the back of the leg and occur-

1. Ruptured Intervertebral Disks. *Annals of Surgery*, Oct., 1943.

ring in attacks. Nearly always the backache and the pain in the leg are intensified by coughing and sneezing during the acute stage of pain. In 95 per cent of cases with such symptoms a ruptured disk will be the cause; the remaining 5 per cent are caused by spondylolisthesis, congenitally defective fifth lumbar vertebra or tumors of the cauda equina. The first two of these may be recognized by x-ray examination of the lumbar spine and the third by finding xanthrochromic fluid at lumbar puncture. Puncture should be done only when tumor is suspected. Ninety-eight per cent of all ruptures of lumbar disks are of the fourth and fifth. This makes the use of a contrast medium in the spine unnecessary.

The treatment of ruptured disks consists in the removal of the protruding disk and of the necrotic interior by the curette. The surfaces of the bodies of the vertebrae after thorough curettment afford such a large area for fusion that fusion of the lateral joints is unnecessary. When the entire necrotic disk has been extirpated firm union occurs between the vertebrae. No plaster encasement is necessary and the patient is out of the hospital within two weeks.

If Dandy's findings are generally confirmed by accumulating experience, as we firmly believe they will be, he will have done much to simplify the vexing problem of persistent disabling backache and he will have cured a class of patients whose treatment has so often heretofore been unsatisfactory.

PEDIATRICS

HEMORRHAGIC DISEASE OF THE NEWBORN

THIS DISEASE occurs in 0.7 per cent of newly-born infants. The usual time of appearance is between the second and fourth days; extremes—the first day and the second week. The bleeding (oozing) may come from almost any portion of the body; the umbilicus, cutaneous surfaces and bowel are favorite sites; it is often initiated by trauma. There is prolongation of the coagulation time, with less or no lengthening of the bleeding time. Blood transfusion is a therapeutic agent of proved worth, but the efficacy of intramuscular or subcutaneous blood has been largely disproved.[1]

Further this essayist says:

Lack of prothrombin is the cause. The administration of vitamin K to expectant mothers, either during the last few days of pregnancy or during labor, results in normal prothrombin values in their infants and virtually prevents the prolongation in prothrombin time which usually occurs in

1. L. G. Pray, Fargo, N. Dak., in *Jl.-Lancet*, Jan.

untreated cases between the second and fourth days of life. Menadione (2 methyl-1, 4-naphthoquinone) one of the most potent preparations having vitamin K activity was given during the latter part of pregnancy in doses of 2 mg. t. i. d. in tablet form. It is likely that a dosage of 1 or 2 mg. daily would have accomplished the same result.

The dosage used during labor was 20 mg. in most cases; in a few instances in which 10 mg. were given there was an equal prophylactic effect. Again it is quite possible that smaller doses would have been equally effective.

A finding of great practical interest is that formula feedings during the first few days of life, either alone or supplementary to breast feedings, counteract the prolongation of prothrombin time which occurs ordinarily in untreated cases in which the baby is breast-fed.

The prompt curative action of menadione in oil in hemorrhagic disease of the newborn is shown in three such cases. This acted with equal rapidity whether given by mouth or intramuscularly; the dosage was 2 mg. to 6 mg.; within two hours bleeding stopped entirely or almost completely in each instance. There was apparently no need to repeat the initial dose, although in one case of severe bleeding two injections were given an hour apart. The intramuscular route is preferable in severe cases, because of the possibility of loss by vomiting.

Results suggest that the reduction is greatest in the cases in which treatment is instituted before the onset of labor. These findings are of particular interest in their possible relationship to intracranial hemorrhage.

It is considered advisable to administer vitamin K to *all mothers*, either during early labor, or daily during the last few weeks of pregnancy. In case this is not possible, vitamin K should be given to the infant during the first 12 hours of life, either by mouth or parenterally. If none of these courses is feasible, supplemental formula feedings are to be given the baby during the first two or three days.

Treatment of hemorrhagic disease itself should consist of prompt administration of vitamin K, preferably by a parenteral route. Preparations for blood transfusion should also be made, because not all cases of hemorrhage of the newborn are due to lack of prothrombin. There are cases of neonatal purpura hemorrhagica due to lowered platelets. There have also been several reports of congenital lack of fibrinogen causing bleeding. If blood is given, it should be administered intravenously because of ineffectiveness when injected intramuscularly.

UROLOGY

RAYMOND THOMPSON, M.D., *Editor*, Charlotte, N. C.

VENEREAL DISEASES OF THE ARMY

VENEREAL DISEASE accounted for over two million hospital bed days in the army between January, 1942, and September, 1943, although the rate of infection was below peace time levels and less than half that of the first world war. Both preventive and curative measures aim at reducing this manpower loss.

Syphilis: Continuation of treatment (of syphilis) over long periods presents administrative difficulties. A system covering the shortest time, consistent with safety, is much to be desired.

Since 1942, treatment has taken the form of an intensified scheme consisting of forty injections of arsenoxide administered twice weekly with added injections of bismuth, covering a total of 26 weeks. The recommended individual dose of arsenoxide is 60 mg. and of bismuth subsalicylate 0.2 Gm. in oil.

No more-intensive methods (such as intravenous drip or combined arsenoxide and fever therapy) have been adopted as routine by the army on account of the risk, though "the importance of the contribution of Hyman and his co-workers in demonstrating the practicability of the five-day treatment, if one is prepared to accept the risk, must not be minimized."[1]

The army is in a unique position to study the biologic false positive tests. Ordinary precipitation and complement-fixation tests become positive in not less than 15 per cent following vaccination for smallpox (with take) and during a variety of acute febrile diseases. Medical officers have recommended to follow individuals with positive or doubtful vaccination reactions for a period of three months without treatment, and then to discharge from observation those in whom the serologic reaction has reversed to negative.

Gonorrhea: Seventy per cent of persons with uncomplicated gonorrhea respond to one course of sulfathiazole or sulfadiazine, another 10 or 15 per cent to a second course. Penicillin will cure the remainder (victims of sulfonamide-resistant strains) when more readily available. The average number of days lost per case is now under fifteen.

Recommended course of treatment is 4 Gm. of sulfathiazole a day for five days; for hospitalized patients, 33 Gm. given as 4 Gm. initially and 1 Gm. every 4 hours day and night for five days.

For years soldiers were hospitalized for treatment of gonorrhea until treatment on a duty status

---

1. Management of the Venereal Diseases in the Army, Lt.-Col. T. B. Turner and Maj. T. H. Sternberg, *J. A. M. A.*, 124:133-137, Jan. 15th, 1944.

was authorized in early 1943. This treatment calls for "one course of sulfadiazine to be given while the patient is carrying on his normal activities. If symptoms have not subsided in seven days after the beginning of treatment the patient is hospitalized and given a second course of sulfadiazine."

The danger to barracks mates of gonorrhea patients has been exaggerated: ". . we have yet to learn of a case of gonorrhea acquired from toilet seats, towels or by means other than sexual contact."

Fully 50 per cent of days lost from duty due to gonorrhea are accounted for by the ten to twenty per cent sulfonamide-resistant patients. Until the advent of penicillin, fever therapy with sulfonamides by mouth was the preferred treatment. "This remarkable drug bids fair to reduce gonorrhea to the status of an inconsequential infection." The limited penicillin supply is now kept for those places where it is necessary to keep every soldier on the job.

Recently the army has demonstrated that complications of gonorrhea most frequently occur as a result of manipulative procedures which traumatize the urogenital tract. Local treatment is indicated in only a few cases. If a patient with gonorrhea has phimosis or urethral stricture, the condition must be corrected; but meddlesome manipulation serves no useful purpose. Clinical observation is now the principal criterion of cure by sulfathiazole.

More than one clinical entity may be found in those cases of chancroidal lesions refractory to treatment. "Further clinical and bacteriological studies on this problem are needed."

The incidence of lymphogranuloma venereum and granuloma inguinale is low in the army and presents no serious problem.

THERAPEUTICS

J. F. NASH, M.D., *Editor*, Saint Pauls, N. C.

SUCCESSFUL TREATMENT OF GOUT

ALL OF US have patients with gout. Much of it is not so recognized. More than 4 mgm. uric acid per 100 c.c. of blood generally means gout, whether or not the patient has pain in his great toe and tophi in his earlobes.

Bartels[1] has no fear of cinchophen, and he says nothing about colchicum. The plan of treatment utilized consists of a diet low in purine and fat and high in carbohydrate, to which is added the periodic administration of cinchophen. Purine restriction relieves the overburdened purine-metabolizing mechanism, the low-fat intake prevents retention, and the high-carbohydrate element tends toward the diuresis of uric acid. Cinchophen 7½ grains t. i. d. for three days a week furthers uric acid elamination. Alcohol is not permitted.

Periodic determinations of the uric acid are made at one- to three-months intervals, and when a reduction in uric acid occurs the intervals are reduced from three days a week to two, to one, and omitted entirely when the uric acid reaches normal or near normal. Patients understand that the diet is basis of treatment and that it is to be somewhat restricted indefinitely. However, if the uric acid continues at a normal level, a more liberal diet is given.

Acute attacks of gout have been treated by the intravenous injections of glucose in addition to the plan outlined. Since the diet is low in vitamins A and B, these vitamins are added. At times in gouty arthritis physiotherapy is helpful and large tophi are removed, if troublesome.

Indisputable benefit was obtained in a group of 31 patients with gout who carefully adhered to this plan of treatment, which gave the desired results of reducing the blood uric acid level and the number and severity of further attacks. Even patients in the phase of chronic gouty arthritis responded to this plan of treatment.

* * * * *

NEW TREATMENT OF HIGHLY FATAL HEART DISEASE SEEMS PROMISING

REPORT has been made[1] of the apparently successful treatment by use of penicillin in conjunction with heparin, an anticoagulant, of 7 patients with subacute bacterial endocarditis.

Further observation will be required to determine the permanence of results, but the immediate effects suggest uniformly successful sterilization of the blood and relief of clinical manifestations.

The penicillin was given in requisite dosage by continuous intravenous drip (1 patient also received it by injection into a muscle).

Heparin was deposited beneath the skin in most instances but occasionally was given by injection into a vein.

Six of the 7 patients suffered from a bacterial endocarditis that was engrafted on a chronic rheumatic inflammation of a valve of the heart. The other had a congenital heart defect. In 5 of the 7 cases the organism causing the condition was a streptococcus viridans; in the sixth a hemolytic streptococcus and in the seventh a pneumococcus type 27.

In a few of the cases the efficacy of the therapy may have been enhanced by the preliminary use of sulfonamide (given to all 7 patients.)

"In experimental thrombotic bacterial endocarditis," the authors explain, "the disappearance

---

1. E. C. Bartels, Boston, in *Jl. Tenn. State Med. Asn.*, Jan.

1. Leo Loewe et al., Brooklyn, in *J. A. M. A.* for Jan. 15th.

of vegetations requires the use of a suitable chemotherapeutic agent and an anticoagulant. The clinical application of this principle in subacute bacterial endocarditis has been disappointing; the technics of therapy are cumbersome, the toxicity of treatment has been excessive even for an otherwise fatal disease and the successes have been few and irregular. Early efforts made with sulfonamides, with or without heparin, have been mostly abandoned. The introduction of penicillin proved equally disappointing; the commission appointed by the National Research Council has already reported unfavorably anh discouraged the use of the at present inadequate supply of the drug for the treatment of viridans endocarditis. . . ."

HOSPITALS

R. B. DAVIS, M.D., *Editor*, Greensboro, N. C.

MOST HOSPITALS WOULD DO WELL TO BUILD ADDITIONAL ROOMS NOW

IF ANYONE mentions putting up a new building or adding to or remodeling an old building, he is immediately met with the exclamation, "Not now; labor is too high and material unobtainable!" The law of supply and demand has always been the greatest stabilizer of economics. If the demand for hospital service is increased to the extent that the writer believes it has, something should be done about supplying this demand. Practically all hospitals are running to capacity load. This means that with any epidemic hospitals are overcrowded and in many instances cannot take care of all those applying.

In some instances, priorities on building material for hospitals are obtainable. In others, a substitute will serve the purpose. The second opposition that looms mightily before the eyes of the would-be builder is that of labor. Immediately we say we cannot compete with the United States Treasury. However, a reasonable number of workmen, skilled and unskilled, remain at home and are willing to do good work for much less money than war workers are now making. It is true that any building program will have to set aside a larger amount for labor than would be necessary in normal times. However, for an institution to make an expenditure of $1,000, the directors or owners want to know first how much dividend will $1,000 bear if spent in this or that particular manner. The writer believes that any reasonable increased capacity expense will give a very large dividend return. There is more money among the working class of people than there ever was, and there are more working people than there are all other classes.

At one time a hospital could be built and equipped for $2,000 per room, x-ray, kitchen, operating rooms, coldstorage equipment, everything included. Most of the institutions could take care of an increase of from 10 to 50 beds without increasing the other facilities. In many instances no increase in the personnel, particularly that of the business office, laboratory and dietary supervision, would be necessary. The cost per patient per day for the additional rooms would not be more than 50 per cent of that spent in the original institution. The average hospital is probably making more profit today than it has ever made. This is not because of the increased rates, for they have advanced very little. It is because they are collecting their bills and because they are running practically full all of the time. Patients are being denied hospital treatment who are able to and would occupy private rooms. An addition of 10 to 20 per cent of bed occupancy would be an exceedingly good investment for most hospitals. When material and labor return to its normal state, hospitals in turn will return to their normal states. With this one exception, and here lies the keynote to the situation, when a hospital is built in any particular community, its size is based upon the population in the community in which it is located. However, every year that rolls by sees many more people born than die in that particular locality, so the population increases rather rapidly. More and more of our women are being delivered in the hospital, so that the new citizen renders his first service to the community by contributing to the support of the hospital and in most instances, the last community contribution by those who pass out during the year, is one to the hospital.

Let us assume that we can add a bed to the present operating institution for $2,250. If the present income of a bed in a private room that rents for $6 a day is $2,190 at full capacity per year and the average occupancy of the institution is 85 per cent, then this would mean 85 per cent of $2,190, which would be $1,861.50. Now the per capita cost of hospitalization is $4.90. This figure could be lowered by adding bed capacity but we will leave the figure at $4.90. This would mean that this added room would make an overhead cost on the institution of $1,520.22. Therefore, the difference between income and the outgo on this room would be $341.28 profit, which is more than 33 1/3 per cent on the investment. This does not include the income from laboratory, x-ray and operating room services, which were added to the per capita cost at $4.90 a day. If the present rate of increased demand is continued for two years after your addition is opened, you will have paid for almost 70 per cent of your annex. Then if things return to normal and your income is cut in half, you will still have an investment which is paying over 16½ per cent. If this condition exists for two more years, the addition to your hospital will be paid for.

I do not believe any of this is exaggerated or reckless thinking and figuring. At any rate it is well worth the time and effort necessary for hospital trustees and owners to sit down and figure this matter out for themselves; they will be surprised and I believe will give serious thought to enlarging their institution if the demand exists in their community.

INSURANCE MEDICINE

H. F. STARR, M.D., *Editor*, Greensboro, N. C.

1943 MORTALITY INCREASE DUE TO WAR

THE HEALTH RECORD of America in 1943 is a reliable indication of the excellent job the health authorities and the medical profession are doing.

According to preliminary reports of insurance companies' experience among policyholders, there was an increase of 5 per cent in the death rate, the increase almost wholly due to deaths due to enemy action or causes arising out of the war. In spite of the increase, the death rate for 1943 among insured lives the country over was lower than for any year prior to 1938.

A great part of the increase was accounted for by deaths due to heart disease, which caused one-third of all deaths among policyholders during 1943. Heart disease is customarily the leading cause of death, but this reached a new high. The higher average age of the population, and a larger proportion of older people would be expected to cause an increase in heart deaths, but the rise was somewhat more than this would warrant. The war effort, increased strain, and the return of older persons to work may have contributed to the causes of the increase in deaths due to heart disease.

War deaths due directly to enemy action increased materially over the previous year. There was a decrease in merchant marine losses, but there was an increase among the armed services. All war deaths amounted to 5 per cent of total policyholder deaths. In some individual companies the proportion was twice that. A higher mortality due to war losses is to be expected during 1944.

The greatest percentage increase last year was due to deaths from pneumonia, but compared with the experience prior to the use of the sulfa drugs the rate was still low. During the last month of the year there was a sharp increase in the death rate due to the effects of influenza, but this affected but little the aggregate results for the year.

With industry fully employed and working under war production pressure, an increase in occupational deaths was expected; but, on the contrary, there has been a reduction in the occupational death rate. This experience is splendid evidence of the value of the safety and health programs widely employed by industry. Home accidents, however, showed a slight increase. Automobile accidents decreased, yet they still account for as many deaths as direct war causes.

During war tuberculosis generally shows an increase, but fortunately the death rate continued to decline and reached a new low last year. Cancer showed little change from recent years. Sugar shortage and rationing seems to have had had no effect on the increasing diabetic deaths, for the rate was unchanged.

The health of the nation has come thus far in the war in excellent condition. For this we can be thankful; but never let us forget for one moment that disease has always been the constant companion to war and it is only by eternal vigilance that he can be prevented from striking with an epidemic far more destructive to life than war itself.

ORTHOPEDIC SURGERY

JOHN T. SAUNDERS, M.D., *Editor*, Asheville, N. C.

HIP FRACTURES

FRACTURES OF THE HIP are a frequent finding in general practice. Surgery on these elderly patients is often the best choice of treatment even though the outlook is poor. The solution of this problem requires careful thought since the average age at its occurrence is sixty-eight years and they are often seen in patients who have complicating conditions making them poorer risks than in those with robust health.

It is distressing to see these elderly patients rapidly go into a decline following this accident as many of them do. We all know that patients in this age group do not tolerate confinement well, that they often fail to eat, develop cerebral symptoms as shown by mental meandering, and gradually lose ground despite the best treatment and nursing care.

It has been my experience that those suffering with the trochanteric type of hip fracture have more shock and are a more difficult problem all through treatment, even though the fracture itself responds well to many types of simple treatment. Maintenance of sufficient length, internal rotation and moderate abduction are all that are required to obtain a good result provided the patient survives. There is always a strong tendency in this type of fracture for coxa vara and resultant shortening to recur. There are many ways of preventing this recurrence of deformity, but the only one not requiring confinement of at least the lower extremities is open operation with internal fixation.

The more this problem is observed, the more it is realized that it is the patients who are poor operative risks who most require operative reduction since the healthy patient will usually recover by any recognized method of treatment. Poor-risk patients for the most part do not survive this type of fracture by more than six weeks unless the fracture is adequately fixed. Operative reduction with internal fixation requires a gadget such as the Neufeld nail or a "blade-plate." The three-flanged nail alone or multiple wires will not hold properly a comminuted trochanteric fracture.

In the reduction of the intracapsular type of hip fracture as well as in the trochanteric type it should be thoroughly realized that the fracture must be reduced before abduction is started, because abduction does not reduce the displacement, but locks the fragments in whatever position they lie and renders further reduction impossible.

A carefully placed three-flanged nail will usually hold an anatomically reduced intracapsular fracture and with proper simple precautions the surgery is done with remarkably little disturbance to the patient. It is a pleasure to see an elderly patient thus treated the day following this nailing procedure and to anticipate his smooth convalescence as compared to methods requiring confinement.

I do not believe that all fractures of the hip unite if they are properly reduced and immobilized, either by abduction methods or by internal fixation, but I know that incomplete reduction accounts for many failures.

GENERAL PRACTICE
D. HERBERT SMITH, M.D., *Editor*, Pauline, S. C.

THERAPY OF COMMON SKIN DISEASES[1] *

Ringworm
The patient with ringworm should be told that he must continue treatment long after he is apparently well. The acute stage is treated by incising lesions and letting the infected fluid drain out. Potassium permanganate soaks or baths of 1-4000 dilution are used during the acute stage. The dry type is treated by Castellani's paint.**

Chronic ringworm is treated with a strong desquamating ointment, using up to 50 per cent salicylic acid, such as:
Lanolin
Salicylic acid, equal portions

[1]. C. S. Wright, Philadelphia, in *Clinical Med.*, Jan.
*Taken and abstracted by R. L. G. during the Chicago meeting of the Interstate Postgraduate Medical Assembly.
**Castellani's paint is manufactured by Handley Laboratories, Somerville, Mass.

Scabies
This is the third most common skin disease and should be thought of first in all patients who complain of generalized pruritis. It is readily cured by U. S. P. sulfur ointment, except in those patients with sulfur sensitivity. Benzyl benzoate, applied after a bath, rubbed over the entire body, except face, and allowed to remain for 24 hours will frequently cure scabies. Pruritis stops almost at once.

Eczema
Nummular eczema appears on the forearms as coinshaped lesions, which weep at first and then become thickened and scaly. Use silver nitrate ¼- to 1-per cent by compresses during acute stage, followed later by 5 per cent crude coal tar in chloroform; vitamin A is given in large doses by mouth.

Eczema on the cheeks of an infant is often atopic, and is incurable like hayfever. If seborrheic or caused by external contact, learn which substance is causative by using a simple patch test.

Any simple treatment, such as 1 per cent tar ointment or boric acid salve, will cure, after removal of the irritating substance responsible for the contact dermatitis.

Facial Eruptions
Seborrheic dermatitis spreads from the scalp; it is not curable. The scalp should be attacked with sulfur or U. S. P. crude oil.

Impetigo is often cured in 5 days by local applications of sulfathiazole.

Herpes zoster is somewhat improved by the injection of 150 mg. of thiamin (vitamin B_1) intravenously or intramuscularly. The intravenous injection of 30 gr. of sodium iodide twice weekly is of value in painful cases.

Lupus erythematosus is made worse by sunlight. Gold thiosulphate injections cure many cases; they may be used if white blood count is normal. If the white blood count is less than 6,000 it should not be used because of the danger of causing leukopenia. Bismuth salicylate injections should then be used.

Dermatitis herpetiformis is much improved by sulfadiazine given orally.

Generalized Eruptions
Chronic urticaria is based on nervous instability. Histaminase relieves a number of patients, especially if the wheals appear following cold or other physical cause. Chronic hives in children often respond to parathyroid injections.

Psoriasis is of frequent occurrence (one out of each 18 patients with skin disease). If such patients can be hospitalized, they may be cleared up by the routine of crude coal tar applied at night and strong ultraviolet or sunlight the next day. A few patients are permanently cured by this treatment. An occasional case responds to massive doses of vitamin D (not considered a safe treatment).

Nevi: If of the port wine type, they are best covered with Cover-Mark as treatment is ineffective. If of the strawberry type carbon dioxide snow applied for 10 to 40 seconds on two or three occasions will usually cure. As the birthmark grows with the child, treatment should be started during the first week of life. One may also inject sodium morrhuate as a sclerosing solution or treat with x-rays.

Warts: When one wart appears remove it at once. For warts on the sole of the foot, cut off the extra skin and treat with x-ray. If acids or electric fulguration are used, a slow-healing, painful ulcer often results.

Epitheliomas of the skin may be cured in the office if seen in the early stages, by electrofulguration, x-rays or radium.

EVALUATION OF MEASURES FOR THE PREVENTION OF IVY DERMATITIS

FEW INDEED are the doctors in this country who have no need to be concerned about the annual occurrence of cases of dermatitis from plant poisoning. Many of the accounts of early explorations in the Western Hemisphere contain descriptions of maddening itchings and burnings and breaking-outs from contact with beautiful leaves. And these symptoms from this cause have afflicted large numbers of us every summer since that time.

All will agree with Howell[1] that the present status of prevention of this affliction is confusing. After concluding that no protection is afforded by the two to four injections of commercial ivy preparations, he conducted a series of controlled investigations, and it is on the basis of this research that the article under review is written.

Howell reports:

Soap and water did not prevent or mitigate ivy dermatitis in an extremely sensitive person, even if used within one minute of exposure; and in a person of average sensitivity only if employed within 10 minutes of contact.

Applications of 10-per cent ferric chloride were without effect.

A freshly-prepared 10-per cent solution of potassium permanganate applied within 10 minutes prevented the development of dermatitis in most instances and greatly reduced the severity in others. Even after 30 minutes some reduction of severity was accomplished in three persons only mildly sensitive.

Sodium perborate ointment (10%) gave little if any protection and tended to spread the resinous poison and so increase the area of dermatitis.

Petrolatum caused wide spreading of the skin inflammation and gave no benefit.

We are left wondering whether there be any truth in the popular belief that protection is afforded by rubbing exposed surfaces of the skin with kerosene or alcohol before hieing away to mossy hill and dale.

It's worth something to know that those painful injections do no good to compensate for the putting out of commission of the part into which they are injected.

[1.] J. R. Howell, in *Archiv. Derm. & Syph.,* Oct., 1943.

OPHTHALMOLOGY

HERBERT C. NEBLETT, M.D., *Editor,* Charlotte, N. C.

RHEUMATIC FEVER OR SYPHILIS IN CHILDREN?

NOT INFREQUENTLY one sees a child between the ages of 5 and 16 years who has lost weight, is pale, has general lassitude, poor appetite, painful swollen joints, fever, leucopenia, secondary anemia and, occasionally, pathological notching of the permanent teeth. Many of these children have a good family background, are above the average economic and social level and the moral character of their parents would appear to be above reproach. Such a status of the child might serve to delay arousing the suspicion of the attending physician to rule out syphilis first, rather than proceed along other lines of diagnosis. Hence one probable cause of the not infrequent diagnosis and treatment of rheumatic fever until much time has been lost and other complications have arisen which produce serious consequences especially in the eyes of the victim.

It has been said, and truly, that syphilis is the great imitator of many diseases and we should keep this thought constantly in mind that we may surely make a correct diagnosis and prevent the embarrassing consequences of an incorrect one to say nothing of the lamentable effects upon the child when syphilis is present and its diagnosis and treatment delayed.

In the South rheumatic fever being rare, as compared to its incidence in the Northern and Eastern States, is another reason that in cases simulating that disease in this area syphilis should be first suspected and exempted.

In many of the cases the writer sees annually the diagnosis of rheumatic fever had been made and treatment for it instituted over a period, until symptoms in the eyes had suggested an eye examination. The condition then present in the eyes is one of an initial or fully developed keratitis with its attendant symptoms of severe pain, photophobia, lacrymation and almost total visual disability of many weeks. After prolonged systemic antisyphilitic treatment and intensive local treatment to the eyes the keratitis subsides, leaving, in the majority of cases, scarring of the corneae which results in a permanent defect in vision of a greater or lesser degree.

Inherited syphilis stands among the first five major causes of permanent partial or total blindness in the population. An incidence of such magnitude and of such disabling consequences applicable to one of the main special sense organs of the body demands our constant awareness of the possibility, and the immediate use of appropriate tests.

GENERAL PRACTICE

JAMES L. HAMNER, M.D., *Editor*, Mannboro, Va.

CORONARY DISEASE: ITS RECOGNITION AND MANAGEMENT

THE DIAGNOSIS of coronary disease associated with angina pectoris is usually made on the basis of the history alone. In some of the atypical cases the diagnosis will tax one's skill to the utmost. Electrocardiography, physical examination, and x-ray examination often are of little help. The most important symptom, and usually the only one, is pain, usually substernal; may be substernal and epigastric, rarely is it precordial. Pain frequently extends to one or both arms, may extend up the sides of the neck to the jaws or cheeks.

In this matter-of-fact way Smith[1] begins a clear-cut discussion of coronary-artery disease.

The patients feel as if they had something inside of them which they cannot get rid of. The pain is brought on by physical exertion, excitement or sexual intercourse and relieved by rest. If it lasts longer than 30 minutes one should be suspicious of coronary occlusion.

The pain can be distinguished from pain in the thoracic wall by the site and duration of the pain and by the local tenderness of the latter.

Cardiospasm and spasm of the esophagus are associated with eating or drinking and cause regurgitation. Diverticulum of the esophagus, gastric ulcer, and duodenal ulcer are distinguished by röntgenographic examination, disease of the gallbladder by the history and x-ray findings. Scalenus anticus syndrome shows vasomotor disturbances in the arm and hand, and the pain is aggravated by rotation of the head and depressing the soulder. A normal ecg. does not rule out the presence of coronary disease. In atypical cases 10 per cent oxygen is administered for 20 minutes. If coronary disease

is present, a change will occur in the S-T segment or the T wave will be inverted. If substernal pain and dyspnea should develop in the course of the test, 100 per cent oxygen should be administered immediately.

In coronary occlusion the pain is much more severe and of much longer duration than is the pain of angina pectoris, shock is evident, b.-p. usually falls, t. 100 to 102°. The leucocytes increase and the sedimentation rate rises after a few hours or a day or so. A friction rub may be heard if the infarction involves the anterior surface of the left ventricle. In acute coronary occlusion, the ecg. is more important in establishing the diagnosis than in other types of heart disease.

Mild coronary sclerosis requires that one work less and under less emotional strain, have 10-11 hours of sleep at night, small meals, rest 30-60 minutes after eating. Overweight should be reduced. As a rule, no medication is required.

Severe coronary disease and angina demands a much more rigid program. Nitroglycerine to relieve the pain, in some instances to 1½ grains of aminophylline t. i. d. If does not sleep properly, small doses of phenobarbital. Often necessary is complete rest in bed for 10 days to two weeks. It is important to instruct them how to rest, read interesting books on a book-rest or listen to the radio.

In acute coronary occlusion give morphine, enough to control the pain; digitalis for symptoms of heart failure or gallop rhythm or auricular fibrillation. Frequent extrasystoles require quinidine. It is dangerous to administer quinidine to patients who have large and dilated hearts. We usually give oxygen for pain, dyspnea, cyanosis and restlessness. Keep patient in bed from three to six weeks. Very old patients often are allowed to sit up in a chair one week after the acute occlusion. With the aid of a skilled nurse and an orderly, there is less strain on the patient when a commode is used than there is when the patient uses the bedpan.

* * * * *

PEPTIC ULCER, AN ENDOCRINE DISEASE

IN 1927 a demonstrator for a pharmaceutical house stated that his company's extract of the parathyroid gland was being used to promote the healing of *varicose* ulcers. I[1] began to use it in all of my case of *peptic* ulcer. The results have been prompt and almost universally gratifying, the ulcer usually healing and the gastric distress and pain disappearing within a few weeks.

I have been using this therapy for 16 years, at first falteringly. During the first few years there were several recurrences coming within 12 to 18 months after treatment had been discontinued.

---
1. H. L. Smith, Rochester, Minn., in *Jl. Iowa State Med. Soc.*, Dec.

1. J. A. Crabb, Topeka, in *Jl. Kansas Med. Soc.*, Nov.

They would yield to treatment promptly. In later years, I have advised my patients to come in for a small dose of hormone every two or three months and have had very few recurrences.

There are chronic cases of duodenal ulcer where scar tissue obstructs the pylorus in which operation is the only solution. In other cases a dense ring of scar tissue may prevent an adequate blood supply to the ulcer and thereby retard or prevent healing, but acute and subacute, and most chronic cases, respond to parathyroid therapy and heal promptly.

My usual method: Give one c.c. of parathyroid extract every third day for three doses, then 10 minims every 5-7 days for from 6-12 doses according to the results obtained.

I also use a palliative, such as bismuth and paregoric mixture, or an alkaline powder, to be taken 20-30 minutes before the expected pain to protect the ulcer from the gastric juice.

Foods allowed are milk, cream, cereals, milk toast, meat juices, soft eggs, custards and many other foods which the resourceful doctor may select.

* * * * *

ABOUT IMMUNITY TO COLDS

THE EXPLORER of the arctic and antarctic, exposed to excessive cold, humidity in crowded shelters, and physical strain to the point of exhaustion, catches anything from chilblains to frozen limbs, but he doesn't catch cold. Yet the moment he makes port on the home journey sneezing, sniffing and coughing remind him that he is to share the blessings of civilization in symbiosis with the microbes and viruses of the common cold.

This seems to be proof of the loss of immunity through prolonged absence from contact with the antigens of respiratory infections. On a larger scale, if not as clean-cut an experiment, we observe the first epidemics of colds early in autumn, when children and adults return from summer vacations in the prime of health.

All these are strong arguments of a competent observer,[1] who goes on to say:

The occupational group which shows the lowest incidence of acute respiratory infection is the general practitioner and the pediatrician. Although receiving day in and day out massive and virulent cold inoculations, these show a lower rate of absenteeism due to colds than any lesser exposed group of workers. Evidently this immunity is conferred by a higher titre of immunity.

The persons who train and harden themselves to withstand inclement weather are less likely to succumb to the recurring cold epidemics. It is a common experience that graduates from a tuberculosis sanatorium, after having acquired the health hab-

[1] K. F. Kastowitz, Milwaukee, in *Milwaukee Med. Times*, Jan.

its of breathing and enjoying fresh air, disdaining the fear complex of drafts and chills, are less likely to become chronic cold sufferers than the average, normal, coddled winter underwearer.

CLINICAL CHEMISTRY and MICROSCOPY

J. M. FEDER, M.D., and EVELYN TRIPBLE, M.T., *Editors*, Anderson, S. C.

A NEW HOPE FOR THE ALLERGIC?

THE MAIN DIFFICULTY that lies before the allergic individual is not so much one of diagnosis as it is of effective treatment. The dermal, intradermal and patch application of suspected substances, backed up by properly performed and interpreted leucopenic indices and passive transfer in certain cases will positively identify the offending items in fully 90 per cent of the cases.

If the tests incriminate one or two unimportant foods or inhalants or possibly pollens, the road to recovery is well sign-marked. Undoubtedly here, especially in pollinosis, the orthodox allergic regimen will prove to be efficacious. In another and much more difficult group we have to deal with basic food sensitivity; *i.e.*—wheat, egg, milk etc. The most intelligent patient will find difficulty in avoiding all foods containing portions of these substances, while those in the lower I. Q. rating group will be unable to understand instructions. The successful treatment of an allergic (or diabetic) patient must presuppose an intelligent, coöperative individual.

Viewed from the angle that not all of our patients are either intelligent or coöperative, it is not to be wondered that a high percentage of failures are noted in treating the chronic allergic. The hayfever victim is immunized by the doctor with excellent results, while the asthmatic, left more or less to his own devices, is sent home to carry out the provisions of a great many complicated dietary instructions, mostly prohibitory, and frequently reports, "No results."

Recognizing these shortcomings, numerous investigators have sought some substance that would strike at the root of the difficulty and eliminate the back-door approach to the atophic state now generally practiced.

A year ago we began following the work that was being done with the substance *ethylene disulphonate* in the treatment of allergy; and the distributors for the United States—Spicer, Gerhart Company of Sunland, California—sent some of the material to our group for trial. No conclusive data are at hand concerning our own work as the number of cases is too small, but the report of Wasson[1] from the Children's Allergy Clinic of the City Hospital Dispensary, New York, is convincing. Their problem was essentially that of any group dealing with the usual dispensary patients, many of them neither coöperative nor intelligent. Further, there was the complicating problem of multiple sensitivity which would subject already undernourished children to an indefinitely prolonged denatured diet. Many of these people would have been unable to obtain the required supplemental vitamins without outside financial assistance.

Wasson's series consisted of 40 patients, 20 of whom received ethylene disulphonate, while 20 were treated in the customary manner but received none of the drug. In tabulating his results, eleven of the treated cases are shown to be completely relieved, while only six in the control group are so designated. In those treated with the chemical, only two are listed as unrelieved, while this designation is applied to ten in the other group.

The modus operandi of the substance has been explained by British and Belgian observers on the basis of restoration of the cellular carbohydrate metabolism of the allergic individual. Whether or not this hypothesis is correct, there is one reassuring fact that stands out prominently in all of the reports reviewed. It is the absence of any untoward effect except a moderate amount of pain at the site of injection, and many of the patients were infants who received the same dose as an adult.

It is necessary to carry out the routine allergic investigations even if treatment by this substance is contemplated and its use does not preclude a thorough physical investigation. Routine stool examination for the presence of parasites has been stressed and positive findings have been reported more often in the case of the allergic than the non-allergic. Elimination of parasites must be accomplished before the specific medication (ethylene disulphonate) is started.

From available statistics, ethylene disulphonate appears to be worthy of a trial in all severe allergic conditions. We are especially impressed by its potentialities in intractable allergy, in multiple sensitivities, especially to the basic foods, and certainly where a doubt exists in the doctor's mind about strict adherence to his instructions for dietetic or other mandatory routine.

1. Wasson, V. P.: Archives of Pediatrics, New York, 60:511-517, Sept., 1943.

* * * * *

ON THE IMPORTANCE OF MALARIA AS A CAUSE OF FALSE POSITIVE SEROLOGIC REACTIONS

It is obvious that reporting to a person that he or she has syphilis when this is not true, is doing that person a very serious injustice and injury.

From numerous studies it has been shown that yaws, leprosy, infectious mononucleosis and malaria are diseases in which positive serologic tests for syphilis can be frequently expected. In occasional instances other conditions; e.g., pneumonia, vaccinia, measles and other acute febrile diseases give rise to false positive tests.

Since yaws and leprosy are extremely infrequent diseases in the United States infectious mononucleosis and malaria will be the chief causes of biologic false positive serologic recations. Both of these diseases are common and often are present in a subclinical state.

Latent malaria may produce positive tests easily mistaken for latent syphilis and the distinction between the two conditions not always easy. In a review of all the cases of naturally occurring malaria seen at a U. S. Marine Hospital between July, 1936, and July, 1940, the following facts were established.[1]

Total cases of malaria	64
Total cases with positive serologic tests	19
Cases diagnoses as syphilis	7
Cases probably due to syphilis	4
Cases with false positive serologic reactions	8

A 20-year-old white boy's Kahn reaction was 3 plus, Wassermann strongly positive. On June 28th (three days after admission) he had a chill and a t. of 40.2° C. A blood smear showed tertian malaria. Treatment with quinine was begun.

On 7/1 Kahn—3 plus; Wassermann—strongly positive
7/8 Kahn negative; Wassermann—negative
7/12   "   "   "   "
7/19   "   "   "   "

Prior to the development of the chill this patient was considered syphilitic and would have been treated as such had he not fortunately developed clinical malaria. A smear had not been taken in this case prior to the chill so that it cannot be stated that he had no evidence of malaria prior to onset of chill. It is the writer's belief that he had chronic malaria, the only manifestation of which were the positive serologic tests.

The longest period of positivity of serologic reactions with quinine therapy was 18 days after the last chill. This occurred in only one case. The other cases all had negative reactions within a period of 10 days following the last chill.

It would then appear that if one allows a month to elapse following malarial infection, the serologic reactions should certainly have become negative, assuming that adequate therapy has been given.

In this very week this case came to my attention: A young man, after being given a report of "positive blood," was discharged from the Army, probably from some other cause. He went home, told his story to a physician and requested treatment. This physician found no evidence of syph-

1. T. R. Dawber, in Annals Internal Med., Oct.

ilis, blood or otherwise, and declined to give treatment. The young man went to another doctor, with the same result.

Then he wrote the letter. He was much perturbed. Possibly his mind may never be at rest again.

The fact should never be lost sight of that a positive Wasserman or Kahn reaction is not infallible proof of syphilis.

HUMAN BEHAVIOUR

James K. Hall, M.D., *Editor*, Richmond, Va.

ILLITERACY AND WARFARE

Killing one's fellow-human has become one of the high arts. The illiterate may kill any other animal than man and do the killing thoroughly and well. But the unlearned man is not permitted to kill his enemy in warfare. The American soldier must be able to read and to write, otherwise he cannot be commissioned to indulge in human slaughter. The reason for the necessity of literacy in the soldier is that killing in warfare is now performed by science. Now the soldier merely operates the machinery that does the killing. The illiterate may be able to manipulate rather complicated machinery in war and in peace; but most of the instruction in the mechanisms utilized in killing and in destroying property in warfare is proffered in printed language, and the illiterate neither reads nor writes any language. Because the illiterate is helpless in the interpretation of written and of printed words, the most robust and valorous and ambitious young man must first acquaint himself with letters if he aspires to the reputation got sometimes at the mouth of the flaming cannon.

Modern Mars refuses admission to his battalion all those who are defective or diseased in structure or infirm in attributes; nor can the god of war instruct the young man how to twang the bow and to interpose the shield against the darts of the enemy unless the young man can understand the meaning both of the printed and the spoken word.

It was not so in more distant days. No typewriters and no pens and no telephones were made use of during the long siege of ancient Troy. Achilles moved the Greeks and struck terror to the heart of the lovely wife of Hector by his death-defying spoken words. Mahomet, the prophet and the founder of a mighty empire, remained unable, did he not? to read either the morning or the evening paper. And the brave, appealing Joan of Arc was illiterate and probably additionally handicapped by hallucinosis. Yet she still lives as no mean figure in the art of war.

An illiterate has been defined somewhat technically as a person ten years of age or older who cannot write in any language. We pay great deference to written and to printed language—and also to spoken words. But man speaks, even if his lips are immobile, and if he forms no words. Man insists upon expressing himself, unless he is engaged in repressing his ideas.

Forever and always man is wondering whether to say it nakedly, as he thinks it; to repress it entirely; or to modify it by paint and mask so that when released his idea may be neither recognized nor understood. One of the purposes of the use of language is to conceal thought or to cover up ignorance. Warfare has always made use of language either to inform or to deceive. The modern soldier must be as able to interpret printed words as to identify and to use the military mechanisms.

In the ancient Commonwealth of Virginia more than 28,000 drafted young men have been refused admission to the armed service because of illiteracy. Almost enough men to constitute two divisions are kept out of the army because they cannot properly interpret typed and written words. In their stead many fathers of children have been taken into the service; and the father of children, however valiant, is an expensive soldier. In the county in Virginia in which I write these words a Negro father of eleven children has lately been taken into the army. His services will cost the public treasury almost $200.00 a month in compensation to him and in guardianship of his family.

If the state would have its young men to do the killing incidental to warfare, it must first give them adequate instruction in the art of making and of interpreting visible words. The man who would aspire to kill his fellow-man with some degree of artistry must first develop some appreciation of linguistics. Even an enemy might object to being killed by an illiterate. I am unwilling to enter upon a discussion of the relationship between illiteracy and ignorance. The usual assumption is that the two words illiterate and ignorant are practically synonymous. But I have known keen-minded individuals who could not read and write.

The educational processes may be too firmly founded upon the belief that all learning must come through the printed page. We would be much more validly educated if less of our learning were derived from printed words. The arts and the crafts are almost completely neglected by the schools. Yet they possess pedagogical worth as well as economic value. We still have little understanding of the educational process. Not infrequently much more would be learned if words, printed or spoken, were not used at all.

RHINO-OTO-LARYNGOLOGY

CLAY W. EVATT, M.D., *Editor*, Charleston, S. C.

CONTROL OF NASAL HEMORRHAGE

ALMOST EVERYONE has seen epistaxis continue despite skilful postnasal and antenasal packing. I have seen several such hemorrhages stopped by the intravenous administration of a solution of oxalic acid.[1] This phenomenon has not been explained. This chemical has not been found to be toxic when administered properly and in no way endangers the status of the patient. It appears that contraindications to its use are essential hypertension, peripheral vascular disease, thromboangiitis obliterans and allied conditions. If the hemorrhage in any given case is deemed more important than any of these conditions, its use should still be considered.

After extensive primary or secondary hemorrhage a patient may be a candidate for transfusion.

For the patient whose condition after operation would be endangered by any type of thrombosis this substance is contraindicated.

As a prophylactic 2 c.c. (0.1% sol.) may be given one to one-half hour prior to operation, followed by the same amount immediately afterward.

In cases of profuse hemorrhage 3 to 5 c.c. intravenously, followed in one-half hour by 2 c.c., is to be given intramuscularly, with the addition of 2 c.c. at hourly intervals for three doses if the hemorrhage does not stop.

Its action is almost immediate, and one adequate dose will persist in its activity for several hours. It contains no alkaloids or proteins, and side effects are not to be expected.

It is economical, easily administered, nontoxic and efficient.

All I know about oxalic acid is that it is supposed to be poisonous, it is used as a bleaching agent, rhubarb is said to contain it; and sodium oxalate is placed in tubes into which blood is to be collected for certain tests, the purpose being to cause the calcium in the blood to unite with the oxalate radical, forming insoluble calcium oxalate, which precipitates from the blood and so makes it incapable of clotting.

This measure is put before you for what it is worth. The sponsor comes from a first-clas school and publishes in a first-class journal.

Write him for a reprint.

[1]. W. F. Hulse, Cleveland, in *Arch. of Otolaryngology*, June, '43.

IN THE GERMAN ARMY wounds of the eyeball are sutured in layers, in some of which sterilized women's hair is used.—*Australian & New Zealand J. of Surg.*

SURGICAL OBSERVATIONS
OF THE STAFF
DAVIS HOSPITAL
Statesville

PTOSIS OR PROLAPSE OF THE KIDNEY

THE RIGHT KIDNEY is more subject to displacement than the left. Downward displacement is apt to produce kinking of the ureter and so, obstruction to the flow of urine from the kidney to the bladder, and the consequent collecting of urine in the pelvis under pressure tends to destroy the kidney substance.

There may be prolapse when standing or sitting, and the kidney return to its proper position when the patient is lying down, this often relieving the obstruction. Where there is pain from the obstruction this may also relieve the pain, due to the fact that the obstruction is relieved and the urine which has collected in the kidney pelvis will drain down into the bladder.

The hydronephrotic kidney may be very large, an enormous amount of urine collecting in the kidney during the day and draining out at night, although in some cases the kidney pelvis remains over-distended for long periods of time. The drainage of large collections of hydronephrotic urine explains the unusual amount of urine passed by some patients at night.

Any pain complained of in the side may indicate renal trouble especially on the right side.

With the patient lying on a table on the left side a loose kidney can sometimes be felt by gentle palpation. With the patient standing a kidney can be felt fairly well and, since this causes the prolapse to become more pronounced, it may be associated with the characteristic pain of ptosis of the kidney.

Undue mobility of the kidney is caused by absorption of the fat pad in which the kidney lies, due to disease, sickness, or possibly to injury; laxity of the abdominal walls from any cause; congenital absence of the peritoneal support of the kidneys; ptosis of the other abdominal viscera; repeated jars and jolts as from jumping or falling from a distance.

I know a test pilot who says that he and others in his profession have ptosis of the kidneys. As they pull out of a dive there is a tremendous downward pull upon all the abdominal viscera. Doubtless, also, the rough riding in jeeps and tanks over rough terrain would tend to produce ptosis of either or both kidneys.

Usually the kidneys are more mobile in women and ptosis is far more frequent in women. The greater frequency of this mobility and prolapse of the right kidney is explained thus:

1. The heavy liver, moving with respiration, constantly pounds on the right kidney.
2. The right renal artery is the longer and this gives the right kidney more latitude of movement.
3. The right kidney is naturally a little lower than the left and so more exposed to the application of force.

Pain in the kidney region may be mild or severe, sometimes agonizing. Nausea and vomiting sometimes occur. The continued pain and dragging sensation cause extreme nervousness in many cases.

Traction upon the gastro-intestinal tract may cause gas on the stomach or indigestion, possibly enough obstruction of the duodenum to give pronounced symptoms. Traction on the bile ducts may produce symptoms. Rotation with torsion of the vessels might cause hematuria and if long-continued, serious renal lesions.

Traction and an angulation of the ureter causes intermittent obstruction, which later may be continuous. Hydronephrosis may result with degeneration of the kidney substance with great impairment of the function of the right kidney. Such a kidney is more subject to infections.

In undertaking the diagnosis the following examination should be made:

1. A cystoscopic examination, with ureteral catheterization.
2. Collection of specimen of urine from each kidney. Measurements of the urine drawn off from each kidney pelvis.
3. An x-ray picture made with catheters in place aids greatly in locating calculi. This should be done before the pelvis is injected for pyelogram.
4. A pyelogram shows position, shape and size of the kidney pelvis, and often yields other valuable information in regard to tumors and other conditions of the kidney.
5. With the patient standing or lying an x-ray picture of the kidneys with the radiopaque solution still in the renal pelvis will demonstrate just how far the kidneys come down.

Among the pathological conditions causing prolapse of the right kidney are:

1. Nephroptosis.
2. Aberrant blood vessels.
3. Calculi. (It must be remembered that some calculi are sometimes non-opaque).
4. Infections of the kidney pelvis or the ureter or the kidney itself.
5. Spasms of the ureter.
6. Congenital stenosis of the ureter, especially at the uretero-pelvic junction.
7. Abdominal tumors pressing on the ureter.
8. Inflammatory conditions about the cecum and appendix, causing pressure on the ureter or even obstruction from combined pressure and inflammation.
9. Tumors of the cecum and ascending colon.
10. Back pressure from prostatic obstruction.
11. Back pressure from bladder hypertrophy, especially where there is obstruction to the urethra, such as in prostatic disease or other similar conditions.
12. Fibrous bands.

Relief is afforded in some cases by an abdominal support, with or without a kidney pad.

Our advice to patients who have any great degree of prolapse is that the kidney be anchored in its proper position. The standard operation gives good results and recurrences are extremely rare.

Within the past two years in this clinic we have operated upon patients who had kidney suspensions as far back as fifteen years ago and some more recently. These patients were all operated upon (the second time) for pelvic conditions which had no relation to the former prolapse of the kidney. We have found in every instance the kidney had remained in proper position all these years; and they all stated that they had no further attacks of trouble such as they had had before the kidney was fixed in the correct position.

I feel that patients may be reassured about this operation since many of them have been told that recurrences are the rule rather than the exception. Recurrences in our experience have been almost nil.

DUKE PSYCHIATRIST TO HAVE CHARGE OF CHARLOTTE MENTAL HYGIENE CLINIC

Dr. R. Burke Suitt, new psychiatrist of the Charlotte Mental Hygiene Clinic, by an arrangement perfected in January, now conducts two Mental Hygiene clinics each month in Charlotte.

Dr. Suitt, a native of North Carolina, attended Trinity College and the St. Louis College of Arts and Sciences. He was graduated from the St. Louis School of Medicine in 1932; was instructor in psychiatry at Henry Phipps Psychiatric Clinic of Johns Hopkins School of Medicine; associate in neuro-psychiatry at Duke University, and assisting neuro-psychiatrist at Duke Hospital since the opening of the department in 1940. In July, 1942, he joined the 65th General Hospital as psychiatrist and served there until released from military duty late in 1943.

He is a Fellow, American Medical Society; a Diplomate, American Board of Psychiatry and Neurology; a member of American Association for the Advancement of Science, International League Against Epilepsy, Southern Medical Association, Allied Regional Societies, Tri-State Medical Association, American Psychiatric Association, National Committee for Mental Hygiene, Association for Mental Deficiency, and Southern Psychiatric Association.

DIABETES.—In families with a predisposition to the disease starchy food and sugar should be restricted by way of prevention.—*Christian*.

DIABETES.—Only the unusual case requires the care of a specialist.—*Christian*.

CLINIC
Conducted by
FREDERICK R. TAYLOR, B.S., M.D., F.A.C P.,
High Point, N. C.

A 6-YR.-OLD BOY from an orphanage was brought to me on June 9th, 1925. His chief symptom was fever. Three months before this he was believevd to have had a mild attack of influenza which kept him in bed 3 days. He seemed well a week later except for weakness, but then one night had a violent attack of spasmodic croup, lasting only a few hours. A week later Dr. H. L. Brockmann saw him and said his left lung was congested. At that time his t. went to 104 and stayed there 3 or 4 days. Dr. J. T. Burrus then saw him and prescribed mustard packs, and his fever was not so high afterward, he had a cold sweat as soon as he would get to sleep at night, and by midnight his t. would get to 100-102, falling some by morning, but reaching normal only by afternoon. No nausea or vomiting till the day before I saw him—he was nauseated all that day. Then he ate an orange and had a severe abdominal pain ending with vomiting the orange. He ate a good breakfast the day I saw him, without pain. His bowels usually moved normally, but 3 days before I saw him he passed 2 or 3 spoonfuls of fresh bright blood per rectum. This seemed to weaken him, and the next day he would tremble like a leaf when picked up. Never had any other hemorrhages. No sore throat or cough. He breathed hard during his night sweats. No edema. He complained of aching in his calves, and they would stay cold when his feet were hot. No headache or earache. He complained of lumbar pain the night after the rectal hemorrhage, but never before or since. No urinary symptoms. Urinalysis at hospital negative. Pulse reported very irregular at night. Rectal examination by Dr. Brockmann negative.

He had never had typhoid fever, scarlet fever, diphtheria, malaria, rheumatic fever, chicken-pox, whooping cough or mumps. He had a mild pneumonia the winter before coming to me, a very severe influenza in the epidemic just after he was born, another mild attack 1½ yrs. before I saw him. The attack the winter before he came to me seemed mild, but he did not seem to regain his health. He had measles two years before I saw him. He had never been vaccinated against anything and had had no operations or serious injuries. His father died of influenzal pneumonia, his mother and 1 brother were well.

He showed adenoid facies, faucial tonsils moderately enlarged, lingual tonsil the largest I ever saw. He was a mouth breather. He showed a generalized pallor. His neck, chest, abdomen and rectum were negative. His station was normal, gait slightly ataxic, no knee-jerks unless reinforced—perhaps due to voluntary fixation. No clonus or Babinski. Rough tests of sensation gave normal findings. He had been referred by Dr. Brockmann for a neurologic examination, and was referred back to him with a negative neurologic report and the suggestion that he have a special otologic examination, an x-ray study of his chest, and perhaps a gastrointestinal x-ray study after having a barium enema. To be considered in diagnosis were a simple post-infectious weakness and possibly epidemic encephalitis. His blood findings were normal including a negative Wassermann test.

The next day his walking got worse, and if he tried to run fast his feet would tangle. T. 99.6 at 3:00 p. m., though it was said to be usually normal at that hour, t. record for the preceding 24 hrs.: Noon, 99.4; 3:00 p. m., 98.0; 9:00 p. m., 97.0; 6:00 a. m., 99.0; 9:00 a. m., 99.4; noon, 99.4. He never complained of headache, but almost cried when he would have to walk a little distance because his legs and ankles ached, though they showed no tenderness or redness. Knee-jerks decreased now—absent except with reinforcement and then very weak. Pupils reacted promptly. A von Pirquet tuberculin test was negative. An otologist gave a negative report. Dr. Jean V. Cooke of St. Louis, who was holding a University of North Carolina Extension Postgraduate course in Pediatrics, saw this boy and advised x-ray study of the paranasal sinuses, pointing out that hemiplegia had been attributed to antral infection and cleared up in two weeks after treating the antra. He thought the development too slow for epidemic encephalitis. The boy certainly had an infection. Though he had not had a cold or a cough for 2 months, Dr. Cooke suspected the upper respiratory tract involvement. He felt that brain abscess was unlikely. He suggested removal of the tonsils and adenoids and repeating the von Pirquet test.

The boy was under my observation no further after this, but a note dated December 31st, more than 6 months after I had last seen him, states that Dr. Brockmann had been called to see him and found a large psoas abscess in the right side! It seems clear in retrospect that with the complaint of lumbar pain with the rectal bleeding, an x-ray study of his spine would have been in order.

BRITISH MEDICAL ASSOCIATION ON BEVERIDGE PLAN
(From *Lancet*, Oct. 2nd, via *J. A. M. A.*, Nov. 20th)

The annual representative meeting of the British Medical Association, which is comparable to the House of Delegates of the American Medical Association, met September 21st-23rd. The attitude of the meeting was shown by a vote of 200 to 10 in favor of the resolution that "In the opinion of the Representative body the creating of a whole-time salaried state medical service is not in the best interest of the community."

SOUTHERN MEDICINE & SURGERY

Official Organ
JAMES M. NORTHINGTON, M.D., *Editor*

Department Editors

Human Behavior
JAMES K. HALL, M.D. ....Richmond, Va.

Orthopedic Surgery
JOHN T. SAUNDERS, M.D. ....Asheville, N. C.

Urology
RAYMOND THOMPSON, M.D. ....Charlotte, N. C.

Surgery
GEO. H. BUNCH, M.D. ....Columbia, S. C.

Obstetrics
HENRY J. LANGSTON, M.D. ....Danville, Va

Gynecology
CHAS. R. ROBINS, M.D. ....Richmond, Va.
ROBERT T. FERGUSON, M.D. ....Charlotte, N. C.

General Practice
J. L. HAMNER, M.D. ....Mannboro, Va.

Clinical Chemistry and Microscopy
J. M. FEDER, M.D.,
EVELYN TREBBLE, M. T. } ....Anderson, S. C.

Hospitals
R. B. DAVIS, M.D. ....Greensboro, N. C.

Cardiology
CLYDE M. GILMORE, A.B., M.D. ....Greensboro, N. C.

Public Health
N. THOS. ENNETT, M.D. ....Greenville, N. C.

Radiology
R. H. LAFFERTY, M.D., and Associates ....Charlotte, N. C.

Therapeutics
J. F. NASH, M.D. ....Saint Pauls, N. C.

Tuberculosis
JOHN DONNELLY, M.D. ....Charlotte, N. C.

Dentistry
J. H. GUION, D.D.S. ....Charlotte, N. C.

Internal Medicine
GEORGE R. WILKINSON, M.D. ....Greenville, S. C.

Ophthalmology
HERBERT C. NEBLETT, M.D. ....Charlotte, N. C.

Rhino-Oto-Laryngology
CLAY W. EVATT, M.D. ....Charleston, S. C.

Proctology
RUSSELL VON L. BUXTON, M.D. ....Newport News, Va.

Insurance Medicine
H. F. STARR, M.D. ....Greensboro, N. C.

Dermatology
J. LAMAR CALLAWAY, M.D. ....Durham, N. C.

Pediatrics

Offerings for the pages of this Journal are requested and given careful consideration in each case. Manuscripts not found suitable for our use will not be returned unless author encloses postage.

As is true of most Medical Journals, all costs of cuts, etc., for illustrating an article must be borne by the author.

BRITISH DOCTORS ON THE BEVERIDGE PLAN

MANY STATEMENTS have been made in this country by those favoring socialistic government that the British doctors were highly pleased with such legislation.

Editorially, the *Medical Times* (New York) reports to the contrary:

At the annual meeting of the British Medical Association September 21st-23rd the following resolution regarding the Beveridge plan was passed by a vote of 200 to 10:

In the opinion of the representative body the creating of a full-time salaried state medical service is not in the best interests of the community.

Another resolution was passed by a vote of 149 to 37 which declared that a comprehensive medical service should be available to all who need it, but that it is unnecessary for the state to provide for those who are willing and able to provide for themselves.

The principles adopted placed the prevention of disease above sickness insurance; declared for free choice of physician; adequate nutrition and security from fear and want to precede or accompany any future organization of health services, since the health of the people depends primarily on environmental conditions; it is not in the public interest that the state should convert the medical profession into a salaried branch of central or local government service.

The Wagner-Murray-Dingell Bill is even worse than the Beveridge Plan.

Doctors are at a great disadvantage in speaking up for themselves. They have not the effrontery of lawyers and other boasters.

Let a priest[1] speak for us.

I am an honest man—I hope—but I would not like the responsibility for over 110 million people and 48 million dollars a year! It would not be fair to any physician who might be appointed as Surgeon General, either. I trust more in many—average, intelligent and honest men in an honorable profession. I prefer to confine the superman to the funnies. In real life he would be a menace—like Hitler —or any other dictator.

Better and better medical care has continuously and more widely been distributed, and made more generally available. Many of the formerly fatal diseases have been conquered; and most of the more dangerous and deadly of the other diseases have been or are being brought under control—all under the system by which all our scientific victories have been won.

Let us keep medicine unshackled—as free as religion, the press and honest speech.

Let us preserve the personal relationship between doctors and patients which now contributes so largely towards recovery and healing.

Allow me to inject a personal note. I was desperately hurt 200 miles from Atlanta and taken to a small hospital near the scene of the accident and given splendid service.

[1] The Very Rev. R. de Ovies, Litt.D., LL.D., D.D., Dean of the Cathedral of St. Philip, Atlanta, in *Jl. Med. Assn. Ga.*, Dec.

WSB put the story on the air within minutes, and my personal physician here in Atlanta obtained the best brain specialist available and they immediately drove that 200 miles to make sure that everything needful was done for me.

Money—fees—schedules—cannot buy such service as that; nor could any system of security administration guarantee such kindness and personal consideration.

But it wasn't Social Security, you see. It was the Physician's Oath and Creed put into practice, for medicine serves with the heart as well as with skill. LEAVE IT FREE TO DO SO!

* * * * *

MARRIED MEN SHOULD BE DRAFTED FIRST

Addressing the New York Academy of Medicine on November 18th, Sir Gerald Campbell, British Minister and Special Assistant to the British Ambassador, declared that there was some incongruity in our seeking to postpone the advent of old age and death at the same time that we restrict births. He thought that thereby science might be hindering progress. He advocated an increase in births and suggested that we cease allowing older men to become a nuisance to everyone and to hinder ambitious younger men attempting to advance themselves, but who, thus thwarted, lost zest and efficiency. He proposed "if wars there must be," that the older men who produce them be the first ones drafted, youth to be brought in to finish them off, thus allowing the great majority of those in the prime of life to live, not die, for their country. Finally, he thought that the older men in all countries should be prevented from adopting policies and croaking shibboleths which can only keep the world under such stress and strain that wars become inevitable.

My father always maintained that in filling the ranks of the fighting forces married men with children should be taken first. His sound reasoning was on this wise: The most valuable asset of a nation is its citizenship; indeed, the citizenship is the nation. Without continuation of reproduction of citizens the nation ceases to be. Men who have married and begot children have continued themselves, even if they lose their lives. If a single man is killed, that branch is forever cut off. Besides, the man with children has more chips in the game, more to fight for.

What's wrong with it? Except that there are more married than single men in authority?

* * * * *

THE EFFECT OF SPECIALIZATION ON THE EDUCATION OF THE MEDICAL STUDENT

The general practitioner is fast becoming a revered memory. Some time ago, a physician entered a particular specialty only after years of general practice.

A man who intends to specialize learns best that which he believes is requisite to the particular specialty. There is even unconscious rejection of other subject matter.

Before the instructor can help the student he must help himself. He must be impressed with the unity of medicine. We tend to forget that all the fields of medicine are interrelated and none can stand alone. We are even guilty of emphasizing our particular subject and placing all other subjects on a lower level.

The time to begin stressing the unity of medicine is on the very first day of college. The integral place of a subject in the general scheme of things must be made clear, and stressed not only once but over and over again. Medicine can be a strong and beautiful edifice if it is built strongly and according to plan on solid bricks with fine mortar, or it can consist of a number of scattered and isolated outhouses.

We would like to postpone choice of a specialty as long as possible. Preferably, the student should be encouraged to wait until after his rotating internship before deciding on a specialty or on general practice. As the years go on, we shall consider the general practitioner a specialist who is becoming so rare only because his is the most difficult and sacrificing job to perform. A student does not know what he can do best until he has done everything.

Surgery and surgical specialties have been glamorized because of the excitement and action which are always found in the operating room. The drama in the other branches of medicine must be demonstrated to the student. A student may want to be a surgeon, and not see of what use a knowledge of rheumatic fever will be to him. If we begin by showing him how the abdominal pain in rheumatic fever is often confused with acute appendicitis we will learn, because purposefully.

Thus a teacher of medicine[1] gloomily views the status of the general practitioner. But it is not as bad as he thinks, though, Heaven knows, that it is not worse, no thanks are due medical schools or hospitals. These institutions, along with the lay press, and too much of the medical press, have missed no opportunity to belittle the group which does most good for sick folks—not the least of this great service being saving their patients from unnecessary and expensive hospital and specialist treatment.

Medical schools can go a long way toward remedying the evil they have done, and atoning for it.

Make a general practitioner Dean of every Faculty of Medicine and Surgery in the country.

---
1. L. B. Slobody, New York City, in *Jl. Assn. Amer. Med. Col.*, Nov.

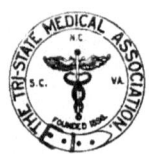

FORTY-FIFTH ANNUAL MEETING
CHARLOTTE, N. C., FEBRUARY 28th-29th

PRESIDENT'S ADDRESS—GEORGE BEN JOHNSTON, PIONEER SURGEON—
Dr. FRANK S. JOHNS, Richmond
NAVAL WARFARE CASUALTIES—
REAR ADMIRAL J. J. A. McMULLIN, M.C., U. S. Navy
ADDRESS—
LT. COMDR. WM. J. MARTIN, M.C., U. S. Navy, U. S. Naval Hospital, Bethesda, Md.
A NEW TECHNIQUE FOR THE TREATMENT OF PILONIDAL CYST AND FISTULA—
LT. COL. WILLIAM FRANCIS MARTIN (Charlotte), M.C., U. S. Army, Langley Field
SPLENIC RUPTURE WITH CASE REPORT—
LT. WM. A. JOHNS, M.C. (Richmond), U. S. Navy, United States Naval Hospital, New Orleans
SOCIAL ADJUSTMENT IN OBSESSIVE TENSION STATES FOLLOWING PREFRONTAL LOBOTOMY—
DR. JAMES W. WATTS & DR. WALTER FREEMAN, Washington
PREFRONTAL LOBOTOMY WITH SPECIAL REFERENCE TO INVOLUTIONAL MELANCHOLIA—
DR. J. G. LYERLY, Jacksonville (Fla.)
MEDICO-LEGAL ASPECTS OF CORONARY THROMBOSIS—
DR. J. M. HUTCHESON, Richmond
SOME MILITARY CONSIDERATIONS OF THE ALLERGIC INDIVIDUAL (Illustrated)—
THE TREATMENT OF INTERTROCHANTERIC FRACTURES OF THE NECK OF THE FEMUR—
DR. JAMES W. DAVIS, Statesville
THE POLITICO-ECONOMIC SITUATION IN REFERENCE TO MEDICINE—
DR. H. F. STARR, Greensboro
PITUITARY DISTURBANCE IN ITS RELATION TO NEUROPSYCHIATRY—
DR. BEVERLEY R. TUCKER, Richmond
PENETRATING WOUNDS OF THE HEART (Lantern Slides)—
DR. DANIEL L. MAGUIRE, JR., Charleston

THE IMPORTANT ROLE OF BRONCHOSCOPY IN THE OCCASIONAL CASE OF ASTHMA—
DR. V. K. HART, Charlotte
AN APPRAISAL OF THE CLINICAL LABORATORY (Technicians Invited)—
DR. J. M. FEDER, Anderson
NEUROPHYSIOLOGICAL ASPECTS OF GASTRO-INTESTINAL FUNCTION: PRACTICAL PSYCHOSOMATIC CONSIDERATIONS—
DR. FREDERICK H. HESSER, Duke University Medical School
THE PREVENTION AT SUPRAPUBIC HYSTERECTOMY OF POSTOPERATIVE CYSTOCELE—
DR. G. H. BUNCH, Columbia
STATUS PRAESENS OF THE RAPID TREATMENT OF SYPHILIS—
DR. J. LAMAR CALLAWAY & DR. RAY O. NOOJIN, Duke University Medical School
SOUND AND COLOR MOTION PICTURE "THE RIGHT TO HEAR"—
DR. CLAY W. EVATT, Charleston
THE LOCAL TREATMENT OF SURFACE BURNS—
DR. WM. H. PRIOLEAU, Charleston
THE PHYSICIAN AS TEACHER—
DR. KARL SCHAFFLE, Asheville
PELLAGRA sine PELLAGRA—
DR. E. L. COPLEY, Richmond
INSULIN RESISTANCE—REPORT OF TWO CASES—
DR. WILLIAM R. JORDAN, Richmond
TREATMENT OF HIP FRACTURES OF THE INSANE (Illustrated)—
DR. JOHN R. SAUNDERS, Morganton State Hospital, and DR. YATES S. PALMER, Valdese
A RESEARCH IN SURGICAL WOUND ANTISEPSIS—
DR. T. C. BOST, Charlotte
HOLD THE LINE—
DR. E. J. WILLIAMS, Monroe
THE AID THAT MAY BE HAD FROM THE ELECTROCARDIOGRAM—
DR. PAUL D. CAMP, Richmond
MENINGOCOCCEMIA—
DR. ROY S. BIGHAM, JR., Johns Hopkins Hospital, Baltimore
THE GENERAL HOSPITAL AS THE PLACE FOR TREATING MOST NEUROLOGIC AND PSYCHIATRIC PATIENTS—
DR. ARCHIE A. BARRON, Charlotte
PENICILLIN—
DR. E. McG. HEDGPETH, University of North Carolina Medical School

NUTRITION AS AN ETIOLOGICAL FACTOR
IN CHRONIC DEGENERATIVE DISEASES
OF THE NERVOUS SYSTEM—
 Dr. James Asa Shield, Richmond
PREVENTION & EARLY TREATMENT OF
PROSTATIC DISEASES—
 Dr. Raymond Thompson, Charlotte
FUNCTIONAL HYPOGLYCEMIA—
 Dr. G. L. Donnelly, Valdese, N. C.
RECONSTRUCTION OF THE LOWER JAW—
 Dr. Austin T. Moore, Columbia
BENIGN RECTAL DISEASES—
 Dr. R. B. Davis, Greensboro
CARCINOMA OF THE BREAST—
 Dr. Robert P. Morehead, Bowman Gray Medical School, Winston-Salem
MEDICINE IN CHINA & EXPERIENCES
AS A PRISONER OF THE JAPANESE—
 Dr. R. T. Shields, University of North Carolina Medical School
FATALITIES FROM THE USE OF NEOARSPHENAMINE IN LATE PREGNANCY—
 Dr. John Z. Preston, Tryon, N. C.
PUDENDAL BLOCK IN OBSTETRICS—
 Dr. M. Pierce Rucker, Richmond
THE INTERPRETATION AND TREATMENT
OF THE DISCHARGING BREAST—
 Dr. J. D. Gilland, Charlotte

This is incomplete. Finished programs will be mailed within a few days.

Fatality From Air Embolism Following Attempted Abortion
(R. R. Killinger & C. C. Collins, Jacksonville, in Jl. Fla. Med. Assn., Jan.)

A 40-year-old quadripara, seven months in her fifth pregnancy, was found dead in bed with the described apparatus inserted tightly into the cervix. The bag and tubes were new, clean and dry. The bag was collapsed, the cap connected to the tubing screwed in airtight, the stopcock open. A 24 catheter had been rubber-cemented airtight to the end of the tube. With the cap screwed in place and the stopcock open, the bag was easily distended retrograde by mouth. No pump or other apparatus was found.

We visualize that she had inserted the tube in the cervix, where we found it tightly wedged, opened the cock and squeezed the bag between her hands, thereby injecting into the uterus a considerable amount of air under pressure.

Immediate autopsy showed a 7-months' pregnancy, a distended crepitant uterus, all lacunas and uterine appendages filled with air. The placenta had been perforated by the catheter and rent asunder by a powerful air blast. Air was in the venae cavae. The right side of the heart was distended with a foamy blood froth, and air globules and columns in the sections of vessels of both lungs indicated a blocked pulmonary circulation from massive air emboli.

For the treatment of Scabies:
 Unguentum Sulfuris Composition, N.F.,
 also known as Wilkinson's Ointment.

NEWS

Patrick-Henry Counties (Va.) Medical Society

Dr. Rowland H. Walker, of Martinsville, was elected president of the Patrick-Henry Medical Society for 1944 at the quarterly supper meeting of that group January 14th, at the Broad Street Hotel, Martinsville. Other officers chosen are: Dr. J. T. Shelburne, of Critz, vice-president, and Dr. Henry Dickinson, Martinsville, secretary. Following the business session, Miss Louwilla Honaker, local Red Cross nurse, spoke of her work in Henry County. Guest speaker was Dr. Robert L. McMillan, associate professor of medicine at the Bowman Gray School of Medicine, Winston-Salem, N. C., who spoke on Rheumatic Heart Disease.

First Year of Eastern North Carolina Sanatorium

January 15th was the first anniversary of the Eastern North Carolina Sanatorium at Wilson. Dr. H. F. Easom, superintendent, reported that during the first year 353 patients had been admitted, that 178 of the 353 had been discharged. The hospital, throughout the year, averaged 180 patients.

Dr. Easom examined 1,510 "out patients" in the clinic for the past year and interpreted 915 x-ray pictures for outside doctors and hospitals.

University of N. C. Medical Faculty Entertains

The faculty of the University Medical School entertained the afternoon of January 30th at a tea in the Keesler Memoral Library for new members of the medical faculty and for the new freshman class. New members of the faculty are Dr. James P. Hendrix of the Duke Medical School, lecturer in pharmacology; Dr. Fred W. Ellis, formerly with the Jefferson Medical College in Philadelphia, assistant professor of pharmacology; Dr. Alex Webb of Raleigh, lecturer in surgery; Dr. W. W. Vaughan of Watts Hospital, Durham, lecturer in radiology; and W. R. Straughn, formerly of Maryland State Teachers College, instructor in bacteriology.

Dr. Crowell Gives Dinner

For the evening of the 26th of January, Dr. L. A. Crowell, Sr., Lincolnton, invited a number of his friends for dinner and discussion of hospital problems, especially the desirability and feasibility of a flat hospital rate to include laboratory services.

Those enjoying Dr. Crowell's hospitality were:
Dr. Glenn R. Frye, Richard Baker Hospital, Hickory
Mr. S. K. Hunt, Administrator, Grace Hospital, Morganton
Mr. Carl I. Flath, Administrator, Charlotte Memorial Hospital
Dr. John R. Saunders, Supt., State Hospital, Morganton
Mr. Harry Riddle, Director, State Hospital, Morganton
Dr. Yates Palmer, Valdese
Mr. D. W. Alexander, Administrator, Valdese Hospital
Dr. J. D. Rudisill, Lenoir
Dr. Verne H. Blackwelder, Lenoir Hospital
Mr. Crawford Poag, Administrator, Reeves Hospital, Lincolnton
Dr. J. R. Gamble, Lincolnton
Dr. L. N. Glenn, City Hospital, Gastonia
Mr. Harold L. Bettis, Administrator, Shelby Hospital
Dr. J. M. Northington, Charlotte
Dr. J. Q. Myers, Charlotte
Dr. J. W. Davis, Davis Hospital, Statesville
Dr. F. M. Houser, Cherryville

Dr. F. W. Jones, Newton
Dr. L. M. Caldwell, Newton
Dr. L. M. Faulk, Ellen Fitzgerald Hospital, Monroe
Mr. Frank H. Crowell, Administrator, Crowell Hospital, Lincolnton
Dr. W. F. Elliott, Lincolnton
Dr. L. A. Crowell, Jr., Lincolnton
Dr. A. M. Cornwell, Lincolnton
Dr. J. H. Fitzgerald, Lincolnton

UROLOGY AWARD—THE AMERICAN UROLOGICAL ASSOCIATION offers an annual award, not to exceed $500, for an essay (or essays) on the result of some specific clinical or laboratory research in Urology. The amount of the prize is based on the merits of the work presented, and if the Committee on Scientific Research deem none of the offerings worthy, no award will be made. Competitors shall be limited to residents in urology in recognized hospitals and to urologists who have been in such specific practice for not more than five years. All interested are requested to write the Secretary for particulars.

The selected essay (or essays) will appear on the program of the forthcoming meeting of the American Urological Association, June 19th-22nd, 1944, Hotel Jefferson, St. Louis, Missouri.

Essays must be in the hands of the Secretary, Dr. Thomas D. Moore, 899 Madison Avenue, Memphis, Tennessee, on or before March 15th, 1944.

Dr. Funsten's Home in Albemarle Burns

Padoboja Farm, country home of Dr. Robert V. Funsten, Professor of Orthopedics at the University of Virginia, was destroyed by fire in January together with its contents.

There was no one at the residence when the fire was discovered, Mrs. Funsten being critically ill of pneumonia at the University, and the other members of the family were away. Responding to an alarm, turned in by Dr. Oscar Swineford, of Pine Knots, members of the City Fire Department went at once to the scene, but upon their arrival the dwelling was found in ruins.

After using what water they had in the tanks of the apparatus on hand, the firemen took out a tank of water on a truck.

The residence was located on the Barracks Road, a-mile-and-a-half northwest of the city. The loss, estimated at $20,000, is only partly covered by insurance.

Merger of High Point Hospitals

Final merger of High Point's two hospitals, the Guilford General and the Burrus Memorial, became effective January 15th, under the name High Point Memorial Hospital, with the Burrus Memorial designated as the Boulevard unit, the other as the Washington Street unit.

For some time plans for combining the two hospitals have been under consideration, and to date, according to the chairman of the Executive Committee of the High Point Memorial (Burrus Memorial) Hospital, a total of $102,975 has been placed in a trust fund for building a modern hospital when materials and manpower are available.

Named as members of the new executive board are Judge D. C. MacRae, Tom J Kearns, Myron H .Folger and Fred Ingram.

Under provisions of the merger J. P. Richardson, administrator of the Burrus Memorial Unit, will become director of the combined unit, and W. R. Peters, holding a similar position with the Guilford General Hospital, will become business manager of the new institution.

MARRIED

Miss Catherine McMillan, of Vass, N. C., and Dr. Norris M Burleson, Lt., M.C., U. S. Navy, at present stationed at the Norfolk Naval Base, January 6th.

Dr. John Ransom Lewis, Jr., of Louisville, Georgia, and Miss Katherine McQueen Palmer, of Albemarle, North Carolina, were married on December 30th, 1943.

DIED

Dr. Virgil Hamner, 66, former coroner and health officer of Page County for 30 years, died at his home at Luray, Va., January 1sth, from a relapse from an attack of influenza. A graduate of Richmond College, he was for 43 years a practicing physician in Page County. Among the survivors is a doctor brother, Dr. James L. Hamner, of Mannboro, Va.

Dr. Philip D. Kerrison, 72, a specialist in ear diseases, suffered a heart attack in the subway January 24th, and died a short time later.

A native of Charleston, S. C., he had practiced in New York for 45 years and formerly was a lecturer at New York University.

Dr. William B. Peters, of Appalachia, Va., died January 6th in a Baltimore hospital.

Medical College of the State of South Carolina

The Refresher Course held November 5th and 6th was a great success with more than 150 physicians attending from South Carolina and other states. Dr. G. W. Thorn of Boston was one of the highlights of the course, and Dr. Henry Meleney of New York the speaker on tropical diseases at the Founder's Day banquet.

Forty-one men and two women were graduated on December 22nd. Those in the Army and the Navy at the presentation of their diplomas received certifications. Forty-two nurses received degrees, 11 affiliate nurses their certificates. Dr. W. K. Green, president of Wofford College, delivered the annual address.

At the time of graduation, Dr. Robert Wilson retired as Dean of the College. He had served for 35 years as Dean and taught for 51 years. He will continue as Dean Emeritus and Professor Emeritus of Medicine and Special Lecturer in Medical History. Dr. W. H. Kelley was announced to succeed Dr. Wilson as Professor of Medicine.

Dr. Kenneth M. Lynch, Professor of Pathology, who has served the College since 1936 as Vice-Dean, is the newly-elected Dean and opened the 117th session of the College on January 3rd. Some 190 students registered for the coming session, 54 being new students, 50 of whom entered the freshman class, while four transferred from other colleges.

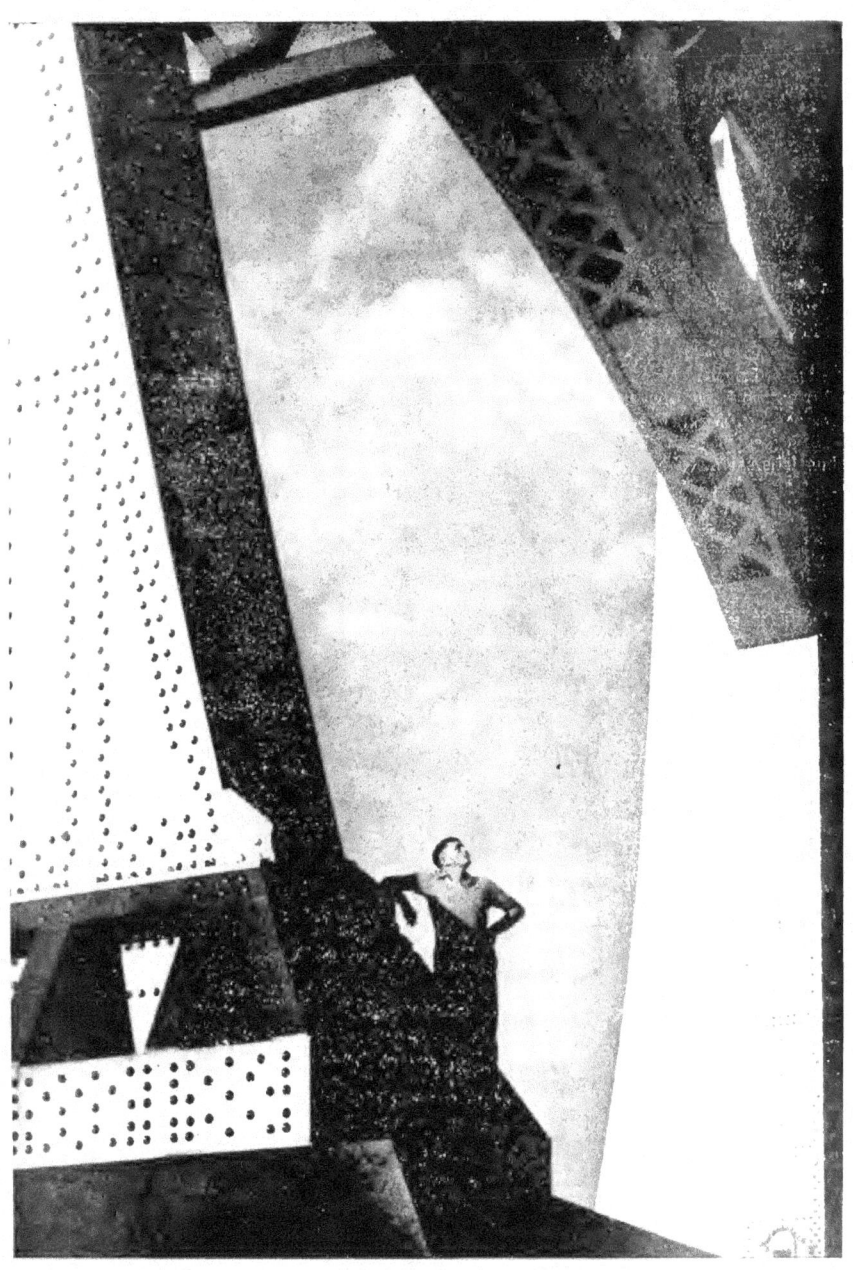

RIVETS TO ENSURE STRENGTH......*Vi-Penta Perles* *Vi-Penta Drops* 'ROCHE'

Dr. M. D. Wheatley has joined the Faculty in the Department of Anatomy. He is a graduate of the Universities of Kansas and Iowa and has published a number of articles in scientific journals. At present he is working on the subject of the hypothalamus and affective behavior in cats which will be published shortly.

UNIVERSITY OF VIRGINIA

On December 16th and 17th Dr. Vincent W. Archer, Professor of Röntgenology, gave two talks on Gastro-intestinal Diagnosis, was Leader of an X-ray Conference, and was one of a panel of four in a round-table discussion on Diseases of the Chest at a War-time Graduate Medical Meeting, LeGarde Army Hospital and the Naval Hospital, New Orleans.

Dr. Fletcher D. Woodward attended a meeting of the Eastern Section of the American Laryngological, Rhinological and Otological Society in New York on Friday, January 14th, and a meeting of the council of the same society on Saturday, January 15th. As Vice-President of the American Broncho-esophagological Association, he attended a council meeting of that organization on Sunday, January 16th.

The Personnel of the Eighth Evacuation Hospital, sponsored by the University of Virginia, now on duty in Southern Italy, recently presented to the Medical School a collection of 75 replicas of surgical instruments discovered in the ruins of Pompeii and Herculaneum. The originals from which these reproductions were made were on exhibition in the National Museum of Naples. The reproductions, the handiwork of the Neapolitan Cavalier Guglielmo Gallo, were made by hand from the same metals as the originals, usually bronze. They will be put on display in an appropriate museum case in the Medical Library.

MEDICAL COLLEGE OF VIRGINIA

Dr. C. C. Coleman, Professor of Neurosurgery, attended the annual meeting of the American Academy of Orthopedic Surgeons in Chicago, January 23d, giving a paper on Surgery of the Peripheral Nerves.

Major Joseph M. Dixon, an alumnus of the college, has been appointed Professor of Military Science and Tactics, in the stead of Colonel Paul L. Freeman, who is being retired as commandant of the 3313th Unit of the A. S. T. program under the army at the college.

Dr. Erling S. Hegre has been appointed Assistant Professor of Anatomy effective January 1st. Doctor Hegre received his bachelor of arts degree from Luther College of Montana State University, his master's from the same university, and his Ph.D. from the University of Minnesota Medical School.

Dr. Helen J. Ramsey has been appointed Instructor in Pharmacology. She received her bachelor's and master's degrees in science from Purdue University and her Ph.D. from Duke.

A grant in the amount of $1,000 has been made by C. C. Haskell for research in biochemistry. The Office of Scientific Production and Research of the Federal government has made an additional grant of $4,000 for continuation of the research work in shock and burns. A gift of $10,000 has been received for the North Campus project.

Mr. Samuel Bemiss has been appointed to the college Board of Visitors to fill the vacancy caused by the death of Mr. Julien Hill.

President W. T. Sanger visited the research laboratories of R. C. A. at Princeton, those of General Electric Company at Schenectady, and also visited Saratoga Springs, January 21st-23d.

Dr. R. J. Wilkinson of Huntington, West Virginia, was a recent college visitor.

WITH OUR ADVERTISERS

EVERY MOTHER DOESN'T KNOW HOW TO GIVE COD LIVER OIL

Some give cod liver oil in the morning and at bedtime when the stomach is empty; others give it after meals in order not to retard gastric secretion. If the mother will place the very young baby on her lap and hold its mouth open by gently pressing the cheeks inward between her thumb and fingers while she administers the oil, all of it will be taken and the infant will soon take the oil without having its mouth held open. It is important that the mother administer the oil in a matter-of-fact manner, without apology or expression of sympathy.

If given cold, cod liver oil has little taste. As any "taste" is largely metallic from the spoon, a glass spoon has an advantage.

On account of its higher potency in vitamins A and D, Mead's Cod Liver Oil Fortified With Percomorph Liver Oil is to be given in one-fourth the dosage of ordinary cod liver oil, and is particularly desirable in cases of fat intolerance.

NEW ESTROGEN DEVELOPED

Ethinyl estradiol, the most orally-administered estrogen yet developed, has been announced by the Schering Corporation. The new drug is a derivative of alphaestradiol, the natural follicular hormone. Clinical evidence indicates that the new estrogen is 5 to 20 times as potent as stilbestrol when given by mouth. Because of its extremely high potency, the new drug is given in minute doses, .02 to .05 mg., and this small dosage makes treatment with the drug inexpensive.

The new estrogen, which will be known as Estinyl, is less toxic, in therapeutic doses, than the synthetic estrogens. Nausea and vomiting following its use are uncommon. When they occur, they usually indicate overdosage, and in most cases can be corrected by decreasing the dose. Clinicians report that patients receiving Estinyl enjoy the general sense of well-being characteristic of naturally derived estrogens and not generally produced by synthetic compounds.

Estinyl is indicated in the treatment of such estrogenic deficiencies as the menopausal syndrome, juvenile and senile vaginitis, hypo-ovatianism, and certain disturbances of the menstrual cycle.

Physicians who would like to receive clinical samples of this new drug sufficient for trial in an average menopausal case, and reprints covering its clinical investigation, are invited to address a request to the Medical Research Division, Schering Corporation, Bloomfield, N. J.

THE SCHOOL-CHILD'S BREAKFAST

Many a child is thought dull when he should be treated for undernourishment. In hundreds of homes a "continental" breakfast of a roll and coffee is the rule. If, day after day, a child breaks the night's fast of twelve hours on this scant fare, a small wonder that he is listless, nervous, or stupid at school. A happy solution to the problem is Pablum. Pablum furnishes protective factors especially needed by the school-child—especially calcium, iron and the vitamin B complex. The ease with which Pablum can be prepared enlists the mother's coöperation in serving a nutritious breakfast. This palatable cereal requires no further cooking and can be prepared simply by adding milk or water of any desired temperature.

Mead Johnson & Company, Evansville, Indiana, U. S. A.

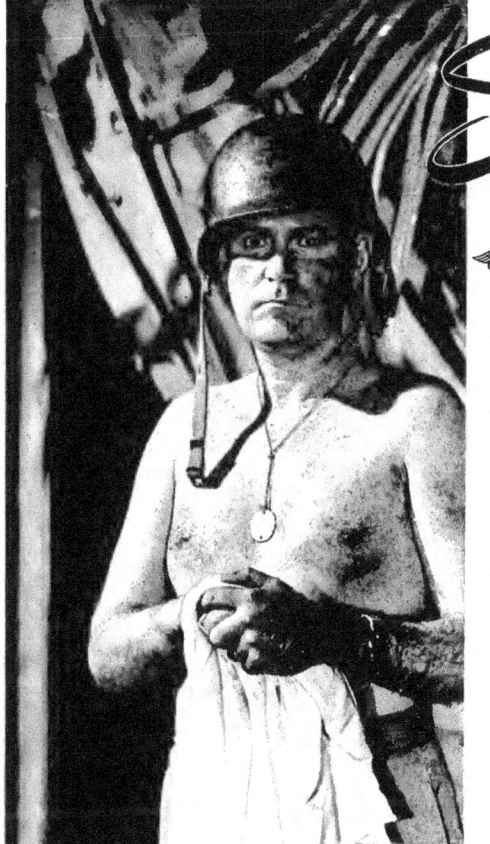

Sleep?...

WHAT'S THAT?

Now—a delicate brain job... then another... and another... to the tune of mortar fire... blast... shock! Steady... steady—easy now. "O. K.... clear the table! Next!" Operating... treating... night and day... Two hours sleep in seventy-two!*

• • •

Yet that's just a side glance into a war doctor's life. When does he relax? Seldom, but that's when he's eager for a cheering smoke. Camel his likely choice—the fighting man's favorite**—for mildness, sheer good taste.

Friends, relatives in service? Remember them often—with a carton of Camels—the gift of gifts for service men!

*From actual experiences of U. S. doctors in war.

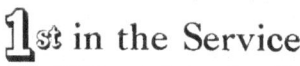

1st in the Service

**With men in the Army, Navy, Marine Corps, and Coast Guard, the favorite cigarette is Camel. (Based on actual sales records.)

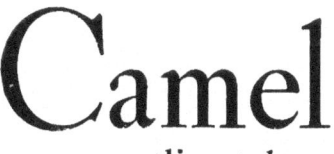

Camel
costlier tobaccos

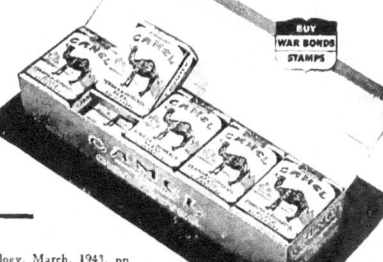

New reprint available on cigarette research—Archives of Otolaryngology, March, 1943, pp. 404-410. Camel Cigarettes, Medical Relations Division, One Pershing Square, New York 17, N. Y.

BOOKS

TRAUMATIC INJURIES OF FACIAL BONES, by JOHN B. ERICH, M.S., D.D.S., M.D., Consultant in Laryngology, Oral and Plastic Surgery at the Mayo Clinic, Assistant Professor of Plastic Surgery, The Mayo Foundation for Medical Education and Research, Graduate School, University of Minnesota; Diplomate of the American Board of Plastic Surgery; and LOUIE T. AUSTIN, D.D.S., F.A.C.D., Head of Section on Dental Surgery at the Mayo Clinic, Associate Professor of Dental Surgery, The Mayo Foundation for Medical Education and Research, Graduate School, University of Minnesota. In Collaboration with Bureau of Medicine and Surgery, U. S. Navy. 600 pages with 333 illustrations. *W. B. Saunders Company*, Philadelphia and London. 1944. $6.00.

It would seem that a team made up of an oral surgeon and a dental surgeon would be a proper pair to write a book on trauma of the facial bones, in so many such cases do these two have to work together for the cure.

An excellent dealing with general considerations leads up to discussions of the different problems in diagnosis and treatment of traumatic injuries to the several bones of the face.

The book's essential conservatism may be illustrated by quoting a sentence: "Open operations are never to be undertaken; one should rely on, and have enough ingenuity to construct, intra-oral or external appliances . . . . . . to supply adequate immobilization."

A statement that stands out from the page is: The patient's lower denture [in case of fracture of the toothless mandible] may be employed as a splint. The many ingenious mechanisms for holding the fragments in place are the natural result from just this kind of teamwork.

The descriptions are clear and concise, and, as supplemented by skillful illustration, cover the subject in an admirable manner.

MINOR SURGERY. By FREDERICK CHRISTOPHER, S.B., M.D., F.A.C.S., Associate Professor of Surgery at Northwestern University Medical School, Chicago; Chief Surgeon at the Evanston (Ill.) Hospital. Fifth Edition. Reset. 1006 pages with 575 illustrations. *W. B. Saunders Company*. 1944. $10.00.

The author does not say, as does a distinguished North Carolina surgeon now retired, that there is no such thing as minor surgery; but he begins the preface to this edition: "All minor surgery is potentially major surgery, a distinction between the two often being impossible."

Certainly this is an excellent approach to the very fine consideration of the subject matter, which includes a good deal larger part of the whole of surgery than used to be dealt with under the title, "Minor Surgery and Bandaging."

Certain measures described and advocated in previous editions are omitted from this one, because, as the author explains, they have not meas-

BIPEPSONATE

Calcium Phenolsulphonate	2 grains
Sodium Phenolsulphonate	2 grains
Zinc Phenolsulphonate, N. F.	1 grain
Salol, U. S. P.	2 grains
Bismuth Subsalicylate, U. S. P.	8 grains
Pepsin, U. S. P.	4 grains

Average Dosage

For Children—Half drachm every fifteen minutes for six doses, then every hour until relieved
For Adults—Double the above dose.

How Supplied

In Pints, Five-Pints and Gallons to Physicians and Druggists only.

Burwell & Dunn Company

Manufacturing *Pharmacists*
Established in 1887

CHARLOTTE, N. C.

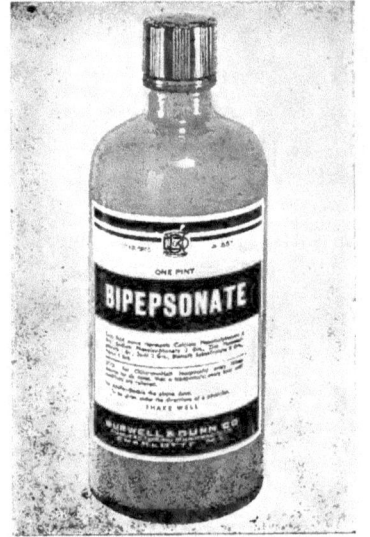

Sample sent to any physician in the U. S. on request

ALBEE'S
BONE GRAFT SURGERY

I   The General Principles of Bone Grafting
II   Armamentarium of the Orthopedic Surgeon
III   Spine Fusion
IV   Bone Graft Surgery of the Hip Joint
V   Bone Graft Surgery of Ununited Fractures
VI   Bone Graft Surgery for Replacement of Bone
VII   Plastic Bone Graft Surgery
VIII   Orthrodesing Bone Graft Operation
IX   Bone Block Operations

A VERY OPPORTUNE BOOK

It is now twenty-five years since I set myself to the task of writing the first book published in any language upon the sole subject of bone graft surgery.

Since that time, the trustworthiness of such work has been amply proven. Bone graft operations were then relatively new, but have been since adopted by the surgical profession the world over, much to the benefit of the patient.

In the present volume there are incorporated those procedures which have stood the test of time, namely: those which I have used myself, and those which I have not elected to use myself but have included because of their employment by experienced surgeons of mature judgment.

—FED H. ALBEE

BONE GRAFT SURGERY in DISEASE, INJURY and DEFORMITY
by
Fred H. Albee, M.D., LL.D., F.A.C.S., F.I.C.S.
assisted by
Alexander Kuschner, M.D., B.Sc.

Copyright, 1940, by D. Appleton-Century Company.

D. Appleton-Century Company, New York, N. Y. SMS
Please send a copy of Bone Graft Surgery (Albee), $7.50.

☐ Check enclosed   ☐ Send C. O. D.

Name..

Address .... City.............................. State..................

ured up to expectations, or because they have been superseded by better techniques.

A book deserving the fullest praise—and use.

GASTRO-ENTEROLOGY, by HENRY L. BOCKUS, M. D., Professor of Gastro-enterology, University of Pennsylvania Graduate School of Medicine. In three volumes, totaling about 2700 pages with about 900 illustrations, many in colors. Volume II—"Intestines and Peritoneum." 975 pages with 176 illustrations—12 in colors. *W. B. Saunders Company,* Philadelphia and London. 1944. Price—3 Vols. and separate desk index, $35.00.

Vol. II, just off the press, carries the sections covering diseases of the small and the large intestine; and diseases of the peritoneum, mesentery and omentum.

Common and rare conditions are dealt with in the same detailed fashion. Reading the differential diagnosis of spastic colon one cannot fail to be impressed with the breadth of knowledge, the experience and the judgment of the author. And that is only a subject taken at random. The whole volume will grade to sample.

It is gratifying to see this heading: "So-called 'Chronic Appendicitis.'" Also, such sentences as these:

Although the causes of chronic diarrhea are many, there are few symptoms which lend themselves so readily to a critical diagnostic study.

Most of the organic causes for chronic diarrhea are associated with changes in the mucous membrane of the lower ten inches of the large intestine, an area which can be directly inspected through the sigmoidoscope.

From our review of Vol. 1:

Such great advance has been made in klowledge of disorders of the digestive tract in the past quarter century as to demand a work on an encyclopedic scale. Bockus has provided such a work, dedicating it, fittingly, to the "student physicians of the University of Pennsylvania Graduate School of Medicine," who have stimulated him to better and better teaching over many years.

The second volume confirms the impression made by the first:

From this, the first, volume, one may learn that this is a monumental treatise on gastroenterology which will exercise a commanding influence in this field for decades to come.

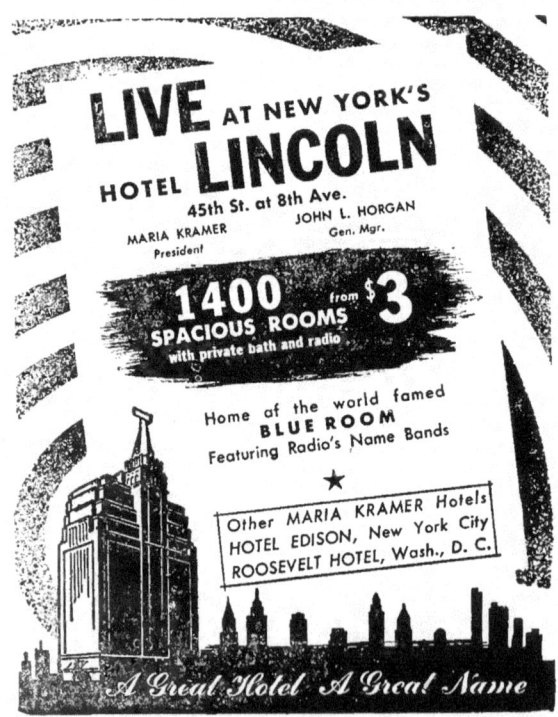

TEXTBOOK OF MEDICINE, by Various Authors, edited by J. J. CONYBEARE, M.C., D.M. Oxon., F.R.C.P., Physician to Guy's Hospital, London. Sixth Edition. *The Williams & Wilkins Company*, Mt. Royal & Guilford Aves., Baltimore. 1942. $7.50.

This is our first acquaintanceship with this textbook—and it in its Sixth Edition! It has been our loss.

There is no vagueness, no prolixity, in the book. It is chockfull of meat from cover to cover.

What physician would not be enthusiastic about a book which makes this unequivocal statement: The most certain indication of organic heart disease is cardiac enlargement?

It may be that there is some error on the side of dogmatism; but this is infinitely preferable to the exaltation of mechanical, diagnosis, and the so-and-so may occur and this-and-that may be tried, of the great majority of the books now coming out.

A book worthy of the Old Guy's tradition.

THE 1943 YEAR BOOK OF GENERAL SURGERY, edited by EVARTS A. GRAHAM, A.B., M.D., Professor of Surgery, Washington University School of Medicine; Surgeon-in-Chief of the Barnes Hospital and of the Children's Hospital, St. Louis. *The Year Book Publishers, Inc.*, 304 S. Dearborn Street, Chicago. $3.00.

From year to year, in going through the Yearbook of General Surgery, one is impressed with the fact that the editor consistently takes the wheat from the chaff and accepts only the valuable for inclusion.

PAIN, by THOMAS LEWIS, M.D., F.R.S., Physician in Charge of Department of Clinical Research, University College Hospital, London; Fellow of University College, London. *The Macmillan Company*, New York. 1942. $3.00.

Sir Thomas is not at all ashamed to write about a symptom, or to say he has been unable to define pain. His chief purpose, to review modern ways of the mechanism of human pain and to publish the work in this field of his own laboratory, is accomplished with great thoroughness; yet the resultant book is hardly too large t o be called a booklet.

Pain remains the chief warning that al lis not well within us, and the chief complaint for which people demand of us relief. Pain is worthy of the time and study Sir Thomas has devoted to it, and of his admirable setting forth.

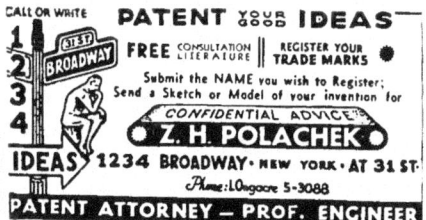

CHUCKLES

Being Dead Yet Speaketh

The *Texas State Medical Journal* says (and who are we to question):

"Glasses, if properly fitted and adjusted, never create any defect or weakness of the eyes or cause the muscles to deteriorate from nonuse," the late John Oliver McReynolds, M.D., Dallas, Texas, *contends* in *Hygeia, The Health Magazine.* "They simply supply the deficiency already existing, and the muscles still have their normal work to do," he says.

Doctor: "I can't tell you how delighted I am, Mrs. Smith. My son has won a scholarship."

Farmer's Wife: "I can understand your feelings perfectly. I felt just the same way when our pig won a blue ribbon at the county fair."

Prolonged exercise after forty is harmful if you do it with a knife and fork.

Nurse (to housemaid): "Baby's got her mamma's complexion."

Father (from next room): "Nurse, are you letting that child play with its mother's cosmetics?"

Now Little Red Riding Hood meets the wolf at the door and comes out with a fur coat.

"What's inertia, Dad?"

"Well, if I have it it's laziness; but if your mother has it it's nervous prostration."

An optimist from official Washington declares we should pay our taxes "with a smile." We've tried that, but the collector demands cash.

The farmer looked up from his magazine in the dentist's waiting room.

"Well, well," he said, "I see there's a new child actress. Mary Pickford, they call her."

"Where can one find a doctor honest enough to tell a man there is nothing wrong with him?" asks a novelist. There are said to be quite a number in the Army.

In giving her girdle to the rubber drive, Gertie says it is more important for the government to be in good shape

---

Jonathan Swift told his wife that it was best not to celebrate their Silver Wedding Anniversary, but to wait five more years and observe their Thirty Years War. *Roche Review.*

Manager: "Did you put 'Handle with Care' and 'This Side Up' on that carton of glassware?"

New Clerk: "Yes, sir. And to make sure everyone would see it, I printed it on four sides."

Teacher: "Why must we always keep our homes clean and neat?"

Little Girl: "Because company way walk in any minute."

Dog Catcher: "Little boy, do both of your dogs have licenses?"

Little Boy: "Oh, yes, sir, they're just covered with them."

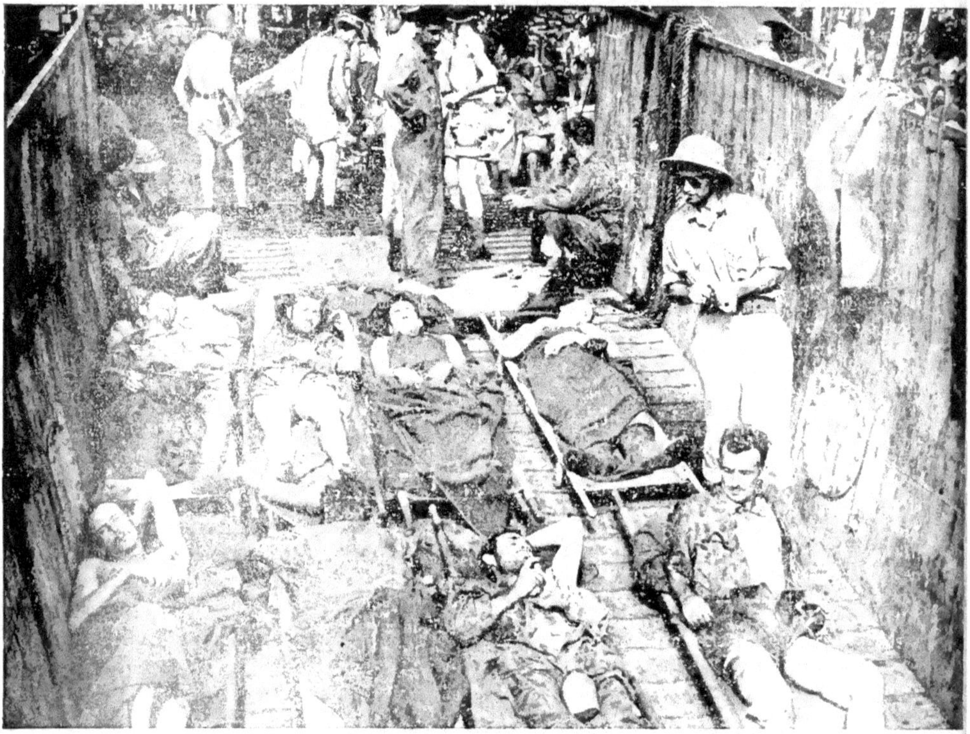

Pin-up picture for the man who "can't afford" to buy an extra War Bond!

YOU'VE heard people say: "I can't afford to buy an extra War Bond." Perhaps you've said it yourself... without realizing what a ridiculous thing it is to say to men who are dying.

Yet it *is* ridiculous, when you think about it. Because today, with national income at an all-time record high... with people making more money than ever before... with less and less of things to spend money for... practically every one of us has extra dollars in his pocket.

The very *least* that *you* can do is to buy an *extra* $100 War Bond... above and beyond the Bonds you are now buying or had planned to buy.

In fact, if you take stock of your resources, and check your expenditures, you will probably find that you can buy an *extra* $200... or $300... or even $500 worth of War Bonds.

Sounds like more than you "can afford?" Well, young soldiers can't afford to die, either... yet they do it when called upon. So is it too much to ask of us that we invest more of our money in War Bonds... the best investment in the world today?" Is that too much to ask?

Let's all BACK THE ATTACK!

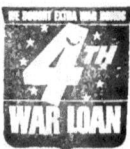

"Who was that man you just raised your hat to?"
"That was my barber. He sold me a bottle of hair restorer a year ago, and whenever I meet him I let him see what a fake he is."

This inscription is found on the tombstone of an Army mule:
"In memory of Maggie, who in her lifetime kicked one general, four colonels, two majors, ten captains, 24 lieutenants, 42 sergeants, 454 privates, and one bomb."

Hermann Goering accompanied the Fuehrer on one of his vits to Rome. On the crowded railway platform filled with dignitaries and troops, the massive Marshal roughly jostled past an Italian gentleman of aristocratic bearing, who turned and haughtily demanded an apology. Fiercely the Marshal turned upon him and snapped, "I am Hermann Goering." The Italian bowed and replied, "As an excuse that is not enough, but as an explanation it is ample."

At a house party a maiden lady of vinegary mien would not be deterred one day from her proposal to take a stroll with the Irish wit Sheridan. He begged off on the pretext of the threatening weather.
Shortly afterward, sneaking out by a back entrance to walk alone, Sheridan was accosted by his nemesis.
"So, Mr. Sheridan," said she, "it has cleared up."
"It has cleared up just a little, Madam," said Sheridan hastily, "enough for one, but hardly enough for two."

Sugar Daddy: A form of solidified sap.

THREE WORKERS in the country at large are killed in off-the-job accidents for every two that are fatally injured while on the job.—*Bul. Met. L. I. Co.*

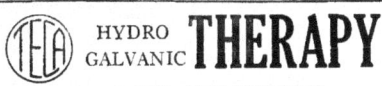

HYDRO GALVANIC **THERAPY**

FULL BATH TREATMENTS
in any available bath tub
TANK TREATMENTS
IONTOPHORESIS

— FOR HOSPITAL AND OFFICE USE —

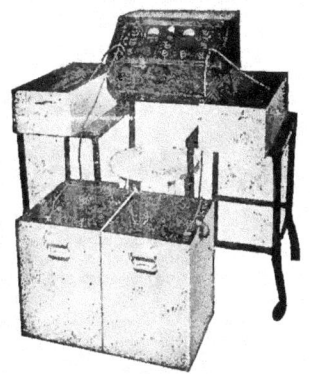

For full information and literature write to
TECA CORPORATION
220 WEST 42nd STREET   NEW YORK 18, N. Y.

FOR
FULLY EFFECTIVE THEORY
B COMPLEX
derived from
RICE BRAN CONCENTRATE

"BEFACLIN*" Rice Bran Concentrate is a natural source of all known B factors observed but not yet positively identified.

Deficiencies in the B vitamins usually occur together.

No single B vitamin, such as Thiamine, will control the deficiencies adequately.

High Thiamine content of so-called B complex preparations is not necessarily a true index of therapeutic value, since all the various B factors must be supplied in properly balanced amounts (1).

"BEFACLIN"—Tablets and Elixir supply the whole Vitamin B Complex.

(1) L. B. Pett, J. A. McKirdy and M. M. Cantor, Canadian Medical Journal, 46:413, 1942.

*"BEFACLIN" is a trademark of Tablerock Laboratories.

TABLEROCK LABORATORIES
GREENVILLE, SOUTH CAROLINA, U. S. A.

GENERAL

Nalle Clinic Building   412 North Church Street, Charlotte

THE NALLE CLINIC
Telephone—C-BVDN (*if no answer, call 3-2621*)

General Surgery   *General Medicine*

BRODIE C. NALLE, M.D.   LUCIUS G. GAGE, M.D.
GYNECOLOGY & OBSTETRICS   DIAGNOSIS

EDWARD R. HIPP, M.D.
TRAUMATIC SURGERY   LUTHER W. KELLY, M.D.
*PRESTON NOWLIN, M.D.   CARDIO-RESPIRATORY DISEASES
UROLOGY

                         J. R. ADAMS, M.D.
Consulting Staff   DISEASES OF INFANTS & CHILDREN

R. H. LAFFERTY, M.D.
O. D. BAXTER, M.D.   W. B. MAYER, M.D.
RADIOLOGY   DERMATOLOGY & SYPHILOLOGY

W. M. SUMMERVILLE, M.D.
PATHOLOGY   (*In Country's Service)

C—H—M MEDICAL OFFICES
DIAGNOSIS—SURGERY
X-RAY—RADIUM

DR. G. CARLYLE COOKE—*Abdominal Surgery & Gynecology*
DR. GEO. W. HOLMES—*Orthopedics*
DR. C. H. MCCANTS—*General Surgery*
222-226 Nissen Bldg.   Winston-Salem

WADE CLINIC
Wade Building
Hot Springs National Park, Arkansas

H. KING WADE, M.D.   *Urology*
ERNEST M. MCKENZIE, M.D.   *Medicine*
*FRANK M. ADAMS, M.D.   *Medicine*
*JACK ELLIS, M.D.   *Medicine*
BESSEY H. SHLBESTA, M.D.   *Medicine*
*WM. C. HAYS, M.D.   *Medicine*
N. B. BURCH, M.D.
      Eye, Ear, Nose and Throat
A. W. SCHEER   *X-ray Technician*
ETTA WADE   *Clinical Laboratory*
MERNA SPRING   *Clinical Pathology*
(*In Military Service)

INTERNAL MEDICINE

ARCHIE A. BARRON, M.D., F.A.C.P.

INTERNAL MEDICINE—NEUROLOGY

Professional Bldg.   Charlotte

JOHN DONNELLY, M.D.

DISEASES OF THE LUNGS

Medical Building   Charlotte

CLYDE M. GILMORE, A.B., M.D.

CARDIOLOGY—INTERNAL MEDICINE

Dixie Building   Greensboro

JAMES M. NORTHINGTON, M.D.

INTERNAL MEDICINE—GERIATRICS

Medical Building   Charlotte

THE JOURNAL OF
SOUTHERN MEDICINE AND SURGERY

306 NORTH TRYON STREET, CHARLOTTE, N. C.

The Journal assumes no responsibility for the authenticity of opinion or statements made by authors or in communications submitted to this Journal for publication.

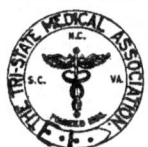

JAMES M. NORTHINGTON, M. D., Editor

| VOL. CVI | MARCH, 1944 | No. 3 |

President's Address*

George Ben Johnston
Pioneer of Modern Surgery in the South

FRANK S. JOHNS, M.D., Richmond

IN 1879 Dr. George Ben Johnston performed the first operation "under Listerism" in Virginia. He was twenty-five years old, and a newcomer to Richmond. Less than two years before, he had moved there from his native southwest Virginia, after a single notably successful year of country medical and surgical practice, in and around the town of Abingdon.

Listerism was a bold departure. Its pioneer technique was awkward, time-consuming, laughable—to some; although to the keen mind of his first Virginian partisan, Surgeon Lister had built soundly upon "the germ theory of putrefaction," laid down since 1857 by the French chemist, Louis Pasteur. Listerism in Virginia would shake the whole citadel of "Confederate medicine and surgery." Its fearless and devoted adoption by an enterprising upstart from the provinces would not endear him to his established colleagues. On meeting the new Dr. Johnston, these gentlemen had also to reckon with the most formidable personal charm, the most brilliant mind and magnetic spirit to enter their profession in many a day.

Richmond was not alone in its reluctance to follow the new star of Lister's troublesome antiseptic method. This was long before a modest man, late of Edinburgh, was named Lord Lister by his grateful Queen. 1879 was only a dozen years from the first, epochal report of a small series of compound fractures—13 cases in 18 months with only two deaths, and two cases of "hospital gangrene," both of which had recovered. It was then only nine years since Saxtorph, Professor of Surgery in the University of Copenhagen, gave his first "outside testimony" to Lister's antiseptic system. It was less than three years since Von Nussbaum in Munich, having transformed the appalling conditions of his State-hospital there by "the sternest and minutest Listerian regimen" had published his tribute to "Lister's Great Discovery"; this, the first statistical proof of the results of antisepsis, appeared in the *German Journal of Surgery* for October, 1876. Richmond, like Joseph Lister's own London, like many medical centers here and abroad, was largely unmoved—or frankly hostile to the "turning-point in all surgery." Recent political miseries of Reconstruction, and the ghastly glories of Confederate surgical defeats were of greater moment still—to many surgeons, if not to their patients.

But thanks to Dr. George Ben Johnston, Virginia ranks well in American surgical history. The year 1879, in which Dr. Johnston became our pioneer "dispenser of the benefits of antiseptic surgery" is also well known in medical annals as "the decisive year in the history of Listerism." It is the year "from which the final acceptance of the antiseptic system may be dated": the year of Lis-

---

*Presented to Tri-State Medical Association of the Carolinas and Virginia, meeting at Charlotte, Feb. 28th-29th, 1944.

ter's first great international triumph, his reception at Amsterdam "with an enthusiasm that knew no bounds" by the triennial International Congress of Medical Science." Working in another world, but with equal enthusiasm and inspired confidence, with a passion for truth and a genius for leadership, young George Ben Johnston had brilliantly placed his native State and region in the van of revolutionizing medical progress.

Dr. Johnston's early assumption of a great preeminence was no accident. His prompt grasp of the profound significance of Lister's work was characteristic of his own intellectual calibre. It evidenced in him the flowering of a long and noble heritage, from men and women of courage and able minds. He stood on the threshold of his great career endowed with many gifts, not the least of them the blood of illustrious forebears, quickening his own.

Back to the thirteenth century, to a Scottish town on the English border, goes the authentic record of "the brave and powerful Johnstone family." Back to Sir John de Johnstone, Marquis of Annandale and Lochwood Castle, whose resounding title, "Warden of the West Marches" was given him by the king of Scotland. Sir John's broadly defined duties were simply "to defend Scotland against the inroads of the English." For 400 years, from that doughty warrior, his Scottish line is studded with Johnstone soldiers, scholars and—always—patriots. Finally, in 1727, his descendant Peter Johnston, an able and interesting young man of the Annandale family, emigrated to Virginia. At home he had a friend named Walter Scott, whose namesake would some day write the Waverly Novels.

In Virginia, where he had settled first on the lower James River, the first Johnston grew rich and prominent in the merchandising trade. He married late and moved up-country to Prince Edward County. His home, near the town of Farmville, is known today as "Longwood"—or the Farmville Country Club. But Peter Johnston's great-grandson surmised in writing his family annals that the name was "a corruption for 'Lochwood,' " the ancestral 13th Century Castle left behind in the West Marches of Scotland. Besides a notable posterity, Peter Johnston's enduring monument is Hampden-Sydney College to whose founders he gave 100 acres of land on which to build it. He was progenitor of many distinguished Virginians, none worthier of their country's honor than the courageous great-great-grandson whose pioneer service to southern surgery I present to you today.

In the three intervening generations of Dr. Johnston's direct line in the Society of the Cincinnati stands first Peter Johnston, son of the immigrant. Born in 1765, he is the family hero of the American Revolution, the "blue-eyed, curly headed boy" of intrepid courage and patriotism, who slipped away from Hampden-Sydney—pursued in vain by parental and college authorities—to become a lieutenant in Lee's Legion at sixteen. His company ranks included the legendary Virginia giant, Peter Francisco. After the war Captain Johnston became a distinguished lawyer, orator, statesman. He was an ardent follower of Jefferson and Madison, the great "Republicans," as democrats of their day were called; and in 1788 he married Miss Mary Wood, a niece of Patrick Henry. As Speaker of the Virginia Legislature he helped notably to pass the famous Resolutions of 1789. In 1810 Peter Johnston was elected a judge of the General Court. But he exchanged circuits with his friend Judge Brockenbrough, who "preferred to stay east," and moved to Abingdon. Thus the Johnston family became identified with southwest Virginia.

Dr. John Warfield Johnston, born in 1790, only son of Judge Johnston and future grandfather of the great modern surgeon, was himself a young man of great abilities and promise, and also, it is said "of charming manners and temper." To study medicine, his father sent him to Philadelphia, then the greatest medical center in America. He returned to practice in Abingdon, where he married Miss Louisa Smith Bowen. But the diary of his son relates that "he died before he was 28 and yet, in that short period, he had acquired a reputation equal to that of a successful practitioner of fifty." He died for others, victim of "an epidemic disease then very fatal in the country," which he contracted while attending his stricken neighbors.

The second John Warfield Johnston, who became the father of George Ben Johnston, also grew up in Tazewell County, Virginia. At 8 he entered Abingdon Academy, where for six years he says, "I distinguished myself more as a bandy-player than any other way." At 15, he rode horseback 350 miles to enter South Carolina College at Columbia. Afterwards, he studied law at the University of Virginia and, on October 12th, 1841, he happily married Miss Nicketti Buchanan Floyd, daughter of the ex-Governor of Virginia. The young couple began life in Jeffersonville. From Commonwealth's Attorney "at the magnificent salary of $100 a year," Mr. Johnston rose rapidly to State Senator, and Bank President, to leading lawyer and foremost citizen of that region. After the War Between the States he was one of the first two representatives from Virginia to be re-admitted to the United States Senate. He was re-elected twice, and states quietly that "it has always been a source of great satisfaction to me, that in all three elections, I never lost one vote in my own section of the State—the great Southwest. I uniformly received every vote, west of Lynchburg."

Mrs. Nicketti Floyd Johnston had two older brothers of already distinguished names. They were George Rogers Clark and Benjamin Rush Floyd; and for them her third son and seventh child would be named "George Benjamin" at Jeffersonville, on July 25th, 1853. Mistress Nicketti's own odd Christian name bore no reference to the bold Indian blood claimed proudly by her father. But, as she could tell you, names were scarce when the youngest of twelve, and a seventh girl was born in Burke's Garden in 1819. One day a great friend of her father's came magnificently to their home. This Indian, of un-savage bearing, stopped near her cradle. "Nicketti, nicketti—" he said gently, which being interpreted means "pretty baby" . . . and thus a new Floyd-family name was coined.

Of the young lady herself, her husband's record states proudly that "her appearance was very striking. Her hair, then a very dark brown, curled naturally and was worn in ringlets . . . " A country girl, who could ride and shoot well and fearlessly, she knew and loved the beauties of her noble countryside. She was gay and sympathetic, charming and deeply spiritual. And she had a way of nursing the sick . . . "walking a mile out of town . . . to sit up all night—night after night—with a sick family." Later, during the war years, she "devoted several rooms to a hospital for sick soldiers." We see a small eager boy, who loved his mother, deeply impressed by the hospital in his own home, and by her ministry to and interest in the victims of disease and wounds.

Mrs. Johnston's flair for helping sick people was already inherited. Her father, Dr. John Floyd, twice Governor of Virginia, had begun his medical studies in Louisville in 1802 with a Dr. Ferguson of that city. Three years later he went to Philadelphia to complete his training under a greater teacher. Besides his vast practice and constant lecturing, Dr. Benjamin Rush of the University of Pennsylvania had found time to be a statesman. John Floyd's career would emulate that of his famous preceptor. During the war of 1812 he left his already large practice to serve as surgeon in the Army. Returning, he settled at Thorn Spring in Montgomery County, and from there "for his prominence and abilities" he was elected to Congress. He served continuously for 18 years. In 1828, the unhappy year of Nat Turner's dark fame, Dr. Floyd became Governor of Virginia. For his wise and able handling of that grievous business, he was returned to office. It is written of Dr. Johnston's grandfather that he "was a remarkable man in all respects . . . As a Doctor he had no superior, and as a public man was most conspicuous, during a period very fertile of great men."

But by far the most colorful career in our great surgeon's tremendous heritage was his maternal great-grandfather, the first John Floyd. He was second of his name in the New World, his father William Floyd having emigrated from Wales to the Eastern Shore of Virginia. John Floyd was born in 1751 in the "wild region" of Amherst, Virginia. From his Catawba Indian maternal grandmother this bold and virile pioneer inherited useful traits for the life of violence and adventure that lay ahead. He married first at 18, but his wife died in childbirth. The bereaved infant daughter was duly named "Mourning" Floyd. Briefly, thereafter, John Floyd became a school-teacher and writer in a surveyor's office. In 1775 he visited and surveyed a great tract of lands in Kentucky, whence he returned safely "after unparalleled suffering," and shortly afterwards won the promise of beautiful Miss Jane Buchanan. But a war intervened. As skipper of the Privateer *Phoenix*, returning with a rich prize from the West Indies, John Floyd was captured during the Revolution by a British warship. He was put in irons and imprisoned in London; but the jailor's daughter helped him escape. In Paris, where the refugee had barely survived an attack of smallpox, the American Minister, Dr. Benjamin Franklin, saw him safely off to the United States. With a scarlet wedding-coat, and silver shoe-buckles for his betrothed, he got back in time to marry her—the day before she, thinking him lost, would have wed his rival! In 1779, taking his family, Col. John Floyd led a group of Virginia pioneers to settle a vast principality in the little-known "dark and bloody land" of Kentucky. The place was named Floyd's Station, and the lands are now a part of the city of Louisville. In his own words he had "set foot upon the threshold of an empire." A giant in strength and courage, Col. Floyd survived many personal encounters with the Indians. But he lost his life, wearing his scarlet coat through the forest near Louisville, in 1783. His third son, John, the little Kentucky-born future governor of Virginia, began life 12 days after his father's death.

This survey of Dr. George Ben Johnston's direct lineal ancestry is vital to our study of the man himself, and his great contribution. We find the pattern of his brilliant personality set in noble fabric. His keenness of intellect, his extraordinary abilities, his integrity, courage and enterprise, besides his compassionate interest in human suffering, and a vital concern for the public good—all these fine qualities were his inheritance. They were "in his blood," like the dark curling hair that framed a splendid brow, like the powerful physique of the best wrestler at Abingdon Academy, where his father was the foremost "bandy-player" years before him.

As a boy Ben Johnston was "a fair student," not so good as his elder brother Willie. But Willie, who was drowned during their first college year together in Wheeling, West Virginia, was "confessedly the best scholar; and the best, the Professors said, they ever had." After two years at Bishop Whelan's School, Ben took the collegiate course at the University of Virginia. And for one year there his father "put him to the study of the law." But "he did not take kindly to it, and indicated a very strong inclination to Medicine." Seventy years later, Dr. Johnston's sister remembers that "he did try to study law to please his father, but he always wanted to be a doctor—and a good thing too!" Once in medicine, the young man hit his stride as a student. "At the end of the session," writes his father, "he was elected Final President of the society to which he belonged—the highest honor and greatest compliment the students can pay a fellow-student."

From the University of Virginia Ben Johnston went for his final year of medical study to the New York Medical College. He received his degree there in 1876. Interesting is the visit of Joseph Lister to Philadelphia and New York in that same year. Did his coming focus the fertile mind of his first Virginian follower on the great Englishman's enormous discovery? Was young Johnston present, that October day at the Charity Hospital in New York, to see and hear for himself an address entitled "The Antiseptic Treatment of Open Wounds?" If he was not there in person, certainly many of his classmates did attend that momentuous presentation, or the one in Philadelphia on "Antiseptic Surgery"; so we may be sure that the future Richmond surgeon was directly influenced by the founder of Listerism. And the great new word fell on good ground in the receptive mind of George Ben Johnston. In an amazingly short time it would bring forth its fruit there, a hundred fold.

If all surgeons may be judged by their "end-results," the earliest operative work of Dr. George Ben Johnston, without a fatality during his first year of practice, is an impressive record. We quote his father:

"He only remained in Abingdon a little over a year, but in that short time acquired a great reputation as a surgeon. The principal operations performed by him were: one in Russell County upon a man who had suffered for some years with an obstruction in the throat; this Ben removed and the man got well. The other was the amputation of both legs of a brakeman whose feet had been mashed in an accident and who also got well."

In 1877 Dr. Johnston's decision to move to Richmond was heartily endorsed by his parents, "as giving him a better and larger field for the talents they believed him to possess." They recognized the early evidence of his genius and fostered it. Already his father's advice had been the turning-point of a noble life. After graduating in medicine Ben Johnston received two attractive offers, one to settle in New York, one in Philadelphia. With filial affection and respect he consulted his father.

"Virginia needs her sons," said Senator Johnston. "You should come home to practice your profession."

Now, at the State Capital, the Virginia profession of medicine witnessed a strange and perhaps not too welcome phenomenon—the immediate, startling success of a new arrival, a full-fledged master surgeon, suddenly taking his place in their front ranks. He had not come gradually into surgical prominence from years of medical practice. Within a single year he had fearlessly and firmly established himself as a master in the art and practice of modern surgery.

In later years Dr. Johnston admitted that he had decided never to let himself be called the "young doctor." Youth, he knew, was no asset to a surgeon opening his practice in a strange competitive city. But a surer key to Dr. George Ben Johnston's instant and singular success was his masterly comprehension and meticulous application of the new phrase, "antiseptic surgery."

One spring evening in March, 1879, Dr. Johnston told his mother and sisters that he had a very serious operation to perform the next day, for the first time, and he wanted them to be praying for him. At 11 o'clock next morning, Mrs. Johnston and her daughters knelt devoutly with their rosaries; for them, the beads slipping through their reverent fingers were symbols of sterner instruments in the skillful hands they sought to bless.

Meanwhile, at some antique Richmond hospital, with strict new Listerian antisepsis, Dr. Johnston was successfully removing an ovarian tumor weighing forty-five pounds. His patient recovered without infection; and the news of that miracle, and of others that followed it, spread rapidly through the state and nation, as the marvelous skill of Dr. Ben Johnston made his name a household word in Richmond, in all Virginia, and far beyond her borders.

On October 12th, 1880, he married Miss Mary McClung, "a sweet and lovable young lady" of Tazewell. But in less than a year she was dead of typhoid fever. "After her death," writes his father, "he went home with me to Eggleston and spent some time"—poignant inference to shock and sorrow. But soon Dr. Johnston's fine heart had steadied and he turned back to his active and growing surgical practice in Richmond.

Twelve years later he married Miss Helen Rutherfoord of Rock Castle, Virginia. She was a charming girl, a beloved, delightful wife, and with her there now began for him a lifetime of family happiness, in a home of princely hospitality.

The years had passed, busy and work-filled. In 1885 he was elected Professor of Anatomy at the Medical College of Virginia. In 1888 he resigned at the end of the session "finding that the duties of his place interfered too much with his practice." But Dr. Johnston's earliest affiliations with the Medical College of Virginia were but straws in the wind of a life-long devotion to and ennobling influence upon medical education. It is interesting that in 1893 he was made Professor of Didactic and Clinical Surgery, but accepted the appointment only "on condition that a properly equipped teaching hospital under the control of the College be established." The first hospital, therefore, that owed its existence to Dr. George Ben Johnston was the Old Dominion Hospital, adjacent to the Egyptian Building of the Medical College in Richmond. It was the first modern teaching hospital to be established in Richmond.

Dr. Johnston's surgical work in the '90's commands our full respect today. I present to you one series: a report of three cases of cancer of the cervix complicated by pregnancy. All cases were beyond the fourth month: on two of them he did a pan-hysterectomy on recognition. The third case was allowed to go to term. A live baby was delivered by Caesarean section, and a complete hysterectomy was done. All three cases had complete operative recovery, and the follow-up showed them to be cures. With all our improved surgical procedures few of us today would underestimate the magnitude of this type of surgery.

Within one five-months period during the same decade, a report from the old Dominion Hospital shows that Dr. Johnston performed 71 abdominal operations there. They were: 18 appendectomies, 7 appendiceal abscesses, 2 nephrectomies, 1 nephrotomy, 4 operations for hernia (3 of them double), 8 salping-oöphorectomies, 1 hepatotomy for abscess, 12 hysterectomies, 1 exploration of tuberculous peritonitis. There were only two deaths in this series; one of them in a case of suppurating appendicitis, the other in tuberculous peritonitis.

A partial bibliography of Dr. Johnston's reported work during this period includes eighteen titles: Imperforation of the Anus; Comparative Frequency of Stone in the Bladder in the White and Negro Races; On Movable Kidney; Osteofibromyoma of the Uterus; Splitting the Capsule for the Relief of Nephralgia; Acquired Umbilical Hernia in Adults; Symptoms and Treatment of Hepatic Abscess—Report of 17 cases; Retroperitoneal Fibrolipoma; Some Abdominal Cases; Gastrostomy for Traumatic Stricture of the Esophagus—Report of Case; Progress of Renal Surgery; Report of Two Successful Nephrectomies; The Limitation of Conservative Surgery of the Female Generative Organs; Report of a Case of Uretero-ureteral Anastomosis ('02); A Case of Bilateral Diffuse Virginal Hypertrophy of the Breast (1903); A Case of Uterus Dydelphys (1904); Hermaphroidism ('07); Diverticulum of the Intestine with Report of Case. In discussions before the Southern Gynecological and Surgical Association alone he is recorded on appendicitis, aseptic surgical technique, cholelithiasis, rectovaginal fistula, splenectomy, fibroid tumors of the uterus ('07), ovarian cyst ('02), postoperative complications in abdominal surgery ('07), prolapse of the rectum in women (1900), surgery of the bladder ('07).

We may also remember that in this fertile period of a great career, general surgery included many operations now in the province of the consulting specialist. Besides his tremendous work in abdominal surgery and gynecology, Dr. Johnston was long his own orthopedist, his own neurological surgeon.

In all Dr. Johnston's forthright opinion recorded for us on the current surgical problems of his day, we note an interesting fact. It is a proof of his genius. Rarely, if ever, had he cause to reverse himself. He was consistently *right*, as in his pioneer work in asepsis, from his earliest words on the fundamentals of modern surgery. Many of his statements, daring and provocative when he made them, are axiomatic today: "The essential thing is the proper preparation of the patient preceding operation." "The minimal amount of the anesthetic agent and briefest possible time in administering it." "In regard to complications, the most important thing is prompt recognition of them . . . they must be quickly diagnosticated and energetically treated." "Among all practitioners, for any bowel trouble in very young children they try to clean out the bowels with a dose of oil. I look upon this as a pernicious practice . . . It is our duty to preach a crusade against purgation in acute abdominal conditions." "In my experience (with dilatation of the stomach) . . . after the first thorough lavage the slightest amount of vomiting is an indication for a second stomach-washing, and this should be continued as long as there is any vomiting." "The treatment should be governed not so much by ourselves as by the action and condition of the patient." "Surgical daring is a matter of the *when* and not the *what*."

These are the pronouncements of a wise philosopher, and thoughtful man, who was also a master clinician.

In a discussion of a paper on "Aseptic Surgical Technique" in 1895, Dr. Johnston said, "I am convinced along with Dr. McMurtrie that the greatest source of danger to the patient is through the surgeon and his assistants." In his own paper on "Movable Kidney" that year he concludes, "Nephrorraphy is not indicated in every case of dislocated kidney, but only in such cases as manifest distressing symptoms."

Notably discerning is Dr. Johnston's discussion, also in 1895, of appendicitis in the Negro. He observes that when the Negro is eating in his master's kitchen, appendicitis is common. When he is living in the rough he has no digestive disturbances and appendicitis is infrequent. And, with more seriousness, "Negroes are mostly in the hands of less capable practitioners of their own race; therefore, they do not get as good medical attention as whites, and many cases of appendicitis in the Negro are overlooked."

In 1896, at the ninth annual meeting of the Southern Surgical Society and the year he was elected president of that body, Dr. Johnston discussed appendicitis. He said, "Every case of acute appendicitis should be operated on as soon as the diagnosis is made, during the first 48 hours. After 48 hours, one should be governed by the severity of the disease and the general condition of the patient. If an abscess has developed, drain the abscess but make no effort to remove the appendix, unless it is in the operative field." We should do well to follow this advice today.

"A physician," he adds, "in my opinion has but one duty in the matter of dealing with appendicitis, and that is to call in a surgeon of experience and not undertake to treat cases medically."

As tenth President of the Southern Surgical Society in 1897, Dr. Johnston selected for his presidential topic "The Prevalence of Specialism and Who Shall be Specialists." In a brilliant analysis, he divides the specialists of his day into two classes, the true and the pseudo specialist. The true specialist is a man especially distinguished for his learning and skill in a given pursuit. The false is one having merely a special occupation. Dr. Johnston firmly believed that a specialist should be a doctor of real learning, a man of broad medical education, in order to be able to discuss medicine and surgery intelligently when called in consultation. Above all he must have proved himself efficient in the practice of medicine. The author had in mind the giants of his profession in that day; men who were "broad, learned and wise, owning a mine of experience which fitted them for the high calling of 'specialist.'" "To fix the standard and lay the proper requirement for specialism, the colleges and societies must act," added Dr. Johnston. ". . . that the public may know the specialist is sanctioned by a proper body qualified to judge his fitness to execute the work he seeks." Fifty years later, there is evidence that Dr. Johnston's timely discussion of specialism had a great and beneficent influence on the course of our profession.

At the turn of the century, Dr. Johnston's fame was nationwide. At fifty-one he was elected President of the American Surgical Society, and he already seems to have received every honor in the gift of his profession in the United States. His local, State and Tri-State medical societies, the Southern Surgical Association, the American Surgical all conferred on him their highest offices. As invited guest he appeared on distinguished programs of surgical societies as far apart as Boston and the Mississippi Valley. He was the beloved and honored friend and peer of the leading men of his day, and ever welcomed into the hierarchy of the great in surgery.

Even so, Dr. Johnston's chief influence on the medical profession stemmed from his constant interest in and loyalty to the welfare of his home city and its medical institutions. In 1903, the year of his election to the International Surgical Society, he secured from his friend, Mr. John L. Williams, of Richmond, a memorial gift of $200,-000 to build and equip an adequate teaching hospital for charitable purposes, in connection with the Medical College of Virginia. For many years, the Memorial Hospital was the finest in the South, a model of all that was newest and best in modern clinical facilities. Dr. Johnston was also a founder of Richmond's excellent hospital for Negroes, St. Phillip's.

Dr. Johnston's long and self-sacrificing service to the Medical College of Virginia is important to every alumnus of our institution. From his early refusal to accept a chair in surgery there unless better clinical facilities were provided, he always insisted upon the highest possible standards both in the teaching services and equipment for the Medical College. He obtained an annual appropriation from the State Legislature, and ever afterwards successfully defended that appropriation against all comers. Certainly he was no orator; his voice was rather too high-pitched, and lacking in resonance, but when Dr. Johnston rose to speak before any assembly, scientific or otherwise, his arguments were more than convincing; they were unanswerable. His words carried authority as the eloquence of few men could do. When he differed from an opponent in a discussion, he spoke with a gracious formality, an urbane courtesy that only enhanced the cutting irony and convincing logic of his argument. So the records prove that whoever braved the self-less force of Dr. George Ben Johnston's tremendous energies in behalf of medical education in Virginia, they always did so at their peril.

In 1903, as chairman of the Legislative Committee of the Medical Society of Virginia, he sponsored the first Virginia statute that really governed medical practice—a law so far-seeing and effective against charlatanism that it has required few amendments during the past forty years.

But, with his keen wit and ready interest in public affairs, his championship of truth and fair play, medical politics was not the only realm that felt Dr. Johnston's fine, energizing hand. In a long-dead but ardently waged struggle between two distinguished Virginia politicians, the issue is said to have been decided in favor of the incumbent by *A Fable*, written, printed and circulated in behalf of Senator Martin by a well-known Richmond surgeon! I commend to you "The Fable of the Martin and the Woodpecker" as a masterly bit of strategic satire, and a fine example of its author's unerring wit and wisdom.

Today in Richmond, more than one distinguished elderly physician or surgeon began his success with Dr. George Ben Johnston. His interest in young men was beautiful. He delighted in training them; and the beginning of that training was never easy. It did not take the Chief Surgeon long to decide an interne's fate.He knew rather promptly whether you were just "run of mine," or an interne with potentialities for advanced training. He felt that every young surgeon should have a foundation in medicine. Once having selected them, he believed so firmly in his young men that he soon put real responsibility on them and backed them to the limit in that responsibility. It was hard to fail him. But woe be unto him who did not measure up to that trust!

As a clinical teacher, Dr. Johnston had an uncanny ability to bring out the essentials and to place little emphasis on the negative findings. He went into the greatest detail in discussing his cases before, during and after operation. Certainly he was a great surgeon, a smooth operator, a dissector with few equals. And always, for any operation, there was the greatest dignity in his operating room. If there was a discussion, he led the discussion and he closed it. He was never in a hurry during an operation. Nor was he time-consuming, and he always operated with little lost motion. He wanted his assistants to anticipate every move; otherwise he felt them to be liabilities.

His most promising follower, the "assistant" whose name is linked in surgical history with Dr. Johnston's was my distinguished preceptor, the late Dr. A. Murat Willis. The partnership between these two brilliant and gifted men was happy and productive. Together, with a great clientele, they did much original work, including the well-known operation which they devised and perfected jointly, the Johnston-Willis suspension of the uterus. Together in 1909 they founded the Johnston-Willis Hospital in Richmond. Three other excellent Southern hospitals today owe their existence to the far-flung vision and enterprise of Dr. Johnston and his able partner, Dr. Murat Willis. These institutions are the George Ben Johnston Memorial Hospital in Abingdon, Virginia, the Park View Hospital in Rocky Mount, North Carolina, and the Nassawadox Memorial Hospital on the Eastern Shore of Virginia.

Dr. Johnston's presidential address before the American Surgical Association was entitled "A Sketch of Dr. John Peter Mettauer of Virginia."

It was entirely typical of his passion for truth and justice, that Dr. Johnston should determine to bring before the leading surgeons of America the accomplishment of this great Southern pioneer in surgery, the man who—perhaps because he was a Southerner—had been sadly neglected or forgotten by his surgical beneficiaries. Dr. Mettauer of Prince Edward County was also a neighbor of Dr. Johnston's family some three generations back, so this writing satisfied another leading trait of the essayist: his devoted loyalty to places and people.

In his own words, Dr. Johnston presents Mettauer "in the black and white of simple truth . . . as one of the builders of that foundation which has made the present superstructure of medicine a possibility." He points to Mettauer's great surgical skill "marvelous for his day and well-nigh marvelous for any day"—and, lapsing for a moment into poetic metaphor, he recalls how that great man's reputation "growing as his fame, was spread in widening circles on the sea of human misery." But the crux of this "biography" re-established the fact that in 1838 Dr. Mettauer was the first American surgeon to cure vesico-vaginal fistula with lead-wire sutures, thus antedating Dr. Marion Sims' accepted claim to priority by many years. In 1833, Dr. Mettauer had already accomplished the repair of recto-vaginal fistula using lead-wire. Dr. Johnston also stated that Dr. Mettauer's operation for cleft-palate was the first in the western world. And I am sure Dr. Johnston would heartily applaud Dr. M. Pierce Rucker, who has lately published an original excellent work on Mettauer. Dr. Rucker concludes strongly that Sims must have been familiar with Mettauer's report in the *Boston Medical & Surgical Journal* of 1840; but Sims failed to acknowledge that priority. Twelve years later, Rucker states, Sims ignored Mettauer's published work, dismissing the success of the first American user of the silver catheter and metal suture, to claim that signal historic honor for his own.

No man ever had more staunch friends than Dr. Johnston. In every walk of life, from his honored colleagues to his white cobbler and his negro office girl, all his people loved him with a worshipful attachment. He returned their affection. Particularly, his patients loved and admired him.

From certain doctors today we often hear the remark, "I see patients only at certain hours, only at my office." This was not Dr. Johnston's method of ministering to the sick. I have heard him say, and I know it to be true, that he never turned down a call, from rich or poor, from white or black. He always said that when he got to the point of not looking after his charity practice, he would retire. With such a spirit and such an example before us, there was no place or need for "State Medicine" in that day.

No surgeon ever lived closer to the Golden Rule than Dr. Johnston.

But with all his lovable and winning qualities, he was a man of strong convictions, and utterly fearless in expresing them. I think his pioneer spirit enjoyed opposition; for he did not believe in straddling fences; he was not to be found on both sides of any question. If ever his misguided opponents presented an argument not based on clear facts and simple truth, they were hardpressed from the beginning! In all issues it soon appeared where Dr. Johnston stood. And there he stood foursquare. Particularly if "the question" concerned his friend—if he felt his friend's cause was just, he seemed to revel in the contest. He was willing to go all the way for his friends. On the other hand, it was hard for a man to be "all things to all people" and still keep Dr. Johnston's respect and friendship. Against the rock of that clear-eyed, affirmative integrity, such a man would surely fall.

Notable tributes to Dr. George Ben Johnston are already on record: to the magnitude of his life and work, and the singular charm of his rare personality. Dr. Beverley R. Tucker and more recently Dr. J. Morrison Hutcheson have done him honor. There is also a just eulogy by his friend, the late W. Gordon McCabe of Richmond. To all these, I would add my personal tribute.

I remember well Dr. Johnston's striking appearance, for he was the handsomest man we knew. His hair and mustache had grown white, but his fine high-colored face was never old. He had a lofty forehead, keen brown eyes and noble features; with a smile that won and held his friends. I remember his impressive, though modest bearing; his great physical strength, and the beauty and power of his hands. I remember the warmth of his most casual greeting, and his immediate, unfeigned interest in every human being. I remember also the example of his faith and piety, his devotion to the Church, and his courageous Christian fortitude to the last.

As his interne and resident I was privileged to spend much time with Dr. Johnston. And on two occasions, during the last years of his life, I became his traveling companion. Always such a journey was like a royal pilgrimage. Wherever he stopped, at the Mayo Clinic, in New York, Chicago, or Philadelphia, or as guest of Mr. Wilson in the White House, Dr. Johnston was the center of attraction in every gathering. He had something men liked. They delighted in him for it, although it was a quality that evades a name. They felt only the power of an amazing yet understanding mind, of a heart's natural warmth, a geniality and courtly graciousness rarely met. Equally impressive and characteristic of him to me was his courteous consideration of his young companion. Wherever he went, however grand the function, he took me with him, with a tact and generosity impossible to describe or to forget.

When Dr. Johnston died, at 63, on December 20th, 1916, he left no son to carry on his name. But his four beloved and loving daughters could always more than compensate him for such an omission of fate. Today his immortality goes on. There are 12 living grandchildren, of whom seven are boys. In 1941, a brave and wonderfully handsome young man named George Ben Johnston Handy left his medical course at the University of Virginia to volunteer in the United States Army. He was killed on Bataan Peninsula in January, 1942, the first graduate of V. M. I. to fall in this war, and a grandson of Dr. Johnston worthy of his illustrious name.

Dr. Johnston's own closing tribute to Mettauer is strangely applicable to the man we honor: "great he was . . . untiring, bold, resourceful, zealous, a prodigy in his own age and a prophet of the time to come . . . a character so unique, picturesque and masterful, that if this presentation fail to interest you—*mihi defectus*—the fault is mine and not my subject's."

REFERENCES
Lord Lister, His Life and Work, by G. T. Wrench.
The Life of Pasteur, by Valery-Radot.
The Johnston-Floyd-Preston-Bowen Families, Mss. by John Warfield Johnston.
Southern Surgical Transactions, Vols. 16, 17, 8, 22, 9, 13, 19, 20, 6, 14, 12, 4, 7, 10 and 15.
A Sketch of Dr. John Peter Mettauer of Virginia, by George Ben Johnston, M.D.
Some Medical Men of Mark From Virginia, by George Ben Johnston, M.D.
Dr. John Peter Mettauer, an Early Southern Gynecologist, by Pierce Rucker, M.D.
George Ben Johnston, M.D., LL.D., by J. Morrison Hutcheson, M.D.

(*To page 86*)

The Politico-Ecnomic Situation in Reference to Medicine*

H. F. STARR, M.D., Greensboro

EVEN WHILE ENGAGED in a world war, planned and being carried on to glorify everything low and hateful and destroy everything decent in life, it behooves us all to be watchful of our domestic concerns, lest we find that, having preserved our institutions against foreign assault we have lost them from sabotage from within. The threat is of disaster to every one of us, first as a citizen, second as a physician.

THREAT TO AMERICAN WAY OF LIFE

Post-war planning should not be allowed to distract our attention from during-the-war planning, so much of which is designed to destroy what we have all regarded as the essentials of our civilization. The plan has been unfolding step by step for the past 10 years. We must not allow the international scene to blind us to what is going on here. It is now Medicine's turn to be made over to fit into the general plan.

Americans freely exercise the right of criticism, but seldom have they felt called upon to question fundamental motives of their Government. But when men of high intelligence and patriotism such as Senators Byrd of Virginia, Bailey of North Carolina, Smith of South Carolina, O'Mahoney of Wyoming, and Congressman Summers, Speaker in the House of Representatives, and now Senator Barkley, the Democratic majority leader, have laid before the American people the bare facts showing that constitutional democratic government is fast vanishing, it is time for the private citizen to think and act.

Those who are changing the government and our way of life say in substance that "We get the majority of votes, we have a mandate from the people, and majority rule is democracy." Is it? In the last election in Germany over 90 per cent voted for Hitler. In Italy 80 per cent were behind Mussolini. A majority of votes for a leader does not necessarily make his administration democratic. The test is, what is the relation of the government to the people and how does that government deal with unorganized citizens and minorities?

Mr. Malcolm McDermott, of the faculty of Duke University Law School, after spending the years 1936-1937 in Germany studying National Socialism, told the 1943 meeting of the N. C. State Bar Association that "we are having foisted upon us National Socialism, that is, none other than the German system of government." No one who has read *Mein Kampf*, that self-written case history of the madman Hitler, can help but be struck by the parallelism of what took place in Germany and what has been taking place here. Hitler in his book set down in detail for the world to read what he proposed to do and exactly how he proposed to do it. The following observations were made by Mr. McDermott. Full details are laid down by Hitler in his book:

To gain control and establish National Socialism certain procedures must be followed. They are the same for Fascism, for the two differ in name only:

1. The people must be made to feel helpless and unable to solve their own problems. Then there is held up before them a benign and all-wise leader to whom they must look for relief from all their misfortunes. This state of mind is most readily developed in a time of economic stress or national disaster.

2. Local self-government must be destroyed, so that all political power will be readily at hand.

3. The central government will appear to represent the people but will really register the will of the leader or group in control.

4. Constitutional guarantees and precedents must be swept aside. They can be made to appear ridiculous, out-moded, and as obstructions to progress. The end justifies the means.

5. Public faith in leaders who will not conform and respect for the courts must be undermined if they disagree.

6. The law-making body must be intimidated and rebuked on occasion so as to prevent the development of public confidence therein.

7. The people must be highly taxed. Thus they are brought to a common level. In this manner economic independence is kept to a minimum, and the citizen must rely more and more upon the government that controls him. Capital and credit are thus completely within the control of the government.

8. Large public debt must be built up. This makes government the virtual receiver for the entire nation.

9. Distrust of private business and industry must be kept alive, so that the people may not begin to rely upon their own resources instead of upon the government.

*Presented to Tri-State Medical Association of the Carolinas and Virginia, meeting at Charlotte, Feb. 28th-29th, 1944.

10. Governmental bureaus are set up to control practically every phase of the citizen's life. These bureaus issue directives under authority of the leader to whom they are responsible. It is a government of men and not of laws.

11. The education of the youth must be under control, to the end that all may at an early age be inoculated with a spirit of loyalty to the system and of reverence for the leader.

12. In support of the foregoing there is kept flowing a steady stream of governmental propaganda extolling all that bow the knee, and villifying those who dare to dissent. Propaganda of course is not to be handicapped by restrictions of truth and fact. But Hitler sounded the warning that when you find it expedient to tell the people a lie, tell a big one and continue to repeat it over and over, and never resort to petty lies, for the people are in the habit of indulging in them and will recognize them as such immediately.

They are the features that made the Nazi machine work. Many sensible Germans were drawn into its clutches not realizing what they were getting into until it was too late to extricate themselves. One German said of Hitler's accomplishments "He has brought us all to a common level," and then in a whisper he added "But, my God, what a low level."

The leveling process makes the less fortunate think they are getting something; it keeps efficient, thrifty and self-willed people from rising and possibly getting out of hand. And at the same time it enables the treasury to support the system.

Recent Changes in America

Mr. McDermott then points out the parallel between all this and what has taken place in our own country during the past ten years. You will recall the fight to make the Supreme Court of the United States subservient to the Chief Executive. At the outset of this decade the country was in the depths of an economic depression, but it had pulled through such depressions before. But this time the people were convinced that they must look to Washington for salvation. It was handed down from above, a fact which the people were never allowed to forget. A grateful populace soon formed the habit of turning over all local problems for solution to Washington. More and more the central government insists upon doing for the people what they should do for themselves, and the right of local self-government is being destroyed. The legislative branch of the Government as well as the judiciary fell into line under the executive. Broad powers were granted and huge sums appropriated for an existing "emergency" which never ceased. It was only for a year ago that Congress even made a show of asserting its constitutional functions. The Constitution was regarded with disdain.

Congress was told to pass the Guy Coal Act regardless of its unconstitutionality. The principles upon which the Constitution was based as well as the "nine old gentlemen" of the Supreme Court were held up to ridicule.

The public debt was pushed far beyond what had been considered a safe limit long before the war was upon us. The new ten-billion-dollar tax bill recently submitted by the Treasury Department was designed not to equitably distribute the tax load but, as it was avowed, to bring incomes generally to about $2,500 per year. The bill has just been defeated, but that is a sample of what the rulers have in mind. Industry is to be taxed to the limit, and with no money left for expansion, is expected to employ the eight million discharged from the services at the close of the war. If private industry cannot do it, the Government is to furnish the jobs, private industry derided as out-moded and taxed out of existence to pay for jobs much more political than economic.

The Administration is now supporting a bill providing 300 million a year to the States for public education. With a public debt soon to reach 300 billion, the interest 9 billion annually—which is more than ever collected in federal taxes in any year prior to this war—the nation engaged in a world war, with a creditable school system in every State, imagine proposing to add on another 300 million annually to the cost of education.

I ask you, what do you make of it? In the early days of such carryings-on, when crops were being destroyed, little pigs killed, and farmers paid not to produce, all a part of the program based on the theory that scarcity made plenty, Senator Carter Glass predicted that history would record the times as a period of insanity in government. Many now see it as worse than temporary insanity, a deliberate plant to make America over into a totalitarian State.

With the record before us, is there any wonder that a bill is pending sponsored by administration leaders, calculated to bring the practice of medicine under control of the bureaucrats in Washington. It is just another detail of the general scheme.

Mr. Geo. E. Haws, President of the Virginia Bar Association, in 1942-3 in a guest editorial for the *Virginia Medical Monthly* said of the Wagner-Murry Bill: "This Bill under the cloak of an amendment to the present Social Security law, contains a proposal, which if enacted into law will strike at the very root of those liberties vouchsafed to us under our Bill of Rights, in that it will place practically the entire profession, as well as the hospitals, research laboratories and medical colleges, under governmental control, and regulate the medical service and treatment of the larger part of our population."

The people are to be taxed 12 billion dollars annually for Social Security and medical care. As Mr. Haw states, "three billion will be placed under the control of the Surgeon General of the Public Health Service, a political appointee, who will, through regimentation of the medical profession, of the hospitals, research laboratories and medical educational institutions administer medical service and treatment as well as hospitalization to an estimated 110 million people."

"The menace of this bill to our free institutions is apparent when we visualize the tremendous power which will be placed in the hands of this one man, who has three billion dollars to administer, and who will hold in his hands not only our doctors and hospitals, but the education of our future physicians, as well as the life, death and health of over a hundred million persons.

"The power is too great to be wielded by one political appointee or by any one man or group of men.

"To the unthinking its menace is not apparent, but those who give thought will discern within its supposedly benevolent frame-work, the spectre of absolutism in government reaching out to snatch from us those liberties for which our fathers died."

EFFECT OF ECONOMIC POLICIES ON LIFE INSURANCE

Your program chairman suggested that you will be interested in a discussion as to the effect which present economic trends may have upon life insurance policies, because savings of physicians go largely into life insurance and life insurance makes up the greater part of the estates of physicians.

Low interest rates, threat of inflation and taxation are problems to be met by most businesses, including life insurance.

Earnings of life insurance companies are from two chief sources, excess interest earnings and savings in mortality. The Government has been forced to borrow huge sums. Other sources of investment having been dried up, and the Government being the chief borrower from the banks and insurance companies, it has been able to drive the interest rate down. This tends to eliminate one of the sources of earnings. The other source of earnings, mortality savings, has stood up well, for the mortality has remained favorable in spite of the war.

The huge government debt, full wartime employment and scarcity of goods leads certainly to some degree of price inflation, that is, depreciation in the true value—the buying power—of the dollar.

Life insurance companies are very fortunate as regards inflation, in that the policies call for payment in a specified number of dollars and the premiums are for a specified number of dollars. Life insurance companies have invested heavily in Government bonds and those who have taken care to stagger the dates of maturity of the bonds are in an excellent position, for even if Government bonds should sell for only 50 cents on the dollar, something difficult to imagine, the insurance company could collect 100 cents on the dollar by simply holding the bonds to maturity.

As far as meeting its policy obligations is concerned it is immaterial to the company whether a dollar will purchase a dollar's worth of goods or ten cents worth, except that under the latter condition the cost of doing business would be greatly increased. Money value is not expected to fall rapidly enough to impair the solvency of a sound company on that account. If, as some fear, the present economic practices will go so far as to render life insurance policies worthless, it will be because the dollars paid by the companies when the policies mature will be worthless and not because of failure of the companies to pay. In that case there would be financial chaos and money in the bank, sock or anywhere else would also be worthless.

American companies have ample reserves to meet any foreseen contingency and the owner of a policy need have no anxiety as to whether it will be paid. The present trend if continued will have the effect of reducing dividends on participating policies, thereby increasing the net cost of insurance.

The effect of taxation of life insurance depends entirely upon what taxes might be levied in the future. Life insurance expects to pay a reasonable tax, but it should be kept in mind that any tax on life insurance is a tax on thrift, and it is the policyholders' savings and foresight that are being taxed.

This is one example of how physicians, as citizens, have a stake in the preservation of American institutions and must be vitally concerned in what is happening aside from the proposed changes in the American system of medical care.

TIME TO ACT

Organized medicine opposes regimentation of physicians. But that is not enough, it is the duty of every doctor as an individual citizen to examine the facts, make up his mind as to whether he wants to preserve the way of life and system of practice of medicine that has been found best by test, or adopt some foreign or radically different system. Then he should speak out. The time is late, it is later than you think. You and I and other responsible citizens should have used our influence to call a halt long before the care of the sick bid fair to become a political football.

Discussion

DR. JAS. M. NORTHINGTON, Charlotte:

Dr. Starr has presented a subject of the utmost importance to us all. As citizens we are concerned along with all other members of the body politic with the departures from the fundamentals of our government. As doctors we are concerned for very existence.

Dr. Starr draws a striking parallel between the early stages of Hitler's taking over Germany and what has gone on so far in our country.

When the present Administration in Washington went into power the economic crisis was so acute that all of us realized that drastic measure should be adopted. So we applauded drastic measures. There was general approval when 40 hours was legally made a week's work. Although we knew it was not a week's work, it seemed the best way of spreading the work available so as to reduce the number of idle. It was a lesser evil than having an enormous number idle all the time and supported by taxation.

But our acceptance did not mean that we approved of the 40-hour week, with time-and-a-half for any number of hours on the job beyond the 40 hours, after the coming of the time when an excess of work was available—even necessary to be done to supply our soldiers in the field and sailors on the sea, and our people at home, lest we be defeated and enslaved.

Everybody knows that two whole days of loafing each week would be bad for those who have, because of better education, far more capacity for spending leisure profitably and productively. What would we members of this association do with the time left over, if we were occupied with professional duties for only 40 hours each week? That the idle brain is the devil's workshop has been well known for centuries, and recent events amply attest its verity.

Labor unionists tell us they have sons at the front, too. So they do, and the most damnable evidence against the labor unionists is that they are not only willing to risk the loss of the war, with certain enslavement, but they had rather leave their own sons to be killed for lack of weapons and ammunition, than to pass up the opportunity to extort higher and higher pay in our time of direst need.

And these are the pets of the Administration.

For a long time I have wondered what justification there is for the Government charging an extra fee to insure that in case it loses or destroys a parcels post package, the sender may be paid for it. Every other agency engaged in hauling for profit pays for articles lost or destroyed without such an additional fee. I inquired for the figures, and the P. O. Department gave them to me. In round numbers, here they are in dollars:

Parcels post insurance paid, 6 million; payment to insurers, ½ million.

And I got the further information that it cost the Government (that is, us all) 8 million to operate this insurance feature of the parcels post.

It seems never to have occurred to anybody that 7½ million dollars could be saved to the people by the simple expedient of doing away with this insured parcels post feature and paying for articles lost or destroyed just as every other agency in the hauling business does.

That's a sample of the way business is conducted by the group that is daily taking over more and more of the business of the country, and is undertaking to take over bodily one of the professions, our own.

All the years I have been in Medicine I have talked, written and worked that doctors exert themselves in politics. But we have been too sanctimonious and pecksniffian to "dabble in the dirt of politics."

Dr. Starr says it is time to act. Let us hope it is not past time to act. Anyhow it would be manlier to go down fighting than to sit quiet while the manacles are being fitted on us.

HISTORY OF NEEDLES AND SYRINGES
(Oscar Schwidetzky, Rutherford, N. J., in *Anes. & Analg.*, Jan.-Feb.)

In 1856 Lafargue, of France, invented a needle trocar for depositing morphine in paste form. Up to that time the drugs were rubbed into a previously made incision. In 1939 Taylor and Washington, of New York, used for the first time a solution of morphine in the Anel syringe. This syringe is the real progenitor of the present hypodermic instrumentarium. A small syringe, silver with a leather piston and a fine elongated tapering nozzle that was originally intended for the lachrymal duct. A small incision had to be made for the insertion of the nozzle. Alexander Wood, of Edinburgh, described the Ferguson syringe in 1843, and in 1859 Charles Hunter, of London, made a cutting point on the small nozzle. In 1853 Pravaz, of Lyons, France, first employed a separate needle with the slip joint.

In 1856 Fordyce Barker, of New York, while in Edinburgh, was presented with a Ferguson syringe. From this model Geo. Tiemann & Co. produced the first hypodermic syringes made in the United States.

In 1888 Koch introduced in his work on tuberculosis a syringe of the bulb type having a stopcock between the bulb and barrel. The first all-metal syringe with "ground-in" piston was apparently the Detmers-Robinson made in Boston in 1894. In 1906 Dewitt and Herz, of Berlin, invented the Record syringe, which consisted of a metal plunger and glass barrel ground to a snug fit.

The most radical change in syringes came with the all-glass syringe, invented and made about 1896 by Karl Schneider, instrument maker for Luer, of Paris.

All the early needle makers used carbon steel which will rust and break. Research resulted in the adaptation of platinum-iridium, gold, and nickeloid stainless steel and rustless steel needles.

About 1911 Dr. James T. Greeley, of Nashua, N. H., invented the Greeley unit. This was improved and is now used by our armed forces under the name "Syrette." In 1918 Dr. R. H. Riethmueller, of Philadelphia, invented the Security needle, with security bead fastened to the needle. In 1932 Dr. Herbert Busher, of St. Paul, invented the Busher automatic injector for the automatic insertion of the needle at the proper depth and angle. The injector was designed for insulin users and other patients who use prescribed self-medication. It makes injection practically painless.

JOHNSTON
(From Page 82)

Biographical Sketch of John Peter Mettauer, by Wyndham B. Blanton, M.D.

George Ben Johnston, M.D., of Richmond, by W. Gordon McCabe.

Clipping from an Abingdon paper of March, 1879.

Reply by George Ben Johnston, M.D., and Christopher Tompkins, M.D. Committee of the Faculty of the Medical College of Virginia to a Protest Against the Use of State Funds for Professional Education.

Reprints of the following papers by Dr. Johnston:
Value to the Public of State Medical Societies.
Acquired Umbilical Hernia in Adults.
Symptoms and Treatment of Hepatic Abscess.
Some Abdominal Cases.
Gastrostomy for Traumatic Stricture of the Esophagus.
Progress of Renal Surgery—Report of Two Successful Nephrectomies.
The Limitations of Conservative Surgery of the Female Generative Organs.
Treatment of Cancer of the Cervix of the Uterus Complicated by Pregnancy.
Splenectomy: Report of 6 Cases with a Statistical Summary of all the Reported Operations up to 1908.
Diverticulum of the Intestine, with Report of a Case.

DEPARTMENTS

HUMAN BEHAVIOUR

JAMES K. HALL, M.D., *Editor*, Richmond, Va.

RUM AND WAR

THE MORNING NEWSPAPER of Richmond that carried a first-page account of the temporary cessation of activity in the manufactory that turns out daily one hundred and fifty thousand pounds of cardboard and coarse paper, displayed also advertisements of several brands of alcoholic beverages. Why are these two statements associated? The plant's products spoken of are fabricated out of waste paper. The incoming supply of waste paper had fallen to such a low level that the machinery was brought to a stop.

Why should paper and ink and labour and all those other consituents of an advertisement, and its distribution through countless hands to the American people, be utilized in these troubled, tragic days in efforts to induce people to drink alcohol? I should like to hear the response to the interrogatory in a court of inquiry.

The local press carries a story almost each day of some human tragedy that came in consequence of indulgence in alcohol. Not many months ago a soldier of the United States, far from his home, was killed by the commonwealth in the electric chair in the State Penitentiary in Richmond for the commission of a capital crime. He said that he was drunk and knew nothing about the crime. Associated with him in the alcoholic debauch were two women, now spending their days and nights in the Penitentiary. Is there doubt that the whiskey was legally procured from a store in Richmond operated jointly by the United States, by the Commonwealth of Virginia and by the City of Richmond?

The *Atlantic Monthly* for March flaunts on its cover the advertisement of a bottle of whiskey; and it intersperses such advertisements throughout the text of the magazine. That dignified and historic publication, coming into my home for many a year, is now lowered immeasurably in my esteem. So are all other publications that waste paper in efforts to increase the use of beverage alcohol. The paper, the ink, the labour, of myriad people, and the alcohol, too, are badly needed for helpful purposes in the great war.

Publications carry advertisements of alcoholic beverages for the same reason that religious publications formerly carried commendations of magic electric belts—to make money. There is no authority, scriptural or otherwise, that money is the root of any evil. Sin results, we are Biblically informed, only if the love of the medium becomes inordinate, obsessing, dominating; causing one to be willing, for example, to bring about the intoxication of one's fellow-mortal for a consideration.

During or after every great war in our national history our federal government has been scandalized by alcohol. Almost immediately after the national government was organized there was a whiskey rebellion in Pennsylvania. Grant's administration would have been stigmatized by the whiskey ring, if it had been possible for that administration to be scandalized. If the biography of present-day alcohol could be written with the candor with which old Samuel Pepys talked about his own rascality, prohibition would probably be reinstituted by Presidential decree—not to save the Nation, but the status quo.

SURGERY

GEO. H. BUNCH, M.D., *Editor*, Columbia, S. C.

PERITONEAL TRANSPLANTS AFTER TRAUMATIC RUPTURE OF THE NON-MALIGNANT SPLEEN

A TOTAL OF THIRTEEN CASES of splenic transplants found incidentally in the abdomen at laparotomy, done years after the operative removal of the spleen for traumatic rupture, have appeared in the literature. At first surgeons were loth to accept this explanation of the presence over the peritoneum of multiple, dark-red parenchymatous masses grossly and microscopically identical with splenic tissue. At first these node-like masses were thought to be accessory spleens that had undergone compensatory hypertrophy after splenectomy. The transplant and the accessory spleen could not be distinguished by microscopic study. The location, however, was not common for accessory spleens and the distribution pattern in most cases strongly suggested that transplants had developed from loose bits of splenic tissue that had been deposited over the peritoneum by the extravasated blood at the time of rupture. From contact these had adhered to the peritoneum and in time acquired a blood supply which, as it became adequate, made hyperplastic regeneration of the splenic tissue possible.

One of the reported cases was found at autopsy to have a transplant in the lung, splenic tissue having escaped into the chest through a rent in the diaphragm at the time of traumatic rupture of the spleen years previously. Embryologically an accessory spleen in the lung could not have been possible.

There may be hundreds of the intraperitoneal transplants in an individual case. Some of the nodules are as large as a hickorynut. They are as a rule sessile but may be pedunculated. They are found over the pelvic peritoneum and along the mesentery of the small intestine. They may also be found attached to the great omentum or to the large intestine. Irregularity of distribution suggests their mode of origin. Causing no symptoms they are believed to be of no clinical significance.

Several facts about their incidence, however, are of interest. Only in children or in young adults is rupture of the spleen followed by transplants. With aging of the patient the splenic cell apparently loses the power to live and to grow as a transplant after rupture. Most cases of transplant have been in young boys. Cells from grossly diseased spleens that have ruptured spontaneously have not survived as transplants.

It is believed that the spleen is the only organ with cells capable of being transplanted by rupture. The splenic transplant is somewhat comparable to the endometrial transplant and has to be differentiated from it in young females who have had traumatic rupture of the spleen. The essential differences are that the splenic transplant is not subject to ovarian influence and requires no treatment.

DERMATOLOGY

For this issue RAY O. NOOJIN, M.D., Durham. N. C.

LUPUS ERYTHEMATOSUS

THIS is one of the more serious dermal affections, making it essential that recognition and proper management of its varied manifestations be made as early as possible. Two general clinical forms are recognized: (1) a *chronic* type in which the lesions are limited largely to the face, known as chronic discoid lupus erythematosus. If these chronic lesions become more widespread to involve the trunk or extremities then the disease is called the desseminated discoid form; (2) the *acute* type is a severe toxic disease and is called acute lupus erythematosus disseminata.

The chronic discoid form, the only type to be discussed here, in most cases runs a benign course. The etiologic factors of all types remain obscure. The fact that the chronic form may suddenly acquire characteristics of the acute form hints strongly toward a common denominator present in both types, varying only in intensity. Heredity apparently is not an etiologic factor. Women are more often affected than men, the common age group being twenty to thirty years.

The common or localized discoid form usually begins as an erythematous macule upon the exposed areas, particularly the cheeks, nose, forehead, or neck. The oral mucous membranes and lips are less commonly involved. One or several lesions may occur. The primary lesion ordinarily progresses peripherally to form plaques characterized by erythema, scaling, keratotic epithelial plugging of dilated follicles, a slightly elevated border, atrophy, pigmentation, depigmentation, telangiectasia, and later a tendency toward healing in the central portion of the lesion. Ulceration does not occur. Where hairy surfaces are involved alopecia may result. Not infrequently contiguous spread across the nose and cheeks results in the butterfly lesion.

. The patient may complain of burning or pruritis locally. The fact that exposure to sun and sometimes trauma produces an exacerbation of the lesion is an important diagnostic point. Atrophy, erythema, scaling and the keratotic adherent follicular plugs are fairly characteristic objective findings. These findings, plus microscopic study of a biopsy specimen (the pathologic picture is fairly characteristic), are important diagnostically.

The course of the chronic discoid form is variable, depending upon exposure to sunlight and other irritants, response to therapy, and other factors as yet indeterminate. Usually there are spontaneous remissions, particularly in the winter months. The explanation for the photosensitization is unknown. Even with regression, moderately advanced lesions ordinarily leave scarring and atrophy. Carcinoma is sometimes an unfortunate complication of the older lesions. Acute exacerbation may occur particularly following prolonged or intense sunlight exposure.

Other dermatoses which may simulate chronic discoid lupus erythematosus include rosacea, pellagra, erythema multiforme, seborrheic dermatitis, erysipelas, syphilids, lupus vulgaris, lupus pernio, as well as the acute form of lupus erythematosus.

Acute lupus erythematosus disseminata, in contradistinction to the chronic form, is characterized by leucopenia, acute or chronic nephrosis, hyperthermia, chills, prostration, malaise and arthralgia. The cutaneous manifestation may be similar to the chronic discoid form, but tend to show more erythema and facial edema, and are usually more widespread, purplish and polymorphic. The acute form leaves no doubt that it is a grave constitutional disease. It is usually fatal. Fortunately this syndrome is uncommon. It may follow the chronic type or may be the first manifestation of lupus erythematosus. The acute type occasionally follows a subacute or a less severe fulminating course. The Libman-Sachs syndrome is considered as a variant of the acute type plus an associated endocarditis.

Treatment for the chronic type should include the following regimen:

1. Search for and remove (*with caution*) all foci of infection.
2. Insist upon strict avoidance of sunlight and all unnecessary trauma or exposure.
3. Take every step to improve the general health of the patient. Adequate mental and physical rest are important.
4. Röntgen, radium or ultraviolet radiation therapy should *not* be administered. Shock therapy is contraindicated.
5. The patient should wear a widebrim hat when going out of doors and apply the following preparation locally to screen out sun rays:

Rx Salol	(5%)	3.0
Titanium dioxide	(5%)	3.0
Zinc oxide paste q.s.a d.		60.0

Sig.: Use as protective creme against sunlight.

6. Avoid local destructive means as electrocautery or solid carbon dioxide as cosmetic aids, since these may increase the local disfigurement. Although a lesion may be excised, apparently in toto, it may recur within the edges of the surgical scar. Surgery, therefore, is not ordinarily indicated.
7. Avoid soap and other irritants locally. Cleanse the affected areas with cold creme or olive oil.
8. Administer bismuth subsalicylate 0.2 gm. intramuscularly at weekly intervals for ten weeks. (A standard serologic test for syphilis should be made before starting heavy-metal therapy. The gums, urine, leucocyte count and hemoglobin should be checked before institution of therapy and should be followed.)
9. If no improvement occurs gold and sodium thiosulfate may be tried. The drug is given for ten weeks starting with 10 mgm. intravenously and increasing each weekly dose by 10 mgm. until a 50 mgm. dose is reached. That amount should not be exceeded. This is the most potent drug available for treatment of chronic lupus erythematosus and, if indicated, courses of the drug may be repeated. It should be noted, however, that this medicament may in some instances produce evidences of severe toxicity. It is essential that the *liver* (jaundice), *kidneys* (hemoglobinuria and albuminuria), white blood cell count and differential formula (agranulocytosis), and skin (dermatitis medicamentosa) be checked carefully and persistently throughout the period gold therapy is being administered. If evidence of toxicity appears the drug should be discontinued.
10. Quinine sulfate is sometimes efficacious. If tolerated it may be administered in dosages of 0.6 gms. t. i. d. for from one to three weeks.
11. Mapharsen in courses of ten weekly intravenous injections is to be tried if other measures fail. The same dosages as those used in antisyphilitic therapy are administered—.03 gm. the first dose, .04 gm. the second dose and .06 gm. each dose thereafter.

It is well to disclose to the patient that his disease can be controlled in some cases although a cure cannot be promised. Where atrophy results there is little to offer the patient except the use of some cosmetic preparation to cover the affected area.

The disease is not to be considered lightly at any time and if questions arise regarding its clinical appearance, course or therapy, immediate consultation with one experienced in its management should be regarded as obligatory.

PEDIATRICS

BREAST MILK FOR EMERGENCY FEEDING

IN MANY cases there is no satisfactory substitute for breast milk. Learn how it is being provided[1] in Newark.

Today, when statistics from many parts of the world show an alarming decrease in maternal nursing, breast milk may be termed a therapeutic agent.

Believing that a constantly available supply of breast milk would materially aid in reducing the mortality rate in newborn infants, the Child Welfare Committee of the Essex County Medical Society set up a breast milk station at the Coit Hospital in Newark. The milk was kept frozen and sold upon a physician's order to hospitals and to individuals throughout the area. For the most part the milk was obtained from the Mothers' Milk Bureau of the Children's Welfare Federation in New York City. This milk was received in tablets, having been pasteurized and frozen by a quick-freezing process using dry ice.

The milk was widely used by the profession throughout the country. It became impossible to obtain a sufficient amount of milk to maintain an adequate supply on hand.

We devised a plan of our own. The plan necessitated a wholehearted coöperation of pediatricians and obstetricians of the two nursing staffs. Without the enthusiastic support of the obstetric nurses potential donors are not found. The obstetricians must be convinced, if we expect them to give consent for the use of the breast pump, that the removal of excess milk from congested breasts insures continued lactation in their patients.

We have not attempted to obtain milk from mothers who have left the hospital. The quantity of milk salvaged by our plan has been ample to supply the needs of the hospital, and also we have

[1] Warren Richter, Montclair, in *J. Med. Soc. N. J.,* Feb.

in the past year supplied several hundred ounces for use in other hospitals and in the home. The majority of the babies needing breast milk are premature for whom early milk would seem to be the best.

Our maternity service consists of 41 private beds and 19 ward beds. The pediatric service of 60 bassinets and six incubators. There are also private and ward cribs. The beds for older children are not pertinent to this discussion. During the 12 months covered by this report there have been 1278 deliveries. The number of premature infants (birth weight less than 5½ lbs.) was 48. The number of babies who needed breast milk from the "bank" was 22.

Our equipment at the start was one electric (Abt) breast pump, one ice-cream storage box capable of maintaining a t. of $-10°$ F., a few dozen 4-oz. nursing bottles with rubber caps, and the facilities of the formula room. The procedure is as follows: As soon as the mother's breasts become engorged the baby is put to breast and allowed from 3 to 7 minutes on each breast at 3- to 4-hour intervals. After each nursing or at four-hour intervals during the day (not at night) the pump is applied and all remaining milk is collected. This milk is fed to the baby by bottle if needed, but if an excess over the baby's requirements it is pooled with the excess from other mothers. The pooled milk is taken to the formula room on the pediatric floor where it is measured, and boiled for 10 minutes, cooled and placed in a sterile graduate and brought to its original volume by adding sterile distilled water. It is then poured into sterile 4-ounce nursing bottles, 3 ounces to a bottle, and capped. These bottles are dated, placed in racks, and put into the freezing box at $-10°$ F. until used. When taken out for use the milk is thawed at room temperature, boiled again, evaporation replaced and the proper amounts measured into feeding bottles according to the prescription for the individual baby who is to be fed.

It takes 15-20 minutes to freeze these 3-ounce quantities. This slow method we have found satisfactory. Supplemental vitamins are easily supplied. Rapid thawing is apt to separate butter fat. A brief and vigorous shaking brings about a sufficient emulsification.

We have salvaged an average of 132 ounces of breast milk a month which, without our "bank," would have been lost.

We started with the idea that to be successful we must have the full coöperation of all concerned, the physicians, both obstetricians and general practitioners, the nurses and not least the mothers. This was obtained gradually by what we meant to be a diplomatic approach. We contended that it was not only unnecessary but unwise to pay the mothers for the excess milk obtained. We believe that we are rendering a distinct service to the mothers by relieving the discomfort and danger of the early engorgment of the breasts, and at the same time increasing the probability of continued breast feeding after discharge from the hospital.

In order to safeguard a limited quantity of breast milk from wasteful use, and to assure a supply in cases of dire need, a price per ounce may be set which is high enough to accomplish this end in a given locality. Our initial price was 35 cents. This is adjusted to the means of the purchaser by the financial department of the hospital. That part which is supplied free of charge is prescribed only by a member of the pediatric staff so that unnecessary use is closely controlled. There is a tendency, however, among the physicians of private cases to continue the use of breast milk longer than sometimes seems necessary even at a high cost to the patient. The gross income from the sale of breast milk has averaged $80 a month. Out of this income we have bought a third breast pump, another freezing unit, and all of the supplies used. We are now gradually reducing the charges made so as to determine the lowest price that will suffice to cover expenses and prevent the wasteful use of this valuable therapeutic agent.

ORTHOPEDIC SURGERY

John T. Saunders, M.D., *Editor*, Asheville, N. C.

BRACHIALGIA

Nachlas[1] has recently published a thorough discussion of pain in and about the shoulder and arm. Brachialgia means pain in the arm, and has no reference to the causative factor. It is essentially a sensory disturbance being rarely associated with muscular weakness.

Sensory nerve tracts somewhere between the cortical sensory cells and the areas in which pain is felt are irritated and the sensation is projected peripherally as radiations—that is, it is interpreted by our cerebrum as coming from the distal ends of the nerves.

"Theoretically it is possible to produce these symptoms by irritating the nerves (1) within the skull, (2) where the skull joins the spine, (3) within the cervical spinal column, (4) in the intervertebral foramina, (5) in the supraclavicular region, (6) in the shoulder, and (7) in the thorax."

It is in their passage through the intervertebral foramina that the nerves are particularly subject to irritation. The nerves pass through notches just in front of the articular processes and just behind the bodies of the vertebrae and are partially pro-

---
[1] *Jour. Bone & Joint Surg.*, v. xxvi, Jan., 1944.

tected by a sort of bony "conduit." When the neck flexes, the upper and lower walls of the notches are pushed closer together because the hinge action is just behind them at the lateral articulations. When the neck is extended, the bony portions of the foramen are separated and so the foramen is enlarged. The posterior wall of this "conduit" consists in great part of the capsule, so that when the capsule is swollen or distended by intra-articular fluid, there is a protrusion into the lumen. Also if the intervertebral disc in the front part of the channel should be compressed, so as to produce a herniation postero-laterally, there must be a reduction in the size of the passage for the nerve.

The sensory neurons are much more vulnerable in the region of the intervertebral foramen because the posterior roots are in close approximation to the capsule of the joint and here lose the protective myelin sheaths of the axons. Severe compression in the foramen is necessary to produce a motor disturbance.

The "backache" that is so often the chief complaint of our patients generally has reference to the lumbar region, but the cervical portion of the spine is likewise a frequent source of symptoms. Like the lumbar region of the spine the region of the anterior curve in the cervical spine is most susceptible to strain and wear and tear.

Surgical attack on cervical ribs and the scalenus anterior syndrome fails to relieve brachialgia at times; for this reason and to think of another more common cause for these distressing pains, a careful reading of the entire article by Dr. Nachlas is advised for those interested. Extension of the neck without tilting the head back usually gives relief. Exercises to improve posture, stretching, etc., are also used in treatment.

OPHTHALMOLOGY

HERBERT C. NEBLETT, M.D., *Editor*, Charlotte, N. C.

VERHOEFF'S METHOD OF ENUCLEATION WITH BALL IMPLANT

SINCE reading Dr. F. H. Verhoeff's article in the *A. J. of O.* for October, 1943, entitled "Improved Technique for Implantation of a Ball in Tenon's Capsule" the writer has used his method with excellent results in all of his enucleations; with the exception that a form (as recommended by him) was not used beneath the lids in all cases, principally because it was desired to determine if edema of the conjunctiva were a factor of importance without it. For this purpose five cases were selected. Two of these had phthisis bulbi, three had severe lacerations of the bulb with loss of contents and lacerations of the lids, and one of the latter was complicated with a fracture of the nasal wall of the orbit into the ethmoid sinuses and a comminuted fracture of the outer rim of the orbit. In none of these cases was edema of any consequence. In fact it was less pronounced than in enucleations performed by the old method of suturing the muscles together with capsule and mucous membrane over all. Dr. Verhoeff's technique of dissecting and suturing was carefully adhered to, a dry socket assured before implanting the ball, and a firm pressure bandage applied. In no case was the dressing disturbed until the end of the third day after operation.

These subjects were white, four males and one female. The writer has had no occasion to use the method on a Negro. A year or two ago the writer wrote an article in this department of this Journal on "Edema of the Conjunctiva in the Negro Following Enucleation" and set forth his theory as to the preponderance of this complication in the Negro as compared to the white. The use of Dr. Verhoeff's method may be the answer to this problem when such a case is presented.

In the writer's brief experience in the use of Dr. Verhoeff's method it appears that the good results obtained are predicated upon exact adherence to his technique of dissecting and suturing and the paucity of sutures for the desired result which limit trauma, necrosis and foreign material in the tissues, and their firm approximation with a minimum of strangulation of their blood supply. A thorough study of his method and its intelligent application in enucleations is productive of better results than heretofore experienced by other methods. Further observations on this method will be discussed in this department when greater experience has been had in the use of it.

DENTISTRY

J. H. GUION, D.D.S., *Editor*, Charlotte, N. C.

THE PRACTICE OF ORAL SURGERY BY THE GENERAL PRACTITIONER OF DENTISTRY

IN MOST dental schools the teaching of operative dentistry is stressed and oral surgery is neglected. The dental graduate should take an internship upon his graduation and if he is going into surgery he ought to become connected with some hospital clinic where he can continue treating surgical patients and the study of disease.[1]

The dentist should make a careful examination and record it on a sensible chart, to enable him to make a correct diagnosis and to give the patient a painless and aseptic operation in office or in hospital.

---
1. H. S. Dunning, New York, in *R. I. Med. Jl.*, Feb.

We should be prompt in referring patients with medical symptoms to the proper physician. The dental surgeon must know when to send his patient to the hospital for surgical care. If the operation is to be done under local anesthesia, be kind and firm and keep talking to the patient about anything that has nothing to do with the operation.

If general anesthesia is desired, a good anesthetist should administer the drug and the patient should be surrounded by all the precautionary measures possible, whether in office or in hospital.

The operation must be performed with the best surgical technic possible, painlessly and with as complete asepsis as can be maintained. There should be a minimum of shock and trauma and all wounds should be left in the best possible condition for early healing. We must know when to suture and when to drain. We should guard against accidents, lacerations of the soft parts; fracture of the roots, alveolar process or tuberosity; dislocation of the mandible, openings into the antrum, roots in the antrum, sharp edges of bone, injury to adjacent teeth, breaking of instruments, needles, and so forth. We should have all pathological tissues examined carefully under the microscope and keep a record of the findings.

Postoperative care of the patient is in many cases almost as important as the operation. Rest in a quiet room should be enforced, whether the patient has been given a local or a general anesthetic, not allowed to leave the office unless discharged by the operator with full instructions as to what to do. The reaction of each person to drugs and anesthetics is different, and we must endeavor to guard each patient individually.

The surgeon will surely see the patient not longer than two days after an operation of any importance. If he does not return, he should be communicated with and the surgeon should call upon him if he cannot come to office. The patient should be able to get in touch with the doctor day or night and week-ends.

GENERAL PRACTICE

D. HERBERT SMITH, M.D., *Editor*, Pauline. S. C.

PRACTICAL POINTS IN INTRAVENOUS THERAPY TECHNIQUE

WHEN MANY of us were graduated nobody needled a vein. When saline solution was to be put into a vein, the vein was cut down on and a cannula inserted. So it is not surprising that not all of us are adept at puncturing a vein with a needle and so giving medication.

[1] S. G. Stubbins, Greenville, S. C., in *M. S. C. Med. Assn.* Feb.

With thanks to a Greenville doctor[1] his valuable article on this procedure is abstracted at length.

A little time spent in selecting a good vein pays dividends. Examine both arms carefully and in a good light and allow enough room at the bedside or operating table. Although the antecubital veins are usually selected, in case they are not prominent a good vein may be found on the dorsum of the hand or wrist, and an especially good vein can be found running along the lateral aspect of the wrist and distal forearm. The great saphenous vein is on the ankle anterior to the internal malleolus. It is as a rule advisable to use the veins on the hand and wrist first in a patient who is apt to receive repeated intravenous therapy. Once the more proximal branches become thrombosed, the most distal tributaries are thereby rendered unsatisfactory.

The best site for inserting a cannula is in the great saphenous vein on the medial aspect of the leg two inches above and anterior to the medial malleolus. A transverse incision has advantage over a longitudinal one in that it allows more room to explore laterally if necessary; besides leaving less scar. Cutting down on a vein is seldom necessary except when a cannula is to be inserted preceding an operation or in cases of circulatory collapse. Veins which are not visible or palpable, or small veins on the hand and wrist may be made to increase 3 and 4 times by applying the tourniquet and slapping the tissue with the palm of the hand and applying hot wet towels over a 10-15 min. period. In difficult patients, alternate slapping and hot towels may be employed by the nurse.

A few drops of procaine solution is well before inserting a large needle. Inspect needle for sharpness and possible hooked end, test by drawing the needle point across a piece of sterile cotton or gauze. Also test patency of the needle by forcing air through it with the syringe. Proper care of the needles (cleaning, sharpening and inserting stylets in them prior to sterilization) is important.

After preparing the arm with soap and water followed by alcohol sponges the arm is grasped firmly with the left hand so that firm counter-traction and pressure with the left thumb over the vein immobilizes the vein, keeping it and the skin from folding when the needle is thrust through the tough tissues, and the vein from being pushed to one side by the needle.

A fairly large needle is best for giving therapy, especially with blood transfusions and plasma—18- or 20-gauge or even larger, when giving whole blood. The angle should be 10° in direct line and directly over the central portion of the vein; as soon as blood is obtained, angle decreased 5° for further insertion.

The needle may be secured in place with small adhesive strips and a sponge under its butt end and the arm splinted in a comfortable position.

A common mistake is making pressure with a sponge directly over the point of insertion as the needle is being withdrawn. Following the withdrawal of the needle from the vein there is ample time to place a sponge over the needle hole and apply pressure for a few minutes.

After the needle is inserted and while it is being made secure and the arm is being splinted, allow the fluid to run freely to tell whether the needle has stayed in the proper position. A few bubbles of air given intravenously is of no consequence. After the system has been connected a final test of its patency may be made by pinching off the tubing several feet away and watching for slight return of blood-tinged fluid into the tube.

No serious concern need be given to the t. of fluids given intravenously, especially when given at the usual 20-30 drops per minute. Even cold fluids are occasionally employed in cases of heat prostration. There is some danger of a reaction if fluids are given at a faster rate. There is danger of giving 10 per cent glucose solutions and more concentrated solutions in appreciable amounts, except under very careful supervision; because, should the needle slip from the vein and the fluid become deposited in the subcutaneous tissues, a serious slough and infection are apt to follow. Five per cent glucose solution, however, may be given subcutaneously with no untoward results. In case the subcutaneous tissues become infiltrated with concentrated solutions or toxic drugs, dilute these substances by injecting fairly large amounts of normal saline into the area.

In drawing blood from a donor it occasionally helps to point the needle distally into the lumen of the vein, since in doing this the blood will flow directly into the needle.

Ordinarily, dressings over needle wounds are not necessary, but where large needles have been used a small dry sterile dressing should be applied, to be removed in a half hour.

OBSTETRICS

HENRY J. LANGSTON, M.D., *Editor*, Danville, Va.

THE CARE OF THE FETUS DURING LABOR

DESPITE improvements in surgical technique operative delivery should not be done except for definite reasons.[1] Further:

Paramount in the management of labor is the possession of a distinct and inclusive definition of a test of labor. Some technically trained experts glibly license themselves to do all sorts of operative procedures on the defenseless parturient.

After six years of study in 6,000 deliveries the test evolved thus: Test of labor includes uterine contractions lasting 40 seconds every two to five minutes over a period of 20 to 24 hours with noticeable progress, the parturient being supported meanwhile with water, dextrose, vitamins and oxygen if necessary, plus proper sedation. At the end of this period in most instances the fetus will have been born; or the head will be at least in mid-pelvis, where it may be delivered by forceps; or still floating, when low or extraperitoneal cesarean section may be done safely. By following this rule, one can reduce operative delivery to 3 per cent—forceps delivery 2½, cesarean section .5.

Because of the ever present possibility of necessity for cesarean section, no vaginal examinations were done and a watery solution of an antiseptic was instilled into the vagina q. 4 h. during labor.

During the course of labor there are two important considerations, 1) the degree of progress and 2) evidences of exhaustion of either mother or fetus. The progress may be determined by rectal examination and expressed in terms of dilatation and effacement of the cervix and the descent of the presenting part. Exhaustion of the mother is made evident by dehydration, rapid pulse rate, undue restlessness and alterations in uterine contractions and, very rarely, development of a contraction ring in the lower uterine segment. For fetus, changes in the heart rate, especially slowing or irregularity, indicate hypoxia. All types of exhaustion in either of the patients are best treated by hydration, dextrose, vitamins, oxygen and sedation rather than by forced delivery, as is far too often employed.

Some sort of amnesia, analgesia or anesthesia in labor is necessary as well as prudent. Morphine and scopolamine has gained a notorious reputation for its blue babies, caudal analgesia for a high incidence of forceps deliveries.

* * * *

INDUCTION AND STIMULATION OF LABOR WITH ERGOT

WE have been earnestly admonished to give no ergot until the uterus is void of fetus and afterbirth.

Administration of carefully standardized powdered ergot for induction or stimulation of labor is recommended. In the dosages used ergot has not the pressor nor the antidiuretic action of posterior pituitary extract nor has it the intravascular hemolytic effect of quinine.

Medical induction of labor can be accomplished as follows: One ounce of castor oil in one-half glass of root beer is taken in the morning before a

---
[1]. Richard Torpin, Augusta, Ga., in *Jl. A. M. A.*, Feb. 5th.

1. C. J. Ehrenberg & J. A. Haugen, in *Jl.-Lancet*, 63:209 (1943)

light breakfast, and a 12-gr. "ergot equivalent" capsule is taken after breakfast. The ergot is repeated in two hours if painful contractions do not occur. Induction of labor within 20 hours after ingestion of castor oil may be attributed to the procedure. Surgical induction is done by rupturing the membranes under surgical asepsis one hour after administration of a 12-gr. ergot equivalent capsule.

The latent period in induction of labor is shortened by the addition of ergot. Slow and lingering labor may be accelerated by a 6-gr. ergot equivalent capsule, given as often as every four hours up to four doses. Posterior pituitary extract or intravenous calcium and parathormone may be used with ergot.

A 12-gr. equivalent capsule of ergot contains 6 mg. of ergotoxine and 11 mg. of ergonovine.

* * * * *

A TWO- AND SIX-HOUR PREGNANCY TEST

Two to six vs. 48 hours for a pregnancy that is offered:

Ascheim-Zondek and Friedman tests for pregnancy involves expense and difficulty of procuring animals. Of 86 samples of urine tested, 48 from pregnant and 38 from nonpregnant women, only two yielded undecisive results; later tests on these two patients were strongly positive.

Two-hour pregnancy test.—Immature rats were injected intraperitoneally with 1.5 c.c. of a morning sample of the urine. Divided doses of 3/4 c.c. are injected into both the right and left lower abdominal quadrants. The animal is killed with ether two hours after injection of the urine and the appearance of the ovary and the ovarian capsule is noted.

Redness of the ovary and capsule is considered a positive reaction. Until one is able to distinguish between the normal appearance of the ovary which is white or pinkish and that of the ovary stimulated by pregnancy urine, it is advisable to kill an uninjected animal at the same time so that a comparison may be made.

Six-hour pregnancy test with immature rats.— Two c.c. of urine is administered by subcutaneous injection and the animal is killed six hours later. The end-point is similar to that observed for the two-hour test.

Six-hour pregnancy test with adult rats.—Before the urine is administered, vaginal smears are taken and only those animals in metestrus or diestrus are used. Five c.c. of urine is injected subcutaneously and the animal is killed six hours later. The recent corpora lutea of animals injected with pregnancy urine appear dark red to purple and, microscopically, show considerable vascularization. Again it is best that control animals in the same stage of the cycle be killed simultaneously, for comparison with the rats injected with urine. A more definite reaction is observed two to three minutes after the animal has been killed and the viscera exposed for inspection.

In addition, the reaction of the corpora lutea of the adult animals may be more easily interpreted when the ovaries are placed in formalin. The control ovaries and corpora lutea remain pale while those from animals injected with pregnancy urine turn dark brown or a decidedly darker shade than the controls after being placed in formalin. By means of this simple procedure a convenient set of standards may be prepared and kept indefinitely for comparison with the results from unknown samples of urine.

HISTORIC MEDICINE

WILLIAM HEBERDEN AND THE AGE OF REASON[1]

IN THE 18TH CENTURY in medicine the gold-headed cane symbolized the rise in social status and wealth of the physicians. Men like Radcliffe and Mead lived in a style unequalled even in the palmy days of Victoria, and one which will seem incredible in the future.

It did not help medicine at Cambridge that for 93 years of the century there were only two occupants of the Regius Chair. Christopher Green appointed in 1700 held office until his death in 1741, at the age of 90, but during the last two years he had a deputy who became his successor. During Green's reign occurred the famous controversy between the Royal College of Physicians and the Universities, the former demanding their license before a medical graduate could practice in or within seven miles of London, and the Universities had to undertake to make their medical degrees strictly conformable with the statutory qualifications. And with good reason, for the results of examinations were biased by favouritism and the granting of degrees by royal mandate was rife. Neither Green nor his successor, Russell Plumptre, who held office for 53 years, seems to have published anything or to have held much of a position in the medical world. The mistake of Plumptre's appointment to the Chair was all the more glaring as the brilliant William Heberden was available.

In the year after Queen Anne came to the throne, Richard Bentley, Master of Trinity, established what he described as an "elegant chymical laboratory" for Francis Vigani, who had just been

---
1. H. S. Kupperman et al, in Jl. Clin. Endocrinol., 3:548 (1943).

1. Sir Walter Langdon-Brown, in Proc. Royal Soc. of Med. (Lond.), Dec.

appointed the first University Professor of Chemistry. Vigani, who was born in Verona, settled in Cambridge in 1683 and gave private tuition in chemistry and pharmacy. His drug chest may be regarded as the first physiological laboratory, for here Stephen Hales applied his training in physics under Isaac Newton to physiological problems. He was the first to measure blood-pressure and made many other important observations in animal and plant physiology. When a vacancy occurred in 1764 Mr. Watson of Trinity was appointed through the influence of the Duke of Newcastle, then Chancellor, although it is recorded that "he had never read a syllable on the subject, nor seen a single experiment in it." After holding office for seven years during which time he does appear to have acquired a real knowledge of the subject, he became Regius Professor of Divinity and finally found his proper vocation as Bishop of Llandaff. The first professor of anatomy, George Rolfe, was appointed in 1707. At first dissections seem to have been carried out in the Old Schools, and it is to be feared that the body-snatchers made their contribution, for Laurence Sterne, who died in London from tuberculosis in 1768, appeared a week later on the dissecting table there. A grim return to his old University!

Dr. Walker wrote: "About 15 years ago the learned physician, Dr. Heberden, was so kind as to oblige the University with a course of Experiments upon such plants as he then found amongst us in order to show their use in Medicine." William Heberden was the first man to try to rationalize pharmacology and materia medica, while in clinical medicine he insisted on observation without slavish adherence to tradition. He entered St. John's College in 1742 at the early age of 14, subsequently becoming a Fellow. He resigned his Fellowship, however, as soon as he could afford to do so, in order to allow someone poorer to take his place. He gave an annual course of lectures for 10 years.

His Commentaries were prepared from notes collected at the bedside and revised every month in light of fresh cases, but without borrowing from other writers.

"Many physicians appear to be too strict in the rules of diet and regimen," said he—a remark which is still applicable today. Again "very few remedies have justified their promises. However, the title of 'specific' may be justly claimed by Peruvian bark for ague, quicksilver for venereal disorders, sulphur for the itch and perhaps opium for some spasms." On the gout he says: "People are neither ashamed nor afraid of the gout, but rather ambitious of supposing that every complaint arises from a gouty cause and even try to contract it by means which happily for them are generally ineffectual . . . . the belief that it is antagonistic to other diseases is fallacious."

And further: "The belief that strong wines and in no small quantity are beneficial for gout arises not so much perhaps from a reasonable persuasion of its truth as from a desire that it should be true because they love wine."

He attributed the value of the treatment at Bath to the change of surroundings and habits and to the suspension of business and cares rather than to something subtle in the waters.

He believed in fresh air: "No cordial is so reviving and many persons have been stifled in their own putrid atmosphere by the injudicious."

Of the idea that epilepsy was likely to cease at puberty he wrote: "I should think [it] was founded on theory or in the hopes of the physician rather than on fact." On venereal diseases he commented: "Interested persons have endeavoured to exaggerate [the patient's] fears in order to make an advantage of them by the sale of their silly books and insignificant medicines." He described dyschezia, as it is now called, and realized the connexion between fistula-in-ano and pulmonary tuberculosis. "A little grume of blood," said he, "often forms the nucleus of a stone."

Of all the wit and wisdom of these commentaries only one thing is generally remembered, his description of the nodes which still go by his name.

In 1768 he gave the first real account of angina pectoris to the Royal College of Physicians in a paper which was based on 20 cases. He earnestly wished "that writers would not confine themselves to relate only their successful practice but would have the courage to tell us the ineffectual and hurtful."

Heberden moved to London in 1748. He apparently colaborated in preparing a new edition of the London Pharmacopoeia. From this many useless drugs were deleted, but in some respects the purge was too drastic and several useful drugs had to be reinstated. In London, although he declined the post of Physician to the King his practice became very large indeed. His second son, also named William, who became Physician-in-Ordinary to King George III and Queen Charlotte, declined a Baronetcy, but I do not know whether, like a physician of a later age, he asked for a fur coat instead!

Heberden, Brocklesby, Warren and Butter all attended Samuel Johnson in his last illness without any fee, and in his will he asked each of them to take a book "at their election" from his shelves as a memento.

Heberden's sceptical attitude of mind did not extend to religion. On the death of a certain Dr. Conyers Middleton whose orthodoxy was much suspect, his widow consulted Heberden about the publication of a manuscript he had left on the inefficacy of prayer. Heberden said that though it might be worthy of her husband's learning, it would be injurious to his memory. But as it appeared that a publisher would give 150 pounds for it, he bought it from her for 200 pounds and then burnt the manuscript.

In his 70th year he decided to restrict his practice, so he bought a house near Windsor where he resided in the summer but practiced in London during the winter for several years longer. He was a great walker until his 86 year, when he met with an accident which disabled him for the rest of his life. Yet when he was nearly 90 he said he did not know that he had ever passed a year more comfortably than the last. His mental power and memory remained unimpaired to the end and he was quoting Latin within 48 hours of his death which occurred peacefully and painlessly in 1801 in his 91st year.

A man who had considerable importance in 18th century Cambridge, John Woodward, had been elected a Fellow of the Royal Society in 1693, but was expelled in 1710 for conduct unbecoming a gentleman. He next became notorious for his controversy with Richard Mead and John Freind on the treatment of smallpox. Mead, then at the height of his fame, resented Woodward's attack with the air of a St. Bernard faced by a mongrel puppy. Encountering one another at the game of Gresham College, each drew his sword, but Woodward stumbled on the steps and fell. "Take your life," said Mead contemptuously. "Anything but your physic," was the retort.

The most extraordinary medical alumnus of 18th century Cambridge was Thomas Dover, who, despite his remarkable exploits, was a friend of the great Sydenham. After obtaining his M. B. he practised in Bristol, where he became fascinated by shipping and took to buccaneering! In the course of his voyages with Captain Woodes-Rigers, they touched at the island of Juan Fernandez in 1708-9 and rescued the original of Robinson Crusoe. Next they took a town in Peru by storm and a few months later captured a ship of 20 guns and 109 men. Dover transferred to this ship, with Selkirk as Master; they reached England again in 1711, and Dover quietly resumed his practice in Bristol, becoming so successful that he removed to London in 1721, where he was admitted L. R. C. P. His fondness for prescribing mercury as well as his hasty temper led to his being nicknamed "the quicksilver doctor," but his principal medical claim to fame is his well-known powder. He retired to his beautiful mansion of Stanway House in the Cotswolds, where with his friend Robert Tracy, he spent the closing years of his life, dying in 1742, aged 80.

Richard Warren, born at Cavendish, the son of the Archdeacon of Suffolk, and physician to George III, was one of the first to discard the pompous manner hitherto considered appropriate to the physician of the gold-headed cane epoch.

DISCUSSION
(From Page 86)

PRESIDENT JOHNS: The paper is open for general discussion.

MEMBER: I think nobody ought to discuss this paper who voted for Roosevelt.

DR. WM. W. RIXEY, Richmond: Mr. President and Members: It is the Doctor's business to see both sides of a subject, all around it and through it. My ideas are old-fashioned ones, but some old-fashioned things are not so bad, at that.

I have given much thought to the broad subject of socialized medicine. Anyway, the Doctor still has a good deal of liberty. He may quarrel with his colleagues and expect their forgiveness if he confines the quarrel to the Doctor's own house. It is very important to confine our quarrels. Also, almost anything can be said when the Doctor speaks to his colleagues.

The politico-economic situation in reference to medicine may lead us on into complete state and federal control. I have picked the brains of my Doctor friends and I am assured that when this stage is reached, good Doctors and some mediocre ones, like me, will quit; quit, not because we are lacking in appreciation of the spirit of medicine, but simply because we will be unable to function under such a program.

The Doctor has some talent, else he would not be a Doctor. He can display his talent in other fields and prevent hunger in his home. Perhaps it would be better, even if hunger should enter in, that his children should know that he could be deprived of his freedom but nothing could dim his spirit of the profession most Doctors adorn.

DR. KARL SCHAFFLE, Asheville: With all respect to Dr. Starr and the fine gentleman I had lunch with, Dr. Northington, I would like to say that it is rather absurd to compare what we have, what we are likely to have, with what is going on in Germany. The so-called National Socialism is not true socialism and hasn't been. Hitler backed the capitalists of the younger group or he wouldn't have gotten where he did. Socialized medicine goes back sixty years. Bismarck introduced it for political reasons. He wanted to satisfy the laboring class. He did satisfy them and the protection of the laboring man was an example to other countries so that Lord George in 1911 adopted it for Great Britain. When the medical profession attacked it after it proved successful, a great majority climbed on the band wagon and found receipts twice what they were under the private, competitive system. It was said that 60 per cent of the wealth of this country was in the hands of 2 per cent of the population. That was some time ago. Then it was said that 60 families control America. Recently that has been reduced to 13 families. Senator Wagner is like the President, a humanitarian. He has introduced legislation in New York State for the benefit of the laboring class. He set up this bill, not to be adopted as a blueprint, but as something for discussion with probable improvement.

(To P. 106)

GYNECOLOGY

ROBERT THRIFT FERGUSON, M.D., *Editor*, Charlotte, N. C.

THE USE OF OCTOFOLLIN IN CONDITIONS OF ESTROGEN DEFICIENCIES AND IN GONORRHEAL VULVOVAGINITIS

THE PRINCIPAL objection to diethylstilbestrol, whether administered parenterally, or by mouth, is the resulting nausea which is so frequent. Any estrogenic substance which eliminates this objectional feature is preferable.

Jaeger discusses[1] an encouraging experience:

The practicing physician endeavors to find better methods of therapy, and as his facilities for gathering clinical data are unlimited, accurate records should be kept and report of clinical results should be made.

An effort has been made to develop a synthetic estrogen of low cost and oral activity and without side reaction. For the last year and a half I have been using in my private and clinic practice a new synthetic estrogenic substance, octofollin.

SUMMARY OF CASES TREATED WITH OCTOFOLLIN
Cases usually classed as menopausal:
Recent surgically-induced menopause 42
Active natural menopause 15
Recurrence of menopausal symptoms several years after oöphorectomy in which there has been longer or shorter symptom-free periods 7
Recurrence of symptoms several years after x-ray treatment which had been followed by complete cessation of menses 2
Endocrine dysfunctions in women under 40 years old, with no appreciable pelvic pathology, and in whom menopause could seemingly be ruled out:
Menorrhagia 7
Various symptoms indicating pluriglandular dysfunctions—amenorrhea, irregularity, slight, dysmenorrhea 15
Cases in which the predominating and major symptoms were severe headache, usually of the migraine type 8
Senile vaginitis: Severe vulvovaginal and anorectal pruritus 5
Acute mastitis: following weaning of infants, resulting in solid, painful breasts with usual symptoms 2
Gonorrheal vaginitis in children 30

Total number of patients treated with octofollin.... 140

The results have been uniformly satisfactory. The material has been administered by mouth in daily doses of 1 to 10 mgs.; in oil by intramuscular injection of 2 to 5 mgs., one to three times a week; and in $\frac{1}{2}$ to 1 mg. suppositories or tablet inserts daily or twice daily to children—without a single case of nausea, vomiting, dizziness or any of the other side reactions reported as following diethylstilbestrol therapy.

The average daily dose orally, in conjunction with thyroid, was 2 mg. In certain patients omission of the thyroid raised the daily need for the estrogen to 5 mg. per day. When octofollin was given in oil the dose was 2-5 mg. once to three times a week, or less frequently after the symptoms were under control.

---
1. A. S. Jaeger, Indianapolis, in *Jl. Indiana Med. Assn.*, March.

A better response was obtained with this estrogen when thyroid in varying amounts was used as a supplement.

Octofollin is an excellent estrogenic agent and is to be preferred to diethylstilbestrol.

In the treatment of gonorrheal vaginitis in little girls, octofollin $\frac{1}{2}$ to 1 mg. per day either parenterally in tablet form, or locally in suppositories, or vaginal inserts, produced a rapid maturation of the vaginal mucosa, and in conjunction with the sulfonamides and local therapy yields negative smears somewhat sooner than when the other estrogenic substances, natural or synthetic, were used.

It is well known that thyroid extract has a marked influence on many patients suffering from lack of estrogenic substance.

The cost of any estrogenic substance has to be considered for many patients are unable to bear the expense of prolonged treatment.

The treatment of gonorrheal vaginitis in little girls has truly been revolutionized with the use of estrogen.

The character, or type, of estrogenic substances used is dependent largely on the experience of the practitioner, and on the records kept. Complete records in a large series of patients will reveal remarkable results if followed to their ultimate conclusion. Without such records your statements are purely guess-work.

GENERAL PRACTICE

JAMES L. HAMNER, M.D., *Editor*, Mannboro, Va.

SIMPLIFICATION OF THE TREATMENT OF DIABETES

IT SEEMS that every writer on diabetes has his own method for writing a diet. All this has made for confusion among the practitioners. In despair, most of the diabetic patients are referred to a specialist. A simple but satisfactory formula for computing a diabetic diet is a necessity.

The foregoing paragraph introduces a practical argument[1] for the general practitioners' management of their diabetic cases.

The essential thing is that the diabetic diet be based on known values of the normal diet. The total daily caloric allowance is divided into carbohydrate, 65 per cent; protein, 15 per cent; and fat, 20 per cent.

The diet is calculated for the patient's normal weight, derived from actuarial tables for age-height-weight. It never fails if one keeps in mind that, once the diet has been prescribed, it be maintained until the patient's metabolism has become adjusted to the diet. This will invariably come about in the course of a few days. Then, if the patient still continues to show sugar, insulin is given in sufficient amounts to control the hyperglycemia and glycosuria without changing the diet as a whole.

---
1. Capt. Lazarus L. Pompey, M. C., U. S. A., in *Jl. Lab. & Clin. Med.*, Feb.)

Requirements are: for an average male diabetic patient 30 calories, for a female 25, per kilogram normal body weight. This is for persons whose work is of the business and professional and the housewife character.

Protein.—For a man, 1 gram; for a woman, 3/4 gram per kilo.

Fat.—A maximum of 90 grams per day (as low as 70 grams).

Carbohydrate.—Having determined the protein and fat in the diet, the remainder of the calories are prescribed as carbohydrate.

Such a calculation takes about a minute or two for any patient.

Assuming we are dealing with a patient who is 42 years old, 67 inches tall, and is a salesman by occupation (not heavy labor):
1. Normal body weight 154 pounds (75 kilograms).
2. Caloric allowance 30 calories per kilo.
3. Total daily caloric allowance 70x30—2100 calories.
4. Protein (1 gram per kilo)—70 grams
   Fat: 90 grams
   Protein calories—70x4—280 calories
   Fat calories—90x9—810 calories

   280 calories (protein) plus 810 calories (fat) 1090 calories
   Total daily caloric allowance—2100 calories
   Calories supplied by protein and fat—1090 calories
   Calories to be supplied as carbohydrate—1010 calories
   Carbohydrate (grams)—1010 divided by 4 = 250 grams

Diet: carbohydrate, 250; protein, 70; fat, 90.

The patient is given his maintenance diet, as outlined, for four or five days, without insulin if possible, to evaluate the degree of severity of diabetes; mild, requiring no insulin; moderate, requiring up to 40 units daily; severe, requiring more than 40 units.

One-third of the cases are in the mild group.

The patient is taught to test his urine for sugar before each meal and on retiring, and to keep a record. He collects and measures his 24-hour urine output daily, and a quantitative analysis of the sugar present is done. The volume of urine in c.c. multiplied by the percentage of sugar present yields the amount of sugar in grams that the patient is excreting daily.

All patients requiring insulin are started on protamine zinc only, one unit for every two grams of glucose excreted. It is a good policy not to prescribe less than 10 units daily. A patient excreting less than 20 grams of glucose per day usually can be made sugar-free by readjusting the carbohydrate among his three meals. Ordinarily the patient receives three meals equal in carbohydrate, protein and fat content. For the patient who is showing considerable sugar persistently after any one of the meals, shifting ten to 20 grams of carbohydrate from that meal to another, to a time of day when he is sugar-free, has saved many a patient from taking any insulin.

In many cases, an additional dose of crystalline insulin is necessary. Two main requirements are: (1) that this additional insulin dose never be more than one-third of the total insulin dose per day, and (2) that the additional insulin be given at breakfast time with the protamine zinc insulin. We have always given the two kinds of insulin in the same syringe, drawing the clear insulin into the syringe first, followed by the protamine zinc insulin, so as to avoid injecting protamine into the other insulin bottle. All patients taking protamine zinc insulin receive a small meal at bedtime containing milk, to prevent depression of the blood sugar during the night to the reaction level.

Blood sugar tests are made three times weekly, before breakfast, in all diabetic patients.

* * * * *

SLEEP PARALYSIS

THIS SHORT ARTICLE[1] is abstracted because paralysis always suggests a very serious condition, and having this unusual "sleep paralysis" in mind may serve us and our patient well.

Sleep paralysis is a benign, transient paralysis at the beginning or end of sleep and usually associated with distressingly clear consciousness. Sleep paralysis is probably not uncommon, but it has received slight recognition.

A young man, 23, was referred to the Clinic because of headaches and downward displacement of the left orbit, the latter present since childhood. Attacks of sleep paralysis which began when he was 22 were a secondary but distressing complaint. These attacks would occur one to three times a month, usually when he was lying down for a nap after supper. As he went to sleep or awakened, he suddenly would realize that he was completely paralyzed. He would be unable even to open his eyes but was usually able to moan. This would gain his wife's attention. She merely had to touch him in order to dispel the paralysis. Similar spells might occur if he were to awaken in the night but he never experienced them on awakening in the morning. During the period of paralysis which he estimated as lasting less than three minutes, he was acutely aware of everything about him. On recovering he would lie quiet for five to 10 minutes, for if he were to arise immediately, he would get a headache. These attacks of paraly-

---
1. T. G. Rushton, in *Proc. Staff Meetings of The Mayo Clinic*, Jan. 26th.

sis were always made harrowing by the fear of dying during an attack. On recovery this fear would pass away quickly.

A woman, 54, would awaken at night fully conscious but unable to move, talk or open her eyes. She could make a gurgling noise in her throat which would awaken her husband. During the attack she had great fear of dying but this passed off with the paralysis. On being aroused her husband would rub her arms vigorously and she would regain the use of her muscles within a few minutes. In a period of four years she had had 12 of these spells at irregular intervals. They usually lasted five to 10 minutes. The duration of the spell was largely determined by the length of time it took for her husband to wake up. All had occurred on awakening at night except one. This occurred when she lay down for a nap. Her child by shaking the patient's head would dispel the attack but the patient felt weak for the rest of the day.

Enough reports have now been published to give a fairly definite picture of the disorder.

The attacks of paralysis always occur in association with sleep either on awakening or less commonly on falling asleep. The paralysis is usually complete though movements of the eyes and rarely ability to speak may be retained. The duration of the paralysis may vary from a few minutes to two hours or more. Recovery may be spontaneous or induced. If the latter, it is always by bodily contact varying from a light touch to vigorous shaking. Loud noises appear to have no effect on dispelling the paralysis. During the period of paralysis the patient is acutely aware of his surroundings and of his paralyzed condition. This awareness is often associated with considerable anxiety and even fear of impending death. Occasionally the patient's altered respiration or a moan will warn those about him of an attack. The condition may begin in childhood and persist to old age without serious impairment of health. As a rule the family history is negative for any similar complaint.

It is not proper to establish the etiology of this condition on the basis of the material we have.

The combination of sleep paralysis and the usual manifestations of epilepsy is exceptional. Epileptic seizures run their course and usually are not interrupted by the simple means which stop attacks of sleep paralysis.

Is sleep paralysis a symptom of conversion hysteria? is asked. The hysterical trance is usually not as colorless and it usually is not dissipated by simply touching the individual. The close similarity between sleep paralysis and the narcolepsy-cataplepsy syndrome should make physicians wary of calling the former hysterical without better evidence than is at hand at present.

THERAPEUTICS

J. F. NASH, M.D., *Editor*, Saint Pauls, N. C.

MENSTRUAL PROBLEMS OF ADOLESCENCE

A WISE MOTHER will have prepared her child for the beginning of menstruation[1]

Special attention is called to the influence of the development of muscles on the growth and the shape of the bones. Habitual gum chewers may be recognized by the great development of the masseter muscles which gives them a queer cat-like expression. Now in the pelvis we have the great groups of muscles which require proper exercise to develop. Exercise and exertion are necesary to develop the bony pelvis of a woman into a structure proper for child-bearing.

Among our own people that normal beginning of menstruation is around 14 years of age; although I have seen girls begin at 10 or at 18. It is the usual thing that those girls who begin early will continue to menstruate until late in life, while those that begin late will reach their menopause at an early date. Girls that begin at 12 will frequently menstruate until 55 while the girls who begin at 17 will frequently reach their menopause at 40.

The normal interval in a woman is by no means the same for all—28 days, 21 days, 35 days—then there is a bizarre group who menstruate at any irregular time—sometimes 6 weeks; sometimes 8; then again 5. None of these groups, however, is abnormal. It is dangerous for a physician to try to change or regulate the periods of children. When a child comes with her mother it is generally the mother who is worked up about her child's irregularities. The first thing to do is to set the mother right. She may have a notion that menstruation is some sort of excretory function. When it is explained that menstruation is simply the discharge of the lining of the uterus with a little blood, and why this lining must be discharged periodically to prepare a fertile bed for possible pregnancy, she will be reassured and you will save the child a psychological upset. The period of menstruation in children is a law unto itself, not to be interfered with.

Dysmenorrhea in children requires an abdominal-rectal examination. The position of the uterus varies from day to day, and even from one hour to another. Never come to a conclusion that, because the uterus happens to be retroverted, it is consequently abnormal. An acute flexing of the fundus on the cervix is a possible cause of dysmenorrhea. The canal of the cervix, if stenosed, should be relieved by dilatation under anesthesia, repeated to

---

1. Gerritt Hetzinkveld, Denver, in *Southwestern Med.*, Nov.

assure a permanent result, by passing a sound weekly or monthly for several months. After the initial dilatation the cervix frequently clamps down harder than before, and may easily form scar tissue causing a permanent damage.

Chronic appendicitis is another common cause of dysmenorrhea. If there is an appreciable swelling of the right ovary and there are signs of appendicitis, the appendix should be removed because in young girls chronic appendicitis is destructive to the pelvic organs.

Occasionally one will see a child with menorrhagia. There has been much said in favor of various endocrine preparations, but I do not know of any that give sure results. It may be due to pelvic congestion, and strangely enough, anemia; also to hypothyroidism. I have better success with small doses of thyroid in these cases than all other methods together. Many annoyances and bizarre symptoms of puberty are due to deficient thyroid activity. The acne of puberty, the greasy skin, especially over the bridge of the nose and the forehead and under the eyes, the scraggly hair, the listlessness of some girls, all respond promptly to the administration of small quantities of thyroid extract.

AMBULATORY TREATMENT OF CEREBRAL CONCUSSION

WE HAVE been taught to keep a patient in bed for 24 to 48 hours after severe blows to the head or abdomen, however loud the protest that he is all right and however insignificant the symptoms; and it is easy to recall cases which proved the wisdom of the practice.

However, military practice,[1] at least some of it, seems against this concept.

The time-honored procedure of keeping patients with cerebral concussion quiet for long periods may not be necessary. Seventy-two of 90 male patients who had sustained cerebral concussion after various kinds of head injuries were allowed to walk within 24-48 hours after drowsiness or disorientation had disappeared. Some with drainage from the ears or nose were kept in bed until the discharge ceased.

Unconsciousness averaged in the patients without fracture 3.1 hours, in those with fracture 10.7 hours.

The longest period of bed rest was eight days and most of the patients were allowed out of bed during the first day of hospitalization.

The presence of skull fracture did not alter the management. All patients without skull fracture left the hospital with no headache, vertigo or tinnitus; none returned, and none died.

Post-concussion symptoms are apparently reduced by early ambulation, possibly because of more complete rest of the brain and quicker adjustment of the vegetative centers when the patient is erect. Prevention of, or a favorable influence on, the formation of adhesions within the cerebrospinal fluid pathways, and the prevention of psychogenic difficulties, such as may occur when the patient has time to brood over his injury seem to be demonstrated.

---

[1]. E. W. Shearburn & D. H. Mulford, in *Bul. U. S. Army Med. Dept.*, 69:36, 1943.

CHEWING-GUM FEVER
(H. B. Searcy, Tuscaloosa, in *Jl. Med. Assn. Ala.*, Feb.)

I had forgotten that muscular effort produced a local rise in temperature until last summer when, after tests for undulant fever, typhoid, malaria, etc., on a child, I discovered that on discontinuing the use of chewing gum the temperature became normal. A whole family troubled with fever became normal when the chewing gum habit was discontinued.

On September 20th, 1943, each of 10 nurses was given a piece of chewing-gum and requested to record her own temperature at the beginning of the hour and for every five minutes thereafter. For 30 minutes she was to chew the gum, then to discard the gum but continue the record. The thermometer interfered with the chewing of the gum one minute out of every five.

Chewing produces a physiologic elevation of oral temperature. The amount of elevation depends on the amount of muscular effort used in the chewing. Chewing gum can produce a false fever that may confuse a diagnosis.

LIVER EXTRACT IN ACNE ERUPTIONS, ABSCESSES AND SCARS
(Wallace Marsall, Mobile, in *Jl. Med. Assn. of Ala.*, Feb.)

Various liver extracts produced clinical improvement in patients with acne vulgaris. Certain refinements in the laboratory preparation of these materials may improve the clinical results.

This article is based on a five-year laboratory and clinical study on this topic.

This LYO-6 material has been given to some patients orally. Two capsules of two grains each daily. The results obtained through the alimentary route were adequate. This method was costly and, therefore, not practicable.

One weekly dose of one c.c. of this material is injected subcutaneously in alternating arms; two or three injections per week in obstinate cases. One case required 14 c.c. per week to prevent recurrence. Some patients need continued therapy to prevent a relapse.

Results with an experimental liver extract preparation, Al-3, on 25 unselected cases of acne vulgaris produced a moderate or marked improvement in 68% of the cases.

With the use of a further improved medication (LYO-6) on 27 unselected cases of acne vulgaris, 89% showed a moderate or marked improvement.

Two well-qualified dermatologists used the LYO-6 material in 23 cases of acne vulgaris in their private offices; 85% of these cases were "cured" or moderately improved. Seventeen show slight improvement, and there were no failures.

At this time it is impossible to supply other interested workers with our preparation. However, we shall be happy to grant requests for this material at a later date, when routine requirements are met satisfactorily.

Write Author a postal card requesting Reprint.

A PATIENT'S reference to an odor of burning flesh may be the only diagnostic sign that a central brain lesion exists.—*Pharmacal Advance*, Jan.

SOUTHERN MEDICINE & SURGERY

Official Organ

JAMES M NORTHINGTON, M.D., *Editor*

Department Editors

Human Behavior
JAMES K. HALL, M.D..................................Richmond, Va.

Orthopedic Surgery
JOHN T. SAUNDERS, M.D. ....Asheville, N. C.

Urology
RAYMOND THOMPSON, M.D..................Charlotte, N. C.

Surgery
GEO. H. BUNCH, M.D.................................Columbia, S. C.

Obstetrics
HENRY J. LANGSTON, M.D.........................Danville, Va

Gynecology
CHAS. R. ROBINS, M.D...............................Richmond, Va.
ROBERT T. FERGUSON, M.D. ....Charlotte, N. C.

General Practice
J. L. HAMNER, M.D....................................Mannboro, Va.

Clinical Chemistry and Microscopy
J. M. FEDER, M.D., }
EVELYN TREBBLE, M. T. } ....Anderson, S. C.

Hospitals
R. B. DAVIS, M.D..Greensboro, N. C.

Cardiology
CLYDE M. GILMORE, A.B., M.D................Greensboro, N. C.

Public Health
N. THOS. ENNETT, M.D..............................Greenville, N. C.

Radiology
R. H. LAFFERTY, M.D., and Associates........Charlotte, N. C.

Therapeutics
J. F. NASH, M.D...Saint Pauls, N. C.

Tuberculosis
JOHN DONNELLY, M.D...............................Charlotte, N. C.

Dentistry
J. H. GUION, D.D.S......................................Charlotte, N. C.

Internal Medicine
GEORGE R. WILKINSON, M.D....................Greenville, S. C.

Ophthalmology
HERBERT C. NEBLETT, M.D......................Charlotte, N. C.

Rhino-Oto-Laryngology
CLAY W. EVATT, M.D.................................Charleston, S. C.

Proctology
RUSSELL VON L. BUXTON, M.D................Newport News, Va.

Insurance Medicine
H. F. STARR, M.D.......................................Greensboro, N. C.

Dermatology
J. LAMAR CALLAWAY, M.D. ....Durham, N. C.

Pediatrics

Offerings for the pages of this Journal are requested and given careful consideration in each case. Manuscripts not found suitable for our use will not be returned unless author encloses postage.

As is true of most Medical Journals, all costs of cuts, etc., for illustrating an article must be borne by the author.

THE TRI-STATE MEDICAL ASSOCIATION'S SPECIAL PLACE IN MEDICINE

THE TRI-STATE MEDICAL ASSOCIATION has, throughout the near half-century of its existence, consistently and determinedly maintained the thesis that the general practitioner is the foundation stone of the medical profession.

A distinguished ex-president of the Medical Society of the State of North Carolina once paid the official journal of this Association the compliment of saying it had held to this position when to do so required as much faith and courage as would have been shown by establishing a chain of barber-shops in Russia.

Because of its fundamental belief in the unity of Medicine and the general practitioner as its main man, the Tri-State continues to meet in one body and arrange programs such as the one presented the last of February.

It is gratifying to see that, in the troublous days for Medicine, a great many medical men are speaking and writing for this neglected unit of our profession.

By a happy coincidence, while the recent Tri-State meeting was being held there came across the Atlantic a mighty pronouncement in support of our position.

In the *Proceedings of the Royal Society of Medicine* (England) for January, the President of the Section of Epidemiology and State Medicine, Sir Weldon Dalrymple-Champneys, makes An Examination of the Place of the Doctor in the State from Ancient Times to the Present Day and Certain Speculations Regarding the Future:

Among these Speculations:

Few people familiar with the conditions of general practice before 1911 would doubt the benefit conferred by the Act of that year on the general practitioner.

It can hardly be doubted that the ideal arrangement would be continuous medical supervision of the individual from conception to death *by the same person* [Italics ours.—S. M. & S.], and the preservation of the family unit as the basis of the general practitioner's work.

I hope to give some indication of what I believe to be the need that should be met, or in other words what position the general practitioner should occupy in the State of the future.

We have noticed how during the most advanced and humane phases of many civilizations, the State has appointed medical officers to care for the poor, to guard against epidemics, and to protect, and even prescribe, the food and drink of the people—in other words to practise preventive medicine. Progress must be continuous if we wish to avoid decay and that progress cannot be left to Public Health officials or enthusiastic laymen: it depends for its success on the active, intelligent, day-to-day coöperation of the general practitioner.

We have been struck by the way in which decadence in medicine has coincided with over-specialization on insufficient knowledge. Can we feel so safe against the recurrence of this danger? You may say that modern medicine is truly scientific and that a high degree of specialization is necessary if we are to reap the benefits of new discoveries and expert procedures. But even in these enlightened days we know of new remedies backed by extravagant claims, being snatched at by harassed practitioners in the hope that they may benefit patients whom nothing seems to cure or even alleviate; we know that there are specialists whose outlook is so cramped that they tend too often to attribute their patients' ailments to some unusual condition in their own sphere.

The only sure defence is to give the general practitioner a dominant share in the care of the patient, and to fit him for this important position in the State, we must see to it that he is rightly educated. All of us who have been medical students know the fascination of the study of fully developed disease, the care of dangerous illness, and the dramatic appeal of difficult operations. But the prevention of disease and the achievement and preservation of perfect health, both physical and mental, also have a compelling appeal if presented by teachers who have the right outlook on health and disease, and I refuse to believe that the medical student of today is incapable of feeling the fascination and satisfaction of detecting the first glimmering of ill-health in his patient and defeating it.

The general practitioner, if he is to do his duty as the guardian of the patient's health, must know his patient's heredity and environment, his medical history and present condition; and all the agents, including not merely methods of treatment, but also all the public and private organizations, which can be invoked to restore him to his normal or a condition better than this.

The general practitioner has established himself in the esteem and affection of his patients as a guide, philosopher and friend, though recently certain social tendencies and the growth of specialization have tended to undermine this position, to the detriment of the people's health. We must not only reëstablish him as the trusted confidant and guardian of the patient and of the family, but we must strengthen his position in every possible way, placing in his hand all the weapons that modern science and State organization have provided.

I am convinced that the general practitioner is today presented with a wonderful opportunity—which, if neglected, may never recur—of occupying a key position in medicine and in the State, and from that position exercising an incalculable influence for good on the health and happiness of his fellow-countrymen, thereby ensuring to himself, a life of absorbing interest and abiding satisfaction in the greatest of all professions.

Let us promote the private practitioner to be a general practitioner, a real general marshalling all the forces of the State and voluntary organizations for the capture of health.

Is there missing from this list a one of the points we have made in favor of the exaltation of the general practitioner, not only as a matter of right, but as a matter of reason and of the highest expediency?

It seems to me that I can read between the lines of Sir Weldon's address—"lest we perish."

The official journal of the Tri-State Medical Association has besought its readers, over and over again, to bestir themselves politically.

Read what the Editor of the *Nebraska Medical Journal* has to say as to this:

In his address before the National Conference on Medical Service in February, Congressman Walter Judd of Minnesota says that "physicians, by virtue of their training, habits and analytical inclinations, are better equipped than any other group to help lead this country out of its economic and social maze, by active participation in political and governmental affairs." He cautions, however, that in doing so they will serve their country best by entering this field as citizens first and as doctors only to aid in the interpretation of the origin and the nature of the deteriorating social processes which are now plaguing this earth, and help evolve a system of therapeutics before the hopeless stage of destruction makes its final appearance.

Dr. Judd is talking about general practitioners. He is a general practitioner.

Can any thinking doctor doubt the soundness of the reasoning of Sir-Doctor Dalrymple-Champneys, or of Congressman-Doctor Judd? Or that by these means only can mankind be best served and Medicine as we have known it be saved from extinction?

Is the stone rejected of the builders to become the head of the corner?

We trust so. It is the right way; it is the only way of salvation for Medicine.

MENTAL HEALTH

IN THE Proceedings of one of our most learned societies we read a searching inquiry[1] into the status quo, and urgent suggestions as to the future.

---
1. Goeffrey Evans, in *Proc. Royal Soc. of Med.* (Lond.), Dec.

Science has established the organic unity of the universe. We can look back to something like 3,000 million years ago, when matter in a form smaller than atoms was more or less evenly distributed through space. The universe was in darkness, its temperature that of melting ice. Out of this were created the heavenly bodies and the Milky Way, the sun and its planets, this world of ours and its moon—and all this by the operation of natural laws. There is a pattern in everything, from the infinitely small, such as atomic and molecular form, and nuclear structure to the vastly great: it would seem that our sun with its planets is but a part of a pattern on a large magnificent, and that ours is not the only planetary system in the universe.

There is ceaseless movement within the atomic structure of even cold steel.

In the understanding of the mind we are concerned only with function and this function is feeling.

Humanity lives under the delusion that it is acting on a rational basis, whereas its actions are largely determined by instinctive feeling. The primitive instincts which are common to animals and man are those of Self-preservation, Creation and Destruction. To these three basic instincts must be added the herd instinct, which Trotter regarded as an acquired function of the mind. To his interpretation the mind of the gregarious animal "possesses a specific sensitiveness to external opinion, and the capacity to confer on its precepts the sanction of instinctive force."

Infancy and childhood are largely animated by the instinct of self-preservation, and so for the fullest development of personality and character a child requires above all things security and love. In adult life the impulse of creation supersedes the instinct of self-preservation, and self-sacrifice is born. Some measure of security is required, and for its greatest achievements some measure of isolation too. Home life is the essential unit of a society that has reached the highest level in the evolution of mankind. The Church, politicians, educationists and doctors ,must make this the foundation of their plans for mental health. We must be slow to interpret self-interest in terms of selfishness. Self-interest determines self-preservation. It provides the material background of a home, and maintains its existence. Self-interest is only harmful when it expands to the detriment of others.

Creative activity in its widest sense is the real purpose of life. It is to the restriction and limitation of creative activity that much mental ill-health is due. The absence of children is a well-established cause of married unhappiness and an only child, or perhaps only two children, may not satisfy the needs of human nature, at least in later life. Creative activity demands self-sacrifice. Generally speaking, a woman is ultimately responsible for the activities of a man. She may find the outlet for her creative function in his life's work. A man must be ready to sacrifice himself to his work or for an idea.

Before the war people looked forward to living on income, inherited or earned. Idleness was encouraged by provision of pensions at an earlier age. The birth-rate was falling. Machines did the creative work. An interest in life was found in playing the gallery game, in cinemas, in horse and dog racing, in watching cricket and football matches. The purpose of life, even if the occupation was in creative activity, was holidays or leisure away from work. The war has contributed to show the poverty of all this. In spite of stress and strain, discomforts and anxieties, the health of the community has improved with war, and this may be due to the outlet provided for the basic needs of human nature by the opportunity for creation and destruction on a great scale. In our planning for mental health in the future, ample opportunity for creative impulse must be found by the encouragement of home life and larger families, and by finding opportunity for creative activity in art and literature, in allotments and gardens, and other such occupations, for those who cannot find expression for their natural instincts in their daily work. Creative activity is not open to all, nor has everyone the energy or courage for its undertaking. This service may be performed for an individual, for an institution or for the State. Service has another advantage. Most people require a constant supply of appreciation for their mental health and happiness. For the attainment of mental health when there is no opportunity for creative activity an opportunity for service must be found to take its place.

The instincts of self-preservation and creation up to the present time have beaten the spirit of destruction by but a narrow margin, unless the strength of the destructive instinct is fully realized human nature will destroy itself. There are many occupations in which there are opportunities for its display.

Uncontrolled destruction must be met and overcome by greater force, or even controlled by fear. This war is not, he thinks, "a sporadic outburst of barbarism"; it has its origin in the basic forces of the human mind.

The herd instinct is all pervasive in human life. Fashion in clothes is an obvious example. Fashion in thought and feeling is just as common. Our individualistic outlook must be preserved if an endo-psychic conflict on a national scale is to be prevented, a conflict between the instincts of self-preservation and the herd. Such a conflict would sow the seed of widespread mental ill-health and could lead to revolution.

In the super-sensuous sphere it is commonly imagined that intellect and rational thought reign supreme, but primitive impulses still remain the basis of feeling and action. In this sphere of thought and feeling human beings conceive their standards of truth and justice and their ideals of honour and virtue and human nature has reached its highest level on the winding stair of evolutionary change. This dual nature of man belonging at one and the same time to both sensuous and super-sensuous spheres must be completely realized if human nature is to be understood. The mind is dyed with the instincts of self-preservation, creation, destruction and the herd. These instincts give feeling tone to the highest thoughts conceived in the super-sensuous sphere by the human mind.

A man's activities are the expression of the purpose of life, and the objective best contributes to mental health when it is outside himself and seems to the individual to be worth his while.

Mental ill-health is due to a failure of adjustment of the mind to its surroundings and to a disharmony or conflict in the working of the components of the mind. This disharmony may be due to an endo-psychic conflict within the sensuous sphere, or to a conflict between the sensuous and super-sensuous. In ordinary life the commonest causes of mental ill-health are lack of outlet, exhaustion, and frustration; and even when conflict results from defeat or frustration it is best resolved by acceptance, or it is often better sublimated by diversion and direction to the level of the super-sensuous sphere than by its analysis on the sensuous level.

The future of mankind depends on the development and growing power of activity in the super-sensuous sphere, under discipline and control. It must be developed in conjunction with activity in the sensuous sphere. To develop it alone is to encourage mysticism a dangerous doctrine. A healthy mind is better cultivated by the development of human nature at the same time in its sensuous and super-sensuous spheres. It should be the objective of every man and woman to fulfil his duty towards life completely as a vital member of society in every respect.

The universe, it seems, has increased 100 times in size within the measure of calculable time. This movement, this change in the direction of ordered elaboration, is evolution. Just as science brings all measurable things into an organic unity or whole, so religion brings all these basic scientific conceptions into one conceptual whole. Religion teaches mind control and concentration by prayer. It inculcates discipline of body and mind by religious observance. When to all this is added a firm belief in the beneficence of The All-prevailing Power, mortal man finds peace of mind. All this, or much of it, is the interest of religious bodies, and they must bestir themselves to provide the outlet for the vital impulse in the super-sensuous realm. Educationists and doctors can take a part by teaching how to harness thought and set it in the right direction. Tennyson said: "Think well—Do well will follow thought." Thought can initiate emotion. Thought can be thought-controlled. It can also be mind-controlled. In this doctors have their opportunity; for, not only the attitude of the body, but also its physical condition, affects the mind.

* * * * *

A LETTER (IN ABSTRACT) OF AN N. C. DOCTOR OF 100 YEARS AGO

Smithfield, N. C.
May 22, 1826.

Mann Patterson,
Orange County, Chapel Hill.
Dear Uncle:

Today is the first time in two weeks that I have been able to write, having been taken tomorrow two weeks ago with a pain in the substance of my lungs, connected with the pectoral complaint you know I have been from infancy afflicted with. I had myself bled six times in three days, two Blister Plasters on my Breast and legs, beside other medical treatment that my case required, has reduced me extremely but has been successful. Pressure from my business has induced me to undertake more than my strength was competent to, the day I was taken I rode 40 miles into Wayne County to Tap a man who has the Dropsy. It is not uncommon for me to drive 50 miles in the day and night. The measles and Influenza and the numerous train of diseases arising from them has kept almost the whole country prostrate, but fortunately for the people and for me it was subsiding very fast at the time I was taken down.

I had no medical aid to myself, my student was constantly at my bedside. I told him what to do if I should lose my senses, but thanks to a Kind Providence they were continued as good as when in health. Though it cannot but detract from me I must say to you that I could think of no physician, neither in Raleigh or elsewhere convenient to this place, who I could place confidence in. It is known to you perhaps that there is a fashion in medicine as well as other things, which I hold to be destructive of its fundamental principles. I do not mean to let these fashionable gentlemen practice on me. I had other medical men to see Chesley when he was sick and I believe he owes his life to my having pursued my own course to the entire exclusion of others.

I know not that I ever shall see you again though it would be a great pleasure, had I leisure to come up. I am concerned about my brother Wesley. I am afraid he is mis-spending his time. If he comes in your reach, do give him a lesson. I disapprove of his attempting to teach. Mention me in kind feelings to your family. You will ever have my warmest affections.

Jno. T. P. Yeargain.

NEWBORN BABIES may be immunized against pertussis by vaccinating pregnant women with whooping cough vaccine during the last trimester. Total dosage of organisms advised by authors in 150 billion given in six injections at two-week intervals.—*Cohen & Scardron, Jl. A. M. A.*, 121: 656, 1943.

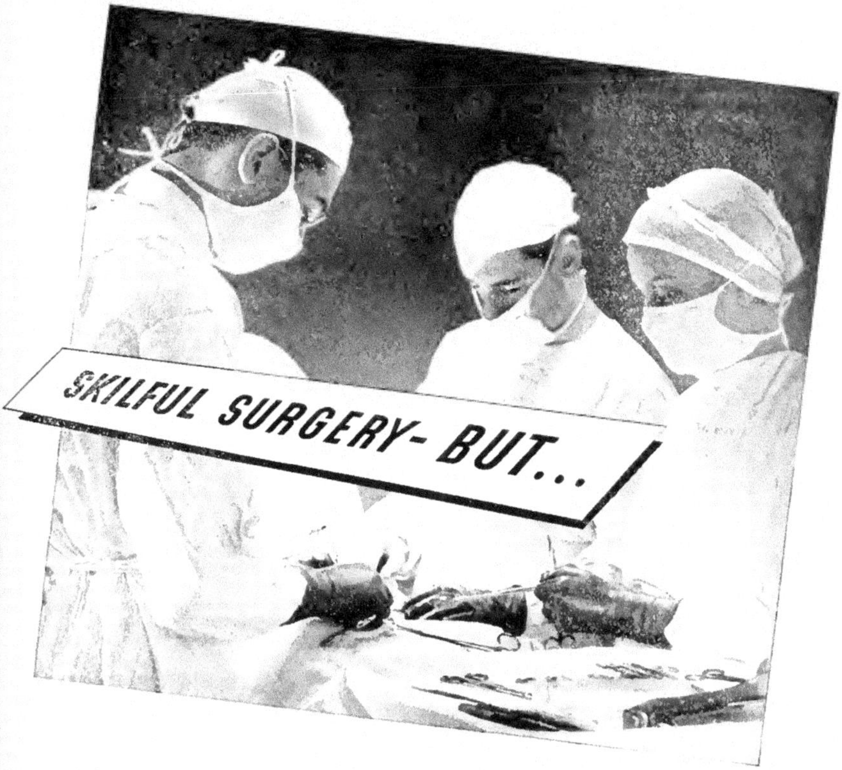

SKILFUL SURGERY – BUT...

—POSTOPERATIVE DISTRESS may mar the clinical picture to a discouraging degree. Abdominal distention and urinary retention, following surgery, are frequently the cause of complications necessitating troublesome procedures that are apt to retard the patient's recovery. The routine use of Prostigmin Methylsulfate* 1:4000 provides a convenient and effective means of preventing intestinal and bladder atony, minimizing the likelihood of "gas pains" and the need for catheterization. Try Prostigmin 'Roche' for a smoother, uninterrupted convalescence. Inject 1 cc (1:4000 solution) at the time of operation. Follow with 5 similar 1-cc injections at 2-hour intervals after the operation. HOFFMANN-LA ROCHE, INC. • ROCHE PARK • NUTLEY, N. J.

*Dimethyl-carbamic ester of m-oxyphenyl-trimethyl-ammonium methylsulfate.

PROSTIGMIN 'ROCHE'

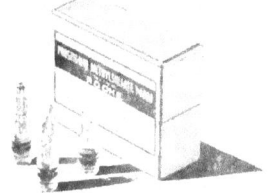

STARR
(From P. 96)

DR. PAUL D. CAMP, Richmond: I don't want to make a prolonged discussion. I want to congratulate Dr. Starr and say that I think such a paper was very, very timely and greatly needed and I want to congratulate him on having the courage to get up and say what he did. I agree with him entirely that the present administration is comparable to National Socialism.

In regard to panel patient practice of socialized medicine in England, I was over there fourteen months and I don't believe that we want the type of medicine practiced in this country that is practiced on panel patients there.

PRESIDENT JOHNS: Dr. Starr, I understand, is running for Mayor.

DR. STARR (closing): That is a mistake. I have never run for anything. I have never taken any interest in politics. I was born and raised North Carolina Democrat and was always proud of it, so I have no political aspirations whatever. I don't want anything to do with politics and it makes me mad that medicine is about to be dragged into politics.

I thank the gentlemen for discussing the paper. I would be very much surprised if all of you agree with me entirely.

THE TALCUM POWDER PROBLEM IN SURGERY AND ITS SOLUTION

(M. G. Seelig et al, St. Louis, in *Jl. A. M. A.*, Dec. 11th)

Our purpose in this report is to emphasize the very serious surgical hazard incident to the use of talc as a dusting powder for rubber gloves and to recommend potassium bitartrate as a substitute powder.

After the technic of dry gloves was adopted, a quarter of a century elapsed before surgeons recognized the evil agency of talc, and even now many are unaware of its harmfulness. Talcum powder is still in almost universal use in preparing gloves aseptically.

Talcum powder is, under any circumstances, a grave menace in surgery. Once having gained entrance into the animal organism, this powder sets up a reactionary, productive inflammation.

Even meticulous care in washing off the surface of rubber gloves before operating does not guarantee against contamination of the operative field with talc.

Potassium bitartrate meets the physical requirements imposed by steam sterilization. It is readily and harmlessly disposed of by the body tissues and fluids. It causes no consequent peritoneal adhesions. It possesses a certain degree of bacteriostasis for the colon bacillus and staphylococcus aureus.

It is important that in the process of sterilization the potassium bitartrate should be subjected only to the now standard and accepted technic for sterilizing rubber gloves —15 minutes of autoclaving under 15 pounds of steam pressure.

Since this paper was submitted for publication, we have received reports indicating that potassium bitartrate shortens the life of rubber gloves. On making tests, we found that tartrated gloves would stand from 7 to 10 separate sterilizations, whereas talcum powdering permitted from 12 to 20 sterilizations (pure rubber gloves). This insignificant economic factor should not be permitted to weigh against the grave disadvantages attributable to the use of talcum, which raises both postoperative morbidity and mortality rates.

VINCENT'S INFECTION of the gums and throat may be satisfactorily treated by giving nicotinic acid. Dose employed is 25 to 50 mg. three times a day for adults and 10 mg. or more according to age for children.—H. M. *Johnson, N. C. Med. Jl.,* 4:51, 1943.

NEWS

THE
American Physicians' Art Association

will have its seventh annual exhibit at the A. M. A. convention, Stevens Hotel, Chicago, June 12th-16th.

Through the courtesy of Mead Johnson & Co., Evansville, Ind., there will be no fees for hanging and no express charge seither way. The type of art to be exhibited includes a personal work of the following types of medium: oil portraits, oil still life, landscapes, sculpture, water color, pastels, etchings, photography, wood carving, leather tooling, ceramics and tapestries (needle work). All pieces should be sent preferably by railway express collect, automatically covered with $50 insurance.

Exhibitors should send NOW for entry blanks to *Dr. Francis H. Redewill, Secretary, A .P. A. A.,* Flood Building, San Francisco; one entry blank should be used for each medium in which it is desired to exhibit.

There will be about 100 trophies, including medals and plaques.

DR. FREDERICK KREDEL, Professor of Surgery in the Medical College of the State of South Carolina, was elected Treasurer of the Society of University Surgeons, in a meeting held at Nashville in February.

COMMANDER RAYMOND S. CRISPELL, M.C., U.S.N.R., who has been serving as Chief of Neuropsychiatry in the Medical Department and Naval School of Aviation at the Naval Air Training Center at Pensacola, Fla., since his leave of absence from Duke University in June, 1941, is under orders to the Pacific area.

DR. WALTER L. BARNES, recently named coroner of Petersburg, Va., has been appointed city physician of the same city to fill the vacancy created several months ago when Dr. C. W. Lynn resigned.

Dr. Barnes, who has been with the United States Public Health Service, located in Petersburg several weeks ago to begin private medical practice.

Work on a new nurses' home at NORFOLK GENERAL HOSPITAL is expected to get under way as soon as the contractor can move his equipment to Norfolk.

Successful bidder for the job, which will cost more than $180,000, was L. B. Gallimore, of Greensboro, N. C. The amount of the successful bid will not be made public until the contract is approved by the Federal Works Agency this week.

DR. J. C. FORBES, Associate Professor of Biochemistry at the Medical College of Virginia, has become a member of the organization, Charles C. Haskell & Co. For the present, Dr. Forbes will continue to discharge his teaching duties at the Medical College but will actively participate in the determination and execution o fthe policies of Haskell & Co.

UNIVERSITY OF VIRGINIA

The Phi Beta Pi Medical Fraternity presented Dr. Karl Menninger, of the Menninger Clinic, Kansas City, Missouri, in a lecture on January 14th. His subject was Psychiatry in Medicine.

Dr. Fletcher D. Woodward attended a meeting of the Subcommittee on Otolaryngology, Division of Surgery, of the National Research Council in Washington on January 21st. He recently accepted appointments to the National

Healers
on the heights

Crawling the crags at dawn ... Exposed on rocky ledges in the blistering noonday sun ... Fighting pain and death through the freezing night ...

Unarmed and unafraid, the medical officer on mountain duty is often marooned amid harrowing hardships for days on end, unrelieved except for an occasional cigarette ... a cheering Camel most likely ... the soldier's favorite smoke.

Camel is first choice of the armed forces* because Camel rates first for mildness, first for fine flavor. Remember that—when you send cigarettes to friends and relatives in service. Send Camels—the brand that's sure to please.

1st in the service

*With men in the Army, the Navy, the Marine Corps, and the Coast Guard, the favorite cigarette is Camel. (Based on actual sales records.)

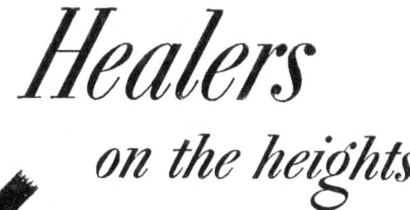

Camel
COSTLIER TOBACCOS

New reprint available on cigarette research — Archives of Otolaryngology, March, 1943, pp. 404-410. Camel Cigarettes, Medical Relations Division, One Pershing Square, New York 17, N. Y.

Faculties in Broncho-Esophagology and in Otolaryngology of the War-Time Graduate Medical Meetings organized for medical officers in the Armed Forces and civilian doctors under the auspices of the American Medical Association, The American College of Physicians and the American College of Surgeons.

On January 24th at the University of Virginia Medical Society Meeting, Dr. C. H. Mann of New York spoke on Lymphogranuloma Venereum.

Dr. Henry B. Mulholland spoke on February 2nd to the Augusta County Medical Society at King's Daughters' Hospital in Staunton. His subject was Federalized Medicine. On January 12th he spoke on The Diagnosis and Treatment of the Pneumonias at the James River Medical Society Meeting at Dillwyn.

The annual Sigma Xi lecture was given on February 9th by Dr. K. C. D. Hickman, research chemist of the Eastman Kodak Company, on the subject, Low Pressure Distillation and Vitamin Production.

Dr. E. P. Lehman and Dr. W. H. Parker attended the meeting of the Society of University Surgeons at Vanderbilt University, February 9th through 12th.

MEDICAL COLLEGE OF VIRGINIA

The annual McGuire Lectures will be delivered at the College in April, the first on the evening of the 5th by Dr. Winfred Overholser, Superintendent of St. Elizabeth's Hospital, Washington, on Modern Trends in Psychiatry; the second on the next evening by Lt. Col. William C. Menninger, M.C., Chief of the Division of Neuropsychiatry, United States Army, on Psychiatric Problems in the Army.

The annual address will be given to the Section on the History of Medicine of the Richmond Academy of Medicine on March 14th by Major Manfred S. Guttmacher, of Baltimore, on The Insanity of King George III.

BOOKS

THE 1943 YEAR BOOK OF DERMATOLOGY AND SYPHILOLOGY, edited by MARION B. SULZBERGER, M.D., Commander, M.C., U.S.N.A.; Assistant Clinical Professor of Dermatology and Syphilology, New York Post-Graduate Medical School; Assistant Editor, RUDOLF L. BAER, M.D., Assistant Attending Physician, Skin and Cancer Unit, New York Post-Graduate Hospital. *The Year Book Publishers, Inc.*, 304 S. Dearborn St., Chicago. $3.00.

The editors consider that the year just past has seen signal advances in this specialty, and are enthusiastic as to future advances.

In the section devoted to Investigative (surely a more acceptable term than Experimental) Studies, many of us will be surprised to see several articles on the toxicity of tannic acid; to learn that sulfonamides may be absorbed by the intact skin, and that a group of patients with severe acne tended to show weaker tuberculin reactions than did patients with mild acne.

The admirable coverage of the field entitles the book to a place among your books for daily use.

STROPHANTHIN: Clinical and Experimental Experiences of the Past 25 Years, by BRUNO KISCH, M.D., Formerly on the Medical Faculty of Cologne University (Germany), Visiting Professor to the International University in Santander (Spain), Research Fellow at Yale University. *Brooklyn Medical Press*, New York City, 1944. $4.00.

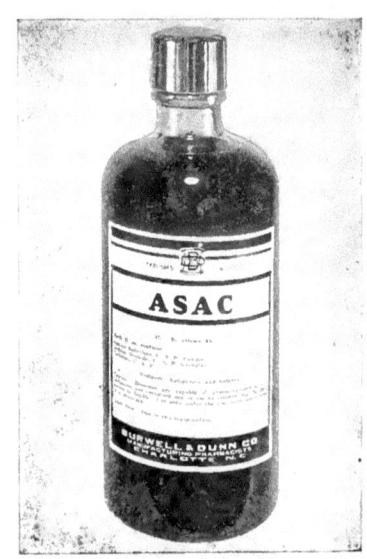

ASAC

15% by volume Alcohol

Each fl. oz. contains:

Sodium Salicylate, U. S. P. Powder........40 grains
Sodium Bromide, U. S. P. Granular........20 grains
Caffeine, U. S. P. ....4 grains

ANALGESIC, ANTIPYRETIC AND SEDATIVE.

Average Dosage

Two to four teaspoonfuls in one to three ounces of water as prescribed by the physician.

How Supplied

In Pints, Five Pints and Gallons to Physicians and Druggists.

Burwell & Dunn Company

Manufacturing   *Pharmacists*
Established   *in 1887*

CHARLOTTE, N. C.

The purpose of the author is to urge the profession of this country to reconsider the subject of the clinical usefulness of strophanthin. The reader is reminded of the esteem in which the drug is held on the continent of Europe and in England, and much evidence is adduced to show that strophanthin deserves a better reputation than it bears with us.

The book opens with a historical note. Then follow chapters on the drug's chemical nature, the history of its modern clinical use, its pharmacology, and its general and special clinical application.

Among the concluding remarks, in which the reviewer concurs:

In many cases it [strophanthin] cannot be replaced effectively by any other treatment.

An obligation exists for every physician to become acquainted with this life-saving treatment.

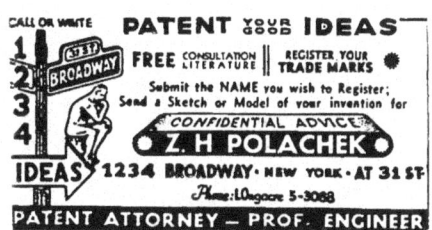

Obesity....!

FHJ
THYRAMINE

Composition

Thyroid I gr. Amphetamine sulphate 5 mgs. Thiamin chloride 1 mg. in suitable combinations with physiological reinforcements.

No. 1—One Capsule before breakfast
No. 2—One Capsule before lunch
No. 3—One Capsule at 4 p. m.

Contraindications
Hypertension .... Hyperthyroidism

Supplied
Capsules: Packages 21 and 42 (one or two weeks supply).

—Professional samples on request—
Available: Any professional pharmacy
F. H. J. PRODUCTS
977 East 76th St., New York 60, N. Y.

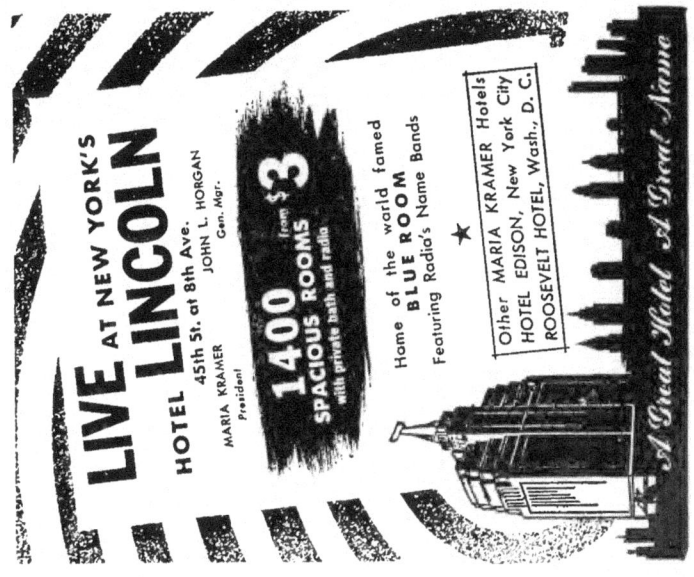

NEUROLOGY and PSYCHIATRY

(*Now in the Country's Service*)
*J. FRED MERRITT, M.D.
NERVOUS and MILD MENTAL DISEASES
ALCOHOL and DRUG ADDICTIONS
Glenwood Park Sanitarium   Greensboro

TOM A. WILLIAMS, M.D.
(*Neurologist of Washington, D. C.*)
Consultation by appointment at
Phone 3994-W
77 Kenilworth Ave.   Asheville, N. C.

EYE, EAR, NOSE AND THROAT

H. C. NEBLETT, M.D.
OCULIST
Phone 3-5852
Professional Bldg.   Charlotte

AMZI J. ELLINGTON, M.D.
DISEASES of the EYE, EAR, NOSE and THROAT
Phones: Office 992—Residence 761
Burlington   North Carolina

THOMAS H. HALSTED, M.D., F.A.C.S.
Otologist
Practice limited to the Selection and Fitting of Hearing Aids. Hours 9:30-4:30 daily. Saturday 9:30-1:00. By appointment. 475 Fifth Avenue (Cor. 41st St.), New York City. Phone LE. 2-3427.

UROLOGY, DERMATOLOGY and PROCTOLOGY

THE CROWELL CLINIC of UROLOGY and UROLOGICAL SURGERY
Hours—Nine to Five   Telephones—3-7101—3-7102
STAFF
ANDREW J. CROWELL, M.D.
(1911-1938)
*ANGUS M. MCDONALD, M.D.   CLAUDE B. SQUIRES, M.D.
Suite 700-711 Professional Building   Charlotte

RAYMOND THOMPSON, M.D., F.A.C.S.   WALTER E. DANIEL, A.B., M.D.
THE THOMPSON-DANIEL CLINIC
of
UROLOGY & UROLOGICAL SURGERY
Fifth Floor Professional Bldg.   Charlotte

C. C. MASSEY, M.D.
PRACTICE LIMITED TO DISEASES OF THE RECTUM
Professional Bldg.   Charlotte

WYETT F. SIMPSON, M.D.
GENITO-URINARY DISEASES
Phone 1234
Hot Springs National Park   Arkansas

ORTHOPEDICS

HERBERT F. MUNT, M.D.
ACCIDENT SURGERY & ORTHOPEDICS FRACTURES
Nissen Building   Winston-Salem

THE JOURNAL OF
SOUTHERN MEDICINE AND SURGERY

306 North Tryon Street, Charlotte, N. C.

The Journal assumes no responsibility for authenticity of opinion or statements made by authors or in communications submitted to this Journal for publication.

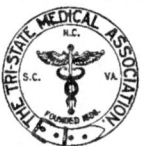

JAMES M. NORTHINGTON, M. D., Editor

VOL. CVI   APRIL, 1944   No. 4

Medicine in China*

RANDOLPH T. SHIELDS, M.D., Chapel Hill, North Carolina
University of North Carolina, School of Medicine
Formerly Cheeloo University, School of Medicine, Shantung, China

IT MAY BE OF INTEREST to mention early Chinese Medicine beginning with the legendary Emperor Sheng Ming in the 29th Century B. C. and the Emperor Huang Ti 200 years later. The latter is supposed to have written of the diagnostic value of the pulse and is said to have described acupuncture. Medicine at that time was mixed up with religion, doctor and priest being the same individual as was the case with other primitive peoples. In the Chou Dynasty, 12th century B. C., medicine was still dominated by philosophic speculations. In the middle of this dynasty (500-300 B. C.) Lao Tze, Confucius and Mencius, the greatest Chinese philosophers, lived. During this period the "science" of medicine was mixed up with the principles of "yin" and "yang." All the universe is made up by the union of "yin" and "yang." All life consists of "yin" and "yang" principles. Some organs of the body are "yin" and others "yang," and therefore diseases are classified as "yin" and "yang" diseases. In addition to "yin" and "yang," the "five elements"—metal, wood, water, fire, earth—all entered into the composition of all substances. The body was a harmonious mixture of the five elements. It is interesting to note that the Nei Ching, or canon of medicine, states that "the heart regulates all the blood of the body" and "that the blood flows continuously in a circle and never stops." In these ancient times there was evidently an attempt to divide doctors into physicians and surgeons and there is a suggestion of preventive medicine in the sentence "the sage does not treat those ill, but those well." In the Han Dynasty, 206 B. C.-220 A. D., there were physicians whose names are revered today. They used drugs, acupuncture, and hydrotherapy.

Hua T'o, often called the God of Surgeons, was credited with a great many operations and the use of anesthesia, probably species of datura, aconite or other herbs. Acupuncture has been practiced from ancient times and is now used extensively by the old-style doctors. It is said to have been used also in Japan and to have been introduced into Europe in the 17th century. Was it brought to Europe from China? Inoculation for smallpox with human virus has been practiced by the Chinese since 1,000 A. D. In 656 A. D. the Emperor appointed a committee of 22 to revise the ancient "Pen Tsao Ching," or materia medica, and they produced a work of 53 volumes. The study of materia medica then must have been as difficult and unsatisfactory as it was when I was a student.

Medicine was one of the many phases of Chinese culture which greatly influenced the other nations of Asia. Translations of books were made in Japan and one of these of 982 A. D. is said to be the oldest book in Japan. The coming of Buddhism into China in 67 A. D. brought many medical as well as new religious ideas to be mixed in with the Taoist practices of incantations, magic, etc. Medical schools were set up in the T'ang Dynasty (619-907 A. D.) Though there may have been

*Presented to Tri-State Medical Association of the Carolinas and Virginia, meeting at Charlotte, Feb. 28th-29th, 1944.

ethical standards at first, they were apparently lost sight of. Old women and incompetent men took up medicine as a business and there were no government regulations to control them. There has been a decline in medicine since the Ming Dynasty (1368-1662 A. D.) In recent times anyone might prescribe drugs, which are accessible in the old style shops dealing in various preparations of animal, vegetable or mineral origins.

But we are interested more in recent medicine. A Jesuit, Father Ricci, introduced medicine along with science and religion and Kang Hsi the Emperor (1655-1723 A. D.) was cured of malaria by quinine. But modern medicine really began in 1805 when Dr. Pearson of the East India Company came to Canton. Dr. Livingstone of the East India Company helped Morrison, the first Protestant missionary, by opening a small dispensary. In 1834 Dr. Peter Parker, a Yale graduate, went out as the first medical misionary and following him there were 195 medical missionaries up to 1890. The work these men did in the face of ignorance, conservatism and indifference, if not active opposition, is something of which our profession can be proud. They built hospitals, treated an increasing number of patients, trained assistants and made books. They laid the foundations upon which it was possible to make the great advances which have been made by their successors. When I went to China in 1905 there were a number of so-called medical schools in the larger hospitals, and they did a very fine job and turned out many efficient physicians and surgeons. But 40 years ago there were probably not a dozen properly qualified Chinese doctors who had studied abroad, and so far as I know there was not a single Chinese nurse, although there were more or less efficient orderlies, men and old women.

The Peiping Union Medical College was started by several missionary societies in 1906. As you may know, it was taken over by the Rockefeller Foundation in 1916 and became the outstanding medical school of the East (until Pearl Harbor). Other schools were started or improved in the next few years, and medical education along with the development of better hospitals and clinical work went forward rapidly. In these early years practically all modern medicine was in the hands of medical missionaries. There were a few foreign practitioners in some of the ports, and as I have said a very few Chinese.

By the early 1920's six Protestant mission medical schools were in existence. The full-time faculties of these schools were small, but so also were the student bodies. The undergraduate instruction would compare favorably with that given in schools in this country. Our School of Medicine of Cheeloo University, Tsinan, Shantung, in 1937 had a staff of 34, 18 of whom were Chinese, five being heads of departments, and nearly 400 M.D.'s had been graduated in a period of 20 years. There was the Rockefeller Foundation School in Peiping; the British Government had a school in Hongkong, and the Japanese one in Mukden. By this time there were many Chinese doctors trained locally and abroad and the government was setting up schools faster than they could man and equip them. By 1937 two or three had grown to be very good schools. To go back a few years—in 1886 the Chinese Medical Missionary Association was formed and by 1915 there were enough young Chinese doctors to start the National Medical Association. By mutual agreement these bodies remained separate until 1932 when they both went out of existence, and then united to become the Chinese Medical Association. A fine example of real international coöperation. A few figures will help to bring out some important facts. In 1935 there were 230 missionary hospitals which employed 325 foreign doctors and 500 Chinese doctors, 270 foreign nurses, approximately 1,000 Chinese graduate nurses and 4,000 student nurses. Dr. Sze, Secretary of the Chinese Medical Association, now in Washington, says in his book published in 1943 that there are 310 hospitals in China, of which 235 are Protestant mission hospitals and 60 Government hospitals. Dr. Lennox, now of Harvard, made a survey in 1931 for "Fact Finders" and reported that there were 178,000 in-patients treated annually by mission hospitals and that there were 3,000,000 treatments given in the out-patient departments. Dr. Sze thinks there are now approximately 12,000 doctors (half of whom are well trained), and 38,000 hospital beds in the whole of China.

There is no need to emphasize the medical needs in China. Great progress was being made by the Chinese Government, with the coöperation of medical missionaries, in public health, health education, and the training of midwives. It was an encouraging picture and though of course there was room for improvement, real and rapid progress was being made. And then the Japanese attacked Peiping on July 7th, 1937, and the work was broken up in the East. Most doctors and educators have gone west and set up as well as they could their old institutions, separately or united *pro tem.* with others.

I will now say something about the diseases of China, many of which are also found in the United States. All three forms of malaria are very prevalent in the southern and central parts of the country, but there is very little of it in the north. I lived in the Yangste Valley for twelve years so saw something of the worst malarial area. The plasmodium falciparum was very common and the mortality from the malaria it transmitted was high.

That was before the days of atabrin or plasmochin, but we used intravenous quinine on cerebral cases which is still considered the best treatment.

Tuberculosis is very prevalent throughout the country. General vital statistics do not exist, but I have figures for two cities, Peiping in the north and Hongkong in the south, where the mortality was estimated to be well over 300 per 100,000. Carefully recorded statistics from various mission hospitals ten years ago gave the incidence of tuberculosis in all hospital patients as approximately 5 per cent. Respiratory and non-respiratory were about equally divided. It is interesting to note that there is no evidence that any of the tuberculosis in China is of the bovine type. The ordinary textbook statement that children are infected by drinking tuberculous milk is absolutely not true in China. Until very recent years practically no children drank any milk except their mother's.

The incidence of heart and arterial diseases is probably not as high as it is in this country, but I have not been able to get the facts on this. Rheumatic fever I think is not so prevalent but one sees arthritis in the clinics. The ordinary contagious diseases of childhood are about as they are in this country, but smallpox is much more common. Gradually vaccination is lowering its incidence. Syphilis and gonorrhea are fairly common, but I cannot give you any comparative statistics. Of course there are more untreated cases of syphilis than one would see here.

Rabies is more common than it is in the United States because there is practically no legal control of dogs. I have personally known a number of people who died of this disease. Tetanus is common and large numbers of infants die of it in their first two weeks of life. This is due to the methods used by the midwives in cutting the cord. I had one post-partum case, infected by a midwife, die of tetanus.

It has been estimated that there are a million lepers in China. There are special endemic areas in various parts of the country, but it is a disease that anyone practicing in China must be prepared to meet in his clinic. We had connected with our hospital one of the few leprosaria. The treatment of this disease is very unsatisfactory. Some claim a number of cures with chaulmoogra oil esters, but few doctors will discharge patients as more than "apparently cured." Some authorities consider the environmental conditions, food, exercise, etc., as more important factors in the treatment than the chemical.

Dysentery, both bacillary and amebic, are found in all parts of the country. There are other diseases which are practically non-existent in the United States. Cholera is endemic in many areas and breaks out in epidemics every now and then. I have never seen anything more dramatic than the resuscitation of apparently moribund cases by large quantities of intravenous saline. Cholera vaccine is now considered to be helpful and is used very generally. Kala azar is found in several areas in North China, and in these areas the percentage of infected cases is very large, making it one of the most serious diseases to be combatted. Though a great deal of work has been done on this disease, up to the present I think there is no positive evidence as to the method of transmission. The Phlebotomus, or sand fly, has been the suspect. The geographical distribution of this disease is difficult to explain. Untreated and constantly reinfected cases probably all die. Years ago the treatment was by intravenous sodium antimony tartrate, which was very effective but painful, and not without danger. In recent years the use of neo-stibosan and other antimony drugs has greatly improved the treatment and cut down the time of it from a few months to weeks. There are almost no complications and cases that are not too far gone can be cured. Schistosoma japonicum, the blood fluke, is very common in the Yangste Valley, but is practically never found north of the Yangste River, as Kala azar is never found south of the river. This disease presents one of the big public health problems of central China, similar to the problem that Egypt has with Schistosoma haematobium. The difficulty of course is with the snail which is the intermediate host of the fluke. Various drugs have been tried and I notice that fuadin has been advocated.

Typhus fever is endemic and is liable to break into epidemic proportions whenever there are famine conditions. So far as I know the type in China is the Asiatic variety which is carried by lice and has a heavy mortality rate. Relapsing fever is not so serious from the standpoint of mortality. It is also louse-borne. In South China bubonic plague is fairly common. In the north there is occasionally the pneumonic form brought from Manchuria, and primary pneumonic is fatal in every case. The organism is the same, Pasteurella pestis, and starts from rat fleas. In the north it seems to have a predilection for the lungs, and if the lungs are affected no rat flea is needed to disseminate the disease.

Probably all of the helminths found in North America are also found in China. Ascaris is common everywhere and unusual conditions sometimes arise from these infestations. Hookworm is common in the south and the Yangste Valley where the temperature and moisture are suitable for development, but it is very rare in the dry north. Clonorchis sinensis, a liver fluke, is common in cats and sometimes in dogs in the south-central portions of the country, but human infestations are rare, as the Chinese as a rule cook their fish, which is the second intermediate host of the fluke. Fasciolopsis buski, an intestinal fluke, is very common in a limited area in central China. The second intermediate host is the water nut. Infestation is often very heavy but the mortality is not high. Filariasis from Wuchereria bancrofti is very common in the south-central portion of the country but unknown in the far north. Diseases due to vitamin deficiencies are fairly widespread. Shansi Province in the northwest is notorious for osteomalacia. I have no statistics on malignant tumors, but my impression is that they are certainly as common as they are in the United States. China has not had yellow fever. The diagnosis of some of these diseases, especially malignant malaria and kala azar, may become of practical importance in U. S. A.

This paper is not supposed to be concerned with the war, but a word might be said in regard to it. You all know the general facts, and that after nearly seven years the Japanese hold only the ports and other important cities and the railway lines. Chinese regular troops or guerrillas are operating even now near the coast. The two puppet governments in the north and the south have very little authority and I am sure that large numbers of those who make up these governments are at heart patriotic, and are only acting as puppets due to force and the necessity for self-preservation. The Japanese method of conquest is based on terrorism and destruction of industries, especially of education. I am sure that all of the atrocity stories of which you have heard are essentially true, but you must know that the treatment of different cities varied tremendously. Where the Japanese did not have to fight to capture a city the place was occupied with very little disturbance of the usual life of the people. Where they had to fight they usually turned the captured city over to their soldiers to do as they pleased. I could give you many instances of brutal treatment, and I could also give you a very few instances where the Japanese have showed a kindly spirit. But one thing I would like to emphasize—we cannot predict what the reaction of the Japanese is going to be in any particular circumstance that may arise. Their actions are motivated by "face," and by the defense mechanism of an inferiority complex. Are they going to continue to fight to the last man? And what is going to be their attitude towards the prisoners whom they hold when their own situation becomes more desperate? Many of us are deeply concerned over this last question, and I sincerely hope that no hot-headed acts are going to be perpetrated in our country which will react in endangering the safety of allied prisoners. I am sure our government realizes the importance of fair treatment of Japs in this country.

Discussion

VICE-PRESIDENT PACE (presiding): I don't know whether any of you have been to China or not. The paper is now open for discussion.

DR. KARL SCHAFFLE (Asheville): I'd like to ask if hypertension is seen extensively in China, and if so, if it is due to some racial disease or if it is environmental or hereditary?

DR. SHIELDS: My impression is that it is not nearly as common as in this country. I know the average blood pressure is 'way below what it is in this country. I have never, in all my thirty-seven years in China, seen pipestem arteries like I saw at Blackwell's Island when I was a boy in medicine.

DR. SCHAFFLE: What about nervous diseases?

DR. SHIELDS: I don't know whether the proportion is greater than in this country or not. I doubt it. Nothing was done for insanity until the missionaries went in and established schools and hospitals.

ICE AS A LOCAL ANESTHETIC
(H. H. Friederwitzer, Bronx, N. Y., in *Med. Rec.*, Jan.)

Whether or not the area is infected, ice is an indicated anesthetic that does not tend to spread infection. Its first action of cold causes an ischemia of the area involved, prevents a spread of the infection, as well as freezing the nerve endings of the epidermis.

For home use, or emergencies, or when the area is badly infected and an injection of novocaine is unwise, or where ethyl chloride causes too much pain because of its burning sensations, ice is the method of choice for anesthesia.

I have found ice to be useful in the following types of cases:

1. Infected toenails: Keep ice in sterile gauze to a previously sterilized skin for 20 min.
2. Carbuncle or boil: Ice works best in these cases; keep ice on area for 20 min.
3. Paronychia: Keep ice on for 10 min.
4. Dislocations of wrists, fingers and elbow: Keep ice on area with little pressure for 20-30 min.
5. Abscess anywhere on or near the skin surface. Keep ice on area 15 to 20 min.
6. Skin growths (nevi and the like): Keep ice on area for 10 min. and remove growth by knife or cautery.

MORTON'S METATARSALGIA
(L. D. Baker & H. H. Kuhn, Durham, in *Sou. Med. Jl.*, Mar.)

Neuralgic pain in the fourth metatarso-phalangeal articulation, usually more prevalent in women, in the early stages a burning sensation in the region of the fourth metatarsal head, which may radiate into the adjacent sides of the third and fourth toes and may be accompanied by paresthesia and numbness constitute the syndrome. In the more severe cases there is a sharp sudden pain usually while walking with the shoe on, radiates to the outer three toes, relieved or lessened by the removal of the shoe and the manipulation of the forefoot. By exerting firm pressure over the third web space one may at times feel a mass and may initiate severe pain. In the cases reported, deep pressure over the tumor did not reproduce the syndrome, but an area of great tenderness has been present in every case.

Three of the patients had bilateral pain. Of the 11 patients, 10 were females.

The characteristic history of the syndrome and a localized tenderness to deep palpation in the third web space or between the third and fourth metatarsal heads on the dorsal surface make the diagnosis simple. Excision of the tumor relieves the symptoms.

The Pituitary in Relation to Neuropsychiatry*

BEVERLEY R. TUCKER, M.D., Richmond, Virginia
Physician in Chief to Tucker Hospital

MY FIRST ACQUAINTANCE with the hypophysis, or pituitary body, was at medical college when one of the professors told us that it was situated in the sella turcica (Turkish saddle) in the sphenoid bone at the base of the brain. He said the function was unknown, but that the ancients considered it the seat of the soul. He remarked that it was situated in the most protected part of the human anatomy and, therefore, must be of considerable importance. Then and there my interest was aroused, and I determined to try to find out something about it.

Next, in Philadelphia, when I was working under Dr. Weir Mitchell in 1905-1906, I learned that one of his recent disciples, Dr. Guy Hinsdale, had won the Boylston Prize for an essay on the pituitary body. At the Infirmary for Nervous Diseases in 1906 we had a case of acromegaly, Marie's disease, who had not only the enlarged features and extremities common to these cases, but clavicles measuring several inches in breadth and a spine six inches wide in the cervical region. Acromegaly is due to a hyperfunction of the pituitary, especially the anterior lobe, after the epiphyses are closed and causes enlargement of flat and short bones as well as of concomitant soft tissues. Longcope once very well described the hands in these cases as having the appearance of "gloves filled with dough."

Acromegaly usually occurs in middle age. It has been my experience that as the anterior lobe is enlarging, frequently the posterior lobe is compressed and symptoms of lowered blood pressure, low blood sugar, and emotionality may occur. At times, at any age, a pituitary tumor or neighborhood tumor pressing on the sella may cause symptoms resembling acromegaly.

On the other extreme, occurs Simmond's disease in which there is a hypofunction of the anterior lobe in the adult with emaciation, cachexia, loss of body hair, amenorrhea in the female, and, in either sex, temperature, blood pressure, blood sugar, basal rate, pulse rate are all low and poor appetite and insomnia occur. These cases are often mistaken for food deficiency diseases.

Hypopituitary obesity is due to adult hypofunction of the posterior lobe and is marked by great increase in shoulder girdle and pelvic girdle fat with huge, fat, pendulous abdomens. It is probably connected with, but should not be confused with, adiposis dolorosa, Dercum's disease, in which more or less the same areas are marked by cakes and rolls of fat very painful to pressure and there is often a low grade neuritis caused by a combination of syphilis and alcoholism.

In early life a deficiency of the anterior lobe secretion coupled with gonadotropic difficulty produces a condition known as dystrophia adiposis genitalia, or Frölich's syndrome, in which the child is undersized, fat, slow in development, often defective, and has infantile type of genitals.

Pituitary tumors usually give varying symptoms of anterior or posterior lobe disturbance and can only be barely mentioned here. Attention should be called to the fact that many of them, because of upward growth, give pressure symptoms on the optic chiasm with, usually, bitemporal hemianopia.

There are many less obvious conditions due to pituitary disturbances, which we shall now briefly consider.

From 5 to 8 per cent of all cases of recurrent convulsions have hypopituitarism as the causative factor. In 1914 I published a paper on hypopituitary convulsions and later gave three criteria for their diagnosis:

1. First attacks appearing during the extreme ages of adolescence—9 to 25 years.
2. X-ray evidence of lessened capacity of the sella turcica.
3. Clinical evidence of hypopituitarism.

There might also be added a fourth dimension—the therapeutic test of pituitary feeding.

In 1933 in a paper reviewing 500 pituitary cases, 104 cases were classified as hypopituitary recurrent convulsions.

Personality Traits.—Certain racial characteristics may be connected with personality changes. There is a considerable difference in the shape of the sella turcica in the white, negro, red and yellow races. War and other difficulties have prevented me from carrying out certain studies I had started in x-ray measurements of the sella in the American Indian, the Chinese, the Japanese and in the Malayan races.

The study of the measurement of the sella in fowl and animals is confusing—I have studied a good many. For instance, the elephant has a smaller and the duck a larger sella than might be ex-

*Presented to Tri-State Medical Association of the Carolinas and Virginia, meeting at Charlotte, Feb. 28th-29th, 1944.

pected. In the human race the shape and size of the sella has a direct relationship to the size of the individual and to the measurements of the head.

The normal sella in an Anglo-Saxon adult should be from 14 to 15 mm. in length, 9 to 10 mm. in height, and 4 to 5 mm. between the clinoid processes. A confusing factor is that at times distinct clinical evidence of hypopituitarism may be observed with an average sized sella and occasionally the same is true of hyperpituitarism. This is due to over or under secretion of the bodies without concurrent bony conformation. Then, too, it is difficult from sella studies alone to estimate the influence of deformed and erroded sellas.

The usual clinical signs of hypopituitarism are shoulder girdle and pelvic girdle excess of fat, rather tapering, flexible fingers, spaced teeth, high arched palate, lowered blood pressure, blood sugar, and pulse rate, lessened body hair and smooth skin, also upper temporal restriction of the visual fields.

The chief signs of hyperpituitarism are excessive length of long bones giving increased height, large teeth, hyperactivity, and sexuality, and at times giantism but with muscular weakness.

The pituitary is the chief gland whose secretion changes, in adolescence, the youth into the adult. It must be remembered that its changed secretion which accomplishes this transition is often transitory and that the secretion may be either hypo-, hyper-, or chemico-hormonic. The latter is designated dyspituitarism.

The pituitary during adolescence is the lead horse of the endocrine system, and its changed secretion may cause personality change, as I have previously shown, or conduct disturbance or psychoses to both of which I have also called attention in the past. I have seen truancy, hoboism, dishonesty, sex aberrations, slothfulness, hyper-excitability, lying, and asocialness corrected during adolescence by treatment directed toward regulation of the pituitary secretion.

Twice I have been called to hold commissions of lunacy on adolescents who showed clinical evidence of hypopituitarism. I asked for a postponement of the commission and had the satisfaction of seeing the psychosis clear up in a few weeks in both instances with pituitary feeding. There have been many more or less striking examples. Recently I have had a young woman who had been in a state mental hospital for two years for supposed schizophrenic insanity and who, after she was brought to us, failed to recover with shock therapy but on pituitary and thyroid extract recovered and is now holding a responsible position.

Attention should be called to the bitemporal headaches first described by Pardee, which quickly responds to pituitary (whole gland) administration, and to diabetes insipidus which frequently adjusts under pituitary feeding. Somnolence and narcolepsy are often due to a combination of hypopituitarism with hypothyroidism and hypoglycemia. Also amenorrhea in the young female may yield to pituitary medication alone. Many cases of obesity, especially of the shoulder and pelvic girdles, yield only to pituitary administration. Aggressiveness and hypersexuality in selected cases subside under x-ray flashes to the pituitary.

Pituitary extract may be given in various forms and by various routes and for various purposes. These extracts are frequently given incorrectly. Pitressin is useful in surgical shock, obstetrics, and in diabetes insipidus—it is the pressor extract of the posterior lobe. Pitocine, a posterior lobe extract without the pressor substance, is used in undersecretion of the posterior lobe especially for the reduction of pelvic and shoulder girdle fat and to constrict the uterus. Pituitrin S (anterior pituitary-like sex hormone) is used in amenorrhea and sexual underdevelopment and antuitrin (anterior lobe extract) to stimulate growth. These preparations are given intramuscularly.

Anterior lobe, posterior lobe and whole gland extracts are also made in tablet form. Some clinicians, arbitrarily I think, decry the oral administration of these. But there is no reason that I know of which justifies this view. My experience is that they are exceedingly effective by mouth and save the patients much running back and forth to the doctor's office and also much expense. There is no reason why pituitary extract given by mouth is not as effective as thyroid extract given by mouth. I fear sometimes that we lean too much to the prick of the needle and not enough to the prick of the conscience.

Addenda

Cushing called attention to convulsions occurring in animals and human beings who had partial extirpations of the pituitary. In 1913 he suggested to me that I might investigate the presence of signs of hypopituitarism in epileptic cases. This I did and my first and further publications are as follows:

A Preliminary Discussion of Pituitary Disturbance as Related to Some Cases of Epilepsy, Psychoses, Personality and Other Obscure Problems. *Jour. So. Med. Assn.*, Vol. V, No. 8, August, 1914.

Hypopituitarism in Its Relation to Epilepsy. *Va. Med. Semi-Monthly*, April 7th, 1914.

Pituitary Disturbance in Its Relation to the Psychoses of Adolescence. *Jour. Am. Med. Assn.*, Vol 71, August 3rd, 1918.

The Role of the Pituitary Gland in Epilepsy. *Archives of Neurology and Psychiatry*, Vol. 11, August, 1919.

Therapeutic Uses of Pituitary Gland Substance. *Medical Record*, August 20th, 1921.

Some Hypopituitary States. *S. Med. & Surgery*, September, 1921.

Consideration of the Classification of Recurrent Convulsions. *So. Med. Jour.*, Vol. 14, No. 11, November, 1921.

Internal Secretions in Their Relationship to Mental Disturbance. *Amer. Jour. of Psychiatry*, Vol. 11, No. 2, October, 1922.

A Resumé of 500 Consecutive Pituitary Cases Occurring in General Neurological Practice. *Va. Med. Monthly*, June, 1934.

Hence the present is my tenth paper on the relation of the pituitary gland to various nervous and mental diseases.

Discussion

DR. R. BURKE SUITT, Duke University Medical School: I am sure that those of us who have been fortunate in being able to attend today consider ourselves particularly so in having heard this paper by Dr. Tucker, likewise to look to the time when this appears in the Journal of the Association so that we may review what we have heard and share this with others.

After so comprehensive a presentation I think it natural that any discussant is properly inhibited; this should be particularly so of one whose perspectives in approaches to these disorders is somewhat limited.

In considering any case where one suspects pituitary dysfunction we need to take into account anatomical and/or physiological symptoms, along with the behaviour, and those things which come from the clinical laboratory, as responsible in sending the individual case to a physician.

With this framework we are able to distinguish with fair clarity those conditions in which the pituitary is architecturally involved, directly or through disturbances in neighboring structures; with the aid of the neurosurgeon and the radiologist we can soon have a diagnosis closely followed by effective teratment for a given patient.

Those syndromes in which the pituitary is primarily disordered in elaboration of secretion are certainly not so readily identified, nor in the same high percentage, in other than classical instances. In this connection, I think that Dr. Tucker's comments with reference to the therapeutic use of endocrine preparations might very helpfully include his thinking and practices in treating premenstrual tension in adult life. As a fairly clear-cut entity, this syndrome not infrequently plays a role in bringing a patient to the physician or to the neuropsychiatrist.

I think it is interesting, in passing on to the less well-known things in which the pituitary position is involved, to call attention to the commonplace way in which some patients whose complaints are considered "purely mental" respond to specific experiences, localizing them in "the seat of the soul," with outstanding fear of an anatomical significance which does not exist, as perhaps best illustrated in the psycholeptic attack.

DR. J. W. WATTS (Washington): It was my impression that while enlarged sella was significant of pituitary tumor or tumor in the neighborhood of the pituitary, a small sella had no significance at all, and I know that I have had patients sent in who have what is called bridging of the sella and the question came up whether that had any significance as to cause of headache or some other symptom, and again it was my impression that it had no significance, and I'd like to ask that you say a little bit more about that, Dr. Tucker.

DR. JAMES ASA SHIELD (Richmond): Those of us who have had the privilege of working with Dr. Tucker have been impressed with the results that he has been able to obtain, particularly in these youngsters who have recurring attacks and those youngsters who have personality disturbances, and the other group is in adolescence that he has been able to get definite results with pituitary.

Today we have heard a pioneer in pituitary study talk to us. He published the first paper on pituitary convulsions, the first paper on pituitary personality variations, and one of the first papers on pituitary in the psychotic, and it has been a real privilege to have heard his presentation.

DR. TUCKER (closing): I want to thank these gentlemen.

In regard to this first question about an adult woman's menstrual tension, I think I am wise enough to pass the buck. I usually refer those cases to Dr. Rucker. I have gotten some lessening of the disagreeable menstrual features by various forms of pituitary administration, but I think my failures would outstrip my results.

Then in regards to Dr. Watts' question, if I understand him right, I said that as a rule the pituitary tumors had large sellas. That has been my experience. Although we have seen pituitary tumors with small sellas, the ones we have had operated on turned out to be suprapituitary cysts, as a rule.

I certainly appreciate what Dr. Shield said, but he is a prejudiced witness. Many others have done more work on the pituitary than I have. I happened to get into the game early because of Dr. Cushing. In 1913 he asked me to go back and gather up the epileptics I had as patients, and see if there were any x-ray disturbances of sella or other clinical evidence. Many of them have gotten well with pituitary findings. If we follow the criteria I gave, convulsions will cease in the majority of the cases.

Thank you.

TREATMENT OF MENINGOCOCCAL MENINGITIS WITH SULFADIAZINE AND SULFAMERAZINE (SULFAMETHYLDIAZINE)
(M. H. Lepper & E. D. Stanley, Washington, in *Med. An. D. C.*, Feb.)

In the treatment of meningococcal meningitis adequate doses of sulfadiazine or sulfamerazine seem equally effective.

Well chosen laboratory examinations are to be made, fluids as indicated, lumbar puncture if needed, and serum in a limited number of cases.

With this therapy 140 cases have been treated with 15 deaths (10.7 per cent). The average duration of fever was 2.8 days. Nerve palsies have persisted in nine cases, six of whom are deaf.

Age and the presence or absence of coma are two of the most important clinical factors in determining prognosis, whereas the number of organisms and level of sugar in the spinal fluid are the laboratory tests of most value.

VACCINATION AGAINST INFLUENZA VALUABLE
(By Members of the Com. on Influenza, Office of the Surgeon General, U. S. A., in *Jl. A. M. A.*, April 1st)

In the autumn of 1943 members of the Commission on Influenza, and associates U. S. Army, undertook a controlled clinical trial of the prophylactic efficacy against epidemic influenza of a concentrated, inactivated vaccine containing the viruses of influenza types A and B.

The influence of subcutaneous inoculation of a concentrated inactivated vaccine on the incidence of clinical influenza in a series of 12,500 men was studied during the recent epidemic of influenza A. Vaccination done shortly before or even after the onset of the epidemic was found to exert a protective effect with a total attack rate of 2.22% among the 6,263 vaccinated, and 7.11% among the 6,211 controls, a ratio of 1 to 3.2. The influence of vaccine was most clearly evident at the height of the epidemic prevalences. The duration of the effect has not been determined.

Neurophysiological Aspects of Gastrointestinal Function: Practical Psychosomatic Considerations*

FREDERICK H. HESSER, M.D., Durham

THE increasingly popular term "psychosomatic medicine" has been an outgrowth of the realization that general medicine and neuropsychiatry must work hand in hand in terms of structure and function as we expand our knowledge of the central nervous system and its role in regulating biological activity. The concept is not a new one, and the holistic psychobiological approach, sponsored by Adolf Meyer, embodies its fundamental principles. Essentially, therefore, all medicine becomes psychosomatic medicine as soon as the physician sees the patient in entirety as an individual capable of certain emotional reactions and more or less able to adjust to his various problems. Potentially, the most skillful student of psychosomatics is the experienced practitioner who "knows" his patients and treats them accordingly.

Perhaps no field of internal medicine has offered a better opportunity for psychosomatic investigation than that of gastroenterology. The interest of man in his stomach is obviously compelled by the constant source of satisfaction and great sense of security that organ can provide on the one hand, and by the many complaints it can produce on the other. In recent years, knowledge of gastrointestinal function and its regulation has improved tremendously with the expansion of study techniques. Neurophysiology, in particular, has provided noteworthy contributions.

The concept of "levels of function," propounded largely by Hughlings Jackson, has been applied to the visceral as well as to the somatic divisions of the nervous system. Hence, "visceral function" must be regulated at different levels of increasing complexity and has been shown to involve even the highest cortical levels in the neuraxis. Our understanding of the part played by the autonomic nervous system with its arbitrary division into sympathetic and parasympathetic must, therefore, be retained according to the concept of "levels of integration" rather than in terms of sympathetic or parasympathetic influence. The position of the hypothalamus, as the autonomic relay station, has been substantiated. Hence, the posterior hypothalamus contains predominantly sympathetic representation; the middle and anterior nuclei are predominantly parasympathetic. The function integrated clearly involves both systems with all levels of the hypothalamus subject to regulation at thalamic, striatal, and cortical levels. There is ample reason to feel that the ability of the individual to adjust to his environment and to regulate his primitive instincts and emotions accordingly is intimately associated with the performance of these structures. Hence, any studies that would contribute to our knowledge of their relation to organ function would necessarily have profound psychosomatic significance.

Experimental studies on animals, employing stimulation and ablation techniques, have provided ample evidence of gastrointestinal as well as vasomotor, vesical and many other forms of autonomic representation in the cerebral cortex. Time is insufficient to enter into an adequate discussion of these. A few examples drawn from the literature and from our own work may be of interest.

In 1876, Bochefontaine stimulated the dog's sigmoid gyrus and produced gastric contraction, pyloric relaxation, and increased peristalsis in the small intestine and colon. The more recent work of Watts and Fulton (1935) gave evidence that cortical representation for the gastrointestinal tract contains both excitatory and inhibitory components. They were able to delimit the more excitable cortical foci to Area 6 in monkeys and showed that bilateral partial or complete ablation of the frontal lobes caused morbid hunger and occasionally intussusception.

Our own studies (1940) on gastric activity released from cortical control gave analogous results (lantern slides). Utilizing a balloon-tambour system, graphic studies of stomach activity in the cat were made before and after successive removal of the cerebral motor cortices. Definite alterations in gastric activity followed ablation of the motor cortices and were demonstrable as greater persistency, consistency and strength of stomach contractions along with increased tone throughout distention. This was interpreted as evidence of release from a regulating influence by the motor cortex. A marked stretch reflex with delayed relaxation of the stomach wall after sudden distention was also apparent. In the esophagus, similar changes occurred after ablation and were seen as increased wave

---
*Presented to Tri-State Medical Association of the Carolinas and Virginia, meeting at Charlotte, Feb. 28th-29th, 1944.

amplitude, regularity and persistency, and as an elevation of the tone baseline. It was felt that tone and contraction in the stomach wall were dependent primarily upon afferent stretch stimuli arising in the smooth muscle itself. We were able to correlate these studies to some extent with our earlier work (1936) on micturition released from cerebral control.

These and other data have shown that gastrointestinal representation in the cortex can be indicated both by changes in smooth muscle activity of stomach and intestines produced by faradic stimulation and by the disturbances of motility which follow bilateral ablation of the frontal region. In the latter case, hypermotility is prone to develop along with associated morbid hunger, causing the ingestion of many times the normal amount of food and failure of adequate digestion of food consumed. Furthermore, it has been shown that the representation of autonomic motor function in the cortex is closely associated topographically with that of corresponding somatic function. The existence of such dovetailing of representation makes possible an integration and unification of response, which is undoubtedly the basis of fundamental adjustments (cf. "homeostasis" of Cannon) or maladjustments of the organism and gives clues to an adequate and definitely patterned relationship between certain "mental" states and the visceral disorders which often accompany them as "functional" symptom complexes. Ultimately, these constitute many of the problems which the practitioner is called upon daily to manage. They may appear as more or less psychogenic in relation to situational or emotional difficulties or as an exaggerated admixture of complaints superimposed upon real organic disease. Most striking is the remarkable consistency in the pattern of these complaints, both in the same patient and in patients presenting similar problems. The "pattern," of course, represents real neurophysiological dysfunction, involving specific organs and definite nervous pathways. Hence, the individual's ability to adjust to psychosomatic injury depends upon the limitations of his own neurophysiological responsiveness, which can vary only according to individual constitutional and temperamental endowment.

A wide variety of clinical observations have contributed to our understanding of the nervous control of gastrointestinal function. Harvey Cushing was among the first to initiate interest in the relation of organic disease to neurophysiological dysfunction and demonstrated that stimulation of interbrain structures was conducive to the development of peptic ulcer. More recently, the studies of Wolf and Wolff (1943) have brought together even clearer evidence on the genesis of peptic ulcer in man and of the part played by the emotions.

They found that depression of acidity, motor activity and vascularity of the stomach was associated with a reaction of flight or withdrawal from an emotionally charged situation. An acceleration of these functions accompanied internal conflicts and unsatisfied aggressions. If the latter disturbances were prolonged and accompanied by marked and sustained increase in gastric motility, secretion and vascularity, a picture of gastritis resulted.

The subject of cardiospasm presents another problem which is best approached as a psychosomatic disorder. In the course of routine esophagoscopic examinations, Faulkner (1941) was able to observe esophageal spasm produced by directing the patient's attention toward his own emotional conflicts. Quite recently, Weiss (1944) reported detailed psychosomatic observations on nine cases of cardiospasm and indicated the need for combined physical and psychological study in this disease.

Other pertinent observations include those of Watts and Frazier (1935), who asserted that the abdominal aura often preceding epileptic convulsions coincides with abnormal gastrointestinal motility. The syndrome of morbid hunger and restlessness was described by M. Levin (1936) in relation to brain tumors, cerebral degenerative disease, trauma and other processes damaging the frontal cortex. A similar condition was found by P. Levin (1936) in association with cortical diplegia in children. The ravenous hunger of certain idiots and general paretics is seen frequently in state hospitals, and schizophrenic or chronic encephalitic patients may develop polyphagia some time in the course of their illness. Unfortunately, gastrointestinal motility in these cases has not been studied.

Some of our own investigations, still unpublished, have attempted to evaluate stomach activity in relation to certain diseases of the nervous system which produce lesions localizable according to levels of function. A balloon-tambour method, similar to that used in the animal experiments already described, was employed. Some evidence has been obtained to suggest a degree of hypermotility and increased response to sudden stretch in individuals suffering from bilateral cerebral vascular damage resulting in quadruplegia and pseudobulbar palsy. However, since no records could be obtained before these patients became ill, results must remain inconclusive.

Psychosurgery has opened still inadequately explored possibilities for investigation of human gastric function. Freeman and Watts (1942) have noted the immediate effect of prefrontal leukotomy in producing nausea, retching and sometimes vomiting after their final cuts were made. Often loud borborygmi were heard. Later the patients showed increased appetite and gained weight as their psychosis improved.

We have had the opportunity to study stomach movements in patients receiving electroshock therapy. The immediate effect of the electrical convulsion was to bring all gastric motility to a complete standstill as clinical signs of an overwhelming sympatheticotonia appeared. Observations carried out several days after a series of six or more shock treatments demonstrated a tendency to increased gastric motility, heightened response to sudden stretch, and some elevation of the tone baseline in comparison to the preshock records. Changes in each case coincided with improved appetite, weight gain and clinical improvement.

Finally, the effect of hypnotic suggestion in producing changes in hunger motility of the normal human stomach was demonstrated by Scantlebury and Patterson (1941). Suggestion given for eating a meal produced temporary or complete cessation of gastric movements. When suggestion was stopped, contractions resumed normal vigor. They suggested that these effects were produced by causing irradition of inhibitory impulses over the motor cortex.

From a practical viewpoint, therefore, it is possible to recognize certain types of psychosomatic gastrointestinal disorder. These may appear in relation to structural, inflammatory or metabolic disease of the nervous system or occur as more purely functional or conditioned disorders at the highest levels of integration. Chronic dyspepsia sometimes proceeding to gastritis and even ulcer formation is seen frequently in anxiety tension states where uncertainties, insecurities and aggressions with relation to the environment are outstanding. Accessory disorders are seen in cardiospasm, pylorospasm, spastic conditions of the hepatobiliary system, and ulcerative colitis alternating with constipation. In the opposite direction, poor appetite associated with gastric atony may progress to protracted anorexia ("anorexia nervosa") in neurasthenic, depressed and schizophreniform illnesses featuring withdrawal from the environment. In any event, gastrointestinal malfunction can be attributed directly to states of hyper- or hypokinesis with associated vascular and secretory change resulting directly from disturbances at various levels of nervous regulation.

The management of psychosomatic problems in gastroenterology includes a rather extensive armamentarium. Considering, along with Sheehan (1944), that many functional disturbances, if sustained, may actually lead to organic change, it is essential that careful physical studies accompany neuropsychiatric evaluation. As a result, the use of supportive measures, such as amphojel and tincture of belladonna in gastritis, must be accompanied by progressive psychotherapeutic formulation if optimum results are to be obtained. In addition, stimulating or depressing drugs such as benzedrine or barbiturates may be employed in conjunction with drugs aimed at counterbalancing autonomic dysfunction, i.e., the atropine series for parasympatheticotonia and the prostigmin-like drugs for sympatheticotonia. Although widely used, various hormone preparations have found little usefulness in our experience, unless some definite endocrinological disturbance can be substantiated.

In conclusion, it is hoped that the practicing physician may be just as aware of patterns of psychosomatic development as he would be of the cardinal symptoms and signs of various organic disease entities. More important still is the estimation of how far he should go to exclude organic disease when he suspects a fundamentally psychoneurotic disorder. All too often, the anxious and highly suggestible patient, whose sufferings are just as real as, and often more incapacitating than, those due to organic disease, is told without further elaboration that his complaints represent a "functional" or "nervous" disorder. The patient then has the choice of deciding (1) that his troubles are imaginary, (2) that his case is so hopeless that the doctor is keeping the truth from him, or (3) that he is losing his mind. In such an instance, the physician can determine one of two courses of action. If he feels that he has the time and ability, he can proceed with further elaboration and psychotherapeutic formulation of the psychosomatic problem. On the other hand, he should specify to the patient as clearly as possible the facts of physical make-up with an indication that certain parts or organs are functioning more or less below par as the result of an imbalance in their nervous regulation. Thereafter, referral to a competent neuropsychiatrist may be accomplished readily when the patient is reassured that he will retain primary contact with his local physician in the psychosomatic relationship.

BIBLIOGRAPHY

1. BOCHEFONTAINE, L. T.: Etude expérimentale de l'influence exercée par la faradisation de l'écorce grise du cerveau sur quelques fonctions de la vie organique. *Arch. Physiol. norm. path.*, 1876, 8:140.
2. CUSHING, H.: Peptic ulcers and the interbrain. *Surg., Gyn. & Obst.*, 1932, 55:1.
3. FAULKNER, W. B., JR.: Esophageal spasm: observation of emotional influences by means of esophagoscope: report of a case. *J. Nerv. & Ment. Dis.*, 1941, 93:713.
4. FREEMAN, W. J., and WATTS, J. W.: Psychosurgery: intelligence, emotion and social behavior following prefrontal lobotomy for mental disorders. Baltimore, Md., C. C. Thomas, 1942.
5. FULTON, J. F.: Physiology of the nervous system. New York, Oxford University Press, 1943.
6. HESSER, F. H., LANGWORTHY, O. R., and KOLB, L. C.: Experimental study of gastric activity released from cortical control. *J. Neurophysiol.*, 1941, 4:274.

7. LANGWORTHY, O. R., and HESSER, F. H.: An experimental study of micturition released from cerebral control. *Amer. J. Physiol.*, 1936. 115-694.
8. LEVIN, M.: Periodic somnolence and morbid hunger: a new syndrome. *Brain*, 1936, 59:494.
9. LEVIN, P. M.: Restlessness and morbid hunger in man. *Science*, 1936, 84:463.
10. SCANTLEBURY, R. E., and PATTERSON, T. L.: Hunger motility in hypnotized subject. *Quart. J. Exp. Physiol.*, 1941, 30:347.
11. SHEEHAN, D.: Physiological mechanisms involved in gastrointestinal dysfunction. *Psychosomatic Med.*, 1944, 6:56.
12. WATTS, J. W., and FRAZIER, C. H.: Cortical autonomic epilepsy. *J. Nerv. & Ment. Dis.*, 1935, 81:168.
13. WATTS, J. W., and FULTON, J. F.: Intussusception: the relation of the cerebral cortex to intestinal motility in the monkey. *New Eng. J. Med.*, 1934, 210:883.
14. WATTS, J. W., and FULTON, J. F.: The effects of lesions of the hypothalamus upon the gastrointestinal tract and heart in monkeys. *Ann. Surg.*, 1935, 101:363.
15. WEISS, E.: Cardiospasm: a psychosomatic disorder. *Psychosomatic Med.*, 1944, 6:58.
16. WOLF, S., and WOLFF, H. G.: Human gastric function. New York, *Oxford University Press*, 1943.

Discussion

DR. J. W. WATTS (Washington): I followed Dr. Hesser's work with Drs. Langworthy and Cole for a good many years and it is interesting to know that he is now applying in the clinic some of the things he did in the laboratory.

I notice in looking over the first slide that he threw on the screen that 35 per cent of the patients exhibited hypochondriacal symptoms and the patients showing those symptoms were relieved by prefrontal lobotomy. Hypochondriacal symptoms are not necessarily prominent, but they do show relief of nervous symptoms and relief of hypochondriacal symptoms.

Dr. Hesser being with the Armed Forces his concluding remarks were not available for this issue. They will be published later.—Editor.

HOW TO LIVE LONGER

Most civilian physicians are working too hard for comfort. The average age of doctors on the home front must be well up in the fifties.

They would be serving their country and their families better—and longer—by taking a little time out to follow an artistic hobby such as sketching, photographing, water coloring, painting, even whittling.

Art may be easier to take than exercise, yet affords you respite from strain and worry, at the same time offering limitless opportunities for self-expression and the joy of achievement!

Now is a good time to get ready to exhibit your artistic handicraft at the annual exhibition of the American Physicians' Art Association which will be held with the A. M. A. session, June 12th-16th, 1944, in the gallery of the Grand Ballroom, Stevens Hotel, Chicago.

You can get full particulars by writing to the Secretary, Dr. F. H. Redewill, Flood Bldg., San Francisco, Calif.

Regardless of how long you've dabbled in art, you can win a prize—and lighten the war's burden on your heart and arteries.

SYMPOSIUM ON WAR MEDICINE IN "THE HEBREW MEDICAL JOURNAL"

The attention of the medical profession is directed to the appearance of Volumes I and II, 1943, of *Harofe Haivri* (The Hebrew Medical Journal), a semi-annual publication, edited by Moses Einhorn, M.D.

Both volumes are dedicated to a timely symposium on war medicine. Among the subjects discussed of particular interest are "The Treatment of Gunshot Wounds of the Head and Brain During the Present War," by Dr. Leo M. Davidoff; "The Early Treatment of War Wounds with Emphasis on Prevention of Deformities," by Dr. J. W. Maliniac; "Newer Conceptions of the Treatment of Burns," by Dr. Jesse Bullowa and Dr. C. L. Fox, Jr.; "The Status of Anesthesia in Military Surgery," by Dr. S. D. Ehrlich; "Shock Syndrome and Its Treatment," by Dr. S. Standard; "Ocular Injuries in Chemical Warfare," by Dr. Ed. B. Gresser; "Physical Therapy in War Medicine," by Dr. Wm. Bierman; and "The Importance of the Proper Prosthesis in Post-War Rehabilitation," by Dr. H. M. Wertheim.

The sections on Palestine and War contain three articles which present a vivid picture of the medical contribution by the Palestine Jews to the war effort.

In addition to an English-Hebrew medical dictionary, the original articles are summarized in English.

For further information, communicate with the editorial office of *The Hebrew Medical Journal*, 983 Park Avenue, New York 28, N. Y.

HISTAMINE BY MOUTH IN THE TREATMENT OF VASOMOTOR RHINITIS

(J. C. Gant et al., Boston, in *New Eng. Jl. of Med.*, Oct. 7th)

Since the effect of histamine is almost immediate and is transient, the drug should be given at frequent intervals Histamine given by mouth is absorbed promptly. We have seen flushing of the face, abdominal cramps, severe headache, and tense menstrual pain in patients shortly after histamine has been administered orally.

The effective dose varies greatly among patients, but for each it remains quite constant over a long period. Start with a 1:1000 dilution, dose 1 drop in a glass of water. The patient is asked to observe the reaction closely. Too large a dose aggravates his symptoms and too small a dose causes no change, but that the correct dose relieves him within 15 or 20 minutes. If there are no bad effects increase by adding 1 drop each day until toxic effects appear. Thereafter he is maintained on the dose that is just below the toxic level, and this dose is repeated as often as is necessary to control the symptoms.

The dose may vary from 1 drop of a 1:1000 dilution to 25 drops of a 1:100 dilution, the average is 5 to 7 drops of the 1:1000 dilution, before meals

ANALGESIA AND PREMATURITY IN RELATION TO NEONATAL MORTALITY

(E. C. Sage, Omaha, in *Jl. A. M. A.*, Feb. 5th)

All known analgesics and anesthetics to the mother have a degree of injurious effect on the fetus (in proportion to the amount administered) with the exception of continuous caudal anesthesia. The ultimate evaluation of any given method of anesthesia will depend on the price paid for the mother's comfort in terms of infant mortality.

Prematurity is one of the most potent contributory factors in neonatal and infant mortality and is the most important single factor in the causation of neonatal asphyxia. Prematurity in itself should not be considered an acceptable cause of death until other possibilities have been excluded. The incidence of premature births is usually between 5 and 6 per cent. Obstetric analgesia with morphine, scopolamine or phenobarbital should be avoided when dealing with a premature infant, as it interferes seriously with the respiratory function of the infant.

OBSERVATION OF 72 cases suggests that early ambulation following cerebral concussion is not only safe but is also associated with fewer post-concussion syndromes.

Prefrontal Lobotomy With Reference to Involutional Melancholia*

J. G. LYERLY, M.D., F.A.C.S., Jacksonville, Florida
Department of Neuropsychiatry, Duke University School of Medicine

IN PREVIOUS REPORTS it has been shown that an operation could be performed on the prefrontal lobes of the brain which would enable the patient to recover from a severe mental depression as seen in involutional melancholia and agitated depression. These reports corroborated the work of Moniz,[1] Freeman and Watts,[2] who accomplished their results by section of the association pathways of the prefrontal lobes. In order to determine the extent of section and then to control any bleeding which may arise it was felt an open type of operation should be devised which would enable it to be done under direct vision and this operative procedure was first done by me in June, 1937[3].

From an anatomical study we learn that the tip of the frontal lobes are connected with the rest of the cerebrum as the parietal, occipital and temporal lobes by deep association pathways. Likewise they are connected with the diencephalon and the hypothalamic region, as well as with the pons and cerebellum.

In doing this operation the incision was made about the hair line in the upper part of both frontal regions. A button of bone was removed with a trephine and this bone was saved and put back in place to prevent a depression in the contour of the scalp. The operation has been done in bald-headed individuals without any visible deformity except for a short transverse scar which might look like a wrinkle.

The point of entrance for cutting the association pathways was about middle of the second frontal convolution, or halfway between the tip of the frontal lopes and the Fissure of Rolando. The anterior horn of the lateral ventricle was located with a needle and the section of the association pathways was made just in front of it which should cut the fibers coming from the front half of the prefrontal lobe. Since all operations were done at this point of entrance it should be equivalent to amputation of this part of the prefrontal lobes. From the post-operative and subsequent study of these patients one can obtain some idea of the functions of this particular brain tissue.

The Diencephalon has been considered to be the seat of the emotions and the autonomic nervous system which controls many of the somatic states. These hypothalamic and subcortical centers are controlled and regulated to a great extent by a higher group of neurones of the cerebral cortex found especially in the frontal lobes. By severing these connections in the frontal lobes one can bring about an improvement of certain emotional and affective disorders as well as the anxiety and nervous tension states. This should prove that there resides in this part of the brain a function which has a controlling influence over certain mental symptoms.

After the operation the patient was changed almost immediately after he awoke from the anesthetic. He was more relaxed, cheerful, and had a smile, which was the opposite of his former state. There might be a period of mental confusion and impairment of memory for a few days as to be expected from an operation on the frontal lobes, but this subsided in a few days with no alteration of the mental capacity. The psychometric tests showed no impairment of intelligence after the operation. Most patients stated they could concentrate better than before the operation. In about half the cases there might be involuntary urination, in a few cases defecation, for a few days. The hands might need restraining to keep from pulling off the dressing and to keep the patient in bed. The patient was forgetful and could not remember that he had an operation. This mental confusion would disappear within a few days and recovery would be sufficient in two weeks to allow the discharge.

In the present study there were 65 cases observed over a period of time from nearly one to seven years after operation.

Table I gives the total number of cases operated on during each year. It has been observed that the operative results produced during the first year were similar to those after five or six years. The changed mental and personality states were immediate and usually permanent as far as the patient was concerned. In other words, after the first few months we could predict what the permanent mental state would be as a result of the operation.

Twenty of the patients operated on were in the Florida State Hospital and were classified as institutional cases as seen in Table II. Even though the other cases were not strictly in the State Hos-

---

*Presented to Tri-State Medical Association of the Carolinas and Virginia, meeting at Charlotte, Feb. 28th-29th, 1944.

pital most of them were candidates for the hospital, some of them being operated on just after their commitment to the State Hospital and before their transfer, while others were transferred from other State Hospitals to Jacksonville for the operation. Of the twenty cases operated on at Chattahoochee nine have been discharged and are apparently well, five others have been discharged and later returned because they were not fully adjusted. Six of the twenty have never been discharged because their recovery was not sufficient for social adjustment on the outside, and in several instances because they did not have any home to go to even though they were socially adjusted.

In the selection of patients for operation it was felt from the beginning that the patient with an affective mental disorder and depression would be the most suitable for the procedure. The symptoms benefited by the operation were severe nervous tension states, emotional instability, apprehension and anxiety and various somatic delusions. The operation tended to convert an individual from an introvert to an extrovert. It was observed that involutional melancholia and agitated depression had the train of symptoms benefited, and therefore they were most frequently selected for the operation.

It was felt that before the operation was done other medical and psychiatric measures should be utilized as far as possible, such as glandular therapy and shock treatment. If the patient did not respond to the treatment mentioned and did not become socially adjusted the operation should be done in preference to a permanent commitment and deterioration in a State Hospital. In this way we have operated on the ones which seem to be the most hopeless and as a last resort in bringing about a remission. It may be mentioned that some of the cases operated on were considered too old, or, because of cardiovascular disease, were not suitable for convulsive shock treatment.

In arriving at a conclusion of the results of the operation we have attempted to classify the patients according to the degree of improvement. The ones coming under the class of greatly improved made the nearest approach to normal. They have become socially adjusted and have returned to form of occupation. Next was the moderately improved group which became socially adjusted but for various reasons have not gone to work. A few of these cases have remained in the State Hospital because they did not have a suitable home for their discharge. In the slightly improved group the patient was no longer a problem for feeding and management even though he remained in the institution and in some cases stayed at home. In the temporarily improved group or failures were the ones which showed slight improvement at first and later reverted to a mental state approaching the previous condition. In some instances the patient went from a depressed phase to a hypomanic state.

It is observed in Table III that the improvement somewhat varied according to the age of the patient. The older the patient the greater was the improvement and vice versa for the younger ones. The patients in the involutional melancholia and agitated depression group were beyond 45 or 50 years of age and since they were most frequently selected for operation the average age would necessarily be raised. Likewise the duration of symptoms before the operation had a bearing on the degree of improvement. The shorter the period of symptoms the greater was the improvement and more nearly was the patient restored to normal. The gain in weight after operation was most pronounced in the cases that showed the greatest improvement. This gain in weight is probably true of most mental cases which respond favorably to treatment. The ones showing slight improvement and the failures actually had a loss of weight. It was not unusual for some patients showing great improvement to double their weight. For example, one frail woman about 65 years old weighed only 71 pounds who was diagnosed as having tuberculosis in addition to a severe mental illness, doubled her weight after operation and has remained in excellent health doing her own housework as well as looking after the business of renting apartments.

The classification of the patients according to diagnosis and the degree of improvement is seen in table IV. It is seen that the greatest number was forty-four cases of involutional melancholia. The number of manic-depresive cases was 8, schizophrenia 5, and psychoneurotic depression was 7. If these cases were eliminated and only the involutional melancholias were included the total percentage of greatest improvement would be much greater than shown in the table. If the operation improved the patient to the extent that he could be discharged from a State Hospital to become socially adjusted and restored to his family even though not gainfully employed the operation would be judged worth while. The patients showing this degree of improvement coming under the greatly and moderately improved group would show a percentage of 78.5. There is no other form of treatment that can show this degree of improvement for the mental case of such extreme degree pointing to a hopelessness and permanency of symptoms. This statement is made with the knowledge that most of the patients showing this degree of improvement after the operation had the trial of other forms of treatment and in many instances over a long period of time.

Since the patients selected for operation were mostly involutional melancholia and agitated depression a few schizophrenias were selected. At the present time the tendency is to include more of this type since there are a large number falling in this group which would be benefited by operation as shown by Freeman and Watts,[2] Palher,[4] Strecker,[5] Tarumianz,[6] Bennett,[7] Woltmann,[8] and others.

A few recent cases operated on were schizophrenias having had shock therapy and other treatment in an institution over a considerable period of time without much improvement and without a great deal of deterioration. It does not make any difference if the diagnosis is schizophrenia or some other class as long as the train of symptoms are the ones which are relieved by the operation. It is important that the intelligence be preserved and that there be no great amount of deterioration, which is so often seen after a prolonged stay in a State Hospital. It is suggested that if it is to be performed, the operation should be done preferably one or two years after the onset. This may be too short a time for some cases and too long for others. Some mental diseases are rapid in onset and progress and may show rapid loss of weight with exhaustion in spite of the usual measures to prevent it with an early fatal termination. These cases may need the operation at an earlier date provided other methods have failed. Old people with cardiovascular disease who cannot withstand convulsive shock therapy may tolerate the operation satisfactorily since it may be done under a local and a basal anesthetic. The post-operative course is usually smooth and the patient is relaxed with a slower heart action and a lowered blood pressure. Several patients have been operated on between seventy and eighty with excellent results.

In the 65 cases there have been no deaths from the operation. No patient has developed a post-operative complication as paralysis, aphasia, or other unexpected neurological signs. An occasional convulsion may be seen in a small percentage of cases as might be expected following any mild traumatic brain lesion.

Table I

YEAR	NUMBER
1937	11
1938	15
1939	8
1940	5
1941	8
1942	9
1943	9
Total	65

Table II
INSTITUTION CASES

Discharged	9
Discharged, then returned	5
Never discharged	6
Total	20

Table III

Average	Greatly Improved	Moderately Improved	Slightly Improved	Temporarily Improved or Failures
Age	51.7	52.9	43.7	41.4
Duration of symptoms years	2.7	4	4.3	8.6
Gain in weight pounds	29.5	27	—4	—8

Table IV

Diagnosis	Greatly Improved	Moderately Improved	Slightly Improved	Temporarily Improved or Failures	Total	Employed
Involutional Melancholia	27	10	5	2	44	26
Manic depressive	2	4	1	1	8	3
Schizophrenia	1	2	1	1	5	1
Psychoneurosis with depression	4	1	2	—	7	4
Psychopathic personality	—	—	—	1	1	—
Total	34	17	9	5	65	34
Percentage	52.3	26.2	13.8	7.7		52.3

CONCLUSIONS

1. The work is based on 65 cases having the deep association pathways severed in the prefrontal lobes. Twenty of these cases were inmates in the Florida State Hospital at Chattahoochee. The observations were made over a period from nearly one to seven years after operation.

2. The operation was done on involutional melancholia cases chiefly, a total of 44 cases. The rest of the cases were manic-depressive 8, schizophrenia 5, psychoneurotic depression 7, and psychopathic personality 1.

3. The greatest improvement was noted in the involutional cases. There was a good response in many of the other cases selected for operation.

4. Of the total cases 78.5 per cent improved to the point that they were readjusted socially and returned to employment in most instances.

5. The improvement was roughly in proportion to the age of the patient, the gain in weight, and the duration of symptoms.

REFERENCES

1. EGAS MONIZ: The First Attempt at Operative Treatment of Certain Psychoses. Encephal., 31:1-29, June, 1936; Prefrontal Leukotomy in the Treatment of Mental Disorders. Am. J. Psychiat., 93:1379-1385, May, 1937.
2. FREEMAN, W., and WATTS, J. W.: Prefrontal Lobotomy in the Treatment of Mental Disorders. South. M. J., 30: 23-31, Jan., 1937.
FREEMAN, W.: The Surgical Treatment of Mental Disorders. Med. Ann. of the District of Columbia, 8:345-353, Dec., 1939.
FREEMAN, W., and WATTS, J. W.: The Frontal Lobes and Consciousness of Self. Psychosom. M., 3:111-119, April, 1941; Intellectual and Emotional Changes Following

Prefrontal Lobotomy. *Zbl. Neurochir.*, 3:1-10, 1940.
WATT, J. W., and FREEMAN, W.: Prefrontal Lobotomy; Six Years Experience. *South. M. J.*, 36:478, 1943.
FREEMAN, W.: Neuro-surgical Treatment of Certain Abnormal Mental States. *J. A. M. A.*, 117:517, 1941.
3. LYERLY, J. G.: Prefrontal Lobotomy in Involutional Melancholia. *J. Florida M. A.*, 25:225-229, Nov. 1938. Transection of the Deep Association Fibers of the Prefrontal Lobes in Certain Mental Diseases. *Southern Surgeon*, 8:426-434, Oct., 1939. Neurosurgical Treatment of Certain Abnormal Mental States. *J. A. M. A.*, 117:517, 1941.
WORCHEL, P., and LYERLY, J. G.: Effects of Prefrontal Lobotomy on Depressed Patients. *J. Neurophysiol.*, 4:62-67, 1941.
4. PALMER, H. D.: Neurosurgical Treatment of Certain Abnormal Mental States. *J. A. M. A.*, 117:517, 1941.
5. STRECKER, E. A., PALMER, H. D., and GRANT, F. C.: Study of Frontal-Lobotomy: Neurosurgical and Psychiatric Features and Results in 22 Cases with Detailed Report on 5 Chronic Schizophrenics. *Am. J. Psychiat.*, 98:524, 1942.
6. TARUMIANZ, M. A.: Neurosurgical Treatment of Certain Mental States. *J. A. M. A.*, 117:517, 1941.
7. BENNETT, A. E., KEEGAN, J. J., and WILBUR, C. B.: Prefrontal Lobotomy on Chronic Schizophrenia. *J. A. M. A.*, 123:809, 1943.
8. WOLTMANN, H. W., SMITH, B. F., MOERSCH, F. P., and LOVE, J. G.: Prefrontal Lobotomy in the Treatment of Certain Mental Disorders. *Proceedings Staff Meetings Mayo Clinic*, 16:200, 1941.

CURE FOR POISON OAK
(Robt. Boyd, Brooklyn, in *Med. Rec.*, Mar.)

Application of a facial mask of thick gauze, and this kept constantly wet with a saturated solution of hyposulphite of sodium, has been demonstrated to my satisfaction to be an excellent treatment for poisoning.

TREATMENT FOR CARBON TETRACHLORIDE POISONING
(*Journal A. M. A.* for March 25th)

Carbon tetrachloride's toxic effects may be produced by absorption through the skin, breathing in its fumes, or by taking it by mouth. The Journal, in commenting on an announcement in a recent issue of the *British Medical Journal*, says:

"An army air force pilot accidentally ingested 30 to 40 c.c. and the immediate onset of symptoms indicating a rapid entry into the circulation. Vomiting was not induced until 45 minutes after ingestion. Enlargement of the liver . . . was demonstrable 19 hours afterward when the patient was given 2 Gm. of *dl*-methionine by mouth. This was retained, and three hours later 1 c.c. of a cascin-digest-methionine solution was injected slowly into an ante-cubital vein. Since this was not followed by any immediate reaction, 5 c.c. more was injected, also without reaction. Continuous infusion of the solution by a drip apparatus was then begun, 2 c.c. per minute. By the end of the next three hours, when 436 c.c. of the solution had been infused, the patient complained of chilliness, intense headache and backache, and some aching of the limb muscles. The infusion was then stopped. The liver at this time was still tender and had enlarged considerably. . . . The next day the liver was no longer tender. . . . On the next day—the third after the accident—the patient complained of dizziness and headache. Abdominal palpation revealed that the liver had again become enlarged. . . . That day the patient was given 2 Gm. of methionine by mouth in the morning and another 2 Gm. in the evening. On the fourth day the patient was alert and made no complaints. . . . The investigators . . . believe that in this case the administration of the methionine was the specific influence that prevented further liver damage. . . ."

LITTLE TUMORS, LARGE SYMPTOMATOLOGY
(J. G. Love, in *Proc. Staff Meet. Mayo Clinic*, March 8th)

The first article on glomus tumors that came to my attention was the one by Mason and Weil published in 1934. Others, however, were published prior to this. In 50 per cent of these tumors symptoms appear after some trauma which may be trivial. Symptoms are out of all proportion to the size of the lesion. The tumor is usually not more than a few mm. in diameter, is most frequently encountered in the extremities, particularly in the digits; most typically under the nail. Usually there are severe paroxysms of pain which seem to originate at the site which subsequently is proved to be the site of the lesion. Neuralgia-like pain may involve half of the body, hemiparesis or hemianesthesia may occur on the side of the lesion. The lesions are sometimes extremely small and, therefore, if the typical purplish color is absent, they may not be seen. If it is eroded, severe hemorrhage may occur because an arteriovenous anastomosis occurs in the glomus, generally glomus tumors are considered benign.

The patient is asked to indicate the point of maximal pain or tenderness. The point of a steel pin is pressed into the skin over the lesion and an attack of excruciating pain is projected from the lesion. On many occasions when I could not see the lesion, I have been able to identify its location and make the diagnosis with the help of the pin.

Neurofibromas are much larger by the time the patient presents himself. An angioma may be palpated without producing severe pain. This is true also of melano-epithelioma and other small dermatologic lesions.

The treatment of this lesion is surgical excision—under local anesthesia so that the patient can help in the identification of the tumor; this is particularly essential when the lesion is not visible.

(*Discussion to be published with Dr. J. W. Watts' paper.*)

REMOVAL OF FECAL IMPACTION RELIEVES 10-WEEKS PAIN
(A. A. Landsman, New York, in *Med. Rec.*, Mar.)

An obese mother of three children with a history of chronic constipation but no significant symptoms had complained for 10 weeks of a dull pain in the lower abdomen and back, a dragging sensation in the pelvis, straining at stool with occasional bleeding, distention, anorexia, but no loss of weight. She did not stress constipation because that was her usual state and the bowel movements appeared no worse than before her illness. Blood pressure, urinary examination, hemoglobin estimation and blood picture were normal. Abdominal examination was not satisfactory because of excessive fat.. Vaginal examination disclosed a regularly rounded, globular, dome-like elevation of the posterior vaginal wall extending upwards 2½ inches. The lower limit of the rounded mass the size of a fist could be palpated in the rectum, was freely movable, pitted on pressure about slipped up when any attempt was made to dislodge it by manipulation. A diagnosis of fecal impaction was made.

The patient was catheterized and at operation every attempt to bring down the mass failed because it moved at once into the sigmoid when touched. Several towels were rolled into a firm pad, placed in the center of the abdomen and held down with broad strips of adhesive plaster applied tightly across the abdomen. An assistant made pressure above the pad and the operator, with two fingers in the vagina, hooked them over the upper limit of the mass to steady it, the impaction was broken up and removed piecemeal. 16 ounces of dried fecal material, normal recovery, discharged after four days.

DEPARTMENTS

TUBERCULOSIS

J. DONNELLY, M.D., *Editor*, Charlotte, N. C.

IMPORTANT FACTS ABOUT TUBERCULOSIS

A GOOD many mistaken ideas as to tuberculosis are held by the people generally, and by too many physicians. This is not to be wondered at, since recent advances in our knowledge of the subject have contradicted teachings which were orthodox a few years ago.

Logi[1] writes with a knowledge that carries conviction:

As a result of this second World War in Scotland, the death rate from the disease is 33% higher than it was the year prior to hostilities. During the first World War the mortality rate in the United States rose 15%. Today the downward trend has slowed up considerably. One per cent of selectees is rejected on account of tuberculosis at the induction centers, and an equal percentage is turned down for this reason by the local draft boards.

Tuberculosis is still the leading cause of death in the 15- to 45-year age group, but more deaths occur from the disease in persons between 60 and 70 than in any other age group. At present, for each death two new cases are reported to health departments and it is estimated that there are five clinically active cases for each death.

Abroad, bovine tuberculosis is a rather frequent condition, particularly in children. Recently attention was directed to the possibility of the production of tuberculosis, through the transmission of the avian bacillus from fowl to man.

No longer is the physician satisfied with a laboratory report of acid-fast bacilli, knowing that they occur everywhere and that the majority of them are nonpathogenic. Also, young tubercle bacilli pass through a stage during which they are not acid-fast, and may be the cause of unusual variations of the disease such as sarcoidosis and uveoparotid fever. The bacilli may occur in the granular form, merely a phase of development. Confusing is the persistent absence of the organism in cases in which the syndrome is otherwise characteristic of tuberculosis. Investigation suggests the possibility of involutional forms of the bacillus having ultramicroscopic and filtrable properties.

Rough colonies are usually nonpathogenic; the smooth colonies are virulent disease producers. In Europe and South America, BCG vaccination of children from tuberculous families, student nurses and medical students appears to give favorable results. In this country, however, it has been demonstrated that cultures of BCG, which consist of attenuated bovine bacilli, may undergo variation and can be made to dissociate the smooth form of organism, thereby converting the vaccine into a dangerous infecting agent.

Eight years after the discovery of the tubercle bacillus, Koch introduced tuberculin as a specific remedy for the disease. As a therapeutic measure it has depreciated in value. The chief value of tuberculin lies in diagnosis, but even here its reliability has been questioned lately. The Mantoux intracutaneous tuberculin test is the most accurate method. The Vollmer patch is gaining in popularity; simple application of a plaster impregnated with a synthetic tuberculin to the skin, which has been cleansed previously with acetone. A negative patch test should be followed by a test with a stronger tuberculin. The tuberculin test is of greater value in young children and is being used for adolescents and adults more frequently, as many young people are now reaching the adult stage without ever having had a primary infection. No longer is it true that in over 90% of adults there is a positive reaction. In Florida, of 760 adults tested with PPD in two strengths, only 59% showed a positive reaction.

How much confidence can be placed in the tuberculin test is questionable in the light of recent findings? In certain conditions, particularly the acute exanthemas, it elicits no response; several observers have reported its failure in ordinary cases of active tuberculosis. Sensitivity to tuberculin usually fades with healing of the lesion, and anergy exists when the bacilli in the body are no longer viable. It has been reported that tuberculin in testing doses may light up latent foci of malaria.

The manner in which the reinfection type of tuberculosis arises is not clear.

Six week after the t. b. makes its initial entrance into the body, the tuberculin test will give a positive reaction indicating that allergy has been established.

So long as a tuberculous cavity in the lung remains patent, the patient will cough up bacilli. In only 40% of cases is the cavity seen on the röntgenogram. Less than 10% of these cavities can be diagnosed with the stethoscope. Occasionally, one is puzzled by the sudden disappearance of cavities. If a ball- or check-valve obstruction exists, the cavity may grow larger or smaller almost before one's eyes, or it may be visible on a röntgenogram today and invisible on one taken a few days later.

No diagnosis of pulmonary tuberculosis is absolute until the t. b. has been demonstrated; but one should not wait for the discovery of the organism before arriving at a tentative diagnosis and

---

1. A. J. Logie, Miami, in *Jl. Fla. Med. Assn.*, March.

instituting precautionary and therapeutic measures.

The röntgen-ray examination has surpassed by far all other means of diagnosing the disease, revealing early lesions in the chest from 2 to 3 years before the characteristic symptoms of tuberculosis appear. Single flat films of the chest are suitable, but stereoscopic plates are preferable when the lesions are complex, multiple, or superimposed. Frequently, the lesion is concealed in the mediastinal shadows, necessitating lateral, oblique, or lordotic views. In case the chest röntgenogram is negative, but there are bacilli in the sputum, bronchoscopy often reveals tuberculous involvement of the trachea or bronchi. In a patient with asthmatoid wheezing and frequent spasms of violent coughing, and who expectorates copious sputum, though a röntgenogram usually shows no lesion in the lung fields, bronchoscopy reveals the true story.

Sputum cultures and guinea pig inoculations may be required. Fluorescent microscopy reveals more tubercle bacilli than any other method of examining the sputum; the bacilli, stained with carbolauramine, are viewed through ultraviolet light. If no sputum is obtainable, examination of the gastric contents by the concentrate method should be made, as patients unconsciously swallow sputum through the night.

Pleurisy with effusion is usually tuberculous and should be treated by prolonged bed rest.

In active tuberculosis the blood platelets show a thrombocytosis. If a thrombocytopenia with increase of megalothrombocytes occurs, the prognosis is unfavorable. The patient with the exudative type usually recovers; the one with the caseous pneumonic lesion requires immediate and prolonged collapse therapy; the one with the proliferative or fibroid type dies eventually of some complication or superimposed condition, such as the overloading of the right heart with the production of cor pulmonale and progressive cardiac failure.

The prognosis in cases of pulmonary tuberculosis has not been improved for the individual patient in the last 20 years. Today the disease develops in fewer persons, but the proportion of fatalities is the same as in 1915. Patients do not receive treatment soon enough. In less than 20% of the cases reported to health departments or admitted to sanatoriums has the disease been diagnosed at a minimal stage. Pneumothorax is employed skillfully by a minority of those who work in this field. Too few physicians realize the futility of continuing pneumothorax when the sputum remains positive after three to six months of such treatment.

In the treatment of tuberculosis, climate no longer receives serious consideration. No longer does the physician employ sunshine when treating active cases. Rather than an overabundance of milk and eggs, he prescribes a regular diet of 2 to 3 thousand calories with a high content of vitamins A, C and K. A chilled mixture of orange or tomato juice and plain cod liver oil administered daily has inhibited the development of the former frequent complication of intestinal tuberculosis. The use of promin, a sodium salt of dextrose sulfonate, holds great promise for the future.

Many will disagree with the author's advice to administer pneumothorax in every case of tuberculosis as soon as diagnosed. Many minimal cases will recover on bed rest alone. However, every case should be closely watched for possible spread or beginning cavitation, on which indications collapse of the lung would be attempted. If minimal lesions show evidence of healing on a reasonable period of bed rest, it is possible that the annoyance of repeated pneumothorax refills can be spared the patient. Even the lung with a considerably advanced lesion will occasionally collapse satisfactorily. It should be continued for at least two years before reëxpansion of the collapsed lung is considered. As a complication pleural effusion develops in 20% of cases. If the disease spreads to the other lung bilateral pneumothorax may be indicated.

If pneumothorax is unsuccessful, thoracoplasty should be considered while the patient has fairly good general resistance.

Pneumoperitoneum has a place in the treatment of extensive bilateral disease, usually with phrenic nerve block.

The article freely abstracted and commented on is not entirely orthodox; but it states our present knowledge of tuberculosis accurately. The author is not optimistic; he is not pessimistic. He is informed and truthful.

HISTORIC MEDICINE

GUNSHOT WOUNDS OF THREE PRESIDENTS OF THE UNITED STATES

Three of the 32 Presidents of the United States have died from gunshot wounds while holding office. There has been speculation all along on what might be done for these wounds had they been inflicted at a later date.

The wounds of all three, with their management, and the attendant circumstances, are described by Harper,[1] and his account, which will prove interesting and instructive to all readers, is herewith given in abstract.

President Lincoln: The bullet entered the occipital bone at the level of the transverse sinus an inch to the left of the midline, obliquely forward across the brain, ending in the right frontal lobe, causing extensive comminuted fractures of both orbital plates, apparently the result of contrecoup since the dura over the frontal lobe was not penetrated, across the upper surface of the pons and through the aqueduct of sylvius. Lincoln lived nine hours after the shooting. In view of its central location near vital centers, it is surprising that the wound was not instantly fatal. Taft, one of the attending army surgeons, noted a deep coma, pulse rate of 48 beats per minute, unequal pupils finally becoming widely dilated, bilateral jacksonian convulsions, shallow respirations becoming Cheyne-Stokes in character, exophthalmos with extensive ecchymosis of the sclera and periorbital tissues. The wound was probed several times to its entire depth and fragmented pieces of the orbital plate were felt by the end of the probe.

With such an extensive wound across the base of the brain, it seems doubtful if the outcome would have been altered by any measures available today.

President Garfield: The second of our martyr Presidents was shot at close range on July 2nd, 1881, by Charles Guiteau, a disappointed office-seeker. The bullet entered the tenth intercostal space three inches to the right of the midline and fractured the 11th rib. The lead ball was deflected down and across the body of the first lumbar vertebra, passed completely through the body but missed the spinal canal, then buried itself under the peritoneum near the spleen after grazing the edge of the splenic artery. President Garfield died 2½ months after the shooting, from sepsis occurring along the course of the bullet wound and rupture of an aneurysm of the splenic artery which developed at the site where the bullet grazed the vessel. As was customary at that time, attention was centered on determining the location of the bullet. Reconstruction of the scene and the shooting of bullets into cadavers was done in an attempt to reproduce the wound. Alexander Graham Bell was requested to conduct electrical experiments to determine the location of the bullet. Many elaborate instruments on the order of modern bronchoscopic forceps were devised to follow a tortuous path and grasp the bullet for extraction. The general public became concerned over the location of the bullet although it was apparent to a few experienced military surgeons of the time that the presence of a bullet in the body was entirely compatible with life. Letters from doctors all over the world poured in to plague the attending physicians. Esmarch, Professor of Surgery at the University of Kiel, offered his analysis of the case before the Physiological Society of Kiel. In spite of all the turmoil, D. W. Bliss, with the assistance of Frank Hamilton and Hayes Agnew, managed to supervise what must have been very good treatment for that time.

A month after the shooting several subcutaneous abscesses appeared around the wound of entry. On two occasions the sinus tract was incised to promote better drainage. Later, severe suppurative parotitis developed which necessitated incision and drainage.

One of the first air-cooling machines was arranged to cool the bedroom in the White House. The heat of the Washington summer was distressing the President so much that he was moved to the seashore in New Jersey where after a period of improvement, he became much weaker and died after sudden hemorrhage from rupture of the aneurysm of the splenic artery. At the time of his death his weight had fallen from 210 to 125 pounds.

The next year White published an article defending the treatment given, which stood against any further criticism. In reviewing the official bulletins issued on the case, several things appear to have been done, which are not done now. The wound was explored digitally by unprotected fingers three times in the first 24 hours and then repeatedly during a collective examination of the patient by many prominent doctors. Probes which were not sterile were used repeatedly during the first five days in an attempt to follow the course of the bullet. It seems likely that this was a factor in the production of the subhepatic abscess and the abscess in the right iliac fossa found at necropsy. It was recorded that a catheter could be passed into the abscess cavity in the right iliac region. The fractured vertebra was not suspected during life since apparently there was no displacement.

Surgical intervention immediately following the shooting does not seem to have been indicated. It is possible that better drainage for the subhepatic and iliac abscesses should have been provided.

President McKinley: The third of our Chief Executives to fall from an assassin's bullet was shot twice on September 6th, 1901, by Leon Czolgosz, an anarchist. One bullet inflicted a superficial skin wound over the upper part of the sternum. The other entered the left upper quadrant of the abdomen, perforating both walls of the stomach at the greater curvature and then, after grazing the upper pole of the left kidney, apparently buried itself in the deep muscles of the back. The President was attending the Pan-American Exposition at Buffalo and was taken to a small emergency hospital on the grounds. Within 90 minutes of the shooting an exploratory laparotomy was begun by Dr. Matthew Mann, a prominent Buffalo surgeon. Light for the operation was provided in part by reflecting the rays of the setting sun into the wound with a hand mirror. The instruments were those carried in a small pocket case by a local physician. Drop ether anesthesia was employed. The perforations on both walls of the stomach were closed with a double row of silk sutures. The shooting occurred several hours after the President had eaten and there was little contamination of the peritoneal cavity from gastric contents. The path of the bullet into the retroperitoneal tissue was found, but, because of the shock attending the operation, the abdomen was closed without further exploration. No drainage was employed.

Dr. Mann's decision to operate would be considered entirely correct today; under the circumstances of the time his decision was remarkable. During the week following operation, the President made satisfactory progress and was beginning to take a little solid food in addition to small amounts of liquids. Fluid balance had been maintained as much as possible by nutrient enemas and on several occasions the injection of small amounts of physiologic salt solution under the skin. Urinary output of 270 c.c. for the second day and 420 c.c. for the third day were recorded. The urine was concentrated (specific gravity of 1.026) and it seems likely that dehydration was present. Frequent irritating enemas and castor oil were given to bring "elimination." These did not aid in maintaining a positive fluid balance.

At noon on the 7th day after operation, shortly after an official bulletin announced the favorable progress, something happened. From the reports issued it was not entirely clear what took place, but the President suddenly became weaker. In 36 hours, the Nation, which had been led to believe that he would recover, was shocked by the announcement of his death. At necropsy no anatomic explanation for his sudden death was found. It was attributed to the presence of a localized region of necrosis near the pancreas in the retroperitoneal tissue along the track of the bullet. There was no general peritonitis. The sutured holes in the stomach were still closed and the slight wound to the upper pole of the left kidney was healing. Although no embolus was reported to have been found on examination of the lungs, the sequence of events suggests a pulmonary embolism. At the time it was suggested that the bullet had been poisoned with curare or smeared with virulent bacteria. These suggestions were officially refuted.

Harper comments:

It seems doubtful if anything different would be done today at operation on such a gunshot wound. While some surgeons might employ a drain into the lesser omental cavity, it was apparent from the report of the necropsy that drainage would not have altered the outcome. Dr. Mann stated that his reason for not draining the abdomen was that there was nothing to drain. This is still sound reasoning. It is doubtful whether failure to remove the bullet had anything to do with the President's death. Although necropsy was continued for four hours, the bullet was never found. This would indicate that further search at the time of operation was not justified.

It would seem that lack of some of the modern therapeutic measures rather than faulty judgment made adequate treatment impossible. Lincoln probably could not be saved today. Garfield would have been helped materially by the use of sulfonamide compounds and blood transfusions. His wound would not have been probed as extensively today and perhaps some of the infection could have been avoided. McKinley might have benefited by intravenous administration of adequate quantities of fluid and blood transfusion. However, gunshot wounds of the abdomen still carry a high risk.

The editor entered medical college right on the heels of McKinley's death. The professor of anatomy, who was but an indifferent surgeon, at our first meeting, went into this case in great detail. A classmate, much impressed, whispered in my ear: "If Billie had been there, the President would have been saved."

OBSTETRICS

HENRY J. LANGSTON, M.D., *Editor*, Danville, Va.

OFFICE DELIVERY IN RURAL OBSTETRICS

THIS paper[1] presents the advantages of office delivery of obstetric patients in rural areas and offers it in lieu of: (1) Home delivery of which there are several types; a) by midwife; b) by physician with little equipment; c) by physician with sterile outfit similar to a hospital set-up, and d) by physician with a private or a public health nurse assistant. (2) Hospitalization in a nearby town or city.

Bloss is quoted that 2/3ds of total obstetric practice of the physicians of the Southern Medical Association is carried on in the homes of the patients. It is agreed that lack of sterile gowns and sheets may not mean non-sterile technic. "Intensive aseptic technic includes proper sterilization of the operator's hands and the patient's shaved perineum. These physicians do not drape the patient, but they do wear wet boiled sterile gloves. Delivery is conducted with the patient in bed unless operative procedures are done; then on the kitchen table.

Any physician who has engaged in rural obstetrics knows that labor, after hours of progress, may suddenly cease and the baby not be born for a week or so. Other objections bear indirectly upon the fetal and maternal mortality and morbidity. The physician's waiting is often taken as a sign of

1. Richard Torpin et al., Augusta, in Jl. Med. Assn. Ga., Feb.

indecision or of timidity in the use of pituitrin or of forceps. In few home deliveries is the equipment necessary for insurance against all eventualities.

The Plan Offered: The physician obtains the use of two or three extra rooms, and puts in ordinary single or hospital beds equipped with legholders. He has a steam sterilizer, or the use of one at a nearby hospital. He has the help of a personally trained assistant, be she nurse or secretary, who is in attendance in the daytime, and he may employ another for the occasional night duty. Such assistants, in addition to maintaining the sterile equipment, are taught to aid in administering the analgesic and other drugs used, and in observing the progress of labor by head stethoscope and by rectal examination with a view to conserving the time of the physician; who then is not tempted to hurry delivery to the detriment of the mother and child, and is able to conduct his regular office practice. The patient, with shaved and thoroughly scrubbed perineum (10 minutes) is placed in stirrups across the bed, or on a nearby delivery table. Under the influence of barbiturates and hyoscine the delivery may be completed without further anesthetic unless an episiotomy is necessary. For this, infiltration of the mesiolateral incision line by sterile 1 per cent procaine solution is done, maintaining an aseptic technic, having drapes, instruments and sutures under the constant care of a trained assistant. Mother and child are sent home by ambulance in a few hours or a day or so.

The main causes of maternal death, in or following labor are: a) puerperal infection; b) postpartum hemorrhage; c) placenta praevia; and d) premature separation of the normally implanted placenta. Equipment to anticipate and combat each of these complications, although rarely necessary, is easy to maintain available in sterile condition at all times in the office.

An automatic uterine packer is kept loaded and sterile for employment at a moment's notice.

The treatment of placenta praevia (excepting centralis, which is rare) is usually the same as that of premature separation of the normally implanted placenta—simple rupture of the membranes under sterile technic and the application of a tight abdominal binder. Blood transfusion in either of these conditions is always in order and is far easier done in the office than in the home.

Cervical laceration, extremely rare in the practice of conservative obstetricians, demands suture. The first hemostatic suture, under good exposure, should be placed above the apex of the tear. Rupture of the uterus, rare in good obstetric practice, demands hospital care, hysterectomy usually.

Apnoea neonatorum is managed by introduction of a tracheal catheter and administration of air or oxygen by use of an electric-lighted infant laryngoscope and a modified Flagg insufflator.

It is suggested that the governmental agencies might do well to investigate the possibilities to employ rural physicians to administer prenatal care, delivery and postnatal care in their offices. In addition, it would be an added inducement for better trained physicians to practice in the rural communities where their services are so much needed.

Comment

Here is recommended and described for the rural practitioner a means of managing his obstetrical cases with greatest advantage to patients and doctor.

Nor need it be restricted to rural practice. We all know that very recently, when few there were who did not have to count expense, many a woman was taken to hospital only after labor had well begun and returned home by ambulance within 24 to 36 hours; and that mother and baby were just as well off.

Putting our patients to unnecessary expense is a large factor in the present threat of medical services paid for by taxation.

The plan of Dr. Torpin and associates deserves adoption by all doctors who do any considerable amount of obstetrics. And those beds may well be used for the accommodation of other classes of patients.

PEDIATRICS

THE LESSONS TO BE LEARNED FROM A STUDY OF INFANT DEATHS

The saving of infants' and children's lives chiefly accounts for the great increase in life expectancy brought about in our time. A chapter in the history of this accomplishment well worthy of our study comes from Chicago.[1]

Prematurity is a direct cause of one-fourth of all deaths occurring under one month of age and is a contributing factor in at least an additional one-fourth. Preventing the premature onset of labor is the ideal treatment. It is necessary to improve the environment into which the premature infant is born.

Even at the normal time of birth, lung development is very incomplete and in the premature period the infant is handicapped by greater immaturity of the tubular system.

In order to provide the infant with the greatest chance of survival it is necessary to place it in an environment which will compensate as far as possible for the incompleteness of development. The

---
1. E. L. Potter, Chicago, in *Jr. A. M. A.*, Feb. 5th.

higher the percentage of O which is present in the inspired air, the greater the absorption which is possible. Human milk is the food choice for all premature infants.

Incomplete development of the body's defenses against infection make the premature infant more apt to succumb to bacterial invasion.

Intracranial hemorrhage is the most common fatal injury and is almost always due to abnormal pressure on the head—from cephalopelvic disproportion, abnormal position of the head, abnormalities of uterine contractions or the improper application of forceps.

Any attempt to decrease the number of birth injuries must be primarily directed toward improved education of the physician and improvement of the environment in which birth is accomplished. When a normal fetus dies during labor when hemorrhage has not occurred the cause is usually anoxia, and, although at times due to cord and placental disturbances, at other times they are associated with excessive maternal sedation or the mismanagement of complications.

In infection the lungs are most frequently involved, although where delivery does not take place under sterile conditions there is still a high incidence of umbilical and cutaneous infections. Epidemic diarrhea takes an annual toll of lives which might be prevented if greater care were exercised in preparation of all material taken into the gastrointestinal tract.

The elimination of all pathogenic bacteria from the environment of the infant during delivery and after birth should be attempted.

Syphilis accounts for few deaths; with proper coöperation of patient and physician all these could be prevented. Abnormal fetal development, in our present state of knowledge, is almost the only condition which is not susceptible to amelioration.

The Chicago Health Department, in coöperation with the physicians of the city, drew up a set of rules governing the physical equipment and conduct of delivery rooms and nurseries and the medical and nursing care of all parturient patients and their offspring. There have been a few minor revisions since the original code.

All such infants have been cared for in especially equipped and staffed nurseries. An incubator ambulance is available when the infant is born at home or needs to be transported from one hospital to another. Human milk can be obtained through the health department if it is not otherwise available. Home conditions are investigated to make sure adequate care can be given the infant before it is discharged from the hospital. Public health nurses, if desired, are available to help the mother learn to care for her child.

Each hospital staff has arranged to have men with adequate training available for obstetric consultation; all physicians without specialized training in obstetrics are required to obtain consultation before undertaking any type of operative procedure. Antepartum care has been stressed, and early treatment of various abnormal conditions that arise during pregnancy, labor and delivery.

Hospitals caring for maternity cases have delivery rooms and rooms for convalescence of patients which are used for no other purpose. The nurses in an obstetric service and in the newborn nursery must limit their attention to such patients. The possibility of infection through the gastrointestinal tract, skin or lungs is reduced to a minimum. An attempt is made to observe an aseptic technic comparable to that used in an operating room.

While a small percentage of infants die in the absence of any discernible cause, the etiologic agent, in the great majority, can be discovered without difficulty.

Our greatest need is for greater disemination of information already available.

The 1942 death rate for Chicago was 40 per cent less than that for the country as a whole.

What has been accomplished in this city can be accomplished anywhere if a sufficient number of people have a great enough desire.

* * * * *

BLOOD IN THE STOOLS OF INFANTS AND CHILDREN

When a child passes blood from any part the mother is alarmed.

A Portland, Oregon, surgeon[1] gives pertinent information on this subject.

The commonest cause found for bright red rectal bleeding was anal fissure; the next, intussusception. The commonest cause of large intestinal hemorrhage in infants and children was Meckel's diverticulum. A rare case of chronic intestinal obstruction causes occult blood in the stools. Strangulated hernia may do the same. Banti's disease may cause tarry stools. Polyps of the colon have been the source of gross blood in stools, and ulcerative colitis or regional enteritis may account for slight to moderate amounts.

Bearing these facts in mind and making a rectal examination may save us embarrassment and make us more useful to our patients in remedying the cause of the trouble without the expense and inconvenience of consultation and hospital care.

[1] M. S. Rosenblatt, in *Northwest Medicine*, March.

Thought Treating Patients on Sunday Might be Sinful

Dr. John Allen, who practiced at the pioneer settlement of Salem, Ill., from 1830 to 1840, worried about treating patients on Sunday, but solved the problem by turning over all Sabbath fees to the church.—*Modern Medicine.*

SURGERY

Geo. H. Bunch, M.D., *Editor*, Columbia, S. C.

THE RIGHT OF THE SURGEON TO BE GOVERNED BY HIS JUDGMENT AT LAPAROTOMY

When laparotomy is advised by the surgeon and is accepted by the patient they enter into a contract, unspoken, unwritten and unnotarized, but nevertheless legally binding. A provision of this tacid relationship which has not been generally understood by surgeons should be emphasized.

Recently a pregnant woman, complaining of lower right abdominal pain, nausea and vomiting, was found on bimanual examination to have a tender mass the size of an orange in the right pelvis. Her physician diagnosed the condition as ectopic pregnancy and immediate operation was performed by him with the patient's permission for the removal of the tubal pregnancy. At operation a double uterus was found with a normal pregnancy. An inflamed appendix, which was the cause of her symptoms, was removed. "Subsequently, at normal term and in a normal way, the patient gave birth to a normal child." Later the physician sued the patient's husband to recover compensation for the performance of the operation." The husband resisted the surgeon's claim on the sole ground that the appendix had been removed without the consent of himself or his wife and that the operation, having gone further than was authorized, constituted a trespass or assault on the wife."

From a judgment in favor of the surgeon the defendant appealed to the Municipal Court of Appeals for the District of Columbia, which confirmed the judgment of the lower court. (Barnett *v.* Bachrach, 34 A. (2d) 626, District of Columbia, 1943.)

Justice Cardoza in a somewhat similar previous case announced the rule: "Every human being of adult years and sound mind has a right to determine what shall be done with his own body; and a surgeon who performs an operation without his patient's consent commits an assault, for which he is liable in damages. . . . This is true, except in cases of emergency where the patient is unconscious, and where it is necessary to operate before consent can be obtained."

As in the case cited, it is often impossible to make an accurate preoperative diagnosis of intra-abdominal pathologic states. The surgeon should operate only on the understanding that he have permission to do what in his judgment seems best for the patient. Only in this way can the welfare of the patient be safeguarded. This fact is understood and accepted by most patients. It is the disgruntled patient who tries to rob the surgeon of his reputation and of his money. A suit for trespass and assault is poor reward for the surgeon for doing his best. At operation the surgeon should be duty conscious rather than litigation conscious.

UROLOGY

Raymond Thompson, M.D., *Editor*, Charlotte, N. C.

DYSURIA AND NOCTURIA IN THE FEMALE

Treating females with sick bladders must be based on an accurate history of all previous ailments, and a survey of habits such as smoking and drinking, and previous medication. Too often the medical profession shows only a half-hearted interest in these patients.

Answer to pertinent questions (such as, "Do you have the frequency both day and night?") should be obtained, and an examination, aided by an intelligent and sympathetic nurse, should follow.

Abnormalities of the labia and surrounding structures, even of the anal orifice, should be noted, also pathological changes around the rectum. A thorough bimanual examination should complete the physical examination, and in many cases the advice of a gynecologist should be used on such matters as cystoceles and abnormalities of size or position of the pelvic organs.

Where a caruncle is discovered, hospitalization is indicated and study continued under a light anesthetic (low spinal). An examination of 202 cases[1] showed urethral strictures present in 8 cases, urethritis in 81. In 111 cases the bladder urine showed infection, in 20 cases the bladder contracted to less than 6 ounces. "In 54 cases of cysts at the vesical orifice cystic degeneration of the mucosa of the vesical orifice was easily demonstrated." In 2 cases interstitial cystitis was found and in 2 cases bilateral pyelonephritis. In 5 cases the bladder symptoms were caused by a relaxed perineum. "As a result of the frequency of involvement of the urinary tract above the caruncle it was concluded not only that urethral caruncle should be regarded as an important etiologic factor in the production of bladder symptoms, but that in many cases they act as true obstructions to the urinary outflow and produce the complications of urinary obstruction."

Though the female urethra may harbor organisms, a catheter may be passed if it can be done aseptically and without trauma and thus a catheter specimen of urine obtained for microscopic examination.

In the presence of inflammation of the bladder,

---
1. Dysuria and Nocturia in the Presence of the Normal Urine in the Female. G. F. McKim, P. G. Smith and I. W. Rush. *J. A. M. A.*, Nov. 6th, 1943.

rest in bed is advisable (with 8 or 10 glasses of water daily, soft diet and sulfathiazole) and further investigation should be postponed.

Cystoscopy was done in each of the 152 cases reviewed by McKim. Cystic degeneration was found to be a common cause of symptoms. Frequency was recorded in all cases and in cases with residual urine there was burning, straining and occasionally hematuria in addition. Of the bulbous type cases three gave a history of urinary retention.

"The cause of cyst at the vesical orifice has never been definitely proved"—but it is suggested that ". . . any condition that will produce an alteration of the normal blood stream supplying the vesical orifice should be given consideration as an etiologic factor in the production of cystic degeneration of the mucosa of the vesical orifice."

The best results in the treatment of such cysts are by hospitalization and, under light anesthesia, the high frequency spark, "it being necessary not only to cauterize the base of the protruding cyst, but to cauterize gently all of the mucosa of the vesical orifice."

In 72 cases where attention was first directed to the bladder by frequency, burning, pain, etc., pelvic disease was demonstrated, for ". . . If any organ or organs of the female pelvis becomes deranged, either functionally or pathologically, interfering with the normal bladder function, the bladder will signify this interference with a symptomatic response such as frequency, straining, burning or retention of urine."

McKim's paper amply demonstrates ". . . How varied causes of dysuria may be and how they can be discovered only by careful study and examination."

OPHTHALMOLOGY

HERBERT C. NEBLETT, M.D., *Editor*, Charlotte, N. C.

MYOPIA SINE MYOPIA (INCIPIENT MYOPIA)

THE THEORIES of the etiological factors in the production of myopia will not be discussed here. There is, however, a phase in its development in a few cases in which the visual status is that of myopia without the refractive error to justify its presentation as a clinical entity. During this phase via a cursory examination it might be diagnosed as amblyopia, unilateral or bilateral as the case might be, or as an initial or mild arrested type of retrobulbar neuritis or the result of some other d'sease condition of the eyes or of the brain.

The differential diagnosis from other conditions with which it might be confused is based upon the absence of any pathological changes in the media and eye grounds, in the fields of vision or any specific signs or group of symptoms suggestive of intracranial disease.

The condition when found is usually present in the early or middle period of adolescence in an individual of either sex. He is usually mentally brighter than his fellows, a keen student, a stickler for good grades in school. He is psychoneurotic, introspective and little given to indulge in the normal activities of youths of his age and environment. He is usually frail, has a haunted look, and appears to be constantly on the defensive. His main complaint is that for several months he has had moderate to severe episodes of dimness of vision, distant and near, without clear vision at any time since the initiation of his condition. The symptoms are augmented by the stress of school work and more particularly during prolonged periods of reading. Headache is not a common symptom, pain in or about the eyes is rarely complained of, but early fatiguability is common in use of the eyes for any purpose. Photophobia is frequent.

Upon examination of the eyes it is found that dilatation of the pupils is greater by one-third than normal and light and convergence reaction is slow. Accommodation is lowered and its range varies from day to day and from time to time even during the period of examination. Visual efficiency in the average case in each eye varies between 20/30 and 20/100; Jaeger type 1 and 3, though readable, is blurred. The vision if tested several times on the Snellen chart during an examination will vary all the way from 20/30 to 20/100. With atropine cycloplegia the visual efficiency for distance is usually comparable to that without it and in some cases is even better sustained. The refractive index with the retinoscope will under cycloplegic will rarely give more than $\frac{1}{4}$ diopter of simple myopia to $\frac{1}{2}$ diopter of combined myopia. The acceptance at the trial case will be comparable and vision is usually corrected to 20/30 or 20/40, but never to 20/20, either during or after the cycloplegic effect has worn off. Any part of a diopter of a plus lens or a combination thereof markedly lowers the visual quotient. The same is true of any combination of plus-minus lenses.

The question arises in such cases as to whether or not the small myopic correction as found should be prescribed. It has been the writer's practice to prescribe glasses only in those cases in which vision is consistently below 20/50 if it can be corrected to 20/40 or slightly better. This for the obvious reason that the individual will be less handicapped in distant vision especially in classroom work.

If these patients are examined from time to time the refractive error, in the majority, at the end of several months to one year, will be found to have become one of frank myopia with vision correctible to 20/20. The use or not of glasses in any case has not served to alter the progress of the myopia.

This transition of myopia sine myopia into a frank myopia can scarcely be said to have been brought about through the so-called turnstile of astigmatism, since this type of refractive error in the cases seen played a minor role in the refractive index. This surmise is therefore a reasonable deduction, or the astigmatic error was not found, or was too fleeting in its action to be detected.

DENTISTRY

J. H. GUION, D.D.S., *Editor*, Charlotte, N. C.

THE EFFECT OF TOPICALLY APPLIED SODIUM FLUORIDE ON DENTAL CARIES EXPERIENCE

THE RESULTS of numerous investigations into the relationship between fluorine and dental disease led to the hypothesis that the incidence of dental caries could be reduced by topical applications of a fluoride solution to the teeth.

In March, 1942, parental permission was obtained in three small urban centers in Minnesota to make topical application of fluoride to the teeth of 337 children aged seven to 15 years, and investigative work begun.[1]

Prior to the institution of treatment, each child in the treated group received a scaling and polishing of the teeth and a detailed dental examination. Only the teeth in the upper left and lower left quadrants of the mouth were treated. The treatment consisted of isolation of the teeth with cotton rolls, drying the teeth with compressed air, and wetting the crown surfaces of the teeth with 2-per cent sodium fluoride solution, allowed to dry in air for four minutes. After the cotton rolls had been removed, the child was instructed to expectorate and he was then dismissed.

During an 8-week period members of one group were given two treatments weekly to a maximum of 15 and a minimum of eight treatments; another group were given one treatment weekly to a maximum of eight and a minimum of seven treatments.

A year after the treatments the teeth of the children in both treated and control groups were reëxamined. Of the 337 children originally in the treated group, 289 were reëxamined; of the 392 children in the control group 326 were reëxamined.

The results demonstrate that topical applications of a 2-per cent sodium fluoride solution to the teeth under the conditions of this investigation was effective in reducing the incidence of dental caries

1. J. W. Knutson, U. S. Pub. Health Serv., & W. D. Armstrong, Univ. of Minn., in *Pub. Health Reports*, Nov. 19th.

by 40 per cent. The duration of the effect is not yet known.

Apparently the treatment is not effective in preventing caries attack on the noncarious surfaces of teeth previously attacked. Further, it would indicate that the effectiveness of the treatment is largely limited to the prevention of caries and that it is not effective in controlling active dental caries. Therefore, the validity of this finding will also be an important factor in establishing the procedures to be employed in conducting a program of topical applications of fluoride to the teeth.

Although a 2-per cent solution of fluoride was used in this study, the most effective concentration of this solution or of other fluorides is not known. A 2-per cent solution of sodium fluoride is highly toxic and must be used and guarded with extreme caution. Certainly the optimum concentration of the fluoride solution would be the minimum effective concentration.

GENERAL PRACTICE

JAMES L. HAMNER, M.D., *Editor*, Mannboro, Va.

ANEMIA IN PREGNANCY

BLOOD EXAMINATIONS as a part of prenatal care are not made at frequent enough intervals. The "physiologic anemia of pregnancy" is not a true anemia but simply a result of the increase in blood plasma with dilution of red blood cells and lowering of the hemoglobin. The usual decrease is 15%. Repeated examinations showing hemoglobin under 70% and erythrocytes below 3,500,000 indicate true anemia.

Eighty-seven per cent of an entire series of 75 cases reported[1] showed a hemoglobin of 69 per cent (10 grams) or less at some time during the pregnancy, although only 3.9% were this low on first examinations. The reports of several others cited show marked and immediate response to iron therapy in the microcytic anemia of pregnancy. Dieckman calls attention to the fluctuation of hemoglobin during pregnancy and cautions against attributing too much to therapy. Labate, in a controlled series of 325 patients who received 15 grains of ferrous sulphate daily, found an average red blood count of 4,090,000 and a hemoglobin of 11.61 grams on admission, while 307 patients who did not receive iron showed 3,010,000 and 8.16, respectively. He also showed a significant reduction in morbidity and hospital days in the treated series.

Present series: All patients with a hemoglobin under 70% were given 15 grains of an enteric coated ferrous sulphate preparation daily. If a significant response was not made, the dosage was

1. E. G. Evans, Aurora, in *Ill. Med. Jl.*, Nov.

increased to 30 grains. The average at six weeks post-partum showed a return of the hemoglobin to normal and a moderate increase in the erythrocyte count.

It is pointed out that the entire picture of blood changes in pregnancy is still confusing. There is marked variation in the time of onset of the hemoglobin fall and many examinations are necessary to determine the true incidence. Many investigators have shown there is less morbidity and toxemia, and more rapid recovery from blood loss, in those patients whose blood levels were normal; therefore, the use of simple iron salts in pregnancy is favored.

* * * * *

THE TREATMENT OF ACUTE GINGIVO-STOMATITIS (VINCENT)

THE MOUTH contains diverse forms of aerobic and anaerobic organisms, which may cause or perpetuate stomatitis when the mucous membrane is injured in any manner.

The most common type of stomatitis is Vincent's, an acute disease, usually of children of one to three years, but which occurs in children of any age and in adults; in epidemic form in schools and armies.

Pelner[1] gives a summary of the diagnostic symptoms and reports highly satisfactory results of treatment.

Acute infectious gingivostomatitis begins with fever, general aches and pains, inability to eat food; soon areas of redness are noted throughout the mouth, especially on the gums, which later ulcerate. The tongue, as well as the lips, may show the ulcerations. Sometimes the disease starts with involvement of the tonsils, extends to the gums and mouth structures.

Treatment. — Separate water glasses, dishes, knives and forks, sterilized separately; separate towels and soap. The saliva and mucus from the mouth of the patient should be disinfected before disposal. All articles that are used during the illness should be sterilized or discarded on recovery.

Before attempting to eat he should suck on one of the anesthetic lozenges; following this, juices can be taken without severe pain. Smoking and alcoholic beverages are interdicted, as are all spicy and rich foods. An extremely simple diet with diluted fruit juices is allowed.

Six adult cases of severe Vincent's angina and stomatitis were treated. Neoprontosil was given: 60 grains on the first and second days, 45 grains on the third, and 30 grains on the fourth day. In addition, a solution of neoprontosil, 5 grains in half an ounce each of distilled water and glycerin, was applied to the lesions every two hours; saline irrigations were useful in keeping the mouth clean.

All the cases were cleared up in an average time of four days.

THERAPEUTICS

J. F. NASH, M.D., *Editor*, Saint Pauls, N. C.

THE TREATMENT OF MENINGOCOCCIC MENINGITIS

FOR SO SERIOUS a disease, it is needful to have a schedule worked out in detail in advance. Washburne[1] supplies such a schedule.

The onset is usually preceded by malaise, nausea, aching, often mental confusion, and a headache which tends to increase. The patient may note spots on the extremities and trunk which may be mistaken for atypical varicella.

A toxic individual with fever of 100 to 105, little to considerable mental alteration, general hyperesthesia to touch, stiffness of the neck, opisthotonos, not infrequently small scattered petechiae on extremities and trunk, Babinski, Kernig, and/or Prudzinski signs suggestive or positive, should have an immediate lumbar puncture.

If complete laboratory facilities are not *immediate available*, and the spinal fluid is cloudy, opaque, or purulent, the examiner should do an immediate cell count and stain for predominating organisms. It is unwise to give large doses of the sulfa drugs in the treatment of meningitis, unless clearly indicated.

Before treatment is begun, 10 c.c. of blood should be withdrawn and sent to the laboratory for culture for meningococci.

For a normal sized, previously healthy adult, 4 to 5 Gm. of sulfadiazine constitutes the initial dose. *Orally* unless the patient is a) nauseated or vomiting, b) extremely ill so that a more rapid method must be used, or c) comatose. Crushing before administering hastens absorption.

By nasal catheter or stomach tube, after pulverizing in a small amount of water, when the patient is a) comatose or b) for some other reason unable to swallow.

Intravenously when a) a rapid method of administration is called for, or b) the patient is unable to retain the drug by mouth or tube. Sodium sulfadiazine which must have been previously sterilized is dissolved just prior to administration in 100 c.c. of freshly distilled water. Great care must be taken to prevent the solution from entering the tissues and so producing a slough. Give slowly by intravenous drip. Nembutal, 2 grains, as suppository, may obtain sedation. *While giving intravenous sodium sulfadiazine blood transfusions or in-*

---
1. Louis Pelner, Brooklyn, in *Amer. Jl. Dig. Dis.,* Mar.

1. A. C. Washburne, Madison, in *Wisc. Med. Jl.,* Dec.)

travenous glucose injections are to be avoided.

Subcutaneously: Five Gm. of sodium sulfadiazine may be given in 500 c.c. of sterilized physiologic saline, 250 to 300 c.c. per hour.

One to 2 Gm. q. 4 to 6 h., day and night. In severe cases, larger amounts or q. 2h. After two to three days q. 6 h. for four to five days. In general, the drug should not be discontinued until after the 10th to 12th day.

The first 24 hours should see a fall in t., p. and white count, decreased neck rigidity, and greater mental alertness. If not, one of three things is demanded:

a) Increase in the amount of sulfadiazine if the sulfadiazone blood level and the urinary output permit.

b) Shift to another of the sulfonamides, as sulfanilamide or sulfapyridine.

c) Utilization of antimeningococcic serum.

The urinary output for 24 hours should not be permitted to fall below 1,500 c.c. If the patient is unable to void, catheterize at 8-hour intervals. If the urinary output falls to 1,000 c.c. discontinue sulfadiazine until the output is again normal.

In the first day or two the diet is liquid, then soft and after 72 hours high caloric. Essential vitamins must be given from the first day of therapy. The first three days it may be well to give by hypo. 25 mg. of thiamin chloride, then 10 mg. of thiamin chloride and 10 mg. of riboflavin, daily.

For restlessness with nausea, nembutal suppositories, 2 rgains or 2 to 3 c.c. of paraldehyde *intramuscularly*. For persistent headache, codeine, ½ to 1 grain by hypodermic.

Quarantine period "at least two weeks from the time the case is reported and until temperature has become normal." From those who have been immediately exposed to the patient obtain cultures of the nose and throat, and place the individuals under supervision, with instructions to report at once if they note any of the prodromal symptoms.

Make daily ophthalmoscopic examinations for edema, hemorrhages and exudates, as frequent lumbar punctures are not in order as a check on intracranial pressure.

Examine the neck for decrease or increase in rigidity; ears for otitis media or deafness; chest for pneumonia, bronchitis, or pleurisy; heart for pericarditis, endocarditis, myocarditis, or enlargement; abdomen for rigidity, fulness of bladder, et cetera; genitalia in male or orchitis or epididymitis; skin for petechiae or edema; extremities for arthritic changes, edema, and reflexes.

T., p., r. and b. p. 2 h. for the first 24 W., then t.i.d.

Liquid intake and output should be recorded for each 12-hour period.

For the first week, obtain daily complete blood count and urinalysis.

Daily blood level determination of sulfadiazine, not to rise over 18 mg. per 100 c.c., and is best held at 10 to 12 mg. per 100 c.c. after the initial rise.

Blood chlorides taken before the administration of fluids will be helpful in estimating the initial amount of saline required.

Fluids should be kept at 4,000 to 5,000 c.c. per 24 hours for the first four days; 3,500 c.c. so long as sulfadiazine is being used. If the patient is unable to take them by mouth, normal saline not to exceed 1,000 c.c. may be combined with 2,500 c.c. of 5 per cent of glucose in sterile distilled water and given by hypodermoclysis; or 1,500 c.c. of 5 per cent glucose in sterile distilled water to make a grand total of 5,000 c.c. by vein. Glucose should not be given by vein if sulfadiazine is also being administered by this route.

If there is evidence of acidosis or alkali reserve below 40, give lactate Ringer's solution—available in 20 c.c. ampules (Lilly). Dilution 25 times, estimate 10 c.c., after dilution, per kilogram of body weight, unless the acidosis is very severe.

GENERAL PRACTICE

D. HERPERT SMITH, M.D., *Editor*, Pauline, S. C.

ACUTE VIRUS INFECTION WITH NERVE ROOT INVOLVEMENT SIMULATING APPENDICITIS

THIS REPORT[1] is concerned with acute pain and tenderness occurring in the right lower abdominal quadrant in 50 patients who did not have appendicitis. The admission diagnosis in all patients except two was acute appendicitis. These were young men observed during a six-month period at a station hospital. Of early patients in the group 13 were operated on, and in each instance a normal appendix was removed. All of us want to reduce our errors that subject our patients to unnecessary operations.

The onset was abrupt. Young men at work, playing football, sitting in a classroom or taking a walk were suddenly seized with a knifelike abdominal pain. This pain awakened them out of a deep sleep and on one occasion struck a medical officer just as he was reaching for his alarm clock. This medical officer had undergone appendectomy some years before.

Nausea and vomiting practically always occurred in the first few hours only. Often a full meal had been eaten just before the pain began.

[1] Capt. W. L. Butsch, M. C., and Lt.-Col. J. C. Harberson, M. C., in Jl. A. M. A., Oct. 16th.

This pain struck in the right middle or lower part of the abdomen as a rule. It might also be felt in the right loin, no shifting or localization of initial generalized pain as in appendicitis. Coughing or deep respiration reproduced the pain. Frequently the patient stated that the whole right side of the abdomen was sore and tender.

Pain was always worse at night. The patients said the pain was lessened when they were up and about.

The entire face presented a brick red appearance; conjunctivas heavily injected, drowsy appearance. The soft palate was entirely covered with a salmon pink raised plaque of edematous mucous membrane. Closer inspection revealed small papular elevations with yellow centers interspersed; pharynx not involved; no sensation of sore throat in 48 of the 50 patients.

The patient could always point to a definite area on the abdomen where the pain had its onset and was maximal. In 30 of the cases this was to the right of the umbilicus. The tenderness could often be traced along the course of the 10th intercostal nerve. The patient flinched and tightened the abdominal muscles the moment the skin was touched. When the patient's confidence was gained one could often palpate deeper and deeper without causing more pain. True muscle spasm was not found.

Two of the patients were admitted with the diagnosis of acute cholecystitis. The illness of one later followed the course of a virus pneumonia, and the x-ray appearance was consistent with that diagnosis. In every patient pain and tenderness were elicited all over the right side of the abdomen. Many of the patients referred pain to the right side of the abdomen when the left side was palpated.

During August, September and early October these patients uniformly showed no elevation of temperature or of pulse rate. As the common infections of the respiratory tract became more prominent in the late autumn some had t. as high as 102 F. and a pulse rate of 100, because of associated rhinitis, sinusitis or tonsillitis.

Only 12 patients had a t. above 98.6 and only three with a t. above 100. There were 16 patients with a leukocyte count of over 10,000 and four with a percentage over 75.

Lumbar punctures were done on five patients. No increase in spinal fluid pressure or cell count was found.

Two patients had x-ray findings consistent with a diagnosis of virus pneumonia, which rapidly cleared. The urine was always normal.

The nocturnal pain was sometimes severe enough to require morphine. Costolumbar nerve block was induced with procaine hydrochloride in five cases. Relief lasting six to eight hours was gained from this procedure. Herpetic or other lesions of the skin were not seen.

No syndrome which includes pain and tenderness in the right lower quadrant of the abdomen can ever be safely assumed not to be appendicitis without careful and repeated observations.

We realize that definite evidence that the infection was due to a virus is lacking.

* * * * *

ENCOURAGEMENT AS TO MALARIA

EXPERIENCE OF MALARIA in World War II has revised many ideas on the subject. One of the new teachings is that quinine should not be used as a prophylactic, because such use (1) will not prevent development of the disease, and (2) will make cases which develop much less amenable to the curative action of quinine.

Investigative work on malaria in birds[1] has produced promising results.

In birds the continuous type of treatment effected a *20-times greater retardation in trophozoite development than did the traditional type of treatment*. The senior author therefore suggests where large numbers of hospitalized malaria patients are being seen: a) continuous venoclysis with physiologic saline solution so fortified with a quinine salt that the patient shall obtain 30 grains of the drug in each 24-hour period; b) the same as the preceding but with a reduced amount of quinine; c) the venoclysis maintained for only 12 hours of each day with the quinine content doubled; d) any one of *a*, *b* or *c*, plus a small dose of quinine by mouth or intramuscularly at the beginning; e) the same as any one of *a*, *b*, *c* or *d* except that the saline-quinine solution be administered by intragastric drip as in the aluminum-hydroxide treatment of peptic ulcer.

All this is particularly encouraging in view of the fact that avian malaria in general has proved extraordinarily resistant to intermittent therapy.

1. Credit line has been misplaced.

PHENYL-PROPYL-METHYLAMINE HYDROCHLORIDE FOR ASTHMA
(K. Glaser, Louisville, in *Clin. Med.*, Mar.)

A new ephedrine-like compound phenyl-propyl-methylamine (Vonedrin brand*) hydrochloride, was investigated on a series of patients suffering from bronchial asthma.

In order to determine the clinical efficacy, the general condition of the patient, the number and severity of attacks was used as a standard of comparison. It was found that the efficacy of Vonedrin was equal, if not superior to that of ephedrine. The toxicity and production of undesirable symptoms was certainly less marked than from epinephrine or ephedrine, while it is not as efficient a bronchodilator as epinephrine.

By ecg. studies and studies of the blood-pressure, pulse rate, weight, and observations on central nervous stimulation it was found that there was no insomnia or nervousness from doses of Vonedrin ranging from 75 to 200 mgs. daily.

*Supplied by Wm. S. Merrill Co., Cincinnati.

HUMAN BEHAVIOUR

James K. Hall, M.D., *Editor*, Richmond, Va.

DR. WARREN TAYLOR VAUGHAN

Dr. Warren Taylor Vaughan died suddenly and unexpectedly at his home in Richmond on Sunday, April 2nd. He had probably thought himself to be in robust health. He carried all the appearances of a sound condition and he lived the daily life of a busy physician. The people are too much in need of medical skill to be willing to give up an acceptable practitioner at the too early age of fifty-one years.

Dr. Warren T. Vaughan was a member of an intellectual family. His father was Dr. Victor Clarence Vaughan, one of the distinguished scientists as well as one of the best known physicians and medical educators of this country. In his latter years, after he came from Ann Arbor to make his home in Richmond, I came to know him rather well. Although he was a native of Missouri, I think his parents were both North Carolinians, of the country near Durham, and that descent probably bound him and me somewhat together.

I recall that Dr. Victor Vaughan would occasionally speak to me of his recollections of the Civil War. His native Missouri was a border state, in which families were sometimes divided in their sympathies and in their allegiances. Dr. Victor Vaughan, as a small boy, would sometimes see the Union troops pursue the Confederates one day and a strengthened Confederate force drive the Federal soldiers back on the following day.

The Civil War must have interfered with his early schooling, but his innate hunger for knowledge was so constant and so insatiable that he got the bachelor's degree at about the usual age; and then he became a student of the University of Michigan. His connection in his youth with that soundly developing institution became good fortune both for him and for Michigan's University. From it Dr. Victor Vaughan acquired several degrees, including doctor of philosophy and doctor of medicine. He remained both a student and a teacher practically all the rest of his life after he had matriculated at Michigan. During his long deanship of Michigan's School of Medicine he brought it to the upper level of American medical colleges. He probably became competent to teach almost any course offered in medicine. And not nearly all of his interest was limited to medical education.

He participated as an important medical officer, on leave as dean of the Medical School, in the Spanish-American War, during which he took part in the important scientific observations made about the dissemination of certain fevers. Dr. Victor Vaughan was commissioned a medical officer in the first World War. But he always returned promptly and cheerfully from the field of war to the University campus; for he was fundamentally a teacher, a scientist, a searcher after truth. Dr. Victor Vaughan devoted his long life to the advancement of science.

But he never lost his touch with students, with folks, nor with patients. He thought of the scientist as a minister trained to render beneficent service to mankind. So he lived; so he taught his students; so he instructed his five children—all sons—by precept and by example to live their lives. Each of those sons, rather early in life, became well-known because of acquired skill in some division of knowledge. One of them gave his life for his country in the first World War. And in that War another son suffered serious impairment of health. One of those sons is a teacher of languages in a great university; another is a widely known public health administrator.

Dr. Warren Taylor Vaughan, the youngest of the quintette of sons, was a graduate of the University of Michigan in the School of Arts and in the School of Medicine. He left an internship in Boston to enter the first World War, from which he returned a Lieutenant-Colonel in the Medical Corps of the Army, though in years he was but a lad of twenty-five. One or two years of work at Harvard following that War gave him fitness for diagnostic work; and with such heredity, such education, such training, in peace and in war, he came a stranger into Richmond about 1920. And with him he brought his young wife. They gave of themselves freely and continuously to the life of this conservative but hospitable city of the South.

I should experience difficulty if I should be called upon to designate a doctor of any age, anywhere, who lived a life more evenly balanced between the search after truth in the wide domain of medicine and in daily ministration to folks sick in various ways. Each aspect of his interest seemed to help him better to do the other duty. He was apparently innately compelled to do both. Had he been domiciled in rural practice in the most remote county in this ancient Commonwealth, he could not have kept himself from setting in action some kind of medical investigative activity. Had he been made a member of the staff of any laboratory engaged in only the most abstract medical research, he would soon have been churched for doing at least a little clinical practice. He was obliged to be trying to find out some of the things that neither he nor any other knew. And he could not, or he would not, live without having the opportunity to try to find out what was the matter with some sick folks, so that he might try to help them to be well again. And while he was working with others he was always submitting himself to tutelage.

Although he was scholarly and learned and scientific always in his attitudes and in his professional activities, he was never pedantic or intolerant or arrogant or hostile in his criticisms. He was human and congenial and companionable.

We shall probably remain ignorant of the pathologic and of the philosophic reason for his death. Those phenomena—and they are all but countless in number—that we cannot understand we must respect by uncomplaining submission.

Dr. Warren Taylor Vaughan no longer has citizenship in Richmond and in the Commonwealth of Virginia. But it is not as if he had never lived amongst us. To those of us with whom he laboured he left an example of the doctor's life as it should be lived. And to the people of Richmond, and to those who came to him from afar, he has left an abiding conception of the ideal doctor. And to the widow and to the four sons, half of whom are doctors and all of whom will soon be physicians, he has bequeathed that priceless heritage that resists forever all disintegrative assaults—the memory of an honest mind and a courageous soul.

LARGE DOSES OF ASCORBIC ACID IN ESSENTIAL HYPERTENSION
(N. S. Davis & E. F. Poser, Chicago, in *Clin. Med.*, June)

To a few patients whose pressures were known to have been persistently high or rising ascorbic acid has been administered in doses of 1/3 Gm. t. i. d., except in two instances in which ½ Gm. have been given b. i. d. Some of the patients received vitamin B complex or some of its fractions before the ascorbic acid therapy was instituted, and others have received both vitamins.

The administration of 1.0 gram of ascorbic acid daily to patients with well-established arterial hypertension has *almost invariably caused subjective relief*. In most patients it has caused a marked lowering of the blood pressure levels. In a few it has had little if any effect.

OBSERVATIONS ON PAINS IN THE HEAD OF INTRANASAL ORIGIN
(H. I. Little, Rochester, Minn., in *Dig. Ophthal. & Otolaryng.*, Mar.)

One of the most common causes for pain is a contact between the anterior end of the middle turbinate bone and the septum. There is usually a bulge or deflection of the septum toward the turbinate or the turbinate may have become large and cystic and so press the two surfaces together. If cocainization relieves, the diagnosis of the cause of the pain is determined. Cure is afforded either by doing a septum operation and removing the anterior end of the middle turbinate bone, or by crushing the middle turbinate and pressing it into a more normal relationship with the lateral nasal wall and the septum, thus breaking the contact.

100,000,000 VOLT X-RAYS.—The Research Laboratory of the General Electric Company, Schenectady, N. Y., announces that 100,000,000 volt x-rays were produced on August 21st for the first time in the history of science. The first few observations show that these characteristics differ radically from those with which physicists are familiar.— *Science*, Sept. 3rd.

SURGICAL OBSERVATIONS
OF THE STAFF
DAVIS HOSPITAL
Statesville

PENICILLIN

THE EXPERIENCE of this clinic with penicillin has been extensive, and the results remarkably favorable. As was inevitable of a new remedy which has accomplished such remarkable results in certain infectious conditions which, without this remedy, were apparently hopeless, yet were promptly cured by its administration, the laity has become overenthusiastic and has expected penicillin to cure infectious conditions due to organisms non-susceptible to penicillin.

Unfortunately, the supply of this beneficent agent is limited and it is not available for use in many cases in which it would be of great help. For the present it is necessary to treat many infectious conditions with the sulfonamides which would yield much more rapidly and easily to penicillin. Because of the shortage of penicillin and the necessity of using large amounts of it for the Armed Forces, it has been necessary to limit its civilian use to those cases of great severity and in which it is specifically indicated.

It acts by inhibiting the growth and division or multiplication of bacteria. It is regarded by many as being directly bactericidal, rather than bacteriastatic as is the case with the sulfa drugs.

Penicillin may be given intravenously by the continuous drip method, intravenously by the intermittent method—for example, 10 to 20,000 units every three to four hours—or it may be given intramuscularly. In addition to these, it may be applied locally and can be used in certain types of infections, such as empyema cavities and in osteomyelitis where irrigation is possible. Penicillin is absorbed freely from muscular tissue or even when injected subcutaneously. It goes directly into the circulating blood and on to the most remote cells and tissues of the body, except it does not go from the blood into the cerebrospinal fluid.

Our experience has been that in small children the best method is to give this intramuscularly at regular intervals, usually every four hours. Naturally, in children of this age a continuous drip would not be practicable and the intermittent intravenous method would as a rule not be practicable except in larger children.

By keeping the body fluids continuously supplied to the optimum concentration, by giving the agent intramuscularly, the maximum of benefit is obtained. While penicillin may be given either in normal salt solution or in 5 per cent glucose, we have found glucose far more satisfactory. It is our opinion that this is the ideal method of administering the drug to the majority of adult patients. A point still in doubt is just how much penicillin should be used in the various types of infections. In some types more is necessary than in others. Especially in the sulfonamide-resistant group it is possible that treatment over a considerable length of time will be necessary in order to get the best possible results. It is rapidly destroyed and excreted by the body—in the urine, bile and saliva. For this reason the dosage should be large and preferably continuous. It is necessary to keep a high concentration in the blood.

The method best suited for administering penicillin requires the patient to be in a hospital where facilities are available for administering intravenous medication and where the patient can be observed carefully and where bacteriological and other special examinations can be made at regular intervals.

Penicillin is given in varying dosages, according to the size and age of the patient and the nature of the infection. Our experience has been that by giving penicillin continuously for 24 to 36 hours and then giving it ten to twelve hours out of the twenty-four we probably get the best results.

In order to do this we dissolve the penicillin in 5 per cent glucose and arrange to give this intravenously by the drip method, usually 30 drops to the minute, so that this will be given over a long period of time. The arrangement of this apparatus is very simple.

In a small child with severe infection 5 to 10 thousand units may be given intramuscularly every three to four hours, depending upon the urgency, and the reaction after these gives very little disturbance. Dosages for other types of patients and conditions are arranged according to age, severity, and promptness of response. The treatment in some cases may be discontinued after the first 24 to 48 hours. In other cases it may be necessary to keep it up over a period of days or even a week or more.

The results in cases where indicated are almost miraculous. It is a wonderful drug and will be the means of saving an enormous number of lives in the future.

When once this is made synthetically, naturally the field will be enlarged just as in the case of the sulfonamide drugs and, with the present penicillin as a base, possibly more potent products will be produced in the future so that practically all types of organisms that invade the human body will be susceptible to derivatives of penicillin, or kindred agents.

It is pleasant to contemplate the possibilities. Even infections that are now difficult to manage by any known form of treatment may be relieved in a short while. The possibilities for its use *in the prevention of infection*, especially in surgical conditions, and the elimination of infection if once established promises to be the greatest single factor in the reduction of mortality.

The field of chemotherapy will naturally enlarge and, since we have a product which is apparently harmless to the human body yet is apparently able to kill certain bacteria in the strength of one part to 24 million, we have the possible basis for the production of other compounds even more potent, more powerful germicides.

With the experience that is being rapidly gained in the use of penicillin, we can look forward to a tremendous reduction in mortality from infectious diseases and bacterial infections generally.

Even when given in doses far beyond those required for therapeutic purposes, penicillin is harmless to the human body. There are apparently no untoward results. In our experience there have been no toxic reactions.

At the present time penicillin is available for civilian use only in limited amounts but it is likely that in the very near future large quantities will be available for other than military use and we hope at a reasonable cost.

The chemical composition of penicillin is unknown. With the large number of chemists working on it, however, and other research workers, it will be only a limited time until the composition is found. When this is once done it is likely that this can be made synthetically and in large amounts and possibly at low cost.

SOAP STILL CLEANS
(Edi. in *Rocky Mountain Med. Jl.*, Feb.)

We have a microscope which is getting along in years, but it is still a good microscope.

Four years ago a defect appeared which gradually got worse, and gave us a lot of trouble. We eventually determined that the imperfections were confined to the top lens of the eyepiece. During a period of over three years, we tried to clean the lens with every chemical in the laboratory, short of concentrated acids. But it just got worse and worse.

We called several optical companies to see if they could polish the lens, but we were informed that it would be necessary to send the instrument back to the factory. They thought we might get it back in six months, or perhaps a year.

The other day we decided to wash the lens with soap and water. This wasn't as "scientific" as the other things we had thought of. We put the eyepiece together again, and looked at a smear through it. It was as clear as it had been the first time we used it, 23 years ago.

It seems that there ought to be a moral of some sort in this little story.

Maybe it is that sometimes we got too "scientific," at the expense of just plain horse sense.

Perhaps it is that life itself need not be as complicated as we humans, with our vaunted intelligence, insist on making it.

PRESIDENT'S PAGE

The Tri-State Medical Association's meeting at Charlotte, N. C., February 28th-29th, was one of the most successful meetings we have had. Because of the great increase of professional work and the many outside demands that have fallen on the shoulders of the physicians left at home during World War II, it was thought wise to postpone the annual 1943 meeting. The one held this year was the first in two years but the interest and enthusiasm had not waned, as there was a very large attendance with a goodly representation from each of the three States.

The program was well planned and all papers were excellently prepared and presented. The majority appearing on the program were members of the Society but several were guest speakers. I do not believe I have ever seen better attendance and more enthusiastic reception given to any medical program than was accorded this meeting during the entire two-days' session. The report of the secretary showed a large increase in membership this year and a larger number of members on the roll than in many years.

Among the many scientific papers presented and discussed, a most interesting and timely one was given by Dr. H. F. Starr, of Greensboro, on the subject, "The Politico-Economic Situation in Reference to Medicine." This you will find in the March issue of your Journal and should be read by everyone. Dr. Starr is to be congratulated for the time and energy necessary in obtaining for us these pertinent facts. He has done a great service for the entire medical profession by bringing these thoughts for our consideration.

I wonder if many of us give full recognition to the important place the Tri-State Medical Association fills. The three states, Virginia, North and South Carolina, have many things in common: (1) The same type of people with more or less similar habits make up the population. (2) The same type of physicians, surgeons and specialists are found here. (3) Each state is about evenly divided with farming, manufacturing and other businesses. (4) All three are states with similar geographical outline, mountains, Piedmont and flat lands bordering on seacoast. (5) The climate is similar and most of the same diseases are found here.

It is, therefore, most wise that the doctors from these states come together for friendship and professional conferences. Every physician eligible should heartily support the Tri-State Medical Association.

Both Dr. F. S. Johns, the past president, and Dr. J. M. Northington, the secretary, are due much praise for engineering such a successful meeting.

—K. B. PACE, M.D.

SOUTHERN MEDICINE & SURGERY

Official Organ

JAMES M. NORTHINGTON, M.D., *Editor*

Department Editors

Human Behavior
JAMES K. HALL, M.D....................Richmond, Va.

Orthopedic Surgery
JOHN T. SAUNDERS, M.D. ....Asheville, N. C.

Urology
RAYMOND THOMPSON, M.D................Charlotte, N. C.

Surgery
GEO. H. BUNCH, M.D....................Columbia, S. C.

Obstetrics
HENRY J. LANGSTON, M.D................Danville, Va

Gynecology
CHAS. R. ROBINS, M.D..................Richmond, Va.
ROBERT T. FERGUSON, M.D. ....Charlotte, N. C.

General Practice
J. L. HAMNER, M.D.....................Mannboro, Va.

Clinical Chemistry and Microscopy
J. M. FEDER, M.D.,   }
EVELYN TREBBLE, M. T.   } ....Anderson, S. C.

Hospitals
R. B. DAVIS, M.D......................Greensboro, N. C.

Cardiology
CLYDE M. GILMORE, A.B., M.D...........Greensboro, N. C.

Public Health
N. THOS. ENNETT, M.D..................Greenville, N. C.

Radiology
R. H. LAFFERTY, M.D., and Associates......Charlotte, N. C.

Therapeutics
J. F. NASH, M.D.......................Saint Pauls, N. C.

Tuberculosis
JOHN DONNELLY, M.D....................Charlotte, N. C.

Dentistry
J. H. GUION, D.D.S....................Charlotte, N. C.

Internal Medicine
GEORGE R. WILKINSON, M.D..............Greenville, S. C.

Ophthalmology
HERBERT C. NEBLETT, M.D...............Charlotte, N. C.

Rhino-Oto-Laryngology
CLAY W. EVATT, M.D....................Charleston, S. C.

Proctology
RUSSELL VON L. BUXTON, M.D............Newport News, Va.

Insurance Medicine
H. F. STARR, M.D......................Greensboro, N. C.

Dermatology
J. LAMAR CALLAWAY, M.D. ....Durham, N. C.

Pediatrics

Offerings for the pages of this Journal are requested and given careful consideration in each case. Manuscripts not found suitable for our use will not be returned unless author encloses postage.

As is true of most Medical Journals, all costs of cuts, etc., for illustrating an article must be borne by the author.

THE PRACTICAL MANAGEMENT OF HEADACHE

THE COMMONEST of all symptoms is headache. Headache has made larger fortunes than appendicitis or enlarged tonsils. A St. Louis[1] doctor thinks we could do more and better for headaches. He puts his finger unerringly on a number of the weak points in the management.

First he comes out against the commonly held, but entirely mistaken, idea that most headaches come from the eyes.

How frequently do we hear from patients stories like this as told by Proetz:

The patient with a headache has an idea, let us say, that it is his eyes. When he goes to the ophthalmologist; the ophthalmologist, instead of saying. "headache is caused by some 30 or 40 things; you go to someone who is conversant with those things and let him find the cause of your headache," is likely to say "your eyes are all right. You should go over and see the sinus doctor across the hall, because it looks to me like a sinus headache." The sinus doctor examines him and says, "I think you should see a neurologist." The neurologist sends him to the dentist. The dentist finds no explanation of the headaches. The patient is discouraged, everything is just where it was in the beginning except that the patient is out of pocket and perplexed. The patient should be directed to someone who is essentially interested in headache and who will take the trouble to go through the entire category of things which might cause it.

Dr. Proetz has made a classification which, he says, "is thoroughly unscientific and at the same time thoroughly practical." Class A, headaches of definite, demonstrable origin—regardless of the origin. Class B, headaches of semi-demonstrable, or questionable, origin. Class C, headaches of undemonstrable origin, "at least to me." The demonstrable causes are local and remote. Histamine headaches are demonstrable and they are definite. He has not seen many histamine headaches. A patient may have anemia and a headache, but it is often hard to attach the headache to the anemia.

A great many hereditary headaches he finds can be relieved. He disagrees with those who think all severe headaches are simply a matter of eating onions or lobster or rhubarb.

The "idiopathic" headaches are largely vascular in nature. They may be caused by endocrine disturbances, hypertension, or a number of other things, "but the causes do not become apparent through any laboratory test."

Most important he regards the history—"a complete headache history which is written down according to a definite plan, preferably upon a pre-

---
[1] A. W. Proetz, St. Louis, in Jl. Iowa Med. Soc., March.

pared chart, with symptoms in juxtaposition which ordinarily would seem to have no relationship."

Some of the references are to foods, and some are to contacts, like dogs and face powder and feathers. The patient records his exposures on this chart for two or three weeks. The patient may be subjected to unaccustomed postural strains. He may have a headache because he works long hours, does not get enough sleep or is worried about his boy at the front.

Very few headaches has this doctor, who sees many patients with headaches, found due to nasal causes or to the sinuses. The periosteum, we are reminded, is closely bound to bone, so a sudden pulling or a distortion of the periosteum may cause sinus pain. Certainly a distortion of the mucosa does not. Tugging on the venous spaces and on the arteries of the brain and its covering is another thing.

In patients with hypertension headaches are most common when the pressure is *coming down*.

The first thing Proetz does with a patient with headache of no demonstrable cause is to prescribe ephedrine with a little seconal morning and evening for a few days, or t.i.d. It is surprising the number of people whose headaches disappear, and stay away for some time. If the patient gets any reaction to ephedrine, you should look farther into the vascular causes.

What is the next thing to try? The administration of thyroid extract. There are people whose basal metabolic rates are —5 to +5 who suffer from thyroid deficiencies, with headache. Often they complain of fatigue, even after plenty of sleep, and often headache after too much sleep. It is surprising how many of the patients without a demonstrable thyroid deficiency will recover from their headaches on thyroid extract. He has found people with a basal metabolic rate of +2 or +3 do well on 2 and 3 grains of thyroid extract who will not respond to 1 grain. One can increase the thyroid administration to an extent otherwise inadvisable and cure the headache, by giving thiamin at the same time. The two things Proetz finds most valuable are the ephedrine experiment and the thyroid treatment.

Some of his patients' headaches come on suddenly, often with hunger or in some relation to the ingestion of food—a severe headache across the brow and usually radiating across the top of the eye and down to the occiput. In many such cases an enema stops the headache. A laxative, given in time, may prevent such a headache.

Hunger is a frequent cause in people who wait too long for lunch. They get a headache when they become hungry, but eating does not stop it. It is well to eat something about 11.

About alcohol he asks: Not, do you drink?, but, how much do you drink? what kind of drinks do you tolerate?, and in what relationship to food does your drinking affect your headache?

Patients who have headaches from smoking are usually those with a septal spur or some demonstrable constriction in the nasal fossa, so that eddies are produced which deposit tar in one particular spot. Faulty heating and air conditioning in houses produce the same type of irritation.

There may be two or more causes for the same headache.

There's not a one of us but may learn a good deal from what this doctor, who believes in his methods, is a keen observer, and is good at analysis of a situation, has to say on what to do about this pain that everybody has, with the exception of old man Dick Vaughan, who said when he was 87, "I never have had a headache and my feet never have been cold."

CHARLES WILLIS CALLS MEDICAL COLLEGE OF VIRGINIA ALUMNI

Doctors graduated from the Medical College of Virginia and practicing in North Carolina take as prominent a part in the meetings of the State Medical Society as do those from other schools. We have our parts in the General Sessions and in the Sections. We have our full share in the responsibility for achieving and maintaining a high standard of professional service in this state, in proportion to our numbers, and we are many.

But it seems that the fire of college spirit burns less warmly in us than in graduates of some other schools. For at least two years Dr. Byrd Charles Willis has been working toward correcting this deficiency. Last year's enthusiastic Medical College of Virginia Luncheon Meeting, held in the course of the meeting of the State Medical Society, was due largely to his endeavors. This year he is asking us all to bear it in mind that an even better meeting is scheduled for Wednesday, May 3d, at 12:30, of course at the Carolina Inn.

Modesty is a virtue, but it may be overdone. When the new Medical College of Virginia Hospital was first opened for patients, it was widely proclaimed—not by any one having anything to do with the achievement, but by hospital authorities generally—as the best and most complete in the world. That, perhaps, was laying it on a bit heavy, but it was and is an institution of which we can well be proud. And this is true of all the other departments of the Old School. It may be recalled, also, that when Memorial Hospital opened its doors forty years ago it laid just claim to being the last word in hospital comfort and care.

To Page 151

NEWS

PATIENTS WON'T LET COUNTRY DOCTOR QUIT

The country general practitioner is said to be passing from the American scene, but at 88 Dr. Henry Boardman Stewart is ministering to the ills of the grandchildren of the first babies he delivered in Greenville County, S. C.

"They just won't let me quit," explains Dr. Stewart.

In the 65 years he has practiced, Dr. Stewart estimates he has brought 5,000 babies into the world. Even now, in roughest weather, he gets out of his bed at all hours and drives miles to provide safe conduct into a world he has found, in the main, good.

MECKLENBURG COUNTY MEDICAL SOCIETY, Medical Library, March 7th, 8 p. m.

A New Drug in the Treatment of Hyperthyroidism, with Report of Cases, Dr. Walter B. Mayer. Discussion by Dr. Luther W. Kelly, Dr. Thomas D. Sparrow, Dr. Paul Kimmelstiel.

2. Comments on Surgery and Medical Institutions Seen on a Latin American Mission, Dr. O. L. Miller.

DR. McCAIN HONORED

For Dr. Paul Pressly McCain, who finished his 30th year of service with North Carolina Sanatorium last month, the staff members and directors of the three State Sanatoria arranged a program which began with open house at the Sanatorium the afternoon of March 13th.

At the dinner Dr. Paul Ringer, Asheville, close associate of Dr. McCain, was the principal speaker. Acting as toastmaster was L. L. Gravely, Rocky Mount, chairman of the board of directors. The North Carolina Tuberculosis Association was represented by Dr. R. L. Carlton, Winston-Salem, president, and Frank Webster, Raleigh, executive secretary. Representing the Medical Society of the State of North Carolina, of which Dr. McCain is an ex-president, was Dr. James W. Vernon, Morganton, president, and Dr. Roscoe D. McMillan, Red Springs, secretary-treasurer.

Dr. McCain is also a trustee of Flora Macdonald College, Red Springs, Fellow of the American College of Physicians, member of the Clinical and Climatological Association, American Trudeau Society, Southern Tuberculosis Conference, North Carolina Tuberculosis Association and the National Tuberculosis Association.

DR. JAMES K. HALL, Richmond, was the chief speaker before the meeting of the Charlotte Mental Hygiene Society held at Hotel Charlotte, March 29th.

DR. DU PONT GUERRY, III, has opened his office in the Professional Building in Richmond for the practice of ophthalmology.

MARRIED

Dr. Fay Ashton Carmines, of Richmond, and Miss Lillie Weeks Burns, of Goldsboro, were married on March 4th. Dr. Carmines is serving an internship at the Medical College of Virginia Hospital.

DIED

Dr. Curran B. Earle died after an illness of only a few hours at his home in Greenville, South Carolina, on March 21st at the age of 69. A son of the late Dr. T. T. Earle, he was born on July 27th, 1875, at the old Earle homestead, Deep Creek Plantation, in Anderson County.

Upon graduation at Furman University, he pursued his studies in medicine at the University of Maryland, where he received his degree in 1896. Before returning to Greenville to practice, he served an internship at the University Hospital and at the Woman's Hospital in Baltimore. In coöperation with Dr. T. T. Earle and Dr. J. B. Earle he established the first hospital in Greenville and became renowned as a surgeon and as a physician. He was a charter member of the American College of Surgeons; a member of the American Medical Association, the Southern Medical Association, the Tri-State Medical Association and the South Carolina Medical Association. He had served as president of his State and County medical societies.

During World War I he was commissioned a major in the Medical Corps and was in charge of Camp Wadsworth's Hospital and Surgical Service. In addition to his wide practice in Greenville, he was surgeon for all the railroads at Greenville.

Dr. James Tayloe Gwathmey, founder and first president of the American Association of Anesthetists, died at the U. S. Veterans Hospital, Fayetteville, Ark., February 11th.

Dr. Gwathmey developed the method known as "Gwathmey's analgesia" in the New York Lying-in Hospital, in 1924, in co-operation with Dr. Asa B. Davis to overcome the defects of the anesthesia known as "twilight sleep." The method was accepted by maternity hospitals generally.

He was a native of Norfolk and a graduate of the Virginia Military Institute and of Vanderbilt University Medical School. In 1902 he began the practice of medicine in New York City and shortly began his researches in anesthesia.

In the first World War, Dr. Gwathmey introduced a method of administering ether and oil instillations orally for dressing of painful wounds. He had previously published a book entitled "Anesthesia," which was considered a standard work in 1924.

Dr. Ernest Sutherland Bulluck, 56, prominent Wilmington surgeon who established and operated Bulluck Hospital, died March 13th at the hospital.

Dr. Bulluck became critically ill February 1st. He had shown improvement recently and his death came suddenly.

Dr. Bulluck was born at Whitakers, the son of the late Dr. and Mrs. D. W. Bulluck. As a young man he attended Guilford College and later Virginia Military Institute and the University of Virginia. He was graduated from the School of Medicine of the University of Maryland. At the start of World War I, he entered the Army Medical Corps. Following the war he returned to Wilmington and resumed practice. The hospital was opened in 1922.

Dr. Bulluck was a Fellow in the American College of Surgeons, a member of the American Medical Association, past president of the New Hanover Medical Society and a former vice-president of the North Carolina Medical Society.

Dr. Horace L. Goodman, 63, head of the General Hospital at Ronceverte, W. Va., died March 4th at his home after a brief illness. Dr. Goodman, a native of Campbell County, was educated at Richmond College and the Medical College of Virginia.

Dr. J. L. Jefferies, 77, died at his home in Spartanburg recently. Dr. Jefferies was a graduate of the New York University Medical College in 1889, and began the practice of medicine in South Carolina the same year. He practiced in Spartanburg for 45 years.

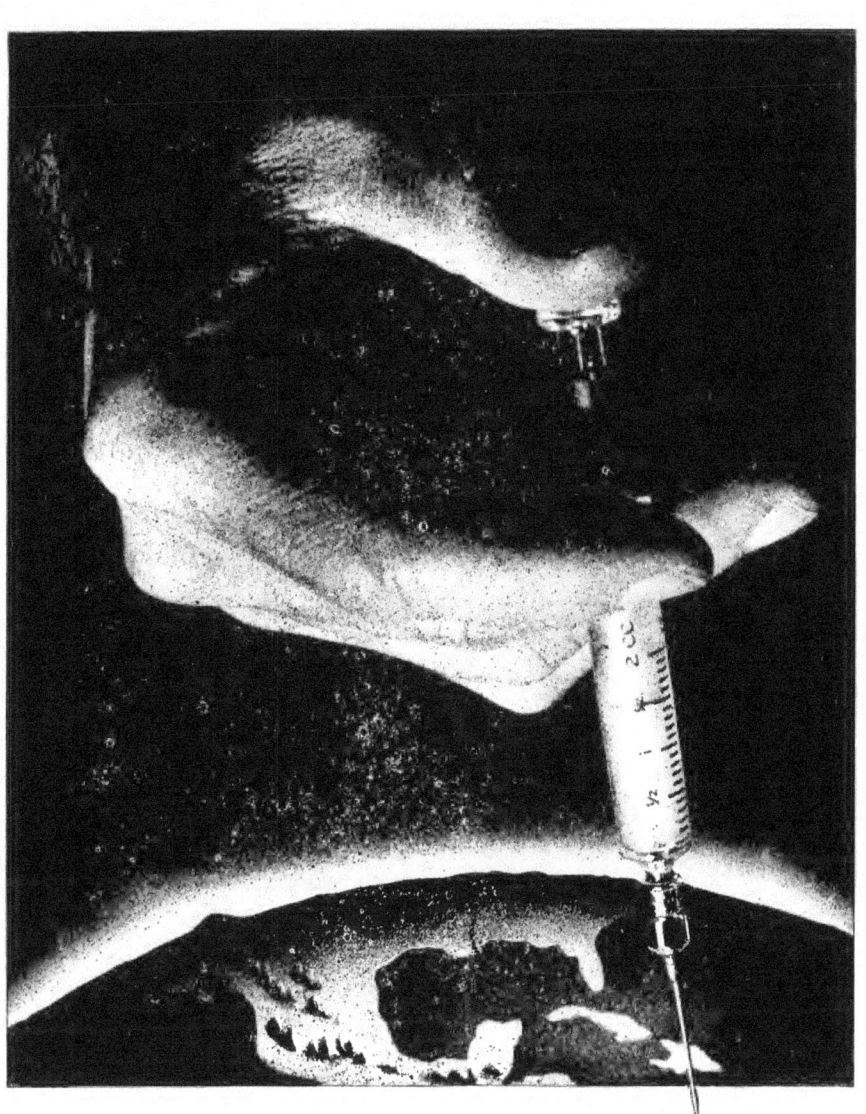

CONQUEST OF PAIN...PANTOPON 'ROCHE'

Dr. William Heyward Furman, 58, for more than 30 years a leading physician of Henderson, N. C., and widely known throughout the state, died suddenly of a heart attack at his home April 3d. For two years he had suffered with a heart ailment. He was born at Louisburg and educated at Wake Forest College and Jefferson Medical College at Philadelphia, going to Henderson in 1910 to practice his profession.

Dr. David Leighton Kinsolving, of Abingdon, Va., prominent physician of Southwest Virginia, died March 13th in the University of Virginia Hospital at Charlottesville.

A graduate of the Medical College of Virginia, he had practiced in that section for almost half a century. Except for two short periods, his entire practice was in Washington County, the latter years in Abingdon, where he made his home. He was with the United States Medical Corps in France during World War I, holding the commission of captain.

UNIVERSITY OF VIRGINIA

On February 18th the Virginia Alpha Chapter of Alpha Omega Alpha presented Dr. Theodore Squier, Associate Professor of Medicine at Marquette Medical School, in a lecture on Hematologic Manifestations of Hypersensitive States.

The University of Virginia Medical Society held a meeting on February 28th. Dr. E. I. Evans of Richmond, Virginia, spoke on the subject, The Mechanism and Management of Traumatic Shock. At this meeting Dr. Samuel A. Vest was elected President and Dr. Carlton J. Casey was elected Secretary.

At the meeting of the American Society for the Control of Cancer in New York City on March 11th, 1944, Dr. Edwin P. Lehman was elected Vice-President.

MEDICAL COLLEGE OF THE STATE OF SOUTH CAROLINA

Dr. Daniel W. Ellis, associate in the Department of Clinical Pathology, is being sent, through the coöperation of the Association of American Medical Colleges and the John and Mary R. Merkle Foundation, to Central America for the study of tropical medicine and parasitic diseases.

Dr. Ellis left on Monday, March 27th, for a period of six weeks. He expects to make observations on in- and out-patients and take part in field trips into rural areas. He has been invited to attend meetings of the Medical Societies of San José and Guatemala City at which he will be called upon to speak.

MEDICAL COLLEGE OF VIRGINIA

Dr. Everett I. Evans, Associate Professor of Surgery, spoke before the University of Virginia Medical Society on the Management of Traumatic Shock on February 28th.

Dr. Harry Bear, Dean of the School of Dentistry; Dr. S .S. Arnim, Assistant Professor of Operative Dentistry; Dr. A. H. Fee, Associate Professor of Operative Dentistry; Dr. Charles F. Vallotton, Assistant Professor of Operative Dentistry; and Dr. P. J. Modjeski, Assistant in Crown and Bridge Prosthesis, attended the annual meeting of the American Association of Dental Schools in Chicago, March 20th-22nd. Dean Bear, Doctor Arnim and Doctor Fee attended also the International Association for Dental Research in Chicago March 18th and 19th prior to the Association meeting.

THE TREATMENT OF CREEPING ERUPTION WITH FUADIN
(J. F. Wilson, Jacksonville, in *Jl. Fla. Med. Assn.*, April)

In this paper creeping eruption refers strictly to the type caused by the Ancylostoma braziliense, the lava of a kind of hookworm.

In five cases, after 1 5-c.c. injection, no further treatment was needed, but in two cases a second injection was required. Two c.c. administered to a baby of 13 months, and the dose was then graduated up to $3\frac{1}{2}$ c.c. in a child of eight years. In no case was there an untoward reaction.

The finding that fuadin is effective in such dissimilar diseases as granuloma inguinale, larva migrans and Vincent's stomatitis suggests that it has a large field of possibilities in diseases of protozoal origin.

Ethyl acetate collodion gives temporary relief from the itching and may be applied as often as desired.

Fuadin appears to be a specific. In the majority of cases one dose is sufficient.

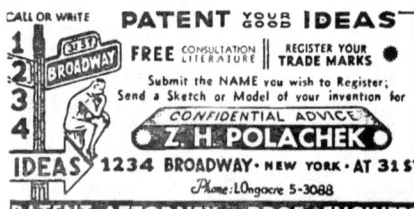

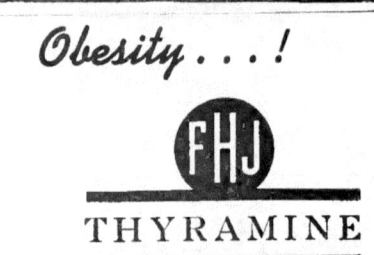

Composition

Thyroid 1 gr. Amphetamine sulphate 5 mgs. Thiamin chloride 1 mg. in suitable combinations with physiological reinforcements.

No. 1—One Capsule before breakfast
No. 2—One Capsule before lunch
No. 3—One Capsule at 4 p. m.

Contraindications

Hypertension .... Hyperthyroidism

Supplied

Capsules: Packages 21 and 42 (one or two weeks supply).

—Professional samples on request—
Available: Any professional pharmacy
F. H. J. PRODUCTS
977 East 176th St., New York 60, N. Y.

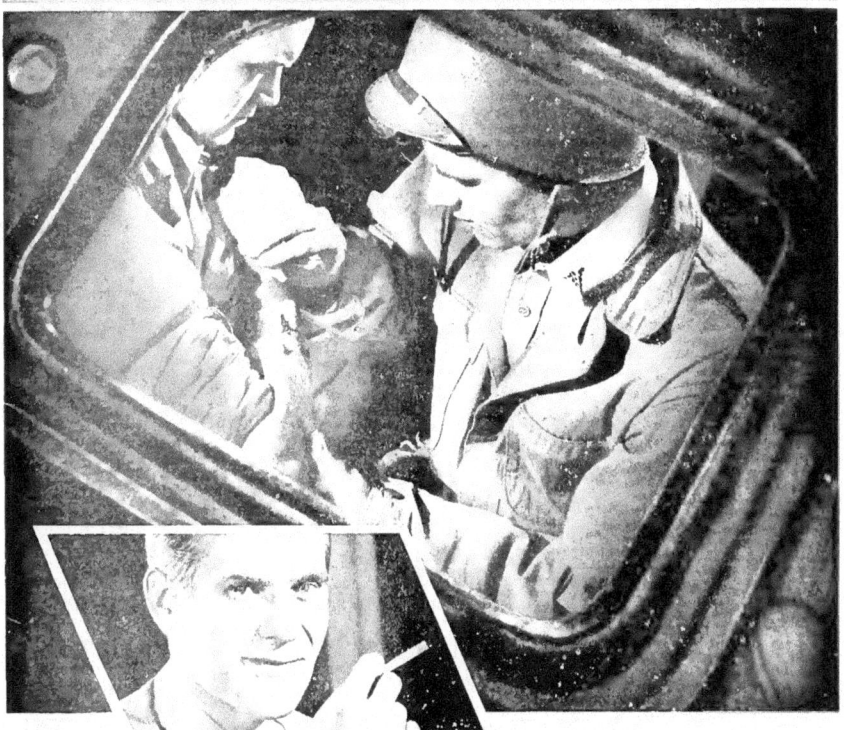

EMERGENCY IN A "FRYING PAN"

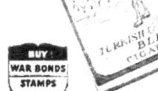

● They call it the hottest spot in war...the blistering gullet of a front-line tank. But medical officers don't hesitate...down they go to the casualties. Tough? Sure—but routine to the war doctor. Heroic risks, exhausting shifts; no special praise. He's thankful for "time off" now and then. Time for a friendly smoke...Camel preferably...the first choice of our men at war.

Camel, they say...for extra mildness, for rare good taste. Camel, for those precious moments of relaxation when a fighting man looks to his cigarette for richly earned comfort.

1*st in the Service*

With men in the Army, the Navy, Marine Corps, and Coast Guard, the favorite cigarette is Camel. (Based on actual sales records.)

CAMEL *costlier tobaccos*

New reprint available on cigarette research—Archives of Otolaryngology, March, 1943, pp. 404-410. Camel Cigarettes, Medical Relations Division, One Pershing Square, New York 17, N. Y.

BOOKS

THE PRINCIPLES AND PRACTICE OF MEDICINE: Originally Written by Sir William Osler, Bart., M.D., F.R.C.P., F.R.S., by Henry A. Christian, A.M., M.D., LLD. (Hon.), Sc.D., Hon. F.R.C.P. (Can.), F.A.C.P., Hersey Professor of the Theory and Practice of Physic, Emeritus, Harvard University; Clinical Professor of Medicine, Tufts College Medical School. 15th edition. *D. Appleton-Century Company, Inc.*, New York and London. 1944. $9.50.

For a textbook to be put out in a new edition within the period of eighteen months is conclusive evidence of its exceptional value.

The name, Osler, was warranty of the best in medicine while he lived. Since his death, more than the revisions and additions necessitating new editions have been made by men whose names have continued the warranty.

In the short period since publication of the next preceding edition great advances have been made, many additions to our therapeutic armamentarium and much clarification as to claims for additions made less recently. All this is presented in a judicious manner. Due cognizance is taken of the practical importance to doctors of this country of a knowledge of disease conditions which are even now being brought to us from far parts by returning members of the armed forces, and by the agency of the airplane; also of the states of impaired nutrition to be expected, the increase of venereal diseases, and other medical problems growing out of the war now going on.

The introduction makes it plain that the author thinks of the sick man as a person, not as a case; that he regards his patient as a diseased or disordered personality, his problem as one of a person who has a disease, rather than a disease which has a person.

There is not a disease called medical which one is likely to encounter in a lifetime of practice, on which Christian does not give all the essentials of diagnosis and treatment—and from his own long and rich experience. And it may fairly be said that Christian's dealing with treatment is much fuller and more satisfying than was Osler's.

HUMAN CONSTITUTION IN CLINICAL MEDICINE, by George Draper, M.D., Associate Professor of Clinical Medicine, College of Physicians and Surgeons, Columbia University; C. W. Dupertuis, Ph.D., Physical Anthropologist, Constitution Clinic, Presbyterian Hospital, New York City; and J. L. Caughey, Jr., M.D., Med. Sci.D., Associate in Medicine, College of Physicians and Surgeons, Columbia University. *Paul B. Hoeber, Inc.*, 49 East 33rd St., New York, London. 1944. $4.00.

The senior author has contributed greatly to our knowledge of the importance of the factor of the human constitution in the study of disease and its management.

Now Available
LEXO WAFERS
SOYBEAN LECITHIN FILLED

For the Treatment of:

PSORIASIS

HYPERCHOLESTEROLEMIA

POOR INTESTINAL ABSORPTION OF FAT AND FAT-SOLUBLE VITAMINS

LIVER CIRRHOSIS

HEPATIC INSUFFICIENCY

BIBLIOGRAPHY

1. **Adlersberg & Sobotka 1943.** (Fat and vitamin A absorption) J. Nutrition, v. 25, No. 3.
2. **Adlersberg & Sobotka.** (Hypercholesterolemia) J. Mt. Sinai Hospital, vol. IX, No. 6.
3. **Goldman.** (Psoriasis) Cincinnati J. Med. vol. 23, No. 4. 4. **Smith, Goldman & Fox.** (Psoriasis) J. Inv. Derm. vol. 5, p. 321.
5. **Gross & Kesten.** (Psoriasis) Arch. Derm. & Syph., vol. 47, p. 159-174. 6. **Kesten.** (Psoriasis) New England J. Med., vol. 228, p. 124.
7. **Hoagland.** (Cirrhosis) N. Y. State J. Med., vol. 43, p. 1041.

Write for free samples and information
AMERICAN LECITHIN CO., INC.
ELMHURST, L. I., N. Y., DEPT. 7

The authors' own methods of approach to the study of the subject are sufficiently detailed. Striking chapter heads are: Personal Inheritance and Personal Disease; Growth, Development, Decline and Death; Problems of Observation, Correlation, and Interpretation; Constitutional Physiology; Problems and Examples in the Clinical Use of Constitution Studies; and Unity of the Organism.

A careful study of this book cannot fail to deepen the understanding of the physician of the problems presented by his patients or to materially increase his usefulness in the management of these problems.

NERVOUSNESS, INDIGESTION, AND PAIN, by WALTER C. ALVEREZ. M.D., Professor of Medicine, University of Minnesota (Mayo Foundation); Consultant in the Division of Medicine, The Mayo Clinic. *Paul B. Hoeber, Inc.*, 49 East 33rd St., New York 16, N. Y. 1943. $5.00.

Dr. Alveraz has been one of the chief among those to lead us back from the too-physical concept of disease which dominated the teaching when most of us were in the medical schools.

A listing of the chapter heads will prove revealing:

Ways in Which Emotion Can Affect the Digestive Tract; The Making of the Diagnosis From a Good History; Importance of Uncovering the Patient's fear or His or Her Real Reason for Consulting a Physician; What Can Be Learned From the Way in Which the Patient Tells the History?; Helps in Sizing Up the Patient; Useful Observations to be Made as the Physician Deals With a Patient; Problems That Come Up in Planning the Examination of the Patient; The Handling of the Nervous Patient; The Problem of Combatting Disturbing Diagnoses Previously Made; On Telling the Truth to Patients; Helpful Points in the Diagnosis of Abdominal Pain; The Chronic "Dyspeptic," and Some of the Things That May be Wrong With Him; Constitutional Inadequacy; The Nervous Breakdown and Its Causes; Insanity and Related Troubles; Types of Neurotic Persons; The Stormy Menopause; Insomnia; Constipation; The Irritable Bowel Syndrome Commonly Called Mucous or Spastic Colitis; Food Sensitiveness or Allergy; Flatulence; Abdominal Bloating, Not Due to Gas; Pseudo-Appendicitis; Pseudo-Ulcer; Pseudo-Cholecystitis and the Postcholecystectomy Syndrome; Regurgitation or "Nervous Vomiting"; Headache; Migraine and Migraine Equivalents; Gastritis; Nervous or Functional or Puzzling Types of Diarrhea; Abdominal Distresses Associated With Pelvic Troubles in Women; Miscellaneous Syndromes; The Treatment of Nervous, Psychopathic, Poorly Adjusted, Much Troubled or Overworked and Tired Persons.

The only statement added is that each of these chapters is written from the amplest experience as analyzed by this master clinician and expressed in forceful language.

BIPEPSONATE

Calcium Phenolsulphonate	2 grains
Sodium Phenolsulphonate	2 grains
Zinc Phenolsulphonate, N. F.	1 grain
Salol, U. S. P.	2 grains
Bismuth Subsalicylate, U. S. P.	8 grains
Pepsin, U. S. P.	4 grains

Average Dosage

For Chi'dren—Half drachm every fifteen minutes for six doses, then every hour until relieved
For Adults—Double the above dose

How Supplied

In Pints, Five-Pints and Gallons to Physicians and Druggists only.

Burwell & Dunn Company

Manufacturing *Pharmacists*
Established in 1887

CHARLOTTE, N. C.

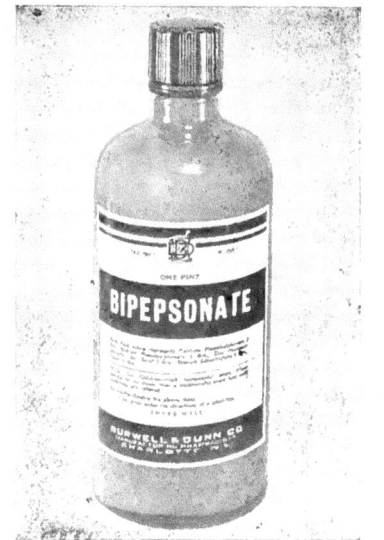

Sample sent to any physician in the U. S. on request

OFFICE ENDOCRINOLOGY, by ROBERT B. GREENBLATT, B.A., M.D., C.M., Professor of Experimental Medicine, University of Georgia School of Medicine; Director, Sex Endocrine Clinic, University Hospital, Augusta; with a foreword by G. LOMBARD KELLY, M.D., Dean, University of Georgia School of Medicine. Second edition. *Charles C. Thomas*, Springfield, Ill., and Baltimore, Md. 1944. $4.00, postpaid.

No physician can read half of what is being written by reputable doctors on this subject. Greenblatt gives us a small book made up of what he, himself, has found to be true. This, the second, edition is a worthy successor to the first as a reliable source of all usable and useful information we have on endocrinologic diagnosis and treatment.

NERVOUS STOMACH TROUBLE, by JOSEPH F. MONTAGUE, M.D. *Simon & Schuster*, New York City. $2.00.

The reader does not have to agree with everything the author says to conclude that the book is one of immense value, that its teaching is sound in content and happy in presentation.

THE 1943 YEAR BOOK OF PEDIATRICS, edited by ISAAC A. ABT, D.Sc., M.D., Professor of Pediatrics, Northwestern University Medical School; with the collaboration of ARTHUR F. ABT, B.S., M.D., Associate Professor of Pediatrics, Northwestern University Medical School. *The Year Book Publishers, Inc.*, 304 S. Dearborn St., Chicago. $3.00.

The reader will find here accounts of recent advances in our practical knowledge of diseases, conditions due to intestinal worms, of childhood asthma, of anemia, of immunity to diphtheria, of rheumatic fever, of poliomyelitis, of burns, of cardiac insufficiency in the newbobrn, of childhood fears—and this is mentioning but a few of the many.

No physician who accepts the health care of infants and children can afford to be without a copy.

HIGH ALTITUDE FROSTBITE

(Loyal Davis *et al*, in *Surg., Gynec. & Obst.*, 77:561 (1943)

The object of therapy for frostbite is release of vasospasm before thrombosis takes place. Heat has been used for dilatation, or cold to prevent extravasation by maintenance of vasospasm, depending upon the conditions thought to be present. Neither agency has been satisfactory. A little better results were obtained by gradually warming the affected part at room temperature; pain and ultimate loss of tissue were less, although blistering was greater as compared with the cooling method of treatment.

Drugs have been ineffective. Sympathetic nerve trunk and stellate ganglion block with novocain caused sudden dilatation of the peripheral capillary bed only when permanent anatomic injury to the capillary wall or thrombosis at the arteriolar capillary junction had not yet occurred.

CRITERIA OF CURE IN GONORRHEA

(R. A. Koch *et al.*, in *Venereal Disease Information*, Feb.)

The patients considered in this report are those who have been treated in a large municipal public health clinic from Jan. 1st, 1941, to July 1st, 1943, and include both men and women with gonococcic infection. Concern has been occasioned by the repeated occurrence of positive gonococcic cultures in individuals who have become promptly asymptomatic on treatment and have remained so for long periods of time.

In many instances those individuals showing no symptoms have been named as sources of new gonococcic infections and have subsequently reached our attention through public health channels. There is a tendency to place too much faith in the asymptomatic state following sulfonamide treatment.

An observation period of three months is required to give reasonable assurance of the elimination of the gonococcus in treated patients. *Even then some patients will continue to harbor the gonococcus despite the absence of symptoms and the consecutively negative gonococcic cultures.*

WORLD WAR'S BEARING ON FUTURE CIVILIAN PRACTICE
(*Proc. Staff Meetings of The Mayo Clinic*, Jan. 26th)

In the war of 1914-1918 disorders of the digestive tract during and after the period of mobilization did not loom as important. Today such diseases are the most important medical problem of the war and dyspepsia represents the single most important prevalent type of disease among hospitalized military patients. Almost without exception contemporary writers convey the impression that the high incidence of gastric and duodenal ulcer has been a development since 1918.

It is a safe rule to suspect every sick person who has recently returned from a malarial country of having malaria, even in the absence of a history of previous attacks, anemia and enlarged spleen, unless some other diagnosis is obvious.

IN MALARIAL DISTRICTS persons who imbibe freely of coffee, tea or cola appear immune during epidemic.—*Anais Paulistas de med e. cire.*, Apr., 1943.

A NEW, SIMPLIFIED TREATMENT FOR SECONDARY AMENORRHEA

Roche-Organon, Inc., announce that they now have available for the medical profession a new, simplified treatment for secondary amenorrhea of less than 2-years' duration.

Zondek found that in cases of secondary amenorrhea of less than 2 years' duration the injection on 2 successive days of a comihnation of 2.5 mg. of alpha-estradiol benzoate and 12.5 mg. of progesterone, mixed in the same syringe, will usually suffice to induce uterine bleeding. Roche-Organon is marketing a special combination package for this Zondek treatment. It consists of 2 ampuls of Dimenformon Benzoate (alpha-estradiol benzoate), each containing 2.5 mg., and 2 ampuls of Progestin (progesterone), each containing 12.5 mg.

Berlind (*J. Clin. Endocrinol.*, 1943, 3:457) states: "This two-day method of treatment inaugurated by Zondek was found to be ideal and the widespread adoption of this simple, short course of treatment will spare to many women the inconvenience of the prolonged therapy of previous days, which is not only time-consuming but also expensive."

This treatment is to be instituted only after ruling out constitutional disorders (tuberculosis, diabetes and syphilis) and local pelvic lesions (neoplasms, degenerative or inflammatory diseases, and malformations). The absence of pregnancy should also be established before treatment is initiated even though the use of Zondek's method will not affect gestation.

When secondary amenorrhea has lasted for more than 2 years, only 5 days are required for treatment in most cases and a daily dose of 10 mg. of progesterone alone, administered intramuscularly on 5 successive days, usually gives satisfactory results. For this treatment Progestin "Roche-Organon" (progesterone) is available in 10-mg. ampuls, boxes of 3, 6 and 50.

CHUCKLES

A gangster rushed into a saloon shooting right and left, yelling, "All you dirty skunks get outta here!"

The customers fled in the hail of bullets—all except an Englishman who stood at the bar calmly finishing his drink.

"Well?" snapped the gangster.

"Well," replied the Englishman, "there certainly were a lot of them, weren't there?"

———

Housewife: "No, I don't want no books or calendars neither. We don't need nothin'."

Salesman: "How about a cheap English grammar?"

———

A Scot who had ordered some meat from the butcher for his cat came rushing in later to cancel the order.

"What's the matter?" asked the butcher. "Lost your cat?"

"No," answered Sandy, "he's just caught a mouse."

———

A colored private, a passenger on a ship crossing the ocean, became seasick. His buddy remarked: "You is jest a lan'lubber."

"That's right," replied the private. "Dey ain't no argument dere. Ah's a lan'lubber and ah's jest findin' out how much ah lubs it."

———

A very thin man met a very fat man in the hotel lobby. "From the looks of you," said the fat man, "there might have beben a famine."

"Yes," was the reply, "and from the looks of you, you might have caused it."

———

IMMUNITY PRODUCED TO TYPHOID, ETC., BY SUBCUTANEOUS AND ORAL VACCINATION
(L. C. Elledge et al. in Quar. Rev. of Med., Nov.)

Subcutaneous administration of typhoid-paratyphoid vaccine was employed in 1,200 cases; oral vaccine in 850 cases. Agglutination tests were carried out four weeks after vaccination on 100 persons, half of whom had been vaccinated by the oral method and half by the subcutaneous method. All of the 50 given subcutaneous vaccine showed some degree of agglutination with all four antigens used (two typhoid strains, paratyphoid A and B); while 35 of the 50 patients given oral vaccine failed to show any agglutination.

———

THE CONCURRENT USE OF SULFATHIAZOLE AND HOT BATHS IN THE TREATMENT OF THE SULFATHIAZOLE-RESISTANT CASES OF GONOCOCCAL INFECTION
(N. Jones & S. L. Warren, Rochester, N. Y., in Am. Jl. Syph. Gon. & Ven. Dis., Sept., 1943)

The previous administration of sulfathiazole even though not curative seems to render the gonococcal infection more susceptible to a short fever treatment, and there seems to be good evidence in the summation of the effects of a sulfonamide and fever when used concurrently. An empirical schedule is presented. Patients receive a total of 4 gm. of sulfathiazole plus 15 gm. of salt and 2,000 c.c. or more of water. Additional fluids should bring the intake up to a minimum of 5,000 c.c. during each daily procedure. Two baths are given each day bringing the patient's temperature up to 104°. This routine is continued daily until the symptoms subside and the cultures and smears become negative. The method of applying such treatment in an army camp is outlined. For stubborn infections a 5-hour fever by radiant energy at 106° F. should be tried, with or without concurrent sulfathiazole.

———

RECENT ADVANCES IN THE TREATMENT OF RUPTURED.... (LUMBAR) INTERVERTEBRAL DISKS
(W. E. Dandy, Baltimore, in Jl. Med. Assn. Ala., Oct.)

Ruptured disks are among the most common lesions coming to surgery. Spontaneous cures must be very rare, although temporary recissions are the rule.

There are two components of a ruptured disk: 1) the necrotic interior of the disk causing backache, and 2) the protruding portion causing sciatica.

The diagnosis is made solely upon the signs and symptoms and x-ray pictures of the spine. Spinal injections of contrast media and spinal punctures are contraindicated; they are unnecessary and they will diagnose only one-third of the total number.

Rupture of two disks occurs in the same patient in about 80 per cent of the cases, occasionally there is a third.

The exposure is unilateral and between the laminae without removal of any bone or removal of a small bite of lamina may be necessary.

Mobility of the vertebra, tested by pressure of the spinous process, will usually determine whether the rupture is at the fourth or fifth lumbar (98% are at these two disks), or at both.

The entire necrotic content of the interior of the disk should be thoroughly removed with curettes; this is the best insurance against recurrences.

Fusions operations are contraindicated. Fusion of the vertebrae occurs after removing the necrotic contents of the disk.

———

UNUSUAL ASPECTS OF CORONARY THROMBOSIS
(H. A. Rurecht, Tulsa, in Jl. Okla. Med. Assn., Feb.)

Not all cases of thrombosis of the coronary arteries are followed by infarction, because there are cases of thrombosis without complete occlusion of the artery.

The syndrome of coronary thrombosis is due to infarction of the myocardium following arteriosclerotic alterations of the coronary arteries and their sequelae, has a strong familial tendency, affects males three times as frequently as females, is fond of diabetics, of the obese, and of those who have hypertension, probably of those who smoke, and much less probably of those who do not drink. It occurs more commonly among physicians than any other occupational group.

Men of 38 to 40 are commonly affected. It has been reported even in the teens.

Most characteristic is pain in the midline of the chest with radiation to both sides, and to the left or both upper extremities, unaffected by nitroglycerine, and the use of this is often suggested to differentiate it from simple angina. Frequently, however, the pain of coronary thrombosis is relieved more or less completely by nitroglycerine, and this is not a reliable differential point.

———

PATHOGENICITY OF INTESTINAL PROTOZOA
(H. W. Soper, St. Louis, in Amer. Jl. Dig. Dis., Oct.)

Intestinal protozoa are pathogenic, producing a low-grade chronic enteritis which is often not diagnosticated. In some cases they become activated by some infectious agent attacking the host, and attain a degree of pathogenicity which results in a regional ileitis which may occur in any segment of the small intestine. This acute stage is amenable to specific treatment by Stovarsol.

If the ileitis advances to the chronic stage, surgical intervention is indicated.

———

CANCER.—Studies made of the skin of cancer victims suggest that breast, colon, uterus and prostate cancer show a high family incidence.—Bul. Am. Soc. Control of Cancer.

WILLIS CALLS
From Page 145

Throughout most of its century of teaching the Medical College of Virginia has devoted itself to the one task—and that it has discharged well—that of making good doctors to take care of the health of our people. Without abating its zeal in that cause, it has in the past score of years taken on more and more work in research, and done that well.

Let every one of us who can possibly do so take part in the meeting May 3d. If you can attend only one day of the State Society meeting, let that day be Wednesday. Alumni from Richmond will be present to tell us many things good for our souls.

PUBLIC HEALTH

N. Thomas Ennett, M.D., *Editor*, Greenville, N. C.

HEALTH WORKERS NOW SUBJECT TO WAR MANPOWER COMMISSION EMPLOYMENT STABILIZATION PROGRAM

This item was taken from the March, 1944, issue of the *American Journal of Public Health*. It is of interest to public health workers and to physicians at large.

"The War Manpower Commission, Washington, has announced that physicians, dentists, veterinarians, sanitary engineers, and nurses who are salaried employees in essential or locally needed activities are hereafter subject to the same provisions of any employment stabilization program as applies to other workers in such activities. Such professional employees may not change their jobs without obtaining statements of availability from the U. S. Employment Service or being referred to new jobs by this Service. It is understood that the U. S. E. S. will make referrals of such employees only after consulting the state chairman of the Procurement and Assignment Service. The W. M. C. state directors may delegate the duty of referring such employees to new jobs to the state and local offices of the Procurement and Assignment Service if this delegation is approved by the regional W. M. C. director."

Dr. Hubert Haywood, Raleigh, is State Chairman of the Procurement and Assignment Service for physicians.

INTERPRETATION OF BASAL METABOLISM TESTS
(F. E. Harding, Los Angeles, in *Med. Rec.*, Mar.)

A series of 13,608 basal metabolism readings is classified. Ninety per cent of all normal basal metabolism readings range from minus 10 to plus 10, but 10% of the normals are taken on persons who have a reading that is at a certain, fairly constant level above or below this group. A metabolic test falling in the hypometabolism or hypermetabolism group may be due to an error caused by a faulty tester, a mistake on the part of the technicians, or a patient not being in a basal state. Eighty-seven per cent of the tests were below plus 11, 30% below minus 10, 15% below minus 15; while 13% are above plus 10 and only 7% above plus 15. This latter 7% includes most of the hyperthyroid cases. It is often difficult to determine the cause of readings between minus 10 and minus 25, and every available diagnostic aid that the clinician knows must be employed. Hypometabolism and hypermetabolism are terms not synonymous with hypothyroidism and hyperthyroidism.

Peptic Ulcer in Children
(L. R. Hutchins, Seattle, in *Northwest Med.*, Feb.)

Peptic ulcer is extremely rare in infants and children; 0.27 per cent have been reported in 1650 admissions at King County Hospital.

A majority of cases are without symptoms. In the remainder, abdominal pain and epigastric tenderness are the the commonest findings.

The ultimate diagnosis is dependent upon roentgenographic studies.

Treatment of peptic ulcer in children is chiefly medical. Surgery must be employed in acute perforations or in obstruction. In general, surgery and especially gastrectomy, are best avoided. Seventeen cases of resection (with two deaths) are noted. One case of a perforated duodenal ulcer in a nine-year-old white female is reported.

Gallstones
(Carl Bearse, Boston, in *Jl. A. M. A.*, Feb. 19th)

Biliary complications may occur at any time in the presence of cholelithiasis. They may be present when the patient is first seen or they may not occur at all even when there are frequent attacks of colic over a long period of years. The occurrence of complications adds to the risk of operation and calls for prompt surgical treatment. Early operation is likewise desirable for cholelithiasis with complications, since delay increases the likelihood of their occurrence.

Operation, however, may be safely deferred in patients with gallstones so long as there is no evidence of complications and provided postponement is not so protracted that it may impair the patient's resistance to the operative procedure.

Explanation for the Absence of Clotting in Bloody Cerebrospinal Fluid
(M. J. Madonick *et al.*, New York, in *Jl. Lab. & Clin. Med.*, Dec.)

We believe the mechanism is similar to that which prevents clotting in menstrual blood.

Fresh bloody spinal fluids of 15 patients with meningeal bleeding were examined to determine the cause of the lack of clotting. It was found that fibrinogen was absent in all cases. This, we believe, is due to the occurrence of clotting in and around the brain during which process the fibrinogen is removed from the fluid.

Hyperhidrosis of the Feet
(R. G. Park, Major, New Zealand Med. Corps, in *Arch. Derma. & Syph.*, Nov.)

Lighter shoes provide some relief, and open sandals are best of all.

In its usual forms this disorder may be controlled by twice daily antiseptic soaks in a warm solution of potassium permanganate (1:4,000). The feet are soaked for 10 to 15 minutes and then allowed to dry thoroughly. Feet and socks next are well dusted with three per cent salicylic acid in talc.

Some ABC stuff about E

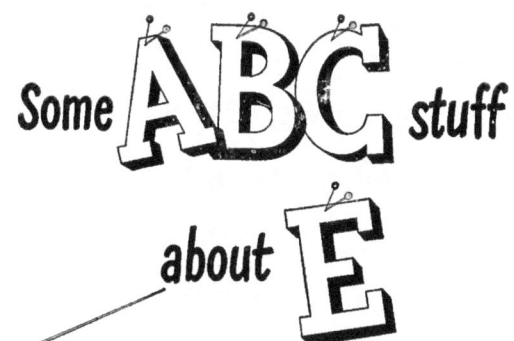

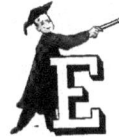 IS A VERY important letter in this war.

It's the name of the War Bonds you buy—"War Savings Bond Series E."

As you know, a Series E Bond will work for you for ten full years, piling up interest all that time, till finally you'll get four dollars back for every

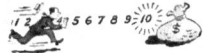

three you put up. Pretty nice.

The first job of the money you put into "E" is, of course, to help finance the war. But it also gives you a wonderful way to save money.

And when the war is over, that money you now put away can do another job, can help America swing over from war to peace.

There'll come a day when you'll bless these Bonds—when they may help you over a tough spot.

That's why you should hang on to every Bond you buy. You can, of course, cash in your Bonds any time after you've held them for 60 days. You get all your money back, and, after one year, all your money plus interest.

But when you cash in a Bond, you end its life before its full job is done. You don't give it its chance to help you and the country in the years that lie ahead. You kill off its $4-for-every-$3 earning power.

All of which it's good to remember when you

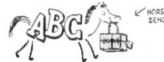

might be tempted to cash in some of your War Bonds. They are yours, to do what you want with.

But . . . it's ABC sense that . .

They'll do the best job for you and for America if you let them reach the full flower of maturity!

WAR BONDS to Have and to Hold

The Treasury Department acknowledges with appreciation the publication of this message by

T-4596   5 1-2 x 8 in.   110 Screen

GENERAL

THE NALLE CLINIC

Nalle Clinic Building   412 North Church Street, Charlotte

Telephone—C-BNDY (if no answer, call 3-2621)

General Surgery

BRODIE C. NALLE, M.D.
GYNECOLOGY & OBSTETRICS

EDWARD R. HIPP, M.D.
TRAUMATIC SURGERY

*PRESTON NOWLIN, M.D.
UROLOGY

Consulting Staff

R. H. LAFFERTY, M.D.
O. D. BAXTER, M.D.
RADIOLOGY

W. M. SUMMERVILLE, M.D.
PATHOLOGY

General Medicine

LUCIUS G. GAGE, M.D.
DIAGNOSIS

LUTHER W. KELLY, M.D.
CARDIO-RESPIRATORY DISEASES

J. R. ADAMS, M.D.
DISEASES OF INFANTS & CHILDREN

W. B. MAYER, M.D.
DERMATOLOGY & SYPHILOLOGY

(*In Country's Service)

C—H—M MEDICAL OFFICES
DIAGNOSIS—SURGERY
X-RAY—RADIUM

DR. G. CARLYLE COOKE—*Abdominal Surgery & Gynecology*
DR. GEO. W. HOLMES—*Orthopedics*
DR. C. H. McCANTS—*General Surgery*
222-226 Nissen Bldg.   Winston-Salem

WADE CLINIC
Wade Building
Hot Springs National Park, Arkansas

H. KING WADE, M.D.	*Urology*
ERNEST M. McKENZIE, M.D.	*Medicine*
*FRANK M. ADAMS, M.D.	*Medicine*
*JACK ELLIS, M.D.	*Medicine*
BESSEY H. SHEBESTA, M.D.	*Medicine*
*WM. C. HAYS, M.D.	*Medicine*
N. B. BURCH, M.D.	*Eye, Ear, Nose and Throat*
A. W. SCHEER	*X-ray Technician*
ETTA WADE	*Clinical Laboratory*
MERNA SPRING	*Clinical Pathology*

(*In Military Service)

INTERNAL MEDICINE

ARCHIE A. BARRON, M.D., F.A.C.P.

INTERNAL MEDICINE—NEUROLOGY

Professional Bldg.   Charlotte

JOHN DONNELLY, M.D.

DISEASES OF THE LUNGS

Medical Building   Charlotte

CLYDE M. GILMORE, A.B., M.D.

CARDIOLOGY—INTERNAL MEDICINE

Dixie Building   Greensboro

JAMES M. NORTHINGTON, M.D.

INTERNAL MEDICINE—GERIATRICS

Medical Building   Charlotte

NEUROLOGY and PSYCHIATRY

(*Now in the Country's Service*)
*J. FRED MERRITT, M.D.
NERVOUS and MILD MENTAL DISEASES
ALCOHOL and DRUG ADDICTIONS
Glenwood Park Sanitarium   Greensboro

TOM A. WILLIAMS, M.D.
(*Neurologist of Washington, D. C.*)
Consultation by appointment at
Phone 3994-W
77 Kenilworth Ave.   Asheville, N. C.

EYE, EAR, NOSE AND THROAT

H. C. NEBLETT, M.D.
OCULIST
Phone 3-5852
Professional Bldg.   Charlotte

AMZI J. ELLINGTON, M.D.
DISEASES of the
EYE, EAR, NOSE and THROAT
Phones: Office 992—Residence 761
Burlington   North Carolina

UROLOGY, DERMATOLOGY and PROCTOLOGY

THE CROWELL CLINIC of UROLOGY and UROLOGICAL SURGERY
Hours—Nine to Five   Telephones—3-7101—3-7102
STAFF
ANDREW J. CROWELL, M.D.
(1911-1938)
*ANGUS M. McDONALD, M.D.   CLAUDE B. SQUIRES, M.D.
Suite 700-711 Professional Building   Charlotte

RAYMOND THOMPSON, M.D., F.A.C.S.   WALTER E. DANIEL, A.B., M.D.
THE THOMPSON-DANIEL CLINIC
of
UROLOGY & UROLOGICAL SURGERY
Fifth Floor Professional Bldg.   Charlotte

C. C. MASSEY, M.D.
PRACTICE LIMITED
TO
DISEASES OF THE RECTUM
Professional Bldg.   Charlotte

WYETT F. SIMPSON, M.D.
GENITO-URINARY DISEASES
Phone 1234
Hot Springs National Park   Arkansas

ORTHOPEDICS

HERBERT F. MUNT, M.D.
ACCIDENT SURGERY & ORTHOPEDICS
FRACTURES
Nissen Building   Winston-Salem

SURGERY

R. S. ANDERSON, M. D.

GENERAL SURGERY

144 Coast Line Street   Rocky Mount

R. B. DAVIS, M. D., M. M. S., F. A. C. P.
*GENERAL SURGERY
AND
RADIUM THERAPY*
Hours by Appointment

Piedmont-Memorial Hosp.   Greensboro

(Now in the Country's Service)

WILLIAM FRANCIS MARTIN, M.D.

GENERAL SURGERY

Professional Bldg.   Charlotte

OBSTETRICS & GYNECOLOGY

IVAN M. PROCTER, M. D.

OBSTETRICS & GYNECOLOGY

133 Fayetteville Street   Raleigh

SPECIAL NOTICES

TWO LABORATORY TECHNICIANS, being graduated from a High-class Hospital Laboratory, services available January 1st, 1944. Address TECHNICIAN, care *Southern Medicine & Surgery.*

TO THE BUSY DOCTOR WHO WANTS TO PASS HIS EXPERIENCE ON TO OTHERS

You have probably been postponing writing that original contribution. You can do it, and save your time and effort by employing an expert literary assistant to prepare the address, article or book under your direction or relieve you of the details of looking up references, translating, indexing, typing, and the complete preparation of your manuscript.

Address: *WRITING AIDE,* care *Southern Medicine & Surgery.*

THE JOURNAL OF SOUTHERN MEDICINE AND SURGERY

306 North Tryon Street, Charlotte, N. C.

The Journal assumes no responsibility for the authenticity of opinion or statements made by authors or in communications submitted to this Journal for publication.

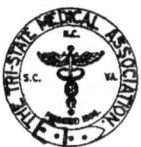

JAMES M. NORTHINGTON, M.D., Editor

Proctologic Practices* **

WILLIAM J. MARTIN, JR., M.D., Bethesda, Maryland
Lt. Comdr. Medical Corps, United States Naval Reserve

KNOWLEDGE of proctology has grown fast in recent years. In part, the recent advances in proctology are due, I feel sure, to the American Proctologic Society, which has striven for years to raise the specialty of proctology to the plane that is enjoyed by other recognized specialties.

The treatment of so-called rectal diseases, as a specialty, was conceived by charlatans who preyed upon suffering humanity, using secret methods and solutions, which, however, might be made known to those who put the proper amount of the coin of the realm in the proper place.

It is no mystery why so many of the laity turn to these rectal specialists who advertise by means of circulars, in newspapers, and more recently over the radio. They are human beings, as you and I, and often they fear medical attention, not only an operation, but even an examination. These people see an easy out in the glowing descriptions of the various painless methods of cure "without the knife." This is a normal response. Is it any wonder that this type of treatment is accepted by the laity when you hark back and remember the type of anorectal surgery that has been approved by many? Consider the lack of equipment for anal and rectal diagnosis and treatment of many of our colleagues. As long as members of the medical profession are willing to pass lightly over anorectal problems they may expect those who are lacking in ethics and are doing this type of work to flourish.

If there were not a need for proctologists, then proctology as a specialty could not exist. The need for proctologists arose, I believe, because the general surgeon did not have the inclination, or did not have the time, or did not take the time to acquaint himself sufficiently with the anatomy and physiology of the lower bowel and the anorectal region, and the pathological conditions affecting this area. Those who have chosen to do this work have done as others have done who have chosen a specialty. They have applied a microscope, so to speak, to that portion of the human anatomy that they have elected to specialize in.

From this lowly origin has arisen the American Proctologic Society and more recently the American Board of Proctology which, I am sure, will guard its doors as zealously as does the American Board of Surgery, the American Board of Ophthalmology, and the other specialty boards.

Proctologists are frequently accused of being too radical in their operative work. This is an accusation which is often directed at any class of specialists. Certainly proctologists, with their knowledge of the parts, do not consider their removal of tissue too radical. Usually it is the one who is not too familiar with the parts involved who is too conservative in his approach. I feel that it is rather more often a question of too many doing too little rather than of a few doing too much at the proper time.

---
*Presented to Tri-State Medical Association of the Carolinas and Virginia, meeting at Charlotte, Feb. 28th-29th, 1944.
** The opinions or assertions contained herein are the private ones of the writer, and are not to be construed as official or as reflecting the views of the Navy Department or the Naval Service at large.

Examination of the anorectum and lower bowel is not difficult if one has the proper instruments and has an adequately clean bowel to examine. A special table is not a necessity for doing this type of an examination although it is an advantage to one who is doing a large number. To my mind there is nothing as important as a clean bowel. The diagnostic instruments necessary are a properly lighted sigmoidoscope fitted with an inflating bulb; an anoscope, preferably of the Hirschman type, the end of which is cut off at a 45° angle; and a flexible probe. With these three instruments, adequate diagnostic aid can be done; or, at least, variations from the normal should be recognized and if desired, should lead to consultation.

Röntgenographic examination is at times a valuable aid to diagnosis of the large bowel and rectal lesions, but when it is recalled that seventy-odd per cent of the malignant lesions of the colon occur within the reach of the sigmoidoscope the use of this indirect type of examination should be called for only after the direct method of sigmoidoscopy has failed. It is indeed difficult, and frequently impossible, to demonstrate early lesions, especially polypoid lesions, of the lower bowel by the ordinary barium enema. Even the double contrast enema or lateral views with the ordinary enema will frequently fail because of the overlapping of other loops of bowel in this area, which is so readily reached by sigmoidoscopic examination.

The most common proctologic disease is hemorrhoids, and the most common complaint of those who present themselves for examination is that they have hemorrhoids or piles. Therein lies the chief pitfall and the most common cause for failure in alleviating the subjective symptoms. A person who says he has hemorrhoids may have anything from a mild pruritus to an inoperable cancer of the large bowel or rectum.

The most common subjective symptom of any anorectal disease is pain of varying degree. Bleeding is the most common sign. These are, as you know, late manifestations of carcinoma of the bowel. It is only in recent years that the percentage of those who are ultimately found to have carcinoma of the rectum, rectosigmoid or sigmoid, and who have been operated on for hemorrhoids since the onset of their symptoms, has fallen below thirty-five per cent. It is a safe rule to suspect every patient who presents himself with an anorectal complaint of having carcinoma until proven otherwise. This argues for more adequate examination.

To understand the symptom pain, as related to anorectal disease, one must understand the anatomy of the anorectal region. For years there was, and in a great many cases there still is, a misconception that the anal canal is lined with mucous membrane. One frequently hears and sees the phrase, "the mucosa of the anal canal." When the anal plate and cloacal membrane meet and disintegrate they leave a true mucocutaneous junction. This leaves, on the ectodermal side, a serrated margin of small elevations known as anal papillae. This junction is variously called the anorectal line, the mucocutaneous line or the dentate line. This is the upper limit of the anal canal. From this point outward the canal is lined with squamous epithelium. The external boundary might be roughly defined as that line formed by the walls of the anus as they come in contact with each other during their normal state of apposition.

It is below this limit, the nerve supply of which is derived mostly from somatic sensory nerves lying in the primary posterior divisions of the first through the fifth sacral and coccygeal nerves, that lesions causing pain usually lie. Above this upper limit of the anus, which is the rectum, the nerve supply is derived from the autonomic nervous system, and there is no proof that a visceral sensory nerve supply is present.

Recollection of these facts in searching for a cause of pain as related to anorectal disease will obviate one of the errors most commonly made, that of looking too high above the anal verge for the cause. This is most frequently the result of the type of instrument used or the position of the patient when examined. The Hirschman anoscope is especially adapted for overcoming this tendency.

Pain or the appearance of blood at the anal orifice brings in most of these patients for examination. The patient almost invariably volunteers the information that he has hemorrhoids or piles after seeing blood from the bowel. Bleeding from, or through, the canal canal may be due to abrasions of the anal margins caused by scratching a pruritus, or vigorous means of cleansing the parts following defecation, or the explosive dilatation as a result of the diarrheal stool. The bleeding resulting from this type of trauma may range from a smear to enough to give the patient the impression that he has had a hemorrhage. A thrombotic external hemorrhoid may erode through and bleeding occur around the partially protruded clot, most frequently preceded and accompanied by pain of varying degree. The most common cause of bleeding from the anal orifice is erosion of internal hemorrhoids, which do or do not protrude. Anal tissue frequently occasions a good deal of bleeding, accompanied or followed by pain which may be extreme.

Among the most important and less frequently discovered causes of bleeding through the anal canal are sessile or pedunculated, polypoid lesions of the large bowel and rectum. These are from a few millimeters to several centimeters in size, and of two main types. The least frequent, and the one most likely to be diagnosed by the occasional peeper through a sigmoidoscope, is the familial type of polypoid disease in which practically the whole colon is studded with polyps, both sessile and pedunculated. The more frequent type is characterized by a single polyp, or perhaps two or three, in the colon or rectum. To men who have specialized in proctology must go the credit for the discovery of the frequency of occurrence of these lesions and the proof of their relationship to malignant growths of the large bowel. Usually for the discovery of these lesions, especially those occurring higher than the rectum, are required: a thoroughly clean bowel, skill in passing a sigmoidoscope, knowledge of variations from the normal and patience to search every fold of the bowel within reach.

In the private practice of the speaker, these two types of lesions have been found in better than five per cent of the patients examined, the majority symptomless and on routine sigmoidoscopic examination. These lesions, amounting to several hundred, have been arrayed against the cases of malignant growths found in the same series of patients. Biopsies from these growths showed that better than seventy per cent were variations from simple adenomatous tissue, ranging from hyperplasia and anaplasia to frank malignancy. The size of the growth was not found to be a determining factor in the variations. The location of these presently relatively benign growths was found to parallel those of the late malignancies. The sex variation was the same. Those who had malignant growths made up a group ten years older than those who had polyps. Such facts have been very widely accepted as incriminating evidence against the polyp and it is a fair supposition that, if a polypoid lesion is allowed to remain for ten years, the chance of the bearer appearing later with a full-blown carcinoma, and frequently an inoperable one, is too great to be lightly passed over.

The diagnosis and removal of those early growths which are within the reach of the sigmoidoscope is easy for those who have the proper equipment. These growths can be permanently destroyed by fulguration with a machine such as the Bovie with no other preparation on the part of the patient than cleansing enemas. No anesthetic is required and hospitalization is rarely necessary.

The proctologist, with the proper equipment, can be of great aid to the surgeon who has to deal with the multiple or familial type of polypoid disease; rather than do a complete colectomy he can, over a period of time, destroy all the growths within reach from below, and, following this, an ileosigmoidostomy, as low as possible, and later the colon is removed in two stages down to the anastomosis. The remaining portion of the sigmoid and the rectum can be examined visually at intervals through the sigmoidoscope and if more polyps appear they can be easily destroyed by fulguration in the office. This is a decided improvement over a total colectomy and ileostomy.

These polypoid growths occur at all ages and usually the first intimation to the patient of their presence is bleeding. Frequently, especially of pedunculated growths, tenesmus is a complaint. In one week recently three cases in widely separated age groups were seen. One was a three-and-one-half-year-old girl who had been bleeding for two years. Another was a physician in his late twenties who had been bleeding for two weeks. The third was a woman in her fifties who, a year ago, was seen in consultation. She had been bleeding profusely through the anal canal for many months. Treatment had consisted of a strict dietary regimen and the usual bismuth mixtures in an attempt to stop the bleeding. Repeated barium enemas had been negative. Her diet, a combination of what had been ordered and one of self-restriction, was so lacking that she had lost fifty pounds. She had been confined to her bed for many weeks, the last few being in an institution because of mental confusion.

A week previous to consultation, a mass had protruded from the anal orifice and she was removed to a hospital. This mass was thought to be a prolapsing hemorrhoid and was ligated.

When seen in consultation this patient was much emaciated, mentally confused, had a fiery red and sore tongue and presented all the signs of a severe anemia and an avitaminosis. The red cells were two million, the hemoglobin in the forties. Sigmoidoscopic examination revealed a bleeding, sloughing mass in and above the internal hemorrhoidal area. The bleeding, though still present, was much less than before the mass was ligated. Because of the inability to differentiate between several things that might have been present before the ligation of the mass, tranfusion with whole blood was advised, and an adequate diet supplemented by large doses of Vitamin-B complex; also hot rectal irrigations, and sigmoidoscopic examination again in two weeks. The mass stopped bleeding and the patient's general condition improved so much that she did not return for examination as requested. In a few months she was well enough to resume her work. Eleven months later this patient was again seen with a complaint of bleeding through the anal canal, and a polypoid growth three centimeters in diameter was found just above the internal hemorrhoidal area at the site of the previously seen sloughing area.

All three of these patients had their growths fulgurated in the office with no preparation other than a cleansing enema. Check-ups three months later showed no subjective or objective signs of the growths. Early discovery and eradication of these growths is of great importance.

Pain as related to hemorrhoidal disease is a sign of complications. Uncomplicated hemorrhoids are painless. The common external, thrombotic hemorrhoid is painful because of the pressure exerted by blood extravasation and clotting putting the skin under tension. One of the common mistakes made is trying to push these lesions up into the rectum in the hope that the pain will be relieved. The mass will not stay reduced because the tension on the anal margin will not allow the mass to stay above the anorectal ring. When internal hemorrhoids swell from infection and thromboses occur they are very frequently protruded. The reaction often extends into the sensitive external hemorrhoidal area, swelling takes place, thromboses occur under the skin and pain results from involvement of the skin of the anal canal.

Another common cause of pain and bleeding which at times are severe is anal fissure—a varicose ulcer confined to the posterior and anterior commissures of the skin of the anal canal, the result of a break in the anal skin becoming infected. In a case of anal pain, if there is no abscess, no acutely inflamed hemorrhoid, and no thrombotic hemorrhoids, almost certainly a fissure is the cause. The term fissure is used by many to denote any break in the anal skin whatever its location. Most proctologists confine its use to an ulcer of the anal canal predominately in the posterior midline, or less frequently in the anterior midline. Due to the peculiar anatomy of the anal canal, breaks in the posterior and anterior midline do not heal readily, whereas those on the lateral walls usually do. Even those occurring in the midline frequently heal when they occur the first time, even though little or nothing is done for them. Once this type occurs, however, they are very apt to occur again and again until the edges of the ulcer become chronic, pile up, the base assumes the characteristics of a varicose ulcer and defies cure other than by operative means. These ulcers occur within the anal verge just a few millimeters from the outside and are frequently overlooked because they are looked for too high up. It is this lesion, which is often accompanied by hemorrhoids, that is most likely to be the cause of one not obtaining relief of symptoms when the patient is treated by injections or other palliative types of treatment.

Still another frequent cause of pain in these parts is abscess—prone to recur in the perianal region. Abscesses in other parts of the body do not tend to recur if adequately drained. Paraänal and pararectal abscess do not begin subcutaneously as do other abscesses. These abscesses are caused, in the great majority of cases, by an infection which starts in a crypt at the anorectal junction whose wall has been broken by trauma. The other causes which allow pus-forming organisms to escape in the surrounding tissue are puncture wounds of the rectal and anal wall and the base of an anal fissure being broken through and allowing infection to be spread to the less resistant surrounding tissue. This type of lesion usually starts in the anal canal, not in an anal crypt. Most patients with an abscess in this region will seek advice on account of the pain. The long-suffering will endure until the abscess ruptures spontaneously and will seek aid only after one or more recurrences caused by the skin healing over the external opening and allowing the resulting cavity or fistulous tract to fill up. The end result, whether the abscess has ruptured or has been incised, is the same—a fistula.

A form of treatment often used in an attempt to alleviate symptoms of the anus, rectum and colon is mentioned only to condemn it. It is that of prescribing rectal suppositories and ointments in tubes. It should be remembered that bleeding and pain, the most frequent sign and symptom of benign afflictions of the anus, rectum and colon, are also the most common sign and symptom of malignant disease of the same areas and usually denote a growth of long duration. Besides, the sites of pain occurring in this region are not where a medicine used for its local effect can reach by being inserted into the rectum. An abscess is outside of the wall of the anus or rectum; thrombosis is on the anal margin; and an anal fissure is within the anal canal, which is closed and will not allow the medicine used to reach the site of the pain. Hence, it would seem that what virtues a suppository or ointment possess would depend on its absorption and systemic effect. More effective, as a rule, are hot sitz baths and an oral dose of something for pain. It is regrettable that many carcinomas of the large bowel and rectum have been treated for a long time by suppositories because of lack of adequate examination.

Another lesion which has recently received renewed attention and which often falls to the lot of the proctologist is that of the pilonidal cyst, or as it is termed in the Navy nomenclature cyst teratoma. It is thought to be congenital. Up until the present it was thought that this lesion was more prevalent in the male, even to being a rarity in the female. Recently the speaker has had to revise his opinion. With the influx of the female into the armed services and as a consequence of the much more rugged activity to which this large number of females has been subjected, the incidence of this lesion has mounted tremendously in the female. Within the past month out of 16 cases of pilonidal cyst—cyst teratoma, sacral, as the Navy terms it—six cases have been in females.

Because its complications occur most frequently in the age group which is now mostly in the armed services, it has become a major problem of war medicine. Much has been written recently about its cure and many strange and bizarre methods of operation have been advocated. Now the usual treatment of a pilonidal cyst or cyst teratoma is the treatment of its complications. There is no more indication for operation unless a complication has occurred than there is for removing an appendix just because there is one present. The cause of the complications is infection, brought on by trauma. Confronted with an abscess in the sacrococcygeal region, or one or more draining sinuses in this area, what should be done? By reason of the time lost to the armed forces, many suggestions as to the ways of closing these wounds primarily following excision have been advocated. This has been done in spite of the presence of gross infection. It suffices to say that I doubt if anyone would thoroughly analyze this situation and remember that he is dealing with an abscess, acute or chronic, and then attempt to close the wounds resulting from the excision of such an infected cyst or the pyogenic wall remaining from infection in such a cyst. No thinking man would carve out an abscess in any other part of the body, close the cavity and expect it to heal by first intention. Why then should one expect a wound in this region to heal by first intention, especially one which, by reason of the anatomy of the surrounding parts, has the added disadvantages of a large remaining dead space and much tension on the suture line.

The speaker has not felt that he can accept the primary closure method of treating pilonidal cysts, certainly not in those which are inflamed, or have been inflamed. If the primary closure has any virtue it would be in those which are totally quiescent and have never been complicated by an abscess. The necessity for operating on this type is questioned. Pilonidal cyst is no new disease. We are now back at the place in the cycle where short methods of cure, which are goals to achieve, are being reached for, but have not as yet been reached. Twenty years ago we were at this same place in the cycle. This type of treatment might be placed in the same class as the injection of para-anal fistulas with paste, in hopes of curing them. It can be done, rarely, if ever.

There is no mystery to the successful eradication of pilonidal cyst. Success comes from adequate drainage and intelligent, frequent and personal observation post-operatively.

The motto of the Medical Department of the Navy is, "As many men at as many guns as many days as possible." As related to civilian practice, this might be paraphrased into "get your patient well quickly and permanently." To achieve this object in the treating of anorectal diseases and pilonidal cysts as well, an accurate diagnosis must be made, adequate drainage of all infected wounds must be instituted, and scrupulously careful and frequent after-care must be carried out to insure quick and permanent cure.

NEPHROSIS
(Maj. W. H. Graham, Kansas City, in Jl. Mo. Med. Assn., May)

With the onset of nephrosis, the patient complains of weakness, tires easily and later shows signs of edema of the lower extremities and about the eyes. Edema, ascites, and in some instances double plural effusion and anasarca insidiously become intensified. The retinas are unchanged. Blood pressure may be normal or slightly subnormal. No dilatation of the heart or other cardiac involvement is noted. The skin is pale. The urine shows a rapid and progressive proteinuria, casts, usually no blood. At times the specific gravity is high. No uremic odor of the breath nor any signs of uremia, early. The blood total serum protein is 4 per cent or lower with a marked reduction in serum albumin and slight if any change in the globulin fraction. The duration is from weeks to years; 76 per cent of all cases recover. In later life, the mortality rate is much higher if the nephrosis is due to syphilis or tuberculosis.

The consensus is that nephrosis is but a stage in the disease of the kidneys.

For weeks and sometimes months there is apparently no involvement except of the proximal and distal convoluted tubules. Nearly always there is an involvement of the other parts of the kidney, more particularly the glomeruli.

The predominating effects on the body are the rapid loss of proteins, large amounts of albumin in the urine with no blood, lipoid bodies in the blood and edema very pronounced.

The condition is more frequently found in children but may be found at any age and as a postoperative occurrence. Death is usually due to uremia and exhaustion.

THE MEDICAL ASPECTS OF HYPERTROPHY AND CANCER OF THE PROSTATE
(H. H. Young, Baltimore, in Conn. Med. Jl., Nov.)

In its early stages prostatic hypertrophy may be largely a medical problem. Hesitation at the beginning of urination, reduction in the size of the stream, and slight discomfort are usually the first complaints. A feeling of dullness, a diminution in potentia and sometimes precocity of ejaculation. For a protracted period there may be very little residual urine, only slight back pressure effects upon the urinary tract and no reduction in the renal function, as shown by the divided phthalein test and blood chemistry. During this period gentle massage of the prostate, perhaps supplemented by diathermy or sitz baths, may prove effective therapy.

As residual urine develops, the problem becomes a surgical one. Strict asepsis in catheterization, the use of sulfonamides and boric acid irrigations will all aid in preventing cystitis. Gradual decompression over the course of 1-2 days should be practiced where retention is marked.

The Role of a Neuropsychiatric Service in a General Hospital*

JOHN M. FEARING, M.D., Durham, North Carolina
Duke University Medical School

I FEEL that it is privilege to be able to talk here today on a subject of such practical value as the role of a neuropsychiatric ward in a general hospital. In this discussion I shall mention briefly something of the physical set-up of such a ward and outline some of the methods used in diagnosis and therapy. In addition, the function of the ward in relation to the hospital and to the referring physician will be discussed. Most of my material is based on experience on Meyer Ward at Duke Hospital. I think, however, that most of my remarks can be generalized to apply with slight modification to the neuropsychiatric service operating, or capable of organization, in any general hospital with 300 beds or so.

First, a few physical details. Meyer Ward is a closed ward of 17 beds in all—14 beds in single rooms with an additional section of three soundproofed, air-conditioned cubicles for disturbed patients. There are also several other rooms especially designed for a neuropsychiatric ward. Most psychiatric patients are ambulatory, but must be kept indoors much of the time. It is necessary, therefore, to have a large recreation room where the patients spend most of their time, always under the supervision of a part of the ward staff. In this recreation room or dayroom, patients are occupied in various activities. I object strongly to the term "occupational therapy," and especially to the initials "O. T." that are so glibly used around most sanatoria. One always thinks of an old man weaving a basket. It is much better if these activities of the patients are used to serve a definite purpose. By close watching and guiding their activities much can be done along lines of diagnosis and therapy. For instance, we find that close observation of social reactions and adjustments of patients in the recreation room in the presence of a group of men and women of various ages, gives usually a much better index of the patient's social capabilities than is given by group or formal psychological tests. These are used also, however, and will be mentioned later.

There is in addition a dining room, used by most of the ambulatory patients. Having their meals together tends to dissipate the hospital atmosphere. It also serves as a test situation of social behavior three times a day.

Meyer is also equipped with a tub room. Here there is an over-sized metal tub so constructed that the patient may be immersed by means of a canvas sling. Excited or agitated patients may be kept in water at 96° F. for as long as eight hours. The entire ward is especially constructed with such safety devices as locking room and closet doors, covered electrical outlets, protected windows and metal mirrors. A ward of this size can be run by a functioning staff of a resident and two interns, with two graduate nurses, three student nurses, and 14 male and female attendants working in shifts.

Before discussing the specific function of such a ward I shall review very briefly our statistics for last year, to give some idea of the volume of work handled. With a 17-bed service operating in a 604-bed hospital, we handled 206 admissions and discharges. Of these only 15 were transferred to state or other mental institutions. Twenty-seven of our admissions were readmissions, and we can expect a proportional number of readmissions in the coming year.

More important in this discussion, however, is the fact that we had no suicides and only two serious accidents—one avoidable when an elderly patient fell and broke a hip, the other unavoidable when an excited schizophrenic woman threw herself to the floor and fractured the radius.

Now something of what such a service is able to offer. To my mind, the principal functions are rather clear-cut. First, definitive diagnosis of the psychiatric problem referred to us. By means of such a ward, we are able to keep the patient under close observation over an extended length of time and to make detailed studies. We usually consider two weeks adequate for complete diagnostic studies—a full history of the patient's background and behavior and the usual physical and neurological examinations, with special studies as indicated, such as x-rays, blood chemistry, electroencephalography, etc. In a general hospital the various consultants in the medical and surgical specialties are available. In addition to a complete work-up from the physical standpoint, the psychiatric patient is subjected to various psychological tests. The Stanford-Binet, Rorschach, Minnesota Personality Test, and the Shipley-Hartford Test for deterioration are widely used. Meanwhile, the patient is studied in interviews with his psychiatrist.

*Presented to Tri-State Medical Association of the Carolinas and Virginia, meeting at Charlotte, Feb. 28th-29th, 1944.

Very important in the diagnostic study and general evaluation of the case is the ward situation itself. The patient is observed as far as possible as a living, reacting organism in a social situation. Much is learned in this way about general elements of his personality and of his difficulties.

Following such a work-up, one of two things is usually done. The patient is given definitive treatment on the ward if the case is such that therapy can be administered in a rather short time. I will give some detail of treatment in a few moments. The other course open is to supply the referring physician with the material obtained by our studies, including a complete opinion on the diagnosis and prognosis, and suggestions for disposition of the case. A good number of our cases are not treated in the hospital, but are handled simply as consultation problems in this way.

Treatment of the psychiatric patient is a complicated business. It begins with protecting the patient. Locked doors and safety windows keep irresponsible or suicidal patients from leaving the ward; locked closets, metal mirrors and other precautions against suicide are also used. The excited patient is protected from harming or exhausting himself by isolation in a bare room, by being put in a continuous tub, or wet sheet pack, or by means of sedatives. The chief protective precaution, however, is constant vigilance on the part of a trained staff that is sensitized to the dangers inherent in mental cases.

Maintenance of nutrition comes next in general therapy and offers quite a problem in some cases, such as stupor states and excitements. Fluid, caloric and vitamin intake must be maintained by tube feeding and fluids by vein, in spite of passive or active resistance on the part of the patient.

I emphasize the protective and physical maintenance phases of therapy because, although they may seem rather dull and uninteresting details, they are an extremely important part of the care of the mental case. It is just this element of care, impossible to maintain in the home or on an open ward, that is offered by a closed psychiatric ward.

The importance of this phase of therapy was brought home to us rather forcibly just a few days ago. An intelligent middle-aged man who seemed to be only mildly depressed was transferred to one of the medical floors because he complained bitterly that being thrown with the patients on Meyer was making him much worse. It seemed that he was not dangerously depressed, and he appeared to be so pleased and relieved to be transferred that it was thought that he could get along all right. That night he cut his throat and wrists severely with a razor. He was, fortunately, seen soon after and is doing well at present. This can hardly be called mismanagement. He appeared to be in good condition; Meyer was over-crowded at the time; and his request seemed well founded. All these points merely emphasize the importance of protection on a closed ward for all mental patients.

I have no intention of entering into the discussion of psychotherapy as such, as it would be entirely outside of the realm of this paper, but I shall say a little about one aspect of it. The definition of psychotherapy given to me by Dr. Greenhill at Duke is: "Psychotherapy is any therapy in which the relationship of the patient with the therapist plays a part in the treatment." This seems to be a pretty good definition. It makes it immediately apparent that not only the formal therapist has influence on the patient, but that a great part of therapy is taken over for good or bad by the attendants and nurses who have almost constant contact with the patient.

We come now to the specific forms of treatment. The neuropsychiatric ward in a general hospital, with its limited number of beds and press of patients needing admission, is forced to treat its patients in a short space of time. An occasional patient may stay as long as three months, but the average stay is six weeks. As we have said, the complete diagnostic work-up takes two weeks, leaving only four or five weeks for therapy.

Two forms of short-term therapy are frequently employed—protracted narcosis, and electric-shock treatment. In protracted narcosis, the patient is kept asleep for eight to twelve days by means of rectally administered Cloetta mixture—principally paraldehyde, with several other hypnotic drugs. The patient gets nothing by mouth during the entire course of the narcosis, fluid intake being maintained by administration of 4 per cent dextrose rectally, 2000 to 2500 c.c. being given in every 24-hour period. Caloric intake is therefore very low, but adequate to maintain the patient through the narcosis. There is always weight loss. Vitamins are administered intravenously. The complete cessation of intake of foods and liquids by mouth cuts down the danger of aspiration pneumonia to a minimum, and we believe that this method of narcosis is much safer than others involving feeding by stomach tube. On our service, this is considered the treatment of choice in manic excitement. In some clinics fair results have been reported with electric shock in manic excitement. We have found final results of shock in these cases to be very poor, especially if the patient is followed over a period of six months to a year. Following narcosis, the patient should be moved immediately to some pleasant and neutral environment for a convalescent period.

Electric-shock treatment has much wider indications and is used in a number of psychotic reaction types. It is definitely indicated and very successful in depressed cases, especially in agitated depressions in the involutional period. It is also used with considerable success in stupor states and catatonic reactions. Electric-shock treatments can be very readily administered in the patient's room by means of a portable machine. The patient simply lies supine in bed with the lumbodorsal spine hyperextended over a hard pillow. The electrodes are applied rather far forward—one and one-half inches anterior to the ear and an inch above the outer canthus of the eye. With this placement we feel that most of the current passes through the anterior portions of the frontal lobes. In addition to hyperextension of the spine, we use a rubber-and-gauze mouthgag to protect the teeth. The movements of the convulsion are not restrained except by the application of pressure to hold the upper arm adducted and thus prevent dislocation of the shoulder in the shallow glenoid fossa. Before shock is begun, routine lateral x-rays of the spine are taken, and during the series any complaint of pain in the spine or other joints is carefully examined and checked by x-ray. A series of shocks usually consists of twelve—given over a course of four weeks. The number and time vary greatly, however, with the individual case.

I would like to go over briefly some of the practical points involved in getting a patient admitted to the Psychiatric Service at Duke Hospital. Because of the limited number of beds and the list of patients awaiting admission, it is practically never possible to admit the psychotic who is sent in directly as an emergency with a note asking for admission. As a rule, it is much better for every patient to be seen in the Psychiatric Out-Patient Department, after which disposal of the case can be made according to the gravity of the disease. In this way patients dangerous to themselves and others can be quickly admitted to the phychiatric ward, while other patients may be admitted to a medical ward, treated as out-patients, or given a deferred admission date. For all practical purposes, it is best to communicate with the psychiatric resident directly by telephone. Through him, arrangements can be made for the patient being seen in the Out-Patient Clinic or by one of the private physicians.

Another important function of the psychiatric service is the training of special personnel. In psychiatry, nurses and attendants have much closer contact with patients than in any other branch of medicine, and are in a position to play a much more important part in their care—diagnostically in the way of careful observation of the patient's activities, and therapeutically in their attitudes toward his behavior. There are also a number of special procedures in the psychiatric management and treatment that hold great potential dangers to the patient and must therefore be carefully and constantly supervised by observers trained to recognize the danger signs; to mention a few—insulin shock, protracted narcosis, and wet-sheet packs. In all of these procedures, there is danger of sudden respiratory failure or sudden peripheral vascular collapse. The attendant must be able to follow the pulse, temperature and blood pressure, also to do a certain number of neurological tests which show the general condition of the patient. The psychiatric attendant must also become attuned to the fact that all psychiatric patients are completely unpredictable in their behavior and realize that each patient is a potential suicidal risk. It is only by such trained supervision that serious accidents can be avoided.

In closing, I would like to put in a word for more propaganda in psychiatry—spreading of sensible ideas about mental disease. At the present time we are getting a good bit of publicity, but most of it is of low grade. For example, the *Reader's Digest's* recent article "20-Minute Cure for Shell Shock." I think that the neuropsychiatric services in our general hospitals should become centers for the spreading of this knowledge. Beginning with such talks as this aimed at acquainting the physician of the community with the facilities offered to aid them with their psychiatric problems, making clear exactly what we are able to do for them, and also the limitations involved; later, concerted effort, not only by psychiatrists but by all interested in medicine, to correct the many misconceptions of the general public concerning mental disease.

TSUTSUGAMUSHI FEVER OR SCRUB TYPHUS MENACES U. S. FORCES

(Maj. Charles E. Alden & Capt. Jack Lipshutz, Army of the U. S., in *Jour. A. M. A.*, April 15th)

Tsutsugamushi fever is a Japanese term meaning "dangerous bug fever." More than forty-five years ago the Japanese learned to associate the disease with mites like chiggers found in the scrub and the brush. The authors saw 70 cases in the South Pacific. Tsutsugamushi fever is apparently identical with the Sumatran fever, K typhus, scrub typhus and Kedani disease found in Sumatra, Malaya and New Guinea.

Most of the American soldiers had been in wooded sections, logging or clearing areas where vegetation is dense along small streams and areas of the damp jungle. These mites attack regions of the human body around the waistline, the groin and the armpits. When they bite they convey the parasite.

Insect repellents have been developed which will keep the Trombicula, or chigger, off the body. This is smeared on the socks and an area up to 6 inches above the trouser cuffs. High boots are worn. The body dusted with equal parts of sublimed sultur and talcum. Larval mites will not pass through the uniform worn in tropical areas, but they can penetrate the mesh of G. I. wool socks. If the sock is properly treated with an insect repellent, the mite is dead before it gets through the sock.

The Important Role of Bronchoscopy in the Occasional Case of Asthma*

V. K. HART, M.D., Charlotte, North Carolina

Charlotte Eye, Ear, Nose and Throat Hospital

THE use of bronchoscopy in the asthmatic patient has received considerable attention in the medical literature of the past decade. I shall not attempt to review all this literature. Time and space permit only of a very brief and practical presentation.

Our approach to any therapy must always be paved with a basic knowledge of the pathology to be treated or corrected. After all, asthma clinically describes only an expiratory type of dyspnea. Lamson, Butt and Strickler[1] use the phrase "paroxysmal dyspnea." Any obstructive lesion of the airway, particularly those below the bifurcation, may give an asthmatic type of labored breathing. It may or may not be an allergic bronchospasm.

It is, therefore, germane at this point to state the causes of this asthmatic breathing. Gompertz[2] (quoting Miller) lists the following causes: 1. Spasm of the bronchial musculature. 2. Thickening of the bronchi and bronchioles from edema, hypertrophy, hyperplasia, and cellular infiltration. 3. Thick and tenacious sputum. 4. Collapse of the bronchi during cough and expiration. 5. Any localized narrowing of the bronchus.

With reference to the latter, Prickman and Moersch[3] reported some degree of stricture in 60 of 140 asthmatic patients bronchoscoped at the Mayo Clinic. They excluded edema and spasm.

For completeness, foreign bodies should be considered in any obstructive mechanism. Chevalier Jackson's famous aphorism, "all that wheezes is not asthma" is still pertinent. A wheeze is very common in foreign body of the airway, and sometimes, too, we may have an expiratory type of dyspnea.

A corollary becomes evident. Any abnormal tissue in the bronchus may produce comparable symptoms. On my service at the North Carolina Tuberculosis Sanatorium asthmatic wheezing and respiration is common in those patients with tuberculomata of the tracheobronchial tree. Likewise, any abnormal tissue may produce such symptoms, viz., benign granulation tissue, benign or malignant growths.

These growths may be extrabronchial and produce the same symptoms. Likewise, for mediastinal tumors.

Lamson[1] and associates list other conditions simulating true asthma. These are interstitial emphysema, distortion of the thorax, cardiovascular disease, syphilitic aortitis with or without aneurysm, and pulmonary fibrosis resulting from tuberculosis and pneumoconiosis. However, they state there is no known pathologic picture, either gross or microscopic, which may be considered characteristic of asthma.

We may now deduce from the above that bronchoscopy has two definite functions in asthma or paroxysmal dyspnea. I say this despite the fact that Unger and Wolf[4] recently reviewed the treatment of 459 of their cases and made no mention of bronchoscopy. The two functions of bronchoscopy are: 1. Diagnostic. 2. Therapeutic.

Diagnostic bronchoscopy should be done on all patients with paroxysmal dyspnea which is not relieved by the ordinary therapeutic measures in the treatment of asthma. In particular would I stress that any inspiratory dyspnea is certainly not asthma. It means an obstruction above the bifurcation. Yet I have seen in the immediate past three cases of this type treated for asthma. In all, the correct diagnosis was dangerously delayed. One of these patients had a bilateral vocal cord paralysis following thyroidectomy. The other two had cylindromas of the trachea. Two were relieved by appropriate surgery, the third is still under treatment.

I recall another most interesting case last year which illustrates the diagnostic value of bronchoscopy. The patient was a white male in his 70th year. He had had asthma for years. He had developed an intractable asthma which defied all the usual remedies. The internist said his cardiovascular system did not account for his symptoms. Bronchoscopy was requested and done. We found only a small amount of mucopus and no intrabronchial pathology. However, a suspicious fixation of the bronchus was noted pointing to extrabronchial pathology. A chest röntgenogram was suggestive but not conclusive as to mediastinal change. Ultimately a gland appeared in the neck. This was removed and proved to be malignant. The case then became one of clearcut mediastinal malignancy and the patient died shortly thereafter.

*Presented to Tri-State Medical Association of the Carolinas and Virginia, meeting at Charlotte, Feb. 28th-29th, 1944.

The moral here is an old one: two diseases may exist in the same patient.

Time does not permit further elaboration of this diagnostic phase. Let us then consider the therapeutic value of bronchoscopy. Its usefulness in obstructive lesions producing asthmatoid symptoms is acknowledged. What about its helpfulness in true allergic asthma? It is of no particular aid in those cases which respond to the usual asthmatic regimen. Bronchoscopy, in treatment of resistant cases, is occasionally useful under these conditions according to Gompertz.[2] 1. When the secretions are copious and the epithelium diseased. 2. When the secretions are very thick, viscid and difficult to evacuate. 3. In those cases where specimens for autogenous vaccine are desired. 4. In collapse of the tracheal and bronchial walls.

I have found it of no value in those cases with little or no secretion and where other intra- and extra-bronchial pathology is not present. I have seen one such patient die in spite of all therapy including bronchoscopy. On the other hand, bronchoscopy occasionally gives dramatic relief by freeing the bronchi of secretions. Bases and Kurtin[5] urge its use in so-called Status Asthmaticus.

Briefly, I shall review two such cases.

CASE 1.—A white married woman, a doctor's wife, was seen in consultation on 4/29/36. She had run the gamut of all allergic and medical care. She was even put in an air-conditioned room. Bronchoscopy was advised and done the same day. Much thick, viscid pus was suctioned from both sides of the bronchial tree. Immediate and spectacular relief was afforded. Moreover, she continued to do well and as far as I know has not had such a severe attack since.

CASE 2.—A married white woman, aged 43 years, was sent to our clinic for bronchoscopy on 11/9/43. The referring physician reported that she had had an asthmatic dyspnea for six weeks. This was her first attack and it had been refractory to all the usual therapy. He had even given her aminophyllin intravenously. She had also had a course of sulfathiazole.

A bronchoscopy was done the day of admission. Definite pus was aspirated from the trachea and both main-stem bronchi. No other pathology was noted. A few c.c. of Mono-P-Chlorophenol were instilled.

She obtained prompt and prolonged relief. No other therapy was necessary.

SUMMARY

The value of bronchoscopy in asthmatic dyspnea has been discussed. The basic pathology was briefly reviewed. Obstructive causes of non-allergic asthma were also reviewed. It was thus emphasized that bronchoscopy had two functions in any intractable dyspnea: 1. Diagnostic. 2. Therapeutic. The only real therapeutic value is in those cases with either copious or thick viscid secretions. In such cases, though few, bronchoscopy may be life-saving.

Illustrative cases were cited.

BIBLIOGRAPHY

1. LAMSON, R. W., BUTT, E. M., and STRICKLER, M.: Pulmonary Pathology with Special Emphasis on Bronchial Asthma. *The Journal of Allergy*, 14:396 (July), 1943.
2. GOMPERTZ, J. L.: Bronchoscopy: Its Role in the Treatment of Asthma. *California and Western Medicine*, 58:10 (Jan.), 1943.
3. PRICKMAN, L. E., and MOERSCH, H. J.: Bronchosteriosis Complicating Allergic and Infectious Asthma. *Annals of Int. Med.*, 14:587 (Sept.), 1940.
4. UNGER, L., and WOLFF, A. A.: Treatment of Bronchial Asthma. *Journal A. M. A.*, 121:323 (Jan. 30th), 1943.
5. BASES, L., and KURTIN, A.: Prevention of Death in Status Asthmaticus. *Archives of Otolaryngology*, 36:79 (July), 1942.

DEMEROL AS A SUBSTITUTE FOR MORPHINE

(R. C. Batterman, New York, in *Conn. Med. Jl.*, Jan.)

Demerol analgesia occurs within 15 minutes when given by the parenteral route, within 20 to 60 minutes for the oral route, and subsides within three to four hours. If the patient does not respond to 150 mg. it is unlikely that a larger dose will be more effective.

Demerol is a potent antispasmodic. Relaxation of smooth muscle spasm whether gastro-intestinal, biliary or renal can be achieved within 10 minutes with 100 mg. intramuscularly. For chronic nerve pain such as neuritis, radiculitis, the shooting pains of tabes dorsalis, intercostal neuralgias following thoracoplasty it is superior to morphine.

Once labor is well established, the administration of 150 mg. intramuscularly immediately alleviates the restlessness and the severe pain without interfering with the course of labor. The majority of patients require no more than two doses. If labor is prolonged 100 mg. may be given every three hours.

Demerol 35 mg. subcutaneously will stop the average acute asthmatic attack within 10 minutes.

Dizziness occurs in 20% of the patients, nausea and vomiting may result, and weakness and syncope in ambulatory patients only.

TOXIC REACTIONS TO THE INTRAVENOUS INJECTION OF MERCURIAL DIURETICS

(J. Wesley & I. B. Ellis, Boston, in *Amer. Heart Jl.*, Jan.)

Experience in general indicates that the common drugs prescribed in heart failure—digitalis, ammonium chloride, nitrites, aminophylline, etc.—have no effect on the toxicity of mercurial diuretics, nor does the type of heart or renal disease. Patients already ill are perhaps more likely to succumb than those in a better state of health, for they are less able to stand the strain of a reaction. A better state of health is, however, no protection against a fatal reaction. The usefulness of mercurial diuretic drugs outweighs their possible danger. They should be administered only when clearly indicated, and the occurrence of danger signals warrants complete reëvaluation of the therapeutic regimen in any given case. No fatalities have been reported after intramuscular injection of a mercurial diuretic, and the diuretic response often compares favorably with that which results from intravenous injection.

PRIMARY OVARIAN PREGNANCY WITH LIVING MOTHER AND CHILD

(L. J. Strumpf, Jacksonville, in *Am. Jl. Obs. & Gynec.*, Feb., '43)

A case of primary ovarian pregnancy in an adult Negro multipara is reported in which a full-term living, normal infant was recovered by laparotomy. Mother and child were discharged from the hospital in good condition on the 14th day.

CLINIC

Conducted by
Frederick R. Taylor, B.S., M.D., F.A.C.P.,
High Point, N. C.

On Nov. 15th, 1935, a 30-year-old man consulted me. He stated that he had been unable to work since the age of 14, at which time he was working in a cotton mill.

His chief complaint was that he had lost the use of himself all over, especially his arms. When about 14 years old, he noticed that his hands were "drawing" and he had difficulty in picking up objects and in talking. This latter difficulty cleared up in 4 or 5 years, but his arms got worse and his legs became involved. The trouble had progressed steadily in his arms and legs. He could still feed and dress himself, but clumsily. He could still walk, but it was hard for him to get up out of a chair. A year ago, he first noticed drooping of his left eyelid. He had no pain. He noted no loss of sensation or paresthesia, but when he sat in one position long he got quite stiff in his muscles. He had no gastrointestinal, cardiorespiratory or urinary symptoms, and no headache or backache.

He had pneumonia when a baby, severe influenza in 1920, measles, whooping-cough and mumps in childhood. He stated that he had had gonorrhea 7 or 8 years previously, and named two good physicians who treated him, but said they did him no good, so he "took 9 bottles of O. K. Specific" and seemed to recover. He denied syphilis.

His habits threw no light on his trouble. He smoked one-half pack of cigarettes a day and denied using alcohol. He slept well 8 to 10 hours a night. His diet seemed sufficient.

He stated that his father had the same kind of disease, only not so badly. His father had been affected only about 10 years—not so long as the patient himself. His mother had been operated on for what was said to be cancer. One sister had "female trouble with flooding." One brother was a patient in the State Hospital at Morganton. He said that this brother had been in the Marine Corps, and one day some of the boys wanted him to drink some liquor and he refused, so they poured it into him, and he cussed them and one of them hit him and knocked him into a rock pile and he was unconscious for several hours, since which time he had been insane. Two brothers were well, one brother was scalded to death as a baby, one brother was born dead. An aunt died of the same disease that he has. Patient was married at the age of 21, but his wife did not know of his condition at the time, and they separated two years later. While the two lived together there was one miscarriage. Patient never had his blood tested for syphilis. He had been examined three years previously at the Guilford County Sanatorium.

Patient's height was 5 ft. 5½ inches, weight 99¾ lbs. (standard wt. 142 lbs.), t. 99.4, p. 84 (weak), r. 20, b. p. 112/84. Moderate ptosis of left eyelid. He stated that he could not smell things well. His pupils reacted well to light. There was some dynamic nystagmus. His hearing was fair. He said he had had a discharging left ear at the age of 15. His cranial nerves in general, except for the ptosis, did not seem to be affected. His head was otherwise negative, as were his neck and chest. His upper extremities showed very marked atrophy throughout their entire extent, from hands to shoulder-girdles. The tendon reflexes were absent. The abdominal reflexes were hyperactive. (No sphincter disturbances.) There was marked, but less extreme atrophy of his lower extremities, more in the legs than in the thighs. The knee-jerks were absent. There was no clonus or Babinski. He had noticed fibrillary twitching in his wasted muscles. He had no Romberg. He had a flaccid gait with toe-drop. His coördination was good. His blood Wassermann was negative.

Discussion: This is a clear-cut example of progressive spinal muscular atrophy of the Aran-Duchenne type, i.e., of lower motor neurone type, with flaccid paralysis and loss of tendon reflexes. A condition similar in every respect, except that the paralysis is spastic, with increased tendon-reflexes, is known as *amyotrophic lateral sclerosis*. The two conditions are probably identical except for the location of the lesions, and mixed types occur, showing, e.g., spastic lower and flaccid upper extremities. If the condition is still higher, involving the medulla, it is usually known as *progressive bulbar palsy*, and here, again, we may have mixed types, some of these patients dying bulbar deaths from dysphagia and choking, or from central respiratory failure.

A factor of special interest in this case is the apparent familial incidence. According to the history, the patient's father had the same disease, though less far-advanced, coming on at a rather late date, and one aunt died of it. There is a definite familial type of progressive muscular atrophy, the Werdnig-Hoffman type, but this is described as occurring only in infants and young children, and as being of rapid course, death occurring as a rule before the 7th year. So, if the history is correct, we must look on this as an interesting familial case of the Aran-Duchenne type, unless we rather strain the facts to consider it as a Werdnig-Hoffman syndrome developing in our patient in adolescence and lasting many years, and in his father at a much later age. The age of his aunt is not given in my record.

A syphilitic type of progressive spinal muscular atrophy has been described, but these cases merely represent a special localization of neurosyphilis, and are amenable to treatment. No treatment of the type under consideration is known to be of any value. Alpha tocopherol, once hoped to be of value, has failed in the experience of most observers, including mine.

CASE REPORT

S-T SEGMENT AND T WAVE CHANGE IN TRANSITORY INSUFFICIENCY— CASE REPORT

Ernest Lee Copley, M.D., Richmond

There is considerable difference of opinion as to the significance of depression or elevation of the S-T segment and inversion of the T wave in an electrocardiogram. While these changes have been generally considered characteristic of disease of the coronary vessels, it is agreed that in many instances this is by no means true. Marvin[1] quotes Sprague who lists 41 different conditions which he maintains produce abnormalities similar to those found in coronary artery-disease, 33 of which he states do not imply heart disease at all.

The alterations due to such familiar factors as digitalis, diphtheria, pericarditis, change of position, axis deviation, and several metabolic disorders which Sprague mentions are quite characteristic, however, and are generally recognized. For instance, one expects to find depression of the S-T segment in a digitalized patient. On the other hand, the alterations due to some of the less familiar conditions listed—trichinosis and Addison's disease, to mention only a few—are rare and seldom encountered in private practice. Obviously, it is impossible to determine from the electrocardiogram, alone, the etiology of certain alterations, and recourse must be had to the clinical signs and symptoms of the particular case for the explanation. I believe careful follow-up examinations will make the diagnosis with reasonably certainty in most instances.

Alteration of the S-T segment and T wave noted in the case herein reported was accompanied by substernal distress and shock, and followed an acute gastrointestinal upset.

Case Report: A colored hotel cook, aged 38, was first seen on January 18th, 1944, an hour after he had suffered an attack of nausea, vomiting and diarrhea. He stated that immediately following the intestinal disturbance, he was seized with a vice-like oppression behind the breast bone and shortness of breath. There was no history of pain in the arms, shoulders or neck, neither had he ever had any abdominal or chest pain. His substernal discomfort was the occasion for seeking medical relief.

He was in shock, his body cold and moist, the heart sounds distant, the radial pulse weak, the systolic blood pressure 100, diastolic 40. An electrocardiogram was advised (Fig. 1).

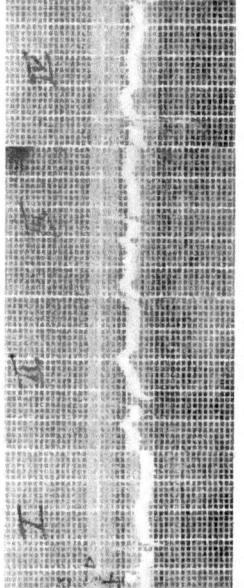

Slightly elevated S-T segment in leads I and IV, slightly depressed S-T segment in lead III. The T wave is upright but flat in lead I, slightly inverted and of coronary type in lead IV.

This abnormal electrocardiogram suggests myocardial involvement due, I believe, to coronary insufficiency caused by spasm of the coronary vessels.

Three days later the temperature was 99.5°, white cell count 8,500 and sedimentation rate 15 mm. for the hour, Westergren method. (According to Todd and Sanford this is the upper normal limit for men.) He was still weak. The heart sounds were normal, however, and there was a moderate rise in the blood pressure. The urine and blood Wassermann tests were negative.

Five days later the blood pressure was 130/80, sedimentation rate 13 mm., white cell count 8,000 and temperature 98.4°. A second electrocardiogram was made (Fig. 2).

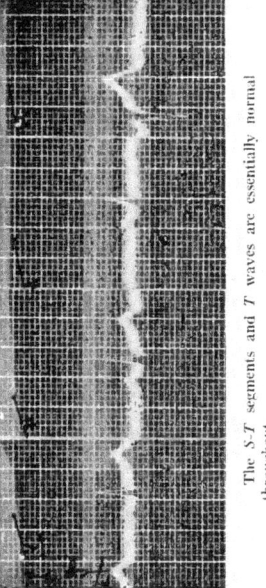

The S-T segments and T waves are essentially normal throughout.

DISCUSSION

The case illustrates the obligation to make repeated follow-up examinations in every heart case in which the diagnosis is at all in doubt. The disappearance of clinical symptoms of coronary artery-disease in this case within eight days excludes the possibility of it having been frank coronary occlusion with infarction. Conceivably, the S-T segment and T wave changes could have been due to an acidosis, one of the conditions which Sprague lists as causing such changes. Also, the shock could have been incidental to the severe vomiting and diarrhea. However, the history of substernal oppression and shortness of breath suggests involvement of the coronary circulation which, I believe, is best explained on the basis of spasm of the coronary vessels.

SUMMARY

Reference is made to the 41 conditions listed by Sprague which he states produce alterations of the S-T segment and T wave of the electrocardiogram. The opinion is expressed that the particular factor causing the alteration can be determined by careful follow-up examinations.

A case is reported in which there were S-T segment and T wave changes accompanied by substernal distress and shock following an acute gastrointestinal upset. The diagnosis was coronary insufficiency believed to be due to spasm of the coronary vessels.
—5701 Grove Avenue

DEPARTMENTS

HUMAN BEHAVIOUR

JAMES K. HALL, M.D., *Editor*, Richmond, Va.

ON THE HISTORY OF MEDICINE

HISTORY is interested in the past, but a biblical passage reminds us that what is to be has already been. And it may be true that the new thing is only the rediscovered forgotten thing.

I cannot easily think of any other domain of human activity in which a knowledge of what has taken place is of more practical value than in the daily practice of medicine. Eliciting a history of the patient, from the patient and from the other available sources, is a high art that few of us are capable of exercising in all of its fulness. Obtaining such a history gives opportunity for the utilization of the most spacious knowledge of medicine, of civilization, of human nature, and of that high gift akin to that made use of by the priest when wayward man comes to reëstablish his peace with God. I often wonder, indeed, if the physician skilled in history-taking may not often succeed in making a diagnosis before the patient lies on the examination table. And it may be equally as probable that the most careful work in the examination room may fail to reveal the nature of the affliction, because the diagnostician was unmindful of the eternal truth that the present always includes the past. The snow of next winter is already in preparation; and the sudden showers of next April are now on their way.

At the annual meeting at Pinehurst two weeks ago of the Medical Society of the State of North Carolina I hoped plans would be formulated for the preparation of a History of Medicine in that state. But I do not know whether or not a Committee on the History of Medicine was created. Within less than a decade that state medical organization will be a hundred years old.

You may be surprised to read that North Carolina was the first state in the Union to establish by legislative enactment a State Board of Medical Examiners. Dr. Hubert A. Royster, whose high intelligence is incessantly active, recently told of the organization of the first Examining Board, in response to the request of the State Medical Society. While I was at the meeting of the Society at Pinehurst, Dr. O'Brian, of Sanford, spoke to me of the medical school that had its brief existence many years ago in a country home in that community. I recall the frequent use made of the so-called madstone in Iredell County in my boyhood days as a diagnostic procedure in suspected hydrophobia

The great herbarium of Wallace Brothers at Statesville has proclaimed for many years the richness of the region in drug-yielding herbs. Much of the curative value of herbs was known by the common people long before drug houses came into existence. Not infrequently pharmacology has been able to demonstrate and to record only what the people had long known.

In the *Journal of the American Medical Association* for April 29th, Dr. R. C. Holcomb, of Upper Darby, Pennsylvania, contributes a letter in which he expresses the wish that the Association may set up a Committee on the History of Medicine. One can only wonder why such a step was not taken long ago. Soon the American Medical Association will be one hundred years old. Within its membership are those competent to undertake the preparation of the history of medicine in our great country. The three-volume *History of Medicine in Virginia* is highly creditable to the Medical Society of Virginia, to medicine and to American history.

Within a few hours I shall be in Providence, Rhode Island, at the centennial exercises of Butler Hospital. Next week I shall be in Philadelphia at the annual meeting of the American Psychiatric Association. In that city the Association was organized in 1844. The meeting next week will be the centennial occasion of the American Psychiatric Association. It is our oldest national medical body.

The existence of a case of pellagra in New York State was reported at the annual meeting of the American Psychiatric Association in 1864. Had our people known that, they would have been less perturbed by the rediscovery of the condition in the Southern States in 1907.

At the centennial in Philadelphia the history of psychiatry in the United States will be in readiness for distribution. The volume—One Hundred Years of American Psychiatry—is the joint creation of the American Psychiatric Association and the Columbia University Press. The hope is being indulged that the book may be worthy of a place in American history.

He who would know the present must know the past; he who knows both may better apprehend the future. What is, has been; what is to be, already is.

---

with histamine orally. In 28 of these cases, within THIRTY CASES OF VASOMOTOR RHINITIS were treated 10 to 20 minutes nasal obstruction, sneezing, and watery discharge ceased. Usually for several hours. In others the relief from a single dose lasts for a full day. When the symptoms recur, another dose is taken, with the same effects. Patients who in the beginning needed 6 or 8 doses of histamine daily, after a few weeks of treatment needed only 2 or 3 doses daily, and later on only occasional doses once every few days.

THERAPEUTICS

J. F. NASH, M.D., *Editor*, Saint Pauls, N. C.

MALARIA TREATMENT TODAY

RECENT experiences, in military medicine and elsewhere, have shown a good deal of what we thought we knew about malaria to be false.

With the increase to be expected as more and more of our fighters come home, all of us will need to know all that is to be known on the subject.

From the authoritative article of Boyd[1] is gained the dealing with this subject which is passed on to our readers.

Until the fever is checked the patient should be confined to bed, while for two weeks subsequently activity should be limited to moderate ambulatory exercise.

If the fever persists it may be suspected that the cerebral heat centers are affected. In this case tepid sponging or cold baths are indicated, their duration being controlled by the rectal temperature, and an abundant intake of cool fluids supplemented by sodium chloride. When free perspiration is begun the patient should be rubbed dry and changed to dry clothing. Subnormal t. calls for covers and numerous hot water bottles, several sinapisms to different parts of the body, and hot beverages. Constipation purgation and daily doses of liquid petrolatum subsequently. For nausea and vomiting cracked ice with or without lime water, 5 minims of tincture of opium, or 5 to 20 grains chlorobutanol. Patients with edema should receive a high-protein diet, those with icterus a high-carbohydrate and vitamin diet.

The specific treatment of malaria must take into consideration the different stages of the parasites in the human host, the infecting or sporozoite stage, the vegetative (trophozoite) stage (to the multiplication of which clinical activity is due) and the gametocytes which render the patient infectious.

Quinine being reserved for military use, totaquin, a standard preparation containing all of the crystallizable alkaloids present in American barks, is the civilian substitute.

Quinine has been routinely taken for years by residents in endemic areas, and of later years atabrine has been similarly ingested, in the belief that it will ward off infection from the bite of an infected mosquito. Quinine, atabrine, nor any other known drug possesses this characteristic. They will check the multiplication of parasites so that few persons will develop active malaria during the period in which they are ingested.

On suspension of treatment many will develop acute malaria two weeks later. As at present prac-

1. M. F. Boyd, Tallahassee, in *Jl. A. M. A.*, April 22nd.

ticed, adults are given 0.1 Gm. of atabrine daily at the evening meal on six days each week. In the specific therapy of the active infection, the civilian practitioner is now practically limited to totaquin and atabrine dihydrochloride. There is little choice between them. Oral administration is the route of choice. Absorption from the stomach is so rapid that no material time is saved by parenteral administration, which should be limited to comatose patients or those with high fever or in whom vomiting is uncontrollable. If required, atabrine rather than quinine should be the choice, and the intramuscular rather than the intravenous route. Injection should be made deeply into the muscles of both buttocks at a point three inches below the iliac crest, with subsequent thorough massage of the site, repeated after 12 hours but should not be continued after the patient can take medication by mouth.

Certain strains of *P. falciparum* require large doses but one may doubt that a parasite strain is likely to acquire a drugfastness. In general totaquin, like quinine, should be administered before meals and atabrine after meals, one of the daily doses should be given an hour before the next anticipated paroxysm in order that a maximum plasma concentration may be available when the young merozoites are liberated. It should not be expected to forestall the next true paroxysm, but paroxysms should not occur on the third and subsequent days. If the drugs are not being absorbed, this will be shown by their absence from the urine. Nothing is gained by administering the two drugs concurrently.

Totaquin dose is not less than 0.6 Gm. (10 grains) daily per 50 pounds of body weight. An adult of 150 pounds and to all over 12 years of age 10 grains t.i.d.; children proportionately large doses. Doses should be given before meals and continued for seven days.

The concurrent administration of plasmochin 0.01 Gm. t.i.d. p.c. is indicated in vivax infections, to lessen the likelihood of a relapse. Tinnitus and deafness are evidence of absorption.

Atabrine dihydrochloride, or quinacrine, is available in 0.1 Gm. tablets. These fractional doses are best given in milk.

It is now recommended that adults initially receive 0.2 Gm. (3 grains) by mouth q. 6 h. for five doses, then 0.1 Gm. (1½ grains) for six days, the early large doses with 1 Gm. (15 grains) of sodium carbonate in 200 to 300 c.c. of water, sweetened tea of fruit juice. For parenteral administration a dose of 0.2 Gm. dissolved in from 5 to 10 c.c. sterile distilled water. Courses of atabrine should not be repeated in less than a month's time.

In case intravenous therapy is imperative, give in at least 200 c.c. of sterile saline solution and at least 20 minutes allowed for the injection. See that the needle is in the lumen of the vein. Give 7½ gr. quinine dihydrochloride, or 3 gr. atabrine to an adult. To the quinine solution may be added 0.5 to 1 c.c. of a 1:1,000 solution of epinephrine hydrochloride. Neither drug should be given more than twice in 24 hours.

Totaquin or quinine is given for two or three days, or until the paroxysms are suppressed, then change to atabrine for five days. If plasmochin is indicated, its administration should await the completion of a five-day rest period.

In those falciparum-infected patients with more than 500,000 parasites per c.m., in addition to the routine therapy, remove parasites by copious bleeding, at the same time transfusing an equal volume of blood from a compatible donor. A liter or more of blood in 24 hours in one or more venesections.

Recrudescences, relapses and recurrences should be treated as primary attacks. In case of vivax or quartan malaria, adequate therapy with totaquin or atabrine destroys gametocytes along with trophozoites and soon the patient is noninfectious. Falciparum patients still remain infectious, as the sexual forms are resistant. Plasmochin overcomes this resistance and makes these patients noninfectious—0.01 Gm. doses t.i.d. p. c. concurrently with each dose of quinine or totaquin during the last five days of the seven-day course, or in the same amounts and for the same period, but subsequent to a course of atabrine, an intermission of five days allowed between the two series.

Infections may be considered latent (a) immediately after treatment has produced a remission in an acute attack and (b) when parasites are discovered in an afebrile patient. Such patients often exhibit an anemia and splenomegaly and may find considerable inconvenience from the enlargement of the organ.

The ultimate extinction of malaria infection probably is more attributable to the activation of the body's resistance than to drugs. Atabrine is given as for treatment of the acute attack as the first course, followed without delay by a course of totaquin and plasmochin as described for 14 days. Dose of totaquin may be reduced to 5 gr. If further treatment is desirable the courses are repeated, allowing a rest period of 10 days between the last day totaquin and the day the second course of atabrine is begun.

If splenomegaly is persistent epinephrine 0.01 mg. is given daily or on alternate days if the reaction is intense. If this dose causes little reaction it is gradually stepped up in 0.01 mg. stages until

0.1 mg. is given. This is repeated 20 or 30 times until the spleen subsides, usually in two months. The reaction to the dose is immediate, the patients manifesting pallor, headache, tremors, sometimes psychic and motor excitation and palpitation.

SURGERY

Geo. H. Bunch, M.D., *Editor*, Columbia, S. C.

TORSION OF THE SPERMATIC CORD WITH GANGRENE OF THE TESTICLE

A boy seven months of age enters the hospital with a tender mass in the right inguinal canal which is said to have appeared for the first time five days previously. There are fever and leucocytosis with the history since birth of an undescended right testicle. At the time of onset the child vomited and cried persistently. Although the condition is thought to be an incarcerated right inguinal hernia, the operative findings are a gangrenous undescended testicle with torsion of the spermatic cord, uncomplicated by hernia. After orchidectomy there is an uncomplicated convalescence.

In 1919 O'Connor could find reports of only 174 cases of torsion from the spermatic cord reported. Up to the present time there has been a total of about 400 cases, two of these by H. W. McKay of Charlotte. There is no record of a case ever having been observed in Columbia. However, atrophy of the testicle is not rare, and torsion of the cord is perhaps the most common cause for it in patients who have not had mumps or who have not been operated upon for inguinal hernia. In most cases the diagnosis of torsion can be made only at operation. Undoubtedly the incidence of gangrene of the testicle from this cause is greater than has been supposed.

Torsion occurs only when the testicle, through development anomaly, is abnormally movable. In cases of torsion the tunica vaginalis is large and the testicle and the epididymis are often widely separated. The gubernaculum is long and lax or congenitally absent. Neither the cord nor the testicle may have any posterior attachment. It is obvious that a testicle freely suspended in a large lubricated sac may readily cause torsion of the cord by rotating upon its own axis.

When torsion begins, as the venous return is obstructed there is swelling of the testicle from passive congestion. When torsion is complete, there is arterial obstruction with destruction of the testicle from gangrene unless the circulation is soon restored by operative relief of the torsion.

Torsion of the cord is more common during adolescence but may occur at any age. The condition has been found to be bilateral in 20 cases. Statistical studies show that torsion is more often associated with incomplete, than with complete, descent of a testis—in the ration of 3 to 2 (O'Connor). It is more common on the left side. When the testis has descended torsion has to be differentiated from epididymitis and orchitis; in undescended cases it is most often confused with strangulated hernia. Recurrent cases have been noted. The prognosis as to life is good, not a single unfavorable case having been reported.

OPHTHALMOLOGY

Herbert C. Neblett, M.D., *Editor*, Charlotte, N. C.

THE MYOPE AT THE BEGINNING OF PRESBYOPIA

Probably the most unsatisfactory patient for refraction is the myope when presbyopia supervenes and his work necessitates the use of bifocal lenses. Since the beginning of the present war the number of such cases is ever increasing because a greater number of people are more and more called upon to enter vocations the nature of which is work of great precision. This further entails quick and accurate alternate seeing in the far and near field of vision. Prior to entering such vocations the vast majority of those now active in such fields rarely used their eyes for much more than getting about comfortably and safely and glancing at the headlines of newspapers, all near work being done at a distance from the eyes that gave clearest vision for detail.

Based upon the amount of presbyopia and the size of the print of object looked at, the print or other object viewed was done with the naked eye at a distance varying from 15 to 25 or 30 inches and without clear perception of detail. The same held for the low-grade myope whose vision for distance was sufficient for his needs without the use of glasses, and the middle- and high-grade myope with his glasses, principally used for distant seeing, which could be removed for near work and fair vision when desired. In the precision work now required of this large group of individuals they find that they cannot qualify for the job at hand without the ability to use the near and far vision accurately. The answer to this problem is the bifocal lenses.

At this point the refractionist is confronted with many "headaches" mainly because the myopic presbyope does not comprehend his visual problem, does not want bifocal lenses, frequently refuses to use them when prescribed despite painstaking and time-consuming effort on the part of the oculist.

The patient insists that all he needs is a close-work glass and will insist upon it, despite the fact that a detailed explanation of its limitations has been given by actual example at the time of the examination. Should the examining oculist subscribe to this viewpoint in sheer desperation and prescribe the proper correction for reading, his troubles begin all over as soon as the patient gets on his job with his new reading glasses. He finds he is all right within the limits of 15 to 20 inches from his eye to his work, but his distant vision is badly blurred with the reading glasses, and if his myopia is of consequence, when he removes his reading glasses his far vision is again badly blurred. After further explanation to the patient either by phone or at office, he agrees in favor of two pairs of glasses—one for correction of his myopia, the other the reading glasses he already has. When again he is shown that neither the one nor the other will meet the visual problems in his vocation he will then argue in favor of a reading hookover for use on his myopic glasses. When shown that this has the same effect on distant vision as the straight reading glass does he is apt to leave the office in disgust, not because he feels he lacks comprehension of a simple problem in vision but because he thinks the oculist is totally incapable of understanding or of correcting his visual defects and should by some sleight-of-hand change his visual quotient or divest his eyes of the inroads of age which he himself is not willing to subscribe to; or he will, finally, but with certain reservations, agree to the use of bifocals.

When this occurs the prescribing oculist is again laying himself open to another episode of return visits and explanations ad infinitum. What is the remedy for this problem? Prescribe the bifocal glasses at the first examination and "take the rap" on this one count rather than on one or more alternatives: or if the patient, as is often the case, refuses to allow bifocals to be prescribed, the oculist may refuse to prescribe any correction and close the case. Whether or not he should charge a fee for his services under the circumstances, that is giving the patient the prescription for bifocals or nothing, rests with him.

In the most intractable of this type of patient a good policy is to advise him to see some other oculist. After he has seen several whose patience may not have been as long-suffering as yours he may have become more inured to the visual infirmities of his age and will return to you, a more sensible, more tractable patient.

These patients, due to the very nature of their refractive error, experience greater difficulty in becoming accustomed to the use of bifocal glasses than do the frank hypermetropes at the presbyopic age because, in the former, clear vision at close range has always been a natural environment, whereas the latter have always had to exert a greater amount of accommodative effort in doing close work and when this begins to waver at the age of presbyopia they more readily give up the effort to accommodate and more easily adjust to the use of bifocals. Even many of these who have excellent distant vision when presbyopia begins find it difficult to understand the necessity for the use of bifocals although the character of their vocation makes their use a vital visual necessity. The writer has rarely found a presbyope who enjoys keen distant vision but who feels that the mere mention of a bifocal is an imposition or an arbitrary ruling of the oculist. No amount of explanation by the oculist can divest him of the viewpoint he has gleaned from a minority of others of the difficulties they have experienced in the wearing of bifocals, until he has tried the straight reading glasses and experienced his visual limitations in using them, as well as the tedium of putting them on and taking them off in the routine of a busy day.

In the final analysis the prescribing or not of a bifocal lens, in many cases, whittles down to one very practical fact, namely, the patient's vocation or his avocation. Many housewives engaged in a limited field of work for specific period of time, and many of the aged for whom distant vision is not a firm requisite, require only a reading glass. Here common sense and good practice dictates against prescribing the bifocal.

Probably most oculists would gladly refer to a fellow oculist the majority of those who apply for examination needing bifocals for the first time. Even among the members of the medical profession it is amazing the paucity of knowledge of the reasons for the use of the bifocal, and their lack of adaptability to its use when the inroads of age have relegated them to the status of the presbyope. Should we then marvel or become exasperated at the layman's attitude toward it?

GENERAL PRACTICE

D. Herbert Smith, M.D., *Editor*, Pauline, S. C.

PRELIMINARY REPORT ON THE CLINICAL USE OF VITAMIN A IN THE TREATMENT OF HYPERTENSION

Every doctor wants to know something he can do for his patients with high blood pressure. A hopeful word comes from the Southwest.

The essential features of the method is the daily administration of 100,000 to 200,000 units of Vitamin A orally. A regimen of rest, avoidance of mental or physical strain, and a low caloric diet was advised in each case but it was felt that the effects of this regimen could be discounted in evaluating the usefulness of Vitamin A since almost all of these patients had previously been given such advice.

Blood pressure readings were made weekly and found in almost all cases to gradually and markedly fall. In some cases when patients discontinued use of the vitamin the pressure rose, falling, however, when use of the drug was resumed. There were no side effects or untoward reactions to the large doses of the vitamin.

A representative case is that of a woman, aged 68. No knowledge of hypertension until cerebral hemorrhage with transient hemiplegia in March, 1943. B. P. 190 110. Placed on 200,000 units Vitamin A daily; April, 1943, b. p. 130/80. Pressure thereafter remained entirely normal for six months and treatment was discontinued. In November, 1943, presure had risen again to 160/90 and treatment was resumed. Again pressure fell to normal and has remained normal on a maintenance dose of 100,000 units daily.

Gratifying results are reported in a case in which potassium thicyanate had proved disappointing.

A small group of esential hypertensives were treated with massive doses of Vitamin A orally. A majority of these responded favorably over long periods of time. This vitamin may prove to be a hypotensive agent of extreme importance and value.

Vitamin A has slight if any potentiality for harmfulness; and, lest the "200,000 units daily" make you think the cost prohibitive, the information is passed on that the ordinary retail price is from 10 to 15 cents per day.

* * * * *

POTASSIUM THIOCYANATE IN HYPERTENSION

TESTIMONIALS as to the benefit to be derived from thiocyanate treatment of hypertension are conflicting. What impresses one as being a fair statement of the case is that[1] which is summarized here.

The initial dose was three grains of potassium thiocyanate by mouth once daily continued for one week. The blood cyanate concentration and blood pressure were determined every week or two. If a sharp drop in blood pressure, toxic symptoms or weakness developed, dosage was decreased. If the blood cyanate level had not reached 12 mg. per cent, if no blood pressure drop occurred and if no signs of toxicity, the dose was increased by three grains daily every week or two until a drop did take place, the blood cyanate level did reach 12 mg.

1. J. S. Blumenthal & M. Wetherby, Minneapolis, in *Minn. Med.*, Mar.

per cent or toxic symptoms developed. When symptoms, blood pressure, dosage and blood cyanate level had been correlated to the best results possible, the patient was observed at one to three months' intervals. A level higher than 12 mg. per cent was lowered by decreasing the dose. The cyanate level is to be kept as low as possible compatible with the well-being of the patient and lowering of the blood pressure. Tolerance to the drug has not developed.

Of the 70 patients treated 58 had headaches, dizziness, weakness, tinnitus. Of these 43 felt much better while under treatment. Too rapid reduction in 10 cases produced weakness, but for a few weeks only. Two developed a rash about the neck which disappeared on withdrawal of the drug. Two had a severe diarrhea which ceased on reducing dosage. One vomited. On giving phenobarbital the drug was resumed with no further difficulty.

The average systolic blood pressure dropped from 192 to 156.

Symptomatic relief was given 43 of 58 patients with hypertension symptoms.

TUBERCULOSIS

J. DONNELLY, M.D., *Editor*, Charlotte, N. C.

DIAGNOSIS AND TREATMENT OF TUBERCULOSIS

ALL of us need to be kept reminded of the essentials of diagnosis and treatment of pulmonary tuberculosis.

Few articles serve this purpose better than the one[1] here given in essence.

For Mantoux test the material must be freshly prepared and it must be injected *into* the layers of the skin. If the first strength is negative (using double strength P.P.D.), the second strength must be used before the test can be considered negative. If the test is negative, it means that the person has not had tuberculosis (almost 100 per cent reliable). If the test is positive, it means that at some time or another, the individual has had a tuberculous infection. It does not tell whether or not the infection is active at this time, nor if it is in the lung or in some other organ of the body.

It is possible to have a minimal pulmonary tuberculosis, and even cavity formation, that does not present any physical signs. If the physical examination reveals the presence of abnormal breath tones, posttussic rales, whispered pectoriloquy, pulmonary tuberculosis is indicated; but if none of these signs are present, and we have reason to suspect from the history and subjective symptoms, we cannot say the disease is not present.

1. W. L. Meyer, Sanator, S. Dak., in *Jl.-Lancet*, April.

A small infiltration behind the heart that does not show upon the usual film, lateral and oblique films, if taken, will show. The x-rays reveal many minimal infiltrations not detectable on physical examination. Stereo chest films are much more reliable than the single flat films and should be resorted to if there is any question of diagnosis. The planographs is more able to outline cavities clearly than even stereo plates.

A single negative sputum sample is not sufficient. At least ten 48-hour specimens should be obtained and concentrated. Tubercle bacilli are proof of tuberculosis; but 20 per cent of the moderately advanced and 50 per cent of the minimal cases do not have a positive sputum.

A very detailed history is essential but it will not rule out a number of other conditions affecting the lungs. It is necessary to detect any signs that might indicate involvement of other organs that will require treatment concurrently with the pulmonary disease.

Every move that the patient makes that someone can make for him increase the length of time that he will have to spend to cure his tuberculosis. Sitting up, talking, laughing, writing letters, etc., all constitute more work for the patient and the lungs. However, physical rest must be sacrificed sometimes for mental rest, and some type of activity, such as reading, or hand work of some kind is allowed.

It is not advisable to stuff the patient with rich food. A balanced diet containing the necessary vitamins, minerals, carbohydrates, fats and proteins, is all that is essential.

In a sanatorium the atmosphere is more conducive to curing than is that of any private home, where as soon as the patient feels well and is temperature-free, with a slight gain in weight, he begins to feel that he should be out of bed and not have anyone waiting on him.

It is probable that there will be a marked change in the treatment of tuberculosis within a short time with penicillin, some modification of it, or even an entirely new one.

A number of surgical procedures assist mainly in putting the lung at rest: phrenic section, pneumothorax, pneumonolysis, extrapleural pneumothorax or an extrapleural paraffin pack, thoracoplasty operations, a lobectomy or pneumonectomy. In a tuberculous tracheobronchitis, bronchoscopic examinations and treatment with silver nitrate in concentration of 20 to 30 per cent, have produced favorable results.

MENINGOCOCCUS CARRIERS can be satisfactorily rendered free of meningococci by treatment with sulfathiazole in dosage of six Gm. daily by mouth for a period of five days.—*Strong & Blumberg*, in *Mil. Surg.*, 92:59, 1943.

UROLOGY

RAYMOND THOMPSON, M.D., *Editor*, Charlotte, N. C.

PROSTATIC DISEASE: PREVENTION SUGGESTED. RECTAL AND CYSTOSCOPIC EXAMINATIONS*

FOR A DISEASE condition as common as prostatic hypertrophy it is natural to ask can it be prevented; and, if so, how? The next question would be, what is the cause?

Many of us recall the time when it was taught that repeated traumatization, *e.g.*, that sustained in horse-back riding, was a cause. Other causes were assumed to be—working both ways—excessive sexual indulgence or the unrelieved congestion produced by abstinence from such indulgence; and, of course, alcoholic drinks and gonorrhea.

No convincing evidence was ever adduced to support any of these assumptions, and they have been abandoned.

Prior to the working out of means of removing the obstructing tissue without a high mortality rate, castration was the favorite operative treatment. It is now established that castration *will* cause the epithelium of prostatic *cancer* to atrophy, that it *may* cause shrinkage of *benign* prostatic hyperplasia, and that eunuchs are almost immune from prostatic enlargement.

But castration could never become popularly acceptable as a means of preventing "the old man's tribulation"; and even for whatever of cure it might offer it could evoked little enthusiasm.

With the development of hormonal therapy over the past twenty-five years, it was inevitable that this form of treatment would be applied to prostatic disease. A great number of men, Alyea, of Duke, among them, have found evidence that an imbalance of the estrogens and androgens may be the cause essential for prostatic enlargement, and that estrogenic therapy may cause atrophy of such overgrowth. Certainly, in many cases this therapy will cause atrophy of the epithelium of prostatic *cancer*.

As *benign* hypertrophy of the prostate is a common condition—afflicting (according to Lowsley) a 5th to a 3rd of all men over fifty years of age—(and these figures do not include the considerable number of cases of malignant growths) it would seem reasonable to administer estrogens in all cases in which increased frequency of urination begins after fifty, in the absence of any demonstrable cause other than prostatic hypertrophy.

It is recommended that stilbestrol be given in small doses, beginning with no more than one mg. daily.

Now as to methods of examination.

A doctor who has had a cystoscopic examination, or witnessed such examination of his father, will not advise or undertake it as a routine measure, or in the absence of plain indications.

There can be no doubt that the routine of "putting the patient through the mill" or giving what is called a "complete examination" is overdone, and this applies to the urological case, as well as to others. And such practice has a good many unfortunate reactions, among them reluctance on the part of the family doctor to refer a patient because he fears that means of investigation will not be chosen with an eye single to the patient's good, and only those done which are indicated on the solid ground of offering a reasonable chance of contributing evidence of value in the diagnosis and management. And the news gets around and causes patients to decline to accept the advice of their physicians.

We all should know the kinds of cases in which cystoscopic examination should be done, and we should know just as well the kinds in which it should not be done. An excellent guide may be had from each of us questioning himself: would I seek, or submit to, such examination if I had the symptoms and signs this patient has?

It is no easy matter to lay down hard-and-fast rules to cover the situation; but we can put into practice, first, the simplest and less painful methods of gaining information, and when these establish the diagnosis, stop there.

One might think that the mention of the importance of making a careful rectal examination as a part of every general examination of a man is superfluous. But the number of cases in which neglect to examine the rectum causes the most important disease condition to be overlooked, and even premature loss of life, remains large.

A simple examination of the rectum will in many cases obviate the need for a cystoscopic examination.

Osler is credited with having said the difference between a poor doctor and a good one is that a good doctor makes rectal examinations.

And in every case in which we find a cystoscopic examination needful we can use an anesthetic procedure, chosen to meet the indications of the instant case; and administered long enough in advance to give genuine anesthesia, i.e., freedom from pain, and supplemented as may be found necessary as the examination proceeds.

A great surgeon once dedicated a textbook to "the heroic man at the point of the knife." But there is no heroism in bearing unnecessary pain; nor has pain any curative value.

When anesthetics were first offered to the profession some surgeons objected that they knew not how to wield the knife without the accompaniment of shrieks of agony. We have come far since that day; but here and there lingers too much of this sadism, and along with it a vague idea that it is unmanly to prevent or avoid pain except that of the severest kind.

There will be too much pain in the world after we have done our best toward prevention and relief.

And it will be well to remember that probably half of us will at some time stand (or lie) in need of a urologic examination, and that there is such a thing as retribution.

A few case reports:

Case 1.—A man, aged 57, married, 4 children, textile worker. Chill and fever four weeks ago followed by frequent and difficult urination, and pus in urine. 18 tablets of sulfathiazole (2 grms.) daily, cleared urine of pus. In a few days, second course of sulfathiazole which cleared urine of pus, but frequent urination continued. The family history was negative.

Usual common diseases of childhood, no complications. General health good. No operations.

Well developed and healthy-looking. Eyes, ears and nose and throat not remarkable. Teeth and gums in good condition. Heart and lungs normal. B. p. 150/85. Abdomen soft. Kidneys not palpable.

No urethral discharge. Scrotum and testicles normal. Rectal: Prostate gland is enlarged 1½ plus. No induration or evidence of malignancy. Large amount of prostatic secretion after massage, 50-60 w.b.c. per h.p.f.

No difficulty in passing No. 16 F. soft catheter. Four ounces of residual urine.

X-ray: Air cystogram. Kidneys of normal size and position. No stone shadows seen. Bladder well filled with air. No stones or diverticula. Definite prostatic indentation at vesical neck.

Urine: Clear. Albumin trace, sugar negative. Sediment: 30-40 w.b.c. per h.p.f. Stained smear, many cocci.

Blood: w.b.c. 8,900; r.c. 4,300,000, hgb. 80%.

Impression: Hypertrophy of prostate gland, benign Prostatitis, nonspecific with residual urine four ounces.

Treatment: Gentle prostatic massage. Urinary antiseptics. Hot sitz baths.

Results: No further chills or fever. Residual urine in four weeks, reduced to 30 c.c. or less.

Patient during past 18 months, no recurrence of symptoms.

Comment: This is a case of prostatitis, producing symptoms of true adenoma of prostate gland.

Case 2.—Farmer, 70, married, 2 children. For the past 8 months has had frequent and difficult urination. Nocturia 4-6 times. Family history negative.

Usual diseases of childhood, no complications. General health good. No operations.

Fairly well developed, fairly healthy looking for age. Eyes, ears, nose and throat not remarkable. Teeth and gums definite pyorrhea. Heart and lungs about normal. B. p. 150/90. Abdomen—no tenderness or masses felt. Ext. genitalia: negative.

The prostate gland is small with marked induration especially right lobe.

X-ray: No bony metastases seen. Kidneys and bladder normal.

Bladder catheterized. 45 c.c. residual, urine.

Urine normal.

Blood normal as to counts, chemistry and psp.

Impression: Carcinoma of prostate gland.
Treatment: Transurethral prostatic resection and castration.

Pathological report: Adenocarcinoma of prostate gland.
Results: 16 months after operation good condition.
Comment: This patient had no further medication or treatment and is getting along well.

CASE 3.—Teacher, 63, married, 3 children. Complaint "prostate-gland trouble" for five years. Has been treated for arthritis for past two years. For the past 8 months has had intermittent pains in left hip and thigh, also pain in back, low. During the past 5 months pain in back and hips and thighs severe and almost constant. Frequent and difficult urination for past 2 or 3 months. Nocturia, at intervals, 4-10 times. Family history negative.

General health has been good until the onset of present illness. Appendectomy 32 years ago.

Anemic-looking and complaining of pain in back and hips. Eyes, ears, nose and throat, no disease. Wears an upper and lower plate. Heart beat is irregular. Lungs are clear. B. p. 140/80.

Abdomen soft. Kidneys not palpable. No masses are felt. Bladder is not distended.

Ext. genitalia normal.

Prostate gland is enlarged, nodular with stony hardness. Bladder catheterized, less than 30 c.c. of residual urine.

X-ray Aircystogram: Kidneys normal size and position. Bladder outline normal. No stones or diverticula. Bony pelvis shows definite carcinomatosis metastases.

Urine clear and negative except 1-plus albumin.
Blood: Reds 3,200,000, whites 8,600, hgb. 68%.
Impression: Carcinoma of prostate with bony metastasis. Anemia.
Treatment: Stilbestrol 1 mgm. daily and deep x-ray therapy.

Patient has had several courses of deep x-ray therapy and stilbestrol 1 mgm. daily for two years and five months and is able to be up and around.

Two essentials in the prevention and early treatment of prostatic diseases are early diagnosis and gentleness in urologic examinations.

In all cases do a rectal examination, especially in men aged 50 or more.

The early diagnosis is the early treatment. The early treatment is the early, perhaps the only, cure.

GENERAL PRACTICE

JAMES L. HAMNER, M.D., *Editor*, Mannboro, Va.

SHORT CUTS IN ENDOCRINE DIAGNOSIS AND THERAPY

THE DIAGNOSIS of some endocrine disorders is difficult and uncertain even with the extensive laboratory facilities available only in research institutions and the larger hospitals. Some of these are, because of their rarity, of little importance; for example, in Illinois with a population of 7,000,-000, Addison's disease causes only 25 deaths each year. Less spectacular conditions are far more common and so of greater importance.

Some of these can be recognized with a fair degree of certainty and adequately treated without recourse to laboratory tests. Disorders are discussed[1] in which this may be done with the facilities possessed by practically all practitioners.

Hypogonadism in non-obese children is due, in great part, to pituitary and thyroid deficiency. Treatment should consist of thyroid in tolerance doses, this determined only by testing the patient's response to gradually increasing doses. BMR determinations are rarely necessary. The patient should be seen once a week and adequacy of dosage controlled by noting tachycardia, tremor of tongue or outstretched fingers, heart consciousness, any complaint of nervousness or insomnia. Should any of these signs or symptoms appear or be reported, reduce the dose 25 per cent and continue.

If thyroid is given to young girls and periods of amenorrhea develop, even without signs of hyperthyroidism the medication should be stopped until the irregularity disappears. Anterior pituitary extracts or gonadotropins should be given in the same way as to the obese.

The opportunity for correcting *obesity and hypogonadism in children* is lost or their chances for recovery greatly lessened by waiting to see what nature will do. Treatment should be started as early as the tenth year—in severe cases earlier—and continued till the defects are corrected. They all require thyroid. Begin with one-half grain per day. See them once a week and at each visit look for signs of over-dosage. Each week the dose is to be increased by one-fourth grain per day till a dose is reached just short of that which produces any of the signs mentioned.

They all need posterior lobe extract. To older children this may be given subcutaneously twice a week in doses just short of those causing annoying intestinal cramps, nausea or faintness. To younger children the posterior lobe may be given in doses of 1/10 to 1/5 grain t.i.d. in enteric-coated pills.

To children of average height or less, give anterior pituitary extract 0.5 c.c. twice a week, in the same syringe at the same time with the posterior lobe extract. Young children may take anterior lobe my mouth in doses of 2½ to 5 grains t.i.d.

Children of more than average height and rapidly growing may have, instead of the anterior lobe extract, some gonadotropic preparation such as A. P. L., Follutein or Antuitrin-S, in doses of 50 to 100 units twice a week, in the same syringe with the posterior lobe extracts.

After two or three months the frequency of injections is to be gradually reduced and finally stopped as the child reaches normal development. Supervision should continue with three or four visits a year until after puberty and it becomes certain that no regression will occur. In case signs of hyperthyroidism develop discontinue thyroid for two or three weeks, then resume in smaller doses.

---
1. J. H. Hutton, Chicago, in *Ill. Med. Jl.*, Feb.

Inspect the genitalia to guard against precocious development; if growth too rapid stop the gondotropin or anterior lobe extract, whichever is being used, for a month or so; longer if growth continues at a normal rate. Examine the urine occasionally for sugar. Glycosuria sometimes follows the administration of the gonadotropins.

These preparations are said to hasten closure of the epiphyseal lines. This danger is probably overemphasized, but in one of the reasons for not using them in children of less than average height.

In pituitary deficiencies the history is most informative; in hypothyroidism the physical findings are more important; while in other endocrinopathies the history and the physical findings plus a therapeutic test may settle the diagnosis. The victim of hypothyroidism gives a history of physical and mental retardation, is sensitive to cold and enjoys hot weather. The administration of thyroid soon brings relief of symptoms. In hypoadrenia the patient is sensitive to cold but is also adversely affected by hot weather. The administration of suprarenal gland by mouth in doses of five grains t.i.d. will often relieve some symptoms within one week. Thyroid aggravates the symptoms.

The obese youngster who has nocturnal enuresis beyond the usual age, or having stopped for a few years and then resumed the habit at eight or 10, will in nearly every case be helped by a course of pituitary and thyroid therapy.

In hypopituitarism the victim is not particularly sensitive to temperature. The injection of 0.5 c.c. anterior pituitary extract will relieve some symptoms within an hour. Hypopituitarism is responsible for an astonishing amount of reduced physical and mental efficiency. It is nearly always associated with some degree of hypothyroidism. Results of treatment are better if the patient is given tolerance doses of thyroid. The woman victim of hypopituitarism, particularly if she is obese, often gives a history of weighing six pounds or less at birth, walked and talked and got her teeth on time or even earlier, was thin, perhaps underweight, until puberty or until after some infection, marriage or pregnancy. Her menstrual periods were a little late in onset; the first period may have been profuse followed by an amenorrheic interval of several weeks terminated by another profuse period. She was unable to nurse her babies or could do so for but a short time, but obesity and the other symptoms of hypopituitarism—headache, fatigue, nervousness, irritability, lack of concentration—were exaggerated after each pregnancy.

A therapeutic test helps confirm the suspicion of hypopituitarism. The injection of 0.5 c.c. of anterior pituitary extract, less often posterior lobe extract, will in most instances relieve headache if one is present and be followed by a sense of strength and well-being and temporary relief of many symptoms.

*Hypo*thyroidism is much more common than *hyper*thyroidism. Most of its victims will have noted some mental and or physical retardation. Often they are tired on awakening, feel better after an hour or two and then soon tire out with the day's tasks. They are sensitive to cold but enjoy hot weather. They are subject to vague aches, pains and disabilities. Hypothyroidism has been mistaken for brain tumor, tabes, neuritis, arthritis, peptic ulcer, cholecystitis, nephritis, pernicious anemia and neurasthenia.

Before subjecting the patient to the expense of a gastrointestinal or gallbladder study or to the ministrations of the neurosurgeon, rule out hypothyroidism. Suppose the patient is a harassed farmer or a busy war worker who can come to the doctor's office only in the evening—when laboratory facilities are rarely available. The history as indicated is helpful. The examination will offer much confirmatory evidence. A therapeutic test will in a few weeks go far toward settling the diagnosis. Give to an adult one grain of U.S.P. thyroid per day. A week later if no signs of overdosage have appeared increase the dosage to 1½ grains per day. See the patient at least once a week, noting the items mentioned. If the symptoms begin to clear up keep the dose just below the amount which causes tachycardia or the other signs. In this way the patient loses no time from his work and no demands are made on depleted hospital or laboratory personnel.

Any woman of menopausal age who consults a physician about her symptoms may need only counsel and advice, or she may need some estrogenic preparation—Theelin, Amniotin, Di-ovocylin, Progynon, etc. Hutton gives 2000 units or 0.1 mg. two or three times a week for two or three weeks. If symptoms are not controlled, gradually increase the dosage. Large doses are expensive, and many women who are made worse by large doses can be relieved by small doses. An aqueous suspension of the crystals is more slowly absorbed than the usual oily solution; one injection lasts longer and the patient needs to visit the office less frequently.

A considerable number of estrogens for oral administration are available, such as Theelol, Emmenin, Progynon-DH, or Premarin. The last-named has been quite useful. The dose is one or two tablets per day or less often.

Hutton's experience with diethylstilbestrol has been disappointing. After the symptoms are brought under control, the frequency of treatments are to be decreased and eventually entirely stopped.

X-ray irradiation of the pituitary and adrenal region or the pituitary and the ovarian region with very small doses (50 r) have sometimes controlled troublesome symptoms not yielding readily to other medication. These treatments should seldom be repeated at intervals of less than a month. The pituitary and adrenals may be irradiated one month and the pituitary and ovaries the next. Treatments should not be given during or within the week prior to an expected period.

A very obese woman complained of backache which was said to be due to a displaced intervertebral disc had been advised to have an immediate operation. Correction of the pituitary and thyroid deficiency with loss of 30 pounds was accompanied by complete relief of the backache.

BMR test supplies only one bit of evidence in any case. Hypopituitarism and hypoadrenia are associated with rates as low as those found in hypothyroidism. The three conditions may be partially differentiated by the history, physical findings and therapeutic tests. Unless the symptoms and physical findings of hypothyroidism are present, the low BMR is usually due to something other than lowered thyroid function. The administration of one grain of thyroid per day will usually aggravate rather quickly the symptoms of hypoadrenia. The administration of 0.5 c.c. anterior pituitary extract will often relieve for several hours the symptoms of hypopituitarism.

The finding of a normal sella turcica is thought to indicate normal pituitary function. Films of the sella have almost no diagnostic value except in cases of suspected tumor.

The editor commends the wisdom here abstracted to the studious attention of every doctor. It offers information promising gratifying results in a large number of discouraging cases, and at a great saving in time and cost.

* * * * *

SIMPLICITY IN FRACTURE TREATMENT

THE REDUCTION OF FRACTURES, says this Northwestern University professor,[1] has become so complicated by the many gadgets advocated for their repair, that we have a tendency to concentrate on someone's method and to forget that all methods should be based on the fundamental principle of traction and countertraction plus manipulation. He reminds us that Hippocrates, 400 years before Christ, designed a heavy fracture table for surgeons who worked in hospitals in large communities, and another table for those whom he called "travelling doctors," this latter made from an ordinary house ladder, to which the patient was fastened by any means at hand, and traction applied between the rungs of the ladder.

As to fractures of different bones, Magnuson goes on:

[1] P. B. Magnuson, Chicago, in Miss. Valley Med. Jl., April.

In the reduction of fractures of both bones of the forearm, the arm may be suspended from a cross-bar by loops of one inch bandage around the fingers, the arm thus suspended with the elbow at right angles, a 4-inch bandage placed close to the elbow on the flexor surface of the upper arm serves as traction against the counter traction of the loops around the fingers. The operator may place his foot in the loop, applying traction to any extent he wishes, leaving both hands free to manipulate, or he may hang weights on this loop and relieve himself of all muscular effort. In reducing fractures it is necessary to do away with muscular effort on the part of the operator or assistants because tired muscles go into clonic contraction and do not apply smooth steady muscle-tiring pull to the fractured member. The operator's hands are free to manipulate and his sense of touch is unimpaired. When the fragments are back in position, the traction may be maintained in exactly the same apparatus without assistants. The doctor, with a pail of water placed at his feet, can then apply a plaster casing, or board splints and strap them in place. All this can be done without skilled assistants. The method maintains steady, smooth traction because the operator is under no muscle strain or tension. Slow, steady traction reduces the fracture, and a dressing that is firm enough to hold but not tight enough to strangulate the tissues, maintains it in position.

Traction always implies countertraction. The patient must be fixed to a table or flat surface in such a way that he will not be dragged off by any amount of traction that is necessary in case of fractured humerus. This stability can be achieved through a bandage placed under his axilla on the injured side and tied to the table leg on the opposite side. Another bandage is fixed around the elbow or wrist, as the case may require, and thrown over the operator's shoulder. The operator can then lean his weight against the pull of the muscles of the arm, leaving both hands free to manipulate, without undue exertion but with all the traction necessary to overcome the pull of any group of muscles in the upper arm. In the forearm this muscle pull is difficult to overcome. Both bones must be perfectly reduced in order to reestablish normal function in the hands and fingers, but in the upper arm the muscles are comparatively weak and require no such traction as do the muscles of the forearm, nor is there so much tendency to displacement of the fracture after reduction. Fracture of the surgical neck or shaft of the humerus, and many times fracture of the lower end of the humerus into the elbow, may be reduced by this method, and may be fixed in position without the necessity of being disturbed until the fracture is healed.

Fractures of the thigh should be immobilized with a Thomas splint for transportation; and in a Thomas splint, with Pearson attachment if possible, for definitive treatment. Some cases will need skeletal traction; others may be held by the Thomas splint without skeletal. Until the patient can be placed under definitive treatment, traction may easily be established with a well-padded notched stick or notched board placed in the groin, the opposite end of this splint being notched so that a bandage may be hitched around it. With a clove hitch around the ankle and a Spanish windlass strong traction may be made for transportation. The clove hitch is commonly called the Collins' hitch, but Hippocrates used it in applying traction to the extremities.

Fracture of the lower leg may be reduced in most cases by using double window pulleys, one attached to the clove hitch fixed around the ankle and the other attached by a rope to the leg of the table, multiplying the strength of the operator 400 per cent. A sheet is passed between the patient's thighs and fastened to the leg at the head of the table to provide countertraction. If the patient is held close to the head of the table, or even to a stake driven into the ground, this countertraction is sufficient to permit reduction of the fracture and application of splints, so that no further treatment will be necessary when the patient reaches the hospital, except possibly the application of a better fitting apparatus to the lower limb.

Magnuson concludes, with practical wisdom:

"If the operator has at hand the mechanical helps that modern surgery has developed, there is certainly no object in not using them, especially if their use makes it easier to reduce the fracture and hold it in reduction; but lack of modern conveniences is no excuse for neglecting a fracture until these aids can be obtained."

Here is help for all of us who have the care of fractures, emergency or throughout; and the words of an authority to encourage and protect against the chance of being haled into court and having a case go against us on the grounds that our management did not have the sanction of an authority.

OBSTETRICS

HENRY J. LANGSTON, M D., *Editor*, Danville, Va.

SOME OBSTETRICAL EMERGENCIES FROM THE STANDPOINT OF THE GENERAL PRACTITIONER

Concise specific directions are given by Schumann[1] for the management of certain of the pathologic features of pregnancy.

---
[1] E. A. Schumann, Philadelphia, in *Med. Clins. N. Amer.*, Nov., 1943.

A continuing elevation in b. p. of 15 to 20, pretibial and facial edema, an increase in weight of a pound per week and the onset of albuminuria constitute the primary signs of pre-eclamptic toxemia. Restrict diet—almost no carbohydrates, but an abundance of proteins, liquids only 40 oz. per day —and free purgation with magnesium sulfate. Kidney function should be studied in detail, urea clearance tests being of great importance. Usually the evidences of toxemia subside in six to 10 days, if they persist induce labor as soon as viability has been reached.

If the toxemia grows worse diet is reduced to skim milk with an occasional bowl of puree of some green vegetable; purgation with saline and the intravenous injection of 1,000 c.c. of 5 per cent glucose solution daily. Vigorous sedation.

In eclampsia most patients go into labor spontaneously, but in those who do not, rupture of the membrane or the insertion of bougies, except in the case of the primagravida with a long cervix and no effacement. If the patient does not improve and when vaginal delivery is impracticable cesarean section under local anesthetic has a distinct place. Elimination of toxins is aided by free purgation by copious colonic lavage and sometimes by sweating with a hot dry pack. Magnesium sulfate, 20 c.c. of a 10 per cent solution is administered intravenously at 4-hour intervals. Morphine sulfate, gr. 1/4 hypo. q. 1 to 4 hrs., depending upon the reaction. Phenobarbital, 6 to 10 gr., is a useful adjunct.

The management of abortion with severe hemorrhage is usually restricted to packing the vagina firmly with gauze or cotton, under aseptic precautions, the packing to remain in place for 24 hours. Ergonovine preparations will do much to contract the uterus and aid in the extrusion of the ovum. Fever requires the sulfa drugs. Curettage may be required for persistent bleeding.

After the fifth month, placenta praevia must be uppermost in the mind when uterine bleeding occurs. As soon as the diagnosis is made, the pregnancy should be terminated either by abdominal hysterotomy or by induction of labor, depending on the degree to which the placental mass covers the cervical canal. On the other hand the desire to conserve the life of the infant, religious objections, and the fact that pregnancy may continue without disturbance makes it wise to explain the situation to both parents in detail and require the final decision to come from them.

A DIASTOLIC MURMUR OVER THE HEART, of peculiar quality and position, and a quick pulse with wide amplitude, the collapsing or Corrigan pulse—when these two features are discovered together the diagnosis of aortic insufficiency is firmly established. The characteristic circulatory manifestations, in the absence of a diastolic murmur over the heart, nearly always mean exophthalmic goitre or arteriovenous aneurysm. Often the degree of insufficiency is too slight to produce characteristic circulatory changes and the diagnosis of aortic insufficiency then must rest entirely upon the presence of a diastolic murmur over the heart.—*Louis Hamman.*

RHINO-OTO-LARYNGOLOGY

CLAY W. EVATT, M.D., *Editor*, Charleston, S. C.

ORBITAL EPISTAXIS

THOUGH I have heard of epistaxis from the eyes I never saw or read of it until the case herein reported was met with. I find five cases reported in *Anomalies & Curiosities of Medicine.** There have doubtless been many other cases yet the condition is relatively uncommon.

A matron, aged 35, was seen in the emergency room of the St. Francis Hospital early on the morning of December 24th, 1943, with nose bleed which began three days before en route from Boston to New York. The nose was packed at the New York Polyclinic. The hemorrhage seemed stopped, so the lady continued her trip south on the twenty-third. The epistaxis recurred on the night of the twenty-third, and continued into the twenty-fourth. She was taken off the train in Charleston, and the nose packed. Immediately two large streams of blood ran down the cheek from the right eye. There was no break discernible in the mucosa of the nose or conjunctiva. The orbital blood did not come through the lacrimal punctum. The red cells seemed in the center of the stream while the periphery was serous, separated as in the sedimentation test. No clotting was seen in the nose. This orbital bleeding stopped of itself in a few minutes without visible clotting or fibrin formation in the path where the streams had been. Sinuses, ears, nose, throat and larynx were normal, except that the mucosa was extremely pale and there were some atrophic changes in the nasal mucosa.

History: Appendectomy 1929. Tumor removed from the womb 1936, and tubes tied at that time. Married five years, never pregnant, divorced. Nose bleed in 1941 not associated with menstruation. No more nose bleed until present attack. Menstruation began at 13, always regular, lasts three days.

Treatment: Nose packed, Vitamin K (Synkamin ampoules) every two hours. Lextron, liver, sedation and forced fluids. Hemoglobin increased from 43 to 56 per cent, erythrocytes from 2,980,000 to 3,130,000, so transfusion was not done. Blood type was III or B, coagulation time 3 minutes, bleeding time 1½ minutes. Slight vaginal bleeding, menstruation, began on the second day, and there was no more epistaxis. The lady left

*Gould and Pyle, 534-535.

the hospital ambulatory, December 31st.

Considering the appearance of the blood streams on the cheek, and the complete cessation of nose bleed when menstruation began, I wonder if this was a case of vicarious menstruation from the nose and eye.

—91 Rutledge Avenue

TREATMENT OF COCCYGODYNIA
(Emil Granet in *U. S. Naval Med. Bul.*, May, '43)

Coccygodynia is simply treated by inserting the gloved finger fully into the rectum, the patient lying on his left side (Sims position), and gently storking the spastic pelvic muscles in the direction of the fibers. Treatments are of 1 or 2 minutes duration on each side and are repeated daily at first, then every second day until about 12 treatments have been administered.

TRANSPORTATION OF SEMEN SPECIMENS
((W. M. Whitehead, Juneau, Alaska, in *Northwest Md.*, April)

A couple unable to have children come to the office. The first thing is to examine a condom specimen from the man and, if this is found normal, then to examine the woman. I advise the man to use a condom and after sliding it off to tie a knot in the neck, then have the wife place the condom specimen in her vagina and put on a pad, bring it to the office at the appointed time. Motile sperm have been found in a specimen 12 hours old but bringing the specimen to the office within three hours is to be advised.

THE DISCUSSION OF THE THERAPY of disease is at best held during the last five minutes of each medical clinic. The orders of the interns in your hospitals almost all are inadequate to the needs of the patients and your desires.—*A. H. Aaron*, in *Penn. Med. Jl.*, Feb.

URINARY TRACT INFECTION.—Sulfadiazine, 2 Gm. daily, in a series of 58 cases of infection (with bacilli, with cocci and mixed)[1] cured in 95% and improved in 5%.
1. Alyea, E. P., & Parrish, A. A., in *S. M. J.*, Nov.

Otitis Media
    Antipyrine .... grs. xxv
    Glycerin qs. ad .... 1 oz.
    Sig. Warm and drop in ear as directed.

DIPHTHERIA-TETANUS-PERTUSSIS, COMBINED, FOR ACTIVE IMMUNIZATION

Diphtheria-tetanus-pertussis is designed to confer adequate protection to infants and pre-school age children. Each c.c. of the preparation contains H. pertussis killed, 10,000 million; diphtheria toxoid, 0.33 c.c. and tetanus toxoid, 0.33 c.c. The toxoids are adjusted to 0.5 c.c. human dose concentration so that in the complete treatment (three injections), the full amount of each toxoid (1.0 c.c.), as recommended by Public Health authorities, is injected. Treatment consists of three 1 c.c. subcutaneous injections with an interval of three to four weeks between injections.

According to the manufacturers, *diphtheria-tetanus-pertussis, combined, "National"* confers simultaneous protection against three diseases with only one series of three injections. Thus it provides quicker protection with fewer injections, and saves time and money for both doctor and patient. It is supplied in single immunization packages of three 1-c.c. vials and five-immunization packages of three 5- c.c. vials.

SOUTHERN MEDICINE & SURGERY

Official Organ

JAMES M NORTHINGTON, M.D., Editor

Department Editors

Human Behavior
JAMES K. HALL, M.D. .... Richmond, Va.

Orthopedic Surgery
JOHN T. SAUNDERS, M.D. .... Asheville, N. C.

Urology
RAYMOND THOMPSON, M.D. .... Charlotte, N. C.

Surgery
GEO. H. BUNCH, M.D. .... Columbia, S. C.

Obstetrics
HENRY J LANGSTON, M.D. .... Danville, Va

Gynecology
CHAS. R. ROBINS, M.D. .... Richmond, Va.
ROBERT T. FERGUSON, M.D. .... Charlotte, N. C.

General Practice
J. L. HAMNER, M.D. .... Mannboro, Va.

Clinical Chemistry and Microscopy
J. M. FEDER, M.D.,
EVELYN TRIBBLE, M. T. } .... Anderson, S. C.

Hospitals
R. B. DAVIS, M.D. .... Greensboro, N. C.

Cardiology
CLYDE M. GILMORE, A.B., M.D. .... Greensboro, N. C.

Public Health
N. THOS. ENNETT, M.D. .... Greenville, N. C.

Radiology
R. H. LAFFERTY, M.D., and Associates ...... Charlotte, N. C.

Therapeutics
J. F. NASH, M.D. .... Saint Pauls, N. C.

Tuberculosis
JOHN DONNELLY, M D .... Charlotte, N. C.

Dentistry
J. H. GUION, D.D.S. .... Charlotte, N. C.

Internal Medicine
GEORGE R. WILKINSON, M D .... Greenville, S. C.

Ophthalmology
HERBERT C. NEBLETT, M.D. .... Charlotte, N. C.

Rhino-Oto-Laryngology
CLAY W. EVATT, M.D. .... Charleston, S. C.

Proctology
RUSSELL VON L. BUXTON, M.D. .... Newport News, Va.

Insurance Medicine
H. F. STARR, M.D. .... Greensboro, N. C.

Dermatology
J. LAMAR CALLAWAY, M.D. .... Durham, N. C.

Pediatrics

Offerings for the pages of this Journal are requested and given careful consideration in each case. Manuscripts not found suitable for our use will not be returned unless author encloses postage.

As is true of most Medical Journals, all costs of cuts, etc., for illustrating an article must be borne by the author.

FACT vs. FICTION AS TO LACK OF HEALTH CARE AND NEED FOR MORE HOSPITALS AND MORE MEDICAL INSTRUCTION IN NORTH CAROLINA

> I speak truth, not as much as I would, but as much as I dare, and I dare the more as I grow older.—*Montaigne (Essays)*.
> The best way to come to truth being to examine things as they really are, and not to conclude they are as we fancy of ourselves, or have been taught by others to imagine.—*Locke (Human Understanding)*.

THE present occupant of the office of Governor of North Carolina has issued a proclamation as to medical care and education in the State, and mailed an expensively printed copy to each of the State's doctors of medicine. The Governor says his concern is that members of the low-income group shall not lack for health care.

The Governor offers no evidence in support of his thesis that members of the low-income group do, in fact, lack for health care. The issue may be met head-on, after the fashion of the intelligent schoolboy who, given his choice of a subject on which to write exhaustively, handed in this:

"Snakes in Ireland

There are no snakes in Ireland."

I have had 30 years of practice in North Carolina (and some years in two other States), and I have never seen, or had trustworthy evidence of, even one instance of a man, woman or child lacking for medical, surgical or hospital care because of inability to pay for such care. All my life I have looked for hants, all my professional life for cases of chlorosis. Not one of either have I been able to find. Long ago I resigned myself to the limitations imposed by the command, "Prove all things;" and contented myself with life within circumscriptions which to the highly-imaginative have no existence.

Every member of the group best qualified to know about any such lack of care who has been queried on the subject has said it had not occurred within his knowledge; and a good many have added comments not at all complimentary to the intelligence of those who assume the existence of such a lack. The group best qualified to know is, of course, made up of family doctors.

There is ground for belief that, as to certain groups far from negligible in point of numbers, those of high-income lack most for medical, surgical and hospital care. Consider the Eddyites, the Anti-vaccinationists, the Anti-vivisectionists. I heard a North Carolina Congressman speak in praise of care he received at the hands of a chiropractor. And a British Ambassador to this country was an Eddyite. There is plenty of evidence that the disciples of Mrs. Eddy are much richer on the average than are the members of any other sect, and that the other vocative antis are in general well supplied with lucre.

The Governor's idea of means of meeting the situation, which he mistakenly assumes to exist, is based on another mistaken assumption—that the place for a sick person is in a hospital.

Hospitals are essentials for certain forms of health care. For the vast majority of illnesses they are expensive luxuries, far beyond the means of ninety per cent of us, even in these affluent times; and beyond possibility of our purchase through taxation, for, be it remembered, payment by taxation is payment by ourselves.

In from eighty to ninety per cent of medical and most surgical cases a patient is better off in his own bed, under the care of his own doctor, with aid of whatever consultative help his own doctor may consider needful. It is interesting and informative in this connection to note that, with the exception of those who die soon after an accident or a major surgical operation, most doctors die in their own beds.

Anyone who goes into hospitals and uses his eyes is bound to see that many patients are kept, or allowed to stay, in hospitals after all need for hospital care has passed. The present excessive demand for hospital beds is due largely to the many women in war work, hospital insurance and the conveniences of the doctor. These conditions will not last.

The plan proposes the erection of a hospital at Chapel Hill of 600 to 1,000 capacity, and other hospitals in various places over the State. Who does not remember the time, since World War I, when hospitals then being operated were no more than half-filled, and all running at a great pecuniary sacrifice? There is every reason to believe that medical and surgical care of the soldiers, sailors, marines, nurses, WACS, WAVES—all those serving in the emergency—and their families—will be given in U. S. Government hospitals.

Those who have provided private hospitals to meet a great health need deserve consideration. Their investments should not be confiscated. It would be far more practicable, more life-saving, and cheaper, for towns or counties having no hospitals of their own to pay operators of near-by hospitals to care for those of their citizens needing hospital care who cannot pay the bills themselves.

There's a great pother about the lack of doctors in rural sections. The lack is nothing like so great as is represented. One doctor can well see after the health needs of at least four times as many persons now, as when typhoid fever, child-bearing, long-drawn out pneumonia, "summer complaint" and pellagra took up half his time; and there were no automobiles, hard-surface roads, telephones or technicians. And there would be lots more doctors in the villages if those in positions of authority in politics, including medical politics, would cease to exalt hospital and hospital doctor service, to the disparagement of the capable services to be had from the general practitioners in the villages.

And we are told that unless we educate our own doctors, have three four-year medical schools in the State, we cannot possibly be amply supplied.

Facts are as stubborn things now as Thomas Gradgrind found them. There was no great lack of doctors in North Carolina when not one was being graduated in the State, and when its population was too poor to make the State very attractive to those graduated outside the State. Opportunity for remunerative employment decides choice of location.

Florida has no medical college within her borders, I believe has never had one, yet there is no record that Floridians have ever lacked for medical care; and for a score of years she has found it necessary to discourage the influx of doctors by refusing to reciprocate with any other State as to licensing for medical practice.

New Hampshire and Vermont are side by side. New Hampshire has no medical school; Vermont has one. The ratio of doctors to population is almost the same in the two States. On the West Coast the States of Washington and Oregon supply the same kind of evidence.

Subtracting the number of doctors of medicine whose homes are just across the Potomac from Washington and others who for various reasons do not minister to the health needs of the people of Virginia, it is seen that the ratio of doctors to population is about the same in Virginia as in West Virginia. There are two graduating schools of medicine in Virginia, none in West Virginia. Is West Virginia alarmed about the situation? Not at all. Within the past twelve-month West Virginia's two-year medical school entered into an arrangement with the Medical College of Virginia to give the third- and fourth-year instruction to all those completing the two-year medical course at West Virginia. Canny West Virginia. She knows giving the latter half of a medical education is an expensive business.

The General Assembly of the State of North Carolina could appropriately provide funds for paying family doctors for services they are now rendering gratis to the needy, and for paying nearby hospitals and specialists for caring for the few who really need such services and cannot pay for them; but, on the whole, it would be better to require each county and town to pay for these services for its own.

He who runs may read. It is to be hoped that he, and a majority of those who make the laws of this State, will read, mark, learn and inwardly digest.

ASPIRIN

It is commonly said that aspirin is a heart depressant and a stomach irritant. All of us know that aspirin is being taken by an enormous number of persons, that it is the most popular of headache remedies, and that headache is the commonest symptom for which medicine is swallowed.

Many of us have wondered why it is that we have not seen some of these cases of heart depression and stomach irritation as untoward effects of the ingestion of large doses; and few would have doubted that the taking into the stomach of 750 grains of aspirin, all of it retained, would prove fatal.

A case report by a Britisher[1] sheds light on the subject.

A European woman, aged 46, living in Kenya Colony, on November 25th, at 2 a. m., swallowed 750 grains of acetylsalicyclic acid (150 5-grain tablets of Howard's aspirin). The doctor called to see the patient 14 hours after found her sitting in a chair, drowsy and disoriented, complaining of tinnitus, r. 40 and deep, p. 30, volume small; sweating and complained of the heat, in spite of the fact that the day was cold. She was not cyanosed and had no rash. Her pupils were small and reacted to light. Examination of the heart and lungs revealed no abnormality.

A catheter specimen of urine was of normal colour had an odour of acetone, sp. gr. 1.030, very acid, nitroprusside test for acetone bodies strongly positive. Gmelin's test for bile pigment positive, moderate cloud of albumin, trace of glucose, several r.b.c. and pus cells, but no casts. In order to test the antiseptic action of the drug, a nutrient agar slope was inoculated with a sample of her urine and incubated—no colonies.

Treatment.—Gastric lavage sod. bicarb. 1 dr. to 1 pint—five ounces of the solution left in the stomach; aperients; much fluid; sod. bicarb. 30 grains q. 2 h.

For ketosis and hepatitis, beginning the second day an injection of 40 units of insulin, combined with oral administration of 40 Gm. of glucose; 20 Gm. of glucose every two hours for 12 hours, then injections of 10 units of insulin morning and evening ½ hr. a. c., followed in each case by 40 Gm. of glucose 3 hrs. later.

A diet of high carbohydrate (with low protein and fat) content, in order to assist recovery from the hepatic damage and to avoid further strain on the kidneys.

There was steady improvement and soon the patient was restored to complete health.

If the experience of one case may be taken as proving any general contention, it may be assumed that aspirin in the ordinary, or even four or five times the ordinary dosage, is entirely safe medication, not depressant nor irritant to any organ.

However much some doctors may scoff at "symptomatic treatment" all of us practice it every day and are sensible in so doing. It is not unlikely that, on the average, doctors of medicine take more aspirin than do the members of any other group. We don't have a "complete diagnostic survey" whenever we have a headache. Far from it.

It was a good day for the race when aspirin was made available. It would be well to remember the exorbitant price charged for as long a time as possible by the original German manufacturers, and the misleading claims still being made by their successors.

Aspirin is aspirin, just as table salt is table salt, and with the law as it now is a purchaser may depend on contents corresponding to label. Besides, a number of firms whose labels have always been dependable are putting out aspirin.

* * * * *

CORRIGENDUM

In our issue for last month by inadvertence the line Dept. of Neuropsychiatry, Duke Univ. School of Medicine which should have been carried under the name of Dr. Frederick H. Hesser (p. 120), was carried under the name of Dr. J. G. Lyerly (p. 124), of Jacksonville, Florida. Our amende honorable to both the gentlemen.

* * * * *

NEWS

SHIPPING ADDRESS FOR YOUR ART EXHIBIT

Artist-physicians desiring to exhibit their works at the June A. M. A. Meeting should ship their works not later than May 20th to the following address:

American Physicians Art Association, Room 1302, 308 W. Washington St., Chicago. Pack carefully and ship by express collect, including $50 insurance.

Mead Johnson & Company have offered to pay the express charges both ways (including insurance up to $50).

Art objects exhibited are automatically eligible for inclusion in the next Paergon, as well as for one of the numerous A. P. A. Association prizes.

Further information may be obtained from Francis H. Redewill, M.D., Secretary, American Physicians Art Association, Flood Bldg., San Francisco, Calif.

Dr. Thomas R. Nichols, of Morganton, has been elected president of the Burke County Medical Society.

Dr. J. Adams Hayne, for many years State Health Officer of South Carolina, has resigned to accept the position of Director of State Health Education established by the recent legislature. Dr. Ben F. Wyman succeeds Dr. Hayne in the duties of State Health Officer.

Dr. Hayne's abilities have won for him a high place in health circles all over this country. He has been the recipient of many honors at the hands of national organizations.

MARRIED

Miss Margaret Elise Ascherfeld, of Baltimore, and Captain William Lowndes Peple, Jr., were married in the Protestant Episcopal Church of the Redeemer, Baltimore, on May 8th. Dr. William Lowndes Peple, of Richmond, was his son's best man.

Dr. Walter Dickenson Woodward, of Richmond, and Mrs. Alice Myrtle Nevins, of Staten Island, New York, married April 20th.

Dr. James Thomas Stovall, of Jefferson, Georgia, and Miss Julia Isabella Cox, of Clarkton, North Carolina, were married April 20.

---
1. A. D. Charters, in *British Medical Journal*, Jan. 1st.

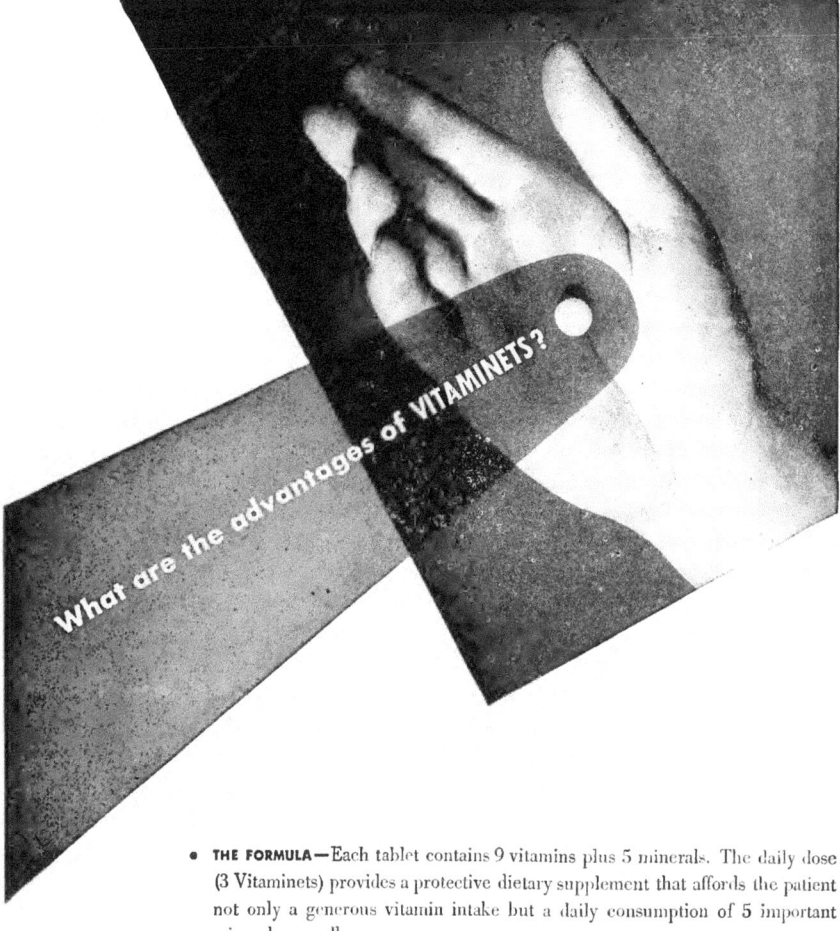

- **THE FORMULA**—Each tablet contains 9 vitamins plus 5 minerals. The daily dose (3 Vitaminets) provides a protective dietary supplement that affords the patient not only a generous vitamin intake but a daily consumption of 5 important minerals as well.

- **PALATABILITY**—Vitaminets 'Roche' may either be chewed or swallowed whole, depending on the patient's preference. The licorice flavor is particularly acceptable to children (and adults, too) who cannot swallow tablets.

- **ETHICAL**—Vitaminets are never advertised to the laity either by drugstore display or other promotional methods.

HOFFMANN-LA ROCHE, INC. • ROCHE PARK • NUTLEY 10, N. J.

Available in bottles of 30 and 100 tablets.

VITAMINETS 'ROCHE'
CONTAINING 9 VITAMINS PLUS 5 MINERALS

DIED

Dr. John A. Drake, Monroe, Va. (M. C. of Va., 1903), died at Lynchburg General Hospital April 14th.

MEDICAL COLLEGE OF VIRGINIA

Dr. Lewis E. Jarrett, Director of the Hospital Division, has resigned effective June 1st, to accept the superintendency of Touro Infirmary, New Orleans. Dr. Jarrett is an alumnus of the College's School of Pharmacy and School of Medicine. He was made director of the hospital division in 1933, succeeding Dr. J. L. McElroy, who went to Paris as superintendent of the American Hospital.

Dr. I. A. Bigger, Professor of Surgery, spoke to the staff of the Woodrow Wilson General Hospital, Staunton, on April 13th, on Drainage of the Pleura with Particular Relation to Chest Injuries.

President W. T. Sanger attended the conference on rural health under the auspices of the Farm Foundation in Chicago, April 10th-14th.

Dr. DuPont Guerry, III, has been appointed Assistant in Ophthalmology. Dr. Guerry has recently opened offices in Richmond.

In April Dr. Bela Schick, Chief of the Department of pediatrics, Mount Sinai Hospital, New York, addressed two meetings at the college—first the faculty and staff meeting on April 20th, when he spoke on Recent Advances in Pediatrics, and the second at noon April 21st, when he addressed the student body, faculty and invited guests on Allergy.

Dr. Sidney S. Negus, Professor of Biochemistry, attended the annual meeting of the American Chemical Society in Cleveland.

UNIVERSITY OF VIRGINIA

A Charles Scott Venable Annual Lectureship in Traumatic Surgery has been established in the Medical School of the University of Virginia. This lectureship is supported by royalties from the sale of an adjustable splint designed by Dr. Charles Scott Venable, Jr. The splint has been made available without royalties or encumbrances to the Red Cross and civilian defense agencies and is now in general use both in the United States and Canada. It is standard equipment for the Canadian National Railway. It is also obligatory equipment for all ambulances in the State of Texas. Dr. Venable was graduated from the Medical School of the University of Virginia in June, 1900. He is chief of staff of the Nix Hospital, San Antonio, Texas, and the seventy-ninth president of the State Medical Association of Texas, and president of the American Association for the Surgery of Trauma. Dr. Venable's father was professor of mathematics at the University of Virginia from 1866 to 1896.

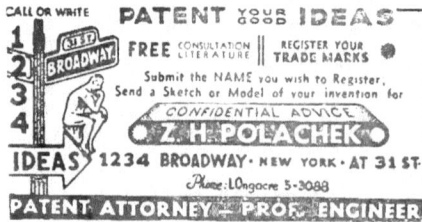

On April 11th, Dr. Henry B. Mulholland spoke at the meeting of the Medical Society of Northern Virginia at Front Royal, on Some of the Newer Drugs and Their Usage."

Major Henzykzi Borowski spoke at the meeting of the Virginia State Medical Society at the University of Virginia April 16th, on Experiences of a Polish Doctor in Peace and War.

BOOKS

TEXTBOOK OF GENERAL SURGERY, by WARREN H. COLE, M.D., F.A.C.S., Professor and Head of the Depart of Surgery, University of Illinois College of Medicine; and ROBERT ELMAN, M.D., Associate Professor of Clinical Surgery, Washington University School of Medicine. Fourth edition. *D. Appleton-Century Company, Inc.*, 35 West 32nd Street, New York City, London. $10.00.

In order to make the text represent all of the rapid advances of the last few years the whole of it has been reset. As was the case in the two previous editions, the physiological point of view is kept to the fore. The inclusion of numerous case histories is a feature of great value. Non-operative treatment is given unusual attention.

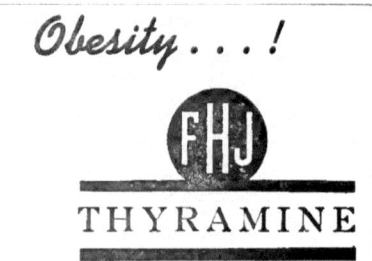

Composition

Thyroid I gr. Amphetamine sulphate 5 mgs. Thiamin chloride I mg. in suitable combinations with physiological reinforcements.

No. 1—One Capsule before breakfast
No. 2—One Capsule before lunch
No. 3—One Capsule at 4 p. m.

Contraindications

Hypertension .... Hyperthyroidism

Supplied

Capsules: Packages 21 and 42 (one or two weeks supply).

—Professional samples on request—
Available: Any professional pharmacy
F. H. J. PRODUCTS
977 East 176th St., New York 60, N. Y.

Marshal of Mercy

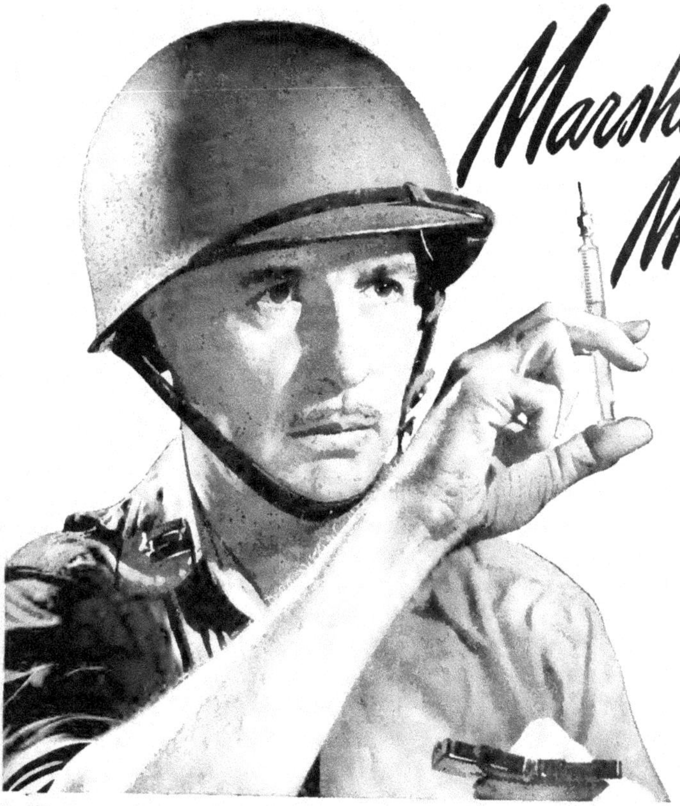

In war, even more than in peace... dispenser of blessed relief... his the precious power over pain.

Long hours the medical officer toils... routinely yet heroically... without thought of citation... grateful for brief moments of relaxation... for the cheer of an occasional smoke. And likely as not, his cigarette is Camel, the favorite brand in the armed forces*... first choice for smooth mildness and for pleasing flavor. It's what every fighting man deserves... that extra measure of Camel's smoking pleasure.

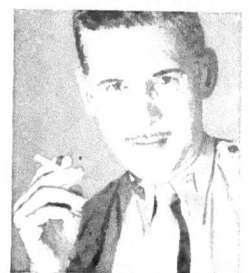

1st in the Service

*With men in the Army, Navy, Marine Corps, and Coast Guard, the favorite cigarette is Camel. (Based on actual sales records.)

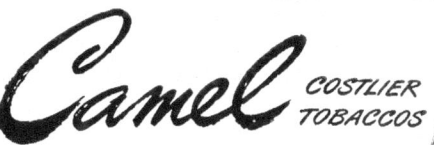

COSTLIER TOBACCOS

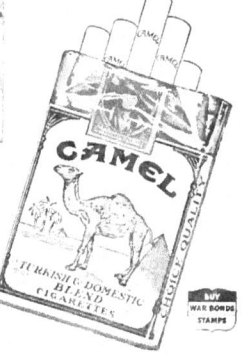

New reprint available on *cigarette research*—Archives of Otolaryngology, March, 1943, pp. 404-410. Camel Cigarettes, Medical Relations Division, One Pershing Square, New York 17, N. Y.

Follow-up examinations and reports are encouraged in all cases. The dealing with acute surgical infections of moderate and slight severity and with acute hand infections is especially good. The importance of reducing to a minimum the amount of pain induced or inflicted is emphasized. Occasional wounds of all degrees of severity are regarded as worthy of careful consideration as to diagnosis and treatment. The chapters on fractures, dislocations and sprains will be found to meet the needs of the general practitioner remarkably well. The same may be said of the chapters on gynecology and the genito-urinary system.

The final chapter is entitled War and Catastrophe Surgery. In this chapter are condensed the best practices of today with all of the improvements that have been learned from the tremendous experiences in the various armed forces engaged in this present war. The importance of first-aid treatment and care in transportation of the injured is emphasized. Wounds of all the different parts involved by every kind of missile including gases are described and appropriate management detailed.

No better text covering the whole field of general surgery has come from the press in recent years.

SMALL COMMUNITY HOSPITALS, by HENRY J. SOUTHMAYD, Director, Division of Rural Hospitals, The Commonwealth Fund; and GEDDES SMITH, Associate, The Commonwealth Fund. *The Commonwealth Fund*, 41 East 57th Street, New York, N. Y. $2.00.

The introduction presents the needs for small-town hospitals and the general plan on which the Commonwealth Fund has proceeded in promoting them.

Subjects discussed are: The Rural Hospital as a Community Institution; The Rural Hospital and the Medical Team; Organization and Administration; Hospital Finances; The Hospital Plant; The Hospital and the Countryside.

An appendix carries suggested rules and regulations, constitution and by-laws, and summary report of medical activities.

INTRACRANIAL ARTERIAL ANEURYSMS, by WALTER E. DANDY, Adjunct Professor of Surgery in The Johns Hopkins University. *Comstock Publishing Company, Inc.*, 124 Roberts Place, Ithaca, New York. 1944. $2.50.

It is news, and welcome news indeed, that intracranial arterial aneurysms are now diagnosable and curable, and that the surgical treatment has a surprisingly low mortality. The book presents a group of 20 cures, truly a record of a triumph for surgery.

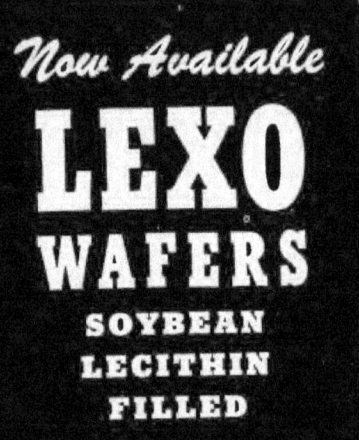

SYNOPSIS OF NEUROPSYCHIATRY, by LOWELL S. SELLING, Sc.M., M.D., Ph.D., Dr.P.H., Director, Psychopathic Clinic, Recorder's Court, Detroit, Michigan; Associate Attending Neuropsychiatrist, Eloise Hospital. *The C. V. Mosby Company,* 3523 Pine Boulevard, St. Louis, 1944. $5.00.

Despite the number of his titles, the author is no despiser of compends. He realizes the value of condensed knowledge, for the student and the practitioner, of "a summary whereby he can see, almost at a glance, the choices in diagnosis and their cardinal signs."

In Part I, devoted to neurology, as a study of each structure is taken up, the anatomy and physiology are given in sufficient detail; then symptoms, diagnosis and treatment of the various disease conditions of the part.

Part II considers mental disorders under these headings: Basic Principle; The General Etiology of Mental Disease; Symptomatology; Psychiatric Syndromes; Immediate Effects, Residuals, and Sequelae of Postnatal Brain Trauma; Neurosyphilis; Alcoholism; Drug Addiction; The Psychoses; The Psychoneuroses; Malingering; Psychopathic Personality; Behavior Disorders of Childhood (Orthopsychiatry); Mental Deficiency.

This synopsis is not intended as a substitute for more elaborate texts, but as a means of presenting the salient features of nervous and mental disorders, their diagnosis and treatment, in the fewest and plainest possible words.

No doctor in general practice could spend the price of this book to better advantage than in its purchase.

SYNOPSIS OF DISEASES OF THE HEART AND ARTERIES, by GEORGE R. HERRMAN, M.S., M.D., Ph.D., F.A.C.P., Professor of Medicine, University of Texas, Director of the Cardiovascular Service, John Sealy Hospital; 3d edition with 103 text illustrations and four color plates. *The C. V. Mosby Company,* 3523 Pine Boulevard, St. Louis, 1944. $5.00.

This book has proved so popular as to necessitate a third edition within a few years. As was the case with the previous editions, the coverage of disease conditions of the heart and arteries is complete as to essentials, and four new chapters have been added covering Nervous Disorders with Cardiac Manifestations, Blood Pressure Abnormalities, Essential Hypertension, and General Systemic Types of Heart Disease. There is an appendix dealing with the new data derived from unipolar central terminal precordial leads.

The whole is a reliable guide to diagnosis and treatment in this important class of diseases.

INDUSTRIAL OPHTHALMOLOGY, by HEDWIG S. KUHN, M.D., with 114 text illustrations including two color plates. *The C. V. Mosby Company,* 3523 Pine Boulevard, St. Louis. 1944. $6.50.

ASAC

15%, by volume Alcohol

Each fl. oz. contains:

Sodium Salicylate, U. S. P. Powder..........40 grains
Sodium Bromide, U. S. P. Granular..........20 grains
Caffeine, U. S. P...........................4 grains

ANALGESIC, ANTIPYRETIC
AND SEDATIVE.

Average Dosage

Two to four teaspoonfuls in one to three ounces of water as prescribed by the physician

How Supplied

In Pints, Five Pints and Gallons to Physicians and Druggists

•

Burwell & Dunn Company

Manufacturing   *Pharmacists*
Established   *in 1887*

CHARLOTTE, N. C.

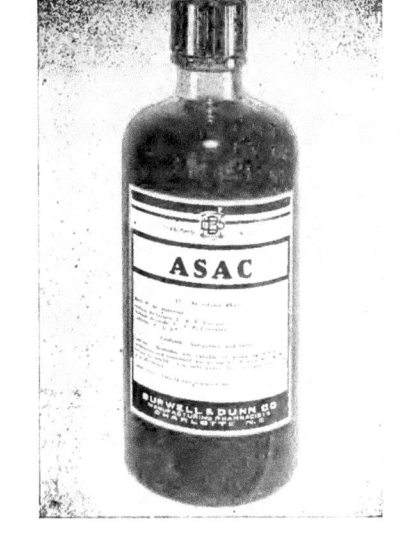

The rapid increase in the number of those employed in industry in the past few years has added tremendously to the importance of this subject. Industrial ophthalmology has features of importance in addition to those covered by ophthalmology in general. It instructs in the screening out of defects in vision and the testing and correcting of these defects, and requires knowledge of proper illumination and ventilation and means of preventing accidents to eyes and limbs and any deterioration of vision from any cause. This book coördinates essential information on the subject, much of it of recent acquisition, which is essential for the rendering of best service by ophthalmologists in this field.

ESSENTIALS OF NUTRITION, by HENRY C. SHERMAN and CAROLINE SHERMAN LANFORD, Columbia University. Second edition. *The Macmillan Company*, 60 Fifth Avenue, New York 11, N. Y. 1943. $3.50.

Although the lay publications do not carry as much information and misinformation on nutrition as they did several years ago, the amount currently carried is tremendous. This circumstance along with the inherent importance of the subject, makes needful a reliable book on the subject. Such a book is this. It is well-balanced; there is not too much emphasis on any item of food; it does not regard any vitamin as endowed with magic; it does not neglect the importance of the food elements that we have recognized over many years.

FEMALE ENDOCRINOLOGY, by JACOB HOFFMAN, A.B., M.D., Demonstrator in Gynecology, Jefferson Medical College; Pathologist in Gynecology, Jefferson Hospital; Formerly Research Fellow in Endocrinology and Director of the Endocrine Clinic, Gynecological Department, Jefferson Hospital, Philadelphia. 788 pages with 180 illustrations, including some in colors. *W. B. Saunders Company*, Philadelphia and London. 1944. $10.00.

It is said that a fourth to a third of ailing women are afflicted with some malfunctioning of the endocrine glands and that many of them require the exercise of profound knowledge of the physiology and pathology of these glands, that they may be cured. The fraction of men and children so afflicted is large.

The foreword tells us of the wonderful training and practice in specialized pathology, so well calculated to prepare a doctor for practice and teaching in this well-nigh boundless field.

Part I concerns itself with the physiology of the different endocrine glands and important physiologic processes as influenced by the secretions of these glands.

Part II, under the general head "Clinic," treats of adolescence, abnormal menstruation, sterility, abortion, abnormal gestation, obesity, and endocrinopathies proper.

In Part III are discussed diagnostic aids, sex hormone findings in blood and urine, and the different classes of hormonal preparations. The chapter on this last-named subject is a reliable source of information greatly needed for appraisal of confusing and conflicting claims.

FUNCTIONAL DISORDERS OF THE FOOT: Their Diagnosis and Treatment, by FRANK D. DICKSON, M.D., F.A.C.S., Associate Professor of Clinical Surgery, Medical School, University of Kansas; Orthopedic Surgeon, St. Luke's, Kansas City General and Wheatley Hospitals; and REX L. DIVELEY, A.B., M.D., F.A.C.S., Colonel, Medical Corps, Army of the United States; Orthopedic Consultant, European Theater of Operations; Orthopedic Surgeon, St. Luke's, Kansas City General, Research and Wheatley Hospitals. Second edition. 202 illustrations. *J. B. Lippincott Co.*, E. Washington Square, Philadelphia, London, Montreal, 1944. $5.00.

Recent experience, the authors say, has not brought to light any evidence requiring changes in their point of view regarding the fundamental causes of foot imbalance, the mechanisms by which foot disorders which cause the symptoms to arise, or the effectiveness of measures advised in the previous editions. Among the additions to be found in this edition are two operations for the correction of flat foot, one for hallux varus, and some two or three for the correction of deformities of the toes. There is a new chapter on Functional Disorders of the Foot in Relation to Military Service, and a second on Foot Disorders in Relation to Industry. The chapter on Constitutional Diseases Affecting the Foot has been entirely rewritten.

This valuable book overstresses neither non-operative nor operative treatment but advises one or the other after a very judicious manner.

SAFE CONVOY: The Expectant Mother's Handbook, by WILLIAM J. CARRINGTON, A.B., M.D., F.A.C.S., Attending Gynecologist, Atlantic City Hospital, etc. *J. B. Lippincott Company*, E. Washington Square, Philadelphia, 1944. $2.50.

This is one of the better books in this field as to subject matter and methods of presentation. It is surprising as well as pleasing to see among the reasons for natural feeding of infants this statement: "Breast feeding offers the best insurance against mammary cancer. Malignant lesions occur three times as frequently in breasts that never have been nursed." This reviewer would like to see that sentence in large letters on a placard in every delivery room and in every room in a hospital occupied by an obstetrical patient.

THE 1943 YEAR BOOK OF GENERAL THERAPEUTICS, edited by OSCAR W. BETHEA, Ph.M., M.D., F.A.C.P., Professor of Clinical Medicine, Tulane University School of Medicine (retired); Member of the Revision Committee of the U. S. Pharmacopoeia, 1930-1940. *Yearbook Publishers*, 304 S. Dearborn St., Chicago, $3.00.

Each of these yearbooks searches out and records significant developments in some special field in each year. The year just past was so fruitful in advances in treatment that the editor of the volume on therapeutics had a full harvest ready to his hand—and he reaped discriminatingly.

RECEIVED

MEDICAL CARE OF THE DISCHARGED HOSPITAL PATIENT, by FRODE JENSEN, M.D., Instructor in Medicine, Syracuse University College of Medicine; H. G. WEISKOTTEN, M.D., Dean and Professor of Pathology, Syracuse University College of Medicine; and MARGARET A. THOMAS, M.A. (Oxon). *The Commonwealth Fund*, 41 East 57 Street, New York 22, N. Y. 1944. $1.00.

TROPICAL NURSING: A Handbook for Nurses and Others Going Abroad, by A. L. GREGG, M.A., M.D., M.Ch., B.A.O. (Dublin), D.T.M. & H. (Lond.), Member of Associate Staff of, and Lecturer to Nurses at the Hospital for Tropical Diseases, London; Lecturer on Tropical Diseases, Westminster Hospital Medical School. Second edition. *Philosophical Library, Inc.*, 15 East 40th Street, New York, N. Y. 1944. $3.00.

STUDIES FROM THE SCHOOL OF MEDICINE, George Washington University, for 1942 to 1943.

THERAPEUTICS

J. F. NASH, M.D., *Editor*, Saint Pauls, N. C.

PSYCHIATRIC TREATMENT METHODS

FAMILY DOCTORS have much difficulty in understanding what psychiatrists in general say as to how patients should be treated. An article[1] just come to my view, I know will be helpful to me, so the gist is herewith passed on.

In addition to being a science, treatment is an art; the two are inseparable. Psychiatric treatment is applicable in some degree by every physician to every type of illness. The physician should view all phases of the patient's existence with the same objective scrutiny—his gastrointestinal life, his love life, his economic problems and his family history and avoid a condescending attitude in which he minimizes the patient's complaints or admonishes him with platitudes.

The patient's avoidance of some subject, his sensitivity about others should be cues in conducting the examination. The patient's response to the physical examination, particularly of the breasts, the genito-urinary system and the rectum, may be of significant diagnostic aid. The physician's approach to examination of heart and blood pressure may be alarming or reassuring.

Suggestion is the most widely used form of psychotherapy. In some instances it is desirable to outline the hours for taking exercise, the type of diet, the amount of rest, the time of arising and going to bed, the amount of application to work, the home situation, taking a vacation.

Substitution is widely used in the treatment of mental illness and is equally applicable to many types of general illness. Occupational and recreational therapy offer opportunities for the patient to find new forms of satisfaction. The physician's prescription to play golf, to bowl or to take in certain forms of social affairs may often be in order. Many patients can profit from some type of educational therapy, invest some of himself in some kind of study such as typing, art, sports ,or types of reading through which the patient can learn a great deal more about himself. Religion may be a substitution therapy.

In psychiatric practice the most widely used is "expressive" psychotherapy. Its most common form is a detailed taking of the history and a discussion with the patient of his history. The fact that the patient gets to tell his tory, that he has a sympathetic listener and that he seems to feel that he is undersood often produces remarkable results in the alleviation of his difficulties. This may require many hours, even many weeks, with the physician listening, occasionally making comments or suggestions or expressing an opinion.

Sedatives are utilized to combat acute excitement and to relieve minor anxieties and insomnia. In the latter situation they are used as a temporary crutch and such an understanding should exist with the patient. Bromide-containing sedatives should never be prescribed for more than a short period of time unless the blood bromide test is frequently made. For mild sedation, small doses of chloral and phenobarbital are best, one barbiturate may work when another fails. Occasionally barbiturates produce excitement and in this case and in post-alcoholic intoxication states paraldehyde is the most practical drug. In neurasthenia syndromes and in disturbances of the peripheral nerves the vitamin B-complex is indicated. Certain pellagra symptoms respond quickly to nicotinic acid medication. Paralysis agitans in some instances responds to pyridoxine. In some instances the female hormone is beneficial in involution states.

In addition to the use of fever in paretic neurosyphilis, the continuous-flow immersion tub, the sitz bath and the wet cold sheet pack are frequently employed for sedative purposes.

Unsung

The dining-car attendant serving the grizzled veteran couldn't conceal his admiration for the several campaign ribbons displayed on the latter's chest. One in particular caught his eye.

"Say, boss," he finally inquired, "what fob is that ribbon?"

"Oh, I got that for gunnery."

"Gee, that's funny," said the puzzled attendant. "I had it twicit and didn't get a damn thing for it!"—*War Doc.*

---

[1]. W. C. Menninger, Topeka, in *Jl. Kansas Med. Soc.*, Nov., 1943.

GENERAL

Nalle Clinic Building   412 North Church Street, Charlotte

THE NALLE CLINIC
Telephone—C-BVDN (*if no answer, call* 3-2621)

General Surgery	*General Medicine*
BRODIE C. NALLE, M.D.	LUCIUS G. GAGE, M.D.
Gynecology & Obstetrics	Diagnosis
EDWARD R. HIPP, M.D.	
Traumatic Surgery	LUTHER W. KELLY, M.D.
*PRESTON NOWLIN, M.D.	Cardio-Respiratory Diseases
Urology	
	J. R. ADAMS, M.D.
Consulting Staff	Diseases of Infants & Children
R. H. LAFFERTY, M.D.	
O. D. BAXTER, M.D.	W. B. MAYER, M.D.
Radiology	Dermatology & Syphilology
W. M. SUMMERVILLE, M.D.	
Pathology	(*In Country's Service)

C—H—M MEDICAL OFFICES
DIAGNOSIS—SURGERY
X-RAY—RADIUM

Dr. G. Carlyle Cooke—*Abdominal Surgery & Gynecology*
Dr. Geo. W. Holmes—*Orthopedics*
Dr. C. H. McCants—*General Surgery*
222-226 Nissen Bldg.   Winston-Salem

WADE CLINIC
Wade Building
Hot Springs National Park, Arkansas

H. King Wade, M.D.	*Urology*
Ernest M. McKenzie, M.D.	*Medicine*
*Frank M. Adams, M.D.	*Medicine*
*Jack Ellis, M.D.	*Medicine*
Bessey H. Shebesta, M.D.	*Medicine*
*Wm. C. Hays, M.D.	*Medicine*
N. B. Burch, M.D.	*Eye, Ear, Nose and Throat*
A. W. Scheer	*X-ray Technician*
Etta Wade	*Clinical Laboratory*
Merna Spring	*Clinical Pathology*

(*In Military Service)

INTERNAL MEDICINE

ARCHIE A. BARRON, M.D., F.A.C.P.	JOHN DONNELLY, M.D.
INTERNAL MEDICINE—NEUROLOGY	*DISEASES OF THE LUNGS*
Professional Bldg. Charlotte	Medical Building Charlotte
CLYDE M. GILMORE, A.B., M.D.	JAMES M. NORTHINGTON, M.D.
CARDIOLOGY—INTERNAL MEDICINE	*INTERNAL MEDICINE—GERIATRICS*
Dixie Building Greensboro	Medical Building Charlotte

NEUROLOGY and PSYCHIATRY

(*Now in the Country's Service*)
*J. FRED MERRITT, M.D.
NERVOUS and MILD MENTAL DISEASES
ALCOHOL and DRUG ADDICTIONS
Glenwood Park Sanitarium   Greensboro

TOM A. WILLIAMS, M.D.
(*Neurologist of Washington, D. C.*)
Consultation by appointment at
Phone 3994-W
77 Kenilworth Ave.   Asheville, N. C.

EYE, EAR, NOSE AND THROAT

H. C. NEBLETT, M.D.
OCULIST
Phone 3-5852
Professional Bldg.   Charlotte

AMZI J. ELLINGTON, M.D.
DISEASES of the
EYE, EAR, NOSE and THROAT
Phones: Office 992—Residence 761
Burlington   North Carolina

UROLOGY, DERMATOLOGY and PROCTOLOGY

THE CROWELL CLINIC of UROLOGY and UROLOGICAL SURGERY
Hours—Nine to Five   Telephones—3-7101—3-7102
STAFF
ANDREW J. CROWELL, M.D.
(1911-1938)
*ANGUS M. MCDONALD, M.D.   CLAUDE B. SQUIRES, M.D.
Suite 700-711 Professional Building   Charlotte

RAYMOND THOMPSON, M.D., F.A.C.S.   WALTER E. DANIEL, A.B., M.D.
THE THOMPSON-DANIEL CLINIC
of
UROLOGY & UROLOGICAL SURGERY
Fifth Floor Professional Bldg.   Charlotte

C. C. MASSEY, M.D.
PRACTICE LIMITED
TO
DISEASES OF THE RECTUM
Professional Bldg.   Charlotte

WYETT F. SIMPSON, M.D.
GENITO-URINARY DISEASES
Phone 1234
Hot Springs National Park   Arkansas

ORTHOPEDICS

HERBERT F. MUNT, M.D.
ACCIDENT SURGERY & ORTHOPEDICS
FRACTURES
Nissen Building   Winston-Salem

SURGERY

R. S. ANDERSON, M.D.

GENERAL SURGERY

144 Coast Line Street   Rocky Mount

R. B. DAVIS, M. D., M. M. S., F. A. C. P.
*GENERAL SURGERY
AND
RADIUM THERAPY*
Hours by Appointment
Piedmont-Memorial Hosp.   Greensboro

(*Now in the Country's Service*)
WILLIAM FRANCIS MARTIN, M.D.
GENERAL SURGERY
Professional Bldg.   Charlotte

OBSTETRICS & GYNECOLOGY

IVAN M. PROCTER, M. D.

OBSTETRICS & GYNECOLOGY

133 Fayetteville Street   Raleigh

SPECIAL NOTICES

TWO LABORATORY TECHNICIANS, being graduated from a High-class Hospital Laboratory, services available January 1st, 1944. Address TECHNICIAN, care *Southern Medicine & Surgery.*

TO THE BUSY DOCTOR WHO WANTS TO PASS HIS EXPERIENCE ON TO OTHERS

You have probably been postponing writing that original contribution. You can do it, and save your time and effort by employing an expert literary assistant to prepare the address, article or book under your direction or relieve you of the details of looking up references, translating, indexing, typing, and the complete preparation of your manuscript.

Address: *WRITING AIDE*, care *Southern Medicine & Surgery.*

THE JOURNAL OF
SOUTHERN MEDICINE AND SURGERY

306 NORTH TRYON STREET, CHARLOTTE, N. C.

The Journal assumes no responsibility for the authenticity of opinion or statements made by authors or in communications submitted to this Journal for publication.

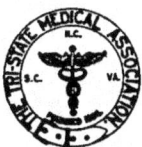

JAMES M. NORTHINGTON, M.D., Editor

VOL. CVI   JUNE, 1944   No. 6

Hold the Line*

EDWARD J. WILLIAMS, M.D., Monroe, North Carolina

THROUGHOUT the recent years the team that believes in Government, of the people, by the people and for the people, has been gradually but steadily pushed back towards their goal line. Our well-wishers stand with mouths open but silent at the thought of what seems to be our inevitable fate. Only we ourselves can try to encourage each other.

There was once a Democratic party and we were glad to feel that we were a part of its rank and file; but we have taken the name for granted and its officers, as it guardians, have allowed Gangsterism to usurp the place of Democracy. Our friends are fearful to encourage us now. We are on our own. Many who are at heart for Democratic Government fear for their livings to raise voice or hand.

It is written that some 2,000 years ago a patriotic Roman exclaimed against the abuser of power of his time: "He doth bestride this narrow world like a Colossus, while we puny men dodge about between his mighty legs to find ourselves dishonorable graves." To use the figure now might be a strain literally, under the petticoat government of Madam President Roosevelt and Madam Secretary Perkins; but in essentials the two times are the same. We are arrayed against a team that delights in grandstand plays. The applause from the bleachers is as sweet in their ears as was that of the Roman rabble when given free bread and circuses in the ears of the tyrant of that age hurrying his country to its destruction.

We are defending against a team that attacks according to no recognized rules. Their coaches are Brain Trusters with fancy ideas and little common sense. We know that their plays are not based on sound principles, but they hope by clamor to upset us so that we will be slow to diagnose and defeat the play.

The first down was made right through our lines when we were accused of being a trust, and thus discredited before our friends. We have made possible longer life, and more ease and comfort when Death finally approaches and will not be turned back. So buck up, brothers, you may still have something to fight with and for. We have done nothing in restraint of trade or competition. Our profession is strictly for the benefit of all the people. Our rules and regulations are for the best interest of certain public-service institutions that cannot be self-supporting unless protected by these rules.

The attacks on us doctors have their origin in the twisted, warped and lopsided dreams of the Brain Trust and certain members of the congress with alien ideas. If they can build hospitals and run them according to such ideas, we will not in any way try to stop them. But it is iniquitous to tax all the people for the especial benefit of the few.

The sick are being cared for, both pay and charity, far better than would be provided by any scheme that they have devised, and a vast amount of that is "charity" simply because the recipients do not want to pay. Thousands, less able to pay, are making their way in life and asking no favors from any one. Many spend their money for pic-

*Presented to Tri-State Medical Association of the Carolinas and Virginia, meeting at Charlotte, Feb. 28th-29th, 1944.

ture shows, liquor and other luxuries, and never pay medical bills. At the wedding feast our Lord didn't tell the foolish virgins to come on in and share equally with the provident. They suffered the consequences of their idleness and folly. On our part we doctors are far exceeding that standard to the indigent.

The coaching team of Brain Stormers is made up of men imbued with weird ideas of economics, based on some such concept as "Evil is the Good we do not understand." In trying out their schemes these hare-brained visionaries risk nothing. They have nothing but an overweening ambition to make over the world and to impose their wills on every man, woman and child of us, and tax us to provide a quart of milk a day for every Hottentot and Bushman; and none of them has figured who's going to make them drink it. The Administration has petted and humored and bowed down to Labor Unions until now these unions hold all the law in contempt, and defy those elected to enforce the laws and those elected to make the laws. We, the public, have to suffer, while they are cajoled, pampered and yielded to. We are told to line up where the line was before the unions advanced.

They set price ceilings on certain items and leave the others to go sky-high. If there was to be price control why wasn't every article pegged at that price as of a certain date? Their Big Brains pay civilians outlandish prices to work in the camps, and so entice that labor away from the farmer that had not already been taken by the Armed Forces, then stop the sale and manufacture of farm equipment which would have made it possible for the farmer to carry on with the small force left. Food will win the war, we are told, but they could not see the need for continuing the supply of farm machinery for the production of food. Not an ounce of horse sense in the outfit. Yet they are calling for more and more tax money to waste in other fantastic schemes and newly-created offices to feed their vainglory. I am backing the war effort to the best of my ability; but it is in spite of, not on account of, the way our domestic affairs are being managed.

The labor unions are given the sanction and support of the government to use gangsteristic methods to get what they want. The rest of us must resort to legal and peaceful methods to obtain what we get. *Just why are the unions exempted?* You know and I know, that it is because of the present gang wishing to stay in office for life and get paid for such wild scheming at the public's expense and to do this they must have an ever and ever larger number with their snouts in the public trough, with power to force this upon us. Did you notice how quickly the unions started to clamor against "inflation" when the farmers wanted their raise to offset the increase in cost of farm labor and everything else he has to buy?

It would be very interesting to know just how many men have been appointed to fill a ten-thousand-dollar job who were never able to make a fourth of that amount in private life. And when he was not able to measure up to the very low requirements, why wasn't he dismissed? His political influence was wanted to help the Gang stay in power, and it cost the Gang nothing to use him in this way. Keep him on the payroll so he won't squeal and so the Gang will not lose the votes he can influence. How many able-bodied men of draft age are being kept in Washington in some so-called important position while your boys and mine hazard their lives in battle and we on the home front—except the pets of privilege—are restricted to the bare necessities? There are plenty of women who could competently fill the places of the pets of the administration. And now we are told that a great many of these men indispensable in their Washington jobs are too psychopathic to be put in the Army or Navy! Well, there's plenty of evidence that if a sane man were to get into high office in Washington, he'd have a mighty lonesome time of it, and have a good chance of being driven insane by daily contact with the Gang.

The other day I heard a man blowing off to a group of self-important women about the accomplishments of one Kaiser that made a little name building ships. His scheme was marvelous. He had hospitals built and employed doctors and his men got the best of every care, free. The cost was seven cents per day taken out of every pay envelope. No one was treated except workers. Let's take a man with seven children, an average family here, making a total of nine in the family. That man would have to contribute $229.95 per year and no family will come anywhere near having to pay that much for regular service in any year. And, be it remembered, these employees of this man Kaiser are young men in the prime of life, a group selected because of exceptional physical fitness, and who will have not more than one-fourth the need of medical and hospital care as will the population at large. Doctors cannot be put along an assembly line and each one cure the ills that fall in his specialty as the patient passes. When the war is over and our outlandish prices cease and most of us are pushed to make a bare living, how will it work? Labor will still strike for higher wages and more shortening of hours thus running the price of any article so high that there will be few sales and less demand for workers. God help us if labor unions are not outlawed by that time and a better way found for giving a man what he justly deserves.

A dramatic, egotistical grandstand player picked

out these Brain Trusters. He loves to show his authority. He depends on his grandstand playing to keep him in a position to carry on. Yes indeed he has done things "different," but what he has done has not by any means always been the thing that should have been done.

We, in America, until the present administration, had found better ways of doing things than any other country, in a legal way, all of us more or less equal before the law. Now the majesty of the law, as well as the law of justice and right, is flouted by labor unions, and the Administration at Washington makes no serious attempt to carry out its oath to uphold the law. If Lewis could get control of all the unions, as he has been trying to do, he could count on enough help to place himself in the highest office in the land and from there take over for all time. Lewis differs from William Greene and Philip Murray only in having more audacity. In greed and power-seeking they are as alike as peas in a pod. If all others must settle our differences under the law why can't the labor union's differences be so settled? The rest of us must present our cases before a judge and jury and abide by the verdict. "Labor" under the leadership of officers not accountable to either the laborers or the Government for what they take in, makes its demands, then quits work on ships, guns, airplanes, rail-roads, munitions, and coal mining, thereby prolonging the war and directly causing additional thousands to lose their lives. We were accused of breaking the law when our organization is solely for preventing sickness and improving the care of those who are sick. That is what we study and discuss in our meetings rather than formulating demands for higher pay and shorter hours, while our soldiers die for lack of munitions of war.

Why can't any man work without having to become a member of some union? Laws passed, even when we are at war, prevent a man from working without a union card. That lacks something of being democratic.

When our forefathers formed the constitution their idea of a unit of government was the individual. The idea has proven its worth in that our country has grown strong financially, socially and industrially. No structure can stand with any other unit for a basis of construction. If we are to preserve the remnants of our Democracy we must fight a life-or-death fight against the policies of the present administration: viz., ignore the rights of all others and give bountifully to their political and industrial pets.

Some States don't allow those who pay nothing to the financial support of the state to vote on anything that has to do with its running. But the Gang say that is wrong. They see lots of votes there to be had by stepping in and telling the State who shall vote. Disregarding States' Rights, the congress passed laws allowing labor unions to impose their will in every State. Those States opposed to union domination were forced to yield to the power-taking gang. Rights of States to govern their inside affairs as seems best to all those who live in their boundaries are being usurped at a rate that Thad Stevens would not have dared. Soon a Governor of a State will not have as much authority as a Federal deputy marshal.

Hitler has convinced his people that he and they are supermen. Those running this government claim this rank for themselves alone. No other person has had the audacity to push himself forward in defiance of the time-honored precedent of not running for the presidency for more than two terms. Was there none other in all this vast country able to fill the office? Just think what a fix this country would have been in if that one person had died. We have ears that hear only that which we want to hear; eyes that see only what we want to see. If it is pleasing to the ear or the eye we are for it regardless of what Reason tells us the end effect will be. I have heard of an employer of many men, who early adopted a rule. "When I find out one of my men thinks I can't get along without him, I discharge him to show him and all the others that I can." Let us do likewise.

Our way is to take the patient's history, examine him and make the diagnosis and then, watching his progress, to advise such changes in treatment as are sound and logical, as will return him to normal health and vigor.

We have here, as you can see, a very ill patient who is growing worse rapidly. It is evident that unless something curative is done our patient will die. A terrific internal strife is going on. Each organ seems to be at outs with every other. Fever is running high.

Twelve years ago when the Head sanctioned groups organizing for compelling compliance with their wishes, there was begun a disease condition that will destroy the entire organism unless stopped soon. There must be great fermentation going on to supply so much gas and distention. Normal bowel passages have been greatly slowed. Witness the strikes.

Labor has, with the encouragement and applause of the Government at Washington, contemptuously violated the laws of right and the laws of the land; and ordered the congress to make certain laws and to defeat others—and had their orders obeyed. The crux of the matter is we are short on statesmanship, short on intelligent and honest leaders that are interested in all of us instead of certain groups. None of this labor trouble would have occurred if those we entrusted with power in making laws for the protection of labor had seen to it that each and every laborer had laws by which he as an individual could obtain justice, instead of having to resort to group force. The unions should have been required to account for receipts and disbursements, just as are all other corporations. When they make a contract they should be compelled by law to live up to it, or to pay to the other contracting party the full amount of loss from breach of such contract. Unions should be compelled to pay for all damage done to property of employers by their members, and the individuals guilty prosecuted for malicious mischief. No man willing and able to work should be forced to pay into labor unions' coffers initiation fees and dues, or denied the right to work wherever and whenever he pleases for the support of his family and his country.

I am not interested in political parties as such. I am deeply interested in saving the ideals of government upon which our country was founded, and up until now, has flourished. It is now an old structure with broad foundations and an architecture that cannot stand radical changing. Our President was careful that our airmen should not destroy the ancient structures of Italy. He has shown great determination in destroying our fundamental governmental structures. So if our beloved Democracy is to be saved it is up to you and me to fight, until its damaged places have been restored, and see to it that it shall never again be tampered with.

It seems that we have lost the spirit of our ancestors. They were tired of the lands of force and privilege. They came where they hoped to live in peace with each other, and have their differences settled under laws knowing no favoritism. They felt the need of each other and gladly would join in standing against odds, that all might thrive and be happy.

I have spoken freely on some of the abuses that affect all the people, us doctors along with them. There are other abuses already realized of doctors as a class, and others threatening which would destroy us.

Poor old Socrates said in the trial which cost him his life that he was at a great disadvantage, because in defending himself he had to speak well of himself "which is hateful to all men."

So I will let non-doctors speak for us.

You all know that the gentle, wise and truthful Robert Louis Stevenson said:

"There are men and classes of men that stand above the common herd: the soldier, the sailor, and the shepherd not infrequently; the artist rarely; rarelier still, the clergyman; the physician almost as a rule. He is the flower (such as it is) of our civilization." Stevenson was an invalid throughout most of his brief span of 44 years and spoke from a full knowledge of experience of many physicians in many lands.

Now hear what a good priest said three months ago for us doctors of today:

"I am an honest man—I hope—but I would not like the responsibility for over 110 million people and 48 billion dollars a year. It would not be fair to any physician who might be appointed as Surgeon General either. I trust more in many average, intelligent and honest men in an honorable profession. I prefer to confine the superman to the funnies. In real life he would be a menace, like Hitler, or any other dictator.

"Better and better medical care has continuously and more widely been distributed, and made more generally available. Many of the formerly fatal diseases have been conquered; and most of the more dangerous and dealy of the other diseases have been or are being brought under control—all under the system by which all our scientific victories have been won.

"Let us keep medicine unshackled, as free as religion, the press and honest speech. Let us preserve the personal relationship between doctor and patient which now contributes so largely towards recovery and healing.

"Allow me to inject a personal note. I was desperately hurt 200 miles from Atlanta and taken to a small hospital near the scene of the accident and given splendid service. WSB put the story on the air within minutes, and my personal physician in Atlanta obtained the best brain specialist available and they immediately drove the 200 miles to make sure that everything needful was done for me.

"Money, fees, schedules cannot buy such service as that; nor could any system of security administration guarantee such kindness and personal consideration. But it wasn't Social Security, you see. It was the physician's Oath and Creed put into practice, for medicine serves with the heart as well as with skill. Leave It Free To Do So."

From such kind expressions we should take heart and line up on the line where men can get their rights as individuals and not have to resort to group force; where every individual shall have the right to work wherever and whenever he pleases without having to pay a royalty for protection; where men can choose the hospital to which they will go for care; and where they can have their own family doctor without any dictatorial strings attached.

Line up there and hold that line.

Discussion

Dr. G. R. Wilkinson, Greenville, S. C.: We have a visitor here from New York State, Dr. H. B. Johnson. It was suggested that I ask him to say a word or two. Dr. Johnson raised George Thorne, who is now a new Professor of Medicine at Harvard.

(To Page 219)

The Local Treatment of Surface Burns*

WILLIAM H. PRIOLEAU, M.D., Charleston
Assistant Professor of Surgery, Medical College of the State of South Carolina

IN DISCUSSING the local treatment of surface burns, it must be borne in mind that the local and systemic conditions are closely related and dependent upon each other. Accordingly, the treatment of one cannot be considered except as in relation to the other. Treatment instituted cannot be by rule of thumb, but must be based upon well established principles. Thus it will vary with conditions present, and to some extent will depend upon facilities at hand. While this discussion deals primarily with the local treatment of burns, the systemic treatment will have to be considered to some extent. These remarks have reference to cases seen soon after injury. The late treatment of burns involves other factors.

The importance of instituting treatment early cannot be over-emphasized from the standpoint of preventing shock, and infection of the burned surfaces. While the systemic treatment should be given prior consideration, the local treatment should be started as soon as possible, and the two administered concurrently. Pain is a prominent feature, and is best relieved by morphine, however, overdosage must be guarded against in the presence of shock, and injury to the respiratory passages. The tendency is for shock to develop soon as a result of the loss of serum protein from the blood by exudation into the burned tissues and to the surface. This should be combatted by the immediate administration of plasma as freely as indicated by the severity of the burn, rather than solely by laboratory tests. This is most expeditiously done by starting a saline intravenous infusion immediately, and adding to it the plasma as soon as it can be prepared. At this stage plasma is the fluid of choice, as it more nearly replaces the fluid lost. Later an anemia develops and the transfusion of the whole blood is indicated. Particularly in the early stages care must be taken not to give more saline than is lost, as an excess is not secreted by kidneys functioning poorly on account of shock, but passes out into the tissues causing edema and various functional disturbances. Fluids and nourishment, especially protein, should be given by mouth as freely as tolerated. The patient should not be subjected to excessive heat, as this increases the metabolic processes and is also harmful to the burned surfaces.

The early local treatment should have as its immediate objectives the prevention of infection, the conservation of remaining viable tissue, especially epithelium, and the reduction of exudation. In these several aspects the different methods of local treatment vary in effectiveness, as will be brought out later in the discussion. However, regardless of the method of treatment employed, the local treatment must be carried out under conditions of surgical asepsis, preferably in the operating room. The average busy emergency room is certainly not suitable for it. Contaminants from the respiratory passages are particularly to be avoided—thus the operating team and also the patient should be masked.

Until recently probably the most popular form of local treatment has been the formation of a coagulum over the burned surface by the application of tannic acid alone, or more lately in combination with silver nitrate which causes the coagulum to form within a few minutes. This method has a great deal to recommend it and still has strong advocates. Before applying the tannic acid it is absolutely requisite that the area must be surgically cleansed so as to prevent the danger of infection developing under the coagulum with possibly serious systemic effects and further destruction of epithelium. Inadequate cleansing is probably the commonest cause of unsatisfactory results with this form of treatment. Generally the preparation of the field and the application of the tannic acid and silver nitrate is best done under a general anesthetic, provided the condition of the patient makes this possible. On the other hand in many cases the treatment can be satisfactorily carried out without anesthesia. Tannic acid should not be applied to the fingers due to the danger of interference with the blood supply causing gangrene; also it is unsuitable for the face, particularly the ears and the nose. Once the coagulum has formed the patient is very comfortable and requires a minimum of nursing care. The coagulum prevents further loss of serum to the surface, which in some cases is of utmost importance. Probably the greatest objection to this method of treatment is the fact that it has the tendency to destroy some of any remaining epithelium, making more likely the necessity of grafting. Also there have been re-

*Presented to Tri-State Medical Association of the Carolinas and Virginia, meeting at Charlotte, Feb. 28th-29th, 1944.

ported a few cases of death resulting from liver damage caused by absorption of the tannic acid. In brief, tannic acid therapy is of most value in extensive but mild second degree burns in which the general condition of the patient permits surgical cleansing of the burned surface and proper facilities for such cleansing are present. Thus it is often not applicable in War Surgery. It may be indicated also in extensive burns where only a limited supply of plasma is available.

What has been said of tannic acid therapy applies in principle to other methods of coagulum formation such as with the triple dye.

A method of treatment which has given very good results is the local application of sulfadiazine in triethanol amine in conjunction with the systemic administration of a sulfonamide. With this method preliminary surgical cleansing of the burned area is not considered necessary. On the other hand, the coagulum formation is slow, requiring application of the drug at diminishing intervals for three days. Apparently it has little if any destructive effect upon remaining viable epithelium. As there is a loss of considerable serum to the surface, this form of treatment should not be used unless there is an adequate supply of plasma on hand. When personnel and facilities have permitted its proper use the results have been excellent.

At present the most generally approved method of local treatment is the application of bland ointment pressure dressings. Sheets of closely woven gauze impregnated with vaseline are placed over the burned surface. Flat gauze is then applied and next a bulk of mechanic's waste or gauze fluff. This is held in place by a circular gauze bandage firmly applied. The original dressing is not disturbed for a period of from five to ten days, according to conditions. Such a dressing provides a bland covering, a firm protection and adequate drainage. The pressure greatly reduces serum exudation into the tissues and on the surface. It protects the remaining viable epithelium. The advisability and extent of preliminary surgical cleansing depends upon the general as well as the local condition. In the Cocoa-Nut Grove cases at the Massachusetts General Hospital no preliminary cleansing was carried out and the results were excellent. It is necessary to give plasma freely by vein as a great deal is lost in the early stages. A sulfonamide is given systemically primarily for local effect. It has been found to be present in considerable concentration in the serum obtained from the surface blebs. This method of treatment is simple in execution and is giving very good results, particularly in reducing the amount of grafting necessary.

In all cases, regardless of the method of local treatment used, the areas devoid of epithelium should be grafted as soon as possible, preferably within three weeks. Removal of the slough should be hastened by soaks and if necessary by excision. Early grafting preserves function and reduces scarring and contractures. As yet no medication has been discovered to have the property of accelerating epithelial growth and avoiding the necessity of grafting. Should grafting be delayed for some unavoidable reason, it is often advisable to excise the granulating surface several days prior to the grafting, so that the grafts may be placed on a bed of newly-formed healthy granulations. Pinch grafts have the advantage of being easily obtained and applied under local anesthesia, which is of great importance in a debilitated patient. By their use, the granulating area can be readily covered in stages in a patient too ill for an extensive procedure. Split grafts are preferable from the cosmetic aspect, as well as from not permanently injuring the donor site. A general anesthesia is necessary for their application, especially if extensive. This precludes their use in a debilitated patient. In spite of these disadvantages, the split graft is the type most generally used in civilian practice; this is made possible no doubt by the great improvement in the care of these cases.

As these patients tend to become anemic and undernourished, no doubt in great part due to absorption of the infectious products from the large granulating surface, particular attention should be paid to diet, and to keeping up the blood volume and hemoglobin by administering plasma and whole blood.

The study of the treatment of burns is receiving a great deal of attention due to its importance in War Surgery. With a better understanding of the changes which take place there is every reason to believe that the treatment will be placed upon a still more rational basis.

DIGITALIS IN THE TREATMENT OF WOUNDS
(Karl Schlaepfer, Milwaukee, in *Jl. Int. Col. Surgs.*, Sept.-Oct., 1943)

Treatment with digitalis compresses at first and subsequently with digalen ointment has proved of special value in the treatment of torpid granulating wounds of the leg following extensive lacerating injuries with or without fracture. Even though the fracture heals, the torpid ulcer persists. The compresses saturated with digalen solution resulted in filling-in the wound with healthy granulations in a few days; then the application of 20-per cent digalen ointment hastened epithelization. Burns have been treated in the same way with good results. Digalen ointment has also been used to hasten healing of third-degree burns after removal of the eschar produced by tannic acid or other dressings. Digitalis compresses used in the operative wound immediately after operation are of value in obtaining primary union in some cases, especially in debilitated persons; in such cases hemostasis must be complete and good approximation of the different layers of the wound must have been obtained.

Treatment of Hip Fractures of the Insane*

J. R. SAUNDERS, M.D., Morganton, North Carolina
Medical Superintendent, State Hospital
AND
YATES S. PALMER, M.D., Valdese, North Carolina
Surgeon, Valdese Hospital

DR. SAUNDERS:

THE MANAGEMENT of any fracture in the insane, from the simplest to the most complicated type, is at least 50 per cent more difficult than is the management of the same fracture in a normal individual.

In the great majority of cases there is no cooperation on the part of the patients. They are much more difficult to treat than children, due to the fact that they are much harder to restrain and, too, a person with a diseased mind seems to have an uncanny knack in devising means of removing casts, splints, etc. One of my patients who had a fracture of both bones of the forearm proceeded to wet the very heavy plaster cast with her own urine until it was necessary to remove it. Another favorite pastime is picking at the padding underneath the cast until the cast becomes loose and is worthless. If he or she can but grasp just a small thread frequently an entire cast will be unraveled over night.

Since this discussion is supposed to deal with the treatment of hip fractures in the insane, I will attempt to confine the remainder of my remarks to this topic.

Since May, 1942, 74 fractures of various types have been diagnosed and treated at the State Hospital at Morganton. Of this number, 33—nearly half—were fractures of the hip. In practically all instances, our hip fractures have occurred in patients past 60 years of age. I am sure all of us will agree that the hip is the familiar site of a fracture in the aged in normal as well as insane individuals. In an attempt to determine why we have had such a large number of fractured hips at the State Hospital at Morganton several factors were taken into consideration. It is common knowledge even among the laity that an old person's bones are brittle. I find that of our 33 patients that have sustained fractures of the hip since May, 1942, the average length of time that they had been in the hospital was 5¾ years. It occurs to me that this number of years of inactive life may readily cause structural changes in the bones and muscles and in a way may account for the large number of fractures that we have had. Incidentally, we have had no fractures of the hip among our patients at the farm colonies where they lead a very active outdoor life; but it is to be borne in mind that these patients do not quite fall in the age group as mentioned above. It appears to me, however, that one must conclude that the inactive life certainly must be a contributing factor in these fractures.

I am sure most of you are familiar with the behavior of individuals suffering with a senile psychosis. They are constantly stumbling about both day and night; many of them become very irritable and disagreeable at times, and with our extreme shortage of help at the present it is impossible to prevent them from occasionally pushing and shoving each other about. Since the hospital was fireproofed in 1939 practically all of our floors are concrete or hard tile. You know that if a floor of this description gets the least bit wet it is rather difficult for a normal person to stand on it and, too, a fall on a concrete floor is much different from a fall on a wooden floor.

The treatment of a hip fracture is a major problem in a normal individual, even under the most favorable circumstances. You can hardly conceive what a problem is presented by an insane person with a fracture of the hip.

Over a period of a number of years the treatment at the State Hospital of fractures of the hip has varied a great deal. We have used sandbags, plaster spicas and modified Balkan frame with weights; also the spread or spraddle splint—the injured hip immobilized by a cast on the injured leg and a brace applied to the normal leg after being fastened to the injured leg; and many other forms of treatment that we thought might prove to be practicable. We were willing to try anything, as none of the above methods proved satisfactory.

As the majority of our patients become very untidy in their personal habits soon after they receive an injury of this kind, you can see what difficulties we run into by immobilizing them. Practically all of our patients developed pressure sores sooner or later and a great percentage of them developed hypostatic pneumonia and died. I can recall working diligently half a day applying a cast to these patients, when I knew from experience we had had practically 100 per cent mortality in these cases.

---

*Presented to Tri-State Medical Association of the Carolinas and Virginia, meeting at Charlotte, Feb. 24th-25th, 1944.

The treatment of fractured hips with metal pins, of course, is not a new procedure, but it is a godsend in the treatment of fractured hips in the insane. It facilitates the nursing care and since May, 1943, when hip pinning was begun more or less as a routine procedure for fractured hips at the State Hospital, we have had only one patient that developed a pressure sore and we have had but one case of hypostatic pneumonia in the 12 cases we have pinned to date. Most of them have been up hobbling about by the time the incision healed and up in a rolling chair even before that time. They are much more comfortable and contented, and no one that has ever dealt with a mental case with a fracture of this kind can imagine what a contrast there is between the treatment that I just described and the older types of treatment. Now, not every fracture of the hip can be treated by inserting pins, and we have not used this type of treatment in all of our cases. In two cases that occurred in patients past 80 the hip was so shattered a pin could not be inserted with any prospect of holding. Both of these patients later died with hypostatic pneumonia. There was another whose physical condition, we thought, would not stand such a radical procedure. She lived and is still confined to bed and probably will be confined to bed the rest of her life.

At the State Hospital at Morganton, we rely on our visiting staff for surgical as well as other forms of medical service. With a population that is near 2,700 patients we are constantly calling on our consultant staff for one cause or another, as it is our intention to render to our 2,700 mentally sick patients the best medical care available. In this connection we are especially indebted to Dr. Yates Palmer as well as many others of the consultant staff for the splendid service that they have rendered our patients.

Dr. Palmer:

Dr. Saunders has not exaggerated the difficulties of treating fractures of the insane where any type of immobilization is required. Immobilization being essential for union and decreasing deformity to a minimum, some type of fixation is necessary.

Treating fractures of insane, we must first realize that we have many problems that we do not have with the sane. These people are not responsible or mentally capable of any coöperation; also, I am more and more convinced we have an obnormal osseous system to deal with; that is, the bones of an insane person who has been in an institution for many years will not stand the same amount of stress and strain as will the bones of an active sane person. It is only logical that people being cared for in an institution where they are confined to wards or court yards, and not mentally capable of exercise or work, will develop an advanced senile osteoporosis from the usual atrophy of disuse. This was very forcibly brought out in a paper titled "Fractures in the Insane," by C. H. Bond, M.D., Senior Assistant Medical Officer, London County Asylum, Bexley. This paper was published in 1902. The cortex beneath the periosteum is thin and very brittle and does not tolerate the abuse of normal bone.

The care of fractures constitutes: (1) diagnosis, (2) reduction, (3) maintenance of reduction. First diagnosis is made and classified as neck or inter-trochanteric fracture. Second, the fracture is reduced under low spinal anesthesia, which these patients tolerate exceptionally well, and to date no accident with this method. The insane patient is an excellent subject for spinal anesthesia and an unsatisfactory one for general; the reason would consume too much time here. Third, we are to do our best to maintain reduction and from Dr. Saunders' statement, external skeletal fixation or immobilization by traction, splints or cast of various types proved far from satisfactory; therefore, some type of internal skeletal fixation is the procedure of choice.

Internal fixation of hip fracture by nails, screws and pegs is by no means a new procedure, as the first report of this method of treatment was made by Langenbeck in 1850. Successful results were reported by Nocolaysen and others prior to the development of the röntgen ray. Thomas, in 1921, and E. D. Martin and A. C. King, in 1922, reported excellent results following the use of steel woodscrews for internal fixation. At that time, internal fixation was not uniformly successful, either because of inaccurate reductions or because of lack of dexterity on the part of the surgeons in introducing the material. As a consequence, this method fell into disuse except among a small number of surgeons, who probably were more expert in properly placing the fixation. Smith-Petersen is responsible for reviving and popularizing the procedure and originating a nail for the purpose. We use the Smith-Petersen nail for fixation and now use the trochanteric fracture plate.

Operations for fresh fractures of the neck of the femur may be divided into two types: (1) exposure of the line of fracture, and reduction and internal fixation under direct vision; (2) insertion of the nail, screw, or pin without exposure of line of fracture. The latter is not strictly an open reduction, and is therefore termed "blind nailing" or pinning. This method is preferable to open reduction and insertion of the nail under direct vision in that internal fixation may be accomplished with less shock.

Conclusion: From the follow-up x-ray films, we find that intertrochanteric fractures of these patients in the institution do not hold well, due to

(To Page 216)

DEPARTMENTS

HUMAN BEHAVIOUR

James K. Hall, M.D., *Editor*, Richmond, Va.

FEAR OF DEATH

Dr. Gregory Zilboorg analyzes man's mental and emotional states as the chemist analyzes matter. Dr. Zilboorg believes that human behaviour is understandable as the manifestation of mind in action. He thinks it not impossible to find out what most behaviour may mean, although the search for the meaning may be long-drawn-out and the discovery of the truth may be made difficult, either by the individual's ignorance or lack of coöperation. Behaviour is energy in action, and energy is governed by natural laws.

At the annual meeting in Detroit more than a year ago of the American Psychiatric Association Dr. Zilboorg presented an essay on: Fear of Death. His thesis began with a discussion of that much-talked-about state called morale. The term rolls off many a tongue and it is written by countless pens, but the word morale is seldom defined.

In Dr. Zilboorg's opinion morale has reference to good cheer; to popular optimism; but in it are implied tenacious courage, steadily maintained and cheerfully demonstrated. But in the final analysis morale has to do with a general sense of security in the face of hardship and danger. And morale may not be so much concerned about such a positive quality as courage as about the negative attributes that interfere with successful action—such retarding influences, for example, as discouragement and depression. Morale insists that the aggression be directed against the enemy destructively and not against the individual.

The fundamental feature involved in morale is the fear of death. How the mortal responds to that universal fear is what designates him as a coward or as a hero. Not many individuals are willing to confess that the fear of death is constantly affecting their emotions and unceasingly influencing their conduct. But man lives in persistent fear of death, however unwilling he may be to confess it. So natural is that fear thought to be that it would seem to be almost absurd to speak of the psychology of that paramount fear. Dr. Zilboorg likens it to the law of gravitation, manifesting itself throughout the world of matter. Yet certain laws govern that mighty force, and mathematicians and physicists devote much thought to it.

Every one fears death. The bravest man would not deny it. In all those conditions that are commonly spoken of as nervousness, the fear of death is the basic feature. Yet the individual is likely to be both unable and unwilling to understand that morbid fact. Not infrequently a psychoneurotic upheaval is nothing more than a fear that the individual is unable to cope with, either by unmasking it and bringing it to light, or by suppressing it entirely and reigning over it.

The lively interest now being displayed in so-called psychosomatic medicine is called forth by the increasing realization that many of the physical symptoms of which individuals complain result from the ineffective attempts to deal with the fear —remotely, of death.

The instinct of self-preservation implies positive action in maintenance of life, but the dangers that threaten life must be constantly warded off. The emotional aspect of the effort to live is fear, unceasing fear. Latent though the fear may be, it is constantly present to guard against personal disintegration. Were the fear not kept in a state of repression, life would be made intolerable for man by its continuing presence. But repressing fear calls for the constant utilization of energy in order that the stored-away fear may be kept in confinement and not be permitted to escape. Such unceasing watchfulness is trying on the individual; tension develops, which must be occasionally relieved. The relief may be afforded by a game of golf, by a week-end of fishing, or by a set-to at the card table. More often than we realize, alcohol is resorted to for surcease. But in this way and in that, a balance may be maintained and personal morale preserved. It is said to be better even to blow-up occasionally than to burst.

We live in normal times as if we were certain of personal physical immortality. We are busily engaged in efforts to conquer death and to make unending physical life certain for the masses. Tables of longevity attract the attention of man. Government and other branches of organized society are increasing efforts to make it possible for man to maintain himself throughout a longer span of years. And that government that seems to concern itself about the preservation and the protection of the lives of the people may expect their support.

Yet man realizes, even in peace times, that life is hazardous and he craves personal protection beyond his capacity to afford it. He turns for help to God the Immortal and the Omnipotent to stand by him. Man seeks solace in religion somewhat in proportion to the danger that he thinks surrounds him. He would commune for comfort and for safety with his ever-living God.

Yet it is difficult for robust man to realize that he is mortal, though he may attend the funerals of many of his friends. Man's ego is maximated by his belief that death is not decreed for him. He exhibits such belief by his frequent participation in dangerous sports—in personal defiance of death. Fatal accidents attract the crowd. The occurrence gives each one of us the opportunity to indulge the belief that death, in such a manner, is not intended for any of us. We are not destined to die at all, certainly not in such fashion. We are different. Each of us seems to say: Death is not for me.

In peace times man's morale is rather-well sustained. The individual manifests no obvious personal concern about death. All the aspects of his government tend to make him feel secure. No foreign foe can reach him, so mighty are the armed forces of his country. Death cannot be brought to him by hostile man's planning.

But when war comes all is different. The personal and the mass morale may be profoundly shaken by the fear of personal death. All is changed. Personal physical immortality may be destroyed in a moment of time by an enemy's bomb. If man would survive and would engage in protective activities that would tend to protect the lives of others as well as his own life, he must direct his energy aggressively against the threatening enemy. Aggressive hostility must replace the utilization of his own energy in ministering to his own comfort. Hatred of the enemy must replace all consideration of personal welfare. Individual and mass morale are maintained at a high level by direction of all the energy against the enemy. Hostility to the enemy and hatred of the enemy displace fear by substituting concern about one's country for consideration of self. In the thick of battle when the guns are roaring, and death is on all sides, there is no fear, because thought about personal safety has ceased to be a consideration.

For those who can deal with life and with death in such realistic, hearty fashion, without a twinge of conscience because of the killings involved, there is no fear; and there will be no neurotic sequelae. Such symptoms result only from half-hearted effort, in which there was always some reservation, some doubt, some self-reproach, some sense of guilt.

The fear of death may be instinctive in all animals. The hero gloriously proffers his life in support of his belief, in defiance of all personal danger. The coward prizes his life as his chiefest possession. But he cannot live his life wholesomely because he lives in the grip of ever-tormenting fear.

Death is a phase of life, whether the final phase one does not know. The instruction intended to guide us in living should be lengthened in order to tell us also how to die. The rites attendant upon man's final encryptment should be deprived of most of the solemnity evolved by the theologians and the morticians. Death is as universal as life. Man should be taught not to fear it, but to submit to it with dignity when it cannot be avoided. If man should lose his fear of his fellow-mortals, there would be no more wars.

Bacon, in his essay on Death, says: "Men fear death as children fear to go in the dark; and as that natural fear in children is increased with tales, so is the other." But children often cease to be afraid of the dark as they emerge into adulthood. Mayhap man could be taught not to fear death.

I wish my readers would request a copy of Dr. Zilboorg's reprint on Fear of Death from his office at 14 East 75th Street in New York. He seldom writes a sentence that is not thought-provoking. I doubt if I know his intellectual superior. And he writes with carefulness and with clarity and with a style and charm of expression that are seldom encountered in medical literature. He is constantly enriching psychiatric literature by his philosophic contributions. Yet less than three decades ago he knew no words in our majestic English language!

HOW A FAVORITE OF OSLER'S THOUGHT OF DEATH

Happening to pick up Sir (Doctor) Thomas Browne's *Religio Medici* a day after reading Dr. Hall's MS, and the book happening to open on that learned knight's disquisition on Death, I am moved to append some passages therefrom.—*J. M. N.*

I am not so much afraid of death, as ashamed thereof. . . . 'Tis the very disgrace and ignominy of our natures, that in a moment can so disfigure us, that our nearest friends, Wife, and Children, stand afraid and start at us; the Birds and Beasts of the field, that before in a natural fear obeyed us, forgetting all allegiance, begin to prey upon us. This very conceit hath left me willing to be swallowed up in the abyss of waters, wherein I had perished unseen. . . . Not that I am ashamed of the Anatomy of my parts, or can accuse Nature for playing the bungler in any part of me, or my own vitious life for contracting any shameful disease upon me, whereby I might not call myself as wholesome a morsel for the worms as any. . . .

At my death I mean to take a total adieu of the World, not caring for a Monument, History, or Epitaph, not so much as the bare memory of my name to be found any where but in the universal Register of God. . . . [But I] commend in my calmer judgment those ingenuous intentions that desire to sleep by the urns of their Fathers, and strive to go the neatest way unto corruption. . . .

If (as Divinity affirms) there shall be no gray hairs in Heaven, but all shall rise in the perfect state of men, we do but outlive those perfections in this World, to be recalled unto them by a greater Miracle in the next, and ru non here but to be retrograde hereafter. . . .

And though I think no man can live well once, but he that could live twice, yet for my own part I would not live over my hours past, or begin again the thread of my days; not upon Cicero's ground, because I have lived them well, but for fear I should live them worse. . . . I find in my confirmed age the same sins I discovered in my youth; I committed many then, because I was a Child; and because I commit them still, I am yet an Infant. . . .

It is a brave act of valour to contemn death; but where life is more terrible than death, it is then the truest valour to dare to live. Were I of Caesar's Religion, I should be of his desires, and wish rather to go off at one blow, then to be saved in pieces by the grating torture of a disease.

'Tis not onely the mischief of diseases, and the villany of poysons, that make an end of us: we vainly accuse the fury of Guns, and the new inventions of death; it is in the power of every hand to destroy us, and we are beholding unto every one we meet that he doth not kill us.

We are happier with death than we should have been without it: we are in the power of no calamity while death is in our own. . . .

That general opinion that the World grows near its end, hath possessed all ages past as nearly as ours. I am afraid that the Souls that now depart, cannot escape that lingering expostulation of the Saints under the Altar, Quosque, Domine? How long, O Lord? and groan in the expectation of that great Jubilee.

HOSPITALS

R. B. DAVIS, M.D., *Editor*, Greensboro, N. C.

AS THE DAYS GO BY

THE REPUTATION that the American people have in other countries is that they do a lot of talking and very little listening. The author sometimes desires to add to that, "but a lot of procrastinating."

The shortage of hospital personnel is continually on the lips of practically every hospital operator in the country.

It has been the privilege of the writer to visit large and small hospitals, in numbers, in the last few years, and there is always weeping, wailing and gnashing of teeth about not being able to get help. When asked, however, to suggest a method by which this condition might be remedied, the hospital operators are as far apart as the East is from the West. Some say, "Increase salaries;" some say, "Decrease working hours;" others say, "Train practical nurses;" other say, "Enlarge the standard training schools;" while still others say, "Let George do it." The only thing that is being done is that of letting George do it through the United States Government.

The story is told that Daniel Webster's father once left home and told his older son to do a certain job and the younger was to help him. When the father returned and no work had been done, the older son was punished for doing nothing. But when the younger son was questioned, he insisted that his job was to help the older brother which he did and that was to help him to do nothing. We hospital administrators are not doing even as well as the younger son did; for we are letting the United States Government run a Nurses Cadet Training School and we are not even so much as allowing them the privilege of working in our hospitals!

The writer of this article does not, by any means, feel that he has a panacea for all of the evils that overtake hospital administrators, but he does feel that there is some benefit to be derived from an honest effort. In a half-hearted manner, many of the hospitals have adopted various remedies, but, so far, I have been able to locate *none* which has gone into the matter in a whole-hearted fashion. If there is one method superior to any other, it will never be discovered until some group of individuals concentrate upon it sufficiently to make a thorough test.

Some of the objections to the plans that have been tried are: the increased cost of raising hospital salaries; said cost being passed on to the patient—the one who is, because of loss of time from work, least able to bear the increase. The method of shortening hours for the nurses might be a good one, but in many instances the ward nurse is carrying on another job, usually that of maintaining a home. She does not feel justified in remaining away from her family twelve hours a day, therefore she stays home and takes care of her household duties and rears her family. She can work from six to eight hours a day in the hospital and so divide her time and energy between the two jobs. This does not always make for better nursing. If there is a baby or any other member of the family sick, she arrives at the hospital physically and mentally fatigued. When the hour comes for her child to return from school, this is on her mind rather than giving treatment to a patient.

Some have argued that practical nurses might solve the problem. In some instances this has helped tremendously. However, it is evident that a good nurse's aide with a reasonable amount of hospital experience will become a good trained nurse's aide. As time goes on, she will assume more authority, coupled with more responsibility in regard to the sick of the community. All too soon, she will become a practical nurse of the community, with hospital training. And when she does, the graduate nurses' status at six dollars a day for eight hours' duty will be rapidly replaced by a four-dollar-a-day, twelve-hour duty. Therefore, from the standpoint of the nursing profession, this does not seem a wise procedure in the mind of the writer of this article.

The Nurses Cadet Corps does relieve the hospital of the financial burden of running a training school. But the red tape attached to it, plus the fact that the government takes these nurses as soon as they are graduated, will not, in the long run, afford any great relief. When the war is over, the Nurses Cadet Corps will probably cease to exist. Besides, these girls are expecting to find charming young soldiers to whom they may attach themselves for the balance of eternity and thereby *absent* themselves from the nursing profession. Eight years is the average professional life of a nurse. I make the conservative prediction that five years will be the average of the Cadet Nurse.

The law of supply and demand has been the safety economic rule for every industry or profession known to mankind. It will not be different in the future with the hospital personnel. All hospitals should become institutions of education. Any physician who has the ability to pilot a patient through a serious illness or operation is capable of teaching an energetic young woman the art and science of nursing. We must have more graduate nurses if we are to supply the demand made upon us today and tomorrow. No matter what plan is devised, in the same of common sense, will those who are determined to try it really go into the matter whole-heartedly and not just talk about it.

As the days go by, the demand is increasing tremendously, the supply is decreasing just as fast. We have been weighed in the balance and found wanting. Let us not repeat that failure. We, as hospital administrators and guardians of nurses' training schools, would do well to do some hard thinking, very quickly, and produce results without further delay. No fly-by-night plan is capable of solving a problem with as much at stake as the shortage of nurses has created. The Nurses Association first must bestir themselves to the nth degree and request the hospitals to open good three-year training schools wherever possible. The hospitals must coöperate to the utmost; giving the best and most attractive training to the ambitious young women seeking to enter that profession which I think is the noblest of all. At the present rate of passing the graduate nurses' exit is all too rapid. We do not want to see her go. We still consider her an "Angel of Mercy" and appreciate the sacrificial services that she has rendered in time gone by. Therefore, we now plea with those who are capable of furnishing us with sufficient nursing personnel not to let us down.

The medical and nursing professions cannot work *contrariwise* in a common cause. I am sure neither profession wishes to try to do so.

CLINICAL CHEMISTRY and MICROSCOPY

J. M. FEDER, M.D., and EVELYN TRIBBLE, M.T., *Editors*, Anderson, S. C.

A SYNOPSIS OF LABORATORY DIAGNOSIS IN GYNECOLOGY

THESE laboratory procedures are in the majority of instances carried out in the physician's office. How well or ill this is done frequently passes in review before a pathologist in a general clinical laboratory.

Gonorrhea: The diagnosis of gonorrhea in the male offers but few obstacles. The organisms if present are usually in pure culture and their identification is easy. Not all cases of urethritis in the male are of gonorrheal origin. All bacteria of the pyogenic classification have been demonstrated as well as trichomonas.

In the female, the examination is much more difficult on account of the multiple coexisting organisms. At least three preparations should be made from every patient examined and these taken only after thoroughly cleansing the urethra, vaginal vault and cervix.

We learned long ago that in many instances in which cervical smears were found to be negative for the specific organism, by swabbing the canal with 10-per cent silver nitrate and then making another preparation within 24 hours, the organism would be demonstrated. Milking of Skeen's glands is another often overlooked procedure.

Regardless of the technique employed, unless the case is acute, it is well to disregard the questionable positive, and many negative, direct examinations. A culture should be made in every questionable case of suspected gonorrhea in the female.[1]

Many of these cases have a potential medicolegal angle and the courts of many states are now demanding the result of a culture and will view with skepticism a report based on a direct examination alone. Even in children, there is no excuse for merely examining mucoid secretions from the orifice. An anesthetic may have to be employed but if the diagnostic information sought is of sufficient importance, its use is justified.

The doctor may obtain from his local laboratory the required culture materials necessary for transporting to the central depot. In one of our Tri-States (North Carolina) notation was seen some time ago to the effect that their laboratory of Public Health was supplying such media. We are not in a position to state whether or not the others are doing likewise. Before any woman is committed to a State detention institution as a gonorrhea victim culture should prove the diagnosis. The Bill of Rights, and damage suits, still exist.

Trichomonas Vaginalis: The appearance of the discharge and of the vagina are characteristic. The secretion has a yellowish-green color with a tendency to be foamy. By aid of the speculum on cervix and vault are seen punctate, superficially ulcerated areas. A drop of the material is placed upon a slide and a cover-glass applied. The high-dry lens facilitates diagnosis but the rapidly moving organisms can be seen under the low power. When they are non-motile their identification is slightly more difficult. Every patient having an intractable vaginal discharge in which gonococci cannot be demonstrated should have the benefit of a search for trichomonas. The diagnosis can be

1. Essentials of Applied Medical Laboratory Technic. Feder. Charlotte Medical Press, Publ., Pp. 187-191.

He won't dodge this—

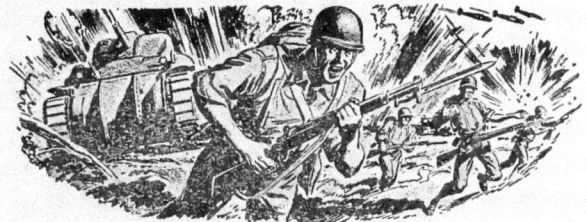

Don't *you* dodge this!

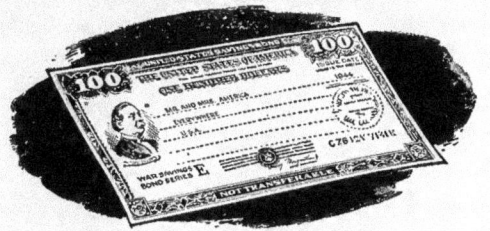

The kid'll be right there when his C.O. finally gives the signal...

There'll be no time to think of better things to do with his life. *The kid's giving all he's got, now!*

We've got to do the same. This is the time for us to throw in everything *we've* got.

This is the time to dig out that extra hundred bucks and spend it for Invasion Bonds.

Or make it $200. Or $1000. Or $1,000,000. There's no ceiling on this one!

Make no mistake! The 5th War Loan is the biggest, the most vitally important financial effort of this whole war!

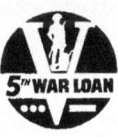

Back the Attack! — BUY MORE THAN BEFORE

This is an official U. S. Treasury advertisement—prepared under auspices of Treasury Department and War Advertising Council

made in a few seconds while the patient is on the examining table, and treatment instituted immediately as indicated.

If essential to transport to a laboratory for examination, these organisms may be kept alive for 30 minutes on a swab which is immersed in normal saline at 99° in a test-tube and kept at that temperature until it reaches the examiner.

The Sedimentation Rate in Gynecological Conditions: Often there is a differential point between subacte, or acute, salpingitis and appendicitis. In many cases the sedimentation rate will serve to aid in making the diagnosis. Uncomplicated appendicitis does not as a rule alter the normal sedimentation, while in the case of adnexal disease it is markedly accelerated. The erythrocyte sedimentation rate is also of value in determining when to operate upon a case of salpingitis. Once the acute inflammatory reaction has subsided, it returns to normal, but much later than the leucocyte count and the polymorphonuclear and Schilling index count.

The Vaginal Smear as a Guide to Estrogen Therapy: This valuable examination is simple and, when its interpretation has been mastered, reveals much information that can be used to advantage.

It is based upon the fact that the adult epithelium shows complete cornification, and this is arbitrarily clasified as grade-4, or normal. Grade-1, on the opposite end of the scale, is a smear showing a marked estrogen-deficiency state. Here the picture is one of small, round cells with deeply staining nuclei and leucocytes. Grade-2 and -3 are improvement steps between 1 and 4. There are many sources of information available upon this subject but the most comprehensive for office use is the excellent little volume prepared for the guidance of the general physician by Greenblatt, of the University of Georgia Medical School, at Augusta.

Technique for making these smears is not difficult. After mopping the vaginal orifice gently, a cotton-wrapped applicator is pressed against the vaginal wall and cervix. Rotation is the proper movement and the material so obtained is placed upon a slide and stained. We have found that the ordinary 1-per cent aqueous safranin used in connection with our Gram stain to be a satisfactory stain.

This method will aid in making the diagnosis of a deficiency state and serve as a control upon the result of treatment once it has been instituted.

EYE HEADACHES
(G. J. Epstein, New York, in *The N. Y. Physician*, May)

The doctor seeking to know if a headache is likely to be of ocular origin, should ask himself these questions: (1) is it associated with use of the eyes? (2) is it associated with diplopia in either near or distance vision? (3) is it a morning headache in a person over 40, associated with transient visual disturbances?

Finding any of these associations indicates a competent ophthalmologic examination.

PROCTOLOGY

RUSSELL VON L. BUXTON, M.D., *Editor*, Newport News, Va

ANAL FISSURE

ANAL FISSURE presents at the same time one of the most painful and one of the most easily curable of ano-rectal conditions. This trouble is due to constipation with a subsequent tearing of the anal mucosa, this followed by infection and pain. The pain causes spasm of the anal sphincters which in turn cause the torn edges of the mucosa to stay apart and not heal promptly. Thus a vicious circle is set up and the condition continues indefinitely. There are remissions in some cases but the condition will ordinarily return promptly if there is even a slight degree of constipation or strain.

The diagnosis can often be made upon seeing the patient who is usually sitting on the edge of the chair with an anxious and tense expression on the face. The history is likewise quite simple, the patient stating, "my rectum hurts." In addition there is exacerbation of pain on defecation and this is usually associated with bleeding.

Digital examination of these patients is almost always impossible due to pain; however, if it is possible, an extremely spastic sphincter is found with tenderness in the anterior or posterior commissure. In a large percentage of patients, there is an associated fecal impaction due to the fact the patient will not defecate because of pain. After the diagnosis is made, the treatment is simple. The patient is advised to enter the hospital for operation, at which time the anal sphincters are dilated. The fissure with the associated sentinel pile is excised and the external anal sphincter is divided. Following operation, large doses of mineral oil and antispasmodics are used. The rectum is gently dilated for two or three weeks.

This may seem to be somewhat radical, but in six years of practice, only one case of anal fissure has healed without coming to operation. If there are no hemorrhoids to be removed at the same time, the patient can be discharged from the hospital in three days and most patients feel much better immediately after operation than they did before.

In case an immediate operation is not feasible, large doses of mineral oil, combined with sedation and antispasmodics and hot sitz baths seem to be the best measures. Added to this, local treatment consisting of suppositories and ointment give temporary relief. However, as stated before, the best treatment is surgery, and the sooner it is done the more quickly the patient is cured.

SURGERY

Geo. H. Bunch, M.D., *Editor*, Columbia, S. C.

LINEN AS SUTURE MATERIAL

There is much discussion about the relative merits of absorbable and of unabsorbable sutures, about the use of catgut and of silk in clean wounds and in infected wounds. Because experience has proved that as a rule there is less tissue reaction to it than to catgut and because of economy more and more surgeons have, until the last five years, used silk whenever feasible.

Indeed, largely because of the teaching of Halstead and of the Johns Hopkins school, silk has up to recent years been generally selected as an unabsorbable suture material. It is easily sterilized, pliable and of fair tensile strength. It is well tolerated by the tissues and was universally available before its importation from the Orient was interrupted by the war with Japan. When dyed black it is readily identified even in a blood-stained field.

In recent years cotton has in many hospitals largely superseded silk as a suture material. It, too, is of good tensile strength and is easily sterilized. If resterilized it becomes weak, however, and unused sutures should be discarded. It is well tolerated by the tissues. It has the great advantage of being the cheapest of all suture materials. It has more body than silk and is easier to work with. Its general use in the place of catgut and of silk has resulted in the saving of thousands of dollars by hospitals. Grown and manufactured in the South, other things being equal, it should be the choice of Southern surgeons and hospitals.

At the risk of being considered unpatriotic and a heretic, the writer has for many years used linen as a suture material in preference to either silk or cotton. Microscopic study after its experimental use in animals is said to have shown more tissue reaction from it. Practically, however, there is no evidence of irritation in wounds in which it has been used and healing is in no way interfered with. It has the great advantage of maximum tensile strength which permits the use of smaller thread for sutures. The surgeon may tighten a linen ligature with the assurance that it will not break under ordinary tension. This adds to the safety of the patient and to the confidence of the surgeon. When wet it is not flimsy like silk and in small sizes is more easily manipulated. It has but little capillarity. It is readily sterilized and even when used in quantity, as in the repair of massive inguinal or incisional hernias, it is well tolerated by the tissues. In our work, whenever much unabsorbable suture material of any kind is used, even in clean wounds, sulfathiazole powder is applied locally. This is almost a guarantee against infection. In our work ties in radical breast removals are practically all of linen. Because of ooze these wounds have to be drained. After the use of sulfathiazole we have not had such wounds become infected and discharge linen ties for weeks until healing is complete.

We have had no experience in the use of stainless steel wire as suture material. It is cheap, well tolerated by the tissues and is easily sterilized, but it is hard to work with.

DERMATOLOGY

J. Lamar Callaway, M.D., *Editor*, Durham, N. C.

RECENT ADJUNCTS TO DERMATOLOGIC THERAPY

For years the efficacy of most remedies used in the therapy of superficial fungus diseases of the skin have depended on their keratolitic action rather than on fungicidal properties.

With the onset of so much dermatophytosis in the armed forces extensive studies were carried out to find a good fungicide that would be effective without causing local irritation. Many preparations have been used but most of the information is restricted and cannot be divulged. However, sodium propionate and related compounds primarily used in the manufacture of bread was found to be a relatively safe yet effective fungicide in the management of the superficial dermatomycoses.

As an adjunct to the usual management of superficial fungus infections of the skin such as dermatophytosis, 10-per cent sodium propionate in alcohol may be sponged on twice daily followed by 15-per cent calcium propionate in talcum powder. At night 10-per cent sodium propionate in a water-soluble base may be applied and left on overnight. The usual care of the skin should be followed, particularly relative to drying between the toes, not exposing naked feet to floors, showers, etc.

Pragmatar ointment is extremely valuable as an effective remedy in the management of the various superficial fungus diseases. It is used in much the same manner as Whitfield's ointment, sodium propionate ointment or other similar remedies.

Metacresylacetate solution (Cresatin) offers help in the treatment of otomycosis, being sponged on two or three times daily to the affected areas.

The "wonder drug," penicillin, when it becomes readily available, will also be a great boon in the management of pyodermias. I have used penicillin, reclaimed from the urine, in a water-soluble ointment base in a strength of 50,000 units per ounce. The penicillin ointment should be kept cold to prevent its deterioration. It has proven invaluable in the management of impetiginous lesions, recalcitrant leg ulcers that are secondarily infected, and pyodermias in general. The lesions are treated with compresses and usual management plus the use of penicillin ointment applied two or three times daily.

Benzyl benzoate in alcohol in strengths from 30 to 50 per cent is an effective remedy against scabies and may be used as a primary treatment for scabies or in patients who are sensitive to the various sulfur preparations.

*Sodium Proprionate ointment and liquid and calcium proprionate powder may be obtained commercially from the Mycoloid Laboratories, Inc., Little Falls, N. J.
**Pragmatar Ointment may be obtained commercially from Smith, Kline, and French Laboratories, Philadelphia.
***Metacresylacetate solution (Cresatin) may be obtained commercially from Sharpe and Dohme, Philadelphia.
****Benzyl Benzoate lotion (Xylate) may be obtained commercially from The Upjohn Company, Kalamazoo, Mich.

OBSTETRICS

HENRY J. LANGSTON, M.D., *Editor*, Danville, Va.

PRESENT STATUS OF OBSTETRICAL ANESTHESIA

THERE are so many good ways of easing the pains of labor as to make the writings on the subject quite confusing. A recent article[1] which fairly states the case is reviewed.

Morphine-scopolamine seminarcosis, the so-called twilight sleep, is little used today except in a few clinics. In small doses, as an analgesic, it is probably the most widely used of any method. We cannot, however, consider this method unless the drugs are given in such concentrations as to abolish pain, or the memory of pain. Twilight sleep, in the opinion of these doctors,[1] is a valuable method which has fallen into disrepute chiefly because it was proposed before the medical profession had advanced far enough to be able to accept it.

Rectal Ether-Oil Mixture is about as effective as paraldehyde or the barbiturates in producing analgesia and amnesia. It is doubtful if a toxic dose of ether could be given with oil by rectum. Delay of the initial respiration in the fetus and somnolence in the first few days of life does occur, but this is of little clinical importance. There is no increase in fetal mortality or morbidity. Restlessness, and even delirium, occasionally occur, and the patients must be closely watched to prevent accidents. It requires 15-20 minutes to take effect. Frequently, by the time the patient has been given

1. J. Kotz & M. S. Kaufman, Washington, in *Arcs. & Analg.*, Mar., Apr.

two or three enemas, and the drug can take effect, it is too late to attain our objective. For this reason, we do not advocate rectal drugs to rapidly progressing multipara. Labor is retarded in only a very few cases. Postpartum bleeding is not increased, nor is the third stage prolonged. Diarrhea is occasionally encountered for two or three days postpartum.

Paraldehyde may be used alone either rectally or orally usually in combination with morphine or the barbiturates. As much as eight ounces of the drug has been given by rectum without ill-effects. Infant apnea is transient, resuscitation not difficult. Somnolence persists for several days, and frequently the odor of paraldehyde may be detected on the babies' breath, but we have been unable to find any ill-effects. Rather lengthy preparation is required, and it takes effect slowly. The drug is better adapted for primipara and multipara in very early labor. An initial dose of barbiturates by mouth, then enemas, and then gas during the administration of the paraldehyde, will give the patient ample relief. Paraldehyde causes a temporary slowing of labor followed by a return to normal pains. Even with sideboards, and head and foot boards, the patient may not be left alone. In our opinion, paraldehyde is the safest of the analgesic drugs.

Barbiturates advantages are the high percentage of amnesia, ease of administration and rapid effect. The safety factor with the barbiturates is not as great as with either paraldehyde or rectal ether; they have slightly less retarding influence on the course of labor and are frequently of great value as a premedication before the administration of the rectal drugs. Restlessness is more marked with any other group of analgesic drugs, the patients require constant supervision. Delirium, and even maniacal states have been observed.

Continuous Caudal Anesthesia is the most recent development in obstetrical analgesia. It is still too early to pass judgment. Relief of pain is almost immediate in the vast majority of cases, complete usually within 5-15 minutes, and may be maintained indefinitely by repeated injections. There is no effect on the newborn. The course of the first stage is hastened somewhat, but the second stage may be slightly prolonged because of the absence of the desire to bear down, the third stage proceeds normally. Consciousness is retained throughout labor, which may or may not be an advantage, depending on the temperament of the patient. The injection of the solution into the caudal canal requires an experienced anesthetist, and the need for repeat doses.

The chief danger is of the needle penetrating the dura, and the drug being injected into the subarachnoid space. This may be minimized by aspiration, and by the use of a test dose; but aspiration may not obtain fluid even though the needle is in the subarachnoid space, especially if the patient is in the knee-chest or knee-elbow position. Injection of large doses into the spinal fluid may result in vascular and respiratory collapse. Another danger is the possibility of injecting the solution into the venous plexus of the caudal canal. Failure to aspirate blood does not prove that the needle is not in a vein. The orifice may be plugged by areolar tissue, or may be against the wall of the vein; the needle may be forced into a vein by the movements of the patient after the initial dose has been given. The injection of the solution into the blood stream will result in severe toxic reactions, collapse, and perhaps death. Anaphylactic reactions may occur. Severe pain in the back of the legs following the recovery from the anesthetic in several cases has been controlled by morphine.

We do not feel that this method is adapted to general usage. The article under review concludes with some general considerations:

Dosage of all analgesic drugs must be fitted to the patient. Body weight has little to do with the dosage. The temperament of the individual, the strength and frequency of the pains, the degree of dilatation, the position of the fetus, parity and whether or not the membranes are intact all must be weighed.

The primipara with intact membranes, a posterior position, a moderately thick cervix, and 1-2 cm. dilated, will almost certainly have an impairment of the progress of labor if given sizable doses of analgesic drugs. On the other hand, a multipara with ruptured membranes may be given large doses even though the pains are slight and infrequent.

The phlegmatic individual will often sleep soundly on a dose that will affect the apprehensive one no more than a drink of water.

The most effective way to combat the occasional delay of labor induced by drugs is early rupture of the membranes. Occasionally in severe secondary inertia, it may be necessary to use small doses of pituitrin to stimulate the uterus.

Amnesia is facilitated by breaking the chain of consciousness. This may be easily accomplished by lightly anesthetizing the patient with gas for periods of 10-20 minutes, especially in apprehensive individuals, and in those who are progressing rapidly. Drugs alone frequently have little effect on these patients, but drugs followed by gas for a short period will usually achieve our purpose of complete amnesia.

All of the methods of analgesia increase the incidence of operative deliveries. Voluntary efforts are inhibited, requiring the increased use of low forceps. Rotation of posterior and transverse positions is impeded. The same is true in caudal block.

I deem it necessary to make this further comment:

It is a rather common practice in these days to rupture membranes to induce labor. Many very good men do it, but I still believe, as all students used to be taught, that the membranes should be kept intact as long as possible because of the value of amniotic fluid in acting as a hydrostatic dilator, and so facilitating the delivery of a live baby spontaneously.

On the other hand, if it has to be an instrumental delivery or a version, the amniotic fluid is of value, particularly in a version. If the amniotic sac is kept intact one will find very little difficulty in doing a version and extraction, providing the baby is not larger than the birth canal.

Also, in some cases where the test of labor is fully met, delivery by birth canal is not possible, and a cesarean section has to be done, one is in a much better position to combat infection if the bag of waters has not been ruptured.

Chloroform is still a valuable anesthesia in the second stage of labor, if properly administered. However, if one doesn't know how to use chloroform he should use ether. I think it is unfortunate that our medical schools and institutions of instruction have gotten away from the use of chloroform, because there are some cases in which it can be used with definite safety and is preferable to ether.

TUBERCULOSIS

J. DONNELLY, M.D., *Editor*, Charlotte, N. C.

OCCURRENCE OF PULMONARY TUBERCULOSIS IN SUPPOSEDLY SCREENED SELECTEES

REGULATIONS exclude active or potentially active tuberculosis from the armed forces, also scarred, infiltrative tuberculosis exceeding a total area of 5 sq. cm. in "flat" films. They permit acceptance of men with scarred, apparently arrested lesions of less than this extent, provided stability has been confirmed by at least six months' observation. They permit acceptance of small, calcified lesions of arrested primary tuberculosis without question and leave to the judgment of qualified medical examiners decision as to acceptance or rejection in the case of large or numerous calcified lesions.[1]

We are informed further that:

The rate of rejection has been one per cent after initial screening by the local selective service board; colored 1.3 per cent higher than for white. Of the registrants rejected for tuberculosis one-

(Col. A. Freer, Washington, in *Dis. of the Chest*, May-June)

half were inactive cases, potentially significant; the other half, including many advanced cases already known or detectable by other means, are made up largely of cases of minimal active tuberculosis that would have escaped attention without x-ray examination.

Re-reading x-ray films or accepted men indicated that during this period 1,500 cases of active tuberculosis per million men were being overlooked.

More than 10 per cent of the total population of the country will have been x-rayed in the physical examinations incident to military service; 150,000 men will have been rejected for tuberculosis.

PUBLIC HEALTH

N. THOMAS ENNETT, M.D., *Editor*, Greenville, N. C

A STEP IN ADVANCE

THE HEALTH of the school child is the concern, first of its parents, next of its family doctor, then of the health officer and the school principal

The need for a better system of school health, especially in the rural school, is a crying need of today. Preventive medicine is at its best when dealing with children for "as the twig is bent so the tree is inclined."

It has been next to an impossibility for all children to receive an annual check-up by the health officer in small towns and in the rural areas. In fact, even in the larger cities, where there is a large corps of school medical examiners, it is seldom that school children are reached annually from the medical standpoint.

Within recent months, the North Carolina State Board of Health and the North Carolina State Department of Public Instruction have, through State funds and through funds obtained from the General Education Board, put on a program in certain counties of the State known as the School Health Coördinating Service. Dr. W. P. Jacocks of Raleigh is the State Coördinator.

Dr. Jacocks and his staff, consisting of nurses, a nutritionist, and a physical educator, have just finished a demonstration program in Pitt County. His staff held a series of meetings and conferences with the teachers of the county, explaining to them how to discover more or less obvious defects and diseases of the children. Following this period of instruction and demonstrations, the teacher "screened" the children in her room. Those children who apparently had some poor vision, diseased tonsils, adenoids, bad teeth, defective hearing, flat feet, etc., were listed and referred to the health officer for final examination. The health officer determining just what sort of note should be sent to the home relative to the defect.

Upon further examination of these children, the health officer was amazed to find that his own opinion, in the great majority of instances, sustained the suspicion of the teacher. It appears to us that this School Health Coördinating Service is one of the most advanced steps in promoting the health of the school child that has ever come to our knowledge.

Of course the teacher will miss some defects but since she grades them 1, 2 and 3—three representing the marked defect—it means that at most border-line cases are referred to the health officer.

We estimate that utilizing the teacher in this way saves 75 per cent of the time the health officer would have to expend in making such examinations unaided.

An important point in the program is that no notice goes to the home except that it bear the authority of a physician.

Another important phase of the School Health Coördinating Program is that it is anticipated that a trained Coördinator take up the work in each community where Dr. Jacocks' staff leaves off.

Now if we can get the Teachers Training Colleges to give more time to training the teacher to teach health, and the State or local governmental unit to subsidize indigent families, in order that defects may be corrected after being found, we will take another advanced step which has been all too long delayed.

UROLOGY

RAYMOND THOMPSON, M.D., *Editor*, Charlotte, N. C.

PROSTATIC AND SEMINAL VESICULITIS: ACUTE AND CHRONIC

CHRONIC prostatic infections occur with more frequency than is generally believed, and, without being dangerous, may cause intense suffering and inconvenience. Pain may be referred to any part of the pelvic region and down the legs, while the effect on the nervous system may be such as to produce true neuroses.

"By far the greatest percentage of cases are not caused by gonorrhea." The prostate may be infected from foci in other areas of the body and may, in turn, infect remote parts. The prostate and seminal vesicles should be considered routinely with the tonsils, teeth or sinuses as foci of infection. Conversely, ". . . one should be constantly aware of the possibility that some other focus in the urinary tract," for example the kidney, "may be responsible for failure to obtain results in the treatment of prostatic infection."

Sexual abuses may predispose to prostatitis by causing congestion of the prostate, and conversely, some sexual disorders are apparently caused or aggravated by chronic prostatitis, for these symptoms may clear up upon treatment of the prostate.

The diagnosis of chronic prostatitis should be based on both rectal examination (this to be done with extreme gentleness) and on the finding of pus in the expressed prostatic fluid. Henline recommends that for examination "the patient kneel on a table, with the buttocks extended and the head down to a level with the knees." A gloved, well lubricated finger may then be gently inserted in the rectum. If rectal palpation gives evidence of an abnormal prostate (enlarged, nodular, boggy, etc.) one should not be misled if, at first, a normal secretion be expressed. Three or four examinations at five-day intervals may be necessary. "The diagnosis of chronic prostatitis is established with the finding of an increased number of leukocytes in the prostatic strippings, particularly if they are seen in clumps."

The finding of a prostate abnormal by criteria outlined above should not conclude an examination. The origin of infection should be established, and an attempt should be made to eliminate factors which may prevent its response to treatment. An infected tooth or tonsil, for example, may by reinfection of the prostate retard its response to local treatment. Infections in the intestinal tract, cutaneous infections, or gallbladder or perirectal infections may all have similar retarding effect, as may also failure to establish normal sexual hygiene.

"The treatment of acute prostatitis is by heat and protection from trauma, that of subacute and chronic prostatitis by prostatic massage. The sulfonamides are often helpful in either condition but cannot be relied on to the exclusion of local treatment." Urethral stricture and other complications of the urinary tract should be sought for and treated.

There are two objectives to be achieved by gentle prostatic massage—the increasing of the blood supply to the prostate and the evacuation of pus, bacteria and debris from the prostatic ducts.

"The use of sulfonamides have been helpful in certain cases"—sulfathiazole 1 gm. 4 i. d. for 10 days, along with prostatic massage. "The sulfonamides are usually very effective in relieving acute prostatitis."

The response to treatment in both chronic prostatitis and seminal vesiculitis may be slow. Massage may be required for long periods, but, "in general, the outlook, in the treatment of these patients is good, provided the coöperation of the patient can be maintained."

1. Prostatitis and Seminal Vesiculitis: Acute and Chronic. R. B. Henline in J. A. M. A., Nov. 6th, 1943.

GENERAL PRACTICE

JAMES L. HAMNER, M.D., *Editor*, Mannboro, Va.

ETHYL CHLORIDE SPRAY FOR FREEZING DONOR AREA IN SKIN GRAFTING

MOST of us have patients whose wounds heal so slowly, even S. S. (since sulfa), as to make advisable the grafting of skin.

We are indebted to a Georgia orthopedist[1] for a one-man technic, and for encouragement to use it ourselves—for most of us "have had some surgical experience."

The method is to use an ethyl chloride spray over the donor area, the tube being wrapped and held in a sterile towel. Only slight freezing is necessary. The frosting is rapidly wiped away and the split skin graft is quickly removed by a razor blade held in a pair of straight forceps. The graft is then transplanted and may be fixed and dressed by the method of operator's choice. I prefer paraffin mesh next to the graft, covering this with sterile gauze and using rubber bath sponge or mechanic's waste for pressure.. The donor area is covered by vaseline gauze and dressed as soon as the graft is removed. As a result of freezing there will be no immediate bleeding from the donor site and if dressed immediately, by a nurse or assistant, the field will be bloodless during the operation.

A protective plaster cast may or may not be used as thought wise by the operator. If the grafted part can be satisfactorily suspended, I prefer a lighter dressing.

Skin grafts, one of our most valuable aids in wound healing, have been used too little and by too few doctors. I am suggesting a method that can be used by any doctor who has had some surgical experience. Its application is simple and the skin can safely stand extremely low temperatures over short periods of time. This is almost a one-man technic; it may make more extensive and late plastic repairs unnecessary.

Even in case in which the transplants did not remain viable the wound always improved and seemed to heal more rapidly.

1. J. H. Gaston, Columbus, in Jl. Med. Assn. Ga., May.

HYPODERMIC MEDICATION SHOULD BE PAINLESS
(F. J. Walter, San Diego, in *Jl. Fla. Med. Assn.*, May)

More and more drugs are given intravenously and subcutaneously. It behooves physicians to keep their patients until they feel they have had sufficient medication. On account of lack of attention to little details they are losing many patients because they hurt them.

With the newer drugs, the sulfa drugs, more transfusions, and penicillin coming along, requiring the use of needles every few hours in their administration, it is of great importance to guard against creating needle-shy patients. When my patients say to me that no one has hurt them so little in giving hypodermic injections, I am complimented and gratified. These patients stay with me and send others.

Infinitely greater results can be obtained in giving vitamin B_1 and scores of other medicines by hypodermic medication. The physician sees his patient as frequently as may be necessary and gets better coöperation by this method of treatment. The nurse and the physician should inspect the points and keep them razor-sharp. Use as small a needle as practicable and insert it as quickly as possible. Find an area away from important nerves. A fold of the skin firmly held and pressed above the point of insertion will make possible the quick and painless jab.

OPHTHALMOLOGY

Herbert C. Neblett, M.D., *Editor*, Charlotte, N. C.

THE HANDLING OF MYOPIA OF INCIPIENT SENILE CATARACT AND THAT OF TRAUMA

When a cataract begins to form the refractive index of the eye becomes myopic and rapidly increases as the cataract develops. In the emmetropic, or the low-grade hypermetropic, eye the patient early becomes conscious of his deficiency for distant seeing, and if he is presbyopic and wears glasses for correction he very soon becomes aware of the increasing difficulty in reading with glasses that heretofore gave him clear vision. If his hyperopia is high and presbyopia present and glasses are used for correction his visual problem becomes more difficult for him than in the foregoing, as the myopia increases lessening his hypermetropia. He is then caught between two greatly divergent and increasing indices of refraction, the one for distance, the other for near, in which case neither in the one nor the other can clear vision with glasses be accomplished. If he were previously myopic for distance and presbyopic also the lens changes (cataractous) greatly augment the myopia and lessen the presbyopic condition so that both far and near vision are seriously curtailed even with the optical lens that corrects his vision to its maximum.

If he has one eye cataractous, which is usual, and the other not until later, and glasses were necessary to correct both far and near vision, his problem is more annoying in the early stages of the cataract than those mentioned, because the refractive indices in the two eyes are diametrically opposed making the size of the images of the two eyes differ greatly, and with the added confusing factor of dimness of vision and dispersion of light in the incipiently cataractous eye. He will continue to be so confused visually until the cataractous eye no longer plays a part in the visual quotient. If both eyes are involved and the progress of each cataract keeps apace the confusion in vision is less pronounced than in the other instances given, but here his total visual quotient is obviously less and becomes increasingly more so as the cataracts progress.

Any one of these conditions presents a problem to the refractionist, not in the technique of doing the refraction but in apprizing the patient of his problem and in satisfying him with the best visual quotient that is possible in his condition. The whole question must be adjudged upon the status of the individual eye problem presented. When one eye is in the early or middle stage of cataract, and the myopic index is equal to or greater than 1.5 to 2 or 3 diopters of correction for distance, and the other eye emmetropic or nearly so, and a presbyopic correction is indicated or is being used, it is more comfortable and less confusing to the patient to correct the vision of the non-cataractous eye and place a plain lens before its fellow and advise the patient of the reason for so doing; or a black hookover or frosted lens may be worn before the eye with the cataract. The majority of patients, for cosmetic reasons, object to the latter. In the case where both lenses are cataractous and vision in neither eye can be corrected to better than 20/50 or 20/60 with glasses, further use of them is contraindicated for those in the professions and trades necessitating good far- and near-vision, and the patient may then be advised of surgical removal of one cataract and later the other.

In the infirm and very aged who have no special need for sharp vision but who begin to develop a cataract, usually in both eyes, their distant vision which prior to that was good and their near vision poor for reading without glasses then find that far vision is blurred and near vision better without their glasses than with them. This condition is the second sight which the layman speaks of with pride when it occurs in one of his 80- or 90-year-old progenitors. In many of these cases when the myopia has reached 2.5 to 3 diopters it is better to advise the patient to read without glasses than to attempt to improve his vision esspecially with bifocals. It will be found that he will read surprisingly well with the naked eye. In some of these cases it will be found provident to correct the myopia with distant glasses largely for their own security in going about, advising these patients to dispense with these glasses when reading.

In the case of uniocular cataract with good vision in the fellow eye, surgical intervention is better deferred if and until a similar condition develops in the latter. If done on the cataractous eye, the difference in the refractive indices of the two eyes is so marked that a cataract optical lens before the eye operated upon causes great confusion in the visual quotient. In such a case the patient should be examined from time to time to detect unusual changes in the cataract and to guard against complications that do occur which, should they arise, no matter at what stage the cataract may be, surgical removal of the cataract is indicated.

Some incipient cataracts markedly reduce the vision to such an extent that no help can be given with glasses, despite the facts that the changes in the lens appear to be slight and a good picture of the fundus can be seen with the ophthalmoscope, and no other pathological changes can be found in the eye. Here surgical intervention is indicated. Such cases suggest the presence of diabetes for which a careful search should be made before surgery is attempted.

Occasionally myopia is caused by trauma to the eye. It is usually transient but may persist for a protracted period. If the vision in the fellow eye is normal or good, no attempt need be made to correct the vision of the myopic eye with glasses. The patient is more comfortable if that is not done.

HIP FRACTURES
(From P. 204)

the thin bony cortex from osteoporosis and senility; therefore, in addition to Smith-Petersen nail an intertrochanteric bone plate should also be applied to strengthen the shaft of the femur. This would not be necessary in the usual patient that would remain in bed for two or three months without undue weight upon the leg. These mental patients as a rule will start walking as soon as they are permitted to have any movement and they should have extra support until adequate callus has formed. There is no definite time for these patients to be permitted up as they will get out of bed at the first opportunity and start walking. Many of them are up and about in two or three weeks without any complaint whatsoever of pain in their hip. It seems that they do not respond to pain as the usual patient; therefore, it is probably valuable to their general condition that they get up, for their remaining in bed without response to sensation would lead to pressure-necrosis of soft tissue in a large percentage of the cases.

HOLD THE LINE
(From P. 209)

DR. JOHNSON: I am just a Yankee from Buffalo. I did have the good fortune to marry a girl from Chattanooga, and she has been trying to get rid of me ever since, but I'm holding on.

I feel pretty strongly about the Magner-Murray Bill. I'd like to take this opportunity to say that it seems a good opportunity for the medical profession to join hands and get the North and the South a little closer together. We have been apart too long and from all I can find out, it is based on a misunderstanding about the negro situation, which is blamed on the North; but as far as I can understand, it should be blamed on Eleanor.

Speaking of the Jewish situation, in the South it is not a big problem. It is a big problem in New York State. We have about 40,000 Jewish doctors, refugees. We feel it is only by joining the forces of doctors in the South and doctors in the North, not Jewish refugees, that we can defeat this bill, and it would seem to me that it is high time that the North and the South, Democrats and Republicans, got together for mutual defense against Socialism of Medicine and everything else. I hope that we can get together. If we do, we are going to beat this bill, and referring to what the essayist said about the fact that sick persons should be taken care of, I believe there is one who is mentally sick should be confined and that would help solve the situation. Women should have a place in our Government, but I don't like to have them run it.

DR. WILLIAMS (closing): I appreciate those kind remarks. I think most of us are lined up about the same. It is time to agree on what we are to do about it, and then do it with our might. One is going in one direction and one in another and few are paying proper attention to the threat to the foundations of our government. It has finally got to the place where we have got to do something or else they are going to do something with us, as doctors and as citizens.

GYNECOLOGY

For this issue EUGENE L. LOWENBERG, M.D., F.A.C.S.
Norfolk, Virginia
From the Gynecological Department of
Norfolk General Hospital

ECZEMA-DERMATITIS OF THE EXTERNAL GENITALIA*

ECZEMA-DERMATITIS is a non-contagious inflammation of the skin, accompanied by itching and burning and characterized by erythema, papules, vesicles or a combination of these lesions, with a varying amount of secondary infection and of infiltration and thickening.

It is most commonly encountered of all skin diseases and as such is rightly a dermatological problem. Our interest comes from the fact that women habitually consult their family physician or gynecologist when anything goes wrong with their "female organs." The dermatologist is hardly better prepared to handle the gynecological aspects of the problem than we are to deal intelligently with the cutaneous manifestations.

ETIOLOGY

Two essential factors enter into the production of eczema-dermatitis of the external genitalia, (1) an especially receptive or sensitive skin or predis-

I am deeply indebted to my close associate, Dr. James Anderson, for direct advice in preparing this paper. Dr. Marion B. Sulzberger, in personal correspondence, has given helpful sources of information. Acknowledgement is also given to W. B. Saunders Company for permissison to quote from their *Manual of Dermatology*, by Pillsbury, Sulzberger and Livingood.

*Condensation of paper presented to the Seaboard Medical Association, meeting at Richmond, December, 1943.

posing cause, and (2) one or more irritant or exciting causes which may or may not be known.

PREDISPOSING CAUSES
(Modified from Stokes)

1. Allergic family background
2. Familial susceptibility to pyogenic infection
3. Personal susceptibility to pathologic synergism between allergy and pyogenic infection
4. The ichthyotic or dry skin—susceptible to soap
5. The seborrheic or oily skin
6. Excessive sweating
7. Skin hydration from high-carbohydrate and high-alcohol intake
8. Skin edema from any cause
9. Obesity—causing chafing
10. Certain medical or constitutional diseases.

EXCITING CAUSES

1. Infection — trichomonas, fungus infection (ringworm), oidium, erythrasma, pyogenic microörganisms
2. Drug allergy (iodides, bromides, barbiturates)
3. Food allergy
4. Emotional upsets, premenstrual tension
5. Intercurrent infections—especially sinus, respiratory and gastrointestinal upsets
6. Contact hypersensitivity to soap, chemicals, rubber, drugs, clothing, dust, plants, leather, toilet paper.

DIAGNOSIS

Contact Allergy: Exhaustively question regarding contacts, using prepared lists of allergens as guide. History of repeated flare-ups is significant. Limits of the lesion may be suggestive. Look for evidence of contact allergy elsewhere on skin—neck, waist-line, wrists, ankles. Patch-test with suspected materials using for this an area close to the affected (localized sensitivity). Prove the cause by removing the suspected contact allergen for 10 days, then using it again.

For the patch test apply a ⅛ to ¼-inch square of the suspected article, or the suspected fluids or greases or powdery scrapings or fillings on a square of white linen or cotton cloth, to ⅛ to ¼-inch of normal skin. Cover with a ¼- to ½-inch square of impermeable matter (oiled silk, gutta percha) and hold both in place with a somewhat larger piece of adhesive tape or scotch tape. Remove and read the tests after 24 to 48 hours. Don't test during acute stage. Clothing and objects of daily use can be applied directly, other substances only in concentrations of known safe dilution.

Trichomonas infestation: The characteristic white frothy discharge and the finding of the organism in the hanging-drop examination.

Pellagrous dermatitis: Symmetrical bilateral lesions, separated from healthy skin by sharp line of demarcation. Look for a sunburn-like rash of face and arms, glossitis and stomatitis, systemic manifestations of "B" complex deficiency.

Fungous infection: a. Tinea (ringworm) characteristically circinate lesion, with central clearing and vesicular or scaly borders; apt to involve the upper, inner surface of thighs, buttocks, interglu-teal folds and perianal region. The diagnosis may be obscured by treatment, giving the picture of contact dermatitis. Ringworm infection may also be found on the feet. The organism can be demonstrated in KOH preparation under the microscope. Technique: Place material scraped from the periphery of the lesion on a glass, add a few drops of 10 to 20 per cent KOH and cover with a coverslip, heat slightly to aid clearing and examine for mycelia and spores in 30 minutes. The monilia or oidium lesion is sharply defined with slightly weeping, deep red, desquamating skin. Inoculation of opposing surfaces is characteristic. Vaginal monilia infection (thrush) may coëxist, with white patches on the mucous membrane and a thick, yellowish white discharge.

Erythrasma: Rare, usually a reddish, yellowish or brownish macular eruption confined to the genitocrural and axillary regions. Resembles tinea versicolor except for its characteristic reddish to yellowish brown color. The vegetable parasite microsporon minutissimum can be demonstrated under the microscope in a KOH preparation.

Seborrheic dermatitis: Eczematous changes in oily areas of skin-scalp, presternal region, interscapular region, gluteal folds, groins. The affected areas are greasy, slightly yellow, scaling. Acne or superficial pyoderma may coëxist. Seborrhea is a background for monilia or other yeast infections, superficial ringworm infection, heat rashes, chronic eczematous dermatitis. Seborrheics do not tolerate greasy ointments well.

Eczematized or seborrheic dermatitis—like psoriasis: Like seborrheic dermatitis except that scales may be dryer and more whitish and lesions of psoriasis may be found elsewhere.

Secondary infection of eczema-dermatitis: There is fever, local pain, lymphangitis and lymphadenitis. Pustules, pus and impetiginization are observed in the lesion.

SYMPTOMS AND SIGNS

Acute stage: The affected parts (labia, mons veneris, clitoris, skin or groin, thigh, perineal region) are edematous and reddened as in acute inflammation. Oozing, even weeping, denudation, blistering are present. The parts are extremely sensitive. Vaginal discharge often.

Subacute stage: Edema is slight or absent. The skin is a dull red. No oozing, weeping or vesicles. Excoriation from scratching in almost every instance. Papules, scales and crusts may be seen. Much of the sensitiveness of the skin is gone.

Chronic stage: The skin is dry, thickened, leathery, hardened, pigmented and brownish. The dull appearance is characteristic.

HISTORY RECORD

Symptoms inquired into as to:
Burning, itching, pain, ardor urinae, duration, family

history of allergy, appearance of eruption at onset, any previous attacks, history of allergy, skin lesions elsewhere on body, recent nervous shock or worry, sugar in urine, skin usually dry, oily, vaginal discharge.

Have you or anyone else applied any local remedies, special prescriptions, proprietary preparations? Which? When?

Do you scratch the parts?

Taken any medicine internally, for bowels, nerves, etc.?

Do you know of any foods that aggravate the condition?

EXAMINATION

Parts involved: external genitalia, thighs, anal region.

Dermatological: acute, subacute or chronic; lesions of other dermatologic entities.

Specificity: a. trichomonas; b. monilia, in vaginal discharge; c. central clearing of ringworm.

Diagnostic lesions: a. ringworm of feet, hands under breasts and elsewhere; b. pellagrous rash on arms, face; c. seborrhea on chest, back, scalp; d. contact allergic rash on wrists, neck.

Special tests: a. of scrapings for mycelia of ringworm; b. intradermal trichophyton test (in chronic stage only); c. culture on special media for monilia; d. patch tests (in chronic stage only); e. urine and blood sugar, glucose tolerance test; f. Wassermann.

TENTATIVE DIAGNOSIS

1. Eczema-dermatitis of unknown etiology.
2. Eczema-dermatitis of known etiology—infestations, allergies, vitamin deficiencies, physical agents.

TREATMENT
SYSTEMIC THERAPY

1. Rest, psychotherapy, catharsis
2. Non-allergic diets (elimination diets)
3. Vitamin therapy
4. Estrogenic therapy, locally or parentally in senile caginitis and pruritus vulvae
5. Dyhydration:
   a. Dilute HCl or acidulin by mouth and acid-ash diet
   b. Reduce carbohydrates
   c. Restrict fruits, fruit juices and soft drinks
   d. Stop alcohol.
6. Calcium gluconate by vein and mouth
7. 10 c.c. of patient's own blood intramuscularly
8. Insulin and diet for diabetes.

DIRECTIONS TO PATIENTS

a. No soap-and-water cleansing; use Tersus (Doak) or Acidolate.
b. Make all tub baths less irritating by the addition of bran or oatmeal (½ lb.) or boiled starch (1 lb.) The bath should be tepid, neither cold nor hot.
c. Cleanse carefully the labial folds and the clitoris.
d. Use "cotton" underwear or none at all. A "T" binder of soft cloth may serve.
e. Absolutely no rubbing or scratching.
f. Insert a cotton plug or tampax into the vagina as needed to prevent any discharge reaching the labia.
g. Use toilet paper from front to back. If paper irritates, use soft cloths instead.
h. No intercourse and keep hands away from the parts.
i. No nail polish, nail lacquer, hair lotions, deodorants.
j. Reduce carbohydrates in diet. Stop fruit juices, soft drinks, alcohol.

THERAPY OF THE ACUTE STAGE

The more acute the lesion the milder and more cautious the therapy. The appearance of the lesion is the guide. Begin with sitz baths, and bland lotions, for a day or so. Then employ sitz baths once or twice daily and wet compresses for 30 minutes or several times daily followed with a soothing lotion. Make no attempt at specific therapy except as to breaking contact with allergens, trichomonas; treating glycosuria, etc. Make no patch, or intradermal trichophytin, tests in this stage. See to it that the prescriptions given for the acute stage contains no possible irritants. If improvement is not prompt, the therapy is too active or the cause has not been removed. Dermatologists get most of their cases because others have applied strong medicaments that have flared up the process. Always test the remedy on a small area before applying it to the entire inflamed skin.

1. The Sitz Baths:
   a. Corn starch baths (soothing)—½ to 1 lb. of corn starch boiled to make soluble and added to a tubful of water.
   b. Bran bath—very hot water is run over a cheesecloth bag containing ½ to 1 lb. of oatmeal bran. Complete the filling of the tub with lukewarm water.
   c. $KMnO_4$ (soothing, disinfectant, toughening). One 5 gr. tablet to 3 quarts water equals a 1:9,000 solution.
2. Wet Dressings:
   a. Milk, or 1 dram of Burow's solution to a pint of milk.
   b. Burow's solution (begin with a 1:20 dilution). Boric acid solution.
   d. $KMnO_4$ solution 1:9,000 to 1:1,000.
   e. $AgNO_3$ solution ¼% to 1%.
3. Bland Shake Lotion:

Rx Phenol 2%	2.5
Tragacanth 1%	1.2
Zinc oxide 6%	7.0
Calamine 6%	7.0
Olive oil 33 1/3%	40.0
Distilled water qs ad	120.0

   Sig: Apply with a flat paint brush every 3 or 4 hours.

Open dressings are more soothing and allay the itching better than closed dressings. Use soft pieces of cloth rather than gauze or cotton, partly wrung-out and applied soppy but not running. Change q 2 to 4 h. It is often advisable to leave off the wet dressings during the sleeping hours, applying a soothing lotion.

LOCAL TREATMENT OF SUBACUTE STAGE

Principle: Shake lotions and bland soothing pastes and ointments, with or without the addition of anti-inflammatory ingredients.

Shake lotion listed for the acute stage, or one of these Rxs.

Rx Zinc oxide	50.0
Talc	50.0
Bentonite	10.0
Petrolatum	60.0
Camphor	1.0
Menthol	1.0
M.	

Sig: Apply to inflamed areas twice daily, cover with a sprinkle of talcum powder.

Rx Boric acid cream	5.0
Menthol	0.25
Phenol	0.5

Ung. Aq. Rosa ps......................100.0
M.
Sig: Apply to inflamed area twice daily.
Rx Liquor carbonis detergens............ 5.0
  Benzocaine 5.0
  Calamine liniment (N. F.) qs....100.0
M.
Sig: Apply to inflamed areas twice daily.
Rx Ichthyol 8.0
  Glycerine 16.0
  Rose water 16.0
M.
Sig: Apply to inflamed areas twice daily.

The pyogenic infections of eczema-dermatitis are apt to yield to $KMnO_4$ (1:20,000 to 1:4,500) as sitz baths or wet dressings, or $AgNO_3$ (0.1 to 0.5%) as wet compresses, or sulfonamide emulsions or ointments.

LOCAL TREATMENT OF CHRONIC STAGE

Principle: Therapeutic applications that contain active ingredients, parasiticidal and keratolytic.

Note: Try medicaments on small area first. Skin may be intolerant to any active medicament.

Calamine liniment, coal tar, benzocaine.
Ichthyol and zinc oxide ointment.
Crude coal tar paste.

Rx Crude coal tar 4.0
  Zinc oxide 4.0
  Castor oil 4.0
  Corn starch 30.0
  Petrolatum 26.0

Mix tar with castor oil and add zinc oxide, mix well and let stand 24 hours, mix corn starch with petrolatum. Combine the two mixtures and triturate until smooth.

Rx Liquor carbonis detergents....drams ½
  Lanolin
  Olive oil   aa ....ounces 1
M.
Sig: Apply locally twice daily.

Refractory cases may require x-rays.

TREATMENT OF CHRONIC FUNGUS INFECTION

Ringworm (Tinea Cruris):

Pragmatar ointment (sulfur, salicylic acid and tar).

Constellani's paint (basic fuchsin and resorcin—use diluted with equal parts of water first).

Rx Thymol ....grs. 5
  Phenol ....m 10
  Ung. picis liquid ....drams 1
  Cold cream ointment qs..........ounce 1
Use to paint area.

Monilia (Yeast Vulvitis, Thrush):

Note: Common in diabetes.

Rx 2% Aqueous solution Gentian Violet
Sig: Apply morning and night for 10 to 14 days until exfoliation occurs.

Rx Lugol's solution ¼ of 1%
Sig: Paint vagina once weekly.

Rx Hesseltine's capsules (0.125 gm. of mixture of potassium iodide and potassium iodate)
Sig: Insert one capsule in vagina nightly.

FLARE-UP UNDER MEDICATION

Bland sitz baths. Wet compresses of dilute Burow's solution or boric acid alternating with application of soothing shake lotion.

PRURITUS VULVAE

This may be a symptom of eczema-dermatitis, or of trichomonas, pin-worm, acarus, pediculus or other infestation. It may be due to atrophy or dryness of skin, senile vaginitis, menopausal pruritus, diabetes, jaundice, leukemia.

Rx Zinc oxide 20.0
  Talc 20.0
  Glycerine 15.0
  Water 70.0
  Menthol 0.5
  Phenol 0.5

$KMnO_4$ (1:9,000) sitz baths are very effective. Subcutaneous injections of 1:3,000 HCl or 95% alcohol.

Estrogenic therapy (in natural or artificial menopause, senile vaginitis, kraurosis vulvae, atrophic vaginitis)

a. Apply locally 30 c.c. of an ointment with lanolin base containing 10 mg. diethyl stilbestrol per 30 c.c. of ointment.

b. Stilbestrol in oil inunctions (Wharton).

c. Estrogen per os or parenterally.

Adequate management of diabetes.

Therapeutic test for pin-worm—Enseals of Gentian Violet (0.06 gm.) t.i.d. for 8 days.

X-ray therapy.

Conclusion

As concomitant gynecological problems cause the patient with eczema-dermatitis of the external genitalia to consult her family physician or a gynecologist, it behooves us all to understand the principles of its therapy.

The guide to treatment is the appearance of the inflamed parts. The more acute the lesion, the milder must be the medicament. All cases are treated similarly during the acute stage, without regard to cause. The dictum should be "do no harm"—soothe the parts into quiescence, and later cautiously apply more sharply focused causal or specific therapy. Consultation and collaboration with a dermatologist should be routine in the more severe cases.

SUMMER DIARRHEA IN BABIES

Casec (calcium caseinate), which is almost wholly a combination of protein and calcium, offers a quickly effective method of treating all types of diarrhea, both in bottle-fed and breast-fed infants. For the former, the carbohydrate is temporarily omitted from the 24-hour formula and replaced with 8 level tablespoonsful of Casec. Within a day or two the diarrhea will usually be arrested and carbohydrate in the form of Dextri-Maltose may safely be added to the formula and the Casec gradually reduced till none remains. Three to six teaspoonsful of a thin paste of Casec and water, given before each nursing, is well indicated for loose stools in breast-fed babies.

Please send for samples to Mead Johnson & Company, Evansville, Indiana.

THERAPEUTICS

J. F. NASH, M.D., *Editor*, Saint Pauls, N. C.

TWO CASES OF INFLAMMATORY AND ARTERIOSCLEROTIC HEART DISEASE

Two cases are outlined[1] in both of which the cause of death as determined by necropsy, escaped clinical recognition while the disease was diagnosed correctly. The lessons taught may well find application in our practice.

A 25-year-old white woman complained of palpitation, muscular pains, fever of 101° for one month. She had been hospitalized on several occasions with the diagnosis of organic heart disease. No history of rheumatic fever. Systolic and diastolic murmurs were heard over the apex. Petechiae were present under the fingernails, a slight anemia, leucocytes 18,850. Blood culture disclosed streptococcus viridans. B. p. 118/50. Sulfadiazine was given repeatedly. A week before death pain was felt in the left leg and no pulsation in the dorsalis pedis. Moist rales developed in the chest and the patient expired.

Diagnosis was subacute bacterial endocarditis.

Autopsy: A few petechial hemorrhages in the conjunctivae, face slightly cyanotic. Pleural cavities 500 c.c. clear liquid, peritoneum 800 c.c. Heart enlarged (350 gms.), mitral leaflets thickening along line of closure, chordae tendinae thickened and in part fused, a few grayish vegetations up to 2 mm. on the thickened areas. On left and posterior aortic cusps luxuriant grayish-brown vegetations up to 1.0 cm. Vegetations also on adjacent endocardium of interventricular septum. Minute ulcerations throughout the free margins of the cusps adjacent to the vegetations, few white fibrous ridges were present on endocardium of the i.-v. septum. Myocardium gray, a few yellowish and white dots irregularly throughout the cut surface.

Liver 1600 gms., chronic passive hyperemia; in middle of the right lobe, a cyst-like structure 1.5 cm. in diameter contained reddish-gray (thrombotic) material, communicated with hepatic artery. Spleen enlarged (300 gms.), firm, several infarcts, chronic passive hyperemia, acute hyperplasia. Kidneys, cloudy swelling and passive hyperemia.

In the left popliteal space was a grayish-brown embolus adherent to the wall and completely occluding the lumen of the popliteal artery.

1. O. Saphir, Chicago, in *Ill. Med. Jl.*, April.

Diffuse cloudy swelling of the fibers of the myocardium, with foci of early fatty degeneration. Several small and larger infarcts. Small emboli in various stages of organization within the smaller branches of the coronary arteries. No Aschoff bodies or remnants of Aschoff bodies encountered, nor any perivascular fibrosis.

Clinical diagnosis subacute bacterial endocarditis likely superimposed upon a rheumatic endocarditis with death from sepsis. The diagnosis was verified but it seems obvious that the patient did not die as the result of sepsis but of heart failure, brought about by the multiple myocardial infarcts and myocarditis.

A 66-year-old white man entered complaining of dull abdominal pain and back pain, vomiting and constipation with cramp-like pain in the right lower quadrant; history of coronary thrombosis six years ago, since then anginal attacks at irregular intervals. Thrombosis of the femoral artery with amputation of the right leg nine months before his death. Partial prostatectomy 13 years ago. Regular heart rhythm, rate 78, b. p. 110/74, heart enlarged to the left. Moderate spasm of the abdominal muscles and tenderness over the right side; 24 hours after admission severe pain in the region of the right hip followed by collapse; b. p. at this time 0. In spite of heroic measures, the patient expired one-half hour later. Death thought to be due to pulmonary embolus, coronary thrombosis, or abdominal hemorrhage.

A large amount of partially liquid and partially clotted blood was found encasing the descending aorta, right kidney and right suprarenal; also along both common iliac arteries. Heart enlarged (450 gms.), an old aneurysm (4 cm.) in the apical portion of the left ventricle, extending to the adjacent interventricular septum. Coronary arteries showed arteriosclerosis with occlusion of the anterior descending branch of the left, a number of severely narrowed portions in other coronary branches, no recent thrombus. The aorta was the seat of a severe arteriosclerosis with many areas of hyalinization, calcification, and atheromatous ulcers. Two cm. proximal to the bifurcation into the common iliac arteries was a large saccular aneurysm filled with lamellated thrombi, communicating with the retroperitoneal space. There were two similar, though smaller, aneurysms in the uppermost portions of both common iliac arteries, and two smaller ones in both internal iliac arteries. Grossly, no changes were found in the residual prostate, but on microscopic examination in one area structures lined by one or two layers of cuboidal cells, which showed marked anaplasia, many atypical mitotic figures—early adenocarcinoma.

(To Page 223)

SOUTHERN MEDICINE & SURGERY

Official Organ

JAMES M. NORTHINGTON, M.D., *Editor*

Department Editors

Human Behavior
JAMES K. HALL, M.D. .... Richmond, Va.

Orthopedic Surgery
JOHN T. SAUNDERS, M.D. .... Asheville, N. C.

Urology
RAYMOND THOMPSON, M.D. .... Charlotte, N. C.

Surgery
GEO. H. BUNCH, M.D. .... Columbia, S. C.

Obstetrics
HENRY J. LANGSTON, M.D. .... Danville, Va

Gynecology
CHAS. R. ROBINS, M.D. .... Richmond, Va.
ROBERT T. FERGUSON, M.D. .... Charlotte, N. C.

General Practice
J. L. HAMNER, M.D. .... Mannboro, Va.

Clinical Chemistry and Microscopy
J. M. FEDER, M.D.,
EVELYN TRIBBLE, M. T. } .... Anderson, S. C.

Hospitals
R. B. DAVIS, M.D. .... Greensboro, N. C.

Cardiology
CLYDE M. GILMORE, A.B., M.D. .... Greensboro, N. C.

Public Health
N. THOS. ENNETT, M.D. .... Greenville, N. C.

Radiology
R. H. LAFFERTY, M.D., and Associates .... Charlotte, N. C.

Therapeutics
J. F. NASH, M.D. .... Saint Pauls, N. C.

Tuberculosis
JOHN DONNELLY, M.D. .... Charlotte, N. C.

Dentistry
J. H. GUION, D.D.S. .... Charlotte, N. C.

Internal Medicine
GEORGE R. WILKINSON, M.D. .... Greenville, S. C.

Ophthalmology
HERBERT C. NEBLETT, M.D. .... Charlotte, N. C.

Rhino-Oto-Laryngology
CLAY W. EVATT, M.D. .... Charleston, S. C.

Proctology
RUSSELL VON L. BUXTON, M.D. .... Newport News, Va.

Insurance Medicine
H. F. STARR, M.D. .... Greensboro, N. C.

Dermatology
J. LAMAR CALLAWAY, M.D. .... Durham, N. C.

Pediatrics

Offerings for the pages of this Journal are requested and given careful consideration in each case. Manuscripts not found suitable for our use will not be returned unless author encloses postage

As is true of most Medical Journals, all costs of cuts, etc., for illustrating an article must be borne by the author.

MEDICINE IS NOT GUILTY

What's come to perfection perishes.—R. Browning.

THE starry-eyed would-be re-e-formers of everything in the heavens above, in the earth beneath, and in the waters under the earth, and of things medical in particular, never tire of pointing to the records of rejection under the Selective Service System. Scandalous is about the mildest word they use in describing the situation, and they accuse Doctors of Medicine of allowing or causing this situation to develop. It is one of their stock arguments for Socialized Medicine. Not a little of this has its origin in absurd reasoning of certain members of the profession, a good many of them on Government payrolls.

Let us consider briefly certain statements of the Chief, Medical Division, Selective Service System, as republished in May.[1]

All of us will agree with the statement that "reliable statistics on remediable diseases are not readily available." The Chief accepts as the best data those of October, 1941, to March, 1942. He gives a chart of "proportion of rejected registrants with correctible defects, by type of defect." According to this chart hernia is responsible for 27 per cent; conditions of teeth, mouth and gums for 19 per cent; venereal diseases for 14 per cent; underweight for 13 per cent. Other percentages: musculo-skeletal conditions 6; nose and throat conditions 4; genito-urinary conditions 4; varicose veins 2½; cancers and tumors 2½. The remainder of the rejections are attributed to eye and skin conditions, and "other."

As he himself says "it is of interest that the first three defects listed—hernia, dental defects and venereal diseases—account for 65 per cent of those regarded as correctible." But he does not call attention to these obvious facts: (1) nobody knows how to prevent hernia, nor how to induce anything like all those having hernia to submit to operation; (2) nobody knows how to prevent dental decay, or to induce all those in need of dental treatment, even all those fully able to pay for it, to have their teeth kept in condition acceptable to the Armed Forces; (3) everybody knows that no human agency can keep young men from contracting venereal disease.

To correct is to free from fault. Underweight for which no causative disease condition could be found, was most likely a family peculiarity, in no sense a disease except to those who do not distinguish between the abnormal and the pathological. The strong presumption is that, despite the cocksureness of the Chief, had the condition been rem-

---
[1] "Correctible Defects at Selective Service Age," by Leonard G. Rowntree, M.D., Colonel, M.R.C., in *Medical Annals District of Columbia*, May.

cd.able (a better word), it would have been remedied long ago. We dearly love to be standardized. From a standardized cradle to a standardized coffin, we are hurried, flurried, worried and buried.

One can but wonder as to the nature of the musculo-skeletal, nose and throat, and genito-urinary conditions which make up 14 per cent of these "correctible" causes for rejection. Most likely most of these are developmental, and about as amenable to human control as the movements of Mars.

Varicose veins in one part betoken a weakness of the veins in general. It is highly improbable that 10 per cent of those rejected could be made acceptable for the Armed Forces by the exercise of the best skill of the surgeon. If anybody knows any way of preventing the development of varicosities he should pass it along.

Cancer still kills most of those it attacks, despite the best efforts of the best doctors. It is axiomatic that the younger the cancer patient the less the chance of cure. Can any one conceive of a greater absurdity than stating that cancer in the selectees is "correctible"? As to the other "tumors," most likely they caused no discomfort, and were therefore disregarded—perhaps wisely.

Obviously, so vague a label as "other" offers no opportunity for refutation.

In a tabulation of "principal causes of rejections of registrants 18-37 years of age in class 4-F as of January 1st, 1944, educational deficiency is given as a cause in 10.4 per cent of the cases, mental disease in 14.5, mental deficiency in 3.3 —non-medical causes 1.1.

The Chief makes this remarkable statement: "illiteracy, while not strickly speaking a medical problem, is to say the least a close relative of disease"; and he excludes the rejections for this cause from the "non-medical" causes in the table! Verily, "Ignorance is the curse of God, Knowledge the wing wherewith we fly to Heaven."

The figures given for rejections because of educational and mental deficiency, and mental disease —all three listed as medical causes, and by implication the fault of Doctors of Medicine—add up to 28.2 per cent. Maybe our vanity should be gratified at having doctors thought to have the knowledge and the power to adequately instruct the whole population, to raze out the written troubles of the brain and to give ripe wits to fools. Certainly nothing in the implication deserves serious consideration or comment.

The Chief arrives at the following conclusions:
1. The present health situation in the Nation is unsatisfactory from the standpoint of procurement of manpower for the fighting forces and, to a lesser extent, for industry.

2. In order to meet their manpower needs, the armed forces in the midst of war have been compelled to shoulder the burden for the remedy of correctible defects of those accepted for military service.

3. Though this country has elected to become the arsenal of democracy, large numbers of defectives, now numbering some four million, are denied military service, and are being turned over to labor and industry without adequate provision for the care of their correctible defects.

Of course the health situation is unsatisfactory. Satisfaction is one of the strong words. Philosophers have always held anything short of perfection to be unsatisfactory. Witness the King James Version, the greatest of authorities on our language: "I shall be satisfied when I awake in His likeness."

Most of these defects are correctible by the Land of Omnipotence only.

This country has not elected to become the arsenal of democracy. Every member of the British Commonwealth, Russia, China and a good many other countries share this burden and this honor. To attempt to claim a higher merit than our allies is as absurd as to say the heart is the most important organ in the body. Life cannot go on without a liver, or without a kidney, or without a pancreas, or without a gastrointestinal tube, or without a suprarenal gland, or without some sort of a brain. Manifestly, no organ can be more important than any one organ without which life could not be continued.

Disparagement of any one of our allies in this life-and-death struggle brings to mind the words of Talleyrand, "It's worse than a crime; it's a blunder."

Medicine is not directly accused; but, inasmuch as these figures have been used over and over again to support arguments for a radical change in the way of rendering medical care, it should have been expressly stated that Medicine is not responsible for these rejections.

Further, the statement that these conditions are medical and correctible naturally suggests that, if Doctors of Medicine did their duty, the conditions would be corrected.

Toward the end of this remarkable article, the author tells us that:

"Experience has demonstrated society's incapacity and failure to solve the problem of correctible disease. Because of the compelling need for manpower, the military establishment has found it expedient to assume responsibilities for leadership in rehabilitation and cure of most of our correctible defects."

Since the military establishment is a part of society, obviously the blame is being placed on Medicine. It is Medicine that is coolly accused of "failure to solve the problem of correctible disease."

It will be interesting and instructive to read about the correction by the military establishment, even under the exercise of the extraordinary powers conferred on and assumed by the Commander-in-Chief, of the defects listed by his Chief, Medical Division, Selective Service System, as "correctible." There is such a thing as self-confidence amounting to the miraculous.

And the same may appropriately be said of pretty nearly every statement in the article under discussion.

Medicine has not been weighed in the balance and found wanting.

Doctors of Medicine have done and are doing their jobs far-and-away better than any other group.

We have never professed to be miracle-workers.

THERAPEUTICS
(From P. 220)

The principle disease in this patient was the generalized arteriosclerosis with coronary sclerosis and resulting myocardial infarction, diagnosed clinically angina pectoris. Arteriosclerosis had produced an occlusion of the femoral and gangrene of the leg had necessitated amputation; atheromatosis in the descending abdominal aorta; atheromatous ulcers and aneurysm had ruptured and caused the death of the patient. A moderate hemorrhage, occurring 24 hours before his death, brought the patient to the hospital. The final hemorrhage occurred ½ hour before death. No evidence of syphilis was found at autopsy.

The early carcinoma of the prostate was of no importance.

Borrowed From the Illinois Medical Journal

A political plum—one result of careful grafting.

Sitizens—those who are not doing much for the War Effort.—*Liberty*.

Sissy—the guy who quits the O. P. A. to join the Commandos!—*Calgary Herald*.

Wickedness—a myth invented by good people to account for the attractiveness of others.—*Hobo News*.

Shot—that which, if some people have more than one, they're half.—*Louisville Courier*.

THE AMERICAN CONGRESS OF PHYSICAL THERAPY will hold its 23d annual scientific and clinical session September 6th-19th at the Hotel Statler, Cleveland. The annual instruction course will be held from 8 to 10:30 a. m., and from 1 to 2 p. m. during the days of September 6th, 7th and 8th. The didactic and clinical sessions will be given on the remaining portions of these days and evenings. All of these sessions will be open to the members of the regular medical profession and their qualified aids. For information concerning the instruction course and program of the convention proper, address the American Congress of Physical Therapy, 30 North Michigan Avenue, Chicago 2.

NEWS

McGUIRE HOSPITAL EVACUATION CENTER

McGuire General Hospital has recently been designated by the War Department as an evacuation center for army sick and wounded returning from overseas. The first consignment of patients, about 250, is expected by June 20th.

The new 1784-bed army hospital, under construction since last August, will serve the Hampton Roads Port of Debarkation, Newport News. Patients will be transported from shipside to receiving wards aboard specially constructed trains and in ambulances. As soon as they have been examined and declared capable of further travel they will be entrained to medical installations nearer their homes or to localities of their own choice, provided that such general hospitals have the necessary bed space and medical facilities to meet the needs of the patient.

Upon arrival at McGuire General Hospital, the patients will be examined to determine whether they are in need of general medicine, general surgery, thoracic surgery, plastic surgery, amputations, neurosurgery, etc. Information regarding the patients' requirements will immediately be dispatched to the War Department in Washington, thus facilitating the routing of men to proper hospitals where specialized medical, surgical and dental treatment will be obtained.

If, upon arrival here, the patient is in need of immediate surgical treatment he will be operated upon in one of the six completely equipped operating rooms. However, when consulting surgeons decide there is no need for an immediate operation, the patient will be readied for transfer to a hospital nearer his home.

SISTERS ACQUIRE NEW BERN HOSPITAL

St. Luke's Hospital, which has been serving New Bern, N. C., and vicinity since 1915, was sold early this month by Dr. R. D. V. Jones and Dr. J. F. Patterson to the Sisters of St. Joseph of Newark, a Catholic order of New Jersey. The Sisters have taken over the operation of the institution, along with the newly-completed annex and nurses' home built under a Federal grant of $210,000.

The purchase price for the old hospital was $60,000, of which half was paid by the Catholic Sisters and the other half by the Duke Endowment, of which Dr. W. S. Rankin is Director of the Hospital Section.

SOUTHERN RAILWAY SURGEONS

Dr. J. M. Cox, of Lake City, Tenn., was elected president of the Association of Surgeons of the Southern Railway System at the closing session of a two-day meeting held at Winston-Salem in the last week in May.

Other officers named were Dr. deT. Valk, of Winston-Salem, first vice-president; Dr. John Wilson MacConnell, of Davidson College, second vice-president; Dr. B. S. Lester, of Birmingham, third vice-president; Miss Lillian Youngmans, of the office of the Chief Surgeon, Washington, secretary-treasurer, and Dr. J. Marsh Frere, of Chattanooga, recording secretary.

Dr. Charles O. Bates of Greenville, S. C., retiring president, was elevated to chairmanship of the executive committee.

STAFF MEETING CHARLOTTE MEMORIAL HOSPITAL

Regular monthly meeting of the Visiting Medical Staff held at the hospital Tuesday, May 30th, at 8 p. m. Program.

Signs and Symptoms of the Eye in General Disease, Dr. H. C. Neblett.
Clinical Cases of General Interest, Dr. Frank C. Smith.

Dr. Carl W. White, a native of Danville, has been elected superintendent of Lynchburg State Colony by the State Hospital Board, to succeed Dr. G. B. Arnold, who resigned January 1st. Dr. A. D. Hutton has been acting as superintendent since Dr. Arnold's resignation.

Dr. White took his premedical training at Washington and Lee University, studied medicine for two years at the the University of North Carolina, and received his medical degree at Jefferson Medical College. Following his internship at Presbyterian Hospital in Philadelphia, he spent 13 years in general practice and internal medicine in Narberta, Penn. and then began a study of neuropsychiatry at the University of Pennsylvania. He has held positions at Moose Lake State Hospital and Rochester State Hospital, Minnesota.

The Hospital Board has under consideration the matter of appointing architects to prepare plans for $6,000,000 in expansion and development of Virginia mental institutions.

Dr. J. M. Northington, of Charlotte, spoke before a Lincolnton Luncheon Club meeting on May 23d, on the Proposed Legislation for Socializing Medicine, as a Feature of the Program for Socialization in General.

MARRIED

The wedding of Miss Mary Catherine Campbell, of Doswell, Hanover County, and Dr. John Alexander Wright, Jr., son of Dr. and Mrs. John Alexander Wright, also of Doswell, was solemnized June 3d. After July 1st Dr. and Mrs. Wright will make their home at Doswell.

Dr. Edward Melton Yow, of Henderson, and Dr. Martha Dukes, of Winston-Salem, were married on May 20th.

DIED

Dr. W. A. Harris, who served three terms in the General Assembly as delegate from Fredericksburg and Spotsylvania County, Virginia, died suddenly at his home at Spotsylvania Courthouse May 25th.

The 66 year old physician was prominent for many years in the civic and political life of this section. He had served as county coroner, as secretary of the Board of Public Roads and as County Health Officer. He was formerly a member of the Board of Visitors of Virginia Polytechnic Institute.

Dr. Harris was graduated from the Medical College of Virginia in 1901. He entered the Army Medical Corps in World War 1 and rose to the rank of lieutenant-colonel. He saw active service in France.

Dr. William Turner Wooton, 67, prominent Hot Springs physician and president of the Southern Medical Association, died May 2nd at a St. Louis hospital, where he underwent an operation.

A native of Pottsville, Md., he practiced his profession at Hot Springs, Ark., for the past 42 years.

He was a member of the Army Medical Corps in the Spanish-American War and the Philippine Insurrection, and was a past president of the Arkansas Medical Society.

Dr. George S. Fultz, 66, died May 16th at his home at Butterworth, Dinwiddie County, Va., several hours after he had suffered a heart attack.

Dr. Fultz, a native of Augusta County, was educated at Hampden-Sydney College and at the Medical College of Virginia, where he was graduated in 1905.

He was a member of the American Medical Association, the Southside Virginia Medical Assciation, the Petersburg Medical Faculty, and the Association of Surgeons of the Seaboard Air Line Railway.

Captain Geo. S. Fultz, Jr., Medical Corps U. S. A., is a son.

Dr. J. Edward Harris, 69, lower Shenandoah Valley physician, died at his home at Winchester, Va., May 30th.

He was stricken while on a fishing trip in the county with a friend and was returned to his home where he died shortly after.

A native of Brunswick County, he was a graduate of the College of William and Mary. After graduation at the Medical College of Virginia in 1900, he began his practice at Berryville in 1901, where he remained for several years before coming to Winchester. He was a member of State and National Medical Societies, secretary-treasurer of the Northern Virginia Medical Society, and was secretary of the Winchester Memorial Hospital for many years.

Survivors include a brother, Dr. William L. Harris, of Norfolk.

Dr. Richard Edward Albert died at his home at Portsmouth, Virginia, on May 30th. He was forty-eight and a graduate in medicine of the University of Virginia in the class of 1919.

UNIVERSITY OF VIRGINIA

Dr. William F. Boos of Boston, former lecturer in Toxicology at Harvard Medical School, spoke on the subject Experiences with Capital Poison Cases on April 24th at the meeting of the University Medical Society

Commencement Exercises of the University of Virginia Hospital School of Nursing were held in the afternoon of April 25th. Sixty-five nurses in the University of Virginia School, four affiliates from the Blue Ridge Sanatorium, and eleven affiliates from the Catawba Sanatorium were awarded certificates of graduation. The graduation address was given by Miss Agnes Ohlson, R.N., of the United States Public Health Service.

On May 4th, Dr. Arnoldo Gabladon, Chief of the Division of Malariology of Venezuela and Chairman of the Pan-American Committee on Malaria, spoke before the University Medical Society on Vectors of Malaria in America. He spoke the following day on the subject Antimalarial Organization in Venezuela.

Dr. Henry B. Mulholland, Professor of the Practice of Medicine, spoke at Camp Lee on May 12th to the Medical Officers on Chemotherapy and Respiratory Diseases. On May 13th, he spoke to the Business and Professional Women's Association of the State of Virginia, meeting in Roanoke, on the subject of Medical Care.

The John Horsley Memorial Prize in Medicine in the amount of $600, founded in 1925 by Dr. J. Shelton Horsley of Richmond, Virginia, as a memorial to his father, Mr. John Horsley, of Nelson County, Virginia, was awarded at the time of the annual initiation ceremonies of the University of Virginia Chapter of Sigma Xi, on Thursday, May 11th, to Dr. William Bennett Bean of the Department of Internal Medicine of the University of Cincinnati. The prize is open to all graduates of the De-

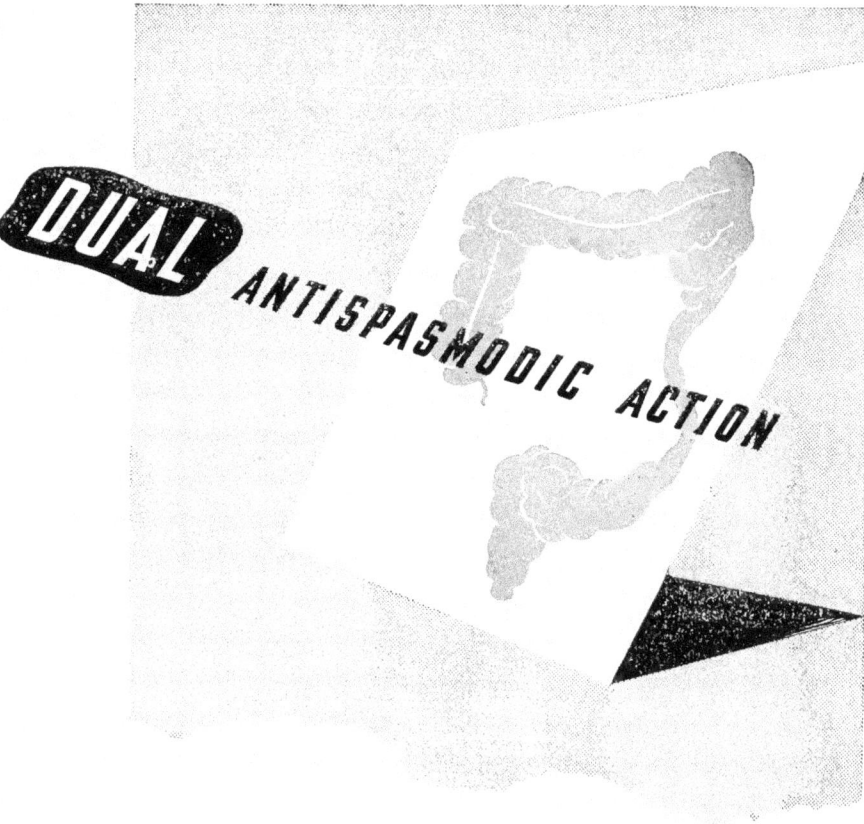

✓ Syntropan 'Roche'—non-narcotic antispasmodic—relaxes smooth muscle spasm by direct action on the muscle cell *and* by exerting an inhibiting influence on the parasympathetic terminations in smooth musculature.

✓ Unlike atropine or belladonna, when Syntropan is given in therapeutic doses, there is very little likelihood of mouth dryness, mydriasis or tachycardia. The dual action plus the wide margin of safety make Syntropan a most effective and desirable antispasmodic. . . . HOFFMANN-LA ROCHE, INC., NUTLEY 10, N. J.

NON-NARCOTIC ANTISPASMODIC *Syntropan* 'ROCHE'

partment of Medicine at the University of Virginia of not more than fifteen years standing, and to former internes of St. Elizabeth's Hospital in Richmond, under the same conditions. Dr. Bean was gradated from the Medical School of the University of Virginia in 1935. He is now on leave of absence, with the commission of Major in the Medical Corps of the United Army, Armored Medical Research Laboratory, Fort Knox, Kentucky. The prize was awarded for a paper on Secondary Pellagra by Drs. William Bennett Bean, Tom Douglas Spies, and Marion A. Blankenhorn, published in the February issue of *Medicine*.

A shy lad wanted to marry the girl, but felt he would choke if he tried to mention the word "marry" or "marriage" to her. So, after giving much thought to the problem, he asked her in a whisper one evening, "Julia, how would you like to be buried with my people?"

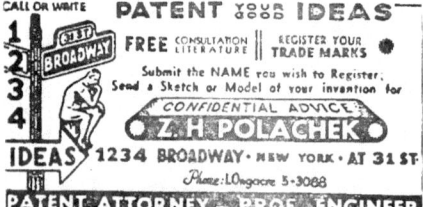

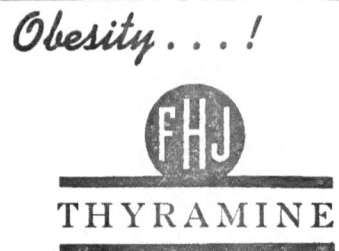

THYRAMINE

Composition

Thyroid 1 gr. Amphetamine sulphate 5 mgs. Thiamin chloride 1 mg. in suitable combinations with physiological reinforcements.

No. 1—One Capsule before breakfast
No. 2—One Capsule before lunch
No. 3—One Capsule at 4 p. m.

Contraindications
Hypertension .... Hyperthyroidism

Supplied
Capsules: Packages 21 and 42 (one or two weeks supply).

—Professional samples on request—
Available: Any professional pharmacy
F. H. J. PRODUCTS
077 East 176th St., New York 60, N. Y.

BOOKS

THE AMERICAN ILLUSTRATED MEDICAL DICTIONARY, by W. A. NEWMAN DORLAND, A.M., M.D., F.A.C.S., Lieut.-Col., M.R.C., U. S. Army; Member of the Committee on Nomenclature and Classification of Diseases of the American Medical Association; Editor of "American Pocket Medical Dictionary." With the Collaboration of E. C. L. Miller, M.D., Medical College of Virginia. Twentieth Edition, Revised and Enlarged. 1668 pages with 885 illustrations, including 240 portraits. Flexible and Stiff Binding. *W. B. Saunders Company*, Philadelphia and London. 1944. Plain $7.00. Thumb-Indexed $7.50.

There was never a time when a dictionary just off the press understanding current medical literature. Since 1900, when the first edition of the American Illustrated received the hearty approbation of the profession, each succeeding edition has better and better met the needs of physicians and surgeons and medical students.

We are told that for the newest edition alterations were found necessary on every page, that many hundreds of entirely new words have been added, with special attention devoted to the vocabulary of war medicine and surgery. The "Standard Nomenclature of Diseases and Operations" has been followed.

However scarce printing materials may be, all of us will rejoice that enough of these were spared for the bringing out of this new edition of "The American Illustrated Medical Dictionary."

MEDICAL DIAGNOSIS, by ROSCOE L. PULLEN, A.B., M.D., Instructor in Medicine, Tulane University of Louisiana School of Medicine; Assistant Clinical Director, Charity Hospital of Louisiana at New Orleans; formerly Fellow in Clinical Endocrinology, Duke University School of Medicine and Duke Hospital, Durham, N. C. With a Foreword by JOHN H. MUSSER, B.S., M.D., F.A.C.P., Professor of Medicine, Tulane University of Louisiana School of Medicine; Senior Visiting Physician, Charity Hospital of Louisiana at New Orleans. 1106 pages with 584 illustrations and 17 colored plates. *W. B. Saunders Company*, Philadelphia and London. 1944. Price $10.00.

As we are reminded in the foreword, most of the books on diagnosis instruct the student in what may be learned by the four classical means of investigation "but the detailed information in the examination of the patient from all other angles is minimal."

The scope and plan of the work may be inferred from the chapter heads: The Medical History; An Introduction to Examination of the Patient; Examination of the Skin; Eyes, Nose, Throat and Ears; Neck; Breasts; Chest; Heart; Abdomen; Extremities; Back, Bones and Joints; Oral; Electrocardiographic; Gynecologic and Obstetric; Urologic; Anorectal Diagnosis; Neurological Examination; Endocrine Survey; Endocrine Survey of Sexual and Reproductive Systems; The Psychiatric Approach; The Differential Diagnosis of Neurosis

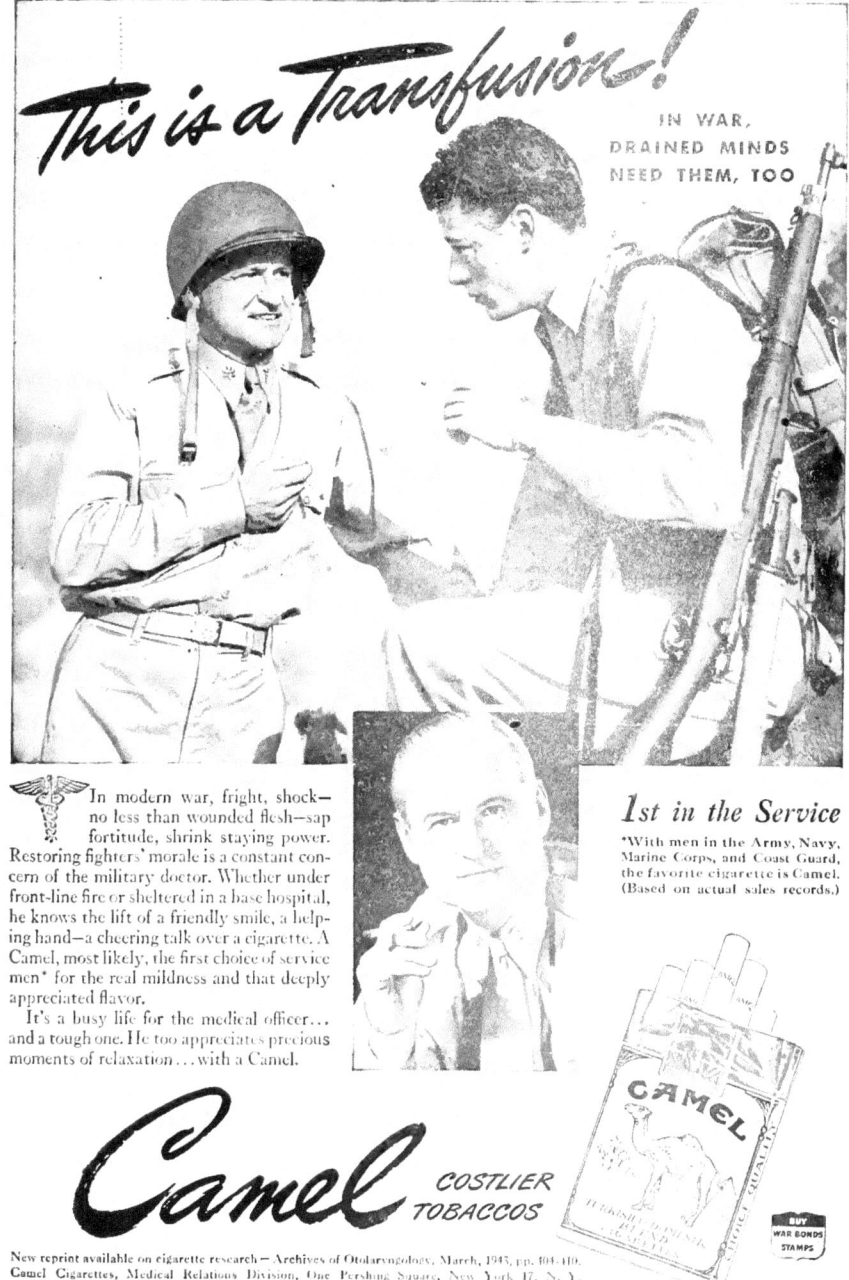

and Psychosis; Practical Mental Measurement; Clinical Electrocephalography; The Differential Diagnosis of the Causes of Coma; Pediatric Physical Diagnosis; The Sterility Survey; Occupational Injury; Military Problems; Determinants of Prognosis.

We can well agree with Dr. Musser that to the doctor who is puzzled by an unusual finding or by unusual association of symptoms, the book is one to be consulted with profit and with the assurance of help in solving his perplexities.

THE MANAGEMENT OF NEUROSYPHILIS, by BERNHARD DATTNER, M.D., Jur.D., Associate Clinical Professor of Neurology, New York University Medical College; with the collaboration of EVAN W. THOMAS, M.D., Assistant Professor of Medicine and of Dermatology and Syphilology, New York University Medical College; and GERTRUDE WEXLER, M.D., Instructor in Dermatology and Syphilology, New York University Medical College. Foreword by JOSEPH EARLE MOORE, M.D., Associate Professor of Medicine, Johns Hopkins University. *Grune & Stratton*, 443 Fourth Ave., New York City. 1944. $5.50.

A survey is made of the various methods now in use in the treatment of victims of syphilis of the central nervous system, and results by the various methods evaluated. The study includes so large a number of cases as to make the conclusions convincing. Diagnostic and therapeutic procedures are detailed sufficiently for the guidance of the practitioner.

Part I describes technic of withdrawal and examination of spinal fluid, with interpretation and evaluation; Part II methods of treatment, application and results.

A study of this book will clarify for the doctor a good deal that is confusingly murky, and bring into agreement a good many seemingly contradictory statements. The robust commonsense as well as the trained experience of the authors is attested by this revealing sentence: "In our opinion the further development of syphilis therapy depends on the close coöperation of the general practitioner, the dermatologist, the internist and the neurologist."

The authors do not paint as rosy a picture as do some, but the picture may be taken as true to life.

THE TREATMENT OF PEPTIC ULCER Based Upon Ten Years' Experience at the New York Hospital, by GEORGE J. HEUER, M.D., Professor of Surgery of Cornell University Medical College and Surgeon-in-Chief of the New York Hospital; assisted by CRANSTON HOLMAN, M.D., Assistant Professor of Clinical Surgery, Cornell University Medical College, and WILLIAM A. COOPER, M.D., Assistant Professor of Clinical Surgery, Cornell University Medical College. *J. B. Lippincott* Company, E. Washington Square, Philadelphia; London; Montreal. 1944. $3.00.

This is a record of the experience of a first-class surgical clinic in the treatment of more than a thousand cases of peptic ulcer, many over a ten-

---

BIPEPSONATE

Calcium Phenolsulphonate .... 2 grains
Sodium Phenolsulphonate .... 2 grains
Zinc Phenolsulphonate, N. F. .... 1 grain
Salol, U. S. P. .... 2 grains
Bismuth Subsalicylate, U. S. P. .... 8 grains
Pepsin, U. S. P. .... 4 grains

Average Dosage

For Children—Half drachm every fifteen minutes for six doses, then every hour until relieved
For Adults—Double the above dose

How Supplied

In Pints, Five-Pints and Gallons to Physicians and Druggists only.

Burwell & Dunn Company

Manufacturing *Pharmacists*
Established *in 1887*

CHARLOTTE, N. C.

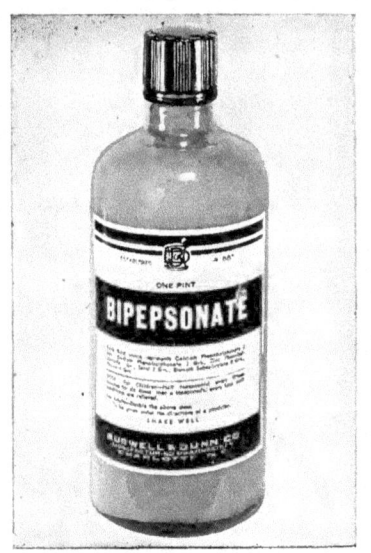

Sample sent to any physician in the U. S. on request

year period, and a summary of the literature on the subject.

The experience is long enough to be of great value in appraising the different methods of management of a condition of interest to every kind of medical and surgical man.

QUARTERLY REVIEW OF SURGERY: HENRY N. HARKINS, M.D., Baltimore, Md., Editor-in-Chief. Published uarterly by *Quarterly Review of Surgery*, 314 Randolph Place, N. E., Washington 2, D. C. $9 per year.

We have received Nos. 1 and 2 of Volume 1 of this timely review. For a surgeon to undertake to read everything that is being written on surgical subjects in the publications of the first order would be to leave himself no time for the practice or teaching of his profession.

As was assured by the personnel of the editorial board, the choice of articles reviewed and the manner of the reviewing proves the wisdom of the decision as to the need, and of the manner of meeting the need.

CHUCKLES

Tempora Mutantur

Sir John Luckley in the latter part of the 17th Century wrote:

Her feet beneath her petticoat
Like little mice stole in and out
As if they feared the light.

If Sir John were alive today, says a distinguished St. Louis doctor, he would have to turn his poetry-writing job over to some modern realist who might say:

Today his best gal's mouselike feet
Mean nothing to her feller,
'Cause even grandma's skimpy skirt
Don't near hide her pateller.

On the Floor

"Bill and Sue were the best looking couple on the floor last night."

"Oh, did you go to a dance last night?"

"No, I went to a cocktail party."

Progress Note

While she was in the knee-chest position she turned to me and said: "Doctor, will you please count my piles carefully; the last doctor told me I had seventeen and I want to know whether I lost or gained any."

"I hear June's marrying a second lieutenant."
"Yeah, the first one got away."

"You told me you had a three-room apartment, but I only saw two rooms."
"Ah, but you didn't see the room for improvement."

In a New Mexico newspaper: "Wanted: Owner of 1940 Buick would like to correspond with widow who has two good tires. Object matrimony. Address 'Old Bachelor' and please enclose picture of the tires."

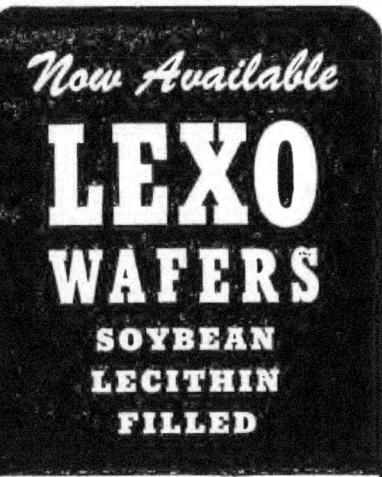

Now Available

LEXO WAFERS

SOYBEAN LECITHIN FILLED

For the Treatment of:

PSORIASIS

HYPERCHOLESTEROLEMIA

POOR INTESTINAL ABSORPTION OF FAT AND FAT-SOLUBLE VITAMINS

LIVER CIRRHOSIS

HEPATIC INSUFFICIENCY

BIBLIOGRAPHY

1. **Adlersberg & Sobotka** (Fat and vitamin A absorption) J. Nutrition, v. 25, No. 3. 2. **Adlersberg & Sobotka.** (Hypercholesterolemia) J. Mt. Sinai Hospital, vol. IX, No. 6. 3. **Goldman.** (Psoriasis) Cincinnati J. Med. vol. 23, No. 4. 4. **Smith, Goldman & Fox.** (Psoriasis) J. Inv. Derm. vol. 5, p. 321. 5. **Gross & Kesten.** (Psoriasis) Arch. Derm. & Syph., vol. 47, p. 159-174. 6. **Kesten.** (Psoriasis) New England J. Med., vol. 228, p. 124. 7. **Hoagland.** (Cirrhosis) N. Y. State J. Med., vol. 43, p. 1041.
8. Pottenger (Dermatoses) Sou. M. J., vol. 37, p. 211.

Write for free samples and information
AMERICAN LECITHIN CO., INC.
ELMHURST, L. I., N. Y., DEPT. 7

GENERAL

Nalle Clinic Building   412 North Church Street, Charlotte
THE NALLE CLINIC
Telephone—C-BVDY (if no answer, call 3-2621)

General Surgery	*General Medicine*
BRODIE C. NALLE, M.D. Gynecology & Obstetrics	LUCIUS G. GAGE, M.D. Diagnosis
EDWARD R. HIPP, M.D. Traumatic Surgery	LUTHER W. KELLY, M.D. Cardio-Respiratory Diseases
*PRESTON NOWLIN, M.D. Urology	J. R. ADAMS, M.D. Diseases of Infants & Children
Consulting Staff R. H. LAFFERTY, M.D. O. D. BAXTER, M.D. Radiology	W. B. MAYER, M.D. Dermatology & Syphilology
W. M. SUMMERVILLE, M.D. Pathology	(*In Country's Service)

| C—H—M MEDICAL OFFICES
DIAGNOSIS—SURGERY
X-RAY—RADIUM
Dr. G. Carlyle Cooke—*Abdominal Surgery
& Gynecology*
Dr. Geo. W. Holmes—*Orthopedics*
Dr. C. H. McCants—*General Surgery*
222-226 Nissen Bldg.   Winston-Salem | WADE CLINIC
Wade Building
Hot Springs National Park, Arkansas

H. King Wade, M.D.   *Urology*
Ernest M. McKenzie, M.D.   *Medicine*
*Frank M. Adams, M.D.   *Medicine*
*Jack Ellis, M.D.   *Medicine*
Bessey H. Shebesta, M.D.   *Medicine*
*Wm. C. Hays, M.D.   *Medicine*
N. B. Burch, M.D.
     Eye, Ear, Nose and Throat
A. W. Scheer   *X-ray Technician*
Etta Wade   *Clinical Laboratory*
Merna Spring   *Clinical Pathology*
(*In Military Service) |

INTERNAL MEDICINE

ARCHIE A. BARRON, M.D., F.A.C.P. *INTERNAL MEDICINE—NEUROLOGY* Professional Bldg. Charlotte	JOHN DONNELLY, M.D. *DISEASES OF THE LUNGS* Medical Building Charlotte
CLYDE M. GILMORE, A.B., M.D. *CARDIOLOGY—INTERNAL MEDICINE* Dixie Building Greensboro	JAMES M. NORTHINGTON, M.D. *INTERNAL MEDICINE—GERIATRICS* Medical Building Charlotte

PROFESSIONAL CARDS

NEUROLOGY and PSYCHIATRY

(Now in the Country's Service)
*J. FRED MERRITT, M.D.
NERVOUS and MILD MENTAL DISEASES
ALCOHOL and DRUG ADDICTIONS
Glenwood Park Sanitarium　　Greensboro

TOM A. WILLIAMS, M.D.
(Neurologist of Washington, D. C.)
Consultation by appointment at
Phone 3994-W
77 Kenilworth Ave.　　Asheville, N. C.

EYE, EAR, NOSE AND THROAT

H. C. NEBLETT, M.D.
OCULIST
Phone 3-5852
Professional Bldg.　　Charlotte

AMZI J. ELLINGTON, M.D.
*DISEASES of the
EYE, EAR, NOSE and THROAT*
Phones: Office 992—Residence 761
Burlington　　North Carolina

UROLOGY, DERMATOLOGY and PROCTOLOGY

THE CROWELL CLINIC of UROLOGY and UROLOGICAL SURGERY
Hours—Nine to Five　　Telephones—3-7101—3-7102
STAFF
ANDREW J. CROWELL, M.D.
(1911-1938)
*ANGUS M. McDONALD, M.D.　　CLAUDE B. SQUIRES, M.D.
Suite 700-711 Professional Building　　Charlotte

RAYMOND THOMPSON, M.D., F.A.C.S.　　WALTER E. DANIEL, A.B., M.D.
THE THOMPSON-DANIEL CLINIC
of
UROLOGY & UROLOGICAL SURGERY
Fifth Floor Professional Bldg.　　Charlotte

C. C. MASSEY, M.D.
*PRACTICE LIMITED
TO
DISEASES OF THE RECTUM*
Professional Bldg.　　Charlotte

WYETT F. SIMPSON, M.D.
GENITO-URINARY DISEASES
Phone 1234
Hot Springs National Park　　Arkansas

ORTHOPEDICS

HERBERT F. MUNT, M.D.
*ACCIDENT SURGERY & ORTHOPEDICS
FRACTURES*
Nissen Building　　Winston-Salem

SURGERY

R. S. ANDERSON, M. D.

GENERAL SURGERY

144 Coast Line Street   Rocky Mount

R. B. DAVIS, M. D., M. M. S., F. A. C. P.
GENERAL SURGERY
AND
RADIUM THERAPY
Hours by Appointment
Piedmont-Memorial Hosp.   Greensboro

(*Now in the Country's Service*)
WILLIAM FRANCIS MARTIN, M.D.
GENERAL SURGERY
Professional Bldg.   Charlotte

OBSTETRICS & GYNECOLOGY

IVAN M. PROCTER, M. D.

OBSTETRICS & GYNECOLOGY

133 Fayetteville Street   Raleigh

SPECIAL NOTICES

TWO LABORATORY TECHNICIANS, being graduated from a High-class Hospital Laboratory, services available January 1st, 1944. Address TECHNICIAN, care *Southern Medicine & Surgery*.

TO THE BUSY DOCTOR WHO WANTS TO PASS HIS EXPERIENCE ON TO OTHERS

You have probably been postponing writing that original contribution. You can do it, and save your time and effort by employing an expert literary assistant to prepare the address, article or book under your direction or relieve you of the details of looking up references, translating, indexing, typing, and the complete preparation of your manuscript.

Address: *WRITING AIDE*, care *Southern Medicine & Surgery*.

THE JOURNAL OF SOUTHERN MEDICINE AND SURGERY

306 NORTH TRYON STREET, CHARLOTTE, N. C.

The Journal assumes no responsibility for the authenticity of opinion or statements made by authors or in communications submitted to this Journal for publication.

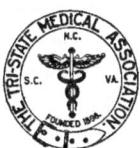

JAMES M. NORTHINGTON, M.D., Editor

VOL. CVI   JULY, 1944   No. 7

Social Adjustment in Obsessive Tension States Following Prefrontal Lobotomy*

JAMES W. WATTS, M.D., F.A.C.S.
AND
WALTER FREEMAN, M.D., Ph.D.
Washington
From the Department of Neurology, George Washington University

OBSESSIVE THINKING and nervous tension are among the commonest symptoms in the neuroses and psychoses.[1] Nervous tension was evident in 98 per cent of the patients upon whom prefrontal lobotomy was performed and obsessive thinking in 94 per cent—and this series includes the involutional depressions and schizophrenias as well as the obsessive tension states.[2] The clinical boundaries of the obsessive ruminative tension states are not well defined. Transitions occur toward schizophrenia on one hand and toward agitated depression on the other.

Wechsler described the compulsive neurotic as "considerably schizoid in character, very little, if at all amenable to persuasion or even suggestion, rather set in his way, meticulous, orderly, punctual, economical if not stingy, and generally of higher intellectual level than the emotionally more labile neurotic."

Prefrontal lobotomy relieves worry, anxiety, apprehension, nervous tension, self-consciousness, and feelings of guilt. Following operation the patient may still have the idea that he has syphilis or tuberculosis or that his ego is contaminated; a woman may look in the mirror and see just as much hair on her face and arms as she had when she thought suicide was the only solution, but if the idea no longer evokes apprehension and nervous tension or self-consciousness, then it loses its importance. The individual can then turn his thoughts and efforts to something useful.

Prefrontal lobotomy consists of cutting the white matter of each frontal lobe in the plane of the coronal suture. This plane passes just anterior to the tip of the frontal horn of the ventricle. Iodized oil has been injected at operation and the depth and extent of the incisions in the frontal lobe have been verified by röntgenograms in nearly all cases. The best results occur when the lobotomy is made in the plane of the coronal suture.[2] When the frontal lobe is incised too far anteriorly, there is usually only temporary relief of mental symptoms. When the incisions are made too far posteriorly in the prefrontal region, there is profound inertia followed by unproductive restlessness. Equally important as the plane of the incisions are the depth and extent of the incisions in the frontal lobe. Prefrontal lobotomy may be performed in the plane of the coronal suture, but if insufficient white matter is cut, then worry, nervous tension, apprehension and obsessive thinking are not permanently relieved. The operation must be done symmetrically on the two sides.[3]

It seems probable that the profound emotional alteration in the absence of any measurable intellectual deficit is the result of section of fibers con-

*Presented to Tri State Medical Association of the Carolinas and Virginia, meeting at Charlotte, Feb. 28th-29th, 1944.

necting the prefrontal region with the thalamus. Anatomic studies in patients who have died some time after prefrontal lobotomy show that there is integrity of the cortical architecture in the frontal lobe, but that degeneration occurs in the nucleus medialis dorsalis of the thalamus. We believe that this bundle is of importance in linking ideational with affective experience and that interruption of this pathway is the greatest factor in producing alteration in emotional responses of the patient.

Having observed repeatedly that a satisfactory therapeutic result occurs when lobotomy produces drowsiness, impairment of memory, and disorientation, this now used as a yard-stick to determine the depth and extent of the incisions. Whenever it is possible, the patient is operated upon under local anesthesia. The neurologist converses with the patient and puts him through various intellectual exercises.

OBSESSIVE COMPULSIVE STATES

The woman whose history follows became germ conscious during the illness of a relative and the idea became an obsession. As time passed, she developed a ritual which guided not only every act she performed, but included every member of the family.

Mrs. M. L., 36 years of age when the prefrontal lobotomy was performed, had been married seventeen years and had two children, one 5, the other 10. Shortly after her marriage her father-in-law developed tuberculosis and it fell to her to take him to a number of doctors. She was told by the doctors not to use the same dishes, not to allow the patient to cough in her direction, and to be very careful about infection. Her sister-in-law also developed tuberculosis and, within the space of two years, both father-in-law and sister-in-law died of the disease.

Mrs. L. then began to wash her hands more often than usual. She would wash her hands several times before opening the refrigerator, and soon required other members of the family to wash their hands before opening the refrigerator. She bathed every night. After five years, things became worse. She would wash her hands hundreds of times a day and make the maid do the same. Because she feared to mingle with other people, she stopped going to the grocery store; her sister would go for her, but had to wash her hands before leaving the house, and was required to hold the bag of groceries up in the air so that it would not come too close to the pavement and get contaminated. About this time, a neighbor across the street developed tuberculosis and it was his habit to spit out into the street from his front porch. Mrs. L. would go in the house and wash her hands every time he spit. She would not allow her boys to play with his boys, and she became so upset about the situation that she sold her home and moved to another neighborhood.

In 1937, Mrs. L.'s father died of liver disease. Since that time she has refused to eat liver. Soon she stopped cooking because she was unable to get things clean enough, so her husband had to wash his hands and go out each morning to get her breakfast. Then he would have to leave work around lunch time, come home, wash his hands and go out and get lunch for her at some restaurant. Mrs. L. and her husband would go to restaurants for meals, but if a waitress so much as dropped a utensil on the floor, all the food was contaminated and Mrs. L. would have to leave the restaurant.

By 1938, when her husband or children would return home, she made them take off all their clothes, take baths and have the clothes laundered immediately. Psychoanalysis was attempted but gave no relief. During 1938, she was given a series of 13 metrazol treatments at the Pennsylvania Hospital, with little or no benefit. In 1939, she was given 14 metrazol treatments at the St. Francis Hospital, in Pittsburgh, without improvement. A short series of insulin treatments were tried with similar lack of results.

The patient and her husband resumed going to restaurants for their meals and she would go to the washroom and scrub up before sitting down to a meal. If a wastebasket were present in the washroom, she considered the place badly contaminated and was unable to eat. For six months prior to prefrontal lobotomy, Mrs. L. had not used the bathtub in her own home because some member of the family broke the ritual and contaminated the bathroom. Because of this, she took a room in a hotel whenever she wanted to take a bath, and would bathe only twice a month. She knew that charwomen sweep floors and empty wastebaskets and the same ones must make up the beds and clean up the bathrooms. Therefore, even the bathrooms in the hotels were not clean.

By the time she consulted us, there were only two restaurants in the entire city of Pittsburgh where she could eat, and sometimes one of these became contaminated. Her average weight was 135 pounds, and at the time of examination she weighed less than 90 pounds. In the preceding six months, she had had four spontaneous convulsions.

After prefrontal lobotomy was performed in April, 1942, she was drowsy and confused for a few days (Fig. 1), then a striking change occurred. Within ten days Mrs. L. had gained eight pounds, appeared relaxed and smiled when spoken to (Fig. 2). She was not even concerned when a trash basket was placed on her bed.

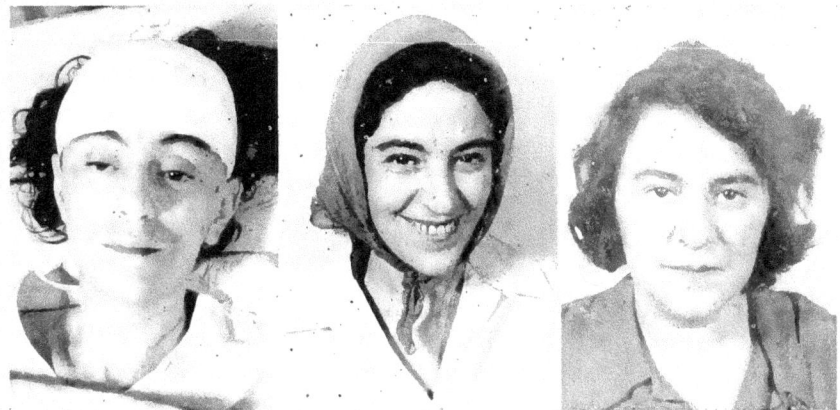

Fig. 1.—Mrs. M. L., on the second postoperative day, drowsy and confused.

Fig. 2.—Ten days after prefrontal lobotomy Mrs. M. L. appeared relaxed and smiled when spoken to and she had gained eight pounds. Her hair has been arranged to cover the shaven area in front.

Fig. 3.—When this photograph was taken three months after lobotomy, Mrs. M. L. had gained 35 pounds and her husband had gained twelve pounds. She still had many of the same peculiar ideas about contamination but they no longer dominated her life.

When she and her husband returned to Washington July 20th, 1942, the patient had gained 45 pounds, and her husband had gained 12 pounds (Fig. 3). Mrs. L. was living with her sister and still had some of her compulsions. She occasionally refused some articles of food because it was contaminated, refused to use a comb which had been dropped on the floor, and would not use a bath towel because bath towels were kept on a shelf next to a bath mat. If her sister passed the trash basket, she must wash her hands before serving food.

When examined October 12th, 1943, Mrs. L. was doing her own cooking, her husband washing the dishes while she wiped them. She refused to clean the apartment, so her son tidied up daily and a cleaning woman came in once a week. The patient would eat something of everything she cooked, no longer considering it contaminated.

She weighed 135 pounds and her general condition was good. She was neatly dressed, her hair well arranged and she laughed often during the interview. According to her husband, she still likes to have her own way, flares up easily over trifles, and criticizes him and the children.

In March, 1944, Mrs. L. wrote that she was continuing to improve and her activities at home were about the same as last autumn.

TENSION STATES

There are other patients who are obviously under nervous tension who have no compulsions and no complaints about any part of the body. Some are disabled by a feeling of inferiority or insecurity or inability to make a decision. Others while still working do so only at a tremendous expenditure of effort, and the margin between ambition and accomplishment is so great that suicide seems to offer the only solution.

The difficulties some patients have making decisions are illustrated by the case of a man of 26, who wrote as follows:

"There is such a vast *mass* of material to be *examined*, and it is often so *devious, subtle,* and *elusive,* in its nature, and, moreover, there are so many *variables* to give due and adequate *consideration* to that I often (or at least sometimes) find myself involved in a sufficiently perplexing preponderance of *seemingly* paradoxical problems to prevent successful and efficient and logical solution and answer to the problem of decision."

A prefrontal lobotomy was performed April 1st, 1942. Soon after operation he was very slow, but once he started something, continued indefinitely. On one occasion he shaved with an electric razor for five hours.

Six months after lobotomy, he became very active- rolled the lawn, cut the grass, and cleaned out brush along the brook. One day he started work at 7 a. m.; at 8 a. m. when told breakfast was ready, he replied he was busy. At noon, his wife called him to come to lunch, and he told her to leave him alone, that he was busy. When she insisted at 5 p. m. that he come in to eat, he became very much annoyed and tore her dress off. When seen March 10th, 1943, all his indecision had disappeared. In January, 1944, he reported

TABLE 1
STATUS OF LIVING PATIENTS ONE TO SEVEN YEARS AFTER LOBOTOMY
PERCENTAGES

Disease	No.	Regularly Employed	Partly Employed	Keeping House	At Home	Institution
Involutional depressions	65	11	6	42	32	9
Schizophrenias	43	26	5	23	32	14
Obsessive tension states	30	47	10	20	17	6
Psychoneuroses	10	50	....	20	10	20
Undifferentiated (Schizoid)	6	33	....	17	17	33
		—	—	30	27	—
Totals	154	25	6	30	27	12

that he had a job as a janitor in a school with a salary of $32 a week, the first money he had ever earned. He still went into detail about everything, about his trip, his job etc., but he did not deviate from the main line of thought as he used to. The patient still wanted to finish high school and go to college. His ambition is to be a psychiatrist or a university president or a professor. For the time being, he is willing to earn a living in a more modest position.

Other patients with tension states know something is wrong but can't put their finger on it. They want to be relieved, but don't know just what they want to be relieved of. This is illustrated by the case of a lawyer 35 years of age, who developed nervous symptoms in the Spring of 1938. At that time he was a partner in a law firm in New York. His work deteriorated so much that, in December, 1938, he was dropped from the firm.

When the patient was asked what he was complaining of, he stated that he was unable to find a job. He had tried two or three times in the past two or three years, but the rest of the time sat around home and worried about not being able to find a position. When his wife suggested that he try to find something, he always found some excuse for not doing it. He had become irritable, slept poorly, and sat around all day worrying about not having anything to do. He weighed every question put to him, and when he finally answered, qualified every statement. When asked if he thought that everyone who could not find a job should have a prefrontal lobotomy, he admitted after some consideration that this would be foolish, and yet when asked immediately afterwards why he came to the doctor, he said it was because he could not find a job.

As he was obviously under nervous tension, it was decided to give him the benefit of a prefrontal lobotomy; so on November 7th, 1940, he was operated upon. This man did not return to work until April, 1941, but he no longer worried about being out of work. In April he opened his office for the practice of law, but after six months closed it because he had no clients. In January, 1942, he got a clerical position with the Government, discharged his duties satisfactorily. He is now employed as an examiner for the Civil Aeronautics Board.

Patients with obsessive tension states come to the doctor seeking operation, in contrast to those with involutional depressions who are virtually dragged in by their relatives. If they can be freed of nervous tension, they believe that they can apply themselves to their task and reach their goal. Prefrontal lobotomy relieves nervous tension and often aids the individual in reaching his objective, but does so by making him more easily satisfied with his accomplishments. It makes him willing to do work commensurate with his ability.

Of the thirty patients upon whom prefrontal lobotomies were performed between one and seven years ago, 15 per cent were employed at the time of operation, and 47 per cent are employed at the present (table 1). An additional 10 per cent are working part time, and 20 per cent are keeping house.

Although the average duration of symptoms in our cases was between ten and eleven years, there was little or no mental deterioration in the majority. Only 11 per cent had been hospitalized except for shock therapy which 35 per cent had received without benefit.

In individuals who are living outside institutions, it is not enough merely to relieve mental pain. Early in our series, we operated upon an insurance man 58 years of age, with a history of nervous tension, numerous abortive suicidal attempts, and several nervous breakdowns. His symptoms, which had been present 25 years, were completely relieved by prefrontal lobotomy, but his aggressive behavior lost him his business and broke up his home. We later learned that when a child he had deliberately kicked his brother's dog to death; he had been cruel to his wife and nagging to his children. In business, his practices had bordered on the shady side and on several occasions he had a nervous breakdown and went to a sanitarium until things blew over. Since that time, it has been our practice to question the family about the patient's sense of responsibility, any tendency toward excessive nagging or teasing, and particularly as to whether he has exhibited evidence of cruelty before the onset of his nervous symptoms. If we suspect that a reduction of self-consciousness and relief of mental pain may give rise to aggressive and antisocial behavior, lobotomy is not performed.

Conclusions

Prefrontal lobotomy has been performed upon thirty patients with obsessive tension states, all of whom were operated upon between one and seven years ago.

Social adjustment is satisfactory and the majority are usefully employed after lobotomy, but care must be exercised in the selection of patients for lobotomy if cases of aggressive behavior are to be avoided. Most of the individuals who were working, or who had been out of work only a short time when the lobotomy was performed, are able to return to their old positions and discharge their duties satisfactorily.

References

1. FREEMAN, W., and WATTS, J. W.: Some observations on obsessive ruminative tendencies following interruption of the frontal association pathways. *Bulletin Los Angeles Neurological Society*, 1938, 3:51-66.
2. FREEMAN, W. and WATTS, J. W.: *Psychosurgery*. Springfield, Ill. Charles C. Thomas, 1942., 337 pp.
3. WATTS, J. W., and FREEMAN, W.: Surgical aspects of Prefrontal Lobotomy. *Journal International College of Surgeons*, 1942, 5:233-240.

Discussion

Note.—Papers of Dr. Watts and Dr. J. G. Lyerly were discussed together. Dr. Lyerly's paper was published in the issue for April.

DR. E. BURKE SUITT, Durham: In Dr. Lyerly's cases both the distribution and frequency of operation and his clear-cut comments indicate that the prefrontal lobotomy needs to be considered in relationship to the therapy benefit in electro-shock. I think all of us who work in psychiatry are interested in what he can tell us in the things which determine the differentiation in selecting patients for the two procedures.

DR. F. E. KREDEL, Charleston: I'd like to ask two questions in relation to other cases suitable for prefrontal lobotomy. We see post-concussion neuroses and also mental defectives who exhibit emotional instability and tantrums. In my own experience is the case of a moron who was a social problem, subject to outbursts of belligerency and emotional upsets. By this operation this patient was relieved of symptoms and able to be kept at home.

DR. JAMES ASA SHIELD, Richmond: I certainly have enjoyed these two excellent papers on a very timely subject. In the practice of neuropsychiatry, certain questions are asked by relatives of patients for whom prefrontal lobotomy is advised. One is, "You say my wife will have no concern. Will she still love me; still have the same sense of responsibility to her daughter or to her son?" And then in regard to the question of these people's mental capacity —our present technic of testing shows people's psychometric level approximately the same before and after. However, those of us who have had opportunity to study these people realize that there are certain definite deteriorations in their capacity to function as a whole personality. That brings up the point that, in recommending this procedure we have to seriously weigh the condition the patient is in and the probable condition afterwards. The operation will certainly be a help to a whole lot of people who are terribly concerned and terribly upset. In my experience, most of these people continue to have concern and hallucinations, but they do not become disturbed by the things they see or the things they hear.

DR. WATTS (closing): In regard to Dr. Shields' remarks, those are important questions. Possibly a patient with involutional depression won't allow her husband to go out of the room and makes a scene every time he does. After the operation she does not make such a scene, apparently doesn't care much whether the husband comes or goes, but she says she still loves him. As to the responsibility to the daughter, that varies. Some of the patients have been a real responsibility to their daughters, rather than assuming responsibility for them, but we do have patients who become too care-free and too irresponsible and are no longer concerned about what time their daughters come in or whether they go to school.

I think you are right about the psychometric tests. They are said not to show any changes, but there certainly are changes in these patients. The only thing I could say is that in obsessive tension cases, 15 per cent were working before and 47 per cent afterwards. If disability is not present or suicide is not contemplated, the operation is not indicated.

DR. KREDEL: I haven't tried it in post concussion. I have tried it on one butting her head against a radiator and it relieved her temporarily. She died of pneumococcus pneumonia after returning home, so we don't have much information.

DR. J. G. LYERLY (closing): Prefrontal lobtomy makes the relationship between the patient and the rest of the family much closer than before. The patient is happier, easier to get along with, not as arritable and fussy as before. The gain in weight may be objectionable and it is very necessary in most cases that the patient be put on a restricted diet. As I stated before ,some patients may double in weight unless restricted. I have some pictures of patients who show great obesity.

In regard to operating on mental defectives, I haven't done that. The ones that I have operated upon have been very carefully selected—involutional melancholia, manic-depressive, schizophrenia, psychoneurotic depression and psychopathic personality. Mental depression, agitation, restlessness, apprehension, anxiety and fears and phobias— all those symptoms will be improved.

In regard to hallucinations, my experience with prefrontal lobotomy is that they do not react to them. They hear voices and have other symptoms of that nature, but they do not react to them and laugh them off. Various hallucinations they tolerate much better and are not disturbed by them.

Two CASES illustrate some of the difficulties in the study of multiple malignant lesions. In one, three primary asynchronous malignant lesions of the colon developed over a period of 17 years; they were removed successfully. The second case involved the removal of coincident primary carcinomas of the rectum and the lung. It is important to evaluate apparently metastatic and recurrent malignant lesions with an eye toward the possibility of their being separate primary lesions.—*A. L. Lichtman.*

NATURE in withholding breast milk for three or four days may be intentionally causing a dehydration program for cerebral edema. Vitamin K should be given to all mothers at the onset of labor and repeated at 12-hour intervals until labor has been completed; this can be supplemented by oral or subcutaneous administration of the vitamin to the baby during the first few days of life.— *Prentice.*

Penicillin*

E. McG. HEDGPETH, M.D., Chapel Hill
Student Health Service, University of North Carolina

WITHIN the past decade we have witnessed wonderful additions to our therapeutic armamentarium. The discovery of the sulfonamide group of drugs has focused our attention in the direction of chemotherapy and has added emphasis to the specificity of therapy. We are increasingly thinking of treatment bacteriologically and chemically rather than in symptomatic and empirical terms.

We now have added to the sulfonamides a group of substances derived from bacteria and moulds which extends even further the horizon of chemotherapy. Of these the most promising at the moment is penicillin, derived from the mould Penicillium Notatum. The following remarks are intended as a brief summary of the literature up to the present, and are not based on any personal experience.

HISTORY

Fleming[1] in 1929, working at St. Mary's Hospital in London, wrote: "While working with staphylococcus variants a number of culture-plates were set aside on the laboratory bench and examined from time to time. In the examination these plates were necessarily exposed to the air and they became contaminated with various microörganisms. It was noticed that around a large colony of contaminating mould the staphylococcus colonies became transparent and were obviously undergoing lysis." He demonstrated also that the mould could be grown in broth, that the filtrate from this broth contained an antibacterial substance effective against a number of gram-positive organisms. He further reported that this substance, which he called penicillin, was non-toxic in experimental animals.

These observations and suggestions were largely over-shadowed by the interest and enthusiasm for the sulfonamides and it was not until 1940, eleven years after the original article, that clinical interest in penicillin became active. In 1940 Chain and Florey[2] and their co-workers at Oxford published their work demonstrating that penicillin inhibited in vitro growth of certain organisms and that it had definite therapeutic value in the treatment of mice infected with streptococci, staphylococci, and cl. septique. In 1941 Abraham, Chain and others[3] reported the use of penicillin in 10 patients with staphylococcal and streptococcal infections. Favorable responses were obtained in all of these patients. At about this time the reports of the British workers were attracting the attention of the Committee on Medical Research in this country. This committee, under the chairmanship of Dr. A. N. Richards, began to urge the American manufacturers to undertake large-scale production of penicillin. Prompted by this stimulation production has steadily increased. Many laboratories and clinics in this country undertook to study and properly evaluate this new substance. In this country the entire production of penicillin has been frozen by the W. P. B. and allocated to the Army, Navy, U. S. Public Health Service, and to civilian research through the Committee on Therapeutic and Other Agents of the National Research Council, Dr. Chester S. Keefer, Chairman.

PRODUCTION

The production of penicillin is a delicate process and influenced by many factors. Of extreme importance is the selection of a high potency strain of the mould. The spores of this mould are inoculated on the proper medium and incubated approximately 7.14 days. As the mould grows there is formed a grayish-green pellicle which is covered with droplets of a yellowish liquid which contains the active principle penicillin. The mould must be grown aseptically and by following the titer of the medium the manufacturer is able to estimate the optimum time for harvest to obtain the maximum yield. When this point is reached the broth-containing penicillin is separated from the mould by filtration or centrifugation and the penicillin extracted with organic solvents. The preparation finally obtained is a dry powder of various shades of orange in color. This is the preparation used clinically and is either the sodium or calcium salt.

The formula suggested for penicillin by Abraham et al.[4] is $C_{24}H_{22}O_{10}N_2Ba$. These authors also show it to be hygroscopic and that it rapidly loses its activity if exposed to the air. It retains its antibacterial power for an indefinite period if not exposed to air. In aqueous solution it deteriorates rapidly if exposed to heat; but may be left at 37° C. for 24 hours at a pH between 5.5 and 7.5 without deterioration. It is inactivated by acids, alkalies, oxidizing agents and certain bacterial enzymes.[5]

*Presented to Tri-State Medical Association of the Carolinas and Virginia, meeting at Charlotte, Feb. 28th-29th, 1944.

MECHANISM OF ACTION

Most investigations adhere to the concept that penicillin is bacteriostatic in its action rather than bacteriocidal.[25] Hobby et al.[26] report in their experiments that penicillin may act either as a bacteriostatic agent or induce active bacteriocidal effect. The fact that the action of penicillin is not affected by the presence of a large number of bacteria, serum, pus or blood, or tissue autolysates[9] is in contrast to the action of the sulfonamides and increases its therapeutic effectiveness. Also in the strength used therapeutically it is not irritating or harmful to tissue.

ASSAY

All administrations of penicillin are accomplished by methods of bio-assay. Several methods[6] [7] [8] have been employed, all making use of the principle of titration against dilutions of known strength. All methods vary rather widely, but the plate-cup method as proposed by Florey et al.[9] seems the simplest and most practicable. Due to impurities in the final product dosage is measured in terms of the Oxford unit rather than in milligrams. Florey and Jennings[10] define the Oxford unit as "that amount of penicillin which when dissolved in 50 ml. of meat-extract broth just inhibits completely the growth of the test strain of staphylococcus aureus." This is sometimes referred to as the Florey unit.

ABSORPTION, EXCRETION AND DISTRIBUTION

Rammelkamp and Keefer[11] studied the absorption, excretion and distribution of penicillin in 22 patients and normal subjects. They administered the drug by oral, intraduodenal, rectal, intravenous, subcutaneous, intramuscular, intrapleural, intraarticular, and intrabursal routes. Oral and rectal doses were poorly absorbed. Intraduodenal administration led to rapid rise in the plasma concentration, with curves comparable to those obtained by intramuscular administration. After intravenous administration they were able to show a high initial plasma concentration of penicillin followed by an abrupt fall with the appearance of large amounts in the urine promptly. They were able to recover from the urine an average of 58 per cent of the dose given. In two of their patients with renal failure excretion of penicillin in the urine was definitely decreased. In their studies absorption and excretion were rapid after intramuscular, slow after subcutaneous injections. Absorption from the joint, bursa and empyema cavities was slow. An average penicillin concentration in the red cells was less than 10 per cent of the plasma concentration. Just what mechanism is involved in the destruction or inactivation of penicillin in the body is unknown.

ROUTES OF ADMINISTRATION—DOSAGE

The maintenance of an adequate concentration of penicillin in the plasma and tissues is essential if full therapeutic effect is to be obtained. Many factors influence this and affect the route of choice. The[11] rapid elimination by way of the kidney when given intravenously, the rapid absorption and excretion from intramuscular use, the slow absorption when given subcutaneously, the destruction by the gastric juice and enzymes of the lower bowel, slow absorption from the body cavities, absence in the spinal fluid when given intravenously, absence of destruction or inhibition by bacteria or tissue autolysates[5] are all factors which must be taken into consideration when penicillin is administered.

Herrel at the Mayo Clinic[12] summarizes his experience as to methods of administration as follows: "It is my opinion that the continuous or nearly continuous intravenous administration of pyrogen-free penicillin is the most suitable method of treating severe infections of the type considered previously. The material rapidly disappears from the blood stream into the surrounding tissues and is rather rapidly excreted in the urine. The continuous intravenous administration, therefore, insures a more uniform and continuous contact between the antibacterial agent and the bacteria invading the blood stream than any other method of administration. Periodic intravenous injections of relatively large amounts of penicillin followed by an interval during which the amount of the material in the blood stream is almost negligible may do much to encourage the development of so-called penicillin-resistant or penicillin-fast pathogens."

Due to the rapid excretion of penicillin when given intramuscularly[11]—and this may be the method of election in the milder infections—it is necessary to administer the drug at frequent intervals for an optimum plasma concentration to be maintained.

Penicillin may be administered intrathecally in meningitis as shown by Rammelkamp and Keefer[13] without toxic effects. They also suggest supplementary intravenous injections where bacterinia is present.

It has been used topically in various types of local infections. Florey and Florey[14] have used it in bepharitis and dacryocystitis, and by injecting solution into chronic wound infections and mastoid infections. They caution also that in local treatment the drug must be applied frequently and treatment continued until all clinical signs have disappeared and cultures are negative.

Dosage of penicillin, as with all therapeutic agents, is variable and depends upon many factors. The age and size of the patient, the acuteness, severity, type and site of infection, and route of administration must all be recognized as important factors. Herrel[12] concludes as follows: "In the treatment of moderately severe or severe infections 30,000 to 40,000 Oxford units per twenty-four hours is in my opinion an adequate amount of penicillin. Half of the twenty-four-hour dose is dissolved in one liter of physiologic solution of sodium chloride. If for any reason the administration of physiologic solution of sodium chloride is undesirable, penicillin may be administered in a 5 per cent solution of glucose in triple-distilled water without any loss of activity of penicillin. Initially between 100 and 200 c.c. of the material is administered at a fairly rapid rate. Following this the rate of injection is regulated to between 30 and 40 drops per minute. The second liter containing penicillin may be attached to the continuous intravenous system eight to ten hours later. Repeated venipunctures may be avoided by allowing the solution of glucose to drip in slowly during the interval in which penicillin is not being administered. A simple arm splint is applied to keep the arm in position. This is tolerated well by the patient and renders the continuous intravenous administration possible and not uncomfortable."

The staphylococcic infections apparently require larger doses than do the streptococcic and pneumococcic infections, and the meningococcic and gonococcic infections require even less.

DOSAGE SCHEDULE IN VARIOUS INFECTIONS[15]

"A. In Serious Infections Due to the Hemolytic Streptococcus, Staphylococcus Aureus or Pneumococcus, with or without Bacteremia.—

1. Five thousand units every hour injected into the tubing of an inlying intravenous set; or

2. Constant intravenous injection of a solution at a rate designed to deliver 5,000 to 10,000 units per hour. In a few cases it may be necessary to use larger doses.

3. After the temperature has returned to normal, the total dose in a twenty-four-hour period may be reduced by half, but it should be continued for at least seven days after the temperature is normal.

B. In Chronically Infected Compound Injuries such as Infected Compound Fractures or Septic Infections of the Soft Parts.—An initial dose of 10,000 Oxford units should be followed by 10,000 units every two hours, or 15,000 units every three hours parenterally, with local treatment as indicated. This schedule may have to be increased or decreased, depending on the seriousness of the infection and the response to treatment.

C. Sulfonamide-Resistant Gonorrhea.—The minimum dosage schedule has not been worked out completely; 10,000 Oxford units every three hours intramuscularly or intravenously for twelve doses has been used with success. It is not unlikely that the same effect may be obtained with 20,000 units every three hours for five doses. The results of treatment should be controlled by culture of the exudate.

D. Empyema—Streptococcic, Pneumococcic and Staphylococcic.—Penicillin in isotonic solution of sodium chloride should be injected directly into the empyema cavity after aspiration of pus or fluid. This should be done once or twice daily, using 30,000 or 40,000 units, depending on the size of the cavity, the type of infection and the number of organisms. Penicillin solutions should not be used for irrigation. It requires at least six to eight hours for a maximum effect of penicillin, so that continuous action is needed.

E. Meningitis — Staphylococcic, Pneumococcic and Streptococcic.—Penicillin does not penetrate the subarahnoid space in appreciable amounts, so that it is necessary to inject penicillin into the subarachnoid space or intracisternally in order to produce the desired effect. Ten thousand units diluted in isotonic solution of sodium chloride in a concentration of 1,000 units per cubic centimeter should be injected once or twice daily, depending on the clinical course and the presence of organisms. Intravenous and intramuscular injections should be carried on at the same time.

F. Pneumonia.—The dosage schedule for pneumococcic pneumonia has not been worked out satisfactorily, but for the present it is well to give between 60,000 and 90,000 units a day for three to seven days. Recovery has followed with smaller doses, but the foregoing schedule seems necessary, at least in some cases."

RANGE OF CHEMOTHERAPEUTIC EFFECT OF PENICILLIN

Fleming[2] in his original article stated that penicillin had a powerful antibacterial effect upon the pyogenic cocci and diphtheria group of bacilli. Many bacteria were not affected by penicillin, principally the colon, typhoid group, the influenza bacillus group and the enterococcus. The antibacterial effectiveness of penicillin has in general been extended to include most of the gram-positive organisms, the meningococcus and the gonococcus, while it has no effect upon the gram-negative bacilli. The following table represents the organisms

Susceptible Bacteria	Insusceptible Bacteria
Pneumococcus	H. influenzae
Streptococcus hemolyticus	E. coli
Staphylococcus	B. typhosus
Meningococcus	B. dysenteriae
Gonococcus	B. proteus
Streptococcus viridans	B. paratyphosus A.
B. subtilis	B. enteritidis
Cl. Welchii	B. pyocyaneus
V. septique	B. prodigiosus
Cl. histolyticus	Friedlander's bacillus
B. sporogenes	Staphylococcus albus (1 strn.)
B. oedematiens	Micrococcus albus (1 strn.)
B. sordelli	Monilia albicans
Lactobacillus	Monilia krusei
Cryptococcus hominis	Monilia candida

studied in vitro by Hobby et al.[8] for susceptibility to penicillin.

It would be hazardous to attempt to predict the ultimate extent that the effectiveness of penicillin may reach. The research on penicillin under the direction of the Committee on Chemotherapeutic and Other Agents of the National Research Council is constantly striving to extend the scope of its effectiveness. While data at present are incomplete, we may well see it become a valuable drug in the treatment of the yeast, virus, spirochetal, and rarer bacillary infections.

TOXICITY

Penicillin has been found to produce remarkably few toxic manifestations.[1,9,11,13,17,18] In fact, the material available for clinical use is an impure product and what few minor toxic effects which have been noticed are generally accepted to be due in large part to impurities rather than to penicillin itself. For all practical purposes, in the strength used therapeutically, it may be considered as possessing an extremely low toxicity. The following reactions have been reported:[15]

TYPE OF REACTION
1. Fever
2. Chills and fever
3. Thrombophlebitis at site of injection
4. Urticaria
5. Gluteal tenderness at site of injection
6. Headache, flushing of face
7. Tingling in testes
8. Pain in muscles

CLINICAL RESULTS

Clinical results obtained by the use of penicillin have been striking. The staphylococcic septicemias are probably the most dramatic.[19,14] However, equally satisfactory results have been reported in many other conditions, for example, cavernous sinus thrombosis,[14] compound fractures,[17] empyema,[21] osteomyelitis,[21,14,17] gonorrhea,[22] in wound infections,[17,12,23] meningitis,[13] pneumonia.[15,57] These conditions represent only a cross section of the conditions in which penicillin is proving to be of tremendous value. As study progresses and knowledge concerning it increases unquestionably penicillin will find many more indications.

BIBLIOGRAPHY

1. FLEMING, A.: On the Antibacterial Action of Cultures of a Penicillin with Special Reference to their Use in the Isolation of B. Influenzae. Brit. Jour. Exper. Path., 10:226-236, 1929.
2. CHAIN, E., FLOREY, H. W., GARDNER, A. D., HEATLEY, N. G., JENNINGS, M. A., ORR-EWING, J., and SANDERS, A. G.: Penicillin as a Chemotherapeutic Agent. Lancet, 2:226-228, 1940.
3. ABRAHAM, E. P., CHAIN, E., FLETCHER, C. M., GARDNER, A. D., HEATLEY, N. G., JENNINGS, M. A., and FLOREY, H. W.: Further Observation on Penicillin. Lancet, 241. 177, August 16th, 1941.
4. ABRAHAM, E. P., CHAIN, E., and HOLLIDAY, E. R.: Purification and Some Physical and Chemical Properties of Penicillin. Brit. Jour. Exper. Path., 23, 103, June, 1942.
5. ABRAHAM, E. P., and CHAIN, E.: An Enzyme from Bacteria Able to Destroy Penicillin. Nature, 146, 837, 1940. No. 3713.
6. FLEMING, A.: On the Antibacterial Action of Cultures of a Penicillin with Special Reference to their Use in the Isolation of B. influenzae. Brit. Jour. Exper. Path., 1929, 10:226-236.
7. FOSTER, J. W.: Quantitative Estimation of Penicillin. Jour. Biol. Chem., 144:285-286, 1942.
8. HOBBY, G. L., MEYER, K., and CHAFFEE, E.: Activity of Penicillin in Vitro. Proc. Soc. Exp. Biol. & Med., 50:277-280, 1942.
9. FLOREY, H. W., ABRAHAM, E. P., CHAIN, E., FLETCHER, C. M., GARDNER, A. D., HEATLEY, N. G., and JENNINGS, M. A.: Further Observations on Penicillin. Lancet, 2: 171-188, 1941.
10. FLOREY, H. W., and JENNINGS, M. A.: Some Biological Properties of Highly Purified Penicillin. Brit. Jour. Exper. Path., 23:120, June, 1942.
11. RAMMELKAMP, C. H., and KEEFER, C. S.: The Absorption, Excretion and Distribution of Penicillin. Jour. Clin. Invest., 22:425, May, 1943.
12. HERREL, W. E.: Further Observations on the Clinical Use of Penicillin. Proc. Staff Meetings Mayo Clinic, Vol. 18, March 10th, 1943.
13. RAMMELKAMP, C. H., and KEEFER, C. H.: The Absorption, Excretion and Toxicity of Penicillin Administered by Intrathecal Injection. Amer. Jour. Med. Sc., 205, 342, March, 1943.
14. FLOREY, M. E., and FLOREY, H. W.: General and Local Administration of Penicillin. Lancet, 244, 387, March, 1943.
15. Penicillin in the Treatment of Infections: Statement by the Committee on Chemotherapeutic and Other Agents. Jour. A. M. A., 122:1217-1224, August 28th, 1943.
16. McKEE, C. M., and HOUCK, C. L.: Individual Penicillin Resistance in a Pneumococcus Type III Culture. Federation Proceedings, 2:100, November 16th, 1943.
17. Penicillin. Statement released by the Committee on Medical Research. Jour. A. M. A., 122:235, May 22nd, 1943.
18. HOBBY, GLADYS L., MEYER, KARL, and CHAFFEE, ELINOR: Chemotherapeutic Activity of Penicillin. Proc. Soc. Exp. Biol. & Med., 50:285, June, 1942.
19. LIKELEY, D. S., and SWIRSKEY, M. Y.: Staphylococcus Aureus Septicemia Treated with Penicillin. Jour. A. M. 123, 15, Dec. 11th, 1943.
20. HERREL, W. E., HIEMAN, DOROTHY H., and WILLIAMS, H. L.: The Clinical Use of Penicillin. Proc. Staff Mayo Clinic, 17:609, Dec. 30th, 1942.
21. RAMMELKAMP, C. H., and MAXON, THELMA: Resistance of Staphylococcus Aureus to the Action of Penicillin. Proc. Soc. Exp. Biol. & Med., 51:386, Dec. 1942.
22. HERREL, W. E., COOK, E. N., and THOMPSON, L.: Use of Penicillin in Sulfonamide-Resistant Gonorrheal Infections. Jour. A. M. A., 122:289, May, 1943.
23. BORDLEY, J. E., CROW, S. J., DALOWITZ, D. A., and PICKRELL, K. L.: The Local Use of the Sulfonamides, Gramicidin (Tyrothricin) and Penicillin in Otolaryngology. Ann. O., R. & L., 51:936, Dec., 1942.
24. REID, R. D.: Some Properties of a Bacterial-Inhibitory Substance Produced by a Mould. Jour. Bact., 29:215-221, 1935.
25. HOBBY, GLADYS L., MEYER, KARL, and CHAFFEE, ELINOR: Observations on the Mechanism of Action of Penicillin. Proc. Soc. Exp. Biol. & Med., 50:281, June, 1942.

Discussion

DR. F. B. MARSH, Salisbury: Dr. Hedgpeth's paper is certainly a very timely one and certainly it was presented in a very fine way. It behooves all of us to learn as much about penicillin now as possible, although we are not able to obtain this drug as yet. As soon as the war is over, perhaps before, it will be available and we should know as much as possible about the application of this drug to the various types of illnesses in which it brings about such remarkable cures. Penicillin is remarkable because of the almost miraculous results which follow its exhibition against infection with a great variety of organisms.

In a recent issue of the *Journal of the American Medical Association* was reported a very severe case of gas gangrene, which had failed to respond to specific serum, x-ray therapy and operative procedures, and it looked as though the patient were going to die. A sufficient quantity of penicillin was obtained and very much to the surprise of those in charge, the patient survived.

Three important and interesting reports have recently come out of Mayo Clinic. One is the experimental work being done in regard to relapsing fever. Those injected or inoculated with the spirochete of relapsing fever have been saved in practically 100 per cent of the cases. There is reason to believe that many of the cases of atypical pneumonias we are seeing will prove amenable to treatment with penicillin. In the experiments carried on at Mayo's a very large percentage have been cured. There in a series of cutaneous syphilitic lesions treated by intravenous administration of penicillin, even better results were obtained from penicillin than from arsphenamines and other methods.

All of that gives an idea of the great variety of the organisms against which penicillin can be used and in which cases it is a specific.

We all appreciate Dr. Hedgpeth posting us to date on this marvelous therapeutic agent.

PENICILLIN.—No evidence of deterioration of any of the preparations was found at room temperature during the first seven days. Beginning with the eighth day slight deterioration was noted with some lots.—*W. M. Kirby*, in *Jl. A. M. A.*, July 1st.

DR. JNO. A. FERRELL

RETIRES FROM ROCKEFELLER FOUNDATION

The following resolution upon the occasion of Dr. Ferrell's retirement was adopted by a rising vote of the Scientific Directors:

John Atkinson Ferrell is soon to retire from the staff of the International Health Division of The Rockefeller Foundation which he has served with distinction for nearly a third of a century.

Perhaps in no like period of time has science made possible a broader opportunity for the conservation and protection of human health. But knowledge must be translated into action before opportunity can become reality. In his capacity as a representative of the Division; through his professional associations with those of us who have come after him; by the maturity and richness of his judgment in organization and public health administration, Dr. Ferrell has achieved a leadership that has enabled him to contribute to that constructive thought which results in action to an extent equalled by but few and excelled by none. His was the job of laying the mudsills and erecting the framework of public health methods and of inspiring others to build for the future. He was the pioneer who blazed new trails.

His untiring energy, his kindliness, vision and foresight have endeared him to all of us who have been privileged to be his professional associates as is attested by the responsibilities which many professional societies have imposed upon him. As a Past President and later Chairman of the Executive Board of the American Public Health Association; as an officer or participant in practically every important public health group and movement of the nation; and as an honorary member in the professional groups of other countries, his influence has been potent for the public good.

Therefore, Be it resolved, that the Board of Scientific Directors of the International Health Division at this, its eighty-fourth meeting, acknowledges with the deepest appreciation the extraordinary influence and service which Dr. Ferrell has contributed to the structure of public health administration and the solution of public health problems both here and abroad. Truly, in his work science found an instrument through which it is being set to the service of mankind.

APPOINTED MEDICAL DIRECTOR MARKLE FOUNDATION

The John and Mary R. Markle Foundation has announced that Dr. John A. Ferrell has been appointed Medical Director effective July 1st. The foundation was established in March, 1927, and since December, 1935, has limited its activities to research in the medical and physical sciences and the area of its operations to the United States and Canada.

The Rockefeller Foundation announces the appointment of Dr. Hugh H. Smith as Regional Director for the United States, Canada and Mexico to succeed Dr. Ferrell.

The regular program of the Markle Foundation does not include a fellowship program or the routine public health services. It does, however, allow aid to research in certain diseases and deficiencies of interest to the health authorities. Its field has been broadened mainly as a war activity in respect to tropical diseases.

In this connection Dr. Ferrell says:

"My association with public health authorities as a representative of The Rockefeller Foundation during the past third of a century has been a joy and a rare privilege. I hope I shall continue to see my public health friends from time to time. Moreover, in the future as in the past I shall watch with keen satisfaction the progress of their work."

His address after July 1st will be 14 Wall Street, New York City.

Dr. Ferrell is a native of North Carolina and a graduate of the Medical School of the University of North Carolina, and he is an ex-Secretary of the Board of Health and of the Medical Society of that State.

FOR ELOCUTION AS A REQUIRED COURSE
(T. B. Johnson, in *Proc. Royal Soc. of Med.*, Eng., April)

Clear enunciation goes a long way to help the deaf part of the audience; it also greatly adds to the comfort of those whose hearing capacity is good. The only cure for this lack of audibility is in the teaching of elocution. Quite apart from broadcasting or acting, our everyday comfort would be greatly increased if people were taught to speak properly. I suggest that elocution should be a standard subject in our schools, for both boys and girls, and not an extra subject, as it is now.

IN THE PAST THREE YEARS two N. Y. doctors treated 40 cases of essential hypertension with potassium thiocyanate. In four cases thrombophlebitis developed.

SMALL QUANTITIES of albumin and sugar are common in the urine of comatose patients, no matter what is the cause of the coma.—*Horder*.

The Physician as Teacher*

KARL SCHAFFLE, M.D., Asheville

IN 1905 a book was published on the subject of rheumatism, by a layman. The title was "Being Done Good." The author had been done—or done in—or done up—financially, in his search for relief from his disease. He had been all over this country and Europe; visiting the famous spas, taking the baths and massage, drinking the waters, submitting to the diets and trying electricity; together with the forms of medication prescribed by various eminent specialists. Moreover, he had had his teeth and tonsils removed, his sinuses drained and his gastro-intestinal tract thoroughly renovated! His observations were both humorous and pathetic and his final attitude one of cynical resignation. Of course the old term rheumatism is now limited to rheumatic fever. Probably the author was suffering from a chronic arthritis of the type which made even Osler say that when confronted by such a case he felt like jumping out of the window!

Another layman, a life-long sufferer from migraine, wrote a very informative book on that subject. His experiences were similar to those of the arthritic patient—and while not so bitter, he expressed a like discontent with the medical profession. Both of these men had been treated by conscientious physicians who had studied their cases thoroughly and had done their best for them, but unfortunately, by other persons who were more or less tinged by a commercialistic charlatanism. Of course the diseases mentioned are still among the incompletely solved problems of medicine. In both cases, however, the patients were subjected to a good deal of unnecessary hocus-pocus.

All of this is cited for the purpose of bringing up the question as to how much medical knowledge should be imparted to the layman. If the family physician or the expert who was first consulted had carefully taught each of these men the nature of his affliction and its unsatisfactory status from the standpoint of treatment, much of their time and money would have been saved and their hopes would not have been raised repeatedly—one to be dashed by disappointment.

The layman reads the columns in the newspapers and occasional articles in the popular magazines by medical writers, most of which are sound. (Woods Hutchinson was among the first and best of these. Stanley Rhinehart was another, who was kind enough to read me several of his articles before publication. Our own Frank Richardson combines a charming style with sage advice.) The layman also sees news items at times (which should have been submitted to a medical censor), the sensational character of which is often misleading. He may also read such books as those by Paul DeKruif whose laudable intention to make science interesting is sadly marred by a hysterical style, causing unfortunate morbid introspection, with alarming phobias and nervous insomnia on the part of some of his readers. Recently there appeared in that widely distributed, reactionary, short cut to culture, the *Reader's Digest*, an article by DeKruif on the treatment of arthritis by vitamin D; the value of which has been questioned by the very men who conducted the experiments, and who greatly resented the gratuitous publicity. This was closely followed in a subsequent issue of the same periodical by another essay entitled "New Hope for White Plague Victims," concerning a product for the treatment of tuberculosis in man, the results of which have not been reported in medical literature. It has certainly been a *plague* to all chest specialists, the *victims* of much anxious inquiry by their patients, their relatives and friends! Again, the experimenter was obliged to write a letter to the *Journal of the A. M. A.*, explaining that "diasone is still an experimental agent and is not ready for distribution until a great amount of investigational work is completed."

Patients also attend certain health clinics and resorts where they are inculcated in the virtues of vegetarianism, put through strenuous exercise, and given frequent formal lectures on "how to keep well." Here again the intention is laudable but the results are frequently deplorable in the manufacture of what have long been known as "Sanatorium Cranks." At a lower level are the devotees of Bernarr McFadden, with his "Physical Torture" and other cheap magazines which pander to the common desire, particularly among the youth, to become "supermen," with all of the accompanying vicious side attractions designed for the moronic mind. Meanwhile it is said that the blatant advertising by the radio in recent years has caused a great up-surge in the use of patent medicines, which previously had begun to show a gratifying decline; to say nothing of the vitamin racket!

---
*Presented to Tri-State Medical Association of the Carolinas and Virginia, meeting at Charlotte, Feb. 28th-29th, 1944.

A step beyond that of the addict to meatlessness, raw food, raw theories and her colonic irrigations to which she euphemistically refers as an "internal bath" (and I say *she* advisedly as those people are largely the females of both sexes!), is the Christian Scientist. The combination of health culture with religion is irresistible to a certain type of person. Of course this harks back to ancient, tribal tradition as well as to more recent biblical sanctions. Here we have the spiritual groping of those who crave something more than they receive from their regular physicians—just as the rise of the osteopath and the chiropractor would not have occurred—if, prior to World War I, the profession had paid more attention to physiotherapy, particularly the "laying on of hands." Perhaps the best thing that was ever said about Christian Science, even including the book by Mark Twain, was the opinion of Mr. Dooley, Peter Dunne's creation of some forty years ago—"if the docthors had more Christ-i-an-ity and the Christian Scintists had more science, the patient would have a purtty good show, providin' he had a good nur-rse!"

As you all know the word "doctor" means literally leader or teacher and of course is applied to other professions than the medical. Its most common application in this country, however, is to the physician. The question which I wish to raise is whether the medical profession as a whole lives up to this title. In the rush of days and nights crowded by many demands and the inevitable routine which becomes a self-protective mechanism, there is little time or effort for much teaching even of the most informal type. Probably we felt more like teachers on that auspicious day when we stood up in our black gowns to receive our green hoods than at any time since! With all of our modern facilities, we have acquired more knowledge than the late, lamented old-fashioned family doctor, but we are inclined to teach less, while handicapped as he may have been, it is generally remembered that he taught more, frequently giving advice on other matters than those of his profession.

Of the three old, so-called learned professions, the medical is the least vocal. An important function of both minister and lawyer is the preparation and delivery of addresses to assemblies of people, while the average physician is notoriously a poor public speaker. Of course, this is hardly true in the territory which this association represents, where American oratory was born and where it continues to flourish in every walk of life and on the slightest provocation! (Particularly in Charlotte, with its Northingtons, Moores and Brenizers!) I am not so much concerned, however, with lectures by physicians, such as the public addresses of health officers and professors of medicine, as with the kind of teaching which we give or fail to give to our individual patients. There are certain specialties in which this is imperative—psychiatry, pediatrics, orthopedic surgery, cardiology, tuberculosis and diabetes. But with most of us it is a matter of getting to the office a little late because of some professional or domestic emergency, to find an air of impatient expectancy in the waiting room, whose occupants must be "run through" rapidly in order to reach the hospital or sanatorium, where hurried rounds are made and most of the instruction is delegated to nurses! A greeting, a few questions, a brief examination, a hastily written prescription or the reaching for a handy sample left by a detail man, a few trite remarks and each, in turn, is disposed of! Have we taught them anything? No wonder they change doctors, to go through the same thing again! On the other hand there are many persons to whom "a little wisdom is a dangerous thing." A few years ago a big, red-faced man asked me to take his blood pressure. He was a physician. As he sat by the machine he said "you notice I am not looking at it and I am not asking you what it is. It's too bad the damn thing was ever invented! It has caused more unnecessary worry than anything I know. If you want me to do anything beside cutting out my smoking, drinking and swearing, which I won't, just say so." Then he said, "I used to know an old country doctor who would examine a patient and when the family crowded around to ask what was wrong, he would look at them over his glasses and say, 'Well, he is sick—*sick!*' And as he reached into his bag, they would ask, 'What you going to give him, Doc?' He would give them another solemn look and say, 'I am going to give him some medicine—*medicine!*' And he had no neurotics cluttering up his office and wasting his time."

Along with such evasion is the old, old question —is a lie justifiable? We often wonder how much truth there may be in the most sober official pronouncements of the preachers and the lawyers and many persons take it for granted that the gentle art of prevarication is an essential part of the doctor's stock in trade.

Often we are unconsciously insulted by patients or their relatives who ask "are you telling me the truth?" Alvarez, in his recent book, describes how he leaves his records in plain sight of such doubters while he steps outside for a few minutes!

I was once associated with a very prominent practitioner who used charts for recording the results of his examinations. These contained a line for the diagnosis, another for the prognosis and a third for the opinion expressed to the patient. On some of these charts there was an obvious discrepancy and I noted in such cases that after the notes on the third line were the initials "e. j. m." I asked him what they meant. He said "end justifies means. If I told them that the outlook was so unfavorable they would lose hope and give up the fight." But this did not appeal to me, whose histrionic abilities atrophied after high school. (I once tried the back-slapping "cheerio" technic on a hopeless case by saying, "never mind, old man, we'll soon straighten you out!" My voice must have had a hollow, hypocritical ring, for the patient looked up and with the grim irony of which the German Jew is master, replied with a sardonic smile—"I know, doctor, you'll *straighten me out*, all right and *soon*"—and we did!) As a beginner in the State Tuberculosis Dispensary in Philadelphia in 1909, I was taught by Alfred Stengel, who was then in charge, to tell patients the truth, even if unpleasant, in order to gain their complete cooperation toward possible improvement; or if the prognosis were bad to allow them to make the necessary social and economic adjustments, which if neglected, renders the inevitable tragedy still more tragic. But a great deal depends upon how it is done. Joking aside, there is such a thing as pulling the trigger gently. Fortunately, people now are generally more frank than those of previous generations. Hospitals are not dreaded as they once were and even the words cancer, syphilis and insanity are not spoken with the bated breath our parents used.

While I am a member of the intelligent minority of our profession who are in favor of socialized medicine, maintaining, of course, that its success will depend upon the choice, qualifications and "esprit de corps" of those who will conduct it, I must admit that years ago, while employed in a government clinic, I had the misfortune to be associated with a member of our profession who was an exponent of the idea of "treat 'em rough and tell 'em nothing." His only greeting to the patient, in a voice redolent with the previous evening's whiskey, was "take off your shirt," with the variation, if the victim showed any hesitancy, of a rise of pitch and increase in volume—"I said—take off your shirt!" At the end of a somewhat cursory examination (and I mean to pun as well as to describe) his final advice consisted of the injunction—"put on your shirt!" This was an extreme example but I observed among others who had been appointed without examination, at a time of great emergency, that there was a tendency with repetitious routine, for them to become perfunctory. They had sacrificed what was laughingly referred to as their "large and lucrative" in the first World War and were now on a regular payroll, undisturbed by telephone and unpaid bills, with at 4:30 p. m. "nothing to do 'till tomorrow." They were not subject to frequent inspections and periodic examinations, as in other departments of the government.

Later when I was in a position to do so, I attempted to correct the attitude of some of these men toward their patients by means of a general order from which I have abstracted the following:

"There is a saying among the craft that a Tb. man first goes through the stage of perfecting and refining his diagnostic technique, but tha tif he develops properly, he will ultimately devote more thought and effort to the subject of treatment. The first phase is subjective, the second objective. During the first period he may develop some original tricks or become enamored of one or more of the special stunts of certain prolific writers, such accomplishments varying greatly in their essential value to him and to his patients. This is an expression of the artistic temperament in the specialist, for the man who devotes the training of his senses to the solution of the problems of vibration is indeed an artist and should have the sensitiveness and enthusiasm inherent in the soul of the highly skilled performer. But to continue with the tradition, sooner or later he turns from his absorption in the reaction of his eyes and ears and fingers to the mechanics and acoustics of the chest in health and disease, to a contemplation of the patient as a human being. With the establishment, at least upon a working basis, of his personal equation to the art of diagnosis, he goes beyond that fascinating field to the less explored region of therapeutics. Here his adjustment will take place more slowly and with less satisfaction to himself.

Our patients, particularly those who have been the subjects of repeated investigation, instinctively appreciate the difference between an inadequate, perfunctory going-over and a thorough examination by an expert. They also have learned through association that a physician of the latter type has the power to apply his knowledge to their further course of action by advice which is detailed and specific. Every examiner should make it a rule to give at least a few words of help and encouragement to each patient after each examination. It is but natural to become impatient at the eternal thumping and listening, if no beneficial results are seen to follow. It is only human to went to know what it's all about and what is going to be done about it. As drug therapy is minimal and success depends upon encouragement and the obtaining of the patient's ready coöperation in living as he should, the successful practitioner in civil life makes a point of having something of value to impart to his patient at each interview. This consists in outlining, in a simple, patient and forceful manner, the procedure to be followed, with the dispensing of as large a portion of the physician's personality as he can spare. He must imbue his patient with his own spirit of optimism, thoroughness and steadfastness. Sincerity and perseverance are fundamental to such purpose. The constant application of such qualities eventually determines the physician's own character and the result is the development of that indefinable element which marks the real specialist and is unconsciously recognized by his patients as the source of their faith in him.

In 1873, Amiel, that gentle philosopher and sufferer from a pulmonary disease, reduced the relation of physician to patient to the following formula: "Every illness is a factor simple or complex which is multiplied by a second factor, invariably complex—the individual who is suffering from it—so that the result is a special problem, demanding a special solution."

We keep saying to patients and to those interested in them that hospital treatment is superior to home treatment because of its "educational value." Have we a right to say that, unless we carefully examine our methods of education and satisfy ourselves that they are effective? General education is suffering at present from mechanical routine and the loss of the personal touch which is incident to over-crowding. (This was twenty years ago.) Our higher centers of learning are obliged to take measures toward effecting a return to small classes with more individual instruction and the inspiration of closer contact between the students and those members of the faculty who are distinguished by positive character and vivifying personality. We should remember the origin and the literal meaning of the term "doctor"—teacher or leader—and not neglect our ancient function of imparting instruction. To be most effective, this should be, as far as possible, individual instruction. A normal human being, placed under a regimen to which he is unaccustomed, naturally inquires into the whys and wherefores. A sick man is more sensitive to changes of habit and in order to adapt himself to conditions should receive his instruction from someone who understands and believes in what is being done. Too often a patient is left to mere surmises as to the reasons for certain procedure from the careless words of an orderly or the cynical comment of a fellow-sufferer who, after weeks of hospitalization, may be as ignorant as he. The nurses, as usual, do their part and more, but they are already overworked. The doctor should be the patient's teacher."

THE CLINICAL USE OF DICUMAROL
(E. P. Eckstam, Duluth, in *Minn. Med.*, June)

In 1940, was isolated from sweet clover or improperly cured silage the active principle dicoumarin; later it was synthesized and called dicumarol.

Dicumarol delays clotting time, clot-retraction time, and red-blood-cell sedimentation rate. It dilates the capillaries, small arterioles, and venules. The bleeding time is not consistently affected because of the tissue factor present when skin is injured. It does not dissolve the clot that has already formed, but it prevents that clot from extending and allows it to be organized.

Clinically there are no toxic effects other than bleeding. Hemorrhages may occur from the nose, lung, stomach, bowel, kidney, bladder, under the conjunctiva, and skin. Kidney and liver function tests are normal after prolonged use of dicumarol. A fresh-blood transfusion, or bank-blood under 48 hours old, is the treatment for bleeding.

Thrombophlebitis and phlebothrombosis in medical or postoperative patients are two of the most common indications especially when the patient has had a previous episode of either. Pulmonary embolism is a definite indication since the embolus has developed from an existing thrombus. It has also been used in the treatment of thrombosis of arteriosclerosis (as in the cerebral and coronary vessels), Buerger's disease, and a few cases of involvement of the cavernous sinus, and retinal veins.

Absolute contraindications are hemorrhagic tendencies and existing low prothrombin time, liver and kidney damage, and subacute bacterial endocarditis. Relative contraindications are the presence of ulcerative or granulating surfaces, gastric decompression tube, and pregnancy plus one week of the puerperium.

The average patient satisfactorily responds to 300 mg. the first day, 200 mg. the second and 0 to 200 mg. daily thereafter, depending on the prothrombin time that day. Allowance must be made for the latent period. The therapeutic level is reached when the blood prothrombin is 25 to 50 per cent of normal as measured by the prothrombin time. Dicumarol is continued until the patient is subjectively and objectively well. After stopping the drug it takes from two to 10 days for the prothrombin time to return to normal, in cases of liver or kidney damage, or bleeding tendencies, even longer. A transfusion of fresh blood is then indicated.

CHARCOAL WOOL FILTER-CLOTH AS A DEODORANT
(J. M. Regan & M. S. Henderson, in *Proc. Staff Meetings of Mayo Clinic*, May 31st)

The problem of eliminating the odor which occurs during treatment of open wounds by the closed plaster-cast has been attacked by many means. Seddon and Florey of the University of Oxford reported the use of wool cloth impregnated so completely with activated charcoal dust that the dust does not sift out of the material in handling. This deodorizing cloth prevents diffusion of the obnoxious odors and since it is made of a lightweight material, it is neither cumbersome nor difficult to use.

The material is effective for from two to five weeks, depending on the amount of drainage. It can be reactivated by steam sterilization and washing in a weak solution of ammonia, but, since the material is so cheap, it is usually burnt after using.

We have used it in 10 cases. In all cases the results were satisfactory.

After patients who were wearing extremity casts became ambulatory, they could be seen at the Clinic without any embarrassment because of the odor. After removal of the wool sock, the odor was noticed for some distance.

The Section on Dermatology and Syphilology has used the charcoal filter-cloth as a covering over dressings in several cases of infected cutaneous ulceration with marked drainage and the odor was greatly lessened after the application of the filter-cloth.

PRESENT OBSERVATIONS suggest that not only does penicillin, by local injection combined with systemic treatment, offer the prospect of cure in severe and sulphonamide-resistant cases of empyema, but that it can even bring about cure without rib resection in cases where the pleural cavity already contains large quantities of pus.—*Bennett & Parkes.*

The Clinical Laboratory: Its Personnel and Some of Their Problems*

J. M. FEDER, M.D., Anderson, South Carolina
Director of Clinical Laboratories, Anderson County Hospital

THIS presentation is not free from controversial issues so complete agreement is not to be expected. It is an expression of my firm conviction based upon two decades of intimate experience and close observation.

The clinical laboratory has existed for a quarter of a century and the history it has written during this period has won for it a lasting place in medicine. Its facilities were not widely used until the close of World War I. The few laboratories that had been established were mostly in the larger teaching centers, manned largely by men who had been trained in Europe during the Golden Age of Bacteriology.

When the first great conflict terminated, many doctors who had received their introduction to the clinical laboratory in military hospitals, returning to civilian practice, demanded laboratories, and these were established; the laboratory physicians being in many instances medical officers who had received their training in this new specialty while in service. Likewise many of their technical assistants were enlisted personnel who had assisted them in their work during the war.

This nucleus proved to be insufficient to meet the growing need and, in order to more effectively meet the need, residiencies in pathology were established in a number of the larger hospitals. The teaching of technical assistants was undertaken by colleges, privately owned schools of medical technology and laboratories of some hospitals. This last method, in my opinion, based upon the study of all three systems, is the most satisfactory.

Only a superficial investigation would seem to prove that despite the years that the clinical laboratory has been with us it is still misunderstood by members of our own profession regarding the type of service that it can and does render.

I was once pointed out to a visitor in our hospital by a staff member as "the fellow who does the blood counts;" and many consider our technical staff as not much above the bottle-washing stage. In most instances in which some clinician has doubted the report of a technician on general principles it has been because of lack of familiarity with the rigorous grind that this girl must undergo before she is even permitted to render a report; if the laboratory service is properly organized.

If we admit that the profession's concept is at times hazy concerning our activities, it is patent that the concept of the general public is opaque. It is not infrequent to have a layman confuse the term pathologist with that applied to some of the "drugless healers." It is not difficult to see why the patient has little or no knowledge concerning the big part played by the hospital's laboratory in speeding him along the road to recovery. What does he know about the long, hard hours keen-witted and nimble-fingered girls have worked on his case behind the scenes in the laboratory? He is fully aware of the glamour that is the nurse's, but the technician is merely a person who comes in occasionally and does something unpleasant to him with a needle. Her story remains yet to be told to the public in a manner that they can understand.

The term pathologist was applied to dead-house investigators back in the days of Virchow, and suggests a bewhiskered German in a malodorous Prince Albert coat slithering about a Berlin morgue. He bears no more resemblance to the modern laboratory diagnostician than Lister does to a contemporary surgeon. Virchow was a dead-house pathologist and Lister's art was confined to a large extent to performing amputations.

The surgeon of today is too busy studying procedures aimed at rendering amputations unnecessary to devote much time to the art of tricky dissections for the removal of a limb. Likewise, the laboratory doctor is spending much more of his time in developing investigative techniques to aid him at arriving at a diagnosis upon real, live patients.

We do perform autopsies when they are required, but they make up a small part of our work—and the surgeon must occasionally remove a mangled leg, for even in this day deaths and accidents occur.

In the early days of the laboratory, there was a trusting group of physicians who were so impressed with the infallibility of the newly-founded institution that they imbued it with some of the legerdemain of the fortune-telling machine in the corner drug store. To them it was something into which a specimen was dropped and with a whirring of wheels a report would thrust itself from the other side complete with diagnosis, treatment and

*Presented to Tri-State Medical Association of the Carolinas and Virginia, meeting at Charlotte, Feb. 28th-29th, 1944.

even prognosis.

There is such a thing as a laboratory diagnosis and in many diseases, noteworthy those of the blood, in which the only possible diagnosis is one made by this means. However, it is one made by a physician who is thoroughly acquainted with other diagnostic methods and, in addition to these, brings to his aid certain instruments of precision in the use of which he is an expert.

The value of this diagnosis bears a direct ratio to the accuracy with which this laboratory physician has been apprised of *all* of the available facts in the case under investigation. Unfortunately, these facts are not always easily obtained. Occasionally, I regret to state, they are deliberately withheld. Witness a conversation that I had with my dinner partner, a surgeon at a Southern Post-Graduate Assembly some years ago. He stated that he never furnished a radiologist or pathologist with more than a minimum of information for fear of furnishing him with a preconceived conclusion.

Not infrequently the value of a laboratory examination is seriously impaired by a demand for too much haste. In no case should time be wasted, but even with the patient under an anesthetic and the surgeon awaiting a report on which will rest the decision between a slight and a radical operation, the pathologist should firmly refuse to be hurried into giving a report until he has arrived at an opinion satisfactory to himself.

Six great evils confront the clinical laboratory; some of them of sufficient magnitude to stifle progress. I will attempt to tabulate them:

1. A volume of work is often thrust upon the laboratory impossible of performance by the few technical helpers available. Reliable work cannot be performed by a harrassed, tired technician. This is a plea for curtailment of the volume of routine work when it becomes a burden, especially the so-called academic. Remember that I am speaking solely of "front-line" clinical laboratories in our smaller hospitals, and not of those in teaching and research institutions. It is a plea for more of the rifle and less of the shotgun.

2. Many laboratories suffer from lay domination and as a result determination of the policies of his department is taken out of the hands of the laboratory director. In such unfortunate situations, he often finds it difficult to maintain the *status quo* of a medical specialist. In fact, in some hospitals, this violation is so flagrant that a lay administrator usurps the prerogative of making appointments to the technical staff, for whose work the laboratory doctor must assume responsibility.

3. In some institutions, the compensation of director and technical assistants is so inadequate as to cause a constant efficiency-disrupting turnover of help. This is especially true where the straight salary basis is adhered to. A salaried job makes for transients while a commission or other arrangement causing the laboratory staff to feel that they are partners in the business makes for satisfaction and permanence.

4. In a few hospitals, the laboratory—and x-ray department—are conducted with a view to the making of sufficient profit to make up deficits of other departments. You know how it is with the football team in college athletics; but the football team is accorded a lot of glory.

5. The average small-hospital laboratory with an ambition to do a certain amount of original investigation is often handicapped for lack of funds. Some of the research of obscure workers has met with national acclaim but, regardless of this, though other departments of the hospital may share the beneficence of locally-made endowments, the laboratory is usually passed unseen—and unendowed.

6. Some of our colleagues have discoursed on State medicine. Probably they should have consulted us for a few points as we have long been made to feel the thrust of state interference with private enterprise. In most States, if a doctor has a container in which to send a specimen to the Board of Health laboratory, they will do the rest free of charge, despite the fact that probably no more than 10 per cent of these examinations are made upon indigents. In some of our great Commonwealths, the State Board of Health even goes so far as to assume control of all laboratories within their domain, sending them trick specimens "to test their efficiency." No other specialized field is subjected to this autocratic and humiliating dictatorship.

In these chaotic times it can be expected that we should be bedeviled by more than our share of problems. That of personnel is one of these. This brings us to the important question; just what should the technician-patient ratio be to maintain peak efficiency?

It is estimated that it should be 1-to-25. This brings us up squarely against the problem of maintenance cost. Obviously the average 100-bed hospital cannot afford to employ four graduate technicians and if the service is at all active, the work will prove too heavy for a smaller number to do properly. The answer is the operation of a training school for technicians: at least it was ours; and by having one graduate technician-instructress and a class of five students who are in varying stages of their course, we are able to render a reasonably good routine service.

In the smaller hospitals, especially those having no internes, much thought is recommended to having a night technician on duty. This eliminates the pernicious night-call system. For an already-tired technician to have to dress and travel for blocks when a transfusion or emergency appendectomy is in the offing may be necessary at times; but I dare say a better arrangement could be worked out in most hospitals with more satisfaction all around. I maintain that it is inhumane to call a girl back on duty who has rendered ten hours service and who must be ready to go on duty again the next morning, regardless of the fact that she had to mill a dozen prospective blood donors at 2 a. m.

There are many technician problems. Among them is the girl who works in a 20-bed hospital, unsupervised and unadvised. Her lot is not an easy one, and it is suggested that whenever possible arrangements be made with a nearby pathologist from whom she may seek guidance when in need of it, possibly having with him a weekly or semi-monthly consultation about her work.

I am led to wonder if the technician is not the forgotten woman of the medical world. Certainly the government forgot her when provisions were made for the organization of the Nurse Cadet Corps. A laboratory girl in training still must pay her expenses and purchase her uniforms. She was forgotten when nurses were commissioned immediately upon graduation although the technician who possibly aided in training them was made eligible only for a private's billet in the WAACS.

There are all kinds of technicians with an equally varying degree of qualifications. At one end of the pendulum's arc are the girls who hold higher degrees from great Universities; at the other end are those who saved their small wages in Woolworth's and took a three-months course in the Big City College of Medical Technology. Gilt-edge Diploma (of gigantic size) $5.00 Extra. With these facts before us, is it not time that something more than a gesture at standardization were undertaken? Fully cognizant of the need, I hesitate to emphasize it for fear of becoming rather dogmatic and thus defeat its very purpose. It is not believed that this will happen at the hands of those who are familiar with our problems and needs; to be more specific, Southern hands, competent to cut the cloth to fit the subject.

As a step in the right direction, I have made the suggestion that the Tri-State Medical Association take under advisement the innovation of adding to it a Technologist's Auxiliary. Were this accomplished, several pages might be added to *Southern Medicine & Surgery* devoted to these coworkers in which ideas and ever-present problems could be brought to the attention of all. Were this accomplished, I would consider it a great honor to be permitted to act, gratis of course, as one of the editors of this new section. Once this suggestion were put into effect, the next step would be to gain the cognizance of a national Technologist's association with the end in view that they consider recognizing this as an official chapter.

I say this to all technicians: All of us are facing soul-trying days in medicine and only by organization will we be able to preserve the American way in laboratory medicine and we want you, our valued associates, right in there fighting with us.

SUMMARY

1. That it may render maximum efficiency the clinical laboratory staff and the clinicians must labor upon a basis of mutual understanding and respect in the realization that the problems of one group automatically become problems of the other.

2. Ills that lie within the laboratory have been diagnosed and in some cases remedies suggested.

3. No laboratory service is stronger than its technical staff. In some instances it appears that lack of organization or other elements have operated against the best interests of these coworkers of ours and to this end—that of remedial affiliations—a new organization has been proposed.

TRICHOMONAS URETHRITIS AND PROSTATITIS
(R. B. Roth, in *Venereal Disease Information*, June)

This study is of unselected male hospital patients in the Johns Hopkins Hospital. All patients, medical or surgical, with sufficient intelligence to void according to directions were utilized.

To date 62 Negro males have been examined, with the discovery of 17 infestations; 100 white males, with the discovery of four cases.

Reliance has been placed entirely on the wet-spread technic.

If the patient had recently emptied his bladder and could void only a few c.c. of urine, identification frequently was impossible, because time had not been allowed for the regeneration of the protozoa.

Whether the organism is pathogenic or "normal" inhabitant of the urogenital tract has not been settled to general satisfaction.

Forty-eight per cent of the patients complained of nocturia; burning on urination 13, frequency 11, itching 11%.

T. vaginalis, some insist, will disappear if left alone. Three patient sare known to have been infested for five years without intervening sexual exposure.

Individual cases have been treated with many solutions; currently we are using either zephiran 1:3,000; or silver picrate 0.5%, or in 0.25% water-soluble jelly.

In only two cases with proved infestation of both the urethra and prostate have we apparently succeeded in eliminating the parasites. In each case this was accomplished by an intensive inpatient regimen consisting of daily diathermy to the prostate, prostatic massage every other day, strong alkalinization of the urine for one week, followed by strong acidification for a week or longer, and the use throughout the treatment of urethral irrigations with zephiran or silver picrate. However, two other patients similarly treated either continued to show parasites or promptly resumed showing them on cessation of therapy.

Three cases were found in which infestation was limited to the preputial sac in uncircumcised individuals; no therapy beyond instruction in cleanliness was necessary. In the remaining 41 cases, only one persistently showed ure-
(To Page 261)

CLINIC
Conducted by
FREDERICK R. TAYLOR, B.S., M.D., F.A.C.P.,
High Point, N. C.

SEPT. 26th, 1939, a 12-year-old colored boy was brought to me for psychiatric examination because of a behavior problem. The chief complaint was general bad behavior. His parents originally lived at Jonesboro. They moved to New York, where patient was born. His mother died when he was nearly 2 years old. His father had disappeared and could not be found. The boy was sent back to High Point to an aunt of his mother's, a colored woman of unusual attainments and character. She cared for him till he was 6 years old, but he gave trouble during that time. He was "contrary" and disobedient from the very beginning and soon got to stealing. He ran away first at the age of 3 years. His aunt would whip him, not brutally, and he would run away 5 minutes later.

When he was 6 years old he went back to Lee County, where he was put in charge of an uncle, but he told white people lies about his uncle, stole eggs, etc., and got into a lot of trouble and after a year he was returned to his great-aunt. Two years later his great-uncle died and his great-aunt said she couldn't manage him, so he was placed in the care of a woman at Mount Vernon Springs. She kept him nearly 2 years, but he killed chickens, broke eggs, ran off at nights, etc. The woman and her husband were good people and had no children. The woman wrote the boy's great-aunt several times about his bad behavior, and finally had to decline to keep the boy any longer.

So, back to his great-aunt, who met him on his arrival by bus. Within a week the boy had run away again. Every morning he would run off and not return till he got hungry. At times he would stay away until 10 p. m. The principal of the colored school advised severe whipping, so the great aunt tried this, but found it wouldn't work. He suggested that she whip him till the blood ran out of him, but she said this was too brutal and refused to do it. Soon after this the boy broke into a woodhouse and stole a large toy wagon, at first saying that another boy (who had no wagon) let him have it, and later that the boy who owned it had let him have it while he was to be away from town. He was made to take the wagon back, and the lock on the woodhouse door was found broken, the door having been locked that morning by the man who owned it. The patient then admitted that he broke the lock and said he did it "just to be doing it."

Four days ago his great-aunt went to see the school principal again, who advised a psychiatric examination. He said he would try to get the boy into a reform school, but that the institution was full at present. The boy was started in school at 6, but did not finish out the year, being sent to his uncle's. Down there he would start to school with his lunch, but wouldn't go to school half the time—just stayed out and got into trouble. At Mt. Vernon Springs he got expelled for throwing rocks, etc. Since coming back here the last time, he started in the second grade when school opened, but has not attended regularly and makes trouble and fidgets constantly. He bullies the little children. He got whipped his first day at school. He doesn't seem to mind being whipped—rather he boasts about it —says with pride that he got whipped for running off. He can read a little, but doesn't stay home long enough to do any spontaneous reading.

On being asked if he likes his home, patient says "Yeh" in a lackadaisical way, but looks away from me. He says he doesn't know why he runs away. (His parents were married. Most of the history was obtained from his great-aunt.)

He cuts screens out of neighbors' houses and says he just wanted to be doing something. Asked if he would like it if someone else cut screens he had worked hard to pay for, he turned his head away and said "I don't know." On repeating the question, he said "No." He says he would be happier if he didn't steal and get into trouble, and doesn't know why he does it. He says he likes his great-aunt and she is good to him—always answers "Yeh" to these questions when he can answer them that way. He says he realizes that such behavior when he is grown will land him in prison ("Yeh"), and that it would be better to stop it before he gets into trouble. While saying "Yeh," he looks away and puts his hand in front of his mouth. Now he says it makes him feel bad to do these things. Asked why he does them, he answers "I don't know, sir" (the first time he said "Sir"). He peered interestedly at the figures on my sphygmomanometer scale, and when asked what he was looking at or interested in, said "the numbers."

Every fall he has impetigo, has it now on his legs. No headache or backache. Some polyuria.

He was never sick except with measles and whooping-cough when very small, and once a small abscess burst (apparently a boil) in his neck. He eats irregularly, drinks considerable water, no milk, no tea, coffee or coca-cola. He stole 2 packs of cigarettes and after denying having them said he was going to smoke them. A boy rooming at his house missed his cigarettes and the great-aunt searched patient and found them. He also stole some from someone's car. Great-aunt says she never saw him smoking. He never got hold of any liquor so far as known. He sleeps well 10 to 11 hours unless out late. Enuresis practically every night—will wet bed when wide awake.

The health and mental condition of his father is unknown. Mother was a trained nurse, had a good mind and was "a good girl." She is said to have died of kidney trouble. Patient is an only child.

Physical Examination. A fidgety Negro boy who turns his back on me much of the time, but otherwise his behavior in my office is fairly normal. Height 4 ft. 6¾ in. Wt. 70½ lbs. T. 98.7. P. 96. R. 24. B. P. 86/60. Head negative. He obeys orders from me promptly and accurately. His great-aunt says he will carry out her simple, immediate requests, but won't stay at home when told to. He came home the other day with his lips swollen, said a girl dropped a nickel and he told a boy he would beat him finding the nickel, and then the boy hit him. His great-aunt does not believe this tale, as he will invent all sort sof lies. His chest shows a number of small punctate and linear scars, cause unknown. None look like severe wounds. There are scars on his left shoulder from running into a hot stove when small. Heart, lungs, abdomen and genitals normal. Shotty inguinal glands, apparently due to impetigo. Legs show marked impetigo. Tendon reflexes normal. Urine negative.

The *diagnosis* here lies between a mental deficiency such as that of a high-grade imbecile or low-grade moron, and that of constitutional psychopathic inadequacy. I am rather inclined to favor the latter, but study in an institution is needed to reach final conclusions. His great-aunt is sensible, kind and intelligent, and not the sort of person to make scenes. She says it would be a sin to whip a boy for what he can't help. She says that at times he will start to school, then she goes to work, locking up the house. He comes back, breaks through a screen, and then runs off and leaves the door unlocked and the house wide-open. Once he tried to set the house on fire, starting a fire in a wood box in the house.

Whichever alternative diagnosis is selected, whether a mental deficiency or constitutional psychopathic inadequacy of antisocial type, the prognosis is bad. I advise his commitment to a reform school. If further study proves him to be feeble-minded, he should be transferred to the State School for Mental Defectives at Kinston when he can get in. If not, the reform school is about the only place I san see for him, though I doubt if they can improve him much.

PHANTOM LIMB.—This name is given to sensations, after amputation, in many instances painful, as if the limb were still *in situ*. It was recognized 400 years ago by Paré, and many others of renown give its rate of occurrence as from 95 to 100 per cent of cases. Resection of portions of the brain cortex has been curative in some cases.—*Edit. Jl. A. M. A.*

DEPARTMENTS

OPHTHALMOLOGY

HERBERT C. NEBLETT, M.D., *Editor*, Charlotte, N. C.

THE RIMLESS AND HALF-RIMMED SPECTACLE AS AN EYE HAZARD

WHEN AN OCULIST has examined a patient and has presented him with the prescription for lenses he has no final jurisdiction over the choice of the type of spectacle frame he may purchase of an optical company, but in the interest of visual conservation he may advise the patient of the economic and visual hazards attendant upon the use of any type of half-rimmed or rimless spectacle. For obvious reasons such spectacles are interdicted for use by the armed forces. For the same reasons the oculist in civil practice may apprize his patients of the dangers of wearing such frames and should discourage their use especially by the industrial worker, the farmer, the driver in the public utilities motor transportation systems, employees in railroad transportation and in other hazardous occupations; the one-eyed, those whose useful visual is entirely dependent upon the use of glasses, children, young adults and mothers with young children.

The danger in the use of such spectacles is that the unprotected lenses therein are easily broken and the fragments often produce severe injury to the eyeballs and to the lids. A fragment of glass penetrating the eye is very difficult to remove. First, because it is difficult to locate, and secondly, it is non-magnetic which adds an additional obstacle to its removal. Further, glass fragments, especially if minute and lodged in the tissues of the globe, in a cul de sac, or in the tissues of the lids are elusive. As result of automobile accidents, industrial accidents, simple accidents at play and in the home the writer has seen many minor and some serious injuries to the eyes where the person was using the rimless type of frame where had he been using the rigid or rimmed frame there would have been no or minimal injury to the eye. It is obvious that should trauma over the front of the globe be severe enough to shatter into fragments a lens inclosed in a rigid frame the eye would have been seriously damaged or lost had no glass been worn. Conversely, most of the force of a blow is expended on a rigid frame, which would have shattered the rimless lens injuring or destroying the eye.

In the past 18 months the writer has seen six patients who, as the result of moderate trauma to the rimless lenses they were wearing, had an eye seriously damaged, whereas had a rigid frame been worn the type of trauma applied would not have resulted in an injury to the eye. Two of these victims, one a young physician and one a young woman, lost an eye.

There is no valid reason for the wearing of any type of frame other than the rigid type. No other gives any added advantage in the visual quotient—the basic reason for the wearing of glasses. To too many this reason, and that of safety and economy, is subordinated to what the wearer considers better cosmetic result.

HOSPITALS

R. B. DAVIS, M.D., *Editor*, Greensboro, N. C.

THE ANNUAL MEETING OF THE CAROLINAS-VIRGINIAS HOSPITAL ASSOCIATION

ON MAY 17TH-18TH the Annual Meeting of the Carolinas-Virginias Hospital Association was held in Asheville. A large and representative attendance was on hand for the opening—nurses, doctors, business administrators and trustees. There was a look of seriousness on the faces of many that I had not noticed at former meetings, due to a combination of causes—war problems, institutional worries, long hours of hard work.

The program ranged from purely military matters, socialized medicine and penicillin, to diets, and back again. Dr. Dailey discussed "Infant Care and Child Welfare," how the Government proposes to "partially" pay for hospitalization for infants and children out of the United States Treasury. It was not hard to see that he was laboring under difficulty in presenting his paper. The difficulty arising from the fact that the politicians were telling him what to do and how to do it, and he in turn was trying to tell the hospitals what they had better do. Many hospital administrators asked him why the Government wanted to insist upon a "cut-rate price" for the hospital services. He made a desperate effort to tell them that his expert political advisors had decided that the rate mentioned in his paper was not less than cost. In the end all parted good friends but the general impression was that he had not sold the scheme as easily as the politicians had expected.

When Dr. Henry Highsmith of the Department of Education of North Carolina was asked about the pre-nursing training requirements, it was brought out that a good many of the applicants could not write legibly nor even spell common English words; also that the Department of Education was thrusting biology, chemistry and other required subjects in the laps of the hospital instructors of nurses, expecting the nurses to learn these subjects after they entered the Practical Training Course. It was pointed out by these hospitals that the high schools are in a far better position to teach many of the subjects required in the nurses' curriculum. Nurses should be taught in the hospitals drugs, solutions and nursing technique with its ramifications including details of treatment. It was the consensus of opinion that high school graduates are woefully lacking in the fundamentals of education, i.e., "reading, writing and arithmetic." Dr. Highsmith insisted that his high school graduates were superior, mentally, to any high school graduates of former days and further offered to pit their spelling ability against that of his audience. It is entirely possible that Dr. Highsmith might be mistaken. At least this was the spoken opinion of those present. Dr. Highsmith's curriculum was planned in Raleigh and not in the classrooms of the high schools over the state.

Another interesting feature of the meeting was the explanation of the Nurses Cadet Corps. There are certain features of it that are attractive but one could not help but feel that it was just another step of the national government taking charge of the medical and nursing profession of our country. The only attractive part of this method of taking training is that the expenses are born by the government and the hospital *jointly* and that the student receives some remuneration during her training.

Every report from the Nurses Asociation was instructive. Some work had been done in trying to organize the undergraduate and practical nurses services as now rendered to the sick people of North Carolina. The feeling seems to be that it is best for them to bring this very large and partially trained group of women under the Graduate Nurses State Requirements. The judgment of this editor is that they would do far better to compete with this group by putting out graduate nurses well and ethically trained to nurse the sick people of the state in which they reside. Unless they do this very soon there will be more partially trained nurses than R.N.'s If the registered nurse even hopes to dominate in the field of nursing over those partially and poorly trained now entering the field, she will be obliged to get this group into some type of organization. When this happens they will demand representation and all consideration as to their own hours and fees. If they outnumber the graduates they will out-vote the graduate nurses. If their voice is not heard and their vote not counted that will mean regimentation without representation. Should the nurses succeed in getting a bill passed through the legislature and then the authority to dictate the fees, the hours and the conditions under which the undergraduates and practical nurses should work, they will find throbbing headaches not relieved by B.C.'s, et cetera, in trying to administer the law in regard to inadequately trained nurses. The wise step for them to take is that of organizing and maintaining as many good training schools as possible. We all know that sick people must be nursed whether excellently, poorly, or miserably. They will always take the excellent nursing if we will but do our duty and furnish them with this type of nursing.

The Legislative Committee of the North Carolina Hospital Association has been helpful in formulating state and national policies concerning the hospitals. It is highly desirable that every state have an active legislative committee. Few legislators are familiar with the hospitals' problems; some do not care. By and large, those making laws, both nationally and locally, would be much more favorably impressed with the difficult problems of our hospitals if they had a picture from the inside explaining this to them. This is done by a legislative committee.

Highlights of the meeting were: The seriousness of the delegates; the scarcity of personnel; the Government taking a hand in the training of nurses; the pre-nursing educational attainments; the Government participating in infant and child welfare through local hospitals; and the graduate nurses' efforts to bring under their control those who are not graduates but who are rapidly filling the places of graduate nurses.

CLINICAL CHEMISTRY and MICROSCOPY

J. M. FEDER, M.D., and EVELYN TRIBBLE, M.T., *Editors*,
Anderson, S. C.

LEUCOPENIC INDEX WITH REFERENCE TO GASTROINTESTINAL ALLERGY*

IN THE FIELD of laboratory research leucopenic index has found its rightful place in the diagnosis of gastrointestinal allergy, although it has been in the background for several years and very little progress has been made.

Some time ago a patient was admitted to the hospital who was suspected to have some type of food allergy. The history gave no definite clue. Seventy-two intradermal tests gave positive reactions to: chocolate, bananas, potatoes (both kinds) and tobacco. The patient did not use tobacco in any form, but said that in the presence of others who were smoking he always developed a severe headache.

Doubtful reactions occurred to pork. In order

*Arthur Beverung, M. T., Ville Platte, Louisiana, in the April, 1944, issue of *Journal of the American Medical Technologists*. Reproduced by permission.

to eliminate this protein beyond a doubt, a leucopenic index was made and the following day three fasting counts were taken with the same pipette (Adam's certified) to obtain the normal. After the ingestion of one portion, counts were taken at 30-minute intervals for two hours. At the end of the two-hour period there was no definite leucopenia. (Chart No. 1.)

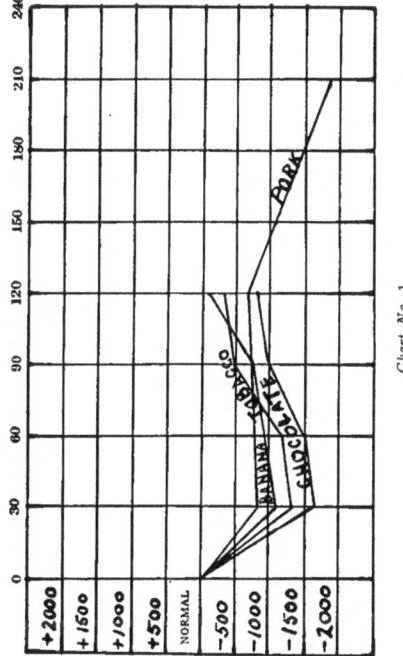

Chart No. 1

After three and a half hours the patient had a slight itching of the skin and a headache. A count taken at this time, always using the same pipette and counting chamber, showed a definite allergic response—a drop of 1800 cells. The test was repeated the next day and the same results obtained. This I termed a delayed allergic response. Pork was excluded along with the other proteins that showed an allergy and the patient no longer had symptoms. With this case in mind in future cases where skin tests are doubtful or where history shows an allergy with a negative skin test a leucopenic index should be done.

Another patient admitted to hospital with suspected food allergy. History was negative with the exception of duodenal ulcer and a stomach resection. Skin tests were negative to all foods except chocolate. Upon the ingestion of beef and eggs the patient would have violent stomach cramps and headache. When ingested separately one for one meal and the other at another, no symptoms would occur. Skin tests (paste, powder, liquids) were negative even when tested in combination. When leucopenic index was carried out there was a leucopenia of 2,900 in thirty minutes. (See Chart No. 2.)

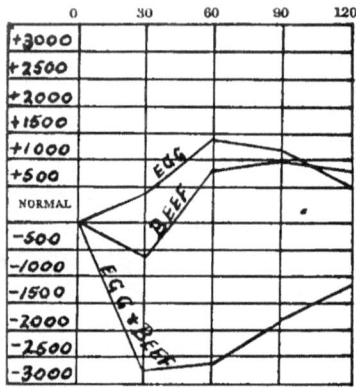

Chart No. 2

A leucopenic index was made for beef alone and for egg. These showed no allergic responses, and there were no symptoms when both were ingested. In this case skin tests were absolutely useless in diagnosing intestinal allergy, where leucopenic index showed definitely positive reaction which dovetailed with symptoms produced.

I can see only one disadvantage of the leucopenic index—it is time-consuming. Although I have only a few cases to report I believe that it was well worth the time and a distinct help to the patient. I further believe that the use of leucopenic index is still in the primitive stage and it is superior to any type of skin test yet devised.

DEPARTMENT EDITOR'S NOTE:

It has long been the belief of this writer that the only approach to some of the food allergies is the leucopenic index. Granted, it has been far from a satisfactory solution in many cases. Probably Mr. Beverung's article clarifies some of these failures.

We also hold the opinion that there are more numerical combinations of the various foods than we can possibly comprehend and that these have the power in combination to form new protein factors, foreign to either of the foods when taken or tested for alone.

Aside from its scientific value, this article is illustrative of the splendid work that our medical technologists are doing and are capable of doing in your own office and hospital.

In the last place, it set us to wondering just what fraction of one per cent of allergic diseases receive a final proper diagnosis.

GENERAL PRACTICE

D. HERBERT SMITH, M.D., *Editor*, Pauline, S. C.

THE INCIDENCE OF HYPOTHYROIDISM

BASAL METABOLISM tests were made on 706 patients:[1] a few had high rates; more fell within normal ranges; 408 had readings from minus-10 down. Many tests were done by our laboratory for other doctors; as a rule these patients were tested once only. We do have complete records of our personal cases which numbered 234 of the larger group.

As symptoms of hypothyroidism: weakness is common, fatigue, muscle tiredness at the end of the day with aching and, not infrequently, muscle cramps; the patients have plenty of desire to do things, but their objectives seem hard to attain. They usually have a good intelligence yet it tires them to use their minds; they become sleepy on reading. They seem nervous largely because of things undone and which they worry about doing; ordinarily, they are good sleepers, often they sleep too much, and many of them wish they could take naps in the daytime; a small minority have insomnia, at least they so state; many are overweight, some are of normal weight, a few are thin, but it is a general rule that the obese ones all complain of how difficult it is for them to lose weight short of very rigid dieting.

Treatment is almost universally satisfactory. Many patients coöperate well and carry on their treatment indefinitely, believing the statement made that, more than likely, they must continue it the rest of their lives. But for some it seems too simple; so much so, that they forget it easily; they are apathetic, anyhow, and perhaps should rather be pitied than blamed. Therefore, they lapse. In a few cases thyroid extract disagrees, causing palpitation and nervousness. A change of brand or the use of thyroxin may help there.

The small-dose method takes longer; the patients respond more slowly, but there is less danger of starting activity in an adenoma which could not be found at examination. Patients should be interviewed frequently at first and their appearance, heart action, blood pressure and weight watched for any signs of over activity of the thyroid.

We have tested the basal metabolic rate of 706 patients. Of these, 408 registered minus-10 or below. Of the latter, 234 are personal patients of whom we have complete records. These 234 pa-

---

1. R. M. Watkins, Cleveland, in *Ohio State Jl.*, June.

tients with hypothyroidism represent 6.8 per cent of the total patients seen over a period of time in a practice limited to internal medicine. Therefore, the disease must be very common and should be watched for.

A great many of our patients would be better off for having thyroid gland preparations. As Dr. Watkins says, it is wise to begin with a small dose. Some whose b. m. r. is "normal" are much improved by thyroid medication.

INSURANCE MEDICINE

H. F. STARR, M.D., *Editor*, Greensboro, N. C.

HEART MURMURS IN LIFE INSURANCE

MITRAL REGURGITATION, the most common of heart murmurs found in applicants for life insurance, is systolic in time, loudest at the apex. It may be soft and blowing, of little intensity, and heard over a very limited area, or transmitted into the axilla, or upward over the precordium a few inches, or rough and loud and heard over the whole heart and around to the back of the chest. The pulse is in no way characteristic, but when decompensation takes place it may become weak and irregular. The exercise test may show abnormal blood pressure if decompensation is taking place. The pulmonic second sound in the second left interspace is sharply accentuated.

THE MURMUR OF MITRAL OBSTRUCTION is diastolic (late) or presystolic in time, rough and rumbling in character. It occurs usually in a limited area, being heard over a small space immediately surrounding the apex. In case the murmur is slight the area of cardiac dullness may not show any enlargement, but with a pronounced murmur the apex beat may be displaced to the left. The dullness may increase to the right. It is usually more pronounced in the erect position and may almost disappear in the recumbent position. Exercise or leaning forward in the erect position intensifies the murmur.

With a history of rheumatism and the characteristic murmur of mitral regurgitation, the presence of mitral stenosis should also be suspected, and tested for by exercise. The pulse is small and may be irregular and the blood pressure is apt to be low. With mitral obstruction plus decompensation the pulmonic second sound is markedly accentuated, but as dilatation takes place, it gradually diminishes in intensity.. The presystolic thrill at the apex is characteristic of mitral stenosis provided it is substantiated by other signs. It should not be confused with a normal forcible impulse found frequently in young individuals with thin chest walls who are often nervous on examination.

THE AORTIC REGURGITATION murmur is diastolic in time beginning when the second sound ends and sometimes obscures the second sound entirely. The point of greatest intensity may be the second right or third left interspace, or over the base of the sternum. Occasionally it is heard over the body of the sternum. It is usually transmitted downward along the left border of the sternum, even to the apex of the heart. It is usually more marked in the erect position. The pulse is regular with a characteristic quality—the so-called water-hammer (Corrigan's) pulse—like a sharp blow falling away without being sustained. The pulse pressure is high—high systolic and low diastolic. Pulsation of the arteries is visible and especially marked in carotid, temporal or brachial. In some cases a pistol-shot sound is heard over the femoral artery. Alternating flushing and paling with each heart beat may be noted in the lips and fingernails.

AORTIC OBSTRUCTION or stenosis is not so common as the other lesions and is often presesnt in combination with aortic regurgitation. In case it exists apparently alone, aortic regurgitation should be sought for. It is more frequent after the age of forty. The murmur is systolic, replacing or immediately following the first sound. The maximum intensity of sound is at the second right interspace and is transmitted upward and it may also be heard over the base of the sternum and over the carotids and subclavians. It is rough and may be very loud and is best heard when the applicant is recumbent. On palpation a thrill is usually felt. The heart is often enlarged to the left and downward. The aortic second sound is usually absent or faint. In many cases a mitral regurgitation murmur is heard all over the precordium, but without transmission into the neck, and it is often difficult to say whether there is only one murmur or more than one. The pulse is slow, small with a slow ascent and descent with a plateau due to sustained pressure between rise and fall.

A FUNCTIONAL MURMUR is blowing, systolic, and best heard over the pulmonic area in the second left interspace. It is not transmitted and may disappear in various phases of respiration as well as with certain postures of the body. It is not accompanied by hypertrophy of the heart or any other evidence of circulatory abnormality. The applicant should be free of past history of infection (rheumatism), personal history of cardiac embarrassment, abnormal reaction to exercise, high or low blood pressure, cardiac enlargement, presence of tachycardia or cardiac arrhythmia. Any of these conditions, in addition to the murmur, should preclude murmur being labeled functional.

The "CARDIO-RESPIRATORY" murmur is heard during systole and diastole, due to the passage of the lung over the heart during its beats. In other

WITHOUT X-RAY OR ORTHODIAGRAM
Distance of left border of heart from mid-sternal line
4 in. to 4½ in.   Over 4¼ in. to 5 in.   Over 5 in. to 5½ in.   Over½ in.

Weight		Add to normal mortality		
130 lbs. or less	50%	75% or more	100% or more	Decline
151 to 175 lbs.	0	50% " "	75% " "	150% or more
176 to 200 lbs.	0	0	50% " "	100% " "
Over 200 lbs.	0	0	0	50% " "

words, the sound is produced in the lung by the tapping of the heart. It disappears at full expiration or inspiration. If the diagnosis is clearly established, this is usually disregarded.

CONGENITAL HEART MURMUR, if accurately diagnosed, generally causes rejection for life insurance. Few persons so afflicted reach adult insurable ages.

HYPERTROPHY: There is a definite relationship between the normal position of the apex beat and an individual's build. It is important that the examiner locate the apex beat accurately and give the exact distance from the mid-sternal line to the left border of the heart. This is especially important in cases with present or past findings of heart or pulse abnormalities, high blood pressure, arterio-sclerosis, etc. It is well to remember that tall, thin individuals are apt to have vertically placed hearts, whereas the short, heavy-set often have transverse hearts. The following ratings, based on applicant's weight and the distance of left border of the heart from mid-sternal line, give a general idea as to the extra mortality anticipated by many companies on account of hypertrophy.

APEX MURMUR, SYSTOLIC, CONSTANT, NOT TRANSMITTED TO THE LEFT:

	Add to normal mortality
Under age 30	10%
Ages 30 to 39	20%
Ages 40 to 49	35%
Ages 50 and over	50%

WITH X-RAY OR ORTHODIARGAM the enlargement of the heart is to be determined by the criteria of Eyster and Hodges. The so-called cardio-thoracic ratio is generally considered much less reliable. If hypertrophy is definitely established by x-ray examination add 75 per cent as the minimum additional mortality to be expected in the group.

UNCOMPLICATED MURMURS:
No Hypertrophy:

	Add to normal mortality	
Mitral Regurgitation—light manual worker	75% to 100%	
heavy manual worker	125% to 150%	
Mitral Obstruction	400%	
Aortic Regurgitation	350%	
Aortic Obstruction	125% to Decline	
Double Murmurs	Decline	
Tricuspid	Rate as Mitral	
Pulmonic	" " Aortic	
Any sign of Failing Compensation	Decline	
Functional Murmurs:		
Under Age 30	10%	
Ages 30 to 39	15%	
Ages 40 and up	25% to 50%	
	Slight Hypertrophy	More than slight Hypertrophy
With Hypertrophy:		
Mitral Regurgitation (Apex, systolic, transmitted, constant)	150% up	250% up
Mitral Obstruction	Decline	Decline
Aortic Regurgitation	400%	Decline
Aortic Obstruction (second right interspace, systolic, transmitted)	250%	300% to Decline

APEX MURMUR, SYSTOLIC, CONSTANT, TRANSMITTED TO THE LEFT WITH HISTORY OF:

Light Manual Labor	Acute rheumatism or chorea			Other Infections
Without Hypertrophy	Under Age 30	Ages 30-49	Age 50 and over	All Ages
within 2 yrs.	Decline	Decline	Decline	Decline
3rd & 4th yrs.	"	"	"	Add 175%
5th & 6th yrs.	"	"	"	Add 140%
7th to 10th yrs.	"	Add 200%	Add 175%	" 110%
11th to 14th yrs.	Add 175%	" 150%	" 130%	" 110%
15th yr. & later	" 125%	" 110%	" 110%	" 110%
With Hypertrophy				
Slight	Decline	Decline	Decline	Add 50% or more to above ratings
Moderate	"	"	"	Decline

Heavy manual labor adds 50% to the above ratings.

EFFECT ON MORTALITY

Many companies provide for an extra mortality in heart murmurs, expressed in percentage added to the normal, as indicated in the following tables:

Consider "slight" hypertrophy where rating under "Hypertrophy" shown above without x-ray is 50 per cent. If rated more than 50 per cent without x-ray consider as more than slight hypertrophy.

EFFECT OF HISTORY ONLY OF MURMURS:
Add the following to the normal mortality:

Functional	Disregard
Mitral Regurgitation	25 to 40%
Mitral Obstruction	75% and up
Aortic Regurgitation	50% and up
Aortic Obstruction	50% and up
Double Murmur	100% and up

A history of a heart murmur found on a previous examination (except functional murmurs) should not be disregarded unless not found on subsequent examinations made by a qualified cardiologist who had knowledge of the previous findings. An electrocardiogram, of course, does not give any information regarding the presence or absence of a heart murmur.

RHINO-OTO-LARYNGOLOGY

CLAY W. EVATT, M.D., *Editor*, Charleston, S. C.

THE TREATMENT OF TONSILLITIS, PHARYNGITIS AND GINGIVOSTOMATITIS WITH THE BISMUTH SALT OF HEPTADIENECARBOXYLIC ACID IN SUPPOSITORIES

THE EFFECTIVENESS OF BISMUTH injections in infections of Spirillar and Spirochetal origin has long been known. Bismuth is also effective in cases of Streptococcal tonsillitis and possess some analgesic properties. Ten per cent acid tartrobismuthate of potassium locally in Vincent's angina has been used with brilliant results. Tonsillitis has been treated successfully by injecting 0.005 gm. of bismuth, with repetitions if necessary. The morbidity was greatly reduced. Patients usually had a drop in temperature to normal within 12 to 24 hours. The earlier in the course of the ailment the bismuth was administered, the more rapid the defervescence. Follicular exudate disappeared in 24 hours in most of the cases.

The effectiveness of the bismuth was most marked in the extensively involved cases. The more profuse the exudate and the deeper the necrosis, the more efficient was the treatment. Prompt relief of pain and disapparance of exudate from the tonsils was noted in twenty-four hours. The average duration of tonsillitis is reduced from six to eight days to 24 to 48 hours. The rapid absorption and penetration of the bismuth, especially by lymphatic tissues such as the tonsillar, is emphasized, also the toxic effects are obviated by rapid elimination.

Lewis treated 40 patients for fusospirochetal tonsillar infection over a six-months period, so severe as to justify "specific treatment." He thought bismuth to be the drug of choice and hoped that its injection could be obviated by giving the drug orally.

Bismuth has been used in the form of suppositories,[1] probably easier than the oral administration and as effective as the injections. Especially absorbable and easily utilized is the bismuth salt of heptadienecarboxylic acid in cocoa butter. Complete clearing up of symptoms in 72 hours is reported in cases of ulcerous angina and upper respiratory infections. Retrogression of symptoms in thirty-six hours is reported in cases of tonsillar and peritonsillar infections. Fifteen cases of ulcerous stomatitis were treated by the daily use of suppositories. High fever, hemorrhagic coated, ulcerated gums, intense pain, and swollen cervical nodes began to improve the first day. Objective signs were definitely less on the fourth day, and complete recovery occurred on the seventh day. Glycerin-salvarsan painted locally in half these patients seemed to make no difference from those not treated. Quite a few cases of tonsillitis, pharyngitis and gingivostomatitis (Vincent's) were treated with the absorbable salt of heptadienecarboxylic acid in cocoa butter suppositories.* Subjective symptoms disappeared within 22 to 48 hours. Temperature dropped and signs of local improvement appeared in 24 hours. No more than two suppositories at 24-hour intervals were required in most of the cases. There were no local ill effects from the use of suppositories. There were no toxic reactions to bismuth.

1. Silber, Samuel; The Treatment of Tonsillitis, Pharyngitis and Gingivostomatitis with the Bismuth Salt of Heptadienecarboxylic Acid Suppositories. *Jour. of Pediatrics*, pgs. 59-68, July, 1943.
*Suppositories used contained 0.0675 Gm. of the Acid and 0.0225 Gm. Metallic Bismuth in cocoa butter. Produced by Specific Pharmaceuticals, Inc.

UROLOGY

RAYMOND THOMPSON, M.D., *Editor*, Charlotte, N. C.

INDICATIONS FOR VISUAL EXAMINATION OF LOWER URINARY TRACT

A CYSTOSCOPIC EXAMINATION made by an experienced and skilful operator yields information (regarding developing pathological changes) which can be gained in no other way. If patients have learned to dread this procedure, their reaction may be regarded as a comment upon the operator, for, correctly performed, it should be ". . . without discomfort or untoward aftermath."[1] It is important to understand under what conditions this form of examination is contraindicated.

A cystoscope is a highly-specialized instrument, and one designed appropriately for the type of work, and of a size fitted to the patient, should be used. The use of the wrong size or type may result in trauma and subsequent infection. "As soon as ureteral catheters are passed the cystoscope should be withdrawn immediately," *i.e.*, before x-ray pictures are made and before discomfort or injury is produced. Exposure of the genitalia during visualization is an avoidable embarrassment.

Use of an appropriate anesthetic produces relaxation and freedom from pain. For the female patient "a cotton applicator dipped in 10-per cent solution of cocaine and placed in the urethra for five or ten minutes," according to the procedure outlined by Bumpus is recommended. A few c.c. of one of the cocaine derivatives may be injected into the bladder to anesthetize the trigone.

For the male patient a solution of $2\frac{1}{4}$ grains cocaine in an ounce of sterile water may be injected slowly into the urethra, and the meatus treated with a swab dipped in 10-per cent solution during which time a penis clamp is applied. If there is any question of idiosyncrasy for cocaine, or in case the urethra hass been recently traumatized, one of the cocaine substitutes should be used.

"If the office affords facilities for recovery from complete narcosis, no anesthetic is as satisfactory for such work as pentothal sodium"—but fortifying it with codeine or morphine is contraindicated.

Before instrumental examination is attempted, in either sex, "the type of infecting organism should be ascertained by stain and culture and every effort made to render the urine bacteriostatic, at least to the specific organisms, before proceeding to investigate the damage they have caused." A microscopic examination of the urine obtained by catheter will supply the evidence on which it may be decided for or against a visual examination.

Overdistention of the bladder or passage of instruments may both cause trauma. The importance of this is obvious when it is realized that in the absence of trauma a normal urinary tract may be exposed to bacteria without infection. Once a lesion is observed an examiner should terminate his examination, thus reducing the possibilities of trauma through protracted examination. The report of cystoscopy consuming from 15 to 30 minutes reflects the inexperience of the examiner and in no way indicates his thoroughness or efficiency."

Some pathological conditions of the lower urinary tract do not require visualization for examination. Presence or absence of stones in the bladder or prostate may be determined by x-ray examination. Injection of the bladder with air will reveal diverticula and the extent of trabeculation. Finger examination per rectum will reveal the type of enlargement and a rubber catheter the amount of residual urine.

Prostatic obstruction is likely to be increased by instrumental examination. "Probably in no condition has instrumentation been more painfully or uselessly employed or yielded less worthwhile information than in routine cystoscopy of the elderly man with urinary obstruction the result of prostatic hypertrophy."

The general use of intravenous pyelography has made evident the need for urethral catheterization and visual examination as a means of furnishing supplementary information. "Unless all possible information from all possible sources is at hand, both diagnosis and treatment are of doubtful validity."

1. Indications for Visual Examination of the Lower Urinary Tract. H. C. Bumpus. *J. A. M. A.*, Nov. 6th, 1943.

DENTISTRY

J. H. GUION, D.D.S., *Editor*, Charlotte, N. C.

THE TEETH AND AGING

THE SLOGAN, "A clean tooth does not decay," should be changed to, "A well-nourished tooth does not decay," well-nourished teeth keep clean. Thus a St. Louis dental surgeon[1] corrects an old misstatement. And he goes on to make other points:

Dental caries is the most prevalent disease afflicting mankind. It is not necessary in every instance for the pulp to be exposed through the decalcification of the dentine in order to become infected. Pathogenic organisms may be carried through the dentinal tubules and infect the pulp any time after the enamel has been destroyed to the dento-enamel junction.

A considerable amount of laboratory research and animal experimentation has been and is being done to explain *how* teeth decay. Not so much has been done to explain *why* they decay.

Active dental caries is observed almost entirely in childhood and youth. Arrested dental caries and periodontosis are observed in adults usually beyond 30 years of age. Correct nutrition and wholesome living for children are the safest means by which to achieve healthful adulthood with sound teeth.

There are but two distinctive disease processes which cause mutilation of the human dentures: dental caries active chiefly during childhood and youth and the destroyer of the crowns of the teeth; and periodontosis, an inflammatory disease process

1. B. N. Pippin, St. Louis, in *Jl.Lancet*, June.

confined to the gingivae, periodontal membrane, cementum and the alveolar bone. If allowed to progress, it will result in the loss of all the teeth. Periodontosis is caused by systemic dysfunctions resulting chiefly from malnutrition. The usual surgical curettage while indispensable in treatment is not sufficient to effect a cure. The cause, systemic dysfunction, must be corrected.

The wholesale extraction of third molars on the assumption, "they are no good anyway," should be discontinued. Adequate nutrition and growth in youth would tend to effect perfect dentition.

Civilized man must adopt methods in his industrial and social relationships that will lead to conservation rather than destruction. The impoverished soils must be replenished, the forests replanted and maintained, the streams purified and made fit for aquatic life, and all the natural resources conserved for use and not exploitation. With the means of rapid transportation and refrigeration, nutritious foods grown upon replenished soils can be, through coöperative handling, placed upon the consumers' tables within a few hours from the time of shipping.

The consumption of natural highly nutritious foods will go a long way toward preventing disease, including dental disease. Food, however, is not alone responsible for malnutrition.

SURGERY

Geo. H. Bunch, M.D., *Editor*, Columbia, S. C.

REFRIGERATION ANESTHESIA

Allen in 1937 found that the survival time of a ligated limb is increased by lowering its temperature to within five degrees of freezing. He also found that limbs kept within this temperature range remain viable after the application of the tourniquet for a much longer time than do those at ordinary room temperature. There is no thrombosis and shock does not follow the removal of the tourniquet in them as it does in those that have not been chilled. The clinical application of these facts to the surgical treatment of peripheral vascular disease has been revolutionary; although Larrey, more than a hundred years ago, noted and recorded the beneficial effect of cold upon the seriously injured limbs of French soldiers cared for by him in Napoleon's tretreat from Moscow.

Metabolism is so slowed by cold in bears during hibernation that they pass the winter months without food and without water. A fish may be frozen in a block of solid ice, and swim as before when the ice is melted. The blood serum of the fish freezes at a lower temperature than does water. If the serum freezes the fish dies.

Perhaps the most practical benefit of Allen's work is in the production of refrigeration anesthesia for the amputation of limbs that have become gangrenous from sclerosis of the peripheral arteries. It has been found that a thigh completely surrounded by crushed ice for two hours, although the tissues are not frozen, becomes sufficiently chilled that it may be amputated without pain and without the administration of any anesthetic. A tourniquet should be applied just above the place of amputation before refrigeration is begun so that chilling of the limb may be facilitated without the body temperature being affected. Stumps heal more slowly after refrigeration but amputation in these aged, seriously-ill patients is without shock or unfavorable reaction of any kind. They hardly know they have been operated upon and are ready to eat when they leave the operating table. Because bacterial activity in the limb is inhibited by chilling, the danger of infection is reduced to a minimum. The mortality rate of amputations of the thigh in this class of patients has been reduced by nearly one-half.

Refrigeration is the anesthesia of choice for amputation on diabetic and senile patients. Another of its fields of usefulness is in the surgical care of the indigent down-and-outs who fill the charity wards of every large metropolitan hospital. In these institutions the clinical material is of sufficient volume to permit perfection of technique. In them special operating crews should be trained to work under refrigeration conditions. These unfortunate patients, some of whom have already lost one or more limbs, are entitled to our best efforts.

THERAPEUTICS

J. F. Nash, M.D., *Editor*, Saint Pauls, N. C.

HAND INFECTIONS

According to modern teaching, few of us carry out as elaborate antiseptic technique in our offices as we should. The following abstract is made from an article[1] which—face mask and all—has my endorsement.

Care should be taken not to further injure structures—sharp, well-placed, purposeful incisions are esential; gentle mechanical cleansing of the part should be done with white soap and water.

Too often injuries and infections of the hand are treated where proper surgical surroundings are lacking, inadequate instruments are used, and no provision is made for masking the nose and mouth and thus the wounds become reinfected. Minor infection may become major.

---
1. R. F. Hedin, Red Wing, in *Minn. Med.*, June.

Early adequate drainage should be carried out with the least possible trauma. It is necessary to visualize clearly the path of the infection. A bloodless field is obtained by placing securely a blood pressure cuff on the arm and, after elevating the hand, raising the pressure in the cuff to 250 mm. of Hg. General anesthesia is essential in order that the patient may withstand the pressure from the inflated cuff.

Rigid drainage material causes necrosis. Soft rubber tissue or vaseline gauze inserted into the angle of the wound for 24-48 hours gives drainage without damage.

Dressings done in the office merit the same antiseptic technique as in operating room. If moist dressings are employed to provide drainage for an infected surface, the patient should be cautioned not to moisten the dressing at home.

Sterile towels are spread to extend from the axilla to beyond the finger tips. "Abd" pads are then placed on the towel to form a trough, and fluff dressings are placed on the pads so that the arm, forearm and hand are completely encased. Dressings put between fingers prevent skin maceration tion of the skin. The dressing is then moistened (not soaked) with sterile, warm saline. After a layer of "abd" pads has been put over the fluffs, the towel edges are fastened with safety pins. Elevation of the forearm and hand by a pillow will prevent edema and provide dependent drainage. The dressing is kept warm by electric light bulbs in a cradle. Such dressing is usually opened only every 12 to 24 hours to moisten with warm, sterile saline and to replace soiled dressings.

Splinting prohibits movement of the part and thereby protects against tearing of granulation tissue. By minimizing muscular movements, it prevents spread of infection through vascular and lymphatic channels. The use of a wooden tongue blade often provides sufficient splint for a finger. In case of extensive infection a metal splint can be quickly made which will hold the hand in position of function.

Exuberant granulations can be dealt with by means of a firm pressure dressing. Cauterization with silver nitrate will open up to infection the small vessels in the granulations. Necrotic tissue is best separated by dressings moistened with freshly made Dakin's solution. All granulating surfaces should be covered with sterile *fine-meshed* gauze.

We are too prone to slackness in asepsis in treating accidental wounds, regarding them as already infected, and not giving proper value to the dangers of additional, more virulent infections. Particularly in treating wounds of the hand should every possible safeguard be taken against infection which so often leads to crippling.

PROCTOLOGY

RUSSELL VON L. BUXTON, M.D., *Editor*, Newport News, Va.

ON THE IMPORTANCE OF MAKING RECTAL EXAMINATIONS

MOST of our egregious errors in diagnosis come, not from lack of knowledge, but from failure to apply our knowledge to the problem in hand. One of the most notorious of the examples of this failure of application of knowledge lies in neglecting to examine the rectum.

A Georgia proctologist[1] presents this thesis convincingly and in no disparagement of the general practitioner.

This specialist deplores the lack of interest in disease conditions of the rectum on the part of recent graduates, general practitioners and general surgeons. He rightly ascribes most of the neglect in this field to the fact that practitioners attach little importance to rectal symptoms and too frequently make an offhand diagnosis of piles without making any examination.

The statement that anything which makes the patient conscious of the fact that he has an anus or rectum is an indication for rectal examination does not put the case too strongly.

Two instructive cases are cited.

A man, 55, applied for treatment with the sole complaint of moderate constipation for the past few weeks. No pain, no bleeding, no anything but constipation. An index finger inserted into the rectum readily felt a growth, biopsy of which showed adenocarcinoma. A resection was done and the patient is well after seven years.

A young lady, 30, came after having two copious hemorrhages from the rectum. The first occurred at night. The patient was sent to hospital by her physician, who, the next morning, found large internal hemorrhoids; and, the bleeding having ceased, sent her home with instructions to return in a few days for hemorrhoidectomy. A week later the whole series of events was repeated. The patient consulted the proctologist who took cognizance of the facts that there had been no bleeding with bowel movements, and that the patient said she "must have lost a quart of blood," sought other explanation of the bleeding. On sigmoidoscopic examination, seven inches from the anal margin a small ulcerated mass was found which proved to be an adenocarcinoma. Resection was done and there has been no recurrence.

These two cases teach us to be on the lookout for dangerous diseases as the explanation of symptoms and to bear in mind at all times the probability of more than one pathological condition existing in any given case.

Phillips counsels digital and proctoscopic investigation of the rectum as part of any general examination, and these, he well says, are within the abilities of the general man. He would not recommend that sigmoidoscopic examinations be made by anyone who has not had some training in the use of this longer scope.

There can be no reasonable disagreement with the statement: "It would be little trouble to the doctor and no particular discomfort to the patients if a rectal examination were made on all patients presenting themselves for general examination." In only a short time the physician would be familiarized with the normal rectum. Both digital and proctoscopic examination should be done for each will reveal what the other will not. For example: small internal hemorrhoids will not be found by the finger, but will be by the proctoscope; and the reverse is true of many an abscess.

Most of us can recall patients dead before their time because of neglect in the diagnosis of rectal cancer. When we realize that 90 per cent of cancers of the large bowel are within reach of the index finger, we can but feel guilty.

By making a rectal examination of every patient any doctor will better serve his patients and himself.

1. A. M. Phillips, Macon, in *Jl. Med. Assn. Ga.,* June.

PEDIATRICS

POLIOMYELITIS PREVENTION

JUNE THROUGH SEPTEMBER is the season when infantile paralysis is most prone to develop in the United States. The National Foundation for Infantile Paralysis has compiled the following suggestions:

1. During an outbreak of infantile paralysis be alert to any early signs of illness or changes in normal state of health, especially in children. Do not assume that a vomiting, constipation, diarrhea, severe headache or signs of a cold and fever are of no importance. These may be among the first symptoms of infantile paralysis. All children and adults sick with unexplained fever should be put to bed and isolated pending diagnosis.

2. Don't delay calling a physician. Expert medical care given early may prevent many of the crippling deformities. Proper care from the onset may mean the difference between a life of crippling and normal recovery.

3. There is no known special prevention or protection against infantile paralysis.

4. Observe these simple precautions:

(a) Avoid overtiring and extreme fatigue from strenuous exercise.
(b) Avoid sudden chilling such as would come from a plunge into extremely cold water.
(c) Pay careful attention to personal cleanliness, such as thorough hand washing before eating. Hygienic habits should always be observed.
(d) If possible avoid tonsil and adenoid operations during epidemics. Careful study has shown that such operations, when done during an epidemic, tend to increase the danger of contrasting infantile paralysis in its most serious form.
(e) Use the purest milk and water you can. Keep flies away from food. Contaminated water and milk are always dangerous and flies have repeatedly been shown to carry the infantile paralysis virus.
(f) Do not swim in polluted water.
(g) Maintain community sanitation at a high level at all times.
(h) Avoid all unnecessary contact with persons with any suspicious illness.

5. Don't become panicky if cases occur in your neighborhood. While infantile paralysis is communicable or catching during any outbreak, there are many who have such a slight infection that there are few or no symptoms. This large number of unrecognized infections is one of the reasons there is no practical way of preventing the spread of the disease. But it is also reassuring to know that, of the many persons who become infected, few develop serious illness and that, with good care, the majority who are stricken will make a satisfactory recovery.

6. Attempts to stop the spread of the virus by closing places where people congregate have been uniformly unsuccessful. The resulting disturbance to community life is a disadvantage.

7. There is no known cure for infantile paralysis. Good medical care will prevent or correct some deformities. But in about every fourth or fifth case there will be permanent paralysis that cannot be overcome. Do not believe those who for one reason or another promise to cure these cases. Be guided by sound medical advice.

TRICHOMONAS—From Page 249
thral infestation without ever showing the organisms in the prostatic secretion.

"Trichomonas genitalis" would be more truly descriptive of the habitat of a parasite which infests as high as 27.4% of certain portions of the male population and at the same time would assist in impressing on the profession that infestations of males as well as females are to be considered.

HUMAN BEHAVIOUR

James K. Hall, M.D., *Editor*, Richmond, Va.

ON AGEING AND ADAPTATION

"The average individual, too frequently the biologist and usually the pathologist, limits his interest and confines his intelligence of ageing to narrow categories of thought. He fails to appreciate the yearning of tissues for life and the amazing chemical and structural modifications they may participate in, even gross structural changes designated disease, in order to bring about organ adaptation and the adaptation of the individual as a whole to those changes which occur as the life span progresses. The certainty of the termination of this life span and the fact that all living things are concerned with it have stimulated the imagination of poets and philosophers. Their inquisitiveness has been either romantic or dominated by resignation and has not been demonstrably helpful. Another period which concerns itself with the facts of life is in its beginning, and as these facts accumulate through chemical, biological and psychical research the romance of life will find sound ground on which to express its related beauty. Ultimate resignation will become lost in an interest in the transitory prolongation and effectiveness of the different periods of the life span. The Browning concept of the 'last of life for which the first was made' will assume tangible significance."

Only a philosopher can look upon the manifestations of disease as constituting fundamental proof of the yearning of the living thing to continue to live, and to make almost unbelievable sacrifices in structure and in function in an effort to make the adaptation to environment successful. The scientist sees in life everywhere purpose. Even in those perturbations of Nature that would seem to most of us to constitute mere chaotic futility, the wise man realizes that cause is followed by effect and that all activity has an end in view.

Those of us who are fortunate enough to enable us to believe that we know him well recognize the initial quotation as the language of Dr. William de B. MacNider, Kenan Research Professor of Pharmacology of the University of North Carolina. The language is excerpted from the first paragraph of his address at the Symposium on Ageing at the Washington University Medical School in Saint Louis on March 24th and 25th of this year. He addressed himself to an elaboration of the thesis: Age, Change and the Adapted Life.

Not since I read Gregory Zilboorg on the Fear of Death have I been so profoundly moved by the rationalizing of one of my medical acquaintances. I do not know that Dr. Zilboorg and Dr. MacNider know each other personally. But how deeply related the profundity of their thinking about life is! What pleasure lies in store for each in coming to know the other! How intimately related each to the other is life and death! One cannot contemplate either without calling into immediate association the other.

Within the last few years a number of volumes have come from the presses in which the ageing processes in man are dealt with; and more than one organization has come into being whose purpose is to develop an understanding of those forces and of those changes that are associated, causatively and symptomatically, with the senescent state that ends ultimately in death.

Occasionally I have been embarrassed when asked while in the witness chair in the court room to proffer a definition of arteriosclerosis. And once, at least, my embarrassment was increased by the Court's expression of appreciation of the clarity with which I defined the phenomenon. But I felt obliged to arrest the Court's attention until I could confess that I was wholly without understanding of the meaning of the anatomical and functional changes associated with the arteriosclerotic process and of the reasons for the changes in the circulatory tubes that tend to interfere so seriously with the blood-flow.

In some such fashion would the biologist, I surmise, confess his limited understanding of those more comprehensive changes that take place progressively in man's body and mind as he becomes older and still older. A certain relentlessness would seem to underlie the processes, yet no one presumes to speak out about the meaning and the purpose of the anatomical and physiological and psychological mutations that tend to mar the last years of every elderly mortal's life.

Dr. MacNider protests against the conception of age as a fatalistically fixed, natural, irreversible process, chronologically determined by the species of animal. He insists that the processes associated with ageing should be looked upon as living, fluid, elastic states of give-and-take for the sake of adjustment as the organism passes through its life span. Those changes indicative of ageing he would interpret as manifestations of the attempt of the organism to effect an adaptation to the years of its life. Not infrequently, however, many of the changes in structure and in function in the organism must be looked upon as failures in adaptation

It is the duty of the student of the processes to consider the reasons for the failure, the causes underlying it, and to discover the biologic necessity for the disappearance of man through death merely because he has become old. How large and how involved and how important the problem is! Perhaps the problem is made up of a cluster of problems.

Age constitutes an associated causative factor in many diseases. Certain infections are so associated with the early years of man's life that they are not improperly spoken of as children's diseases. The infant is apparently disinclined to contract in the first months of life those diseases to which it is exceedingly susceptible afterwards, for a few years. But the child's susceptibility to measles, for example, diminishes with the roll of the years. I should think an attack of measles in the sixth decade of life would be unusual. What changes take place in the cells of the individual, in structure and in function, making him when a new-born infant, non-susceptible to mumps, for example; causing him later to be highly susceptible to that disease; and those changes that still later in life protect him from an invasion by mumps? In years lately gone by, most individuals in this area contracted typhoid fever in that period of life between the age of 20 and 50. What cellular and what biochemical state invited an attack of the disease at 30, but warded it off at 10, and again at 60? We do not know. Acute anterior poliomyelitis is now prevalent in an area in western North Carolina. But the disease will seldom fall upon a babe in arms or upon an individual in mid-life. Why? We do not know. But should we not know? Can we not find out?

The age of the individual must be almost a determining factor in malignancy. The young, so susceptible to many deadly diseases, live in relative defiance of cancer. Why?

It is little wonder that for a generation Doctor MacNider has been one of the impressive medical teachers of our country. He thinks of life, perhaps, as the manifestation of Divinity in declaring itself through law and order, and as affording man the opportunity to exist in harmony with his environment. In Doctor MacNider's world there can be no trivialities and no accidents. Disease does not fall upon man, he might say; but that man, consciously or unconsciously, invites upon and into himself those states and conditions that become a part of him—for weal or for woe. In thought and in language the address of Doctor MacNider at the Symposium in Saint Louis is worthy of American medicine at its best and of him in his most philosophic humor. The address is published in full in *Science* for May, 1944; and from that illuminating weekly it has been reprinted.

The individual, the environment, the remorseless roll of the years—what an impressive trilogy! No wise doctor would think of man or of disease disassociated from time and from environment.

A PUNCTURE WOUND from an indelible pencil often results in a serious infection. Do wide excision, care being taken to remove all of the dye-stained tissue.

OBSERVATIONS
OF THE STAFF
DAVIS HOSPITAL
Statesville

PSYCHOSOMATIC DISORDERS MANIFESTED MAINLY BY CARDIOVASCULAR SYMPTOMS AS SEEN IN THE MILITARY HOSPITAL

DURING THE PAST YEAR medical literature has reflected a tendency to revert to the consideration of illness as disease of the individual as a whole, psychosomatic medicine—disease of psyche and soma—of mind and of body. Renewed interest in this concept has been occasioned in part by the emotional stress of war on armed forces and civilians. The creation and functioning of military hospitals where a complete staff of psychiatrists, cardiologists, internists, general surgeons and surgical specialists, who often studied and reported jointly as a medical board on the soldier-patients' complaints and states, has favored this kind of medical study. To a great extent this is the method employed by the family physician, who, with his knowledge of details of his patients' heredity and environment, is able to arrive at proper diagnosis and prescribe proper treatment often with a minimum of examination. In addition, the present-day physician has the application of the many advances in all lines, including psychiatry, to draw from in arriving at his conclusions and making his applications.

In the psychosomatic approach the physician attempts to fully investigate the soma and the psyche, to determine the relationship between what the individual organs are doing and what the patient as a whole is doing; how the patient's emotions, efforts, hopes, discouragements and anxieties are influencing the symptoms, as well as the part played by physical and chemical agencies.

Various research centers have for the past decade put forth much effort in this field, not only in clinical studies of human illness, but in laboratory studies of lower animals. The reports have dealt especially with cardiovascular diseases and disorders, gastrointestinal disorders, asthma and injury from accident.

Medical thought at about the beginning of the last war differentiated diseases into functional and organic—emphasis on the organic, the disease rather than the patient.

As we near the middle of the 20th century, as a result of research and other studies in psychiatry, we have modified our view a great deal. We consider the patient more at times than his disease and consider that mind and body both play a part, and that often the same group of symptoms in one patient may result from physical causes and in another from psychical causes. It is necessary to be able to differentiate between reversible functional illness and irreversible organic disease, since only thus can the proper diagnosis and treatment be determined.

Almost every individual looks upon any disturbance or disorder of the heart with much concern, if not alarm. During the past decade the public in this country has been too concerned over the high incidence of heart disease as first among the causes of death. Insurance companies, public health authorities, private physicians and the lay press have spread this news until patients coming suspecting heart disease in themselves and requesting ecg. examination take up a large part of the cardiologist's time. In most instances no organic heart disease exists.

Now with the high incidence of real heart disease and disorders, and an even higher incidence of feared heart conditions in the civilian of peace time, it is no wonder that the Army medical officer is confronted with many cardiac complaints and diagnostic problems.

The examinations by physicians for the local draft boards and other preliminary screening of inductees and enlistees have eliminated the more manifest cases of organic heart disease. But the haste and speed with which these screening examinations are done allows some of the cases of actually or potentially disabling organic heart disease to reach the induction stations and some of them get inducted into the Armed Forces before their true condition or disability is determined.

It might be of interest to mention here some of the best means that many of the induction boards have employed in examining some of the borderline problems. The examining board of the induction station arranged with the Station Hospital for admission for a three-day observation and study of any men whose condition could not be determined adequately by the board in the allotted manner and time. Men for induction who were found to have a slight abnormal or suspicious condition of the cardiovascular system—tachycardia, moderately elevated blood pressure, systolic apical murmur, or definite complaints referable to that system—are sent to a special ward of the cardiovascular section of the medical service at the Station Hospital for this three-day study. The medical officer in charge of this ward, who is in most instances a cardiologist, has posted in the office of this ward a routine schedule which the nurse and wardmaster follow in checking and recording special findings. Tachycardia, slightly elevated blood pressure, and abnormal heart sounds are often found exaggerated if not caused entirely by, nervous excitement, homesickness, loss of sleep or overindulgence incident to their leaving home for the Army.

In order to evaluate the effect of such functional factors as contrasted to preëxisting organic disease or potential disability, the administration of nerve sedatives for the first two days is found proper. The inductee is confined to the ward and all stimulants are withheld. The day of admission he is interviewed by the medical or ward officer who designates any special tests or examinations—fluoroscopic examination of the heart, eyeground study, or cold-pressor test for blood pressure—that may appear indicated. Ecg. and urinalysis are usually the only routine procedure. Chest x-ray and serological studies have, of course, already been made the day the men arrived at the induction station. The nurse or wardmaster (an enlisted man) in charge, all of whom have been given special instructions and training, are responsible for taking and recording the pulse rate and blood pressure at least t.i.d., some of which should be made during the night or while the man is sleeping or relaxing. These recordings are made on a special mimeographed form which accompanies the man from the induction station. The duplicate sheets are signed at the top by the senior officer of the examination or induction board, who also indicates the studies to be made. Toward the bottom of the sheet is a space for the ward officer (cardiologist) to write in his conclusions or final diagnosis, which he does about the third day after reviewing the recordings of the three days—the ecg. and other routine or special reports—after making in most cases a brief physical examination. Perhaps in the majority of instances he is able to write in "No Disease; administrative admission for determining state of cardiovascular system." In some cases, such as those with a persistent slightly elevated blood pressure with evidence of arteriosclerosis or other organic disease, he may have to write "Arterial hypertension; slight, functional, from psychic factors." But most often this type of case can be reduced to "No disease of cardiovascular system"; that is, unless along with persistently elevated blood pressure there are positive findings in either the ecg., eyegrounds or kidney studies.

The routine followed in making and recording the results of the cold-pressor test, it is believed, gives indications of the potentially significant hypertensive individuals. The man under study is allowed to lie quiet and relaxed while a blood pressure reading is taken every five or 10 minutes, or until it remains at a basic level. Then, with the man lying still on cot or examining table, his hand and forearm are placed in a bucket of ice water for a period of three minutes. Then, the blood pressure band having remained on the arm, the blood pressure readings are repeated. An elevation of more than 20 mm. above the low average previously recorded is considered evidence of a potentially significant hypertensive state.

The standard diagnostic nomenclature used by the Army Station Hospitals lists a number of different headings under which disposition of the patient with a functional disorder may be made. Some of these might be present along with an organic disease, in which case both diagnoses would be listed. The following are some of these:

(1) 5480—Neurocirculatory asthenia; severity, cause
(2) 1170—Cardiac disorder, functional, type, severity, cause
(3) 1230—Cardiac palpitation, severity, cause
(4) 5520—Neurosis cardiac; severity, cause
(5) 5521—No disease; ill defined condition of (heart or cardiovascular system) manifestations
(6) 5522—No disease; administration admission for determination of state of cardiovascular system
(7) 5740—Other disease of circulatory system
(8) 3930—Hysteria, conversion: severity, cause
(9) 6950—Psychoneurosis; acute or chronic, manifested by, cause
(10) 4800—Malingering; state the disease feigned and method of detection

Neurocirculatory Asthenia—The medical officer frequently sees the various degrees of the condition which has been given this classification of N. C. A. by the U. S. Army. This syndrome was described toward the end of the American Civil War by Stille (1863), Da Costa (1864) and Hartshorne (1864). Especially by the English it has been termed Effort Syndrome and D. A. H. (disordered action of the heart). It is also described as Da Costa's Syndrome, Soldier's Heart and Irritable Heart.

The ancient writings of Galen indicate that he recognized the effect of physical effort and the influence of emotions on the pulse and heart action. More than 100 years ago John C. Williams wrote a book entitled *Practical Observations on Nervous and Sympathetic Palpitations of the Heart, Particularly as Distinguished from Palpitation the Result of Organic Disease*. In modern times apparently the first more complete treatise published was by Da Costa, who had made many observations as a medical officer in the Northern Armies. He published his paper entitled "On Irritable Heart: A Clinical Study of a Form of Functional Cardiac Disorder and Its Consequences," in the *American Journal of Medical Sciences* (LXI, 17), 1871. The term, Neurocirculatory Asthenia, was introduced by B. S. Oppenheimer *et al.* in 1918 and since that time has been the more acceptable term in American medicine and especially for Army diagnosis.

Sir Thomas Lewis made some of the most significant contributions on the subject in a book entitled *The Soldier's Heart and the Effort Syndrome*, in 1918, with a later edition in 1940.

Now for years past the soldier (or civilian) in peace, but more especially in wartime, who becomes dizzy, shaky, exhausted and somewhat breathless, with fast, forceful and painfully-beating heart, upon slight provocation, has puzzled and vexed Army doctors, without the condition having ever been fully understood.

Symptoms and findings observed in patients with N. C. A.:

*Breathlessness (45% to 100%)
Dizziness
*Cardiac pain
*Palpitation
Headache
Nervousness
Sleeplessness
Undue sweating
Tremors
*Fatigue while at rest
Indigestion
Nightmares
Cramps
Numbness
Constipation
Blurring of vision

*After effort; occasionally at rest.

This syndrome of fatigability, dyspnea, tremor and palpitation, with precardiac distress and tachycardia, may be provoked in any man by severe infections, prolonged hard physical or mental labor, or lack of sleep. However, it is only those with a very low threshold for the reaction that are so diagnosed. These men are the ones who during the physical examination present clammy extremities, profuse axillary perspiration, rapid pulse, tremor and dyspnea, and in whom tachycardia will not subside in 30 minutes after excitement or exercise. It is considered that 20 hops on one foot in one minute should not accelerate the pulse rate more than 45 beats per minute, and the rate should return to normal in less than three minutes after completion of the exercise.

Many of these men could be rehabilitated in a judiciously-planned program, but in wartime the Army does not have time or facilities for this.

It has become the conclusion of the authorities from observing the wars of the past that most of such cases upon whom this diagnosis has been properly and correctly made should be excluded from military service.

The British from 1916 to 1921 admitted to their medical units two cases of functional disease of the heart for every three cases of functional disease of the nervous system.

According to their observations in World War I, one patient out of ten admitted to the cardiac hospitals suffered from organic heart disease. Between 1917 and 1919 there were admitted to the American Army hospitals 4,376 cases of neurocirculatory asthenia. This does not include the many thousands of other types of functional cardiac disorder.

The early writers thought the victims of this condition were mostly men with small hearts. It has been considered due to heart strain, infection, tobacco, alcohol, hyperthyroidism, gas poisoning and shell shock.

Hurst felt that this was a manifestation of the combined effects of physical fatigue, mental exhaustion and toxemia (of exogenous origin).

Lewis dismisses tobacco, alcohol and hyperthyroidism as important factors, pointing out that heavy smokers have a better prognosis. In 80 per cent of his cases infectious diseases preceded the onset, though in only 30 per cent *immediately* preceded the onset. He stressed the frequency of the disorder in soldiers who had previously followed a sedentary life. In Lewis' opinion the condition is progressive and in one-half the cases it becomes completely incapacitating.

On the psychological side the patients fall into at least two groups:

One group is of physically and emotionally immature men who have been nervous since childhood. These are perhaps the ones who react more typically to effort.

In the second group are the ones who actually suffer from mild organic disease of the heart in which the symptoms of N. C. A. are superimposed. In these the emphasis seems to be placed on precardial tenderness and pain rather than on palpitation.

Mobilization Regulations No. 1-9 (MR 1-9), War Department, Washington, March 15th, 1942, which sets forth the standards for physical requirements for men procured for general military service (Class 1-a), lists under paragraph 62 as an acceptable condition (1-a): Neurocirculatory asthenia (effort syndrome), if it is very mild; otherwise it is listed as cause of rejection (class 4). It states that the usual symptoms of this condition are exhaustion, breathlessness, heartache and palpitation. The symptoms may follow exertion such as would not produce them in healthy individuals. These and other symptoms, such as dizziness or fainting, may arise without evidence of organic disease sufficient to account for the disability of the individual. It further states that cases of effort syndrome may be divided into four groups (in some cases more than one of these factors is present):

(1) As an accompaniment of organic heart disease
(2) Following infections
(3) In individuals with poor physique or insufficient training for work required
(4) Psychoneurosis.

The MR 1-9, War Department, Washington, October 15th, 1942, lists these standards as previously except that the fourth group, psychoneurosis, is left out and in its place is listed orthostatic hypotension tachycardia.

Then it is seen that were Mobilization Regulations No. 1-9 followed closely and the diagnosis properly made at or before induction, the Army would be spared the necessity for dealing with the more severe forms of this syndrome. However, since some of the cases are more difficult to detect and many do not manifest themselves fully until military training starts or combat duty is confronted, the Army medical officers, and especially those working largely with cardiology and psychiatry, have to examine, treat and make disposition of these cases.

Roughly, the cases, like "All Gaul," are divided into three groups: the mild, the moderate and the severe. Those of the first group after proper examination and reassurance can usually be returned properly to Full Duty. Many of the second or middle group after proper working up will become candidates for presenting to Reclassification Board for Limited Duty. Most of the men in the third group will, in the best interests of the Army, be disposed of by C. D. D. (Certificate of Disability Discharge). But on the disposition of this last group once they are in the Army will come a more prolonged consideration; however, there is no proper reason for it being long once the diagnosis is made.

When the Army cardiologist is confronted with such a problem he goes about working up the case by eliciting symptoms and eliminating the presence of or determining the type of any organic heart disease. If in his opinion the findings are largely or entirely functional, he requests consultation with the psychiatrist who then, if his findings justify, makes the diagnosis of Neurocirculatory Asthenia.

Note: The data given and opinion expressed in this paper were drawn from experience of the writer while acting as assistant and chief of the Cardiovascular Section of the Medical Service of the Station Hospitals at Camp Blanding, Fort Bragg, Camp Pickett and Shenango Personnel Replacement Depot with some observations at other Station and General Army Hospitals during 1942 and 1943.

The data were collected in part in 1942 but were finally written up while at sea and somewhere in North Africa, June 11th, 1943.

—J. S. HOLBROOK, M.D., 0-309413
Captain, U. S. Medical Corps.

PRESIDENT'S PAGE

BATTLE FRONT AND HOME FRONT

IN TIMES like these when duty to country comes to the front more than ever, it is indeed fitting to ask oneself how he is serving his nation. Because of the small number of doctors left on the home front each is fully occupied with his own professional duties and there is not much time left for the reading of world events. It is evident that in some cities and communities such a large number of physicians and surgeons have gone into the armed services that only 50 per cent of the normal number of doctors are caring for the community sick. In spite of any criticism that might arise that some patients have to wait two or three hours for a doctor, it is nothing short of a magnificent job accomplished by these doctors who have had to take on almost a double number of patients. This double duty is being carried on in a majority of instances by the older group of physicians who had dreamed or planned to retire, or at least slow down, at this age rather than work into the late hours of the night as they are now doing.

It is gratifying to know the splendid spirit shown by this group during this emergency. Many who had retired because of age or impaired health have gotten back into harness and are making the rounds regularly. These men show the real spirit of service when they say they expect to do all they can until the younger men return. With these elderly men working long hours we may expect an increase in the death rate in our ranks. Statistics for the past year will confirm this, yet there is no complaining among the ranks of medical men about these added duties and long hours.

There is a spirit of splendid coöperation among the physicians in all the communities as they plan and aid each other in seeing that all the sick may be treated. An excellent job is being done on the home front without any fanfare or publicity. If one reads what the foreign correspondents have to say in reporting the major activities from all sections of the world battlefronts, one cannot help being impressed with the splendid way the army, navy and air surgeons are giving an account of themselves. Many times a member of the armed forces who has returned to this country from the battlefronts has been asked what type of work impresses him most. Almost invariably he at once cites the work of the medical men. There are many instances of medical services in saving lives that seem little short of a miracle. These doctors doing this marvelous work on the battlefronts are identically the same men who were only a few months ago in private practice of their profession back here in the States.

Are we behind in the procession of world events? I don't think so. It would seem from all points of view that we are well in advance and wherever necessary the doctors are going beyond the point of duty to accomplish the task before them.

—K. B. PACE.

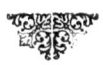

SOUTHERN MEDICINE & SURGERY

Official Organ

JAMES M. NORTHINGTON, M.D., *Editor*

Department Editors

Human Behavior
JAMES K. HALL, M.D. .... Richmond, Va.

Orthopedic Surgery
JOHN T. SAUNDERS, M.D. .... Asheville, N. C.

Urology
RAYMOND THOMPSON, M.D. .... Charlotte, N. C.

Surgery
GEO. H. BUNCH, M.D. .... Columbia, S. C.

Obstetrics
HENRY J. LANGSTON, M.D. .... Danville, Va

Gynecology
CHAS. R. ROBINS, M.D. .... Richmond, Va.
ROBERT T. FERGUSON, M.D. .... Charlotte, N. C.

General Practice
J. L. HAMNER, M.D. .... Mannboro, Va.

Clinical Chemistry and Microscopy
J. M. FEDER, M.D.,
EVELYN TRIBBLE, M. T. } .... Anderson, S. C.

Hospitals
R. B. DAVIS, M.D. .... Greensboro, N. C.

Cardiology
CLYDE M. GILMORE, A.B., M.D. .... Greensboro, N. C.

Public Health
N. THOS. ENNETT, M.D. .... Greenville, N. C.

Radiology
R. H. LAFFERTY, M.D., and Associates .... Charlotte, N. C.

Therapeutics
J. F. NASH, M.D. .... Saint Pauls, N. C.

Tuberculosis
JOHN DONNELLY, M.D. .... Charlotte, N. C.

Dentistry
J. H. GUION, D.D.S. .... Charlotte, N. C.

Internal Medicine
GEORGE R. WILKINSON, M.D. .... Greenville, S. C.

Ophthalmology
HERBERT C. NEBLETT, M.D. .... Charlotte, N. C.

Rhino-Oto-Laryngology
CLAY W. EVATT, M.D. .... Charleston, S. C.

Proctology
RUSSELL L. BUXTON, M.D. .... Newport News, Va.

Insurance Medicine
H. F. STARR, M.D. .... Greensboro, N. C.

Dermatology
J. LAMAR CALLAWAY, M.D. .... Durham, N. C.

Pediatrics

Offerings for the pages of this Journal are requested and given careful consideration in each case. ...Manuscripts not found suitable for our use will not be returned unless author encloses postage.

As is true of most Medical Journals, all costs of cuts, etc., for illustrating an article must be borne by the author.

STOP DISCREDITING AND IGNORING THE G. P. AND DOCTORS WILL LOCATE IN THE VILLAGES

DR. REGINALD FITZ recently presented to the Rhode Island Medical Society his thoughts on the education and distribution of doctors.[1] He finds that there exists a striking need for redistribution of medical manpower: for densely populated areas continue to have plenty of doctors whereas the thinly populated districts with less going on are depleted. How best to encourage returning doctors to enter practice in small towns where they are most needed is an important question which must be answered; "something must be done to make rural or suburban practice attractive."

Another significant finding is the increasing demand by the civilian population for hospital facilities, beyond that due to the desire of persons insured by the Blue Cross or some other insurance plan to get some back for their investment; for in any respectable hospital in any part of the country, the same growth in use is shown. "One may conclude, therefore, that the American people are now hospital-minded and will demand adequate hospital facilities in whatever community they live."

Further pertinent observations are made:

At a meeting of the House of Delegates of the American Medical Association in 1931, Dr. Carl T. Moll of Michigan, conscious of the growing desire for doctors to call themselves specialists, asked the House to appoint a Commission on Qualifications for Specialists. From this beginning our present specialty boards were established and began to function.

The self-taught young doctor acquires, besides bad habits, too much self-confidence and too little knowledge; he needs to be drilled in the art of practice, an art that can only be mastered by hard work intelligently controlled.

Hospital meetings must be conducted regularly and with a certain degree of formality. At such meetings an interne or resident should always present a case, learning to speak from his feet, without notes, and clearly and succinctly. He must be encouraged to write. Medical writing stimulates a beginner to learn to use a library properly, teaches him to read, analyze, criticise and abstract literature, and also something of facility of expression and of the difficulties of composition—all good things for a young doctor's development.

An important step to make rural or suburban practice attractive lies in the encouragement of local hospitals to establish the type of internships or residences ordinarily obtainable in hospitals con-

---

1. Third Chapin Memorial Lecture, published in *R. I. Medical Journal*, June.

nected with medical schools; internships where the work of each department is under the direction of qualified specialists, where the patients admitted are studied carefully and systematically, where staff conferences are active and interesting.

The satisfaction and rewards of rural or suburban practice would be more, better medical work would be done and greater use would be made of qualified specialism if more of the hospitals in our smaller cities determined to become "A" institutions.

A Committee representing the American College of Physicians, the American College of Surgeons, and the American Medical Association has been at work perfecting a variety of short postgraduate courses established all over the country. "Every doctor, wherever he is, must be made to feel that he is an important part of the profession," he must be encouraged to improve the quality of his work, and he must be stimulated to broaden his education continuously. This is the goal which post-war planners should strive to attain.

We heartily agree that something should be done to make country practice attractive. We would go further and say that influential doctors should cease to make country and village practice unattractive.

All Dr. Fitz says in favor of better and better training in medicine and surgery is endorsed; but no matter how well-trained a doctor of medicine may be, so long as the doctors most conspicuously before the public continue the present over-emphasis on the importance of the specialist and the hospital, and the need for their services, the general practitioner will not be accorded the high place he deserves in the profession.

A specialist from a thousand miles away, the distinguished invited guest of a county medical society made up entirely of general practitioners, was heard by this editor to say from the platform of a rather new treatment procedure: "It's not complicated. Anybody can use it. The nurse can use it, or even the general practitioner." And he didn't say it as a joke, either. Indeed, so accustomed is everybody to this belittling of the general practitioner that, apparently, nobody else took note of the statement.

A few well-trained doctors will continue to do village and country practice until such practice is absorbed by the specialists and the hospitals; but the vast majority of doctors, along with the rest of the human race, like to be given recognition as persons of some consequence, by their profession and by the general public.

So long as the public is encouraged to believe in the omnipotence of the specialist and the hospital, and that the general practitioner's function does not go beyond "the pricking out of thistles or the laying of a plaister to the scratch of a pin," most doctors will specialize and do hospital and office practice.

The difference in pecuniary rewards is not the main thing. The great majority of country doctors have incomes satisfactory to themselves. The main reason for getting out of this kind of practice is that it hurts their pride to be regarded by everybody as qualified to treat minor, very minor, conditions only.

An excellent general practitioner, with an M.A. degree, was once asked by me why he never came to meetings of the local medical society. He replied, "because I am tired of having men without education talk down to me, and about educating me."

* * * * *

COMMITTEE REPORTS TO A. M. A. ON THE KENNY METHOD

O, popular applause! What heart of man
Is proof against they sweet, seducing charm?

AN EVALUATION of the Kenny treatment of infantile paralysis, made by a group of distinguished professors appointed by the Orthopedic Section of the American Medical Asociation, the American Academy of Orthopedic Surgeons and the American Orthopedic Association was presented to the 94th Annual Session of the A. M. A. This report was published in the June 17th issue of the *Journal of the A. M. A.*

This committee visited six cities and 16 clinics, some of them two or more times. A total of 740 patients were examined, 650 of whom had been treated by the method advocated by Miss Kenny. Following is an abstract of the report:

It is well known that epidemics vary tremendously from year to year as to severity, type and extent of paralysis. One of the things Miss Kenny has stressed in her writings, talks and newspaper articles is the difference of her treatment from what she calls "orthodox" treatment. It is rather difficult to understand what she means by "orthodox" treatment.

Four major points in her concept of the disease have been stressed by Miss Kenny:

1. Muscle "spasm" — This committee believes that while this does exist in the early phases of the disease it usually disappears spontaneously. There may be residual "spasm" which can lead to deformity, but it is by no means the cause of the residual paralysis. Early contractures have been long recognized and considered an integral part of the acute phase of this disease.

2. Mental alienation — The statement that flaccid muscles are normal is obviously not true. A functional loss of use may result from pain, and in

these instances function is restored as the pain subsides. Functional disuse may also result from stretch in any muscle opposed by muscles in varying degrees of contracture. Temporary paralysis, stretch paralysis and physiologic dissociation would seem a more satisfactory explanation. Mental alienation is not a new discovery, having been well described in 1911 by Robert Jones.

3. Incoördination—The term was used by Wilbur to describe this condition in poliomyelitis as early as 1912. This question is of academic interest and of little importance.

4. Paralysis (denervation now preferred by Miss Kenny—The committee believes that if deformities are prevented the flaccid paralysis caused by destruction of nerve cells is the most important cause of crippling. The institution of treatment directed toward the involved muscles as early as possible is desirable, but the general condition of the patient during the acute febrile stage may be such that the handling necessitated by the Kenny treatment can be detrimental. Therapy during the acute febrile stage is primarily a medical problem. Proper positioning in bed by one means or another has been a standard practice among physicians for over thirty years. It is still a recommended procedure.

Heat, including hot foments, has been used by physicians for many years to combat pain in infantile paralysis. It is the impression of this committee that pain is not an important feature of the disease in most instances. Recovery from "spasm" in most instances takes place spontaneously. Hot packs may relieve this "spasm," but so will adequate rest. Active and passive movement of these extremities has been recommended by many physicians, but this movement should not be forced beyond the point of pain.

Cases have been seen under Kenney treatment in which early contractures were developing, and by application of plaster splints these contractures were controlled after their correction. Braces should form an important part of the treatment during the later stages of this disease. Respirators have saved many lives and should be used for patients with sufficient paralysis to embarrass respirations.

There is no evidence that the Kenny treatment prevents or decreases the amount of paralysis. We criticize severely the oft-repeated statement of Miss Kenny to patients who have come to her after treatment elsewhere that had this case come to her early the disability would have been prevented. Such statements are not founded on facts.

Spontaneous recovery in poliomyelitis occurs in from 50 to 80 per cent. We have seen many patients receiving Kenny treatment who showed no muscle involvement at any time, yet she assumes the credit for their satisfactory results and does not take into account the factor of spontaneous recovery.

Miss Kenny's objection to muscle examinations and hence the lack of accurate records is to be condemned. If this should be followed by all cases no reasonably accurate statistics would be available nor could the results from any type of treatment be determined.

Miss Kenny has repeatedly stated that under "orthodox" treatment only 13 per cent of the patients recovered without paralysis, while under her treatment over 80 per cent recover. We believe that this is a deliberate misrepresentation of the facts of treatment by other methods.

Miss Kenny's statement of 80 per cent recovery under her treatment has not been supported by accurate statistics in a significant number of cases. The figure on "orthodox" treatment is taken from an article which dealt entirely with severely paralyzed patients. Miss Kenny has been told repeatedly that this is not a fair comparison to make and that, if every case in an epidemic is included in the statistics, recovery of from 70 to 90 per cent can be expected from "orthodox" treatment. Miss Kenny made this inaccurate comparison as late as May, 1944.

We have seen enough cases in which the Kenny treatment was instituted very early to be convinced that this does not prevent or even minimize the degree of permanent paralysis. The prevention of these contractures is the primary means by which medical care is able to minimize the effects of the disease.

In the opinion of the committee the continuous hot packs for all patients with minimal evidence of "spasm" is an unnecessary waste of manpower and hospital beds. Judgment should be exercised in determining the cases in which hospital treatment should be instituted or continued.

Miss Kenny has laid claim recently to a new and revolutionary discovery by means of which she can diagnose the disease and determine the involved extremities prior to the onset of the usually recognized diagnostic clinical signs. She also claims that the institution of her treatment at this time will control the pain and prevent paralysis. She has stated that this is her greatest single contribution.

There has been no satisfactory evidence presented to this committee that the institution of early local treatment will alter the course or the extent of the paralysis in any case.

While the committee disapproves of and condemns the wide publicity which has misled the public and many members of the medical profession, it acknowledges that this has stimulated the medical profession to reëvaluate known methods of treatment of this disease and to treat it more effectively.

This report is made by doctors who have a thorough knowledge of the anatomy and physiology of the parts prone to be affected by poliomyelitis. These doctors have studied the cases treated by the Kenny method. These doctors are eager to welcome and applaud any measure which will save the life or the limb of even one child out of a hundred affected.

But they know the wisdom of: "Prove all things; hold fast to that which is good." They do not believe in miracles. They have none of that faith which is ability to believe what one knows is not true. They know the cruelty of holding out hopes for which there is no foundation.

Miss Kenny's honesty is no more questioned here than is her zeal. Her experience of an epidemic of poliomyelitis of a mild form convinced her that she had made a great, life-saving discovery. As she obtained more and more of the limelight she was more and more convinced of the value of her "discovery." She was quoted, consulted and flattered by great and small the country over. It would have been wellnigh miraculous had she been able to weigh judgmatically the evidence as it accumulated. To admit that she had contributed nothing to life- or limb-saving would be to fall, as did Lucifer, from Heaven.

Sad! Sad! But much sadder to sacrifice one life or one limb to keep from hurting an intrinsically good and honest woman, who has perhaps no more love of adulation than the general run of humanity.

A SIMPLE, EFFECTIVE TREATMENT FOR EPIDERMOPHYTOSIS
(W. A. Albert, Clemson, S. C., & R. F. Zeigler, Jr., Seneca, S. C., in *Sou. Med. Jl.*, June)

The following solution was developed over a period of years used by one of us in treating his own frequent infections of "athlete's foot":

10 grams salicylic acid
33 c.c. acetone
33 c.c. 85% ethyl alcohol
33 c.c. glycerol

In a warm room the pressure of the acetone vapor will probably push out an ordinary stopper. Acetone is more volatile than alcohol and is inflammable.

The majority of the cases consisted of the typical vesicular and scaling lesions on the toes, soles and palms, with maceration. Secondary infections were frequently present. Other cases were of the macular type which usually involved the groin, still others of the slightly elevated, ring-like patches which occurred principally on the face, neck and arms (tinea circinata or "ringworm").

The infected areas were freely mopped for two or three minutes, then waiting for drying before replacing socks or clothing. Instruction in foot and body hygiene was given so as to lessen the chances for reinfection. The patients were seen again in from five to seven days and when necessary the treatment was repeated.

Relief from itching was usually a matter of minutes. More than half the patients were completely healed after one application, all after two or three applications at five to seven-days intervals. A few complained of smarting for a minute or two.

AMBULATORY TREATMENT FOR SPRAINED ANKLES
(Lt. Comdr. Jos. T. Webber, M. C., U. S. N. R., New York City, in *West. Va. Med. Jl.*, June)

The common findings in the case of a sprained ankle are: 1) muscle spasm at once or delayed, 2) pain, immediate or delayed, 3) venous stasis with ecchymosis, edema, and tissue anoxia and 4) laceration of the ligaments about the joint.

McMaster reports a series of 500 cases; 200 treated by the use of procaine and elastic bandages, over 200 by adhesive strapping, and a lesser number by bed rest, elastic bandage exercise. His results with the procaine anesthetic method were remarkably good. The only restriction in the cases treated by exercise were running or jumping.

Murphy reports a series of 41 cases of which 28 had, in addition to the procaine, a modified Gibney boot; three had a muslin bandage; 10 had no support. His best results were obtained when the hematoma could be aspirated.

Our technique is somewhat different. The usual x-ray picture was taken, and injection of the tender spots and aspiration of the hematoma (if possible); but for the first 20 cases no support was given and the patients were sent back to full duty including marching, running and jumping. The remainder were given, in addition, an injection in the talocalcaneal joint space.

In a review of the x-ray pictures most cases showed a distinct widening of the talonavicular and cuboidalcalcaneal joint space. The discovery led to the injecting of this space with 2 to 4 c.c. of the procaine after aspiration of any blood. The ache deep down in the foot and up the back of the leg noted in the first 20 cases was absent after this latter injection. No infections occurred. Perhaps the removal of the blood from the joint space was a factor in the prevention of infection.

TREATING BLEEDING PEPTIC ULCER BY FEEDING
(Leon Schiff, Cincinnati, in *Cinti. Jl., of Med.*, July)

In a period of five years we have treated 160 patients with bleeding peptic ulcer by a slightly modified Meulengracht diet. The diagnosis of ulcer was confined in each instance by x-ray examination, gastroscopy, operation, or autopsy. In 12, there was no history of any digestive distress prior to hemorrhage, while in 33 the digestive distress was not characteristic. One-half of the patients had had no previous episode of hemorrhage. In 61, the red cells had been reduced to two million or less. One-half of the patients received one or more blood transfusions, usually 500 c.c. of citrated blood. The gross mortality was 6.8 per cent, a considerable improvement over the figure of 25.6 per cent obtained on the old preliminary starvation regimen.

IT IS A FREQUENT (A. Mueller-Deham, New York, in *Clin. Med.*, June), but always shocking, experience to find that the most severe diseases, such as acute cholelithiasis, stomach ulcers, appendicitis, peritonitis, etc., may take their course in senile cases without any localizatory signs, or only with very slight intimations. In some cases all one can find is a slight tenderness, a minimal rigidity, which seems quite negligible to the inexperienced in geriatrics, and can only with great difficulty and uncertitude be evaluated by the expert.

NEWS

NEW MEMBERS AMERICAN PROCTOLOGIC SOCIETY

Dr. C. C. Massey, of Charlotte, N. C., and Dr. W. H. Poston, of Pamplico, S. C., were made Associate Members of The American Proctologic Society at the recent annual meeting held in Chicago June 12th-13th.

North Carolina did not have a member of the society until Dr. Massey's election to membership. Dr. Thomas Brockman, of Greenville, S. C., President-elect of the South Carolina Medical Association, was made a Fellow in the society at the same time.

Announcement is made in the press that the SHRINERS' HOSPITAL FOR CRIPPLED CHILDREN at Greenville, South Carolina, is the residual legatee of the estate of the late W. T. Shelton, Waynesville, North Carolina. The bequest may eventually amount to more than $50,000.

Dr. FRANK B. STAFFORD has been appointed superintendent of Blue Ridge Sanatorium, near Charlottesville, Va., to succeed Dr. W. E. Brown, who resigned recently because of ill health. Dr. Stafford has been assistant superintendent at Blue Ridge Sanatorium since the institution opened in 1920. Previously he was a member of the staff of Catawba under Dr. Brown for a year, going to that institution immediately after his graduation from the Medical College of Virginia.

Dr. OREN MOORE, of Charlotte, president-elect of the Medical Society of the State of North Carolina, spoke by invitation to the Greenville County, South Carolina, Medical Society on May 29th about Some of the Minor Ailments in Obstetrics.

MEDICAL COLLEGE OF VIRGINIA

Mr. Robert Smith Hudgens, administrator of Emory University Hospital, Atlanta, has been appointed director of the Hospitals of the College, succeeding Dr. Lewis E. Jarrett, who resigned to accept a similar position at Touro Infirmary, New Orleans.

Mr. Hudgens is a member of the American College of Hospital Administrators, a former president of the Georgia Hospital Association, of the Southeastern Hospital Conference, and a member of the American Hospital Association.

MARRIED

Dr. Richard Loomis Oliver, of Raleigh, and Miss Frances Christine Biles, of Troy, were married on June 12.

Dr. Kingley Miller, of Danville, Kentucky, and Mrs. Virginia Tull Ragland, of Kinston, North Carolina, were married on May 31st.

Dr. William Price Spencer and Miss Mary Catherine Waddell, both of the University of Virginia, were married on June 19th. Dr. Spencer, a member of the senior class of the Medical School, will become a member of the teaching staff after graduation.

Miss Evelyn Suter, of Bridgewater, Virginia, and Dr. Ashby Turner Richards, of Harrisonburg, June 4th. Dr. Richards is stationed at the U. S. Marine Hospital, New Orleans, and the couple will make their home temporarily in that city.

Dr. Thomas Lynch Murphy and Miss Virginia Bruton McKenzie, of Salisbury, were married on June 11th.

Dr. Raymond Arwell Adams, of Red Oak, Virginia, and Dr. Jane Ellen Berry, of Richmond, were married on June 10th.

Captain Henry Haskins Ferrell, Jr., Medical Corps, United States Army, of Goochland County, Virginia, and Miss Joan Jamieson Cotter, of the University of Dublin, Eire, were married on May 20th.

Dr. Vance Benton Rollins, of Henderson, North Carolina, and Miss Carrie Lee Laney, of Camden, Arkansas, were married on June 20th.

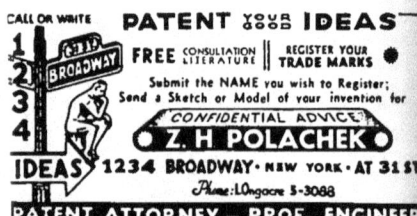

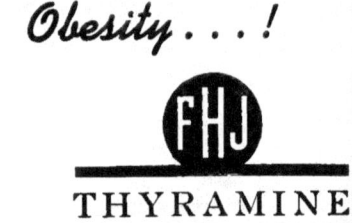

Composition

Thyroid 1 gr. Amphetamine sulphate 5 mgs. Thiamin chloride 1 mg. in suitable combinations with physiological reinforcements.

No. 1—One Capsule before breakfast
No. 2—One Capsule before lunch
No. 3—One Capsule at 4 p. m.

Contraindications

Hypertension .... Hyperthyroidism

Supplied

Capsules: Packages 21 and 42 (one or two weeks supply).

—Professional samples on request—
Available: Any professional pharmacy
F. H. J. PRODUCTS
977 East 176th St., New York 60, N. Y.

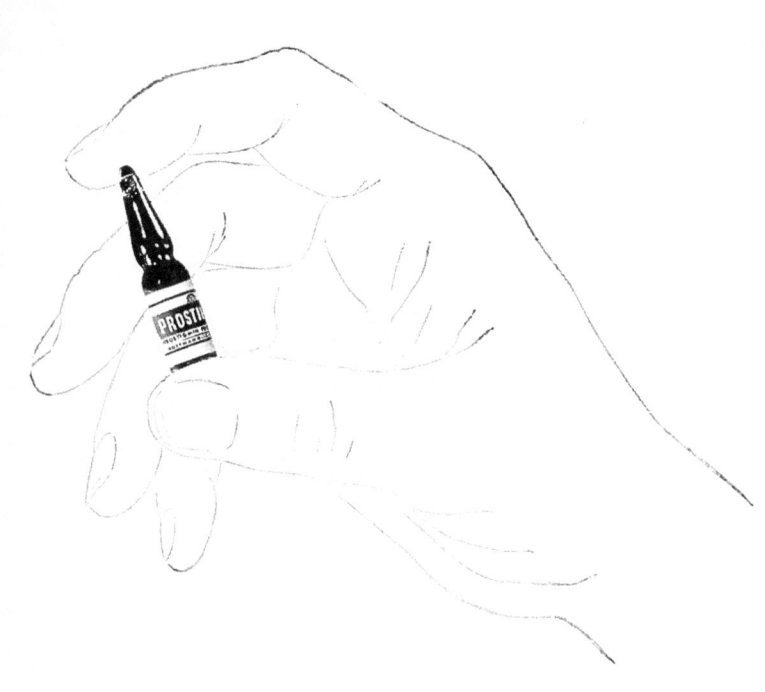

"AN AMPUL OF PREVENTION...

— is worth a pound of cure"... Postoperative abdominal distention and urinary retention — and the troublesome procedures that follow — are often entirely prevented by the routine use of Prostigmin Methylsulfate 1:4000. Convalescence may be hastened — "gas pains" and the discomforts of catheterization can be eliminated by this simple, effective treatment. Inject 1 cc of Prostigmin Methylsulfate 'Roche' 1:4000 at the time of operation and continue with five similar injections at 2-hour intervals after the operation ..... HOFFMANN-LA ROCHE, INC., ROCHE PARK, NUTLEY 10, NEW JERSEY.

PROSTIGMIN METHYLSULFATE 'ROCHE' 1:4000

Major John Tabb Walke, Medical Corps, United States Army, and Miss Evelyn Chamblin Murrell, both of Richmond, were married on July 6th.

Lieutenant Milton J. Chatton, Medical Corps, United States Army, and Miss Mildred Vick, of Richmond, were married in the chapel of Mason General Hospital, Brentwood, Long Island, New York, on June 30th.

Dr. Sarah Hildah Hoover and Mr. George R. Jones of Jacksonville, Fla., were married June 10th. The bride is a graduate of Westhampton College and the Medical College of Virginia. She is now interning at the Medical College of Virginia Hospital. Mr. Jones is a graduate of the University of Florida and is a member of the Army Medical Corps and of the Junior Class of the Medical College of Virginia.

Dr. W. H. Kibler, of Morganton, has gone for several weeks of graduate work in surgery in the University of Michigan. Dr. Kibler is president of the medical staff of Grace Hospital at Morganton.

Dr. Reuben W. Lominack, formerly of Charleston and Newberry, has been commissioned a first lieutenant in the Medical Corps. He has completed a course in Field Medicine and Surgery at Carlisle Barracks, Pa., and is now stationed at Lovell General Hospital, Fort Devens, Mass., with the Department of Surgery.

DIED

Dr. William Alexander Lambeth, for fifty years a member of the faculty of the University of Virginia and former director of athletics, died June 24th in the University Hospital. He was 76 years old.

From 1908 until 1921, Dr. Lambeth was a member of the National Football Rules Committee and was responsible for many changes, among them the division of the game into quarters. He was a member of the council appointed to rewrite football rules when the game's existence was threatened by frequent disabling injuries. Lambeth Field at the University of Virginia was named for him.

He was a teacher of materia medica and hygiene, superintendent of buildings and grounds, and head of the department of physical education. He retired six years ago at the mandatory age of 70.

Dr. Lambeth was born in Thomasville, N. C., and was a graduate of the University of Virginia, with medical and doctor of philosophy degrees. He also held a degree from the Harvard University School of Physical Training.

He was the author of several books, among them, "Thomas Jefferson, Architect," "Trees and How to Know Them," "The Geology of Monticello Area," "The School of Athens" and "Food and Dietetics."

Rear Admiral David C. Cather, 66, who died last week in Los Angeles, where he has resided since retirement two years ago, will be buried in Arlington National Cemetery. He was born in Frederick County and obtained his academic education at the University of Virginia, and his medical degree at the University of Pennsylvania in 1903.

While practicing in the Bronx, I was called one morning very early to Brooklyn. On my arrival an old man asked me to write the death certificate for his wife who had died in her sleep. When I asked him why he hadn't called some doctor in his own neighborhood, he replied: "Doctor, you were so highly recommended to me."—*New York Physician.*

BOOKS

PRINCIPLES AND PRACTICES OF INHALATION THERAPY, by Alvan L. Barach, M.D., Associate Professor of Clinical Medicine, Columbia College of Physicians and Surgeons; Assistant Attending Physician, Presbyterian Hospital. Fifty-nine illustrations. *J. B. Lippincott Company*, E. Washington Square, Philadelphia; London; Montreal. 1944. $4.00.

The physiological principles are gone into as a rational basis for the therapeutic application of remedies by inhalation. The different techniques are presented in sufficient detail to enable the doctor in charge to give the patient the greatest good to be derived.

Among the subjects given in individual chapters are altitude sickness, pneumonia, edema of the lungs, congestive heart failure, coronary thrombosis and sclerosis, shock, pulmonary infarction, atelectasis, asthma, emphysema, asphyxia, hemorrhage, migraine, tetanus, gas poisoning, cerebral embolism and thrombosis, pulmonary tuberculosis, oxygen poisoning, hiccough.

A chapter of exceptional value is that on care of the special equipment necessary for inhalational therapy.

Most of us are fetched up short at having it suggested that there is such a thing as oxygen poisoning. We think of oxygen as life's first essential.

HARDWARE MUTUAL
FIRE INSURANCE COMPANY
OF THE CAROLINAS

offer

NON-ASSESSABLE,

STANDARD POLICIES

at the

ESTABLISHED RATES

with

SUBSTANTIAL SAVINGS TO ALL

POLICY HOLDERS

ESTABLISHED 1912

SAFETY   SERVICE
SATISFACTION

Phone   or   Write
HOME OFFICE
2-2333   118 E. 4th St.
CHARLOTTE, N. C.

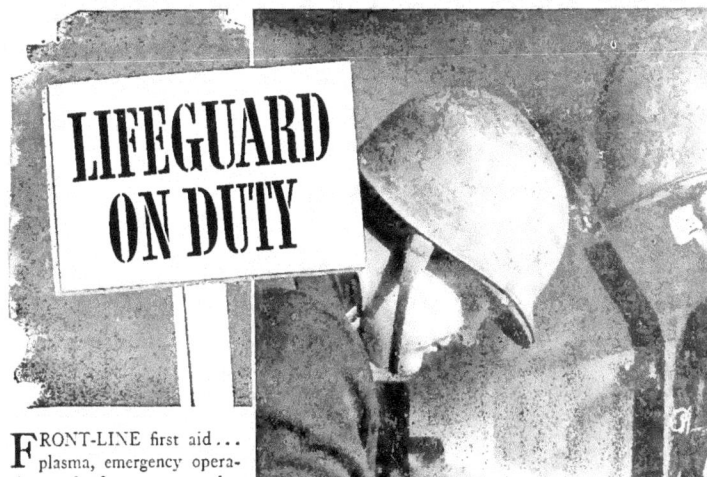

LIFEGUARD ON DUTY

FRONT-LINE first aid... plasma, emergency operations under fire...cuts casualty rates astonishingly. Physicians of World War II constantly face sudden death to bring modern medical miracles to fallen troops. Harrying, the war doctor's life. Weary grinds. Respites rare. Perhaps only a few moments or so now and then... time off for a welcome cigarette. A Camel, most likely—favorite brand in the armed forces.* Camel, first choice for mellow mildness, for appealing flavor... in this war, as in the last, cigarette of fighting men.

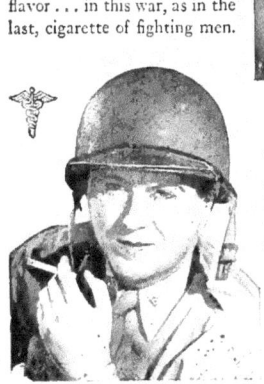

● New reprint available on cigarette research — Archives of Otolaryngology, March, 1943, pp. 404-410. Camel Cigarettes, Medical Relations Division, One Pershing Sq., New York 17, N.Y.

1st in the Service

*With men in the Army, the Navy, the Marine Corps, and the Coast Guard, the favorite cigarette is Camel. (Based on actual sales records.)

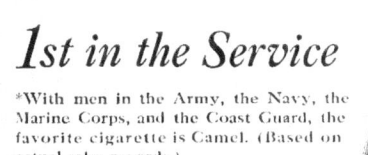

Camel
costlier tobaccos

BUY WAR BONDS STAMPS

But we are given here a new illustration of the fact that there may be too much of a good thing, and we are caused to reflect on the fact that Nature provides us with our O well diluted.

Inhalational therapy has traveled far since our interne days when to see an oxygen tank being wheeled into a patient's room meant that death was imminent.

Dr. Barach's book is made up of his carefully checked researches and experiences in this field over many years. It makes a valuable addition to our therapeutic resources.

THE ELECTROCARDIOGRAM: Its Interpretation and Clinical Application, by LOUIS H. SIGLER, M.D., F.A.C.P., Attending Cardiologist and Chief of Cardiac Clinics, Coney Island and Harbor Hospitals; formerly Instructor in Medicine, New York Post Graduate Medical School, Columbia University. *Grune & Stratton, Inc.,* 381 Fourth Avenue, New York 16, N. Y. 1944. $7.50.

The author tells us plainly that abnormalities in the electrocardiogram do not always mean heart disease, that in many cases no cause can be found to account for such abnormalities. On the other hand, frequent and significant changes in the ecg. in any case, even if each tracing in the series is of normal appearance, are indicative of structural or functional abnormalities in the heart muscle or the conduction system.

Among the extrinsic factors recognized as producing changes in the ecg. are: acute or chronic conditions in other parts of the body, endocrine disease, vitamine lack, metabolic abnormalities and the recent administration of certain drugs.

Disease conditions of the heart producing more-or-less characteristic ecgs. are: congenital abnormalities, inflammations, ischemia and infarction due to coronary disease, parasitic invasion, infiltration by malignant growths, trauma, and hypertrophy of heart muscle from any cause.

The early chapters on the foundations of the electrocardiogram, the recording of the heart current, the normal ecg. and the electrical axis establish a solid basis on which to build the superstructure of the use of the ecg. in diagnosis, prognosis and treatment.

This reviewer has no better book on this important subject. He doubts if there is one so good as this.

RHEUMATIC ORCHITIS.—A case is reported (*Med. Annals Dist. Col.*, Apr.), most likely rheumatic, associated with pericarditis with effusion.

The proud father called up the newspaper to report the birth of twins.

News Editor (not hearing clearly): "Will you repeat that?"

Father: "Not if I can help it."

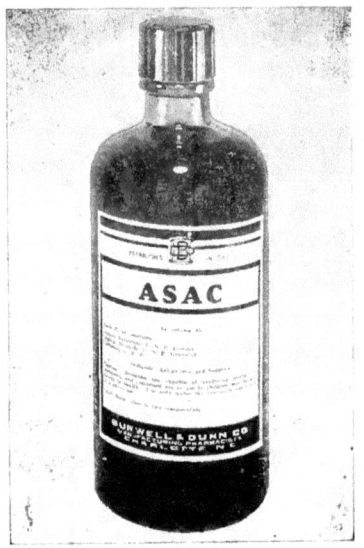

ASAC

15% by volume Alcohol

Each fl. oz. contains:

Sodium Salicylate, U. S. P. Powder..........40 grains
Sodium Bromide, U. S. P. Granular...........20 grains
Caffeine, U. S. P....................................... 4 grains

ANALGESIC, ANTIPYRETIC AND SEDATIVE.

Average Dosage

Two to four teaspoonfuls in one to three ounces of water as prescribed by the physician.

How Supplied

In Pints, Five Pints and Gallons to Physicians and Druggists

Burwell & Dunn Company

Manufacturing Pharmacists
Established in 1887

CHARLOTTE, N. C.

NEWS

HARVARD MEDICO-LEGAL SEMINAR

The Harvard Medical School, Courses for Graduates, with the coöperation of the Medical Schools of Boston University and Tufts College, offers a seminar in Legal Medicine to occupy the entire week of October 2nd-7th. It is planned particularly for medical examiners and coroners' physicians but will be open to any other suitable graduate of an approved medical school.

The course will consist of autopsy demonstrations, technique and interpretation of laboratory tests, study of the day-by-day cases of a medical examiner, round-table conferences, etc. In order that each participant may receive the maximum benefit, the enrollment has been limited to fifteen. For the Seminar the fee is $25.

Application should be made on or before October 1st to *Harvard Medical School, Courses for Graduates,* 25 Shattuck Street, Boston 15, Massachusetts.

THE NEW YORK ACADEMY OF MEDICINE PROVIDES POST-GRADUATE MEDICAL INSTRUCTION FOR PHYSICIANS RETURNING FROM MILITARY SERVICE

The New York Academy of Medicine has created a Bureau of Medical Education to serve all physicians interested in furthering their medical education, but particularly the physicians returning from the war, and the increasing numbers of foreign physicians who come to New York for post-graduate instruction and training.

The Bureau will render its services without charge. It plans to publish announcements of post-graduate courses, conducted by the universities and the hospitals of New York City. Thirty-three of the leading hospitals have been invited to collaborate in this work.

OLD NORTH STATE MEDICAL, DENTAL AND PHARMACEUTICAL SOCIETY

This, the oldest Negro medical society in the world, at its meeting in annual convention at Winston-Salem June 6th-8th:

(1) Approved the plan of his Excellency the Governor for better hospital and medical care for all the people of North Carolina.

(2) Went on record as favoring equal medical training for Negro students within the State; and

(3) That Negro physicians be accorded the same opportunity for self-improvement and service to their people as is accorded other physicians in all state-supported institutions.

UMBILICAL HERNIA IN CHILDREN
(M. J. Bennett-Jones, in *British Med. Jl.*, 4332: 79-79, 1944)

Spontaneous cure of umbilical hernias with support alone occurs in 50 per cent of children under three years of age. To increase this proportion and hasten cure, he injected small umbilical hernias of 42 children, 3 months to 5 years of age; of this number 31 were completely cured; 7 were improving gradually; 2 could not be traced for further observation and 2 subsequently required operation.

No anesthesia is necessary when injecting hernias in young infants, although ethyl chloride may be useful to control voluntary movements. About 4.5 c.c. of 5% phenol in almond oil is injected into the subcutaneous tissue as near the neck of the hernial sac as possible without risk of puncturing the peritoneum. Of the 42 patients, 26 required only one injection; 11 patients had two injections and, of these, two were operated on when the hernia did not become smaller; four patients had three injections and only one needed four treatments.

After injection the hernia was kept reduced by small round pad of gauze held in place with elastoplast applied as a belt at the level of the umbilicus, kept in position after the scar tissue produced has become strain-resistant.

Large umbilical hernias in young children necessitate operative repair.

THE USE AND ABUSE OF BARBITURATES
(H. B. Gardner, Pittsburgh, in *Penn. Med. Jl.*, Feb.)

These four barbiturates—barbital and barbital sodium; pentobarbital sodium; phenobarbital and phenobarbital sodium; evipal sodium (for intravenous anesthesia)—the writer believes are sufficient, with the addition of pentothal for prolonged intravenous anesthesia. The bromides and small doses of chloral hydrate and chlorobutanol may better be used as simple sedatives, pain relieved more sufficiently by dilaudid or pantopon.

When called to treat an unconscious patient known to have taken an overdose of a barbiturate, the procedure is as follows:

1. Gastric lavage with 1 to 5,000 potassium permanganate solution.
2. Saline purgation—sodium sulfate or phosphate by the lavage tube.
3. Colon irrigation with 1 to 5,000 potassium permanganate solution followed by instillation of black coffee.
4. Frequent aspiration of secretion accumulated in the pharynx; insertion of an airway; administration of oxygen by nasal catheter, and artificial resuscitation if necessary.
5. Ten per cent glucose in normal saline intravenously, or 50 c.c. of 50 per cent sucrose if pulmonary edema develops.
6. Picrotoxin 3 mg. or 1 c.c. of the 0.3 per cent solution intravenously every 20 minutes until facial muscle twitch is noticed—then less frequently.
7. Plasma when a high degree of anoxia exists.

In addition external heat, frequent change of position, and best nursing care.

PREGNANCY WITH ACUTE POLIOMYELITIS
(A. L. Wakefield, Louisville, in *Ky. Med. Jl.*, July)

Acute poliomyelitis developed in the 12th week of pregnancy with a febrile period of two weeks, the course of pregnancy was normal, delivery occurring spontaneously at eight and a half months. Labor was normal, the only assistance given being an abdominal binder to reinforce the weak recti muscles, and an episiotomy to enlarge the outlet to recompense for the patient's inability to iron out and stretch the perineum adequately. The baby shows no abnormality.

Onset poliomyelitis August 9th, 1943, with pain in head, back and legs. Four days later patient collapsed and the family physician was called. Both knee jerks were hyperactive and there was slight abdominal pain to deep pressure. Nausea and vomiting developed with increased headache. She slept that night and most of the next day when she lost appetite and had pain in each arm and shoulder.

August 16th, head and neck were hyperextended, pain and stiffness of neck, back, arms and legs, and some headache; weakness of both upper and lower extremities; tightness in hamstring and calf muscles; unable to lift arms to side of head without supinating hand or forearm; back hyperextended.

August 19th, there was pain and stiffness of neck and back with paralysis of both legs—movement only in foot muscles. Involvement of recti muscles.

Two weeks after delivery she resumed her walking with the walker, then with walking sticks. Present condition of leg muscles is rated as poor, left foot muscles four and right foot muscles a trace.

GENERAL

THE NALLE CLINIC
Nalle Clinic Building   412 North Church Street, Charlotte
Telephone—C-BVDV (*if no answer, call 3-2621*)

General Surgery

BRODIE C. NALLE, M.D.
GYNECOLOGY & OBSTETRICS

EDWARD R. HIPP, M.D.
TRAUMATIC SURGERY

*PRESTON NOWLIN, M.D.
UROLOGY

Consulting Staff

R. H. LAFFERTY, M.D.
O. D. BAXTER, M.D.
RADIOLOGY

W. M. SUMMERVILLE, M.D.
PATHOLOGY

General Medicine

LUCIUS G. GAGE, M.D.
DIAGNOSIS

LUTHER W. KELLY, M.D.
CARDIO-RESPIRATORY DISEASES

J. R. ADAMS, M.D.
DISEASES OF INFANTS & CHILDREN

W. B. MAYER, M.D.
DERMATOLOGY & SYPHILOLOGY

(*In Country's Service)

C—H—M MEDICAL OFFICES
DIAGNOSIS—SURGERY
X-RAY—RADIUM

DR. G. CARLYLE COOKE—*Abdominal Surgery & Gynecology*
DR. GEO. W. HOLMES—*Orthopedics*
DR. C. H. MCCANTS—*General Surgery*
222-226 Nissen Bldg.   Winston-Salem

WADE CLINIC
Wade Building
Hot Springs National Park, Arkansas

H. KING WADE, M.D.	*Urology*
ERNEST M. MCKENZIE, M.D.	*Medicine*
*FRANK M. ADAMS, M.D.	*Medicine*
*JACK ELLIS, M.D.	*Medicine*
BESSEY H. SHEBESTA, M.D.	*Medicine*
*WM. C. HAYS, M.D.	*Medicine*

N. B. BURCH, M.D.
    Eye, Ear, Nose and Throat
A. W. SCHEER   *X-ray Technician*
ETTA WADE   *Clinical Laboratory*
MERNA SPRING   *Clinical Pathology*
(*In Military Service)

INTERNAL MEDICINE

ARCHIE A. BARRON, M.D., F.A.C.P.
INTERNAL MEDICINE—NEUROLOGY
Professional Bldg.   Charlotte

JOHN DONNELLY, M.D.
DISEASES OF THE LUNGS
Medical Building   Charlotte

CLYDE M. GILMORE, A.B., M.D.
CARDIOLOGY—INTERNAL MEDICINE
Dixie Building   Greensboro

JAMES M. NORTHINGTON, M.D.
INTERNAL MEDICINE—GERIATRICS
Medical Building   Charlotte

NEUROLOGY and PSYCHIATRY

(*Now in the Country's Service*)
*J. FRED MERRITT, M.D.
NERVOUS and MILD MENTAL DISEASES
ALCOHOL and DRUG ADDICTIONS
Glenwood Park Sanitarium   Greensboro

TOM A. WILLIAMS, M.D.
(*Neurologist of Washington, D. C.*)
Consultation by appointment at
Phone 3994-W
77 Kenilworth Ave.   Asheville, N. C.

EYE, EAR, NOSE AND THROAT

H. C. NEBLETT, M.D.
OCULIST
Phone 3-5852
Professional Bldg.   Charlotte

AMZI J. ELLINGTON, M.D.
DISEASES of the
EYE, EAR, NOSE and THROAT
Phones: Office 992—Residence 761
Burlington   North Carolina

UROLOGY, DERMATOLOGY and PROCTOLOGY

THE CROWELL CLINIC of UROLOGY and UROLOGICAL SURGERY
Hours—Nine to Five   Telephones—3-7101—3-7102
STAFF
ANDREW J. CROWELL, M.D.
(1911-1938)
*ANGUS M. McDONALD, M.D.   CLAUDE B. SQUIRES, M.D.
Suite 700-711 Professional Building
                              Charlotte

RAYMOND THOMPSON, M.D., F.A.C.S.   WALTER E. DANIEL, A.B., M.D.
THE THOMPSON-DANIEL CLINIC
of
UROLOGY & UROLOGICAL SURGERY
Fifth Floor Professional Bldg.   Charlotte

C. C. MASSEY, M.D.
PRACTICE LIMITED
TO
DISEASES OF THE RECTUM
Professional Bldg.   Charlotte

WYETT F. SIMPSON, M.D.
GENITO-URINARY DISEASES
Phone 1234
Hot Springs National Park   Arkansas

ORTHOPEDICS

HERBERT F. MUNT, M.D.
ACCIDENT SURGERY & ORTHOPEDICS
FRACTURES
Nissen Building   Winston-Salem

SURGERY

R. S. ANDERSON, M. D.

GENERAL SURGERY

144 Coast Line Street   Rocky Mount

R. B. DAVIS, M. D., M. M. S., F. A. C. P.
GENERAL SURGERY
AND
RADIUM THERAPY
Hours by Appointment

Piedmont-Memorial Hosp.   Greensboro

(*Now in the Country's Service*)

WILLIAM FRANCIS MARTIN, M.D.

GENERAL SURGERY

Professional Bldg.   Charlotte

OBSTETRICS & GYNECOLOGY

IVAN M. PROCTER, M. D.

OBSTETRICS & GYNECOLOGY

133 Fayetteville Street   Raleigh

SPECIAL NOTICES

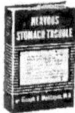

NERVOUS STOMACH TROUBLE—By J. F. Montague, M.D. 49 Chapters. Clear and easy reading about the "facts of life" as presented by stomach ulcer, colitis, gall bladder trouble and appendicitis. Medical facts on treatment comprehensive yet most interesting — even entertaining. Published by Simon and Schuster. Send orders to Joseph J. Boris, Publishers' Representative, 1440 Broadway, New York, N. Y. (Price $2.00)

TWO LABORATORY TECHNICIANS, being graduated from a High-class Hospital Laboratory, services available January 1st, 1044. Address TECHNICIAN, care *Southern Medicine & Surgery*.

TO THE BUSY DOCTOR WHO WANTS TO PASS HIS EXPERIENCE ON TO OTHERS

You have probably been postponing writing that original contribution. You can do it, and save your time and effort by employing an expert literary assistant to prepare the address, article or book under your direction or relieve you of the details of looking up references, translating, indexing, typing, and the complete preparation of your manuscript.

Address: *WRITING AIDE*, care *Southern Medicine & Surgery*.

THE JOURNAL OF SOUTHERN MEDICINE AND SURGERY

306 NORTH TRYON STREET, CHARLOTTE, N. C.

The Journal assumes no responsibility for the authenticity of opinion or statements made by authors or in communications submitted to this Journal for publication.

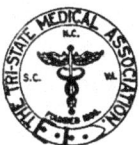

JAMES M. NORTHINGTON, M.D., Editor

"The Mill Cannot Grind With the Water That is Past"*

CARL V. REYNOLDS, M.D., Raleigh
North Carolina State Health Officer

I AM NOT OLD enough to reminisce, but it will not embarrass me to point out that, in 1920, I directed the attention of the Medical Society of the State of North Carolina to the fact that:

"Medicine, as an applied science, has through individual, rather than a collective effort, made marvelous advances through her various avenues of research; this reward of merit through individual attainment should not be lost.

"Then it behooves us for the sake of self-preservation, if not for the higher motive—the preservation of humanity—to have a strong committee to watch, plan and outline for those who are endeavoring to pass Medical Legislation, that we may guide their efforts in the proper way. Never before did we need, as we do now, intelligent leadership."

With the passing of the years there has been an intensification, rather than a diminution, of the necessity for leadership, in view of the increasing complexity of the social order and its growing needs.

In enumerating a few of the important and informative reports on the various approaches to better health, I desire to bring to your attention, for purpose of reëmphasis, the increasing necessity for our taking an active part, as members of the organized medical profession.

While we, as physicians, detest and abhor anything which smacks of advertising, we must not lose sight of the fact that there is a vast difference between what is commonly regarded as advertising and education. We can, therefore, accomplish much through the orderly and dignified processes of education, as advertising for personal aggrandizement would bring upon us that stigma which we so much desire to shun. Through education, then, we can and should participate, as an organized group, in a firm movement to bring about the accomplishment of the aims of those who desire to serve humanity to the highest degree. We can do this and, at the same time, retain our individuality, conserve every right which we have cherished down through the long and honorable history of medicine and neglect none of our assets.

It may be that we have neglected our greatest asset to man in awaiting his call for aid and then attempting a cure, rather than anticipating his ills and preventing them. We advise how to get well; we should advise how to keep well.

Again quoting from the original address:

"Experience has taught us something. We should awaken, ere it is too late, and realize that certain fundamental changes are to be made, and that this is necessary to society, before we are embarrassed by having our duties poorly done by incompetents.

"Our already accumulated knowledge, if awakened and put into active service, can reduce sickness and accident one-half. The philanthropists, the politicians, and the people at large have this interesting knowledge—made possible for them by us and given to them by our press. Do you think for one moment that they are going to sit idly by and see this vast waste of human life?

"Our individual problems may cause us to sit idly by, forgetful of, or, with indifference to, the

---

*Presented to Tri-State Medical Association of the Carolinas and Virginia, meeting at Charlotte, Feb. 28th-29th, 1944.

greater problems of the community, the State or the United States health program, and we will suffer the consequences of the inactive, thoughtless, indifferent citizen, and suffer in consequence of our inactiveness.

"The physician is still an individual, and deals with his patient as an individual, failing to recognize that community interest should and must be conserved, even at the loss of the individual for the good of the many."

Curative medicine is necessarily individualistic in thought and administration.

Preventive medicine is collectivistic in thought and administration.

The two branches are didactically and idealistically the same, and are so interwoven and interlocking that the success or failure of one means the success or failure of the other. This is the period in our history and in the process of our advancement, if we are to advance as we should, when these two schools should not only fraternize but organize together and make this new era "serve us rather than enslave us."

The basic element of any successful endeavor is a sound organization carrying forward intelligently, conscientiously, and concertedly, the issues involved, with "Service Before Self" emblazoned across our banner, as we pursue the march of human progress.

The last war brought us face to face with many hitherto undiscovered, or unrealized facts, chief among which was proof, beyond the shadow of a doubt, that thirty-three and a third per cent of our manhood was impaired, which meant, of course, impaired manpower to that extent.

The startling disclosure brought forcibly to our attention that remedial measures must be put into effect.

But to what extent have these measures been put into force?

The laity—the socially-minded, organized groups, civic bodies, students of public welfare, and others today are seeking concrete information, having been awakened to this necessity by the revelation that with the outbreak and progress of World War No. 2 remedial measures had not been put into effect, as indicated by the fact that conditions are worse than they were during the first World War.

These lay groups are adamant in their insistence that measures for improvement be taken, which brings the members of our profession face to face with the fact that either we must act, and act with a definite plan in view, or the laity, independently of the medical mind, will devise its own plan, and we will find their will superimposed upon us. What will be our decision in this critical moment, and how do we plan to execute that decision? I speak as a physician and not as a layman; as one sympathetic with our problems, and not as a critic—and, above all, as one with an abiding confidence in the sincerity of our purposes; but we must bolster that sincerity with positive action, and not proceed in a reactionary manner. We are living in a new age, whether we like it or not; we are living in a world that no longer will tolerate stagnation. Either we lead the way, or must be carried away with the flood!

Health is essential to human happiness, and to the economic success and safety of the nation. Men and women will seek health through *some sort* of leadership. If the medical profession furnishes that leadership, then *we* shall be the *true leaders*. If not, leadership will be sought and found elsewhere. The choice, I think, lies with *us* rather than with the medically uninformed laity, with its various groups and schools of thought, which might easily build a tower of Babel pointed theoretically toward heaven but, in reality, leading to a confusion not only of tongues but of action also.

When it comes to supplying ways and means for a readjustment as to the best method of approach, we all too often hide behind the cloak of fear of political control, personal relationship with the patient (much desired but little achieved by the younger medicos and specialists), inferior medical service, and lose sight of the most important factor of all—that the doctor makes known the evils that deter the prevention of disease and the preservation of health, and he should not stop there, but furnish a sound plan which will retain the high standards of medical care now enjoyed by the few and make them available to all, regardless of their economic status, as their right, and not administered as charity.

A negative acquiescence—or approval—is not enough. Action must be positive and with a sincerity of purpose, if we are to retain our boasted heritage.

If we fight the social trend for the betterment of man's security in physical, mental and moral fitness, we will be the cause of the objectionable features, and the effect will be the establishment of lay, rather than medical, control: for as surely as night follows day, man is going to have as his right, the medical, social and environmental protection needed to give him security in his effort to compete for his place in this world!

It may interest you for me to review with you just a few of the health protective measures that have been taken, in order that we may see with clearer vision and understanding the problems with which we have contended in the past and which confront us for future determination; also how essential it is that organized medicine participate in the careful survey of a fact-finding nature that must precede sound planning, so essential to the success of any undertaking.

It is pointed out in the Foreword of the Annual Reports of the United States Public Health Service for 1941-1942 and 1942-1943 that the health of our nation since our entry into the war has remained good, as indicated by the fact that, in 1942, we established an all-time low national death rate of 10.3 per 1,000 population, as compared with 10.5 the preceding year. It is probable that final figures will show a decrease in maternal mortality for the thirteenth consecutive year, reaching an all-time low of about or less than three deaths per 1,000 live births. Infant mortality decreased to 40 or 41 per 1,000 live births in 1942, as compared with 45 in 1941. At the same time, the birth rate rose from 18.7 per 1,000 population in 1941 to 20.7 in 1942. It was, without doubt, higher still in 1943 although the national rate has not yet been printed in report form.

We all know that longevity has steadily increased during the past century, with the advance of medical science and the rise of public health and preventive medicine. In 1850 the child born had but 38 years to which he could look forward, whereas the period of longevity at the present time is about 64 years. It took a combination of circumstances to bring this about, as nothing just happens.

Supplemental medicine has played a conspicuous part in the progress we have made, in both health and consequent longevity.

Let us have a look at the record of Federal assistance to the States for a single year, the fiscal year of 1944, which amounts to the almost unbelievable sum of $262,145,260, divided as follows according to information received from Washington on February 17th: Title VI (Social Security), $11,000,000; Venereal Disease Control, $10,276,200; Maternal and Child Health, $5,820,000; Crippled Children, $3,870,000; Emergency Maternal and Infant Care, $23,000,000; Emergency Health Sanitary Activities (General), $2,983,376; Malaria Control, $7,649,314; Industrial Hygiene, $546,310; projects approved covering construction and maintenance of health centers, hospitals, rapid-treatment centers and nurses' homes, $75,000,000; construction of sanitary facilities, $122,000,000.

Statistics, as such, are fit only for the archives; translated into definite action, they can become a source of constructive enlightenment.

Perhaps no problem has given rise to more perplexity than that of venereal diseases.

The number of venereal disease clinics increased during the fiscal year from 3,245 to 3,569, more than 10 per cent. Serologic tests for syphilis totaled 20,500,000 and arsenical drugs for its treatment distributed by State Health Departments continued to increase; a total of nearly 9 million doses of arsenicals was distributed to clinics and private physicians—an increase of nearly 7 per cent over 1941.

The performance of routine serologic tests for syphilis under the Selective Service Act of 1940 proved to be a case-finding procedure of vast importance. The examination of the first 2,000,000 men revealed the presence of syphilis in 45 selectees and volunteers per 1,000 tested. The rate for the entire male population between the ages of 21 and 35 is 48 per 1,000. For whites it is 24 and for Negroes it is 272. The highest rates were found in five Southern States, namely: Mississippi, South Carolina, Georgia, Florida and Louisiana. The lowest rates, less than 10 per thousand, were reported in New Hampshire, North Dakota, Wisconsin, Vermont, Utah and Minnesota.

What has Federal aid meant in this fight? It has meant that the States and localities were able to carry on this fight where, otherwise, they would have been greatly handicapped, because of a lack of funds. In my own State, if we had depended upon State and local appropriations, our position would have been far less favorable than it is today; but this is a question that is bigger than any one State. Hence, we must get an overall picture.

Of the $12,367,000 appropriated by Congress for venereal disease control activities in 1943, plus balances accrued from previous years, $10,170,000, or 81.4 per cent, was allotted to the States of the Union, the District of Columbia, Alaska, Puerto Rico, the Virgin Islands and Hawaii; and of this amount, $3,018,900 was earmarked for State Cooperation with the armed forces and other war needs. State and local funds budgeted for venereal disease control were increased by $472,500 over the previous year, totalling $7,457,100. The total Federal, State, local and other funds for venereal disease control during 1943 was $19,368,458.

What is being accomplished from these enormous expenditures? I am sure I may mention with pardonable pride an excerpt from recent United States Public Health Service reports to the effect that: "In North Carolina definite progress has been made in maneuver extra-cantonment areas, especially at Fort Bragg, where epidemiologic and treatment facilities have been improved."

An outstanding achievement of 1943 was the network of Rapid-Treatment Centers developed by the Public Health Service and War Manpower Commission, in coöperation with State Departments of Health and other public and private agencies. These centers—of which one of the most efficient is located here in Charlotte—are the logical outgrowth of the five-year-old control program, during which new methods of finding, treating and preventing venereal diseases have been studied, with marked progress. The accumulation of evidence points to the fact that the greatest source of venereal diseases among the armed forces, war workers and Selective Service registrants is the prostitute and the promiscuous woman. To quarantine, test, and aid in redistricting these women, 30 rapid-treatment centers were established in the United States, the Canal Zone, Puerto Rico and the Virgin Islands, including two in North Carolina —the one in Charlotte, previously referred to, and one in Durham.

Vigorous venereal disease control activities on the part of the Army and Navy were reflected in a lowering of venereal disease rates, especially during the latter part of the year. It might be added that when houses of prostitution in camp areas are closed, the venereal infection rate is lowered not only among service men in the community but also among the civilian population, which furnishes a strong argument for the elimination of prostitution for the good of the entire population, whether in uniform or civilian clothing.

Reports from State and territorial health departments for that part of 1943 for which complete figures have been compiled indicate a marked acceleration. Better and more thorough reporting naturally led to more effective control. A total of 590,604 cases were reported to State Health Departments, an increase of 20.7 per cent over 1942.

Admissions to clinic service increased from 343,312 in 1942 to 430,302 in 1943, a net increase of 26.3 per cent. The average monthly patient load in clinics increased 11.4 per cent during 1943 over that period reported in 1942. A total of 12,506,784 doses of arsenicals and heavy metals was administered in clinics, an increase of 17.1 per cent over 1942 and 50.4 over 1940, before America's entry into the war.

Approximately 31 million tests were made in all laboratories, an increase of 53.1 per cent over 1942.

These figures leave no doubt in my mind as to where the money is going that is appropriated for venereal disease control. This could have never been accomplished by private practitioners of medicine; it could not have been accomplished by State, communities and localities without Federal aid—and if this be a form of State Medicine, then we can but make the most of it and accept the benefits which, otherwise, would not and could not have accrued to humanity, both that portion suffering from venereal diseases and that portion free of infection but exposed to it. The money expended has accrued to the physicians' financial benefit.

Let us consider for a moment malaria, a great problem in many sections of our own country in peace- as well as war-time, but we had its seriousness impressed upon us in the early stages of the war against Japan, at Bataan and other points. It will continue as a post-war problem until its control is effected and we have eliminated the mosquito of the type that transmits it.

In Puerto Rico the program as to the civilian population has not been so successful; but by excellent coöperation between the Public Health Service and military officials, the rate among military personnel has been reduced from 114 per 10,000 in July, 1942, to 8 in 1943.

On June 30th, 1943, a force of 3,704 persons were engaged in deducing mosquito breeding by drainage operations and larviciding in areas contiguous to 1,161 military, naval and war industry establishments in 18 states, the District of Columbia and Puerto Rico.

One of the most important of the obligations confronting us is that of keeping our people supplied wits pure milk. Some of the factors involved making this undertaking difficult derive from the commercial angle of the business as administered by pressure groups. The medical profession should cry aloud in its denunciation. All possible assistance has been given the Army, the Navy, the Coast Guard and other branches of the service, but until mercenary interests no longer demand to be allowed to sell milk of an inferior quality the protection due the military and civilian population alike will remain in jeopardy.

The public at large should demand Grade A milk and decline milk of doubtful purity. The matter should not be left with pressure groups with axes to grind, whose success might easily spell disaster for the dairy industry, as well as harm for the public. The members of our own profession can render great assistance in this respect by impressing upon those who seek their advice the importance of safe, clean milk for the population as a whole, for every individual should have his quota of milk.

We will, as time goes on, have to deal more and more with tropical diseases. The Government has let no grass grow under its feet in attacking the problem. The importance of this work will be magnified with the return of our military forces from the tropical East. Four fatal cases of plague have occurred in Hawaii and one in northern California. Surveys found plague in rats in California, in Washington and in Hawaii, and in other rodents in California, Oregon, Nevada, Montana, Colorado and New Mexico. Extermination by poisoning and gassing was carried out on military reservations in California and Washington. During the year 140,000 rodents and 4,000 specimens of their parasites were collected and examined; and 110 were found to be infected with plague, and five with tularemia. Laboratory examinations also were performed upon 9,000 field rodents collected by survey units of the Washington, Oregon and Montana State Health Departments on 600 collected from ships by the quarantine service at San Francisco. Rodent control is a coöperative measure and should be aided by public demand.

With present rapid means of transportation germs may span the continent or the widest ocean with the rapidity of the airplane. This calls for nation-wide coördination of effort.

A major tuberculosis project is case-finding in war industries. The newly-developed 35 mm. and 4x5 in. photofluographic x-ray units are used in this work. By the end of the last fiscal year, ten field units were in operation. During the year chest examinations were made of 320,000 workers in 85 war establishments in eleven states and the District of Columbia; and 60,000 migratory workers were examined before entering the United States from Mexico. Tabulation of 125,000 case records showed 1.3 per cent of the workers examined had tuberculosis of the reinfection type. On this basis, it is estimated that 5,000 cases of significant tuberculosis were discovered. Cases found were referred to their family physicians. Is that significant?

The numerous coöperative Government industrial hygiene services reached a new peak in 1942-1943. The impaired were referred likewise to their private physicians.

The facts I have called to your attention are sufficient to lay emphasis on the tasks that lie before us and the progress that has been made through coöperation of existing Federal and State Public Health agencies. The greater part of this progress could not have been brought about except through the application of new social concepts of the importance of mass protection. We could not conquer disease through the individual-by-individual methods of the past. We must now move *en masse* in health matters as in war. The fight against disease is a war of the first magnitude and it will remain a continuing war for centuries to come.

The establishment of blood plasma banks has become an important nation-wide medical service. At the close of the fiscal year 158,290 units of plasma were available in hospitals and reserve depots in 316 communities in the United States and at strategic outposts. Of this amount, 79,500 units were provided by the United States Public Health Service, and 78,790 were pledged by the participating hospitals. Emergency use of plasma reserves were responsible for the saving of lives in such disasters as the Boston Cocoanut Grove Night Club Fire, the wreck of the Congressional Limited at Philadelphia, and various other fires, explosions, etc., to say nothing of the marvelous results obtained on the far-flung battlefields. No serious reactions have been reported on the part of those receiving the plasma, or of the blood donors.

The fight against everything pertaining to segregation, political control, State medicine, contract practice, etc., can only be successfully waged, through a united effort on the part of the medical profession, in looking toward the ultimate goal of devising ways and means—under the supervision of the medical mind—to furnish medical and hospital care to those who need it, regardless of their social or economic status.

In conclusion, let me call your attention to a plan recently promulgated by Governor J. Melville Broughton of North Carolina, who, after the plan received the full endorsement of the Medical Committee of the Medical Society of the State of North Carolina, was unanimously endorsed by the Board of Trustees of the University of North Carolina.

In the words of the Governor: "The ultimate purpose of this program should be that no person in North Carolina shall lack hospital care or medical treatment by reason of poverty or low income."

Briefly, the Governor's program would provide that:

1. The present two-year medical school at the University be enlarged so as to provide a full four-year course. The two other medical schools in the State already on a four-year basis, can never supply the full requirements for physicians to serve adequately the civilian population of North Carolina.

2. That an adequate hospital be erected at the University of North Carolina, with a capacity of not less than 600 and preferably 1,000 beds, to be built by State funds, supplemented by such Federal, private and foundation funds as may be available, and shall be open to patients from all sections of the State, with provisions for free hospital and medical service to all such patients as may be unable to pay for same; that the various counties of the State be encouraged to set up appropriations to provide a substantial portion of the cost of patients who may be sent to such hospital from such county, such funds to be supplemented by funds that may be available from the Duke Foundation or other foundations now in existence or hereafter created for such purpose.

3. That other smaller hospitals to serve as local centers be established in strategic regions of the State for hospitalization of those in need of medical care without means to provide that care.

Governor Broughton's program would carry into some of the smaller counties well-equipped hospitals which would attract the best element of professional service and encourage doctors to leave the centers and work among the 73 per cent of our population who live in rural communities and villages of less than 2,500 population.

Would that the great Commonwealth of Virginia and the Sovereign State of South Carolina might join with the Old North State in leading the entire nation in carrying out this magnificent program of such features as do not now exist in our sister States to the north and to the south.

With such a program in effect, we could not any longer bemoan the fact that:

"Man's inhumanity to man
Makes countless thousands mourn."

Discussion

DR. K. B. PACE, Greenville, N. C.: I hope you got what Dr. Reynolds was driving at—that is, socialized medicine. We have often criticized the plan, and probably the criticism is deserved. Now the time has come when we have got to offer a detailed plan and put our united strength behind it in order that the medical profession can lead in the movement rather than let the Federal Government take charge and lead it. If there is nothing better to be done, the medical profession can join hands with the Health Department and come to grounds where it can be kept well within the medical profession and not have an outsider telling us how and why to do it. Most of you know and I know very well the great governments of North Carolina, South Carolina and Virginia are very anxious to see that something is done before the Federal authorities come in and start it with outside men over which we will have no control. We can't put it off any longer. It would be better to take charge and offer plans and cooperate with each other, rather than have the Federal Government take full charge.

DR. JAMES W. VERNON, Morganton: I am sorry to say your chairman may be mistaken, but I feel constrained to say that I believe we are at a critical point in the history of medicine and in the history of possible progress in medicine.

As the essayist, Dr. Reynolds, has said to you—there are three opportunities offering themselves to us as a profession. They are here. They are now upon us. I believe we are perhaps at a fork of the road as a profession and we may stand still or go backward or lose our leadership. I don't like the idea of a threat that we *must* do something, but apparently it has come to the point where it is pretty much that We have been talking much about socialized medicine. Whatever that means, most of us know that we mean that we don't want the therapeutic side of the practice of medicine taken over by any governmental agency and the doctor-patient relationship destroyed. Briefly and simply, those are some of the things we are afraid of. I think perhaps the time is here when we should go along with the progress of preventive medicine and therapeutic medicine under the control of the medical profession and that we are not capable of stepping out and taking that leadership. I am afraid it will create some dangers to the medical profession.

I am hoping we are going to carry out the recommendations of our Governor which Dr. Reynolds has outlined, and if we do, I believe it will be one of the most significant things in our state that has happened in this generation. I believe we need medical leadership throughout the whole state. I think it exists. The ability is in our state with our profession, but I am frank to say that it is not as expressive and as active as it is needful for it to be. I am hoping that the plan that has been initiated here in North Carolina is going to be the answer to socialized medicine in this state.

DR. REYNOLDS (closing): Mr. Chairman, Patient Followers: I want to thank Dr. Vernon for his supporting remarks and leave with you this thought—that we cannot get anything through rebellion, but through coöperative approach we can control the situation. We can direct and control it through medical channels, without any political interference and belonging to what we term state medicine. I firmly believe it. I have been thinking of it all these years and for the last ten years I have been dispensing the funds that have been coming out of Washington for these purposes and I know from sources and conferences in Washington we are going to have millions in the future where we have had thousands.

If you take the roll call of Republicans and Democrats in the Congress and Senate, they are in favor of this, what I call supplemental medicine, and it is coming, whether the Republicans or Democrats are in power. You take the syphilis bill. I happened to be there when it was brought up. We visited Mr. Bulwinkle of North Carolina and we visited LaFollette, and it did not take those men fifteen minutes to decide that they would introduce the bill. LaFollette is a Republican and opposed to everything; Bulwinkle is a Democrat, of course—and it went through smoothly and the appropriation has been increased each year. The vast majority are in favor of it and it is coming, and for God's sake, let's take a hand and control it.

WHAT TO DO ON DIAGNOSING LATENT SYPHILIS

(Abraham Gelperin, Cincinnati, in *Clin Med.*, July)

The diagnosis of latent syphilis makes imperative examination of any family for evidence of infection. *The disease is not inactive but smoldering.* It is important to treat any existing disease, not the blood serodiagnostic test.

Patients with no serious complicating disease, and with early latency, should receive the same treatment as patients with primary syphilis; arsenoxide three times a week with an insoluble bismuth preparation once a week, for a total of 8 to 10 weeks. A man weighing 120 to 155 lbs. receives 60 mgms., 40 mgms. for the patient under 90 lbs., and a maximum of 80 mgms. for those over 185 lbs. The dose of bismuth is 1 c.c. of any insoluble preparation.

In *late* latent syphilis a series of 4-6 weekly injections of bismuth is in order, prior to starting tri-weekly intravenous medication. If complicating disease such as arteriosclerosis, chronic nephritis or cholecystitis is present initial doses of arsenoxide should be no more than half that recommended, and cautiously raised as close to the desired dose as is tolerated; given twice or even once a week, continued until the calculated total amount of drug has been administered—1500 mg. for a 150 lb. patient. A total of 10-15 injections of bismuth is usually sufficient.

If the physical examination at the termination of treatment is essentially negative, the treatment series is to be stopped whether the blood examination is positive or negative. A recheck spinal fluid examination should be made 1 and 2 years later, and periodical physical examinations with special attention to the cardiovascular and central nervous system.

ULCER PATIENTS, EMOTIONALLY UPSET, SHOULD EAT.

(W. C. Alvarez, in *Jl. A. M. A.*, July 2d)

When a patient who has had an ulcer goes through an emotional crisis he should immediately start taking food every hour or two. He shouldn't wait for the expected flare-up or hemorrhage or perforation. The extra feedings are probably most needed between the hours of 10 p. m. and 3 a. m.

Some Military Considerations of the Allergic Individual*

L. C. TODD, M.D., Charlotte

THE EXPERIENCE of the two World Wars has revealed the greater importance now being placed upon the true place of the allergic individual relative to the physical standards of the drafted and volunteer soldier.

It is my intention at this time to review the general ground work of the subject and make some of the applications to the present military situation.

Though late in recognizing the fact that the allergic person, though symptom-free at his civilian occupation, was apt to break down under military and combat conditions, the changes made in November, 1942, by the selective service system in the physical requirements relative to the allergic person was a step in the right direction.

The most extensive published report which I have found of the incidence of allergic states in selectees comes from Col. L. G. Rowntree's report published in the *Journal of the American Medical Association*, September 25th,[1] concerning the rejection rates of 18- and 19-year-old selectees. Of the 45,585 cases examined the local boards rejected 5.2%, the induction stations 21.3%—a total rejection rate of 25.4%. Of each 1,000, 3.7% were rejected because of asthma, vasomotor rhinitis 0.8% and sinusitis (type not specified) 0.6%—a total per 1,000 of 5.1%, these being the only allergic conditions identified. Major Hyde's reports[2] from the Boston Recruiting and Induction Station in which report it is stated that of the 60,000 men examined (age groups 21-34 and later 21-44), 495 (0.82%) were rejected for allergic states.

All examinations were conducted by a team of civilian internists under the same medical officer in charge and in all instances the standards of mobilization regulations numbers 1-9 were followed which specify:

Class 1-a (qualified for general military service). May include cases of hayfever, unless severe, and of acute eczema.

Class 1-b (qualified for limited service only). May include cases of severe hayfever and chronic asthma which is mild and which has not prevented the registrant from successfully following useful vocations in civil life.

Class 4-f (disqualified for military service). Includes cases of chronic asthma associated with chronic bronchitis and emphysema, except as stated above, and of allergic dermatoses if severe and not easily remediable.

On November 15th, 1942, there were changes in mobilization regulations numbers 1-9 to:

Class 1-a. May include hayfever if mild; acute eczema if mild.

Class 1-b. May include hayfever if moderate.

Class 4-f. Includes cases of hayfever if severe, allergic dermatoses if severe and not easily remediable, and bronchial asthma.

It is to be noted that the latter standards are more strict than the first since they disqualify all bronchial asthma and severe hayfever.

When one considers that the screening tests rule out the great majority of severe alergics and the induction centers uncover a considerable number; that the military hospitals are seeing large numbers who develop active symptoms under service conditions, the incidence of allergy in this age group is important. The change to stricter standards concerning allergics in general was an advanced move.

There are all degrees of allergy in the human—from A to Z and where is the line to be drawn? This question goes back to some of the fundamentals of this condition.

Allergy is a chronic constitutional state, with strong inherited potentialities and while usually functional in its earlier or minor manifestations, it may become secondarily organic.

The allergic reaction characterized by increased capillary permeability, smooth muscle spasm and mucous gland hyperactivity is reversible if not too severe and both the structural and functional characteristics of the shock tissues involved may return to normal. If it reaches a certain point of severity it may become irreversible and secondary degenerative changes occur in the involved tissues. Kline[3] has convincingly demonstrated this in his histologic studies of the induced reaction. Periarteritis nodosa, thromboangiitis obliterans or even erythema nodosum may be examples of irreversible allergic reactions. It is settled that certain changes in the respiratory mucosa—nasal passages, sinus linings, bronchi and alveoli—are irreversible and, with secondary bacterial infections complicating the picture, may become widespread and gross in character.

*Presented to Tri-State Medical Association of the Carolinas and Virginia, meeting at Charlotte, Feb. 28th-29th, 1944.

If a history of past major allergic episodes is to be heeded at all, many more selectees would be ruled out. It goes without saying that these histories must be authentic and have been fully recorded before any beginning of the present war has taken place. A transcript of these pre-war records is usually very helpful in determining the action the examining boards or induction centers are to take with a selectee who presents very little, if anything, upon physical examination but gives a strong past history of asthma, hayfever and eczema. A careful family history, past medical history and physical examination usually picks out the great majority of potential cases. An acquired allergy is always possible and more extended investigation including tests for hypersensitivity could best be confined to these cases.

It is interesting to compare the above figures with the number of men rejected by the draft boards of the last war.[4] Rejections because of asthma associated with emphysema and bronchitis were at the rate of 2.45 per thousand—less than one-fourth of 1%. In the same group there were nine times as many rejections for pulmonary tuberculosis. The medical department of the U. S. army from April 1st, 1917, to November 31st, 1919, admitted 7,445 enlisted men to hospitals with the diagnosis of asthma or about two per 1,000. In 1935, of the World War group, 1.2% of those receiving disability compensation were asthmatics; 62% of these or 4,644 were more than 50% disabled and 29% were totally disabled; 86% of them had established service connection for their asthma.

From these figures, it is evident that even before the medical profession was "allergy conscious," allergy could have been considered an important cause of physical disability.

To date, we do not have complete figures on the total number of allergic individuals revealed by the examinations of the draft boards, the induction stations or in military hospitals but undoubtedly it runs much higher than this.

The incidence of major degree allergy in the population of the United States as a whole is estimated to be somewhere from 5 to 10%. If the incidence of minor allergy and so-called minor food allergy is estimated, the figure is much higher. Several population surveys have been made on the basis of history and 10% is the figure most widely accepted for major allergy. From his survey, Vaughan[5] concludes that in round numbers 1 in 18 have frank hayfever; 1 in 20 have urticaria; 1 in 22 gastro-intestinal allergy; 1 in 30 asthma; 1 in 32 allergic migraine; 1 in 34 vasomotor rhinitis; 1 in 166 allergic eczema; and 1 in 250 angioneurotic edema. Of course, some of these symptoms overlap in the same individual.

If we will review and recollect the development of the scientific ideas on the subject, we will find that *Allergy* in the commonly accepted von Pirquet characterization is any specific alteration in the capacity to react which occurs in living organisms or tissues upon exposure to certain living or inanimate agents or substances. By "specific" is meant that the alteration brought about by an antigen or agent can be only demonstrated by reëxposure to that same agent or one immunologically related. Von Pirquet and Schick pointed out that the individual who has been adequately exposed to tubercle bacilli, spirochetes, horse serum or vaccinia virus, or to diphtheria or tetanus toxin or to certain drugs, foods, pollens, etc., on reëxposure to the same agent this individual will often react differently. Exposure to tubercle bacilli, to trichophyton fungi, to foreign sera are likely to become specifically more sensitive to these agents and their products—namely, the previously exposed are likely to react to quantities which produce no reactions in those not previously exposed. Those exposed to diphtheria toxin or tetanus toxin are apt to become specifically less sensitive to the agent. These are closely related biologic phenomena and are examples of allergy as the meaning intended by von Pirquet although the altered reactions may proceed in opposite directions. Increased resistance may be called immunity, decreased resistance may be called hypersensitivity which is the modern synonym for allergy. Idiosyncrasy is also synonymous. Anaphylaxis is the word first used by Richet in 1902 to describe the experimentally produced reaction in animals by injections of a sensitizing dose and a subsequent shocking dose and he believed that the first dose did something to the animal in the removal of its natural protection—thus anaphylaxis—without protection.

A brief resumé of some of the characteristics of the state of hypersensitiveness follows:

Heredity: It is quite generally accepted that the allergic tendency is in part at least inherited. The children of allergic parents are more liable to develop manifestations and at an earlier age than children of nonallergic parents. It is the allergic tendency and not the specific manifestation that is inherited. Nearly three-fourths of children with bilateral allergic inheritance will eventually develop symptoms, while with unilateral inheritance about one-half do so.

Age distribution of symptoms is best illustrated by the life history of an allergic person.

Allergics may be grouped into three groups as the age of onset and course of the activity of their symptoms are concerned:

Type I—Onset before puberty; usually of bilateral inheritance.

First Year—Foods are the chief allergens; the gastro-intestinal tract and skin being the chief shock tissues with the production of cyclic vomiting where the gastro-epimucosa is involved; colic, diarrhea, colitis if the intestinal epimucosa is involved; infantile dermatitis where the blood vessels of the cutis are involved.

Inhalants—chiefly environmental organic dusts act as allergens with the production or rhinitis, croup and asthma.

Second Year—Frequent so-called "colds," rhinitis, asthma and group are the rule, being exaggerated during seasonal changes of weather and during pollinating seasons.

Third Year—Increase in nasal and bronchial symptoms (dusts, pollens, moulds), especially during seasonal changes.

Digestive upsets, intestinal symptoms with collapse syndrome (foods).

Changes in disposition and temperament—production of irritability and nervous and emotional upsets.

Sixth Year—Rhinitis has become perennial; asthma more constant and emphysematous changes more definite. Lack of development in weight and statute; nervousness, irritability and quarrelsomeness.

Tenth Year—Continuous asthma of some degree; definite emphysema—irrevocable changes in lungs, shortness of breath and bronchitis; symptoms perennial becoming alarming in the seasonal changes of spring and fall; personality seriously affected.

Early recognition and treatment of this type modifies the symptoms and prevents much of the structural change.

Symptoms continue into later life but with usually a marked improvement after puberty or with a change of environment—getting away from environmental dusts and moulds; away at school with change in diet, climate and residence as well as away from certain domestic incompatibilities.

Type II—Symptoms come on at or after puberty whereas they had been previously normal, usually a unilateral inheritance, a typical course is as follows:

At the 13th-15th year—Summer cold in the spring with a persistent rhinitis through the summer and then a severe flare-up in the fall. By the 17th year, the summer and fall colds have continued, starting earlier each spring and lasting until midsummer; severe recurrences in the fall with tightness in the chest and recurrent or persistent cough.

Examination shows a pollinosis—trees, grasses and ragweed being involved.

With specific treatment he or she responds satisfactorily. If allowed to proceed uninterrupted, his symptoms continue getting worse and showing subsequent accessory sinus and bronchial and pulmonary complications unless he "outgrows it" by a change in environment or geographic location.

Type III—Has onset of symptoms in early adult life. He may or may not have an allergic family history.

The nasal symptoms are usually first and usually seasonal—pollens. Seasonal asthma follows. New sensitivities rapidly develop among the dusts, fungi and miscellaneous inhalatants as well as the foods. Asthma becomes more frequent until if not relieved it becomes chronic, obstinate and disabling. Respiratory tract bacterial factors become more important as it progresses.

It is very evident that, while many of the allergic inducted and volunteer soldiers are "getting by" quite satisfactorily, altogether too many have had their allergic balance upset because of training and combat conditions. It would appear that most of these cases occur in Types II and III.

Race: There seems to be a distinct difference in allergic predisposition among the races. In general, it may be explained that one chief reason why races living in the tropics have very little hayfever is that most of the flowers are fertilized by insects and the pollens are not wind-borne. Hayfever is rarely seen in Cuba and Mexico. The American Indians were said not to be sufferers of hayfever and asthma. Thommen stated that the Javanese, Malays and East Indians in Sumatra, Dutch East Indies and the Malay Peninsula never have hayfever, while Europeans and Americans living there do have it. The same is true of India. The Negro in our experience has all of the allergic manifestations. Rowntree's rejection rate for asthma in the Negro was 5.1 per 1,000, which is higher than in the white race.

Climate: Factors of barometric pressure, humidity, altitude, prevailing winds, temperature, amount of sunshine are all important physical factors. Practically all allergics in our experience who have definitely proven extrinsic etiologic factors such as pollens, dusts, foods, etc., have some degree of physical allergy. This is also true of intrinsic cases.

Environment: Environment determines what one becomes exposed to and it follows that it determines most of his sensitivities. His home site, his living quarters, his clothing, his occupation, his recreation and even his diet may be included.

A botanical and atmospheric survey of the vicinity will reveal the possible pollen and mould factors. A knowledge of his exposures at work or under war-time exposures is important in determining possible exciting and irritating factors.

Quarters are extremely important in determining environmental organic dusts and fungi—these are becoming more significant as more is being understood about them.

Specific allergens: These all continue to be operative under service conditions.

I Inhalants
    Pollens
    Danders
    Environmental organic dusts
        House dust
        Moulds
        Cottonseed
        Flaxseed
        Kapokseed
    Miscellaneous
        Orris
        Pyrethrum
        Tobacco
        Glue
        Insects
    Botanical excitants—hay, straw, leaves, fuzz, sawdust, turpentine

II Ingestants
    Foods
    Beverages
    Medicines and chemicals

III Contactants
    Worms
    Cosmetics
    Plants
    Clothing
    Furs
    Many miscellaneous: paints, dyes, oils

IV Injectants
    Animal sera
    Drugs
    Insect bites

V Miscellaneous
    Physical agents
    Parasites
    Bacteria, etc.

By far the most frequent exciting factors under war-time conditions are physical agents and bacterial infection.

Summary and Conclusions: In personal conversations with the medical officers of several of our large induction centers in this area, I have been informed that large areas of the station hospitals are taken up with asthmatic patients especially during or after the seasonal changes in weather or following large-scale maneuvers. In a recent letter from a medical officer in charge of one of our evacuation hospitals in Italy, he stated that their evacuation hospital was burdened by the large number of asthmatics whose symptoms were activated by the strenuous combat exertion, smoke and fume exposure, exposure to inclement weather, etc. As he aptly stated—"they can't take it."

Major allergy, as evidenced not only by the status praesens at the time of induction but by the personal and family history and, in doubtful or selected cases, by actual test with key allergens, should be a denying factor for admission to the combat forces whether they be land, air or sea forces. A compensated symptom-free allergic can be used for limited service. The minor allergic will always get through the bars unrecognized.

There are innumerable instances where the allergic soldier is handicapped seriously by his constitutional state—with him also his special squadron or patrol is handicapped.

One can imagine the ineffectiveness of the chronic asthmatic after any undue and prolonged exertion, exposure to dusts, fumes, restricted rations and inclement weather.

The asthma patient is now left out of consideration by selective service but before changes were made in the physical requirements many thousands were taken in who are hampering the medical departments of the services now; who will be given disability compensation and who will probably establish service connection for their disability because they broke down under service conditions.

Note: Since presentation of this paper, GOLD and BOZEMORE, *J. of Allergy*, 15:279, July, 1944, report from the Station Hospital, Camp Blanding, Fla., on "The Significance of Allergy in Military Medicine" and outline the criteria for disposition of allergic soldiers and inductees which they have found valuable.

BIBLIOGRAPHY

1. ROWNTREE, L. G.: Causes of Rejection and the Incidence of Defects. *J. A. M. A.*, 124:181, 1943.
2. HYDE, R. W.: Distribution of Allergic States in Selectees. *J. of Allergy*, 14:386, 1943.
3. KLINE, B. S.: Cases of Reversible and Irreversible Allergic Inflammation. *J. of Allergy*, 6:258, 1935.
4. VAUGHAN, W. T.: *Practice of Allergy*, p. 57. C. V. Mosby Co., St. Louis, 1939.
5. VAUGHAN, W. T.: *Practice of Allergy*, p. 57. C. V. Mosby Co., St. Louis, 1939.

THE ASSOCIATION OF MILITARY SURGEONS OF THE UNITED STATES

Addresses by the nation's three surgeons general, the chief of the Veterans Administration and the Commanding General of the Second Service Command will feature the 52nd Annual Meeting of the Association of Military Surgeons of the United States at the Hotel Pennsylvania, New York City, November 2nd–4th. Also there will be forum lectures, discussion panels, military and commercial scientific exhibits and medical motion pictures.

Forum lectures will cover War Surgery, Chemotherapy, Communicable Diseases, Neuropsychiatry, Medical Problems in Theaters of Operation, Dental Rehabilitation and Equine Encephalitis.

Topics for discussion panels, which will be integrated with the lectures, are: "War Wounds, Burns and Fractures," "Neuropsychiatric Problems," "Treatment and Prevention of Venereal Diseases," "Penicillin and Sulfonamide Therapy," "Orthopedic and Reconstruction Therapy," "Neuro-surgical Problems," "Tropical Diseases in the Army and Navy" and "Aviation Medicine."

DEPARTMENTS

PEDIATRICS

PAPERS BY A GROUP OF AMERICAN PAEDIATRICIANS*

THE AMERICAN APPROACH TO ALLERGY IN CHILDHOOD[1]

ALLERGY, a term coined by von Pirquet, and meaning specifically "altered reactivity," refers to a broad field of immunology including not only the atopic diseases but also drug idiosyncrasy, serum disease, tuberculous allergy, and a host of other conditioned reactions. Atopy is a term devised by Coca and means specifically "strange disease." In this group of diseases fall asthma, hayfever, eczema, urticaria, and some gastrointestinal disturbances manifested in childhood. They are characterized by a familial predisposition, a multiplicity of manifestations, a blood eosinophilia, the immediate wheal and flare type of skin response, presence of reagins in the serum, and flaring up of the pathological process by contact with specific excitants, usually proteins.

Most important is a careful history, taken primarily from the point of view of specific offenders. Vitamin deficiencies and endocrine abnormalities are rarely encountered. The blood is studied as to the percentage of eosinophils and leucocytosis when there is secondary infection. The urine is examined routinely. Sixty scratch tests including the common pollens, moulds, dusts, animal epithelia, and foods are made. If one or more satisfactory reactions consistent with the history, no further testing is done. If no reactions occur, intracutaneous tests are applied, usually 16 at each of two or more sittings. All suspected offenders are abolished from the child's environment or diet and he is desensitized to those substances such as pollens and house dust which he cannot avoid. During his weekly clinic visit in subsequent months clinical trial of the various specific offenders is made. If suspected that he is sensitive to cottonseed, he will be permitted to sleep on a cotton-stuffed pillow for one night or until symptoms occur.

HERPETIC STOMATITIS IN INFANTS AND CHILDREN[2]

APART FROM affections of the mouth avitaminosis, blood dyscrasias, specific bacterial or fungus infections, there is a common stomatitis among infants and young children called aphthous, membranous, ulcerative or Vincent's stomatitis. The evidence to be presented is sufficiently conclusive to show that these types of stomatitis are really one disease, with a clinical picture varying due to primary infection with the virus of herpes simplex.

It attacks children between the ages of one and six years, onset sudden with fever, which may be as high as 105° F., irritability, anorexia and malaise, which symptoms may coincide with the onset of a sore mouth or may precede this by several days, seven to 14 days of pain and fever, subsiding before the disappearance of visible signs in the mucous membranes. Shallow yellowish painful ulcers on the tongue and buccal mucous membranes, the result of ruptured vesicles occasionally the tonsils which can be seen as such very early in the disease; occasionally the tonsils and pharynx are affected early, leading to a misdiagnosis of follicular tonsillitis. Enlargement of the regional lymph nodes, which may persist for several weeks after the acute phase is over, oral foetor.

Dehydration brought on by refusal of food and fluids by mouth. Impetiginization of accompanying labial herpes. Paronychia in thumb suckers.

The virus of herpes in the saliva or from the lesions rubbed on to the scarified cornea of a rabbit causes kerato-conjunctivitis.

Treatment is entirely palliative and consists of preventing dehydration, by parenteral fluids if necessary, remembering that cold fluids by mouth are more acceptable than warm; the local application of chromic acid or gentian violet to the mouth lesions to alleviate pain; maintaining mouth cleanliness; treating secondary infection and reassuring the anxious mother.

FIBROSIS OF THE PANCREAS IN INFANTS AND CHILDREN[3]

IN FIBROSIS of the pancreas almost all the exocrine portion of the gland is profoundly affected.

During 15 years at the infants' and children's hospitals in Boston 35 examples of this lesion were encountered in examinations of the pancreas in 2,800 necropsies.

Failure to gain in weight in spite of an adequate food intake and a good appetite is usual. A cough and signs of pulmonary infiltration ultimately appear. Diarrhoea or altered stools are a regular feature. When patients are ill a short time (eight months) before death the features are indistinguishable from many disorders causing chronic wasting and terminal bronchopneumonia.

If the illness lasts longer large pale offensive "fatty" stools, abdominal distension, and extreme emaciation. Appearance is similar to that seen in coeliac disease except that by this time the pulmonary involvement is usually conspicuous and gives a clue to the basis of the symptoms.

Symptoms appear at or soon after birth in the

---

*Proceedings Royal Society of Medicine of England, May.

1. Lt. Col. H. N. Pratt, U. S. A. M. C., in Proc. Royal Soc. of Med. (Lond.), May.
2. Major T. F. McN. Scott, U. S. A. M. C.
3. Major C. D. May, U. S. A. M. C.

great majority of patients. Rarely two to four years may pass without any disorder attracting attention, and the child may appear healthy and well nourished. Close inquiry will reveal that from an early age stools have been abnormal, the appetite extraordinarily good, and a chronic cough had developed. No child with this lesion in the pancreas has been reported to have lived longer than 15 years.

More than one sibling in a family is often affected.

The diagnosis can be readily established by estimation of trypsin in the pancreatic juice, easily obby passing a tube into the duodenum.

When no special therapy is available allow the patient an abundance of all types of food to satisfy the appetite regardless of the appearance of the stools. Fats might be somewhat restricted but not if it makes the diet unattractive.

Pancreatin preparations potency is variable and uncertain. The enzymes are inactivated by the acid of the stomach. Enteric coatings may be removed too soon or too late and the enzymes thereby be ineffective. The daily doses required are large (0 to 4 months—6 g.; 5 years—21 g.) Enteric coated tablets or capsules cannot safely be given to infants when proper treatment is most urgent.

Predigested foods offer great promise for treatment during infancy and early childhood. Hydrolysates of casein are now available, composed primarily of amino-acids. Absorbed without digestion and have been utilized to maintain nitrogen balance and a proper nutrition. They can be combined with sugar not requiring digestion like glucose and a minimum of fat and the proper salts and vitamins. Babies have been successfully reared on such mixtures. In a few instances of fibrosis of the pancreas the results are greatly encouraging, in one instance successful. If the diagnosis is not made early and the treatment prompt and efficacious the pulmonary infection is so far advanced as to be irreversible.

Vitamins may be given by mouth in doses four times the daily requirement sto make up for the impairment in absorption. Vitamin-B complex to the usual vitamins A, D and C.

Discussion on Enuresis[4]

Mr. Higgins

A HEALTHY INFANT properly trained, should be dry after 18 months at the latest—many much earlier. Thereafter in frequent flooding something is likely to be wrong. If this is not appreciated, a gross uropathy may well pass unrecognized in its early stages. Enuresis may be a prominent feature

[4]. T. T. Higgins, H. P. Winsbury-White, W. Sheldon, E. B. Strauss.

of certain rare diseases such as diabetes and hyperpiesia. Spina bifida occulta, when unassociated with other neurological signs, is a rare cause and should be borne in mind, particularly in the case of sacral defects.

One case in 10 of enuresis in children has some obstruction in the tract, infection, or a combination of both. Frequent and urgent voiding of small quantities of urine, pain, with or without fever, is likely infection or obstruction. Have child pass its urine under observation.

Vulvovaginitis is a frequent source of infection and enuresis; frequently both are cured with its disappearance. The urethra should be inspected for signs of inflammation, malformation, etc.

In a boy the external meatus should be examined for contraction, ulceration or malformation. A glandular hypospadias is very often unrecognized, contracture of the misplaced meatus almost always.

Phimosis is rarely, if ever, a cause of enuresis. There is no operation in surgery performed with so much frequency yet with such little cause as that of circumcision.

On passing a catheter after the child has voided as completely as possible, residual urine in any quantity means obstruction. Urinary analysis should include culture.

If examination revealed nothing abnormal, the enuresis may be assumed to be "functional," and appropriate treatment adopted. If, after three months, there is no improvement, a complete urological investigation should be made.

Mr. Winsbury-White

CHRONIC INFLAMMATORY CHANGES in the posterior urethra and in the bladder are the commonest cause of disturbances of micturition at all ages and in both sexes.

In so-called functional enuresis the younger the child the more constant the cystitis. In older children and in adults inflammation is commonly localized to the urethra.

This is a group of cases which give a good response to treatment by urethral dilatation.

Inflammation may be present in the urinary tract without corroboration of its presence in the urine.

Many cases respond favourably to urethral dilatation. A general anesthetic should always be used for children.

Fulguration of urethral polypi is necessary in some cases.

Dr. Sheldon

CHILDREN with allergic rhinitis often wet their beds. Desensitization, or ephedrine ½ gr. to 1 or even 2 gr. given at bedtime over some weeks may banish enuresis.

Wetting with an ammoniacal smell buttocks reddened,—reduction of his fat intake may be all that is required.

Enuresis associated with mental retardation is most resistant.

Bribery may be legitimately used. Thyroid is as valueless in this group as in any other. Withhold fluid after the tea meal, and forego supper. Empty the bladder completely on retiring and, if necessary, within an hour of going to bed. After four hours rouse to pass water, and this time of rousing should not vary from one night to the next. Praise for a dry night is infinitely better than scolding for a wet one.

Treatment by suggestion, such as belladonna in increasing doses, or a more powerful suggestion such as stretching the bladder by distension may help to bring about a cure.

Dr. Straus

PRIMARY ENURETICS are curious about the holes of the body and what ocmes out of them, they express themselves in sleep when the restrictive code of standards is lifted. Ideal treatment is through uninhibited play-activities and hypnotic suggestion. The symptom is due to "secondary anxiety," anticipation of the symptom itself.

HUMAN BEHAVIOUR

JAMES K. HALL, M.D., *Editor*, Richmond, Va.

MEDICINE IN NORTH CAROLINA

IN MY NATIVE NORTH CAROLINA neither medical men nor professional historians have given much consideration to the history of medicine in that state. But I often find myself wondering if the intelligent citizens of any other state are so lacking in interest in the history of their own people as the people of North Carolina are in the life-story of that great state. I should not know where to turn for a historic account of medicine in North Carolina.

A good deal has been told about the history of the state's Medical Society, one of the oldest in the Union; and also about the State Board of Medical Examiners, probably the oldest State Board of Medical Examiners in the United States. But of the history of human diseases in North Carolina; of the attitude of the citizens towards their afflictions; of the diagnostic and therapeutic practices of the lay people; of the effects of disease upon the adequacy and the happiness of the people and upon the civilization they have been busily engaged in fabricating, there is no continuing story known to me.

Interesting sketches have been written of the lives of some of the physicians of that state who impressed themselves upon their contemporaries and upon those who have come after them. Although many people are dependent upon their physician for comfort and for peace of mind, I can think of no other citizen of comparable local consequence who is so promptly and so completely forgotten after his terral encryptment as the doctor. The affection and the loyalty of the clients of the dead doctor are transferred to his successor. Perhaps it should somewhat so be.

I am glad to hear that at the annual meeting in Pinehurst of this year of the State Medical Society steps were taken to bring into being a history of medicine in North Carolina. I know only that a Historical Committee for such purpose has been organized with Dr. Hubert A. Royster as chairman. The physicians of the state especially should lend every help to the project. I know of no other effort comparable to it in magnitude, in complexity and in difficulty undertaken in North Carolina within my memory. The work will call for sustained enthusiasm, time, imagination, unceasing energy, diligent searching for data; for sound judgment about truth, and for that literary grace that makes the reading of history both a pleasure and a duty. All good citizens of North Carolina who are interested in their state's greatness should collaborate heartily with the Medical Society's Historical Committee.

Man can have no other possession so valuable to him as an individual or as a group as a knowledge of the history of man. Had the citizens of some of the Southern States known in 1906 and 1907 and in several succeeding years that pellagra was not a new disease even in the United States, their anxiety and suffering would have been lessened. Few doctors knew enough about the history of medicine in our own country to recall that in 1864 at the annual meeting of the American Psychiatric Association in Washington City, Dr. John P. Gray, Superintendent of the State Hospital at Utica, New York, reported the presence of a pellagrous patient in his hospital. And Dr. Pliny Earl was reminded by the report that, in 1844, while he was visiting the Insane Asylum in Milan, Italy, the physicians demonstrated the presence of pellagra in many of the patients.

History, and history alone, perhaps, teaches. Were it possible for the individual to know comprehensively the history of mankind, such an individual would never be buoyed up too much by hope nor cast down too low by doubt. He would realize that life tends to be cycloidal, and that what has been is that which will be.

Hitler must reproach himself bitterly for not keeping his military machine out of the Russian Empire. Hitler must have been ignorant of the history of Napoleon. The vastness of Russia, the bitter cold, and the relentlessness of the Cossacks' assaults sent Napoleon to his doom. In Russsia again another tyrant is being pulverized. A feature of the present is its repetitiousness. He who is without a knowledge of history is fundamentally ignorant; he who lacks interest in history is hopeless.

GENERAL PRACTICE

D. HERBERT SMITH, M.D., *Editor*, Pauline, S. C.

OPHTHALMOLOGY IN GENERAL PRACTICE

GENERALLY, what the general practitioner undertakes is to reach a diagnosis with the limited ophthalmological diagnostic implements at hand, give first aid treatment and advise the patient as to how soon he should see a specialist. Even in this limited practice there may be errors in treatment and advice.

A South American specialist[1] goes into particulars in a helpful article, the gist of which follows.

Chronic blepharitis is curable in a very high percentage of cases; treatment by the practitioner requires an accurate investigation of the intestinal condition, the patient's metabolism and his general condition. The general treatment if necessary, should take place simultaneously with the ophthalmological treatment.

Conjunctivitis chronic which does not subside rapidly with the use of zinc collyria (may be as low as 1 to 1000, but the pH must be low), require some other mild disinfectant, such as colloidal silver or a 10 or 15% solution of some highly soluble sulfonamide. Generally there is simultaneous corneal involvement, which more often than not can only be seen with the aid of the slit lamp and through the corneal microscope.

Perforating wounds of the eye require immediate attention and often the practitioner must give early treatment, and what can be done should be done swiftly and deftly. Soluble sulfonamide or powdered sulfonamide should be put in the cul de sac and both eyes should be occluded with sterile dressing, and the patient sent in a hurry to the nearest qualified eye-specialist.

Slightly blurred vision or seeing dark spots which move about as the eye move may derive from a simple conjunctival secretion gliding down the surface of the cornea; or it may be due to exudates in the vitreous implying a dangerous inflammation of the ciliary body or the choroid or vascular changes in retinal hypertension.

The practitioner should be always on the lookout for symptoms of glaucoma whenever a patient has any complaint involving the eyes. Early treatment is the only way to prevent blindness. Routine measurement of pressure in the eye and visual field measurement are to be performed. A glaucomatous eye is a sick eye in a sick body and the general condition should always be carefully investigated and treated.

Acute non-compensated glaucoma is dramatic and often it devolves on the g. p. to give efficient first aid. Miotics (pilocarpine up to 5%; eserine, or doryl) dropped into the cul de sac every half hour, if necessary; epinephrine, or mecholy, locally; ergotamine tartrate per os or subcutaneously to deplete the uveal vessels; 100 c.c. 50% glucose solution to deplete the fluid contents of the eyeballs; morphine to do away with pain (incidentally to contract the pupils).

Strabismus or squint is merely a symptom, and just as a doctor nowadays would shrink from making a simple diagnosis of "fever," so he should refrain from labelling all his cross-eyed patients with such an indefinite name. In many cases the simple corrector of an ametropia is enough to bring about an early cure. There are some cases in which little can be done at first, but this should be decided only after a proper and careful investigation. More often than not the g. p.'s advice will be asked by the child's parents, and he should be prepared to advise wisely. It is absolutely safe to operate even at an early age whenever such an operation is necessary.

SURGERY

GEO. H. BUNCH, M.D., *Editor*, Columbia, S. C.

PRE-OPERATIVE AND POST-OPERATIVE CARE FOR THE BAD-RISK PATIENT

CONFRONTED by a condition requiring operation on a patient in such state as to make the risk unduly great, there are many things we can do to bring the risk nearer to average.

The staff of the Hospitals of the University of Minnesota has studied this subject carefully and published[1] conclusions of such value that they are passed on to our readers in some detail.

We are all familiar with patients whose pulse and blood pressure fail late or even early in the course of surgical operations, and who require heroic amounts of plasma or blood.

Lowered plasma protein levels and inadequate vitamin C intake interfere with wound healing and favor the development of edema. Water and salt imbalance predisposes to edema. The site of election for the development of edema in the postoperative period is the lungs, a factor which ap-

---

1. M. E. Alvaro, Sao Paulo, Brazil, in *Clin. Med.*, April.

1. Clarence Dennis, Minneapolis, in *Minn. Med.*, July.

pears to play a large role in the development of postoperative atelectasis and bronchopneumonia. All of these factors play a part in some cases of postoperative anuria, thrombophlebitis, and embolism.

In many cases dehydration—5 to 7% underweight due to fluid loss alone—presents the first problem in preparation for operation. Severe dehydration requires administration of 5% of the body weight of fluids parenterally, one-half of this being 0.9% NaCl. Daily weighing is necessary. Gains of 5% above the usual level ordinarily produce clinical edema; of more than 2 or 3% imply impending edema and dictate caution in giving more liquids.

In these patients excessive salt intake favors water retention, ascites, pleural effusion, etc., particularly since the plasma protein level is also usually low. A low level of plasma chloride may lead to fatal drops in blood pressure which may respond poorly to transfusion. Patients with diarrhea, vomiting, or large ulcerating surfaces are likely to arrive in a low-salt state. For those who must be supplied with NaCl other than by mouth the amount of chloride must be given to raise to the normal level of 560 mgms. per 100 c.c. of plasma (expressed in terms of NaCl): "for each 100 mg. that the plasma chloride level needs to be raised to reach the normal, the patient should be given 0.5 grams of salt per kilogram of body weight." Most satisfactory returns of blood levels to normal are obtained in the acutely ill.

Maintenance is usually easily accomplished by administration of 5 to 6 grams daily, with extra allowance at the rate of 5 grams per liter for losses due to vomiting, diarrhea, drainage, or gross sweating. The aim is to keep the daily output between 2 and 7 grams, which assures a safe margin from either over- or under-dosage.

The patient may come in a state of acidosis or alkalosis, but if adequate salt and water are given and an adequate output of urine is obtained, few cases will require other measures.

Many patients suffering the effects of moderate to severe starvation can be well fed through an inlying nasal gastric tube, using a liquid formula high in protein and carbohydrate and low in fat with a value of 1.5 calories per c.c. After the first day or two, many of these patients can take the diet by mouth and dispense with the nasal tube. The liquid formulas can be used as supplements to a solid high-carbohydrate, high-protein, low-fat diet; getting 5,000 to 6,000 calories a day into these patients by this means. Correction of the fatty infiltration of the liver leads to elevation of the plasma protein level and deposit of carbohydrate and protein in the liver. Marked drops in blood pressure during operation, postoperative anuria, ileus, etc., have all fallen greatly in frequency under this regimen. Duration of such preparation—five days if the loss has been 5 to 10% of the body weight, 10 to 12 days if it has been 10 to 20%, and three weeks if it has been 25 to 30%.

An adequate vitamin intake is also provided with the diet.

Those patients who cannot be prepared by the oral route present a very serious problem. After a trial of 10%, then use 20%, glucose solutions intravenously. There is little other choice as yet, but this solution is irritating and leads to thrombosis of the veins very readily. Ten per cent glucose must not be given faster than 6 c.c. per minute because of loss in the urine and almost none of our patients lose over 15% of the glucose administered as 20% solution if given no faster than 3 c.c. a minute—six hours required to give 1,000 c.c. The needle must be placed away from the elbow, preferably in the midportion of the forearm, to allow free movement. By this means it is feasible to get 1,200 to 1,600 calories daily, supplemented by 200 to 300 calories from subcutaneous injections of 5% glucose with or without salt. Spillage in the urine may be reduced somewhat by partial coverage with insulin added directly to the intravenous fluid. We add also 200 to 300 mg. of cevitamic acid, 20 mg. of thiamine, and 10 c.c. of a crude liver extract.

These patients suffer at least as much from protein starvation as from lack of carbohydrate, and human plasma is the only agent by which this may be promptly and safely relieved. The minimum requirement under the circumstance is 300 to 400 c.c. daily.

Most of these patients need transfusion to raise the hemoglobin level, but this is far less important than the general nutrition for the healing of wounds and the general reaction of the patient.

At operation these patients regularly have nasal gastric suction tubes in place, for ileus has not been observed in patients who have not been allowed to swallow and retain large quantities of air during and after operation. Nasal suction is ordinarily maintained 48 hours, or until abdominal sounds, as heard with the stethoscope, have returned to normal, or the patient has passed gas by rectum.

Postoperative anuria is best prevented by establishment of adequate nutrition preoperatively, and giving, in the few hours just prior to operation, a liter of 10% glucose solution in the vein. During the day of operation, nothing by mouth, but a total of 3,000 cc. of parenteral fluids containing 5 grams of NaCl. Judicious use of mercurial diuretics may be necessary.

The patient returns to the floor in steep Trendelenberg position to maintain blood pressure, also to prevent the accumulation of salivary and other secretions in the lungs. This position is maintained the first 12 hours, preferably with the patient turned half onto his face for better drainage, with turning from side to side every two hours, hyperventilation at similar intervals, and encouragement to cough frequently. The Mueller suction apparatus is uned freely to keep the mouth and pharynx dry in the first few hours, until reflexes are normal and the danger of aspiration seems lessened. After the first 12 hours, the foot of the bed is kept elevated 6 inches until the nasal tube is removed on the third or fourth day. Frequent turning, hyperventilation, and encouragement to cough are continued also until the tube has been removed. Most important of all the patient is urged to move arms and legs continuously—1,000 times a day—a measure which, combined with the 6-inch elevation of the foot of the bed, is intended to prevent stasis in the great veins and to lessen the incidence of thrombosis and embolism.

Until normal feeding has been established 1,500 c.c. of 10% glucose to which vitamins and plasma have been added are usually given by vein and subcutaneous injection of 5% glucose in distilled water, some of which is made up in 0.9% sodium chloride, making a total of 3,000 c.c. of fluids for the patient daily.

Day-to-day weighing serves as a guide to fluid administration.

In the first two or three postoperative days the poor-risk patient should have a nurse in constant attendance.

Those who cannot void need inlying Foley catheters for the first three to four days. A half-gram of sodium sulfadiazene subcutaneously in 100 c.c. of normal saline solution twice daily is helpful against urinary-tract infection.

Following removal of the nasal tube, the patient is kept a day on clear liquids, a day on full liquids, a day on a soft diet, and finally passes to a general diet. After gastric resection, the diet is also carefully graduated as to quantity the first few days.

Good preoperative preparation and careful silk closure seems to us to justify getting these people out of bed seven days after such operation as gastric or colic resection and sending them home nine days after operation.

PEMPHIGUS
(W. F. Lever & J. H. Talbott B,oston, in *New Eng. Jl. of Med.*, July 13th)

Six types of pemphigus are recognized—pemphigus vulgaris acutus, p. vegetans, p. vulgaris chronicus, p. foliaceus, p. erythematosus and p. conjunctivae.

In p. vulgaris acutus, p. vegetans and p. vulgaris chronicus, the amount of sodium, chloride, calcium and protein in the blood serum was found to be reduced, more in the first two. The degree of reduction usually corresponded to the severity of the clinical condition and the amount of skin involved.

No etiologic significance can be attached to the chemical changes. They are regarded as a secondary symptom produced by the disease.

Thirty-two patients with p. were treated with adrenocortical extract, dihydrotachysterol or massive doses of vitamin D. Encouraging results were obtained in several patients with p. vulgaris acutus, p. vegetans and p. vulgaris chronicus. The results of treatment in patients with p. foliaceus, p. erythematosus and p. conjunctivae were in general disappointing.

The treatment tends to correct the reduction of sodium, chloride, calcium and protein encountered in such patients. Since it is believed that the chemical changes are secondary to the disease, the treatment is merely symptomatic.

OPHTHALMOLOGY

HERBERT C. NEBLETT, M.D., *Editor*, Charlotte, N. C.

THE PHOROMETER VERSUS THE TRIAL FRAME IN REFRACTION

SINCE refraction comprises the greater part of the work done in the office of the great majority of oculists, and since it is time-consuming and painstaking and therefore tiring to the examiner, comfort, convenience and simplicity of set-up for doing the work should be provided. In this respect the phorometer is a valuable asset. It has been used personally for 18 years to the exclusion of any model of trial frame. The latter instrument should be a part of the office equipment for a specific purpose though it will be rarely used when one has become accustomed to the use of the phorometer with its many advantages over the trial frame.

The phorometer can be attached to the examining chair or placed on a movable stand to either side of the chair as may be desired. In this position its arm can be swung in front of the patient and its head can be quickly and easily adjusted to the patient's position in the chair. When this has been done the refraction can be accomplished with simplicity and in uninterrupted sequence and with comfort to the patient and examiner.

The examiner should be seated with the trial case of lenses and all other appurtenances within easy reach. Once the patient has been properly seated and the phorometer in position all phases of the refraction can be consummated without moving the patient. This will include the muscle balance with the Maddox rod and rotary prisms or the rod using loose prisms and the field of vision on the Bjerrum screen. The latter can be accomplished by swinging the screen in front of the patient at the desired distance.

In doing the refraction for distance and for near the phorometer head can be adjusted to meet the requirements in each position without moving the patient. Unlike the trial frame there is no sliding forward or downward of the phorometer, its stability maintaining its exact position before the eyes of the patient, and at the point in front of the cornea that the finished lenses should be for the individual patient. This is an important point in the final analysis of the refraction and hence of the prescription when the lenses and frames are made. By use of the phorometer the trial lenses are inserted and withdrawn with greater facility and stability than with the trial frame. Application of the cylinders and cross cylinders are likewise accomplished and the position of their axes more readily defined, and the plumb dial on the phorometer assures the examiner that the instrument is at all times at the 180 meridian. The position of the patient's head can be likewise easily maintained.

Precison and accuracy and the time element in doing a refraction is in large part predicated upon the position and comfort of the patient and examiner and the accessibility of the armamentarium necessary to conduct the examination, without the use and abuse of a great many useless accessories. It is further augmented by having the refracting unit-room and all other appurtenances so arranged that, once the patient is seated, the entire examination can be conducted without moving him with the exception of examining the perimetric fields, using the slit lamp and making ophthalmometric readings.

UROLOGY

RAYMOND THOMPSON, M.D., *Editor*, Charlotte, N. C.

SERIOUS UROLOGIC DISEASE MAY BE PAINLESS, EVEN SYMPTOMLESS

PAIN serves as a warning in many serious diseases. Cancer is one of the conspicuous exceptions to this rule, and it seems that cancer of the urogenitals is peculiarly prone to go on to the inoperable stage before giving ony pain whatever.

An article by Davis[1] constitutes the basis of a warning which can hardly be sounded too often.

Neoplasms of the kidney and bladder are usually first evidenced by painless hematuria, and it is fortunate that this is so, as there is no other way to detect or even suspect them. In a few instances a bladder tumor has been discovered while examining cystoscopically for prostatic obstruction. Hematuria, no matter how slight, no matter how transient, should never be neglected but always traced to its source without delay.

Adenocarcinoma of the prostate causes no pain or any other symptom until its very late stages.

---
1. D. M. Davis, Philadelphia, in *Penn. Med. Jl.*, July.

Few physicians are sufficiently aware of this fact. In eight years only two cases of early carcinoma of the prostate were referred to Davis' private office or to his clinic at the Jefferson Hosuital. The diagnosis can be made, he well says, only by performing careful rectal examinations on all male patients over 50 years of age, and repeating these at yearly intervals. Any hard, discrete nodule in the prostate is probably an early carcinoma curable by radical operation. If the diagnosis is not made until symptoms appear, it is too late for cure, and palliative treatment is all that can be given.

Tuberculosis of the kidney seldom causes pain or any other symptom. It is only when the bladder becomes secondarily infected that frequent and painful urination occur, symptoms which have their origin in the bladder, and which, therefore, for many physicians do not bring the kidneys under suspicion. All of us with long experience will agree with this: Suspicion of tuberculosis can be aroused by three things: 1) a positive personal or family history of tuberculosis; 2) pus and blood in the urine with no bacteria on ordinary smear or ordinary culture; and 3) failure of the bladder symptoms to yield to the usual measures for cystitis within at most three or four weeks. Stain, culture, and guinea pig inoculation will quickly give the diagnosis once the doctor's suspicions are aroused.

Polycystic kidney causes no pain. The first symptom is often bleeding, or one or both kidneys may be enlarged so as to be felt on abdominal examination.

Diseases, often painful, which may appear from time to time without pain, are obstructions, particularly those which are congenital or which, if acquired, are of very long standing and slow development; infections, usually associated with the types of obstruction mentioned; and renal stone.

Davis makes brief reports of a number of illustrative cases, which might be duplicated in any large urologic practice. The lessons of a few of these are cited:

A physician, aged 41, reported that he had always enjoyed perfect health with no venereal disease, married six years, one healthy child. For two or three months he noticed hesitancy in starting the urine, a small weak stream, and frequency up to every hour in the daytime. There was, however, no pain or burning, and no night voiding. The urine and prostatic secretion were normal. Cystoscopic examination showed a hypertrophic median bar, evidently congenital, and transurethral resectioning was carried out. One month later, he was perfectly well, voiding three or four times a day, none at night, with no hesitancy, a large forceful stream of perfectly clear urine. He emphasized especially that he was now voiding much more freely than he had ever done before.

A student nurse, aged 19, husky, who had never been ill, a year after beginning her training noticed a slight transitory discomfort in the left side. Three months later the same pain, more severe. Pus and bacteria were found in the urine. An intravenous urogram showed a normal right kidney, but the left side was blank. Retrograde pyelography showed an enormous hydronephrosis. The specimen removed by nephrectomy showed a hydronephrosis due to a pin-point congenitally narrowed ureteropelvic orifice. This worthless kidney had been there all of her life and had never caused any symptoms until, in some obscure manner, it became infected. Even then it would have been easy to say "just an attack of pyelitis."

An apparently healthy young man rejected by the Army on account of pyuria, at work every day, on examination showed large stones in both kidneys.

A woman, aged 68, 29 years ago had an attack of cystitis, followed by what was called acute nephritis; after this pus in the urine for many years. Symptoms were minimal, consisting of a little blood in the urine on one occasion 12 years ago, on another 1½ years ago, and again during the past six weeks. She voided every three or four hours during the day and never got up at night. There was no pain, burning, hesitancy, or straining upon urination. There had never been, during more than a quarter of a century, the slightest pain in either kidney region. The blood pressure was 130 80. The urine contained many pus cells, a few red cells, and a small number of bacilli. Study of the urinary tract showed everything normal except the right kidney, which was converted into a large, infected, and practically functionless hydronephrosis, containing an enormous kidney calculus. The underlying lesion was a congenital stricture at the ureteropelvic junction. The hydronephrosis must have been present through the patient's entire life, the infection for at least 28 years, the stone for many years. She was intelligent and well-to-do, and had seen many competent physicians, all of whom had been misled by the slightness of her symptoms.

The article concludes with a paragraph, which is here heartily endorsed:

"I hold a brief for the physician who is constantly looking for trouble. He alone will find the sort of things I have been discussing, and I submit that he will better deserve the gratitude of his patients than his ever-hopeful colleague who is constantly saying, ' 'It is nothing; it will soon pass.' "

Two sentences which fairly demand repetition are:

"Hematuria, no matter how slight, no matter how transient, should never be neglected but always traced to its source without delay."

"Any hard, discrete nodule in the prostate is probably an early carcinoma, curable by radical operation; if the diagnosis is not made until symptoms appear, it is too late for cure."

---

1. E. F. Mielke, Appleton, in Wisc. Med. Jl., July.

GYNECOLOGY

ROBERT THRIFT FERGUSON, M.D., *Editor*, Charlotte, N. C.

PERTINENT POINTS AS TO PELVIC EXAMINATIONS

THERE is a need for knowledge of what can be, and what cannot be, learned from bimanual pelvic examinations. If we may believe a good deal we read and hear, a few can learn much more in this way than is vouchsafed to the great majority of doctors who see ailing women.

A Wisconsin doctor[1] states the case so well that the gist of his practical article is appropriated.

The normal fallopian tube is not palpable, the normal ovary with difficulty.

Vaginal examinations are useless in young girls and in ueurotics.

A good examining table is needed with proper stirrups and drapes, buttocks over the edge of the table. At times the knee-chest, Sims or standing position is necessary. Local anesthesia of the vaginal wall is often helpful. The pelvic organs, with the exception of the ovaries, are not sensitive to ordinary palpation. Pelvic sensitiveness is often an attribute of neurasthenia. Tubal pain is apt to be constant, while uterine pain is usually colicy. Any office should be equipped for giving enemas. A nervous polyuria frequently fills the bladder in a short time.

The examiner should start to palpate *away* from suspected site of disease.

The ovary may lie anywhere from the midline to the lateral wall of the pelvis, either anteriorly or deep in the pelvis. The ovary is moveable, slippery and sensitive; squeezing gives a sickening sensation. One imprisons the ovary by making a scoop out of the four fingers of the abdominal hand and raking the area from the fundus to the vaginal fingers.

The ovary is freely moveable, the size of a large almond. One may be small and the other large.

If vaginal examination is unsatisfactory, the vaginal-recto-abdominal procedure should be tried.

Examination with instruments is usually indicated. Two sizes of Graves speculum, dressing forceps, Skene's double type tenaculum, Simpson's uterine sound, an endometrial curette, slides, applicators, and often a proctoscope are needed. A Cameron cold light helps to visualize areas that cannot be seen by direct light. The sound in the absence of pregnancy and inflammation tells us the depth, direction and contour of the uterine cavity, patency of the internal and external os and the canal.

A complete history of the patient's life and present illness are of greater importance than the physical. Further, a complete physical examination is often of more significance than the local examination.

A woman in the climacterium, after years of amenorrhea, may begin menstruating due to a feminizing tumor of the ovary which is so small that it cannot be palpated. Bimanual findings in case of submucous fibroids or carcinoma of the body of the uterus may be perfectly normal and diagnosis be possible only from the history, or scrapings or from the abnormal contour of the uterine cavity. Adnexal disease and endometriosis are easily overlooked where fair-size fibroids are present.

When findings are not explanatory, an examination under anesthesia should be made. TeLinde routinely makes a pelvic examination under anestehsia with complete relaxation in any case in which operation is to be done. Pentothal sodium is well adapted, either continuing with it or switching to some other anesthesia if the laparotomy is done.

PEDIATRICS

IMMUNIZATION OF CHILDREN

WITH accumulating experience the ideas of those best informed as to when immunization procedures should be carried out undergo change.

A dependable guide just published[1] is given in brief:

A new baby is born. The parents' concern is how to keep their baby well. This is the time to instruct them.

We advise that he be inoculated with cow-pox vaccine at the end of the third month. If you should not get a successful take repeat in two weeks. One successfully vaccinated should be again inoculated at the fifth and fifteenth year.

The infant should receive the first dose of standardized pertussis vaccine at five months of age. The second dose of 2 c.c. and the third of 3 c.c. at intervals of 30 days. It will take four months for the infant to develop sufficient antibodies to protect him against pertussis. Some claim immunity in 80 to 90%.

Alum-precipitated diphtheria and tetanus toxoid at eight months. Inject 1 c.c. at a new site on the upper arm. Reaction fever which usually subsides

[1] M. W. Beach & B. O. Ravenel, Charleston, in Jl. S. M. Medical Assn., July.

in 36 hours. The local induration remains for two or three months and may cause necrosis. Three months later, the second dose. Two doses should establish more than 90% immunity. Routinely do a Schick test within six months after inoculation. Reimmunize if necessary and thereafter give yearly booster doses during the pre-school age. When an immunized individual is exposed subsequently to possible tetanus germs, inject 1 c.c. of alum-precipitated tetanus toxoid. *Do not give tetanus antitoxin.*

The first half of the second year give triple typhoid vaccine—$\frac{1}{4}$ c.c. for the first dose, $\frac{1}{2}$ c.c. for the second and third doses, at four-weeks intervals. Six months after the third dose determine the amount of immunity by use of the Widal test; then give a booster dose of vaccine each spring as a wise precaution.

Unless some emergency arises, do no further passive or active immunization in second year. In urban areas, in the first half of the third year, give 500 skin test doses of standardized scarlet fever toxin for the first dose, 5,000 for the second, and 30,000 for the third, at intervals of three weeks. The degree of established immunity may be ascertained by the Dick test.

Sometimes it is imperative that an attempt be made to establish active immunity against typhus fever, Rocky Mountain fever, yellow fever, rabies, tularemia.

With convalescent human serum it is possible to ameliorate or prevent measles, mumps, chickenpox, scarlet fever, and some other diseases.

GENERAL PRACTICE

JAMES L. HAMNER, M.D., *Editor*, Mannboro, Va.

MALARIA

MALARIA is the world's most widespread serious ailment. One-quarter of the inhabitants of the globe suffer from malaria. And it is the world's most economically expensive disease.

As our soldiers come home, we can fully expect a great increase over the number of cases of malaria all over our country. So present knowledge of this disease condition, as well presented[1] in a current review, is needful to us all.

Malaria is transmitted by the great family or mosquitoes, the Anopheles—350 species, 90 of them capable of acting as vectors, but, again, only 12 or 15 are of importance. Responsible for the transmission of perhaps 90% of the world's malaria: *Anopheles quadrimaculatus* distributed over most of the United States, is responsible for the malaria in our southern states.

[1] J. B. Rice, New York City, in R. I. Med. Jl., July.

Anopheles superpictus, in the island of Cyprus, is responsible for intense malarial transmission; in nearby Macedonia, although the temperature is only slightly lower, the life process of this mosquito is so altered that it cannot act as an efficient carrier although the mosquito is present in large numbers.

In order to transmit malaria, it is obvious that mosquitoes must bite human beings, inasmuch as human malarial parasites do not live in the bodies of lower animals. One of the reasons why *Anopheles gambiae* is the most efficient malaria vector known is because it bites only human beings. In order to keep the infection alive, it is necessary that susceptible anophelines be present in and around human habitations in large numbers.

In some localities in West Africa, although practically 100% of the adult population harbor *Plasmodium falciparum*, the parasite of the most malignant type of the disease, the adults for the most part are free of fever, do not have anemia unless produced by other causes and their spleens, if palpable at all, are very small. Their blood is swarming with parasites. They have built up a high degree of immunity for many generations. In Macedonia, refugees who came from non-malarious parts of Turkey after the last Greco-Turkish War having little "racial" immunity, suffered greatly from malaria.

Variation in the virulence of different strains of parasites occur within each species. A certain proportion of patients will relapse after treatment, regardless of the drugs used and regardless of the dosage employed. Antimalarial drugs do not prevent, but merely suppress symptoms. In spite of this fact suppressive treatment is well worth while, especially from the military point of view because by it means the army may be kept on its feet and fighting while in an endemic area.

From 10 to 20% of malaria cases will relapse one or more times, regardless of the drug used and of the amounts administered.

Recently the complete synthesis of quinine opens the door to the possibility of the production of related compounds which may have new and unique antimalarial properties.

In treating malaria atabrine and quinine are qualitatively equal.

Much smaller amounts of atabrine are required to produce a comparable result, and cause only minor manifestations of intolerance. The plan recommended by the Surgeon General of the Army is 0.3 Gm. q. 6 h. for 5 doses, followed by 0.1 Gm. t.i.d. for 6 days, with a total of 2.8 Gm. in 7 days—each dose accompanied by 1 Gm. of sodium bicarbonate. The usual dose of quinine is 2 Gm. daily for from 7 to 10 days—a total of 14 to 20 Gm.

Plasmochin destroys gametocytes of *Plasmodium falciparum*, a property which it shares with no other drug. It is of interest from the public health standpoint. In localities where it can be administered at frequent intervals to the entire population, it is capable of greatly reducing or eliminating this infection altogether. The dose required to prevent the transmission of malaria to mosquitoes is only 0.01 Gm. per Kg. of body weight per week. This amount produces no symptoms of toxicity.

THERAPEUTICS

J. F. NASH, M.D., *Editor*, Saint Pauls, N. C.

TREATMENT OF CYANIDE POISONING
WITH A TRIBUTE TO PEDIGO OF ROANOKE

POISONING with hydrocyanic acid and its salts occurs with enough frequency to make it well to here give the latest treatment.[1] Also, we are glad to call attention to the credit for the original work of an enthusiastic member of the Tri-State Medical Association in its early years.

If a person working with cyanide, or in the neighborhood of HCN fumigation, is sudden taken ill, a suspicion of cyanide poisoning is justifiable; if he is discovered unconscious, and a cyanide container is found nearby, suicidal intent is probable. The odor of bitter almond oil in the breath is highly suggestive of cyanide poisoning; on the other hand, its absence does not rule out this possibility. Other signs, while not pathognomic, consist of rapid respiration, later slow and gasping, accelerated pulse, vomiting and convulsions, followed by coma and cyanosis. Suspicion of having taken the poison by mouth demands withdrawal and analysis of stomach contents; of poisoning by gaseous hydrocyanic acid, a 20 c.c. sample of venous blood drawn and similarly examined.

Sodium nitrite and sodium thiosulfate, given separately, is the best therapy. Intravenously injected, the nitrite followed by the thiosulfate, these remedies are capable of detoxifying 20 lethal doses of sodium cyanide in dogs, and are effective even after rspiration has stopped.

Amyl nitrite by inhalation has the same detoxifying value as sodium nitrite by intravenous injection, and is the oldest antidote for cyanide poisoning and is a preliminary adjuvant of the present treatment. Pedigo, the discoverer, described its antagonism aaginst hydrocyanic acid in 1888. His work, however, was not widely known. It was called to our attention by Dr. Pedigo himself at the time of our experimentation (1934).

Cyanide poisoning is rapidly fatal. On the other hand, no case can be considered hopeless unless the

---
1. K. K. Chen *et al.*, Indianapolis, in *Jl. Indiana Med. Assn.*, July.

heart beat has completely stopped.

I. Instruct an assistant how to break, one at a time, pearls of amyl nitrite in a handkerchief and hold over the victim's nose for 15 to 30 seconds per minute. At the same time the physician quickly loads his syringes, one with a three per cent solution of sodium nitrite, and the other with a 25 per cent solution of sodium thiosulfate.

II. Stop administration of amyl nitrite and inject intravenously 0.3 g.* (10 c.c. of a 3% solution) of sodium nitrite at the rate of 2.5 to 5.0 c.c. per minute.

III. Inject by the same needle and vein, or by a larger needle and a new vein, 12.5 g. (50 c.c. of a 25% solution) of sodium thiosulfate.

The patient should be kept under careful observation for at least 24 to 48 hours. If signs of poisoning reappear, injection of both sodium nitrite and sodium thiosulfate should be repeated, each in one-half dose. Even if the patient looks perfectly well, the medication is to be repeated two hours after the first injections.

If respiration has ceased but the pulse is palpable, artificial respiration should be applied at once, not to revive the respiration *per se*, but to keep the heart beating. When signs of breathing appear, injection of the solutions should be promptly made.

If the poison is taken by mouth, gastric lavage should be carried out, preferably by a third person —a physician or a nurse.

A kit composed of the following articles may be installed in emergency cabinets, ambulances, and chemical laboratories, or carried at all times with fumigation equipment:

12 pearls of amyl nitrite; 2 ampules of sodium nitrite, 0.3 g. in 10 c.c. of water, sterilized; 2 ampules of sodium thiosulfate, 12.5 g. in 50 c.c. of water, sterilized; 1 sterile syringe, 10 c.c. size, with a 22-gauge needle; 1 sterile syringe, 50 c.c. size, with an 18-gauge needle; 1 file; and 1 stomach tube (not necessary for fumigators).

By the addition of certain preservatives a lot of ampules kept at room temperature for eight years was found to be of full strength. The nitrite and the thiosulfate may be separately weighed out from bottles into beakers and dissolved in sterile water, or, if that is not available, in tap water. These solutions may then be promptly injected. The urgent necessity of speed in the treatment of cyanide poisoning justifies the omission of sterilization.

A total of 15 cases have been treated by the new procedure. Fourteen of these patients completely recovered.

The following Note is reprinted from the Transactions of the meeting of the Medical Society of Virginia, held at Norfolk, 1888.

*Gram.

ANTAGONISM BETWEEN AMYL NITRITE AND PRUSSIC ACID

By Lewis G. Pedigo, M.D., Roanoke, Virginia

In the May number of the *Virginia Medical Monthly*, I reviewed a case of atropia poisoning which had occurred in the person of a man prominent in the judiciary of our State, and in which that valuable life was saved by the timely and assiduous use of amyl nitrite. In concluding that article I recorded the suggestion that the remedy used would prove to be a physiological antidote to certain other cardiac depressants, such as veratrum viride, aconite, gelsemium and especially *prussic acid*. Since that time I have continued the series of experiments upon which that opinion was based, and as a result, the opinion has been entirely borne out.

CLINICAL CHEMISTRY and MICROSCOPY

J. M. Feder, M.D., and Evelyn Tribble, M.T., *Editors*, Anderson, S. C.

HOW DOES A REGISTERED MEDICAL TECHNOLOGIST GET THAT WAY?

Reading the list of questions recently asked by the American Technologists as a requirements for registration, shows that they cover a wide field, and it is not difficult to draw the conclusion that successful candidates must have considerable knowledge of their subject.

These questions are being published for the benefit of technologists in the states served by this Journal who may be contemplating applying for registration. It is also being brought to the attention of the medical profession for the purpose of demonstrating the rigid requirements imposed upon these people for qualification.

OFFICAL EXAMINATION QUESTIONS

1. Define:
   A. Normal Solution.
   B. Percentage Solution.
   C. Volumetric Solution.
   D. Achlorhydria.
   E. Reagin.
   F. Antigen.
2. What is meant by pH? Why is it important in Bacteriology?
3. Describe the technique for identification of acid-fast organisms. Name 3.
4. Outline the procedure for a Gram's stain.
   Name two pathogenic bacteria that may be found in each of the following and give their reaction to the Gram stain:
   A. Urine.
   B. Blood.
   C. Stool.
   D. Sputum.

E. Spinal Fluid.
F. Infectious lesion on the skin.
5. Name two ketone bodies which may be found in urine and give a qualitative test for one.
Name two methods for the detection of bile pigment in the urine.
6. Describe the technique for an agglutination test for one of the enteric fevers.
7. Name the reagents used in a sulfonamide determination and state the part each plays in the final result.
8. Name two kidney function tests and describe one.
9. Name three liver function tests and describe one.
10. List the indicators used most commonly in the titration of a fractional gastric analysis.
11. Outline the procedure for preparing a Folin's filtrate.
12. Name four tests that may be run on a Folin's filtrate and describe one.
13. Name two methods for concentrating stool for the detection of parasitic ova.
14. Name four of the more common Nematodes found in man.
15. Name three types of Anemia and describe the characteristics of each, using a Wright's stain.
16. What is the blood picture in the case of malaria? When is the optimum time for obtaining the specimen?
17. Describe in detail the procedure for one of the following serologic tests:
A. Kahn Standard.
B. Kline Diagnostic.
C. Hinton Test.
D. Eagle Flocculation Test.
E. Wassermann.
F. Mazzini.
18. Name three solutions suitable for the fixation of fresh tissue for the preparation of histologic sections.
Name one solution for the decalcification of tissue for histologic study.
19. Name three quantitative tests used in the examination of cerebrospinal fluid and give the normals for each.
20. Describe the Benzidine Base Test for occult blood.
Answer each question. Return questions with your examination papers to the examination supervisor.

EDUCATION AND OTHER REQUIREMENTS FOR ADMISSION TO EXAMINATION

Applicant for admission to the membership shall be a citizen of the United States, of good moral character, and shall be a graduate of high school or a graduate nurse. Applicant shall have graduated from an approved school of clinical laboratory technology or shall have had not less than 18 calendar months' laboratory experience under the supervision of a competent physician. Applicant shall obtain not less than 70% in an examination conducted by the board of examiners of this organization.

A registration fee of five dollars shall accompany all applications for membership. Failure to pass examination: registration fee shall be refunded in full.

Applicant will be notified ten days prior to examination, as to date, place and time of same. If practical, examinations will be conducted in the evening and as near to the residence of the applicant as may be reasonable.

The examination consists of twenty routine laboratory questions, to be answered in writing. A copy of typical questions may be had by the applicant upon request.

EXEMPTION FROM EXAMINATION

Technicians who can present documentary evidence of having satisfactorily passed an examination for Clinical Laboratory Technicians, as held by the U. S. Civil Service Commission, or as held by the State Civil Service Commission of any of the several states; or technicians registered to practice by state law in California or Alabama or other states requiring registration by examination or technicians registered by the A. S. C. P.

PROCTOLOGY

RUSSELL BUXTON, M.D., F.A.C.S., *Editor*
Newport News, Va.

HEMORRHOIDS

IT IS VERY DIFFICULT to attempt to compress any statements concerning hemorrhoids into a few lines. There are so many different methods of treatment, any one of which may be adequate in a given case, that I am merely giving a short resumé of the symptoms and the treatment of hemorrhoids. In this issue external hemorrhoids only are to be considered.

External hemorrhoids are dilated veins on the outside of the anus. The usual presenting symptom is pain. The patients ordinarily state that following constipation or straining they begin to have pain in the rectum which has steadily become worse. In addition, there is usually backache, sometimes aching in the legs, and a general bearing-down feeling.* Ordinarily the patient has some relief by application of an ointment and seeks the doctor's assistance when the pain becomes to great to bear. Examination shows a blue, tender mass in the skin at the margin of the anus. Proper treatment is immediate incision and evacuation of the thrombosed veins. This may be done very simply by using local anesthesia, injected at the base of the hemorrhoid, and making a linear incision through the blood clot and removing with a hemostat. Too much trauma must be avoided and bleeding may be controlled by small vaselin-covered packs inserted into the rectum. These patients are seen usually once or twice following operation and ordinarily miss at least one day of work. They are given a sedative and mineral oil, and advised to take hot baths two or three times a day until the soreness is gone. It is well to warn the patient that a skin tag will remain following incision of this type of hemorrhoid.

In case the patient has not consulted a physician until more time has lapsed, the hemorrhoid will usually be gangrenous and the top necrotic. In these cases immediate incision is not advised but bed rest, heat and sedation. This will usually take care of the situation though both may be indicated at a later date.

Addendum.—A good many years ago I had an experience in my person of this disease condition. My associate

---
*You feel a bearing or dragging about the fundament, and as though if you could only sit down the sensation would be relieved; but when you sit the dragging is not relieved at all and other painful sensations are apt to be worsened.
—J. M. N.

being away when the bearing-down sensation* became very troublesome, and remembering that the Lord helps those who help themselves, I proceeded after this fashion:
1. Obtained sketchy local skin antisepsis
2. Placed a mirror, a 1 g.-to-the-oz. sol. of cocaine, a syringe and a sharp knife (on a sterile towel), and a box of absorbent cotton on the floor
3. Squatted over the mirror, injected the cocaine sol. intradermally over the greatest convexity, made incision, gently pressed out the clot, put a half pound or so of absorbent cotton in the seat of my underbritches
4. Went on about my affairs in great comfort.

OBSERVATIONS
OF THE STAFF
DAVIS HOSPITAL
Statesville

PENICILLIN IN THE TREATMENT OF SYPHILIS

OUR EXPERIENCE with a considerable number of cases of syphilis treated with penicillin is that this bids fair to be one of the most effective treatments for syphilis, both early and late, especially the latter.

Due to the fact that it is also a specific for gonococcus infection, it is likely this will be exceptionally satisfactory for treatment of both these venereal diseases.

The final decision as to just how effective and satisfactory it is requires observation of a large number of cases over a period of years rather than just a few months.

In the treatment of late syphilis, especially in those cases where considerable treatment has already been given and there are no clinical manifestations of the disease except a positive Kahn, Kline or Wassermann test, we have a problem which is really a great one both for the doctor and for the patient. In a Wassermann-fast patient who has had extensive treatment over a period of years and still has a four-plus Wassermann, naturally there is a certain amount of discouragement, especially when prolonged treatment still leaves the patient with a positive Kahn or Wassermann.

Another factor in the treatment of late syphilis is that many of these patients are not in good general physical condition. The cardiorenal system is apt to be seriously affected and it may not be possible to give these patients the vigorous treatment that is most likely to give good results.

Since penicillin produces no toxic reaction of any kind this is a great factor in making it suitable for treatment of a disease in which, because of general deterioration of structures vitally important, the reactions induced by arsenicals and bismuth may prove gravely injurious or even fatal.

Penicillin, being highly effective against a great many different organisms, it is believed that this will probably cut down the treatment of syphilis to a period of days rather than years as has been the case heretofore. In early syphilis it apparently produces a cure in the space of a few days.

Just what is the optimum dosage is not known, and can not be known until the remedy has been used in a large number of cases and these cases followed over many years. It seems best to give a considerable amount in the hope of effecting an immediate cure rather than to give an insufficient amount and run the risk of trouble in the future.

The ideal time for beginning treatment of syphilis would be when the initial lesion first appears, when Spirochaetae are found on dark-field examination and before the serological test becomes positive. Penicillin has shown remarkable power in causing the initial lesion to disappear and the early Wassermann test to become negative.

In the treatment of late syphilis it will require a period of years to determine just how effective this is. Our experience so far has shown that in longstanding cases of syphilis, with Wassermann and Kahn tests positive over a long period of time, under penicillin treatment the serological tests have become negative or only slightly positive, and other evidences of the disease have disappeared. Just how effective penicillin is against the spirochetes within the tertiary lesions and in cases of so-called latent syphilis is problematical. Our clinical results seem to offer hope that it will prove to be the most valuable means of treatment of syphilis, especially in those cases in which the general physical condition is much impaired and the cardiorenal condition precludes the usual treatments.

There are many patients who are not able to stand fever therapy and in this type of case we feel that the patient should have a very thorough and prolonged treatment with penicillin. In one case in which the patient had been given treatment before but none in years, there had developed some months back a headache so persistent that nothing gave relief. The patient was put on penicillin and within twenty-four hours the headache ceased and the patient has had no headache since.

While we do not yet have sufficient data on which to base a final statement of the value of the treatment of syphilis with penicillin, yet we do know that it has been very satisfactory so far in a large number of cases.

ARE ANY VITAMINS EFFECTIVE IN VOMITING OF PREGNANCY?—Yes. Pyridoxine, 100 mg., intramuscularly three times a week. In severe cases 100 mg. daily for four days. Relief occurs in 24 to 48 hours.—*Kalb*, in *Jl. Med. Soc. N. J.*, July.

SOUTHERN MEDICINE & SURGERY

Official Organ

JAMES M. NORTHINGTON, M.D., *Editor*

Department Editors

Human Behavior
JAMES K. HALL, M.D. ....Richmond, Va.

Orthopedic Surgery
JOHN T. SAUNDERS, M.D. ....Asheville, N. C.

Urology
RAYMOND THOMPSON, M.D. ....Charlotte, N. C.

Surgery
GEO. H. BUNCH, M.D. ....Columbia, S. C.

Obstetrics
HENRY J. LANGSTON, M.D. ....Danville, Va.

Gynecology
CHAS. R. ROBINS, M.D. ....Richmond, Va.
ROBERT T. FERGUSON, M.D. ....Charlotte, N. C.

General Practice
J. L. HAMNER, M.D. ....Mannboro, Va.

Clinical Chemistry and Microscopy
J. M. FEDER, M.D.,
EVELYN TREBBLE, M. T. } ....Anderson, S. C.

Hospitals
R. B. DAVIS, M.D. ....Greensboro, N. C.

Cardiology
CLYDE M. GILMORE, A.B., M.D. ....Greensboro, N. C.

Public Health
N. THOS. ENNETT, M.D. ....Greenville, N. C.

Radiology
R. H. LAFFERTY, M.D., and Associates ....Charlotte, N. C.

Therapeutics
J. F. NASH, M.D. ....Saint Pauls, N. C.

Tuberculosis
JOHN DONNELLY, M.D. ....Charlotte, N. C.

Dentistry
J. H. GUION, D.D.S. ....Charlotte, N. C.

Internal Medicine
GEORGE R. WILKINSON, M.D. ....Greenville, S. C.

Ophthalmology
HERBERT C. NEBLETT, M.D. ....Charlotte, N. C.

Rhino-Oto-Laryngology
CLAY W. EVATT, M.D. ....Charleston, S. C.

Proctology
RUSSELL L. BUXTON, M.D. ....Newport News, Va.

Insurance Medicine
H. F. STARR, M.D. ....Greensboro, N. C.

Dermatology
J. LAMAR CALLAWAY, M.D. ....Durham, N. C.

Pediatrics

Offerings for the pages of this Journal are requested and given careful consideration in each case. ..Manuscripts not found suitable for our use will not be returned unless author encloses postage.

As is true of most Medical Journals, all costs of cuts, etc., for illustrating an article must be borne by the author.

A POSSIBLE PREVENTIVE MEASURE AS TO POLIOMYELITIS

SAINT LOUIS' veteran teacher and practitioner of pediatrics has something reasonably hopeful to say on this subject:

Thirty years ago Dr. E. W. Saunders proposed his revolutionary hypothesis on the causation of poliomyelitis anterior acuta. Briefly stated it was this: Poliomyelitis is conveyed by the ova or larvae of the green fly from a fowl or other animal which has died from a specific paralytic disease. Experiments of Saunders proved that the larvae of the green fly or other species of the blow fly developing on a fowl dead from limberneck produces symptoms of paralysis when ingested by other animals (young fowls, guinea pigs).

Saunders, it seems, was the first to establish the fact that the green fly may absorb a powerful toxin and convey a toxin-producing microörganism. He believed that this bacterium or virus was identical with the virus of poliomyelitis.

In 1938, Rice declared that organisms found in the larvae of some of the blow flies causes limberneck in chickens.

Trask and Paul (1943) discovered that the blow and green bottle flies may carry the virus of poliomyelitis either on the surface or within the body. Several other investigators have found the virus in flies.

Saunders concluded that the virus of limberneck was non-inoculable from animal to animal. Then he began a series of experiments on the monkey, the only animal then known to be susceptible to the poliomyelitis of children. The monkey was not only susceptible to the toxin but when he survived showed symptomatic and pathologic evidence of a true virus infection. Although the toxin and virus entered the body by the gastrointestinal route, the spinal fluid and emulsions of the spinal cord of such animals were used successfully in transmitting the virus from one monkey to another by intraspinal inoculation. The pathologic specimens were examined by Dr. F. B. Bowman and revealed a distinct poliomyelitis.

The experiments on monkeys appear to prove that Saunders was dealing with a pathogen that was more than a toxin, probably a virus and asks may there be another factor—a toxin—which prepares the way for the development of the virus.

Saunders was compelled to stop his work on account of lack of financial support.

Poliomyelitis occurs in the fly season and most cases arise in the suburban or rural sections. Tracing the source of contagions to another human carrier is only exceptionally successful. *The conta-*

T. John Zahorsky, St. Louis, in Jl. Mo. Med. Assn., Aug.

giousness of the disease has never been established. Across the river from St. Louis, especially in the country districts of Illinois, poliomyelitis has been endemic for several summers and yet there have been only isolated cases of the disease in St. Louis. What is there in the city which prevents the dissemination of this malady? Contacts with this suburban population over the bridges is a daily occurrence.

Two years ago Schultz[2] made a critical review of recent studies in this disease, in which he said:

Until recently, it was widely held that the common natural portal of entry for the virus of the disease is the olfactory portion of the nasal mucosa. It was believed to spread from this area in the nose along the olfactory nerve to the bulbs and from there along the olfactory tracts to the central nervous system. A small minority held that invasion might occur through other mucous surfaces, more particularly through the mucosa of the digestive tract. In addition to finding the virus in the stools of patients on individual occasions, it had been possible at times to induce infection in monkeys by feeding the virus, or by introducing it by stomach tube.

Regarding the prevention of this disease there is little that can be said. It is now generally known that both serums and vaccines have proved ineffective as prophylactic agents. Although it has been established that certain chemical agents applied to the olfactory mucosa in monkeys are highly effective in preventing infection by the intranasal route, such a measure, granting that it could be safely applied in man, would, of course, be applicable only if the virus commonly entered by the olfactory pathway. Until the natural portal of entry is known it seems unlikely that a practical measure will suggest itself for the control of this disease.

Osler said the degree of contagiousness from person to person is slight, comparable to the contagiousness of pneumonia.

All diseases known to be communicable by casual contact—smallpox, scarlet fever, measles, etc.—afflict city populations in much greater numbers than country, and occur in greatest numbers in the cold months.

Poliomyelitis shows a great preference for country folks, and the great majority of its victims come down in the summer months.

The North Carolina county from which the largest number of cases have been reported is largely rural. Over the state the distribution is 10 to 12 rural to one urban. And investigation of the few urban cases might disclose that most of these originated in the country.

2. E. W. Schultz, Chicago, in Jl. Ped., Jan., 1942.

So it is seen that, in these particulars poliomyelitis does not behave like diseases known to be communicable by casual contact, but does behave like a disease known to be communicated by an insect vector; viz., yellow fever.

Here comes to mind the fact that Dr. Josiah Nott, in a *Sketch of the Epidemic of Yellow Fever of 1847 in Mobile*,[3] had this to say: "The disease in Mobile as well as in New Orleans [in its distribution] showed a strong analogy with the habits of insect life."

It would certainly be worth while to protect ourselves and our children so far as possible against contacts with flies—green flies, blow flies, stable flies, house flies, horse flies, deer flies—during the existence of an epidemic; indeed it would be the part of wisdom to provide this protection at all times. And it is plain that if any fleeing is to be done, the part of wisdom would be to flee *from country to city*.

3. Josiah C. Nott, M.D., Mobile, Ala., in *Charleston Medical Journal*, Jan., 1848.

* * * * *

THE RESTORATION OF BREATHING IN EMERGENCIES AND THE MAINTENANCE OF RESPIRATION

THE EXISTENCE of many cases of poliomyelitis in North Carolina and a few in adjoining States makes this an appropriate time to give the substance of an article[1] evaluating the different methods of artificial respiration. Your perusal of this advice may mean the saving of life in your practice.

The success of artificial respiration by manual methods depends on the efficiency of the elastic recoil and this depends upon muscular tone—a property rapidly lost as muscle circulation fails. By the Schafer method a small amount of air may be moved in and out of the lungs during the first few efforts, but the amount rapidly falls to little or nothing. In the Silvester method the patient is served more by the inherent elasticity of all the tissues. This advantage is largely negated by the position of the patient on his back which does not favor drainage from the mouth and throat, and even more by the fact that the inspiratory expansion of the chest attained by arm extension may be too slight to provide an adequate volume per minute.

In 1932, a British physician, Frank C. Eve, called to a child of two with post-diphtheritic paralysis of the diaphragm and dying of asphyxia, tilted its head down, thus clearing the throat of mucus which was rattling there. This clearance was beneficial, and Eve noticed that the tilt produced expiration. The child was laid in a long rocking chair and rocked by the parents slowly

1. C. K. Drinker, Boston, in N. Engld. Med. Assn., July,

over 2½ days. The paralysis passed off and recovery was complete. Any sort of see-saw arrangement could be used. It could not harm the patient, even if continued for a long time. While head-down, pressure applied as in the Schafer method, gives even greater ventilation and still better clearance of air passages. In my opinion this is the best, easily accomplished means of continuous artificial respiration we possess.

The Bragg-Paul pulsator is the best of the many mechanisms which operate by mechanical imitation of the prone pressure procedure.

There are several devices which aim to provide artificial respiration by alternately blowing air mixed with oxygen into a mask covering the mouth and nose, and sucking it out again. A pharyngeal or laryngeal tube may be used instead of the mask. It is hard to appraise the value or dangers of these appliances. My appraisals are at variance with those of the Council on Physical Therapy of the A. M. A.

If such a machine is at hand when breathing stops and if the respiratory passages are clear of obstruction, one can ventilate a patient successfully for sometime and may save life. Few are the instances of successful restoration of breathing following hours of blow-and-suck artificial respiration.

Pure oxygen, or air enriched with oxygen as much as possible, should be given in all cases of asphyxiation. Oxygen will have much wider use in the medicine of the future.

The use of carbon dioxide, under 7%, to stimulate breathing is wholly natural.

The respirator will save the lives of some patients. A larger number it will not save. When poliomyelitis is epidemic, under present popular demand, access to a respirator is almost imperative.

The cuirass respirator gives the patient more freedom and makes nursing care far less difficult, but it does not work well unless the patient retains some ability to breathe. Making the lower seal around the thighs instead of the abdomen makes this a more efficient but less confining respirator.

Drinker emphasizes the necessity for the application *with no delay of the simplest methods* when treating cessation of breathing. Whenever possible, breathing should be aided as it weakens. Anoxia breeds anoxia and physicians often begin to use oxygen or artificial respiration when it is too late. If artificial respiration must be continued for some time special apparatus becomes important. The simplest effective method for hours of use is the tilting technique of Eve, the materials for which are at hand almost anywhere. Next to this, and deserving wider use in this country, is the Bragg-Paul pulsator. As a last reliance we have the body respirator or possibly a cuirass respirator of the sort suggested. We have no reason to be well satisfied with any of these methods. Most of the best are relatively recent which, in a subject of so much medical importance is a healthy and promising symptom of progress. . . . .

MORE ABOUT RELATIVE IMPORTANCE AND EXPENCE IN DIAGNOSIS

A WISE DOCTOR recently lost by North Carolina to Texas[1] has spoken forth for better and cheaper medicine.

The gist of his invaluable and much needed counsel is:

As new objective methods of studying disease are developed there is an increasing neglect of the older and subjective methods. Even useful tests become harmful when applied so as to cause needless expense to patients or are so glorified as to lead to the neglect of simpler and more useful procedures. A five-minutes history followed by five days of special tests in the hope that the diagnostic rabbit may suddenly emerge from the laboratory hat is professionally unwise and economically unsound.

How do the symptoms arise? Often no serious attempt is made to answer this question and the physician assumes that some physiologic variant or even some demonstrated structural abnormality is responsible for the symptoms.

Objective methods alone can rarely reveal the most significant features of a patient's illness. These can come only from a detailed inquiry into the nature of the patient's complaints. Unless the medical schools are going to train men to do this, unless the physicians are going to take the time to apply such training, and unless the people are going to learn to appreciate the importance of such an approach, there is danger that gradual loss of faith in the profession may create in the public a state of mind conducive to undesirable changes in our present system of medical practice.

Modern diagnostic tests are valuable when properly applied and some of them, such as the radiogram of the chest, are being utilized too infrequently. There is serious doubt whether medical schools should persist in regarding diagnostic radiology as a specialty. Probably in the future every young physician will utilize the x-ray, much as he now does the stethoscope. Radiotherapy should remain a specialty in order to protect the patient. There will remain a very important place for the radiologist, who will do all of the radiotherapy and the more difficult diagnostic procedures, and will also serve as consultant for the physician who is himself doing the simpler x-ray work. This would

1. T. R. Harrison, Dallas, in *J. Med. Assn. Ala.*, June.

be an improvement over our present system, whereby many patients are failing to obtain the benefits of the x-ray, and others are being subjected to a large number of unnecessary radiologic procedures, largely because the physicians are failing to obtain and properly interpret an adequate story of the patient's complaints.

The electrocardiograph is valuable in several fields, and of these one of the most important is research. The instrument is also useful in the diagnosis of arrhythmias, although one who has trained himself carefully for a number of years at the bedside in the study of these disorders only occasionally needs to resort to the ecg. for this purpose. Diagnosis and, more particularly, prognosis, when based on the ecg. findings alone, are likely to be erroneous and misleading. Decisions of vital importance to the patient need to be based on *all* the evidence and in the great majority of cases the clinical findings, and proper analysis of the subjective manifestations, are more important than the ecgs. From personal observation many instances could be cited in which unwise restrictions, unnecessary psychic trauma, and even severe anxiety neuroses have been created as the result of misplaced emphasis on electrocardiographic findings.

And now there remain these three methods, the laboratory, the physical examination and the history, and the greatest of these is the history.

Nothing Dr. Harrison says is refutable. This journal is particularly pleased with his ideas on the subject, because they so strongly support us in our steady contention of many years that the function of the specialist is to deal with rare conditions, or common conditions of unusual severity.

A first class Washingtonian[2] on much the same subject:

Since laboratory work constitutes a large part of the expense of medical care, it behooves us to be careful to hold to the essential. It is important 1) to question the accuracy of all laboratory reports, 2) to repeat tests the results of which appear to be erroneous, and 3) to weight carefully reports that do not agree with our clinical impressions.

Ninety per cent of cases of diseases of the heart and of congestive failure may be diagnosed and treated satisfactorily without the aid of any laboratory work. Enlargement can often be determined by physical examination. Distortions in shape are more difficult to determine, but are not so important. Congestion of the lungs can be established by the presence of dyspnea and rales.

"The ecgm. is in many cases a luxury that intrigues the physician more than it helps the patient; its practical value is limited." Sometimes, to be sure, it shows an unsuspected bundle-branch block, or evidence of coronary artery sclerosis in a middle-aged man; but, even so, the handling of the case except for the admonition of moderation in all things will hardly be affected. The ecgm. is of great practical value in the diagnosis of tachycardia of ventricular origin. Here the proper use of quinidine may save life, since this arrhythmia is commonly caused by coronary artery artery sclerosis and, unless it is stopped, it may bring on congestive failure or sudden death. It may be fine to have an ecgm. in every case of suspected or known disease of the heart, but if not readily obtainable, the loss is not great.

"One can make his diagnoses usually in cases of generalized or peripheral vascular disease without the aid of the laboratory. The history and physical examination are usually sufficient. Radiography usually helps very little except in cases of aneurysm of the thoracic aorta."

Both these good doctors place a high value on laboratory tests and make use of them daily. But they use them discriminately, which means after considering whether the aid they are likely to afford is worth the cost to the patient.

* * * * *

PENICILLIN
INDICATIONS—CONTRAINDICATIONS—MODE OF ADMINISTRATION AND DOSAGE

Information prepared by Dr. Chester S. Keefer, Civilian Director of Clinical Evaluation of Penicillin.

INDICATIONS

Penicillin is the best therapeutic agent available for the treatment of:

1. *All staphylococcic infections* with and without bacteremia. Acute osteomyelitis, Carbuncles—soft tissue abscesses, Meningitis, Cavernous or Lateral. Sinus Thrombosis, Pneumonia - Empyema, Carbuncle of Kidney, Wound infections.

2. *All cases of clostridial infections:* Gas Gangrene, Malignant Edema.

3. *All hemolytic streptococcic infections* with bacteremia and all serious local infections: Cellulitis, Mastoiditis with intracranial complications—meningitis, sinus thrombosis, etc. Pneumonia and empyema, puerperal sepsis, peritonitis.

4. *All anaerobic streptococcic infections:* Puerperal sepsis.

5. *All pneumococcic infections* of meninges, pleura, endocardium, all cases of sulfonamide-resistant pneumococcic pneumonia.

6. *All gonococcic infections* complicated by arthritis, ophthalmia, endocarditis, peritonitis, epididymitis, also all cases of sulfonamide-resistant gonorrhea.

7. *All meningococcic infections* not responding to the sulfonamides.

T. W. M. Yater, Washington, in *Penn. Med. Jl.*, June.

CONTRAINDICATIONS

Penicillin is contraindicated in the folowing cases because it is ineffective:

1. *All gram-negative bacillary infections*: Typhoid, paratyphoid, dysentery, E. coli, H. influenzae, B. proteus, B. pyocyaneus, Br. melitensis (undulant fever), tularemia, B. friedlander.
2. Tuberculosis
3. Toxoplasmosis
4. Histoplasmosis
5. Acute rheumatic fever
6. Lupus erythematosus diffuse
7. Infectious mononucleosis
8. Pemphigus
9. Hodgkin's disease
10. Acute and chronic leukemia
11. Ulcerative colitis
12. Coccidioidomycosis
13. Malaria
14. Poliomyelitis
15. Blastomycosis
16. Non-specific iritis, uveitis
17. Moniliasis

Penicillin is of questionable value in mixed infections of the peritoneum and liver in which the predominating organism is of the gram negative flora, i. e.: Ruptured appendix, liver abscesses, urinary tract infections. Also in rat-bite fever due to streptobacillus moniliformis.

TREATMENT OF INFECTIONS WITH PENICILLIN

Penicillin is supplied in ampoules of different sizes—25,000 units and 100,000 units each. Inasmuch as penicillin is extremely soluble, it may be dissolved in small amounts of sterile, distilled, pyrogen-free water, or in sterile, normal saline solution. When large unit sizes are being used in hospitals, the contents of the ampoule should be dissolved in water or saline so that the final concentration is 5,000 units per cubic centimeter. This solution should be stored under aseptic precautions in the ice box, and made up freshly every day. Solutions for local or parenteral use may be diluted further, depending upon the concentration desired.

A. *For Intravenous Injection*

1. The dry powder may be dissolved in sterile physiological salt solution in concentrations of 1,000-5,000 units per c.c. for direct injection through a syringe.

2. The dry powder may be dissolved in sterile saline or 5 per cent glucose solution in lower dilution (25-50 units per c.c.) for constant intravenous therapy.

B. *For Intramuscular Injection*

1. The total volume of individual injections should be small, i.e., 5,000 units per c.c. of physiological saline.

C. *For Topical Application*

1. The powdered form of the sodium salt is irritating to wound surfaces and should not be used.

2. Solutions in physiological salt solution with a concentration of 250 units per c.c. are satisfactory. For resistant or more intense infections this concentration may be increased to 500 units per c.c.

There are three comon methods of administering penicillin—intravenous, intramuscular, and topical. Subcutaneous injections are likely to be painful and should not be used.

Repeated intramuscular injections may be tolerated less well than repeated or constant intravenous injections. In many cases, however, the intramuscular route may be the one of choice.

In the treatment of *meningitis, empyema* and *surface burns of limited extent*, penicillin should be used topically, that is, injected directly into the subarachnoid space, into the pleural cavity, or applied locally in solution containing 250 units per c.c.

DOSAGE

The dosage of penicillin will vary from one patient to another depending on the type and severity of infection. Recovery has followed in many serious infections following 40,000 to 50,000 Oxford units a day, in others 100,000 to 120,000 or even more is necessary. The objective in every case is to bring the infection under control as quickly as possible. The following recommendations are made at the present time with a full realization that revisions may be necessary as experience accumulates.

It is well to remember that panicillin is excreted rapidly in the urine so that following a single injection it is often impossible to detect it in the blood for a period longer than 2 to 4 hours. It is well, therefore, to use repeated intramuscular or intravenous injections every 3 or 4 hours, or to administer it as a continuous infusion.

A. *In serious infections with or without bacteremia*, an initial dose of 15,000 or 20,000 Oxford units with continuing dosage as:

1. Constant intravenous injection of normal saline solution containing penicillin so that 2,000 to 5,000 Oxford units are delivered every hour, making a total of 48,000 to 120,000 units in a 24-hour period. One-half the total daily dose may be dissolved in a liter of normal saline solution and allowed to drip at the rate of 30 to 40 drops per minute.

2. If continuous intravenous drip is undesirable, then 10,000 to 20,000 units may be injected intramuscularly every 3 or 4 hours.

3. After the temperature has returned to normal the penicillin may be stopped and the course of the disease followed carefully.

B. *In chronically infected compound injuries, osteomyelitis, etc*.

1. The dosage schedule should be 5,000 units

every two hours or 10,000 units every four hours parenterally with local treatment as indicated. This dosage schedule may have to be increased, depending upon the seriousness of the infection, and response to treatment.

C. *Sulfonamide-resistant gonorrhea*

1. 10,000 units every 3 hours intramuscularly or intravenously for ten doses. It is not likely that the same effect may be obtained with 20,000 units every 3 hours for 5 doses. The minimum dosage has not been worked out completely. The results of treatment should be controlled by culture of exudate.

D. *Empyema*

1. Penicillin in normal physiological saline solution should be injected directly into the empyema cavity after aspiration of pus or fluid. This should be done once or twice daily, using 30,000 or 40,000 units depending upon the size of the cavity, type of infection and number of organisms. Penicillin solutions should not be used for irrigation. It requires at least 6 to 8 hours for a maximum effect of penicillin.

E. *Meningitis*

1. Penicillin does not penetrate the subarachnoid space in appreciable amounts, so that it is necessary to inject penicillin into the subarachnoid space or intraisternally in order to produce the desired effect. Ten thousand units diluted in physiological saline solution in a concentration of 1,000 units per c.c. should be injected once or twice daily, depending upon the clinical course and the presence of organisms.

These dosage schedules may require much revision as increased experience is obtained. In many cases studied by investigators accredited to the committee, the dosage schedule given has proved to be adequate.

Following is an Editorial from the *Nebraska Medical Journal's* issue for July:

WHEN OUR COLLEAGUES COME HOME

"The following communication was recently received by the secretary of a constituent medical society of the Nebraska State Medical Association. The correspondent is a 42-year-old physician, who, shortly after the outbreak of the war gave up a large city practice to enlist in the United States Naval Reserve.

"'I am now a veteran of some 22 months. I have experienced the sensations of being crouched in a fox-hole with enemy shells exploding nearby. I have been overwhelmed by a feeling of terror beyond description as I realized that my last chip in this violent game was now on the table.

I have discussed post-war conditions for the doctor with perhaps a hundred or more service medical men, including those still safe in the U. S. A., as well as those in active combat. Always we ask each other the same questions:

Do the men at home feel that we are making a sacrifice?

Do they recognize that they can take complete advantage of us by taking over our practices without a plan of ever giving them up?

With so much talk and paper publicity regarding high taxes and long hours for the doctor at home, do they feel that they are the ones who are making the sacrifices; and do they therefore consider that they are justified in keeping all they can get?

Do they realize that they have been afforded unusual opportunities at our expense?

Do they appreciate the fact that they at home have accepted a greatly increased income made inevitable by the sacrifices of their colleagues?

Would they be willing to trade places with us for a while, or do they feel it's good enough for us; we asked for it, they didn't?

More and more the men in the service are expecting definite answers to these vital questions. The only really satisfactory answer can be a concrete plan, submitted soon, and not when the end of the war is in sight. If such a satisfactory scheme fails to appear before peace comes, the service doctor will be forced to support some politically controlled form of medical practice. There appears to us to be no other way to protect what we consider to be our rights.

We expect to continue to give our best, our lives if necessary, for a successful conclusion of this war. We know that without victory there would be nothing to share or hope for; but we are not sure that with victory those who have benefited will be willing to share justly with those who have risked their lives.'"

There is much food for thought in this communication. While we are planning to have every delivery conducted in a hospital by a specialist, every person who consults a doctor given all the different tests afforded by our laboratories (including x-ray examinations), and every person having any disease, medical or surgical, of any consequence, transported to a distant big tax-built and tax-supported hospital, and seen after by big tax-supported doctors—we might do well to devote a little time to reflecting on what this Army doctor and other Army doctors are turning over in their minds.

CANCER OF THE LARYNX
(Max Cutler, Chicago, in *Bul. Amer. Soc. for Control of Cancer*, June)

Each year 1,500 men and women in the United States die of cancer of the larynx; 5,000 suffer from this disease at any given time. Early cancer of the larynx is curable in more than 80% of the cases by a limited operation or by a short series of radiation treatments.

Hoarseness is an early symptom in at least 95 per cent of the cases. Examination of the larynx with a mirror easily establishes the presence of a growth and biopsy readily settles the diagnosis. The outcome depends on early diagnosis and prompt treatment.

Physician-Artists' Prize Contest

The American Physicians Art Association, with the co-operation of Mead Johnson & Company, is offering an important series of War Bonds as prizes to physicians in the armed services and also physicians in civilian practice for their best artistic works depicting the medical profession's "skill and courage and devotion beyond the call of duty."

Announcement of further details will be made soon by the Association's Secretary, Dr. F. H. Redewill, Flood Building, San Francisco, Cal.

COUNTY MEDICAL SOCIETY LIFE MEMBERSHIPS
(Harold Swanberg, Quincy, Ill., in *Miss. Valley Med. Jl.*, July)

This plan affords the member an opportunity for paying his full dues during his most productive years, and while his income is greatest thus avoiding the burden of dues later in life. Since Life Membership fees can be declared a professional expense when filing income taxes their actual cost is not great. The present era of high incomes and high income taxes thus provides an ideal time for making an investment in one's County Medical Society. The net cost of a Life Membership is considerably less than the amount paid since 27 to 57% (depending on the surtax net income) represents tax savings. If Life Membership fees are invested in war bonds and placed in an Endowment Fund it will further help the government finance the war.

Using the successful American College of Physician's Life Membership plan as a basis, a County Medical Society Life Membership should cost as follows:

Annual Dues	Age 45 or less	Age 46 to 50	Age 51 to 55	Age 56 to 60	Age 61 or more
$10.00	$200.00	$165.00	$135.00	$100.00	$ 65.00
15.00	300.00	250.00	200.00	150.00	100.00
20.00	400.00	335.00	270.00	200.00	135.00
25.00	500.00	415.00	335.00	250.00	165.00

A Certified Public Accountant has prepared a table based on net income and present taxes, showing the net cash cost of a Life Membership if $400.00 were paid.

Briefly the changes in the 1944 law as compared with the 1943 rates, are as follows:

	1943	1944
Victory tax	5%	None
Normal tax	6%	3%
Surtax	Brackets generally 7% higher in year 1944	

The cost of a life membership is deductible as a current business expense, to taxpayers reporting either on a cash or on an accrual basis.

Surtax Net Income*	Tax Saving of $400.00 Deduction	Net Cash Cost of Life Merbership
$2,000.00-$4,000.00	$100.00	$300.00
4,000.00- 6,000.00	116.00	284.00
6,000.00- 8,000.00	132.00	268.00
8,000.00-10,000.00	148.00	252.00
10,000.00-12,000.00	164.00	236.00
12,000.00-14,000.00	184.00	216.00
14,000.00-16,000.00	200.00	200.00
16,000.00-18,000.00	212.00	188.00
18,000.00-20,000.00	224.00	176.00
20,000.00-22,000.00	236.00	164.00
22,000.00-26,000.00	248.00	152.00

*Net income from practice plus earnings from all other sources and investments, less personal exemption and credit allowances for dependants.

SOME PHASES OF THE PREVENTION PROGRAM FOR POISON IVY DERMATITIS
(Leon Goldman, Cincinnati, in *Ohio Med. Jl.*, July)

The prevention of cutaneous contact with the oleoresinous material of the poison ivy plant and the removal of this substance from the skin is unsatisfactory. Future work in this field has much promise.

For the investigative study of methods to render the individual less susceptible, highly susceptible persons must be used. Oral antigens which are active and stable are preferred. Dosage is adjusted to the individual to avoid reactions in the early period of treatment, and an adequate dosage continued for long periods.

NEWS

THE AMERICAN CONGRESS OF PHYSICAL THERAPY

The 23d annual session will be held at the Hotel Statler, Cleveland, Sept. 6th-9th. The annual instruction course will be held from 8:00 to 10:30 a. m., and from 1:00 to 2:00 p .m. Sept. 6th-8th. All sessions will be open to the members of the regular medical profession and their qualified aids. For information address the *American Congress of Physical Therapy*, 30 North Michigan Avenue, Chicago, 2.

RICHMOND HAS NEW HEALTH OFFICER

Dr. Jack Berry Porterfield, director of the Virginia Bureau of Industrial Hygiene, has been appointed Director of Public Health of Richmond to succeed Dr. Millard C. Hanson, resigned to enter private practice.

VIRGINIA HELPS NORTH CAROLINA

Dr. I. C. Riggin, Virginia Health Commissioner, has worked in harmony with the Health Officers of North Carolina since the present outbreak of poliomyelitis, which has affected Virginia very little as compared with North Carolina. One feature of this coöperation was the enlistment of ten Red Cross nurses in Richmond for service in Virginia's southern neighbor.

Dr. NELSON MERCER, Virginia tuberculosis specialist, has been named to the $6,000 a year post of chief medical officer in the tuberculosis division of Gallinger Municipal Hospital.

Dr. Mercer, who has served as medical officer at Virginia Polytechnic Institute during the past year, took over his new job August 4th. He succeeds Dr. Charles P. Cake, who resigned early this year.

Born in Richmond 53 years ago, Dr. Mercer was graduated from the Medical College of Virginia. During the first World War he served four years as a captain in the United States Army Medical Corps.

From 1926 to 1937 Dr. Mercer was in private practice in Richmond. For the next five years he served as resident physician at the Home for Consumptives, Chestnut Hill, Pa.

MARRIED

Mrs. Percy Bloxam of Roxboro, N. C., has announced the marriage of her daughter, Barbara Olive, to Lieut. Joe Lee Frank, Jr., Medical Corps, Army of the United States, son of Mr. and Mrs. Joe Lee Frank of Richmond.

DIED

Dr. Richard Fenner Yarborough, son of the late Col. and Mrs. W. H. Yarborough, died on June 22nd, 1944. As a boy he attended the Morson and Denson Private School at Raleigh, from which he entered the University of North Carolina. In 1894 he began the study of medicine at George Washington University, Washington, and four years later he received his medical degree. In 1898 he completed a course in medicine at Columbia University. Following a post-graduate course at the Philadelphia Polyclinic in 1899, he commenced the practice of medicine in Louisburg, N. C., where he practiced until 1918, during

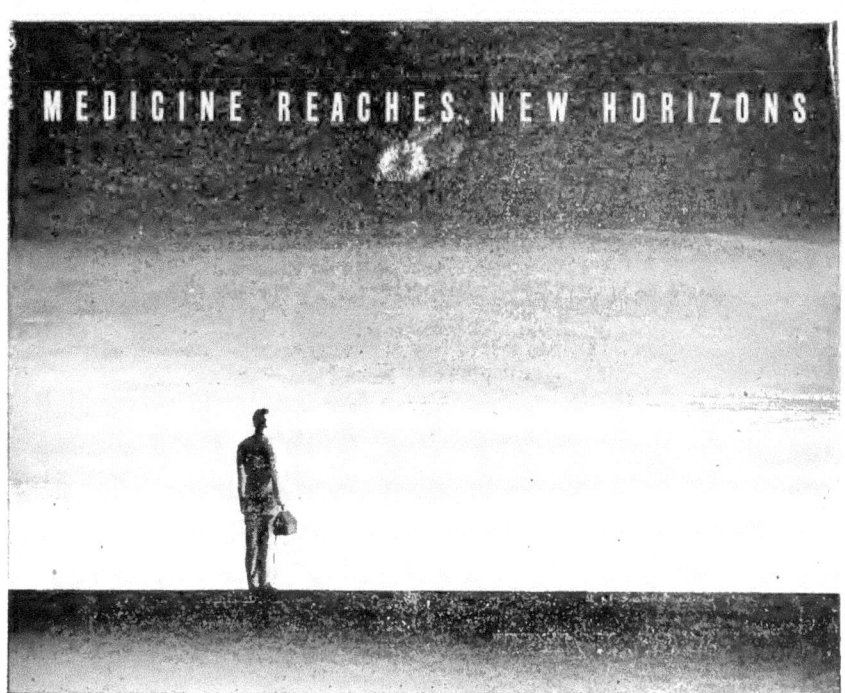

The discovery of penicillin and of its wonderful power to successfully combat death-dealing germs has brought medicine to new heights of ability to cope with many hitherto baffling ills that beset the human body.

The intriguing story of how officials of pharmaceutical concerns gave penicillin production the "green light" and, with the invaluable aid of governmental agencies, feverishly planned for an adequate production — how mycologists, bacteriologists, chemists, and chemotherapists worked day and night — how 22 companies poured $25,000,000 to $30,000,000 into this enterprise — comprises a never-to-be-forgotten episode in the saga of American pharmaceutical industry.

We are proud that Roche has kept in full step with the great march of scientific and engineering progress which ere long will place the wonder drug — penicillin — in the hands of every physician . . . HOFFMANN-LA ROCHE, INC., ROCHE PARK, NUTLEY 10, N. J.

which time he served for a number of years as Superintendent of Public Health for Franklin County.

He was also a member of the Board of Health of Franklin County for several years, and President of the Franklin County Medical Society for several terms.

He was a member of the Board of Directors of the State Hospital at Raleigh during Governor Glenn's administration.

In 1918 volunteering for service in the World War at the age of forty-six, he was commissioned Captain in the Medical Corp of the United States Army. He was ordered to the training camp, Camp Greenleaf, Fort Oglethorpe, Ga., and then to Camp McClellan and assigned as Medical Officer in charge of the 3rd Battalion of 157th Depot Brigade. During the epidemic of influenza in 1918 this Battalion of troops was under his surveillance.

Later Capt. Yarborough was transferred as Medical Officer to the 1st Prov. Co. Q. 98th Reg. and was there when the Armistice was declared.

In 1919 he was appointed Physician to A. and E. (State College), Raleigh, during Governor T. W. Bickett's administration. He served there with efficiency through the epidemic of influenza in 1920.

Resigning this position he returned to Louisburg where he continued general practice. He was again elected County Physician of Franklin County in 1926.

He held the position of Commander of Jambes Post, American Legion, and was also Commander of W. H. Yarborough Chapter of Sons of Confederate Veterans of Louisburg.

In January, 1930, he became the county's first full-time Health Officer under appointment of Governor Gardner, which position he held until his health failed eighteen months ago.

Dr. Yarborough was deeply interested in the health work of Franklin County and was faithful in the performance of his duties. Especially interested in preventive measures against disease, he led the fight which practically eliminated typhoid fever and greatly reduced both the incidence and death rate of smallpox and diphtheria in his county. He made an intensive and continuous fight against pellagra, lecturing throughout the county to schools and P.-T. Associations, writing and publishing many articles, distributing literature on the subject, and composing innumerable letters to parents and teachers. He was on the dfiring line of every phase of health work. He was interested, too, in all civic matters.

In his going Franklin County and his home town of Louisburg have lost a citizen and physician of inestimable value, his family a devoted and faithful husband and father, all the people of Franklin a faithful friend.

MEMBERS OF THE MEDICAL SOCIETY OF FRANKLIN COUNTY,
By Herbert G. Perry, M.D,
Acting Secretary.

Dr. M. E. Street died on the 15th of July at the age of 78. He was a graduate of the College of P. and S. in Baltimore in 1893 and was licensed the same year. He joined the North Carolina State Medical Society in 1902. He settled at Glendon in the western part of Moore County where he developed a large medical practice, mostly office work, particularly in the last few years of his life. On the advent of good roads his office practice developed much wider than in former years; patients coming to his office from far and near, and some parts of South Carolina and Georgia as well as Virginia and all parts of North Carolina.

Dr. Street was a large-scale farmer, devoting much attention to legume plants and doing much experimental work with lespedeza. He was a good mixer, a good talker and a pleasant personality, and had many friends both in and out of his chosen profession. He wrote articles for newspapers and for magazines.

Dr. Street's death is mourned by his many friends, far and near.
—R. G. ROSSER, M.D. (Vass).

Dr. Fred T. Houser, 42, died at his home at Purcellville, Va., after an illness of more than a year. A native of North Carolina, Dr. Hauser was graduated from the Medical College of Virginia in 1933, and served his internship at the Memorial Hospital in Richmond. He practiced medicine in Bland, Southwest Virginia, and later at Fort Monroe with the medical staff of the army.

Dr. Hanser located at Purvellville eight years ago. He was a member of the staff of Winchester Memorial Hospital, member of the Northern Virginia Medical Society, and of Loudoun Medical Society.

Dr. Charles Calvin Hubbard, 76, died at his home at Farmer, N. C., July 18th.

Dr. Hubbard, a native of Wilkes County, began the study of medicine under the direction of the late Dr. Larry Stokes of Wilkesboro at the age of 17. A year later, he entered Jefferson Medical College, Philadelphia, completing a two-year course and receiving his diploma in 1888.

He returned to Wilkes County and began his practice at Moravian Falls and at Wilkesboro, four years later coming to the community of Worthville in Randolph County. He remained there until 1908, when he returned to Farmer.

UNIVERSITY OF VIRGINIA

On Tuesday, May 16th, Dr. W. W. Waddell gave a lecture before the West Virginia State Medical Asociation, meeting in Wheeling, on the subject, Recent Improvements in the Treatment of Purulent Meningitis."

Dr. Dudley C. Smith attended meetings of the Society for Investigative Dermatology, American Dermatological Association, and American Medical Association in Chicago, June 12th to June 22nd. He was elected Vice-Chairman of the Section on Dermatology and Syphilology.

Dr. Samuel A. Vest presented a paper at the meeting of the American Medical Association in Chicago in June on An Inspection Lens-Sheath as an Aid to Transurethral Resection.

At the meeting of the American Urological Association in St. Louis in June, Dr. Vest spoke on the subject, Should Nephroureterectomy Be the Routine Procedure in Tumors of the Ureter? and conducted an exhibit on conservative surgery of the ureter.

Dr. Vincent W. Archer, Professor of Röntgenology, served as chairman of the Committee on Awards, Scientific Exhibits, during the meeting of the American Medical Association in Chicago, June 13th to 16th.

THIOURACIL FOR EXOPHTHALMIC GOITER
(J. P. Kenrick & W. M. Yater, Washington, in *Md. An. D. C.,* July)

The use of thiouracil in the treatment of hyperthyroidism is still in the investigational stage. Preliminary studies indicate that it may be of definite value, probably mainly fo rthe purpose of preparing severely toxic hyperthyroid patients for operation. It acts directly on the thyroid gland, inhibiting the formation of thyroxin in an unknown manner. Thiouracil does not prevent the action of thyroxin administered parenterally.

GLOBIN INSULIN.—In cases of diabetes in which nocturnal hypoglycemia, skin changes, or allergic reactions occur, this insulin may serve well.—*M. Protas.*

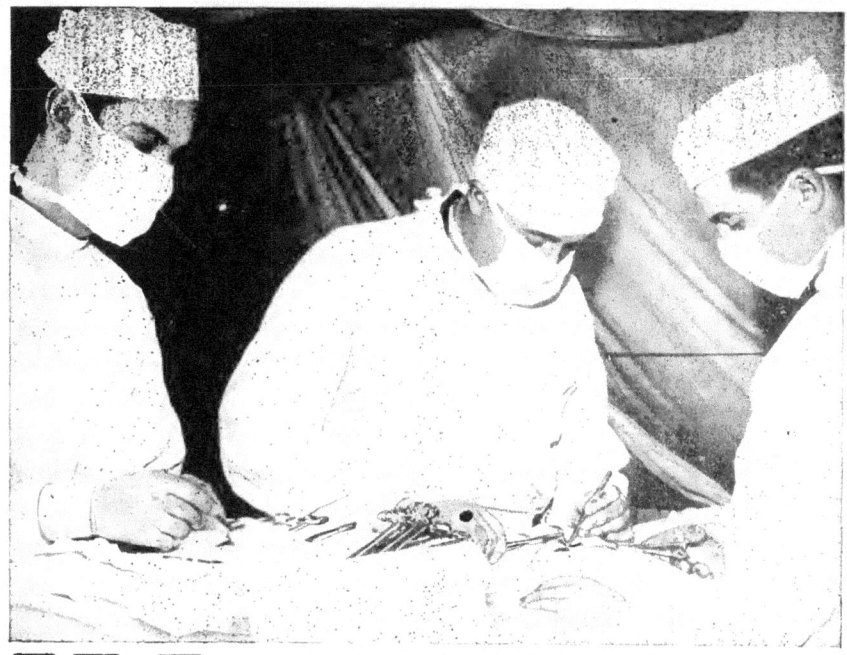

War
...in white

Always exposed to enemy fire, bombing, the field clearing-station surgeons work under the worst hazards ever faced by "soldiers in white." Naturally, their brief respites ... the occasional "breaks" for smokes ... are delightful moments.

More delightful because their cigarette is likely to be a Camel... the milder, more flavorful brand favored in the armed forces.*

Today ... as in the first world war ... Camel is the "soldier's cigarette," every puff a cheering highlight in a fighting man's life.

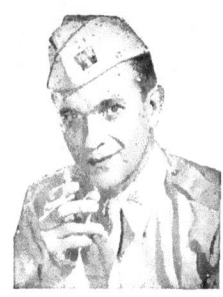

1st in the Service

*With men in the Army, the Navy, the Marine Corps, and Coast Guard, the favorite cigarette is Camel. (Based on actual sales records.)

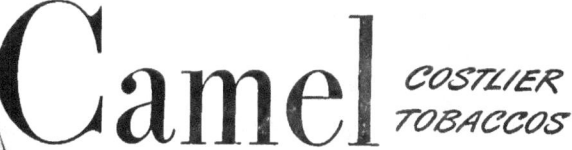

Camel COSTLIER TOBACCOS

New reprint available on cigarette research—Archives of Otolaryngology, March, 1943, pp. 404-410. Camel Cigarettes, Medical Relations Division, One Pershing Square, New York 17, N. Y.

BOOKS

TECHNICAL METHODS FOR THE TECHNICIAN, Third Edition. Published by the author, ANSON L. BROWN, M.D., Columbus, Ohio. $10.00.

No other event could so accurately measure the growing importance of the laboratory technician as the fact that within only the past few years have books been published especially for the use of these workers. For a long time there have been books dealing with laboratory medicine but most of these have been highly technical, many of them lacking in clarity. Doctor Brown has made a splendid job of preparing a text that will be of incalculable value in guiding the footsteps of the laboratory fledgeling. This does not by any means imply that this splendid volume is solely for the beginner. There are many valuable hints within its 700 pages that can be of service to the laboratory physicians and the senior technicians. In the preparation of the text, the author has apparently drawn well upon his extensive experience gained by many years spent in training clinical laboratory technicians.

One of the most laudable features of the book is the step-by-step presentation of each procedure. This saves the busy technician much time that would otherwise be lost in poring over a lot of irrelevant matters. Illustrations accompanying the text are original in most instances and clarify the printed page. This reviewer has much in common with the belief of the Chinese relative to a picture being worth a thousand descriptive words.

A noteworthy feature of the book is the accurate description of the blood counting chamber which faces page 138. Experience has taught us that any diagram that will aid us in teaching this complimated mathematical appliance to student technicians will prove exceedingly valuable.

We are greatly impressed by the code of ethics for technicians embodied in the book; so far as we can recall, it is the first time we have seen any attempt to formulate a set of rules for the government of the technician's relationship with those about her. It would appear to us that these workers trained in places other than hospital laboratories would find the adjustment period quite difficult as when they enter the hospital on their first job they are in reality migrating to a world of different values and rules from that which they have known.

The mottos for technicians with which the book is well sprinkled are to the point and they are aphorisms that all technicians can profit by assimilating. In our own school we have two that are continually impressed upon our students, one of these is: "Precision, Perfection, Speed." The other, a Latin translation of which appears upon the school's diplomas is, "The Art of Doing Things Well, Always."

As contemporaries in his field, we take this opportunity to congratulate Doctor Brown upon a task well done. *Technical Methods for the Technician* is a book that should be in the working library of every clinical laboratory.

As a passing comment, in addition to its appeal as an everyday aid, this book should prove to be a boon to technicians, regardless of their experience, who might be preparing to take the registration examination.

J. M. FEDER, M.D., &
EVELYN TRIBBLE, M.T.

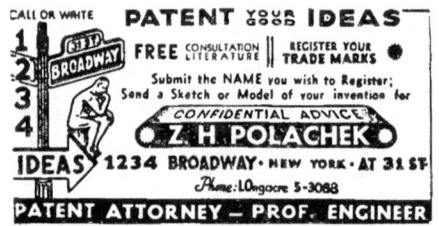

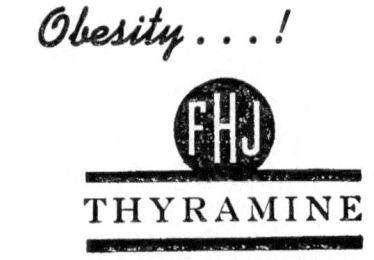

Composition

Thyroid 1 gr. Amphetamine sulphate 5 mgs. Thiamin chloride 1 mg. in suitable combinations with physiological reinforcements.

No. 1—One Capsule before breakfast
No. 2—One Capsule before lunch
No. 3—One Capsule at 4 p. m.

Contraindications

Hypertension .... Hyperthyroidism

Supplied

Capsules: Packages 21 and 42 (one or two weeks supply).

—Professional samples on request—
Available: Any professional pharmacy
F. H. J. PRODUCTS
977 East 176th St., New York 60, N. Y.

HYDRONEPHROSIS AND PYELITIS OF PREGNANCY, by H. E. ROBERTSON, M.D., Section on Pathologic Anatomy, Mayo Clinic, Rochester, Minnesota. 332 pages with 11 illustrations. *W. B. Saunders Company*, Philadelphia and London. 1944. Price $4.50.

The author is a renowned pathologist and a natural philosopher, and is therefore exceptionally qualified to write such a book as this. The introductory chapter constructs a proper background. Unusual emphasis is placed on the influence of anatomical relations, and on the importance of the infected hydronephrosis of pregnancy and pyelonephritis, clinically and pathologically. To ureteral dilatation is ascribed a place of consequence as a factor predisposing to infection.

The chapter on the influence of the nervous system has an interest second to none. The author's conclusions are of great practical value in daily practice in this field.

HYPERTENSION AND HYPERTENSIVE DISEASE, by WILLIAM GOLDRING, M.D., Associate Professor of Medicine, N. Y. Univ. College of Medicine; Chief, Nephritis and Hypertension Clinic, New York University Clinic; and HERBERT CHASIS, M.D., Assistant Professosr of Medicine, New York University College of Medicine; Associate Chief, Nephritis and Hypertension Clinic, New York University Clinic. *The Commonwealth Fund*, 41 East 57th Street, New York 22, N. Y. 1944. $3.50.

The studies here presented represent 15 years of collaboration between the Department of Medicine and the Department of Physiology of an excellent medical school. Certainly no better plan of study could have been formulated for ascertaining the facts that are within our reach as to this common and important disease condition.

From this critical study of hypertensive disease in 6,000 patients, ambulatory and hospitalized, it could not but happen that lessons of immense clinical value would be learned. The results of treatment by various methods, including the so-called specific medical and surgical therapies, are faithfully recorded.

For the doctor who wishes to know not only what to do but why he should do it and what he may expect in this class of diseases, this book will prove invaluable.

TECHNIC OF ELECTROTHERAPY and Its Physical and Physiological Basis, by STAFFORD L. OSBORNE, M.S., Ph.D., Asssstant Professor, Department of Physical Therapy, Northwestern University Medical School; and HAROLD J. HOLMQUEST, B.S., B.S. (M.E.), Lecturer in Applied Physics, Department of Physical Therapy, Northwestern University Medical School, Chicago. *Charles C. Thomas*, Springfield, Ill., and Baltimore, Md. 1944. $7.50.

Perhaps no other therapy has had such ups and downs of popularity as has this form of therapy. A great many have been so enthusiastic as to

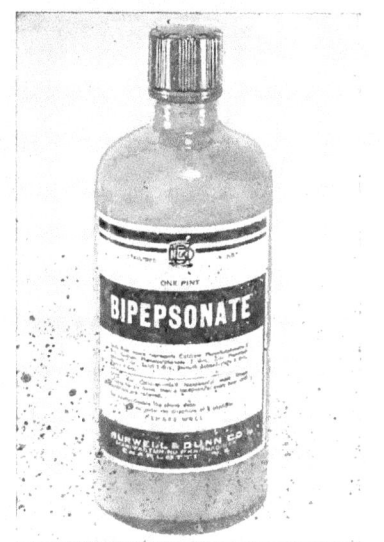

BIPEPSONATE

Calcium Phenolsulphonate	2 grains
Sodium Phenolsulphonate	2 grains
Zinc Phenolsulphonate, N. F.	1 grain
Salol, U. S. P.	2 grains
Bismuth Subsalicylate, U. S. P.	8 grains
Pepsin U. S. P.	4 grains

Average Dosage

For Children—Half drachm every fifteen minutes for six doses, then every hour until relieved.
For Adults—Double the above dose.

How Supplied

In Pints, Five-Pints and Gallons to Physicians and Druggists only.

Burwell & Dunn Company

Manufacturing 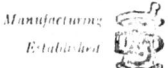 *Pharmacists*
Established in 1887

CHARLOTTE, N. C.

Sample sent to any physician in the U. S. on request

make claims which it did not seem reasonable to the great majority could be substantiated, and so the pendulum swung away over to the skeptical side. Instrument manufacturers by extravagant claims have contributed to this disparagement of this valuable method of treatment.

In the last few years a considerable body of favorable evidence has been adduced from the results of carefully controlled cases, and so electrotherapy is increasing in credit.

This book is devoted almost entirely to the technic which has proven most useful because it has a sound basis.

TECHNIC IN TRAUMA: Planned Timing in the Treatment of Wounds Including Burns, by FRASER B. GURD, M.D., C.M. and F. DOUGLAS ACKMAN, M.D., C.M. J. B. Lippincott Co., E. Washington Square, Philadelphia 5, Pa. 1944. $2.00.

Emphasis is placed on the fact that burns are open wounds of a large area, which should be treated with the most rigid aseptic technique, including dressing no oftener than is demanded by very definite indications.

An in-many-ways improved concept is offered for the treatment of major and minor burns. A report is made on the management using the occlusive, compression dressing with sulfathiazole emulsion.

SPECIALS FOR DOCTORS
★

Letterheads, Envelopes and Billheads on Hammermill Bond—1,000 .... $3.75

Professional Cards, Embossed, Featherweight,
1,000 .... $4.75

2,500 Prescription Blanks $5.00
5,000 for $8.75

Stationery for Armed Forces
50 Sheets, 50 Envelopes $1.98
with name printed and insignia gold stamped.
Army—Navy—Marines—Coast Guard—Air Force
—WACS—WAVES—SPARS

GIFTS FOR THE LADIES
Personal stationery, Deckle-edged, White with blue border, Blue with blue border, Peach with tan border—50 sheets, 50 envelopes $1.98
With 3 letter monogram

All prices are F.O.B. our factory
Terms: Check with order
Orders of $20.00 or over shipped free

JULES PRESS
55 West 42nd Street   New York 18, N. Y.

The final section is devoted to treatment of wounds and infections by means of infrequent occlusive dressings.

FERTILITY IN WOMEN: Causes, Diagnosis and Treatment of Impaired Fertility, by SAMUEL L. SIEGLER, M.D., F.A.C.S., Attending Obstetrician and Gynecologist, Brooklyn Women's Hospital, etc.; with a foreword by ROBERT LATOU DICKINSON, M.D.; 194 illustrations, including 40 subjects in full color on 7 plates. J. B. Lippincott Company, E. Washington Square, Philadelphia, Pa. 1944. $4.50.

Unfertile marriages are becoming more and more of a problem for the sociologist, the statesman, and the doctor. Until very recently it was commonly assumed that the fault is the woman's in pretty nearly all the cases of involuntary infertility. Today it is established that she is responsible in only one-half to two-thirds of the cases.

Among the sub-divisions of the subject as dealt with here are: age index of fertility, effect of contraception, causes of infertility, familial history, and endocrine influence. The importance of the family and personal history is given due consideration. Methods of examination, general and special, are detailed, and the evidence adduced carefully evaluated. General treatment is not neglected, and unnecessary treatment, operative or otherwise, is condemned. Artificial insemination is discussed in a very practical way.

FERTILITY IN MEN: A Clinical Study of the Causes, Diagnosis and Treatment of Impaired Fertility in Men, by ROBERT SHERMAN HOTCHKISS, B.S., M.D., Lt. Com. (M. C.), U. S. N. R. (on active service); Assistant Professor of Urology, New York University Medical College; Instructor in Surgery (Urology), Cornell Medical College, etc.; with a foreword by NICHOLSON J. EASTMAN, M.D., Chairman, Editorial Committee, National Committee on Maternal Health; Professor of Obstetrics in Johns Hopkins University; 95 illustrations. J. B. Lippincott Company, E. Washington Square, Philadelphia, Pa. 1944. $3.50.

This book and the one just reviewed are published as a two-book set.

The various attitudes of the husband in the case under consideration are described as mildly interested, reluctant, much interested, worried, and over-confident. The various methods of investigation to determine the responsibility of the male in any given case, and the most approved methods of treatment, are set forth. The prognosis is in general dubious or worse in most cases.

INFANTS WITHOUT FAMILIES: The Case for and Against Residential Nurseries, by ANNA FREUD and DOROTHY BURLINGHAM. International University Press, 227 West 13th St., New York 11, N. Y. 1944. $2.00.

The observations here recorded have been collected from practical work in three houses of an English nursery. The children taken care of were those of fathers in the armed services, mothers doing full-time factory work or children evacuated as precautionary measures, or after the destruction of homes, etc. The age range is from birth to two years.

The experience in this work under trying conditions carry many important lessons that may be applied to work under conditions less trying.

ARTIFICIAL PNEUMOTHORAX IN PULMONARY TUBERCULOSIS, including Its Relationship to the Broader Aspects of Collapse Therapy, by T. N. RAFFERTY, M.D., Phoenix, Ariz., Formerly Resident Physician, William H. Maybury Sanatorium, (Detroit Municipal Tuberculosis Sanatorium), Northville, Mich. Introduction by HENRY STUART WILLIS, M.A., M.D., Superintendent and Medical Director, William H. Maybury Sanatorium, Northville, Mich. 240 pages. 26 illustrations. Bibliography index. *Grune & Stratton, Inc.*, Medical Publishers, 381 Fourth Avenue, New York 16, N. Y. $4.00.

This is a reliable and valuable coverage of this important means of treatment in a large percentage of cases of pulmonary tuberculosis.

ESSENTIALS OF DERMATOLOGY, by NORMAN TOBIAS, M.D., Senior Instructor in Dermatology, St. Louis University. Second edition. *J. B. Lippincott Co.*, E. Washington Square, Philadelphia 5, Pa. 1944. $4.75.

It may be that a better book on dermatology for the use of the general practitioner of medicine has been written; but, if so, this reviewer has not seen it.

ABOUT "KICKBACKS," REBATES AND ALL SUCH

From a story in the *New York Times* of June 4th:

Industrial Commissioner Edward Corsi of the State Labor Department dealt a blow yesterday at a widespread "kickback" racket by revoking the licenses of nine Brooklyn physicians to treat compensation cases, and suspending 263 others for from one month to two years.

This board heard charges against more than 1,000 Brooklyn doctors accused of accepting "kickbacks" ranging from $1 to as high as $1,127 over a single period of 12 months.

A clean bill of health was given to 10 Brooklyn physicians on the recommendation of the medical society, and it was found in 70 other cases there was no cause for action. Further hearings are to be held in cases of 302 other Brooklyn doctors, while charges against 343 physicians now in the armed services will be "filed" for the time being.

These "kickbacks," the report said, appeared to have been paid to doctors by surgeons, röntgenologists, surgical appliance houses, opticians and specimen analysis laboratories to whom they referred workers.

From the *President's Address* of Dr. Wm. Atmar Smith, to the South Carolina Medical Association, 1944:

The acceptance of fees from optical companies by certain groups of physicians cannot be condoned by the profession. With the complex problems confronting the conduct of medicine at the present time, it is more than ever necessary that we face the public with clean hands.

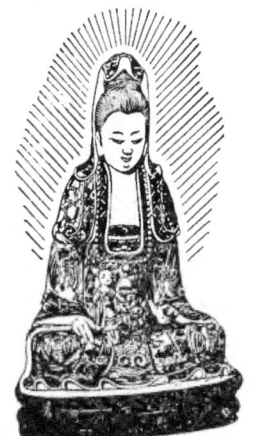

KWAN YIN
Chinese Goddess of Fertility

Hotchkiss and Siegler
FERTILITY IN MEN • FERTILITY IN WOMEN

Since the beginning of time, sterility has been a major concern of mankind. Peoples have ransacked apothecary shops, have sought favor with gods and goddesses, that they might beget and multiply. Even today, the treatment of sterility is a maze of pitfalls and indecision. Cutting clearly through this labyrinth, Drs. Hotchkiss and Siegler bring two thoroughly practical books—*Fertility in Men* and *Fertility in Women*—both heralded as real aids to the medical profession.

FERTILITY IN MEN—
Dr. Hotchkiss handles his subject with charity and perspective. His emphasis on the practical details of treating cases of male sterility makes the volume of great value to the practitioner.

ROBERT S. HOTCHKISS, B. S., M. D.,
Lt. Com., Medical Corps, U.S.N.R. (now on active duty), is widely known and respected for his work as Assistant Professor of Urology, New York University Medical College, and as Instructor in Surgery, Cornell University Medical College.

FERTILITY IN WOMEN—
Dr. Siegler writes from a functional viewpoint, with structure, function, and disease integrated to present a unified clinical picture. Detailed as to procedure and technic . . . completely practical . . . a real, workable guide.

SAMUEL L. SIEGLER, M. D., F. A. C. S.,
is known for his highly successful work as Attending Obstetrician and Gynecologist, Brooklyn Women's Hospital; Attending Gynecologist, Unity Hospital; and Assistant Obstetrician and Gynecologist, Greenpoint Hospital.

Fertility • IN MEN $350 • IN WOMEN $450

BOTH BOOKS IN ATTRACTIVE SLIP CASE $800

J. B. LIPPINCOTT COMPANY, Philadelphia 5, Pa.

Enter my order and send me at once—
☐ Fertility in Men—$3.50   ☐ Fertility in Women—$4.50   ☐ Both Books—$8.00
☐ Cash Enclosed   ☐ Charge my account

Send to: NAME_____
STREET ADDRESS_____
CITY & STATE_____

Under your Guarantee, I may return either book in 10 days, otherwise I will pay in full in 30 days.

GENERAL

Nalle Clinic Building 412 North Church Street, Charlotte
THE NALLE CLINIC
Telephone—C-BVDV (*if no answer, call* 3-2621)

General Surgery	*General Medicine*
BRODIE C. NALLE, M.D.	LUCIUS G. GAGE, M.D.
GYNECOLOGY & OBSTETRICS	DIAGNOSIS
EDWARD R. HIPP, M.D.	
TRAUMATIC SURGERY	LUTHER W. KELLY, M.D.
*PRESTON NOWLIN, M.D.	CARDIO-RESPIRATORY DISEASES
UROLOGY	
	J. R. ADAMS, M.D.
Consulting Staff	DISEASES OF INFANTS & CHILDREN
R. H. LAFFERTY, M.D.	
O. D. BAXTER, M.D.	W. B. MAYER, M.D.
RADIOLOGY	DERMATOLOGY & SYPHILOLOGY
W. M. SUMMERVILLE, M.D.	
PATHOLOGY	(*In Country's Service)

C—H—M MEDICAL OFFICES
DIAGNOSIS—SURGERY
X-RAY—RADIUM
DR. G. CARLYLE COOKE—*Abdominal Surgery & Gynecology*
DR. GEO. W. HOLMES—*Orthopedics*
DR. C. H. MCCANTS—*General Surgery*
222-226 Nissen Bldg. Winston-Salem

WADE CLINIC
Wade Building
Hot Springs National Park, Arkansas

H. KING WADE, M.D.	Urology
ERNEST M. MCKENZIE, M.D.	Medicine
*FRANK M. ADAMS, M.D.	Medicine
*JACK ELLIS, M.D.	Medicine
BESSEY H. SHEBESTA, M.D.	Medicine
*WM. C. HAYS, M.D.	Medicine
N. B. BURCH, M.D.	
	Eye, Ear, Nose and Throat
A. W. SCHEER	X-ray Technician
ETTA WADE	Clinical Laboratory
MERNA SPRING	Clinical Pathology
(*In Military Service)	

INTERNAL MEDICINE

ARCHIE A. BARRON, M.D., F.A.C.P.	JOHN DONNELLY, M.D.
INTERNAL MEDICINE—NEUROLOGY	*DISEASES OF THE LUNGS*
Professional Bldg. Charlotte	Medical Building Charlotte
CLYDE M. GILMORE, A.B., M.D.	JAMES M. NORTHINGTON, M.D.
CARDIOLOGY—INTERNAL MEDICINE	*INTERNAL MEDICINE—GERIATRICS*
Dixie Building Greensboro	Medical Building Charlotte

NEUROLOGY and PSYCHIATRY

(*Now in the Country's Service*)
*J. FRED MERRITT, M.D.
NERVOUS and MILD MENTAL DISEASES
ALCOHOL and DRUG ADDICTIONS
Glenwood Park Sanitarium   Greensboro

TOM A. WILLIAMS, M.D.
(*Neurologist of Washington, D. C.*)
Consultation by appointment at
Phone 3994-W
77 Kenilworth Ave.   Asheville, N. C.

EYE, EAR, NOSE AND THROAT

H. C. NEBLETT, M.D.
OCULIST
Phone 3-5852
Professional Bldg.   Charlotte

AMZI J. ELLINGTON, M.D.
DISEASES of the EYE, EAR, NOSE and THROAT
Phones: Office 992—Residence 761
Burlington   North Carolina

UROLOGY, DERMATOLOGY and PROCTOLOGY

THE CROWELL CLINIC of UROLOGY and UROLOGICAL SURGERY
Hours—Nine to Five   Telephones—3-7101—3-7102
STAFF
ANDREW J. CROWELL, M.D.
(1911-1938)
*ANGUS M. MCDONALD, M.D.   CLAUDE B. SQUIRES, M.D.
Suite 700-711 Professional Building   Charlotte

RAYMOND THOMPSON, M.D., F.A.C.S.   WALTER E. DANIEL, A.B., M.D.
THE THOMPSON-DANIEL CLINIC
of
UROLOGY & UROLOGICAL SURGERY
Fifth Floor Professional Bldg.   Charlotte

C. C. MASSEY, M.D.
PRACTICE LIMITED TO
DISEASES OF THE RECTUM
Professional Bldg.   Charlotte

WYETT F. SIMPSON, M.D.
GENITO-URINARY DISEASES
Phone 1234
Hot Springs National Park   Arkansas

ORTHOPEDICS

HERBERT F. MUNT, M.D.
ACCIDENT SURGERY & ORTHOPEDICS
FRACTURES
Nissen Building   Winston-Salem

SURGERY

(Now in the Country's Service)
R. S. ANDERSON, M. D.

GENERAL SURGERY

144 Coast Line Street   Rocky Mount

R. B. DAVIS, M. D., M. M. S., F. A. C. P.
GENERAL SURGERY
AND
RADIUM THERAPY
Hours by Appointment

Piedmont-Memorial Hosp.   Greensboro

(Now in the Country's Service)
WILLIAM FRANCIS MARTIN, M D

GENERAL SURGERY

Professional Bldg.   Charlotte

OBSTETRICS & GYNECOLOGY

IVAN M. PROCTER, M. D.

OBSTETRICS & GYNECOLOGY

133 Fayetteville Street   Raleigh

SPECIAL NOTICES

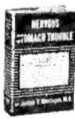

NERVOUS STOMACH TROUBLE — By J. F. Montague, M.D. 49 Chapters. Clear and easy reading about the "facts of life" as presented by stomach ulcer, colitis, gall bladder trouble and appendicitis. Medical facts on treatment comprehensive yet most interesting — even entertaining. Published by Simon and Schuster. Send orders to Joseph J. Boris, Publishers' Representative, 1440 Broadway, New York, N. Y. (Price $2.00)

TWO LABORATORY TECHNICIANS, being graduated from a High-class Hospital Laboratory, services available January 1st, 1944. Address TECHNICIAN, care *Southern Medicine & Surgery*.

TO THE BUSY DOCTOR WHO WANTS TO PASS HIS EXPERIENCE ON TO OTHERS

You have probably been postponing writing that original contribution. You can do it, and save your time and effort by employing an expert literary assistant to prepare the address, article or book under your direction or relieve you of the details of looking up references, translating, indexing, typing, and the complete preparation of your **manuscript**.

Address: *WRITING AIDE*, care *Southern Medicine & Surgery*.

THE JOURNAL OF SOUTHERN MEDICINE AND SURGERY

306 North Tryon Street, Charlotte, N. C.

The Journal assumes no responsibility for the authenticity of opinion or statements made by authors or in communications submitted to this Journal for publication.

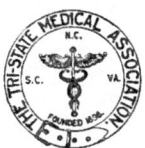

JAMES M. NORTHINGTON, M.D., Editor

VOL. CVI　　　　　SEPTEMBER, 1944　　　　　No. 9

Health Alone Is Victory*

JAMES K. HALL, M.D., Richmond

BY WAY OF INTRODUCTION I shall ask you to commune briefly with me about two events that recently occurred in Richmond. They affected my usual equanimity and they are directly related to the spirit of this symposium. You and I may make free use of the pronouns you and I, because we shall do it unegotistically and without self-consciousness.

Richmond is a serene and stable old city, though she has participated in more than one revolution, for which she makes no apology. Only a few days before the biennial session of the General Assembly of Virginia recently adjourned, a bill was introduced into the state senate proposing to make incurable insanity a ground for divorce. Immediately after the introduction of the bill, one of the senators asked by telephone my opinion of the legislation and he expressed the hope that I might be inclined to discuss in a letter the medical aspects of the proposal. And only two weeks ago I was one of the many members of the Richmond Academy of Medicine to be instructed in certain aspects of the history of some of the most important decades in recent centuries. Dr. Manfred S. Guttmacher, of Baltimore, now a Major in the Medical Corps of the United States Army, is both a busy clinical psychiatrist and a learned historian. He delivered the annual address to the Section on the History of Medicine of the Academy. His thesis was the insanity of King George the Third of England. Some of you are familiar with Dr. Guttmacher's biography of that monarch entitled: The Last American King.

George the Third ascended the throne in 1760, when scarcely more than twenty, and he reigned and ruled until the Boatman bore him away in 1820. During those turbulent sixty years, when the world's history was being re-written, the King became a husband and the father of many children, the behaviour of some of whom did not add to his royal serenity. And during his reign his troubles were not all domestic. Our ancestors entertained him with a revolutionary war, the result of which was the loss of his best colonial possession; and again with the War of 1812. Napoleon and his great cavalryman (who, say some, lies buried only forty miles from Charlotte) shook the world for many years, and probably brought George the Third to unhappy contemplation of the possibility of the dissolution of his Empire and the loss of his throne. Throughout his long reign England was almost continuously engaged in warfare; under him the might of the British Empire became firmly established; Napoleon was sent finally into banishment; and since Trafalgar and Waterloo Britannia has ruled the waves. The prowess of Lord Nelson and of the Duke of Wellington on sea and on land was all the more remarkable, because they were the commanders of a mad monarch.

George the Third experienced during his reign many violent attacks of what was then called insanity, and he was often placed in physical restraint. His last years were spent in blindness and in dementia. But under him the naval and the military might of the British Empire was so firmly established that it stands steadfast today in a tottering world.

*Given by invitation at the Mental Hygiene Institute of the Mental Hygiene Society, of Charlotte, at the Hotel Charlotte, North Carolina, at the dinner on March 29th, 1943.

An analysis of the personality of George the Third and an estimate of his capacity as a ruler cannot be undertaken, of course, on this occasion. But his career illustrates the fact that insanity is a disease, from certain forms of which there may be recovery. And his life may suggest, on the other hand, that positions of great responsibility and power should not be occupied by the mentally unstable. Had George the Third been as wise as some of his prime ministers, there might have been no American Revolution, no Halifax Resolves, no Mecklenburg Declaration, no King's Mountain, no Guilford Court House, no Yorktown, no Constitution, no Supreme Court, no New Deal. Madness has created considerable history and it has brought forth much literature and no little poetry.

No student of history and no one concerned about heredity and hygiene can fail to be interested in the influence of disease upon the course of civilization. Many of the thrones of Europe have been occupied by the descendants of George the Third.

Were I a stranger in a land of strangers, I should not feel apologetic for presuming to believe that my hearers would be with me in my assumption that, aside from his concern about God, man's chief interest is his fellow-man. And man is properly concerned about his fellow-mortal's behaviour, because human history is largely an account of man's ceaseless warfare with his fellow-man. No other phenomenon in a universe filled with things about which man knows little causes him such unending pleasure and such grim despair as much of the conduct of other mortals. Man would seem to be rather hopelessly humanized. He can live neither with man nor without him—and the generic term includes, of course, woman, to make the confusion more completely confounded.

And even if I were in a community that was not in the beginning saturated with that belief in cause and effect that is spoken of biologically as predeterminism and theologically as predestination, I should assume that you look upon human behaviour as not beyond the limits of the operations of those natural laws, through which God performs His wonders and manifests His mysteries. The continuing tragedy lies in the prevalent belief that something so profoundly mysterious inheres in human behaviour as to place it beyond the reach of understanding.

If the term anatomy is used to refer to the structural fabrication, and physiology to indicate the work performed by the individual organ, psychology should be used in reference to the functioning not of an organ but of the individual as a vital totality. Such action of the human being represents the conjoint response of the total mortal to the environmental situation. It must be remembered, however, that in each individual is brought forward from the remotest past all human biological history, and that what is referred to almost glibly as environment may have reference to all else that lies within the boundless stretches of the universe. The purpose is not to make the approach to human behaviour forbiddingly difficult, but to present man as a complex organism whose supremest function is to behave.

For neither man nor any other living thing can escape indulging in behaviour. Freud has said, I believe, that man is inescapably destined to express himself, that he cannot succeed in repressing himself, that if he is silent with his lips he will tattle with his finger tips. The Universe is the Father Confessor to which man constantly tries to pour out his soul. How tragic it is that we seldom thoroughly understand what we ourselves are doing and even less frequently and less perfectly what our fellow-creatures are saying.

The scientist who spends his nights and his days in work and in wonderment about the biological history of man might tell us that the individual in his physical development, within and without his mother's body, portrays all the varied stages and forms through which the human race has passed in the millions of years present-day man has been on the way.

The fact that heredity is and that it exercises profound influence in living things is probably universally known and daily made use of. If like should cease to produce like, chaos would prevail. But man's belief in the transmission through heredity of parental qualities to offspring is somewhat delimited to the physical. By patient observation and by unceasing effort man brings about improvement in certain physical forms—in livestock and in vegetables, in grains and in fruits. Man has found it to be possible to improve the flavour and the palatability of much of the vegetable food. Some weeds and some other wild things have been transformed through domestication and cultivation into nutritious and valuable foods. That fact means that inheritance is not confined always to the physical structure. But the improvement of quality by attention to heredity is not so assured nor so easy as in the physical structure.

We probably do not usually expect the highly useful acquisition in the immaterial domain to be transmitted with certainty to the offspring. The thoughtless speak sometimes disparagingly, if not derisively, of the minister's son. Lord Nelson was a rector's son. But the son of only one of our Presidents has become President.

Heredity it is that gives physical form to the living thing. The directive influence of heredity is transmitted to the offspring through the two parental particles that by their fusion begin the development of the individual—in the human as the embryo within the mother. Even at birth the baby's physical body is old, thousands, perhaps millions of years old. Those of us who hold such an opinion think that we have some degree of understanding of the phenomenon. But not even the scientists who spend their lives in working with living things give thought to the probable, or certain, associated truth that human behaviour is as old ancestrally as the human race and as the physical body of which it is an innate part. Heredity gives the human baby its body. That body can be seen, felt, often heard and sometimes smelt. It is obviously and dominatingly real, small though it is. In structure the baby's body differs little from that of the parent. Within the tiny baby, permeating it and associated with it, is an invisible, imponderable, impalpable structure, as old ancestrally as the physical body, millions of years old; and that immaterial structure has lived in and with the baby always, in safety and in danger, sustaining it and protecting it.

That structure is instinct. It is wisdom of the highest order. It was acquired by attending the ancestral school throughout the ages—primary and grammar school, high school and preparatory school; and university after university. Instinct is inherited ancestral wisdom. It embraces all those qualities that regulate behaviour in a given environment.

Instinct is the faculty of acting in such a way as to produce certain ends, without foresights of the ends, and without previous experience in the performances. Such was the conception of it of William James. The impulse to do the specific thing, to do it in a certain way, and under certain circumstances, is inherited. The doing of the thing requires neither acquired knowledge nor practice. Nay, more, the act does not imply that the performance of it carries with it an understanding of the reasons for the act or the results of it. But the animal may, I should say, come eventually to realize what may come to pass as results of frequent repetitions of the instinctive behaviour.

Why does the animal act instinctively, one may ask? And another might ask, too, why gravitation so affects the universe of matter? Why does Niagara flow downward and not upward? Why does the apple drop to the ground? In stumbling at the half-way landing, why does one not tumble on upstairs, instead of rolling over and over to the bottom? I realize that it is not polite to respond to an interrogatory by another question.

But instinct has no concern about politeness; nor about truth; nor ethics, morals, law, reason, right, wrong, religion, ignorance, knowledge, pride, shame, honour, patriotism, decency; and instinct cares not a snap of its fingers for Mrs. Grundy, nor for Emily Post. Instinct is; instinct represents an urge, a drive, an impulse toward and often into action. Far back in instinct the urge may be a longing, a yearning, a hunger for performance of a kind in keeping with the life of the species. I feel that instinctive behaviour comes in response to a tension that causes discomfort, or unrest, that can be relieved only by the action demanded by the specific urge.

All the instincts may be grouped, I should think, under two headings—self-sustaining; race perpetuating. Instinct, if articulate, might say to the animal: live and beget. Few animals, even human animals, seem to need any encouragement to do either.

Though many instincts are short-lived in children, their disappearances are usually succeeded by others. But the instinct to play in some way probably abides in us throughout life.

Man who would know himself and his fellow-mortal should devote dispassionate study to the primal and fundamental urges. In no other way can one be so impressively and so biologically informed. The same urges are in some degree, perhaps, in all mortals. All human beings are fundamentally alike; much more so than unlike. He who moves the multitudes makes use of that knowledge. If one could know all about instinct, then one would understand, perhaps, all conduct, and especially all forbidden, and much irrational, behaviour. Instinct, as the unconscious automatic adaptation of a means to an end, is the fountain and origin of the doings of most mortals. Many other influences affect the instinctive drives; sometimes by substitution, sometimes by concealment; not infrequently by camouflage, and often, of course, by denial and by other forms of untruthfulness.

Emotion may be thought of as the feeling-tone accompanying behaviour, and usually behaviour of the instinctive kind. It would be impossible to enjoy simulated happiness; and to be grief-stricken on account of affected sorrow. A genuine emotion probably cannot be called forth merely by effort. Nature is not hypocritical, though she may be wholly a-moral. An emotion probably does not cause action. But the behaviour, usually of the instinctive kind, may be enormously influenced by an emotion—in all gradations from complete suppression to the most uncontrollable exaggeration.

I suppose intelligence may be thought of as the capacity to engage in directed thinking. Intellectual activity must be rare if it is thinking unaffected by the instincts and the emotions. If intellectual honesty implies the ability to deal unemotionally and honestly with self, then such honesty is unusual.

I doubt if one can deal honestly with one's self—both because of too limited knowledge of one's self and because one thinks always protectively of self. Discipline—self-discipline—may be defined as purposeful habituation in behaviour. Thorough development of self-discipline keeps one always in complete possession of all of one's personal resources. The disciplined individual is never dominated by fear, nor surprised, nor apprehensive, nor self-condemnatory. Such discipline enables one always to try to live up to the level of one's ideals —not perfectly, not in self-satisfied fashion, but up to one's highest level; if not happy, at least ennobled. So lived Socrates and Jesus and Paul and Joan of Arc and Washington and Patrick Henry and Robert E. Lee and Stonewall Jackson; and some physicians, I hope; and many nurses, and innumerable humble mothers and fathers whose names have never appeared in print, and many also who gave their lives unobtrusively to teaching.

I believe that modern psychiatry does not regard consciousness as a necessary essence of mental life. Yet I suppose that the popular notion prevails that where there is no consciousness there can be no mental life. Psychiatry may feel justified in asserting, indeed, that a decided degree of mental life may exist without concomitant consciousness. In other words, consciousness does not constitute the sole feature of mental life; it is usually an aspect of mentality, but not a necessary feature of it. To the question: Has a sleeping person mental life? Psychiatry answers: Yes. To the question: Is the mind of the person who is unconscious, for some reason other than sleep, active? The answer of psychiatry again is: Yes. The necessary inference is that so-called consciousness and the mind are not synonymous terms. If the mind is to be spoken of structurally, as we are likely to do in these materialistic days, we must not permit ourselves to believe that the only occupant of that structure is consciousness. The mind is much larger than consciousness and much more complex than consciousness.

It seems well always when entering upon a discussion to find out first if the participants all have the same understanding of the meaning of the terms that are to be used. The word mind has already been used. I doubt if it can be acceptably defined, but we may all have the same conception of its function. That phenomenon which directs one in the pursuit of ends and which presides over the choice of methods adopted in the effort to reach the goal probably constitutes the mind. I believe that in our egotism we delimit its possession to members of the human race and deny its possession to all of the so-called lower animals. What those animals may think of our discrimination would be interesting; and we might be enlightened by it.

Involved in such a conception of the mind is the belief that all mental states are always teleological. That rather big and unusual word means that the mind in performing its functions always has an end in view. Every mental states is, therefore, purposeful; and it tends to action. Nature is probably always purposeful in action and never in confusion or in doubt. There are, indeed, mental philosophers who believe that action, movement, indeed, obvious or hidden, is a feature of every mental state. If that be true, it proffers in some degree an explanation of the fatigue and the hunger, too, that follows hard mental work. I am personally inclined to believe that hard physical and hard mental labour cannot be successfully performed at the same time by the same individual.

If we are to consider consciousness, we should define the phenomenon to which the term refers. Consciousness has been defined somewhat mechanistically as the transformation of physical into mental states. There is response, for example, to the pin-prick, because of the pain, in an effort to escape. The injury done to the tissues by the pinpoint is instantly changed into that psychological state known as pain. The response to the call of the telephone represents a higher form of transformation of a physiological into a psychological condition. Unconsciousness is the word used in referring to the situation in which the physical changes are not transformed into mental states. We know, however, that response to a stimulus may take place, and apparently purposeful response, without there being awareness of the response. Sometimes when, in semi-sleep, for example, one may make sensible answer to a call without being aware of it, at the time, or afterwards. In my internship days the superintendent of the hospital made it mandatory that the orders of the internes should always be written. Aroused from sound sleep late at night, the interne's verbal orders might have been lacking in validity.

The word "conscious" is, however, descriptive. We know little of what it implies in the depth of the individual. We do know, however, that an idea, for instance, may be fleeting, and have no fixedness or permanency. Each of you knows that. You know, for example, that three times two are six. Yet that idea abides in your mind only a little while occasionally. Where and what is that idea at all other times, when you are not thinking of it? We say it is latent. That means that under favourable conditions the idea can be called up at any moment; called back from wherever it may be, into consciousness again. The adjective "latent" would seem to imply, then, capable of being called back into consciousness.

But there is another department, so to speak, of

unconsciousness, in addition to the "latent unconscious." It would seem to be true that a powerful mental process, an idea, indeed, may exist without the individual's being aware of its existence; and this process may affect the mental state profoundly. This process may act as a force in cutting certain ideas out of existence as conscious ideas, and removing them from the individual's conscious mental life. Although this is an active process, the individual is unaware that it is taking place. The ideas that are kept out of consciousness are said to be in a state of repression, and the force which initiated the repression and maintains it is spoken of as resistance. The process is not at all accidental or casual, but it is active and dynamic and unconsciously purposeful. This latter aspect of unconsciousness may be spoken of, indeed, as the dynamic unconscious. The content of this division of the unconscious does not easily emerge into consciousness and great difficulty may be experienced by the individual, even with the help of the physician, in bringing into light the dynamic unconscious.

All knowledge is bound up with consciousness. We can know nothing of the unconscious until it becomes conscious. How can the unconscious become or be made conscious? Through the perceptive apparatus. Perceptions received from without are called sense-perceptions. Those from within are chiefly sensations and feelings. And thought-processes that seem to come from deep within may be thought of fundamentally as displacements of mental energy on its way towards action. Does this displaced energy make its way towards the surface of the mind, so to speak, where perceptions are recognized; or does consciousness proceed, so to speak, to meet the oncoming mental energy? It is probable that the moving mental energy, anxious to be in action, comes into association with some memory-residue,—words, for example; and in association with verbal images the unconscious becomes preconscious and then conscious.

We are all conscious of feelings, longings, fears and hopes that never assume the form of words, probably because they never encounter the residues of memory-images as verbal-images. Much mental activity in man must take place far below the word-level. The highest wisdom of the individual probably cannot be spoken. I have no doubt that much purposeful and highly useful conduct has its motivations far beneath the level of words. In such instances the individual, when asked in the courtroom or elsewhere why he did what he did can make no answer in words. Because words did not tell him to do what he did.

The content of the restless unconscious, or the subconscious, as it was once more frequently called, is varied, complex and resentful, because it is repressed, cabined and confined and restrained. And it is without knowledge of itself with which to comfort itself.

It would be presumptuous of me to speak to you of the spaciousness of the mind—of the variety and the complexity and the profundity of its content. I have spoken of it somewhat materialistically as divisible into the conscious, the preconscious and the unconscious. The latter division is by far the larger, the more varied, the more interesting and the more influential in the individual's life, in society and in history.

To the late Dr. Sigmund Freud, of Vienna, we are indebted for that medical philosophy that has come to be known as psychoanalysis. It is based upon Freud's discovery of the division of mental life into the conscious and the unconscious. Freud himself was persecuted and finally banished from Austria by Hitler. Freud's belief was that the major portion of the individual's psyche lies buried in the unconscious, and that there most of behaviour arises. And he taught, too, that the unconscious must be analyzed—dissected, if necessary—in order that the individual may be understood both by his physician and by himself. And Freud practised that form of psychiatric diagnosis and that form of psychotherapy embraced by the term psychoanalysis. His philosophy has affected the mental life of all thoughtful people.

The tendency of human beings is to ascribe the behaviour of the so-called lower animals wholly to instinct and the conduct of ourselves to intelligence. But we mortals were once, probably millions of years ago, almost wholly animals, too, and the behaviour of our ancestors in those distant days was altogether of instinctive origin. We have not succeeded in banishing the instinctual constituent of our mental life. We are probably still richer in instinctual drives and urges than any of the lower animals. But we are unwilling to believe or to recognize that fact.

Such discussion is not of mere academic importance. Knowledge of the origin and the meaning and the value of behaviour is useful in every domain of thought. Within the mind of man conflicts between trends are constantly taking place. The instincts, with which we mortals are still so generously endowed, constitute powerful urges to do many things. And the instincts are interested only in gratifying their own innate yearnings or hungers. They have no concern about the so-called higher things of life—education and law and religion and ethics and right and wrong. The chief concern of the instincts, but of course they are not conscious of the purpose they serve, is to preserve the individual and to perpetuate the race. If the instincts could think, and if they would speak to us frankly about their thinking, they would tell us, of course, that most of their thinking is about sexuality. But the member of modern society is not permitted to think out loud about sex; such thinking is thought to be ugly.

It is easy to surmise that many of the instinctual urges in man are disapproved by some of man's mental acquisitions—by his sense of decency and honesty and by his respect for law and order and public opinion and ethics and religion. In consequence of man's inability to give free rein to many of his instinctual urges, as his remote ancestors did, he finds himself disturbed by the conflict that is taking place within his mind all the time—conflict between the content of the Id and the repressions, on the one hand; and the ego and the super-ego, the conscience, on the other hand. Many nervous and mental conditions are merely manifestations of that unceasing conflict. If the instinctual urge to behave naturally in unhampered response to the drive is interfered with, dissatisfaction is experienced, probably discomfort, mayhap actual disease. Hysteria, for example, arises in the unconscious. The symptoms serve to constitute a protest because of the unwillingness of the individual to liberate the instinctual urges freely through unhampered behaviour; or incapacity to keep submerged so far in the depths of unconsciousness all such instinctual drives that the individual will be unaware of their existence. Most of the neuroses also originate in the unconscious, and in their symptomatology they represent the conflict in the individual between the two trends—the one to behave wholly naturally in response to the instincts; the other, to try to live in conformity to the demands of higher civilization. But to live so, in such distracted times as the present, requires unceasing effort, and the utilization of much mental energy. In consequence of the unending struggle many so-called nervous breakdowns occur. Neurasthenia, psychasthenia, much inadequacy, many life failures, many hurtful indulgences in alcohol and in other drugs, and many suicides have such origins. And the internist and the surgeon are finding out that every complaint of physical discomfort, even of sharp, local pain, does not necessarily imply the existence of underlying pathologic disorder. Such complaints may merely mean that the patient is unaware of or unwilling to confess the existence of the conflict within. The conflict means, of course, that man is fearfully and wonderfully made and curiously wrought in the most secret parts, as the patriarch discovered long ago. And the trouble that man constantly experiences in living with his spacious and complex inner self, about which he neither knows nor wishes to know, illustrates the importance and the difficulty of obtaining a frank history of the individual's life. What medical man possesses either the skill or the patience adequate for such an undertaking?

There are many other aspects of human behaviour about which I would have communion with you. Yet I recall that many of my friends remind me that I have no sense of time. I think it strange that, though a person is never blamed for having organic physical sickness, such for example as Bright's disease or gallstones or tuberculosis, he is often dealt with punitively for being mentally sick. Mental sickness makes itself known, you know, symptomatically through changed behaviour. And nothing takes a person into prison and into the court room so frequently as behaviour. Both society and the law are slow to realize and perhaps unwilling to believe that man is unable to declare his insanity otherwise than through his behaviour.

The great tragedy of human existence probably lies in the assumption that in man intelligence can ever serve as a substitute for instinct. The attempt at the substitution probably always results in failure. I speak merely biologically and not intellectually or moralistically. All pleasures that afford fundamental gratification and satisfaction are probably instinctual. Man may not be civilizable. He may be both unwilling and unable to hold himself steadily in such a plane.

Warfare may represent man's unconscious protest against the demands of sustained civilization; his confession that he is incapable of civilization and his momentary relief from intolerable repression and his sadistic joy in lusty biologic life.

We must take off our ethical lenses and look upon and into man as he is.

Some day your organization may discard the adjective mental, and come to be known as the Hygiene Society. Man's behaviour cannot be separated from man. The act cannot be detached from the actor, though the futile effort is made in the law and in theology. Man is a unit, not part body and part mind; but a living organism. Man cannot be partially well or fractionally sick. Man and his environment are intimately related. It is the duty of society and of medicine to see to it that each is fit for the other.

PLUTARCH, in his Essays, uses an illustration (borrowed from some philosopher more ancient than himself): "Should the body sue the mind before a court of judicature for damages, it would be found that the mind would prove to have been a ruinous tenant to its landlord."—*Isaac D'Isreali.*

A SIMPLE HAEMOGLOBIN ESTIMATION in itself can be of immense help in making an early diagnosis of carcinoma of the stomach. Most malignant areas in the stomach bleed. In 18 successive cases, only three gave a haemoglobin value of 90% at the first examination, and the average value was 65%.—*E. C. Warner* in *Practitioner*, April.

A Practical Introduction to Rorschach Work

VICTORIA CRANFORD, Catonsville, Maryland
Rorschach Worker and Psychotherapist at the Haarlem Lodge Sanatorium
AND
ROBERT V. SELIGER, M.D., Baltimore
Visiting Psychiatrist, Johns Hopkins Hospital, and Instructor in Psychiatry at the Johns Hopkins Medical School

Received for publication May 15, 1944

IN VIEW OF THE FACT that Rorschach analyses and work more and more figure in medical psychology, and in the study of personalities, it seems well to say a few words about this technique—how it originated, what its functions are and can be, and to mention some of the practical uses of the "ink-blot test."

Hermann Rorschach, a brilliant young Swiss psychiatrist, died of peritonitis in 1922 at the age of thirty-seven, only a few months before his monograph, *Psychodiagnostik*, was published.

This monograph, the cornerstone of all Rorschach work, was the result of his eleven years' intensive research, work, and study with the ink-blot in the field of personality diagnosis.

Rorschach's studies were based on earlier pioneer work by Justinius Kerner, Binet and other psychologists of the 19th century who used ordinary ink-blots, made by dropping ink on a piece of paper, folding the paper through the blot, and producing a more-or-less symmetrical, intrinsically meaningless "picture." An individual, looking at this picture, was stimulated to associate with its objective features certain personal memories or thoughts or identifications, and early psychologists saw in the ink-blot possibilities of testing personality traits and trends. Further investigation of these possibilities led Rorschach to evolve the standardized procedure now used by psychiatrists, with certain modifications due to cultural and sociological changes in the course of twenty years.

In our work, we use the Rorschach as a practical tool for personality evaluation, diagnosis and therapy indicator; and we will discuss these and other practical uses a little later on.

The material consists of a series of ten plates, as standardized by Rorschach and remaining unchanged. Selected from thousands of trial ink-blot pictures, they fulfill the various scientific requirements of the experiment, and portray certain fundamental situations sufficiently inclusive and delineable for one to be able to assay, through interpretation, important personality traits, trends, etc.: the degree and level and condition of mental health and of intelligence; the emotional stability or maturity; presence of conflicts, tensions, anxieties; and other factors and facts which will later be summarized.

The value of the Rorschach lies in its being a projective technique which can be measured. A projective technique is any controlled method which supplies objective but intrinsically meaningless stimulus-material (or material capable of various meanings and uses) to an individual and measures what he puts out in interpretation. This is done through analytic study of his projective (interpretive) use of this material, and through comparison with results of other people's use of the same material. Thus certain results and conclusions are derived which constitute the differential analysis of various personality traits and trends. This analysis is accomplished through the use of a methodological procedure of psychological weights and measures which anyone with requisite training, skill and experience can use and so reach equivalent conclusions.

A projective technique, then, to yield most satisfactory results, would be one least dependent on subjective elements, i.e., the interpreter's thinking, attitudes, personal experience, and position of arbiter between satisfactory and unsatisfactory material put out by the individual. It would also have to be flexible and more inclusive than, say, the "yes" or "no" or "sometimes" standards of many quizzes. Excluding other features, on the basis of these two postulates, we can see that certain types of play techniques used in child study and study of psychotics allow for great flexibility but do not, perhaps, sufficiently fence out the examiner's subjectivity, and so are not greatly controlled in the sense of an objective, scientific procedure of measurement.

The Rorschach technique attempts to come as close as possible to a standardized objective method whereby certain personality elements can be accurately measured and revealed by the individual, without his conscious control over concept or words interfering, and so invalidating the findings. In the Rorschach, many factors are of equal importance; no one factor is given a deciding influence in the final interpretation.

All one needs as material for a Rorschach analysis are the ink-blots, paper and pencil. The ten plates standardized by Rorschach measure 7x9½ inches and, as indicated, they attempt to incorporate various distinct situations—easy, approachable;

new, hard to approach; sex in its various phases in the psychosexual field, etc. Therefore, one keeps in mind the fact that the individual is projecting his *total* personality with conflicts, frustrations and so forth in various situations.

In general, the administrator and Rorschach worker desire to score accurately the responses given, along lines of: number of responses, rejections, time-blocking on certain cards, determinants —that is, what caused the individual to make a particular response—content of responses and whether the response is usual, unusual, odd, or rare. These are obtained through the initial responses and through the inquiry.

The material is then tabulated according to various types of movement—human, animal, inanimate, together with the form, and use of vista and perspective responses. These are the *introversive indicators;* and, interpreted with all the other responses, they supply the maturity, capacity and ability, basic drives and trends; and any frustrations, or insight, or anxieties present. On the other hand, the *extraversive responses* having to do with shading, etc., are interpreted as indicating the tact, social adjustment, tendencies to temper outbursts, egocentricity and reaction to external stimuli with or without good emotional brake-power.

It is necessary to mention here that *introversive* and *extraversive*, as used in terms of a Rorschach, do not have the meanings given them by Jung *et al*.

Introversive means, for example, a tendency toward inner creative life and mature thinking ability and a measure of self-reliance and stability. *Extraversive* means a tendency toward needing and wanting contact with other people and various types of social situations, with different degrees of egocentricity and emotional warmth, control, and sensitivity. Further, as a rule, these tendencies are interdependent and serve more as indicators of trends, basic or otherwise, than as evidences of actual dominant traits. They are interpreted always in dynamic terms of interrelationship.

Sometimes these tendencies are in equal balance, and we then say, in a Rorschach analysis, that an individual is *ambiversive;* again meaning that there are more or less equal tendencies toward the *introversive* and toward the *extraversive*, as above defined.

Thus, in a general way, one sees how a personality structure is revealed through the ink-blots. One also — in the Rorschach methodology — ascertains the level and type of intelligence of the individual, obsessive-compulsive trends, perfectionistic attitudes; and, through the content, type of response, position of particular response, one is able to bring out specific material—parental or sibling fixations, latent or overt homosexual trends, conflictual material and also specific hostilities.

By properly interpreting the whole Rorschach analysis, with careful work on each detail of the scoring and relationship, a Rorschach analysis enables one to see whether a personality is deteriorated, neurotic, psychopathic, schizophrenic, epileptic, poorly integrated emotionally, or over-loaded by life and perhaps only temporarily out of the running.

Some workers advocate the use of a Rorschach to determine whether or not electric shock treatment would probably be effective in certain depressive reactions. Other types of illness can also be screened and the type of treatment indicated through means of a Rorschach. One can, with the alcoholic patient, get at some of the underlying mechanisms, possible causes or motivations that helped produce the addiction, and sort out the neurotic-alcoholic from the psychopathic-alcoholic, the schizoid-neurotic-alcoholic from the schizophrenic-alcoholic, and so on. Further, with this, one is supplied with objective data of an individual's stresses, tensions, unconscious attachments, and hostilities, and so enabled to slant and direct therapy at the outset, regardless of the patient's self-appraisal, defensive techniques, blocks in therapy, etc., and, possibly, of one's own feelings about the individual's make-up and problem.

A Rorschach is of practical aid in understanding children's behavior personality problems and those of the aged. It is felt to be helpful in job placement and industrial psychiatry. Likewise, it is of service in criminal-court cases, and is used by various penological groups and at different prisons in this country. In modified forms the Rorschach has been utilized at various army induction stations for screening purposes. Any individual plate can serve as a stimulus for starting a train of free association.

Although many of Hermann Rorschach's findings were based on a European cultural structure and so may be held inadequate for our American type culture, conclusions reached are still derived from the fundamentals set forth by him and are, for the most part, reliable and accurate. We, among others, are, in a practical working way, attempting to adapt the Rorschach to our present-day cultural pattern in this country, taking into consideration different racial and regional backgrounds, economic, educational, and age status, and so on.

We consider the Rorschach as probably the best objective diagnostic scientific method in personality study and borderline difficult cases, and one that will become increasingly useful and important in the field of medical psychology.

Doctors' Responsibility for Expansion of Medical and Hospital Facilities

K. B. PACE, M.D., Greenville, N. C.

ALTHOUGH this article is written with special reference to the situation in North Carolina, I hope it will be of interest to the doctors in other states.

For the past two or three years, we have heard and read much on post-war planning. Of great interest to our profession are the plans as to better surgical and medical care for the low-income group and the indigent. A great deal has been done in providing low-cost hospitalization, operations, better obstetrical care and medical attention through the Blue Cross organizations. This insurance plan provides the best service at unbelievably low cost. All physicians and surgeons should be more alert in promoting and familiarizing their patients with this type of insurance. There are now about 800,-000 individuals in North Carolina who carry this protection in the Blue Cross and other companies. This is all well and good. It gives splendid service at only a fraction of the cost as compared with that proposed on a nation-wide scale, under one control, as expressed in the government proposal.

We laud this work highly; but the time has come when we must branch out and include all kinds of medical and hospital care for cities, towns, villages and country. For this necessary expansion I mean, first, there must be promotion of additional hospital facilities to relieve the over-crowded hospitals and to provide room for numberless undiagnosed cases that might be referred for thorough examination, diagnosis and suggested treatment when they are returned to their family physician.

All of us appreciate thoroughly the services of this nature given by the various diagnostic centers in North Carolina and adjoining states. Every doctor in active practice is, however, only too familiar with experiencing difficulty and delay in finding a vacant hospital bed. Many times it is days and often weeks before a bed is available, especially in the wards at the medical college hospitals. The first need, then, is additional hospital beds. The second need, which is really of equal importance, is more training facilities within North Carolina for providing enough physicians for the people's care. The third need is a program for encouraging physicians to locate in small towns and rural districts. This need cannot be too strongly emphasized.

It is remarkable that so large a percentage of the profession in North Carolina are anxious to be informed on all the needs and proposals before the public and that they are squarely behind the plan for adding to the University of North Carolina Medical School at Chapel Hill the last two years required for a medical degree and for making it a full Grade A, four-year medical college.

This expansion of the Medical School of the University would not only train more physicians but also help meet the need for more hospital beds and another diagnostic center; and to those, if there be any, who are not yet convinced of the need of another diagnostic center, I should like to say that before the present situation we are in was explained to me, I also thought we had enough hospital beds.

But, as previously stated, I am frequently told by other physicians and surgeons of the delay they have in getting a bed in a large hospital for a thorough examination and study of cases where diagnosis is difficult and undetermined. Moreover, on the lists showing hospital beds of the respective states, North Carolina ranks near the bottom in number of hospital beds per thousand population.

Establishing a four-year medical college and a four-hundred-bed hospital with the teaching college would still leave North Carolina lacking sufficient hospital beds. But this would be an excellent beginning and certainly much better than Federal wholesale planning which would attempt to cover the whole country with one blanket law. This latter planned and executed too swiftly and on too large a scale would be unusually expensive in setup and operation; the haste would necessarily cause many mistakes and less efficient service.

At the University of North Carolina the hospital and four-year medical school would be strictly under management of the trustees and the profession. It would be free from all the objectionable features of Federal control. Some might say that the expenses of the last two-year school would be too high, but there are at Chapel Hill so many factors that would work to the benefit of the school that expansion of the present facilities would not be like building in a city where both medical college and hospital would have to be built in their entirety. There are already at Chapel Hill a very large medical building, a small hospital recently built and now being used by the Navy, and full facilities for teaching chemistry and all other sciences necessary to medicine. The main expense to complete a Grade A, four-year medical college would be for only three things: a large hospital, a nurses' home, and additional medical teaching faculty.

I think every physician in North Carolina will agree that we must meet the situation in medicine and hospital care as we did the school program in 1900 and the road-building in 1920. Surely the medical profession is the one body to take the lead and help in every way in promoting the health and happiness of all the citizens of our state. The medical college with its medical hospital would be a much-needed additional diagnostic center and would train thousands of physicians and surgeons essential to the whole health program.

Probably the most urgent need of all for our profession within this state is to see that enough North Carolina boys be given opportunity to study medicine so as to help stop the constantly increasing shortage of doctors in their home state. Statistics show us that for many years we have been falling farther and farther behind in our effort to locate in North Carolina sufficient doctors to supply the population adequately. In recent years we have been getting worse instead of better, and now in some localities there is hardly one doctor to 2500 persons, a shortage that cannot be attributed wholly or mainly to the present war.

Statistics show that from our two four-year medical colleges and other sources we get only two-thirds of the number of physicians needed for replacements by death, retirements and change from private practice to positions in medical college teaching staffs and removals from the state. It is estimated that in order to bring North Carolina up nearer the average for other states in the proper proportion of doctors to population, we need 1500 more physicians. This would require 75 additional physicians each year in addition to the number we already get, and it is estimated that in twenty years we would bring North Carolina up to the ratio of one doctor to a 1000 population. A university four-year medical college is the best solution for providing enough men in the practice of medicine in our state.

That more physicians will be needed not only for replacements is recognized in another change which has already faced us and is becoming more evident. The new graduates when entering practice will not make the mistake we older ones have of working fourteen to sixteen hours a day. Modern teaching for wholesome, most efficient living has trained them to take time off for recreation and vacations. I, for one, rejoice because they will work shorter hours and not make the mistake we older ones have of early exhaustion through too long hours of staying on the job. Nevertheless, more physicians must be trained and ready to cover the field under these new habits.

More accessible training and at less cost because it would be in easy reach bring a partial answer also to the question, How can we get more doctors to locate in the small towns and rural sections? If young men, and young women, too, for that matter, drawn from our rural communities would be fully trained within the state, great numbers of them would return to the localities they know and love, instead of accepting opportunities that may open to them in the distant cities to which many must go if they graduate from medical college. North Carolina's rural population supplies a notable percentage of students in the medical profession; they realize the needs of their people; and if a local university medical college could provide them adequate training, they would serve our modern rural folks.

It is my suggestion I wish to offer that a committee be appointed from the State Medical Society whose duty it shall be to coöperate with the medical college in getting a plan worked out whereby sufficient numbers of doctors may be encouraged to choose rural communities for location.

I recently read a very excellent, timely article in the September issue of the *Progressive Farmer*, on the subject, "How Can We Get Better Medical Care and Hospital Care?" It is written by the editor, Clarence Poe; and I commend it to your attention. The public is being informed by such articles as this. The people are looking to us, the medical profession, to lead the way, to bring this to pass, as we are best informed and qualified to do it. We shall not fail them.

To most of us the idea that deep breathing may be dangerous will be a new thing—

DANGER OF DEEP BREATHING IN PRESENCE OF THROMBOPHLEBITIS OR PHLEBOTHROMBOSIS
(Bul. U. S. Army Med. Dept., May)

The increase of intrathoracic negative pressure in inspiration is an important factor in sucking blood into the chest from venous channels elsewhere in the body. It is of the utmost importance that wherever thrombophlebitis or phlebothrombosis is suspected or established, deep respiration should be avoided.

When a patient has experienced a sharp pain in the chest and has expectorated bright red blood a few days postoperatively, or in the presence of thrombophlebitis, the diagnosis of embolism is likely and the location largely academic. There is a strong risk of *recurrent* emboli and this is markedly increased by deep breathing. The common practice of having the patient breathe deeply or cough during the physical examination of the chest should be omitted. Death has occurred during and immediately after such examinations.

While ligation of a vein proximal to a recognized site of thrombosis may reduce the risk of pulmonary embolism,

DISCUSSION OF INTRAVENOUS THERAPY
(From *Penn. Med. Jl.*, May, 1943, via *Clin. Med.*, July)

Before intravenous medication is given to an ambulatory patient, we should be satisfied that the drug may not be used in some other way with equally good results. Too often the chief reasons for medication by vein seem to lie in the ease of administration, and the fact that the patient will return. Intravenous medication should be given with the patient's stomach empty.

If a patient arrives at the hospital in a state of deep shock and dehydration, the worse possible procedure is to start giving saline or glucose intravenously. The major danger is that plasma proteins would be washed out of the vascular system by adding a diffusable crystalloid. Those who use too much crystalloid solution are in the majority. Since water is generally the element that one desires to replace the ideal method is to give it in isotonic form, that is, either with saline or 5% glucose. More concentrated glucose in certain cases in which a hepatitis plays a part may be justified; but in the ordinary case there is little need for this since if you give it slowly, you might as well give 5%; and given rapidly, it is soon over the kidney threshold and is lost in the urine.

In cases of protracted dehydration and starvation, to oxidize a greater number of ketone bodies, 10% and even higher concentrations are indicated, insulin being given at the same time and in proper dosage.

Many patients will develop edema from isotonic salt solution. Such patients have a critical hypoproteinemia though peripheral edema is not noticeable. In the treatment of nephrosis, a condition in which the blood proteins are low, satisfactory results have not been obtained by giving blood transfusions or ordinary plasma, but results were excellent when lyophilized plasma was given. Recently a boy, a typical hemophiliac, who bled from broken teeth, had 18 or 20 transfusions (ordinarily the proper treatment), but without avail. One dose of lycophilized plasma, and the bleeding stopped promptly.

Where proteins can be fed by mouth or into the alimentary tract lower down, those are the routes of choice for building plasma protein. If these routes are not available the next best way to supply the body with protein is to give plasma in large quantity—perhaps a liter a day.

In a case of renal or biliary or some other colic some individuals receive relief within 15 or 30 seconds if the morphine is given slowly, intravenously. Dissolve ¼ gr. morphine tablet in sterile water and inject *very slowly* until the pain disappears.

THE NERVOUS PATIENT
(G. O. Segrest, Mobile, in *Jl. Med. Assn. Ala.*, July)

The medical profession has been made conscious of organic disease, probably too much so, by medical school teaching, autopsies, and instruments of precision. On the other hand, I well remember two patients with meningitis, in both of whom I missed the diagnosis until late in the disease because both had a typical hysterical reaction. I had seen both of these persons have such reactions to unhappy situations, but the last hysteria they ever had was a reaction to a fatal meningeal infection. One of these was tuberculous.

A patient of mine, a young man, recently died at the age of 23 of a brain tumor diagnosed too late for surgery to be attempted. This patient had had typical migraine attacks with cyclic vomiting since early childhood. The tumor at first only aggravated the migraine headaches.

Especially in the summer afternoon, a temperature between 99 and 100 suggests mild heat exhaustion as the explanation, rather than incipient tuberculosis, cancer or undulant fever.

Many patients with loss of appetite and slight nausea have been treated by me with pituitary extract and in a few instances with gratifying results. In some cases, symptoms of so-called spastic colon have been relieved after learning that the patient was sensitive to one or two foods.

From suspension of a floating kidney I have not seen the first a success, and the number of appendices that have been removed in the name of chronic appendicitis is a disgrace that stinks to high heaven.

Many neurotic people come to the physicians with symptoms referable to the heart.

I often think of these people as having a very narrow comfortable range, a range so narrow that it is impossible to stay out of the rough.

DDT POWDER FOR THE DESTRUCTION OF BODY LICE
(A. L. Ahnfeldt, Lt. Col., Med Corps, & Dir. Sanitation and Hygiene, Div. Office of the Surg. Gen., in *Jl. Tenn. Med. Assn.*, Aug.)

A mixture of 10% DDT in pyrophyllite was adopted for use. Each soldier carries a can in his pack, and the powder is applied by dusting it onto the inner surface of the underwear before he dons the garment, paying particular attention to the seams.

DDT was applied at mass dusting stations which were set up all over Naples. Each station was manned by six to 20 persons. Over a million-and-a-half individuals were deloused with DDT powder in less than one-and-a-half months. Up to the middle of March over two and one-quarter million persons had been so treated. The epidemic was stopped, and to date no case of typhus has been reported in an American soldier in Italy.

The impregnation of underwear with a DDT emulsion has proved effective against lice after the clothing has been laundered eight times over two months.

Production of DDT is moving ahead at an accelerated pace, but is still not sufficient to meet our own requirements. The Geigy Company was the only manufacturer of DDT in this country for the first eight months of the production program.

I firmly believe that the discovery of DDT offers the hope of a new era in insect control and will rank with the great discoveries in medicine of the past century. DDT should close the door forever on those diseases which are companions of death-dealing insects.

TRAUMATIC RUPTURE OF THE INTESTINE
(A. N. Collins, Duluth, in *Minn. Med.*, April)

Sudden trauma to the abdominal wall may cause grave havoc within the abdominal cavity without visible external sign of injury. A man so injured by blunt trauma may, after the first shock of the blow has subsided, return to his work but only when nausea or vomiting appears or abdominal pain recurs does he suspect he may be severely injured. This ability to carry on may mislead the physician when the patient reports for consultation and may result in delay which often contributes to a bad prognosis.

A saving of 96 out of 100 soldier-lives from meningitis death has been achieved by sulfadiazine. The meningitis death rate in our Army in the present war is less than 5%, whereas it was 39.2% in World War I.

DEPARTMENTS

HUMAN BEHAVIOUR

James K. Hall, M.D., *Editor*, Richmond, Va.

BARBITURATES AND BROMIDES AS CAUSES OF MENTAL DISEASE

In the *Journal of Nervous and Mental Disease* for August, 1944, Dr. Frank J. Curran, of New York, occupies almost thirty pages in discussing the barbiturates and the bromides as provocatives of mental disorder, whether taken in an overdose or in medicinal doses over a considerable period of time.

It may be difficult for the physician inexperienced in the toxic effect of a drug so mild as a bromide to believe that it may produce in a mentally normal person the wildest delirium; and that a barbiturate may disturb the psyche almost as decidedly, instead of inducing sedation or sleep. Are medical students of today informed by their investigative work in pharmacology or in the classroom work in materia medica that the bromides and the barbiturates are also delirifacient?

Seven or eight years ago Dr. Curran published his first paper dealing with the neuropsychiatric effects of bromides and barbiturates. Since then he has made a number of additional contributions to the subject. His last paper, to which this review refers, was prepared for presentation to the annual meeting of the American Association for the Advancement of Science in New York, December 28th, 1942, but that meeting was cancelled. In the paper Dr. Curran summarizes his own views on the subject, and in addition, he reviews almost a hundred and fifty contributions to medical literature by English and American authors since 1937. He concludes his article by the report of the condition of a woman made delirious by bromide medication and of another woman made psychotic by taking a large amount of a barbiturate with suicidal intent. Each patient under vigorous treatment was brought back to her normal state.

Balard discovered bromide in 1826. Within ten years the physiological and therapeutic uses of it had been described. Before 1860 it was being used in epilepsy and in the neuroses. Bromide intoxication was described in a patient in 1850; in 1877 Seguin discussed the result of the abuse of it as a sedative, and he catalogued the symptoms of chronic bromide poisoning: debility, cold limbs, memory impairment, and the resemblance of the state to that of paresis. Wuth in 1927 gave an account of a method for estimating bromide, qualitatively and quantitatively, in the blood and in the urine. Solomon describes the pharmacological action of the bromides: They depress all the central nervous system except the medulla, they depress also the psychic functions, the motor cortex and the spinal cord, lowering its reflex excitability.

When hypnotic doses of barbiturates are given, the individual's gait becomes unsteady and he becomes somnolent. The individual may not yield to large doses by falling asleep. On the contrary, there may be periods of purposeless struggle, rage, or muscular tremors or rigidity. In such a predicament, the pulse rate is likely to be increased, respiration slowed, gastro-intestinal peristalsis slowed, blood pressure lessened and body temperature lowered. If death should occur from an overwhelming dose of the drug, it would probably be caused by respiratory failure or by vasomotor collapse. Most investigators believe that the barbiturates are taken up, perhaps almost equally so, by the cells of the body generally, rather than by affinity cells in the brain or elsewhere. Barbital and phenobarbital are said to be eliminated in the urine of normal persons practically unchanged; but amytal and pentobarbital are thought to be decomposed in the body, with little elimination of them in the urine. The barbiturates, synthetic substances, in common use are: allurate, amytal, barbital, ipral, luminal, nembutal and pentobarbital. More than 60 barbiturates are known, and several hundred are chemically possible.

Neurological symptoms occur in persons poisoned by bromides and by barbiturates. Nystagmus is frequently present in barbiturate intoxication, but seldom in uncomplicated bromide poisoning. Babinski's sign is less often found in poisoning by barbiturates, seldom if at all in bromidism. Generalized convulsions are not unknown in barbiturate intoxication. The corneal and the pharyngeal reflexes, lost in deep bromide poisoning, are usually not lacking in barbiturate overdosage. Tremors of lips, tongue and fingers are features of poisoning by either drug. The gait-disturbance in barbiturate poisoning is suggestive of cerebellar disorder. The unsteady walking of the bromide patient is more suggestive of mere awkwardness. The symptomatology of the barbiturate condition may suggest lethargic encephalitis, multiple sclerosis, syringomyelia, or tabes.

Skin rash is rarely seen in association with mental disorder in bromide intoxication. Such a rash is more likely to occur on the face and the neck. It is acneform in appearance. The skin rash due to barbiturate intoxication is more like that of urticaria, or of scarlatina, in appearance; and it tends to spread over the trunks and the limbs. Sometimes the mucous membranes are affected severely by the rash; and the skin may be violently responsive to the toxicity of the drug. One patient lost all his finger nails and toe nails. One patient's skin condition, suggestive of exfoliative dermatitis, immediately preceded death.

Mental disorder may constitute the first manifestation of the drug intoxication, and the cause and the nature of the psychosis may not be recognized. In mental disease due to bromide poisoning the prominent, and often the dramatic, manifestation is delirium. That state may be mild, or wild and violent. Delirium is a symptom in probably two-thirds of the patients. Features associated with the delirium are hallucinations, most often of sight and of hearing. But the things seen and heard are usually not so near the patient as are the snakes, elephants, rats and bugs in alcoholic delirium. The speech is affected, jumbled, mumbled or shouted; and the thought-content is disordered. Often the patient in such condition is lost as to place and time, spatially and temporally, if the technical jargon must be used. The memory may be profoundly impaired. There may be complaints of bodily unsteadiness, as if one were on a rocking boat. Not infrequently speech is a mere medley of messed-up words that carry no meaning.

Barbiturate intoxication may occur in acute or in chronic form, and a single large dose may be taken after medicinal small doses have been taken for some time. But delirium is a rare manifestation of barbiturate poisoning. After too large a dose, taken for suicidal or other purposes, profound coma is likely to develop. Convulsions may occur. The deep reflexes are depressed. Nystagmus may be present. The pulse rate is likely to be quickened, the temperature at first falls and then rises, there is likely to be cyanosis of the moist skin. The pulse may become thready. The patient may emerge from coma in an excited, resistive, or belligerent condition: disoriented, deluded, euphoric and without appreciation of the situation, and be difficult to control. If the drug was taken in overdose with suicidal intent, the self-destructive impulse may become urgent again after the slow return to consciousness. Not infrequently, the comatose and confused condition is followed by excitement, sometimes noisy; and by overactivity associated with impaired memory and defective judgment. There are almost always motor disturbances, manifested in gait, station and in many other muscular activities. But the excited state is unlikely to last more than a few days.

In chronic barbiturate poisoning the condition may escape medical understanding, or result in mistaken diagnosis. Such poisoning may beget euphoria, and a state of feeling altogether out of keeping with the person's apparent poor health. But the chronic poisoning is more likely to exhibit itself in diminished mental alertness, in lessened interest, in more difficulty in understanding, in poor attention, in disturbance of associaton and in memory impairment. But there may be, in another individual, restlessness, talkativeness, irritability, petulance, sarcasm, facetiousness, arrogance, selfishness and a demanding and commanding attitude.

Does drug-taking often cause insanity? is such a question as the man on the street might ask. There are many drugs and the number of them constantly increases. But the piece under review limits the scope of its concern to two groups of drugs—bromides and barbiturates, and to that condition arising in consequence of overdosage in them, and manifesting the symptoms of insanity. It should be borne in mind, however, that generally the person is already nervously affected by taking the drug, and is physically and mentally less adequate, before the psychotic manifestations appear. And it is probable, too, that many persons take bromide or barbiturates to their hurt who never become psychotic, but whose efficiency is lessened.

Between 50 and 100 patients are admitted annually to the Psychiatric Division of Bellevue Hospital in New York who are psychotic because of drug addiction. Bromides and barbiturates are the two drugs most often involved. More than 100 persons are said to commit suicide in the United States each year by taking some barbiturate. Somewhat less than one per cent of all admissions to all mental hospitals in this country are said to be due to drug intoxication.

A section of Dr. Curran's lengthy and thorough study is devoted to the effects of sedatives on brain metabolism. Another division of the contribution details recent experimental work with barbiturates; and another with experimental work with bromides. An exceedingly interesting and enlightening report is made of the clinical uses of barbiturates and of the bromides. Two paragraphs outline the treatment of poisoning by the two drugs.

Dr. Curran believes that bromide intoxication evokes a type of mental disorder so characteristic that it should be recognized as specifically bromidic; and that the psychosis caused by barbiturate poisoning is characteristic.

I hope Dr. Curran's comprehensive survey will assume reprint form and that it may be widely distributed. We physicians probably often prescribe a barbiturate without good reason, and without taking the precaution to see to it that the patient does not take the drug too long. And we should caution lay people against the harm they may do to their health by resorting to the use of drugs said to be mild and harmless. The drug addicts in the United States must constitute a group of several millions.

Dr. Curran is a contribution of Minnesota to the East. He has been doing psychiatric work in Boston and in New York for two or three decades. Now, I believe he is chief of the Department of Psychiatry of the Medical College of New York University and of the Division of Psychiatry of Bellevue Hospital. He has long been interested in the psychotic effect of alcohol and of many other drugs. The Psychiatric Division of Bellevue is the great clearing-house for such conditions in New York City.

It is of the most practical value for physicians to know, for example, that a drug so mild as a bromide may produce the wildest delirium. Without such knowledge the physician might prescribe bromide for the patient in the beginning of the mental unrest caused by the bromide ingestion. And it is probably more important for the physician to understand that the barbiturates also are dangerous drugs and that their continued use may evoke physical and mental symptoms not easily differentiated, without a helpful patient history, from certain organic conditions. Apprehending officers probably arrest occasionally a toxic pedestrian or driver on the assumption that his digressive behaviour is of alcoholic origin. The ataxia may be due to the pharmacologic effect of a bromide or of a barbiturate.

I surmise that a request for a reprint of the study addressed to Dr. Curran at the Psychiatric Division of Bellevue Hospital in New York would reach him.

CLINICAL CHEMISTRY and MICROSCOPY

J. M. FEDER, M.D., and EVELYN TRIBBLE, M.T., *Editors*,
Anderson, S. C.

THE ART OF COLLECTING SPECIMENS AND GETTING THEM TO THE LABORATORY

PROLOGUE

THE VALUE of a laboratory examination depends to a great extent upon two factors. The first of these is the degree of care exercised to obtain a specimen properly; the other is furnishing the examiner with an adequate history of the case. Not infrequently a surgeon removes a bit of tissue from the body and with a wave of his hand instructs a nurse, graduate or otherwise: "Cut a piece out of this and send it to the laboratory." Here it is obvious that only the chance of an all-seeing Providence controlling the thrust of the knife can make her select the right tissue.

A case of a number of years ago: A tumor of the tongue had been removed and a nurse instructed: "Cut this in half. Send one piece to our laboratory, the other piece to Doctor X." Several days later, we delivered our report, "Chronic Inflammatory Reaction." It was extremely disconcerting a few days later to have the operator wave under our nose the findings of Doctor X, "Squamous-Cell Carcinoma. Grade 2." The cancerous portion had been sent to our neighboring pathologist, while the portion we received contained nothing worse than inflammatory reaction. In the event that it is at all possible the pathologist should designate the region from which the specimen is to be taken, or take it himself.

Operating in an area in which a pathological diagnosis is not available, special attention should be given to *marking* suspicious areas by passing a suture through each zone to be examined with special care.

In many cases the specimen should be seen by the laboratory physician in its fresh state, without fixation. In that event if not more than twelve hours is to elapse between removal and the examination, such tissues may be sent in ice making use of a tight-fitting jar or can or a vacuum jug.

TISSUES

The universal reagent for fixing tissues and preserving them during shipment is 10 per cent formaldehyde. Tissues are received unfit for examination because chloroform or alcohol, or even salt solution, has been depended on a preservative. When a large mass is being sent for examination, a number of gashes should be made in order that the formaldehyde may penetrate readily and prevent necrosis in the central portion.

It is necessary that a comprehensive history accompany the specimen. Diagnosis is in the interest of the patient, for on it depends decision as to mode of treatment, and in many a case on mode of treatment depends the patient's very life. For greatest accuracy diagnosis is a coöperative enterprise of clinician and pathologist, not a contest as to which is the more valuable, the bedside or the laboratory examination.

BLOOD FOR CHEMICAL EXAMINATION

The best interest of all concerned can be best served by sending the patient to the laboratory to have blood specimens taken for chemical examination. If this is impracticable, send the specimen *immediately* after withdrawal. Mail or other slow means of delivery spells deterioration in most instances, but a delay of as much as twelve hours will not seriously affect the majority of results. Blood sugar determination is an exception. If a delay in transit is unavoidable, 0.1 gram of powdered potassium fluoride should be introduced into the container for each 2 to 5 c.c. of blood collected. Such a blood specimen can be kept at room temperature for 24 to 48 hours without glycolysis occurring. If the ordinary oxalate is employed, the accuracy is diminished at the rate of 10 to 20 mgs. per hour.

BLOOD CULTURE

Remoteness from a laboratory need not prevent a blood culture being made when needed. Any central laboratory can prepare blood culture flasks in accordance with our technic given in *The Essentials of Applied Medical Laboratory Technic*—Feder, pages 82-84. (Vials of culture media ready for use can be obtained from Lederle Laboratories.) Other than the flask of medium, all that is necessary in a 10-c.c. syringe that has been boiled for ten minutes and an antiseptic such as merthiolate. This is applied to the rubber cap of the vial, the patient's arm is antiseptisised, 10 c.c. of blood is withdrawn and injected into the culture medium through the rubber diaphragm. Then a drop of collodion is applied to puncture in cap as an additional safeguard.

Shipping, in this instance especially, is synonymous with incubation, so no time is lost. It should be borne in mind that during the first ten days of a suspected typhoid, the blood culture is the diagnostic means of election—and we still have some typhoid.

COLLECTIONS OF BLOOD FOR WASSERMANNS, ETC.

Sterile dry tubes and syringes are essential. Lacking these, bacterial contamination and ill-defined, erroneous diagnosis are the reward. If boiling must be the means of sterilization, the tubes and syringes must be washed thoroughly with sterile normal saline solution to prevent hemolysis. The method of choice for collecting blood outside the laboratory for the Wassermann test is by using a vacuum tube of the Keidel type, Sheppard modification. The small-neck, regular Keidel tube is profanity-provoking.

BLOOD SLIDES FOR MALARIA, ETC.

For the physician who is *not sure* that he can make a serviceable film by the usual method, here is *a technic by which he cannot fail to make a satisfactory film*. On a *perfectly clean slide* place a small drop of blood near one end. Holding an ordinary cigarette-paper parallel with the slide let edge just touch the drop of blood. When it spreads across the width of the slide, draw paper to opposite end.

Few of the slides received for examination for malaria parasites are so made as to permit satisfactory examination and report. Of course, one end can usually be used in making a thick-smear examination.

THROAT CULTURE

Attention is invited to the fact that postal regulations require that *bacteriological specimens be* placed in tin containers, well-wrapped with some absorbent material, and this tin container placed in another tin container. Both of these must be very carefully closed.

Direct smears for the presence of diphtheria organisms are worthless, but on the other hand it is mandatory that a swab be sent with culture, for it is impossible to determine the presence of Vincent's organisms other than from the direct smear.

Every doctor who has to make an occasional throat culture should have constantly on hand Brahdy rapid-culture tubes (Lederle). These tubes make a diagnosis possible after 4- to 8-hours incubation. The laboratory receiving them will use them to prepare cultures on Löfler's medium for further study.

URINE FOR FRIEDMAN TEST FOR PREGNANCY

It is best to get an early-morning specimen and see that it reaches the laboratory promptly. During any lag in transportation the specimen should be surrounded by ice and insulated within a container to prevent chilling.

Urines for ordinary routine appraisal are best examined while fresh.

SPUTUM

This material should be sent to the laboratory in a wide-mouth, screw-top 1-ounce jar, and should contain *1 or 2* expectorations from deep down in the chest. One who has never handled filled-to-the-brim sputum containers can appreciate the reason for this insistence.

FECES

If some delay is expected in transit, a cubic-inch of material should be emulsified in 10-per cent formaldehyde in a wide-mouth bottle. This method is suitable for the various parasitic ova but worthless in the case of ameba. When this protozoön is suspected there is no substitute for a freshly-passed stool.

These few remarks are aimed towards the goal of best working together of the various clinicians and the laboratory folks. The methods given for collecting specimens are those used by the laboratories of the Anderson County Hospital and have proven satisfactory over a period of many years. Frequent talks between the laboratory staff and those sending in work are advantageous to all concerned—particularly the "main man," the patient.

SURGERY

GEO. H. BUNCH, M.D., *Editor*, Columbia, S. C.

SKIN CANCER

Attendance upon one of the Cancer Clinics, which are sponsored and operated over the nation by the State Boards of Health though largely supported by Federal funds, must impress any physician with the prevalence and the importance of epithelioma of the skin.

In the ageing process the human skin undergoes characteristic changes which, taken together, are known as senile atrophy. The skin becomes dry and thin, the hairs attenuated and lifeless. The skin is apt to be blotchy from irregular distribution of pigment, some areas pale while others are hyperpigmented. "Wrinkles, time's irremovable footprints," are caused by the loss of elasticity. Senile atrophy is a condition from which cancer frequently develops. Because the ageing skin is more vulnerable to the effects of actinic rays and of exposure to the sun, the wind and the weather, epithelioma occurs most frequently on the face. Contrary to common belief, however, trauma is seldom an etiological factor in the development of skin cancer. Corns do not become cancers.

Epitheliomas of the skin are either basal-cell or squamous-cell, depending upon the layer of the epidermis from which they spring. The characteristic beginning of either type is a small, hard macule or papule with a waxy surface, which is without evidence of inflammation and which remains without noticeable change for a variable period of time. Such a lesion should be removed by knife, by cautery or by radiation *before ulceration begins*. Biopsy examination is of academic interest only and, in our opinion, should be done only upon lesions that have been widely excised. Incomplete removal of a malignant lesion as a diagnostic or a therapeutic procedure, recognized authority to the contrary notwithstanding, may activate the growth so that it becomes rapidly fatal.

Cases in which the lesion is frankly malignant when first seen should be referred for radiation. Almost as a rule radiation destroys the lesion with a minimum of scar and disfigurement. Basal-cell cancer, rodent ulcer, occurs usually as a single lesion. It does not metastasize through the lymphatics and is radiosensitive. Squamous-cell cancer, on the other hand, may be multiple with epitheliomatous changes scattered over large areas of skin. An experienced dermatologist recently referred a patient to an equally experienced surgeon for the operative removal of all the skin from one entire side of the neck. The patient, a feeble old man, and a pronounced blonde, had many small epitheliomas over the lower face and neck. Radical removal was not done. Large areas of involved skin should be treated by radiation, or not at all.

Skin cancer begins as a local lesion. Suspicious lesions should be recognized early and promptly treated by a physician who has had adequate training in cancer work. Such men are available even for indigent patients at the cancer clinics. The clinics, by making the layman and the physician cancer-conscious, are already materially reducing both the morbidity and the mortality rate of cancer. The quack with his cure-all, arsenical paste, has been thrown into the discard.

HISTORIC MEDICINE

THE GREAT CONFEDERATE STATES HOSPITAL

From the Richmond *Times-Dispatch*, August 20th

McGuire General Hospital, in Richmond, is one of the largest military hospitals of the United States. McGuire, however, is not the largest military hospital ever located in Richmond. This credit belongs to Chimborazo Hospital, established 83 years ago in the eastern end of the city in what is now Chimborazo Park, and, at the time it was built, the largest military hospital in the annals of history, either ancient or modern.

Chimborazo Hospital was opened early in 1861 and included 150 well-constructed and well-ventilated frame buildings. It had an average number of patients each year larger than the entire white resident population of the city at the time. Within one week after it was opened 2000 soldiers were admitted, and in two weeks' time there were all of 4,000 patients enrolled. In addition to its 150 buildings with over 4,000 cots, there were 100 Sibley tents in which were put, from eight to 10 convalescent patients to a tent.

Richmond's great hospital of the 1860s had a dairy farm of its own, a soap factory, five large ice houses, its own bakery and its own brewery. It is not known how many barrels of beer were brewed at the brewery. However, from 7,000 to 10,000 loaves of bread from its bakery were issued per day to its patients and staff. Its dairy herd consisted of more than 200 cows, with pasturage nearby, where also were kept some 500 goats to supply the hospital with kid meat for the sick and convalescent patients. The hospital also had a canal boat that plied between Richmond, Lynchburg and Lexington bartering for provisions.

Over 70,000 patients received treatment at Chimborazo Hospital during the period of its existence of less than four years. Complete records are in existence today, upon which the name of every patient is recorded and the cause of every death. The mortality rate was exceedingly low for the time—a fraction over nine per cent.

An extract from the Richmond *News Leader* of Jan. 9th, 1909, reads as follows: "When we consider the size of this great military hospital, the number of soldiers admitted, treated, furloughed, discharged and buried; its successful work for nearly four years; the perfect discipline, order and harmony that existed from its establishment to its close; the immense amount of work done; the difficulties always attending the securing of supplies for such a large body of invalids, especially toward the closing days of the Confederacy, and the low mortality, we cannot but accord to Dr. James B. McCaw, its medical director and commandant, the highest praise."

GENERAL PRACTICE

JAMES L. HAMNER, M.D., *Editor*, Mannboro, Va.

CARE OF THE PATIENT WITH CHRONIC HEART DISEASE

A DOCTOR who thinks of the care of the patient, rather than the treatment of the disease, generally has something worth-while to say. Two Atlantans[1] offer us the best in the care of the patient whose heart is failing him.

Digitalis increases the ability of the failing heart to perform its work. Its action on the myocardium can be counted on in patients with regular rhythm and in those with auricular fibrillation. Indeed, digitalis is beneficial in patients with myocardial failure even in the presence of complete heart block.

Individual requirement of digitalis for complete digitalization is variable, due mostly perhaps to differing efficacy of absorption of the drug from the gastrointestinal tract. The average is about 1.5 Gm. As the point where digitalization can be expected is approached, doses should not be large, and before each the patient should be questioned about early symptoms of toxicity. Loss of appetite often is the earliest symptom.

For rapid parenteral digitalization lanatocide C, a pure glycoside from digitalis lanata, has been used with satisfaction: 1.6 mg. intravenously or intramuscularly in two equal doses, produces good clinical response with low incidence of toxic effect. Soon after lanatocide C has been given, digitalis leaf is started by mouth in doses of 0.1 Gm. t. i. d., continued until the patient has a satisfactory clinical response or shows evidence of toxicity.

Retention of sodium appears to be the primary cause of edema in cardiac failure. This is possible even though salt intake is limited, unless acid-ash foods are selected. If such a diet is followed strictly fluids may be given freely. Many patients will not eat a low-salt, acid-ash diet; in these, and in others with malnutrition, it may be better to increase the salt intake so that the patient will take more food, and then to increase salt elimination by use of diuretics. In case of chronic congestive failure, not relieved by rest and digitalis, the physician must plan a program of active treatment for the rest of the patient's life.

Xanthine diuretics are useful but much less powerful than mercupurin and salyrgan, which, with theophylline are the diuretics in common use. Original dose should not exceed 0.5 to 1.0 c.c. After initial injection they usually are given intravenously in 1 to 2 c.c. at intervals of two days to two weeks, depending on the retention of salt and water. Mercurials should be given in the morning so that the resultant polyuria will not interfere with sleep.

If ineffective, supplement with ammonium chloride in enteric-coated capsules, 6 to 8 Gm. daily for two to three days. At the end of that time the mercurial diuretic is given and the ammonium chloride discontinued. This routine may be repeated p. r. n. to keep the patient free of dyspnea and edema.

Urea 90 Gm. per day is an effective diuretic, but of unpleasant taste.

Fluid may accumulate in the chest in spite of good cardiac care. Then thoracentesis will allow the patient to breathe much more comfortably.

As a result of infection, overwork, ingestion of large amounts of sodium chloride, omission of digitalis, too long intervals between administration of diuretics, or because of progressive myocardial disease, sudden dramatic episodes of pulmonary edema occur during the course of chronic heart disease.

Give morphine 15 mg. hypo. to quiet the patient. If peripheral veins are not already distended and if extremities are not tight with edema, blood can be shunted from lungs to extremities by use of tourniquets applied to the extremities as close to the trunk as possible. Blood pressure cuffs are preferable, inflated to a pressure midway between systolic and diastolic. They are left in place until the acute attack subsides and then are removed *one at a time* to prevent too sudden restoration of blood of the extremities to the circulation. If veins already are distended and extremities already are tight with edema rapid removal of 500 to 1,000 c.c. of blood by venesection may produce great improvement. Recurrences may be prevented by proper use of digitalis, rest, restriction of sodium chloride and *persistent* use of diuretics.

It is pleasing to have the backing of these doctors in giving digitalis in cases showing no irregularity of heart action. Endorsement of blood-letting in pulmonary edema is welcomed, also.

CONTRECOUP LESIONS IN SEVERE CRANIOCEREBRAL INJURIES (Major O. W. Stewart, R.A.M.C., in Proc. Royal Soc. of Med. Med. (Lond.), May)

When a projected head strikes on its side, the major injury is apt to be in the opposite temporal lobe. When the blow is to the occipital, lesions of the frontal lobe the rule—left occipital, right frontal. From a

---

[1]. E. A. Stead, Jr., & J. V. Warren, Atlanta, in *Med. Clin. No. Amer.*, Mar.

blow to the frontal region, no instance of a contrecoup lesion of the occipital lobes.

Only in a certain group of these cases, wherein the contrecoup lesion is relatively localized, is surgical treatment of value.

A 29-year-old slightly inebriated soldier was first seen in another hospital. A half-hour before admission he had received a blow on the right occipital region. He was conscious, had walked in complaining of headache, was very restless but coöperative; transferred to our hospital seven days later, confused, restless and incontinent. Motor, sensory and reflex examinations did not point to a localized brain contusion or compression. X-rays showed a linear fracture in the right occipital bone beneath the site of the blow, the pineal gland well calcified and displaced to right 7 mm., downwards 1 cm. During an hour's observation his condition becoming worse a left subtemporal decompression was made and a solid subdural clot ⅜ in. thick was found. This was sucked and syringed out. Frontal and posterior parietal burr holes were then made and at each site there was a thin subdural clot. The size and amount of the clot did not seem sufficient to account for his condition. For the following 24 hours he remained drowsy but did not change greatly. On the second day following operation he suddenly expired.

At post-mortem a large, solid, subdural haematoma was found surrounding the left frontal pole and beneath the left frontal lobe, clot extruding from a laceration in the cortex and the brain adjacent to the haematoma and laceration was soft and friable. Frontal flap turned down at the first and the entire lesion adequately dealt with would have saved his life.

* * * * *

CARDIOVASCULAR ROUND TABLE

ANSWERS to certain important questions in clinical medicine are derived from a round-table discussion.[1]

What heart lesions contraindicate pregnancy?

Acute rheumatic fever is always a contraindication to pregnancy, also lesions of the aortic valve. Mitral stenosis, the typical rheumatic lesion, if well advanced, is a contraindication. In a primipara interruption is justified. All mitral and aortic combined lesions and all aortic lesions justify interruption. In older multipara a coronary lesion.

How long should a child with active rheumatic fever remain at bed rest?

Good men say a minimum of three months. The white count, the differential, particularly the sedimentation rate, should be guides. A noted cardiologist says he keeps all of his acute rheumatics in bed for one year. Rheumatic infection has a tendency to recur anyway.

What is the most important single finding in the examination of the heart?

Undoubtedly the most important single sign is heart enlargement. A heart that is enlarged is most likely a diseased heart. A heart that isn't enlarged, while it may be diseased, the chances are it is not. A heart may show signs—murmurs, and so on—

1. F. D. Murphy et al., Milwaukee, in Ill. Med. Jl., Mar.

and if the heart is not enlarged, apparently it hasn't suffered great strain. This enlargement can be determined by simple palpation; it is not necessary to make a teleo-röntgenological examination in order to determine this.

What is the value of oxygen therapy in heart disease?

Many people who have serious cardiac disease with dilatation and some pulmonary edema have great difficulty in sleeping. A sedative and 20 to 30 minutes of oxygen will often give sleep the night through.

Of what value are the sulfonamides in the treatment of rheumatic infection? What success has been obtained in the treatment of subacute bacterial endocarditis with the newer drugs?, also with fever therapy.

None. I have seen no convincing reports, have had no success with any of these new products in subacute bacterial endocarditis, and I might add that in one case I feel our enthusiasm for the use of those preparations with heparin proved disastrous.

What is the place for Papaverine in cardiovascular lesions?

Papaverine seems to increase the blood flow in the coronary system rather than diminishing it, as do morphine, codeine and other. In acute coronary papaverine has been used in one-grain doses intravenously every three or four hours; one may use it intravenously or by mouth three or four times a day. Papaverine does not seem to leave the bad effects that other opium derivatives do. A grain by mouth of papaverine is in many places supplanting nitroglycerine in attacks of angina pectoris.

What is your experience with testosterone for angina pectoris?

I gave it a very extensive trial two or three years ago and gave it up. Then I recently went back to it to see if I could do any better, and in both instances I am quite well satisfied that it gave me nothing at all.

What prognostic significance has a persistent 'Q' wave six months following a coronary attack?

The 'Q' in many instances is the only remaining evidence of posterior coronary occlusion. If the myocardium has regenerated and is capable of carrying on the particular individual's activities, not much significance; but for those who conduct themselves as of 25 years of age instead of 50, the 'Q' wave is of far more significance.

The prognosis on persistent 'Q' wave, six months following coronary occlusion, would be poor.

Method of diagnosing auricular fibrillation without an electrocardiogram?

The general practitioner may just forget the electrocardiographic tracing and treat the patient, and he will come out all right. Auricular fibrillation is a disease of older people, apt to occur in hyperthyroidism. If the heart is continuously irregular, if there is a difference of 10 or 15 beats between the apex and the wrist, that is certainly auricular fibrillation and one doesn't need an electrocardiograph to tell it.

What is the minimum time for coronary patients to return to work? Patients with decompensated hearts, especially after recovery from coronary occlusion, rate 90 in spite of digitalis to intoxication, rhythm normal but patients remain dyspneic and ortheopneic even at bed rest, what can be done for these patients?

I routinely use quidinine for the first weeks after the coronary occlusion in the hope that I may prevent a sudden death. There are certain instances in which the damage is so severe, where the occlusion is so extensive, that life continuation is impossible. Those people usually die either at once or within the first three or five days. There is a second group that have enough reserve to carry them through the first four or five days, and treatment will carry them over 30 to 60 days—a gradually losing contest with congestive failure, and they die.

In the third group the shock is survived, there still remains some reserve. My order is not less than six weeks complete rest in bed—they may be expected to go on to recovery. Beyond this six weeks, whatever rest is necessary to put back reserve in the heart: then get them up very slowly, usually with quinidine along with other drugs as a preventive of ventricular fibrillation.

In the case of the patient whom digitalis has not helped there is always a possibility that the old vessel may reopen or a collateral circulation may develop. A number of patients have had to remain down six months to a year, returned to work in full capacity and lived for considerable periods. Those patients give us encouragement to persist with those who have chronic failure over a long time.

There is always a possibility that iodides may give a man enough blood supply and give him enough time to repair his damage. Most of the improvement is made within the first 90 days.

The dosage of quinidine when used routinely is 6 to 9 grains daily.

TORSION OF THE UTERUS
(C. C. Bell, St. Paul, in *Minn. Med.*, April)

Torsion of the uterus is not uncommon in veterinary practice, but in women it is so rare that most textbooks are silent on the subject. It practically always occurs in a pergnant uterus or in the presence of some type of pelvic tumor. The first case, recorded by Virchow in 1863, was discovered at postmortem. The great majority of cases have been in women the subjects of fibroids or ovarian cysts.

The usual symptoms are the sudden onset of severe, acute, generalized abdominal pain with nausea or vomiting and the rather rapid development of symptoms of shock.

Diagnosis is best made by a careful consideration of the history and examination of the uterus, vagina, bladder and rectum.

In the usual case the only treatment is surgical intervention at the earliest possible moment. The prognosis is good if treatment is not delayed.

OPHTHALMOLOGY

HERBERT C. NEBLETT, M.D., *Editor*, Charlotte, N. C.

ASTHENOPIA—"EYESTRAIN"

THE TERM implies weak sight and is the commonest of all eye symptoms. It is accompanied by or results in fatiguability of the eyes, burning of the eyes and lids, blurring of vision, eye ache and headache often after use of the eyes for brief periods at near work and in viewing moving objects at a distance. Sir John Parsons said "The exact pathology of eyestrain is unknown and the rational visual fatigue in the production of ocular systemic disorders is largely a matter of conjecture."

The symptom-complex is complained of in the presence and absence of refractive errors, in the presence and absence of eye muscle anomalies, in the presence and absence of demonstrable focal infections and systemic disorders of whatever nature, in asthenic states and functional nervous disorders. It seems to predominate in the adolescent and at the beginning of the fourth decade of life, especially in the high-strung nervous individual of either the explosive or the suppressive type. These individuals are apt to be obsessed with imaginary fears concerning the status of their eyes and when examined and reassured of their condition their symptoms are more often than otherwise relieved.

Many of these persons have worn glasses for years without relief and have negligible errors of refraction. After being persuaded to discard their glasses, the wearing of which was not indicated, and given reassurance of the normal status of their eyes and advice as to correction of any faulty habits as to their work, rest, recreation and diet, improvement was usually marked without recourse to any other form of treatment. The writer finds asthenopia to be more common among women than men since the advent of the war. The reason appears to be the fact that a far greater number of women from 16 to 50 are now engaged in work requiring speed of action and sustained use of the eyes. Careful questioning elicits the information that the greater number of these workers never or rarely eat breakfast, and their lunch is usually small in amount and inferior in quality. The hours of sleep are usually insufficient, especially in the younger worker. Add to these factors the emotional stress and the tempo of life under which the major portion of the population is living and there is presented what appears an assignable cause for the prevalence of asthenopia in a large class of people. It should be taken into account that the threshold of endurance for sustained eye work varies greatly in different individuals—organically or functionally diseased or normal.

Stephen, in an excellent article on this subject in the *Journal of the Iowa State Med. Soc.*, Feb., 1942 (Excerpt in *Digest of Ophth. & Otolaryngology* for May, 1942) says: "Due to the exactness of the diagnosis in these cases it is certain that the examiner must have a good knowledge of general medicine. The laxity with which general practitioners send their patients to ordinary glass fitters and not to those having a medical education should be duly condemned. There is no department of ophthalmic work in which the ophthalmologist must be more deeply versed in general medicine than in the search for the cause of asthenopia."

DERMATOLOGY

J. LAMAR CALLAWAY, M.D., *Editor*, Durham, N. C.

THE COMMON WART

VERRUCA VULGARIS, the common wart, is seen most frequently in children. It is now well established that this lesion is due to a filterable virus and consequently autoinoculable, which accounts for the multiplicity of lesions seen in some individuals.

The most frequent type of lesion is the seed wart occurring usually over the dorsal surface of the fingers or hands; however, involvement of any portion of the skin, mucocutaneous borders, or mucosae may occur. The location of the lesion tends to influence its appearance.

When involvement of the hands and fingers occurs the lesion is usually dry, elevated, has numerous projections on the surface, round, dirty brown to black in color, pea-sized or smaller, and nontender. When the bearded region, scalp, mucosae, or eyelids are affected the verruca tends to be single, thin, soft, and threadlike or filiform. Involvement of the sole of the foot rsults in a yellowish, translucent, papular lesion with a central core surrounded by zones of cornification. If the top of the lesion is shaved off with a scapel brownish-red specks may be visible in the center of the lesion. This effect is more easily seen when the area is moistened with an alcohol sponge and is helpful in distinguishing the verruca from a callus or a corn. It is called a plantar wart, is usually painful, and tends to occur over pressure areas on the ball of the foot or heel.

Verruca plana juveniles (the flat wart) and condyloma acuminatum (the venereal wart) are other types of verrucae, but are not described here.

Numerous hearsay methods of healing warts are "common knowledge" among the laity. This probably arises from the fact established by Bloch that psychotherapy may effectively cure verrucae. By this method alone he was able to cure 44 per cent of a series of cases of verruca vulgaris. The healing of a virus disease by suggestive therapy alone is difficult to apprehend; however, the validity of this fact is now confirmed by several investigators. The occasional spontaneous cure of warts, although well known, is not readily explicable.

Treatment.—The successful treatment of verruca at times becomes a complicated problem, particularly if there are multiple lesions. The single seed wart occurring over the hand or finger is perhaps most easily removed by electrodesiccation. It is necessary to infiltrate the base of the lesion with 1 to 2 per cent procaine. With a medium spark the lesion is charred, but not too deeply. The body of the lesion may then be removed with a skin curette or small curved surgical scissors. Following this the base of the lesion should be desiccated lightly. The application of 1 per cent gentian violet in 70 per cent alcohol followed by 3 per cent ammoniated mercury ointment and a protective dressing will usually prevent secondary infection. Healing usually requires 10 days to two weeks. The lesion must be kept out of water. If the site is over a joint, splinting will facilitate healing. The patient should be informed that a small scar will result.

If multiple lesions are present, rather than subject each lesion to the specific treatment, it may be well to try 6 to 10 weekly injections of bismuth subsalicylate intragluteally (dosage 0.2 gm.) When successful the lesions usually disappear rather uniformly within 3 to 6 weeks after therapy is begun. Although the method is not invariably successful it is frequently efficacious. There is unfortunately no way to be certain that the method will succeed in any particular case until it is given a trial. Bismarsen may be used similarly instead of bismuth subsalicylate.

Whereas the aforementioned use of bismuth designated its administration at a distant site, it has been shown that another bismuth compound may be injected locally into the lesion with frequent successful results being obtained. An ampule of sodium bismuth thyo-glycollate (192 mgm.) is mixed with 2 c.c. of novocaine solution and approximately .2 to .4 c.c. are injected with a hypodermic needle into the center of the base of the lesion. The needle is introduced into the skin a short distance away from the verruca and inserted until the needle point lies within the lesion's base. A second injection is suggested if the first is unsuccessful.

The use of röntgen therapy is perhaps the most ideal therapeutic method from the standpoint of the cosmetic end result as well as the painlessness on the part of the patient. On the other hand röntgen therapy should only be employed by the expert, and it is impracticable and expensive where multiple verrucae are to be treated. It is by all means the treatment of choice for plantar verrucae which are undoubtedly the most difficult of all types of warts to eradicate without unwarranted sequelae. Röntgen therapy also is the best approach to the subungual verruca.

In general the use of nitric acid, trichloracetic acid or other escharotic agents is interdicted because of the difficulty in controlling the depth of penetration.

THERAPEUTICS

J. F. NASH, M.D., *Editor*, Saint Pauls, N. C.

ANESTHESIA IN OFFICE PRACTICE

NOT NEARLY enough anesthesia is used in office general practice. An excellent presentation of the subject[1] is quoted in extenso, and heartily recommended to general practitioners of this section for daily use.

I. Infiltration anesthesia is useful for:
1. Removal of small tumor masses and foreign bodies.
2. Paracentesis and thoracentesis.
3. Repair of lacerations.
4. Reduction of fractures.
5. Treatment of non-weight bearing fractures, sprains and contusions, low back pain, shoulder disabilities due to sore muscles.

II. Nerve block or regional anesthesia may be used for:
1. Brachial plexus block—for all disabilities of arm and forearm.
2. Tibial block for leg injuries of various kinds.
3. Intercostal block for fractured ribs or rib resection.
4. Wrist block: radial and ulnar block.
5. Caudal and continuous caudal.

1 & 2.—A skin wheal should be raised with a

---
[1] N. E. Lenahan, Columbus, in *Ohio Med. J.*, July.

fine needle and then a 21-gauge needle introduced through this anesthetized area infiltrating below the object, fanning out in different directions as necessary. A pause of three to five minutes, then the incision made.

Novocaine solution of .5 to 1 per cent is used.

3.—Skin edges gaping widely an injection of novocaine is made from the cut surface and fanned out as necessary.

4.—Reduction of fracture with hematoma. A 2 per cent solution of novocaine or metycaine is used. The needle is inserted so that a drop of blood may be aspirated from the hematoma. This blood usually contains fat globules and is darker. Injection is made very slowly so that any signs of toxicity will appear before a large dose is given. For the average Colles' fracture 10 c.c. of solution is used; for a fractured femur 50 c.c. The anesthesia appears in a few minutes and lasts several hours.

Closed reduction of fractures without hematoma a .5 per cent solution of procaine or metycaine with 1 c.c. of 1/2600 adrenalin per 200 c.c. is used. Skin wheals are made and the solution is injected down to the periosteum, where 20 to 50 c.c. of .5% solution is deposited. Anesthesia is usually effective in five to 10 minutes. A preliminary dose of morphine is advantageous.

Fractured rib pain can be relieved by injecting a 1% solution into the line of fracture. If necessary the rib above and below may be injected as well; repeat if necessary—rarely necessary more than two or three times.

5.—Treatment of non-weight bearing fractures. Injection relieves discomfort and edema, thus permitting early resumption of activity, and better blood supply for fracture healing. After skin asepsis a wheal is made over the point of maximum tenderness. A large needle is then introduced and the solution is injected until there is no more pain, the part is massaged, then wrapped with an Aceelastic bandage. Patient may then use the part normally. Weight bearing in ankle injuries is permitted in five days. Fractures of tarsal and metatarsal bones are treated by injection and adhesive strapping; of the toes and fingers by injections and early mobilization.

Open and dirty wounds are a contraindication. A sprained ankle may be so treated, followed by an elastic support. Pain is relieved for two, six, eight hours; may be reinjected several times with the 1 per cent solution.

Contusions of the chest without fracture: severe pain, limitation of motion and breathing are relieved by the injection into the painful area.

As a rule five to 10 c.c. is sufficient but occasionally 15 to 20 c.c. of a 1 per cent novocaine solution or 1/4 to 1/2 per cent solution of pontocaine.

Low Back Pain.

Group A. Pain and tenderness are confined to the iliac crest muscle attachments.

At three points on each side of the crest inject 30 c.c. novocaine in saline—180 c.c. in all. Massage vigorously. The patient is to perform all movements which were previously painful. Then the back is thoroughly strapped in lumbar lordosis with 3-inch tape from tip of coccyx to shoulder girdle. Seven strips longitudinal and after every second strip apply a strip horizontally around the waist.

Group B. Pain and tenderness over one or both sacro-iliac joints.

Feel for iliai tuberosity between transverse process of the 5 lumbar vertebrae and the posterior iliac spine. Insert needle at the points shown tangentially until the rough surface of the tuberosity is encountered, then move needle medially when it is felt to sink into the fascial and ligamentous mass until the lateral edge of the sacrum is reached. At each of these three points on each side introduce 20 c.c. of ½% solution. Forcibly massage as before and then make the patient perform a full range of movement.

The patient lies in a position of lumbar lordosis. Four overlapping layers of 3-inch strapping are used. Commence on the right side at the level of the tip of the coccyx draw the right buttock forcibly toward the midline and then apply the plaster commencing 4 inches ventrally to the great trochanter of the femur and pull strongly to the left. Now draw the left buttock medially and finish off the plaster at the corresponding point on the left side. The plaster remains on the patient 10 days and then a sacro-iliac belt is worn if necessary.

Pain and Disability of the Shoulder Joint.

The minimal criteria for infiltration: a) increase of pain on active motion elicited either by quick or sustained effort; b) tender points in the muscles of the back or shoulder girdle. Let us assume we press on a "trigger point." This is exquisitely tender to pressure which may elicit pain in the reference zone. Maximum point of tenderness is located by putting the muscle on a stretch and by the use of pressure. Blind infiltration is usually ineffective. A small intradermal wheal is made and novocaine is slowly injected to abolish pain—usually 2-5 c.c. The amount injected at one time is 10-20 c.c. of 1% solution. In 40% of cases a transient weakness, dizziness, contraction of throat or thirst occurred.

May be injected daily to weekly. In addition, Vitamin C. 75-200 mg. per day, local heat and encouragement of motion. Complete relief of pain and limitation of motion is found in 60% of cases, improvement in 30%.

Nerve Block or Regional Anesthesia is produced by infiltrating the nerve or an area immediately around the nerve with an anesthetic solution.

Brachial plexus block is very useful in any type of operation involving the upper extremity, particularly in persons who have recently eaten and a general anesthetic would be contraindicated. The patient supine with head slightly turned toward the unaffected side, a wheal is raised ¾ in. above the middle of the clavicle and immediately lateral to the subclavian artery and the external jugular vein and 1st needle inserted through the wheal and down to the first rib; 2nd needle inserted parallel to the first, 1 3 in. from the clavicle; a 3d parallel to the first and 1/3 in. posterior to it. Three to 5 c.c. of 2% solution is injected through each needle on to the first rib and 7 c.c. as the needle is slowly being withdrawn. Then a bracelet injection around the arm near the shoulder to block off any intercostal nerves.

For tibial block, the patient prone on the table, a needle is inserted into the flexion crease behind the knee a little outside the midline. The tibial nerve lies at this point. Five c.c. of sol. injected just beneath the skin blocks sensation from the medial cutaneous branch. Then deeper in same location under the deep fascia, 15 c.c. of 2% novocaine are injected. A needle is inserted on the lateral or posterior lateral aspect of the fibula just below the head and 10 c.c. of sol. is injected.

For ankle block, an imaginary line is drawn between the most prominent points of the internal and external malleoli. A skin wheal is made at the midpoint of this line, a 50-mm. needle is introduced through the wheal and pointed toward the anterior border of the internal malleolus. Just before the needle strikes the tibia 10 to 14 c.c. of 1% solution should be injected. The posterior tibial is injected as indicated and the bracelet injection of skin and subcutaneous tissue made. Anesthesia is produced in 20 minutes.

Intercostal block is used for rib resection, fractured ribs, etc. Morphine gr. ⅛ and nembutal are given beforehand. Three to 5 c.c. of 1% solution is deposited in the intercostal spaces near the inferior border of the rib, at a point between operative site and spine. If the fourth rib is to be blocked a wheal is made over the fifth rib, the needle inserted directly down to the rib to estimate depth, the needle is withdrawn and angled up to the inferior border of the fourth rib where the solution is deposited.

For wrist block, a ½% solution is injected in bracelet fashion around the wrist. The hand is flexed so that the two tendons are prominent, a very fine needle is introduced between them through the skin wheal, fascia offers mild resistance. Needle is passed 3 to 4 mm. deeper and 3 to 6 c.c. of 1% solution injected. Again the needle is inserted through the wheal and down to the styloid process and 3 to 6 c.c. injected. The same technique is used for the radial nerve. Wrist block usually gives two hours anesthesia.

Caudal and transacral anesthesia are office procedures, but very useful in the aged and debilitated and those subject to shock.

GENERAL PRACTICE

D. Herbert Smith, M.D., *Editor*, Pauline, S. C.

MANAGEMENT OF SOME COMMON PHASES OF LATE SYPHILIS IN PRACTICE

All of us know of instances of great harm resulting from too-vigorous attacks on late syphilis. Perhaps nowhere else is it more necessary to treat the patient who has the disease rather than the disease which has the patient.

Some words[1] of wisdom to remind us:

Usually the syphilitic infection becomes quiescent in the months after the invasion of the body without clinical manifestations subjective or objective. Only a positive blood test indicates the presence of disease. This stage of latency may be maintained for the remainder of the patient's life.

In some 50% of untreated patients late syphilitic disease appears in from five to 25 or more years after infection as 1) late benign syphilis, 2) cardiovascular syphilis, and 3) neurosyphilis.

Late Benign Syphilis.—The process is usually that of gummatous infiltration, tissue destruction, scarring. Gummatous involvement has been seen in every tissue and organ of the body—skin and bone lesions most commonly. Next in order come mucous membranes of the nose, throat, and larynx, liver and stomach.

Therapy in late benign syphilis presents a difficult problem. Many multiple foci of syphilitic inflammation are well walled off. The objective of treatment is to obtain healing of the presenting lesion, and to assist the host in the resolution and walling-off foci present or which may arise during the course of therapy. A "long-range" use of the antisyphilitic metals by continuous therapy for two years, consisting of alternating courses of eight once-a-week injections of an arsenical preparation (in full dosage) and bismuth subsalicylate in oil. Potassium iodide by mouth in the early months of treatment. The first course of bismuth should consist of four to six injections.

For practical purposes syphilitic heart disease means aortic disease with at times secondary affection of the heart muscle. The aorta may have

[1]. R. H. Kampmeier, Nashville, in *Jl. Tenn. Med. Assn.*, July.

lost its elasticity and may have become dilated. Uncomplicated aortitis is difficult of diagnosis unless the coronary ostia are narrowed. Then heart pain may arouse the suspicion of syphilitic aortitis and may lead to further study by fluoroscopy. The commonly recognized complication of syphilitic aortitis is aortic regurgitation, dilatation and attendant changes at the root of the aorta. Dilatation and hypertrophy of the left ventricle cardiac failure is certain to follow within a variable period. A livelihood involving little physical exertion offers a better outlook than one of heavy labor. In general, the management of the cardiac failure is similar to that used in failure due to other forms of heart disease. Treatment must do no harm. Bismuth in oil weekly for 10 to 12 weeks, with rest periods of six to 12 weeks, is a promising regimen.

The management of neurosyphilis is so complex, and the need for individualization of treatment so great, that helpful discussion of this subject in a few minutes is not undertaken.

* * * * *

ANOTHER RAPID TREATMENT FOR SCABIES

The procedures here described were instituted at the U. S. Naval Training Station, Great Lakes, and Camp McIntire Dispensary.[1]

The mixture used is:

Benzyl benzoate	250
Duponol C	20
Aqua bentonite, q.s. ad.	1.000

The benzyl benzoate is gently poured over the Duponol C in the bottom of a container. To this the 2.5 per cent aqueous solution of bentonite is added slowly without shaking. The emulsion is then agitated until all of the wetting agent is dissolved.

Technic

1. Remove all clothing, put clothing in bag, either autoclave or send to laundry.
2. Shower, using soap freely. Scrub, with particular attention to the involved areas.
3. Paint entire body from ear-chin line down, covering all folds of body. Use paint brush with long firm bristles.
4. Let dry on skin. Repeat painting in five minutes.
5. Put to bed. Cover sufficiently to make patient warm. Keep in bed for four hours.
6. Shower, dry well. Apply calamine ointment if any irritation is noted.
7. Clean clothes.
8. Return to duty with instructions to report for follow-up examinations.

A number observed between the 14th and 28th day exhibited involuting papules, crusts, scars and

[1]. Lt. (jg) A. H. Slepyan, U.S.N.R., in *Jl. A. M.*, April 15th.

pigmentation, at times suggesting recurrences; however, repeated potassium hydroxide preparations were negative.

Four men were seen on the third day after treatment complaining of isolated new vesicles appearing on the webs of the fingers. A vesicle was removed and a sodium hydroxide preparation examined. In each instance an egg was found undergoing degeneration. Several of the vesicles were marked and observed on the 10th day and found dried and no longer pruritic.

Two patients were concurrently infected with pediculosis pubis. One of them had involvement of the axillary and abdominal hair. The treatment was gratifying in stopping the itching. No live pediculi could be found after the treatment. On the 3rd, 7th and 14th days, nits were plentiful but could be easily slid off the hairs. Twenty-one days after treatment there were no signs of parasitic infection. Under the microscope the pediculus was killed almost immediately on being engulfed with a drop of the scabies lotion.

A clean, simple, nonirritating 5-hour treatment for scabies has been developed. Of the 189 patients followed longer than 14 days, recurrence was noticed in not one.

The lotion presented suggests further trial on patients with pediculosis pubis.

UROLOGY

RAYMOND THOMPSON, M.D., *Editor*, Charlotte, N. C.

MANAGEMENT OF GONORRHEA IN GENERAL PRACTICE

A "NEW CURE" which has any value is certain to be credited with too much, and later, when failures begin to be reported, to be debited with too much.

The treatment of gonorrhea with sulfa drugs has covered enough cases for the indicator to cease its wide swings to right and left and point to actual value.

A sane article on management of gonorrhea in general practice[1] suggests presentation of the essentials of this subject in this department at this time.

As confidence in various techniques for treating gonorrhea rises and falls, it is well to have a clear-cut statement of opinion now and then.

Here is the gist of an advice[1] which avoids extremes.

Prophylaxis should be used by the lay people as well as by our armed forces.

There are plenty of free clinics for all not able to pay.

The sulfonamides will cure 70% of the acute

[1] J. L. Morgan, Memphis, in *Jl. Tenn. Med. Assn.*, July.

cases, only *a very small percentage* of the chronics.

Six or eight days of one gram (15 grains) of sulfathiazole four times a day until he has taken 20 or 30 grams suffices. If discharge still contains gonococci further administration of the drug is of no value; use injections of mild silver salts, and give 10 minims of sandalwood oil after meals.

Until a patient shows that he will not respond to the sulfonamides there should not be anything injected into the urethra or any kind of instrumentation or massage of the prostate gland.

At the onset sit down with your patient and inform him of the seriousness of the infection; to leave off all alcoholics, not to attend any social functions or call on any girls, to get as much sleep and rest as possible, to drink a great deal of water. Even if the discharge stops after two or three days on sulfonamide, treatment must continue for at least a total of five days.

The prostate should never be massaged other than gently, and not oftener than every three or four days. It is necessary in some resisting cases of urethral gland infection, stricture or granular tissue in the urethra to pass graduated sounds, not oftener than four to seven days.

Most gonorrheal prostatic abscesses will drain into the posterior urethra by spontaneous rupture. Such patients should be kept in bed and given hot sitz baths or colonic irrigations with warm water. A few of these cases will have an acute retention, and will have to be catheterized. The catheter should be strapped in for two days. If the patient can void after this, there is no need of placing the catheter back in bladder. The point is that you will do less damage in leaving the catheter in than you will by catheterizing your patient every time his bladder fills up. Most all gonorrheal epididymitis cases should be put to bed and a bridge of adhesive plaster placed beneath the scrotum, and an ice-cap on the swollen epididymis. In all painful complication of gonorrhea good results may be gotten from the use of belladonna and opium rectal suppositories. In women the percentage of cures with sulfonamides in acute or resistant gonorrhea is the same as in men. Women should have cleansing douches; and the physician apply nitrate of silver to the cervix—if she has a cervicitis and doesn't have an acute pyosalpinx. Acute pelvic inflammatory diseases requires bed treatment, with ice cap or hot-water bottle. Diathermy in the subacute and chronic conditions is of value.

Clinical cure means all evidence of the infection has disappeared and there is no discharge, no visible or symptomatic evidence of the disease. It is not an easy matter even with training and the latest equipment to find the gonococcus in every case in which it is present, so a lot of chronic gonorrhea goes unrecognized to spread the disease. Cessation of discharge does not necessarily mean cure. No person who has had gonorrhea should be declared cured on the strength of one examination.

When penicillin is available for civilian use we will have, according to the more hopeful, a specific.

PEDIATRICS

MANAGEMENT OF ACUTE INFECTIOUS DISEASES IN CHILDHOOD
(A. L. Hoyne, Chicago, in *Jl. Kansas Med. Soc.*, June)

Smallpox and diphtheria lead the field of the acute infections diseases which can be prevented by means of active immunization. The average child at birth is vulnerable to an attack of variola. Vaccination against smallpox may be done at three or four months of age, in case of exposure at any age. The reaction is less in the very young than if the primary vaccination is postponed until school age or later. Since the diphtheria antitoxin which most children possess at birth is lost toward the end of the first year, immunization at nine months using alum-precipitated diphtheria toxoid combined with alum-precipitated tetanus toxoid, protects against two diseases with fewer injections, and stimulates greatest antigenic response to each toxoid.

Whooping cough is a serious concern in early childhood and infancy. Because of insufficient antigenic response in the first year of life, vaccination against pertussis is not undertaken until after six months. Then use Sauer's vaccine, 1 c.c., 2 c.c., and 3 c.c. at three- to four-week intervals, in combination with diphtheria toxoid. There is also available a triple antigen including tetanus toxoid. Reactions are no more frequent or severe to such combinations. Four months are required to establish immunity. However, we have no protection for the infant from whooping cough during the first year of life, a period when fatality rates are highest. Human convalescent or hyperimmune pertussis serum might be used for passive immunization, but neither of these serums is easily obtainable, and so artificial means for affording immunity to pertussis continue to be unsatisfactory or difficult to achieve.

Against measles there is no artificial means of bringing about active immunization. For passive immunization human convalescent measles serum in doses of 3.5 to 5 c.c. if given within three days of exposure will, as a rule, afford temporary protection. Pooled adult serum or whole blood in 20 to 30 c.c. doses is less reliable. Immune globulin is less dependable for prevention than for modification of measles. For active treatment we have used amidopyrine during the past years with excellent results and no harmful action.

If tonsils and adenoids were removed before children entered school there would be far less scarlet fever. Not that immunity would be greater but that there would be fewer scarlet fever carriers to transmit the disease. Even if the child is immunized according to the Dick method it may become a carrier of hemolytic streptococci capable of producing scarlet fever. Moreover, a Dick-negative individual is not free from attack by hemolytic streptococci from a scarlet fever patient even though no rash occurs with the infection. Passive immunization may be established either by human convalescent scarlet fever serum in 10 c.c. doses intramuscularly, or by scarlet fever antitoxin, if one of these measures is adopted within 12 hours of exposure. In either instance protection is afforded only for 10 day to three weeks. Scarlet fever is now so mild that the necessity for specific therapy seldom seems indicated; but since severe complications sometimes develop when least expected, it is advisable often not to deny the patient any possible advantage which serum may provide.

There is no reliable immunization against chickenpox, mumps or German measles. Probably it is better for the child to have mumps than to risk acquiring it after puberty.

Most spectacular in responsiveness to the sulfa drugs is meningococcic meningitis, and favorable action is observed in almost all other forms of meningitis except the tuberculous. Erysipelas is a disease curable by sulfanilamide.

The sulfa drugs are of no value in chickenpox, whooping cough or measles. For the toxemia of scarlet fever we feel convinced that nothing is gained by the use of these drugs.

In smallpox, if sulfanilamide is administered during the stage of invasion the eruption may be aborted. There is no doubt in respect to efficiency of these drugs in cases of pneumonia and sinus infections, including the ethmoiditis of scarlet fever. The action of the drugs on cervical adenitis, otitis media, and mastoiditis is not always easily determined and effectiveness in cases of nonsuppurative arthritis is doubtful. We may find penicillin the choice for many conditions for which the sulfonamides are now given.

Acute infectious disease patients should be hospitalized only for the same reason that other ill patients are hospitalized; namely that they require some special care that a hospital alone is able to provide. Most children with acute infectious diseases can be cured in their own homes. Moreover the assembling of large numbers of children with different diseases in the same institution must necessarily present certain hazards regardless of the efficiency of the hospital.

Every general hospital should have a small isolation unit. Fear in respect to the common contagious diseases on the part of hospital authorities can generally be attributed to lack of knowledge. With proper technique there should be practically no danger of spreading infection if such diseases as poliomyelitis and meningococcic meningitis were treated in a general hospital.

THE CLAVICULAR SIGN OF LATE CONGENITAL SYPHILIS
(S. L. Wang, Shanghai, in *Chinese Med. Jl.*, Oct.-Dec.)

Traditionally interstitial keratitis, labyrinthine disease, and Hutchinson's teeth are the most typical stigmata of late congenital lues. Actual interstitial keratitis occurs in from 25 to 50%; the other signs are rarely observed.

In 1927, Higoumenakis, in Greece, described two cases of congenital lues with tumefaction of the inner third of the right clavicle. In a later series of 197 cases, he found that clavicular enlargement in 170 cases—85%—of which 157 were on the right side and 13 on the left side. The latter group was composed of left-handed individuals.

Since then sporadic reports have appeared from various parts of the world. From Oct., 1941, to Sept., 1943, we have been able to collect 23 cases in the Chungking Central Hospital—21 of congenital syphilis, two probable cases of congenital syphilis. Twenty out of 23 cases showed the clavicular sign.

Its extremely big incidence made it a very reliable diagnostic sign of late congenital syphilis. At time it is the only clinical sign with or without serological reactions.

Tripotherapy has not yet been proved to be a cure for choretocavoid, but it is of value in aiding the surgeon in his efforts to attain the ideal operative state which he has so long sought.—*Int. Med. Digest*, Aug.

SOUTHERN MEDICINE & SURGERY

Official Organ

JAMES M. NORTHINGTON, M.D., *Editor*

Department Editors

Human Behavior
JAMES K. HALL, M.D..Richmond, Va.

Orthopedic Surgery
JOHN T. SAUNDERS, M.D. ....Asheville, N. C.

Urology
RAYMOND THOMPSON, M.D............................Charlotte, N. C.

Surgery
GEO. H. BUNCH, M.D..Columbia, S. C.

Obstetrics
HENRY J. LANGSTON, M.D...............................Danville, Va

Gynecology
CHAS. R. ROBINS, M.D....................................Richmond, Va.
ROBERT T. FERGUSON, M.D. ....Charlotte, N. C.

General Practice
J. L. HAMNER, M.D..Mannboro, Va.
J. HERBERT SMITH, M.D. ....Pauline, S. C.

Clinical Chemistry and Microscopy
J. M. FEDER, M.D.,
EVELYN TREBLE, M. T. } ....Anderson, S. C.

Hospitals
R. B. DAVIS, M.D..Greensboro, N. C.

Cardiology
CLYDE M. GILMORE, A.B., M.D..................Greensboro, N. C.

Public Health
N. THOS. ENNETT, M.D.................................Greenville, N. C.

Radiology
R. H. LAFFERTY, M.D., and Associates.......Charlotte, N. C.

Therapeutics
J. F. NASH, M.D...Saint Pauls, N. C.

Tuberculosis
JOHN DONNELLY, M.D..................................Charlotte, N. C.

Dentistry
J. H. GUION, D.D.S...Charlotte, N C.

Internal Medicine
GEORGE R. WILKINSON, M.D.......................Greenville, S. C.

Ophthalmology
HERBERT C. NEBLETT, M.D...........................Charlotte, N. C.

Rhino-Oto-Laryngology
CLAY W. EVATT, M.D....................................Charleston, S. C.

Proctology
RUSSELL L. BUXTON, M.D..........................Newport News, Va.

Insurance Medicine
H. F. STARR, M.D..Greensboro, N. C.

Dermatology
J. LAMAR CALLAWAY, M.D. ....Durham, N. C.

Pediatrics

Offerings for the pages of this Journal are requested and given careful consideration in each case. Manuscripts not found suitable for our use will not be returned unless author encloses postage.

As is true of most Medical Journals, all costs of cuts, etc., for illustrating an article must be borne by the author.

REST POSSIBLE ONLY TO THE WEARY

Man's o'erlabored sense repairs itself by rest.
—Shakespeare.

WHEN I was a little boy one of my teachers had us little folks write each day in a book each of us had for the purpose, a "Quotation," of the teacher's selection. We had to commit this quotation to memory. One of these comes to mind right now. It runs something like this:

"Rest is not quitting this busy career;
Rest is the fitting of self to its sphere."
Rather grandiloquent it is, to be sure; but, as far as it goes, it indicates that rest has a curative effect and that it is not to be long-drawn-out. I don't remember who wrote the lines, or what teacher had me remember them. Paltry as they are, they bear out the contention that if you will save anything long enough you will find a use for it.

There is much difference of opinion as to what rest is. It seems that most of the general public and entirely too many doctors do not distinguish between resting and loafing. A very intelligent lady, past sixty and a great worker, was heard to remark recently that she had never been so tired in her life that one good night's sleep did not rest her. She knows what rest is. The great Oxford English Dictionary defines rest as: 1) a bed or couch; 2) the natural repose and relief from daily activity. Plainly just doing nothing is not resting. Another high authority tells us that the derivation is: L. resto—*re-*, back; *sto*, stand—a standing back or aside (from further work).

The clearest statement of the proper use of the word, rest, with which I am familiar is that of an old colored man, sitting by the roadside with his hoe in his lap, in the late afternoon. A passer-by greeting him with: "Howdy, Uncle; are you resting?," got the reply: "Naw, suh, I ain't 'xactly restin' 'cause I ain' tired. I'm just setting here waitin' for de sun to go down, so I can quit work."

Over the past three or four decades rest has come to be regarded as the greatest of therapeutic agents, aside from surgical measures. That this rest has come to mean something quite different from recuperation from the tiring produced by labor is evidenced by its being prescribed for weeks, months, and years. Oddly, it seems that for those who did least work, most rest was prescribed.

At the last meeting of the American Medical Association a symposium on the abuse of rest was held in which was discussed this abuse in cardiovascular diseases, in obstetrics, in surgery, in orthopedic surgery, in psychiatry, and in general All this may be found in the issue for August 19th of the *Journal of the A. M. A.* All of it is hereby endorsed and recommended for earnest study.

It is also recommended that this be considered as an illustration of the evils (1) of misusing words, and (2) of refusing to be guided by the plain promptings of Nature. Rest, in the proper sense of the word, is demanded by Nature, but only up to the point of disappearance of fatigue. The abuse of rest, as will be seen from the reading of these articles, and as you will realize on looking back on your own experiences, comes from inaction after the patient has inclination for renewing his usual activities.

From Dr. Tinsley R. Harrison's (Dallas) contribution to the Symposium:

There is no proof that rest in bed carried out for many weeks after symptoms have disappeared is of value in the physical management of the patient with congestive failure, angina pectoris or myocardial infarction. The available evidence points to the contrary, and more especially so if the recumbent posture is enforced while the patient is kept in bed. From the psychic standpoint there is disadvantage in the enforcement of a rigid regimen after the acute phase of the illness has subsided.

Tentative suggestions are offered for a plan of treatment with modification according to the status of the individual patient:

Persons with congestive heart failure should be allowed out of bed for several hours a day, as soon as severe dyspnea at rest has subsided. Following myocardial infarction, recumbency should not be prescribed for a longer period than two to three weeks after the more acute and alarming symptoms have subsided. The recumbent position should not be enforced on patients who are more comfortable sitting. Other things being equal, it would appear wise to allow elderly patients out of bed sooner than younger ones. Rest in bed for more than a day or two at a time probably has no place in the treatment of angina pectoris except in those patients who are especially liable to develop in the immediate future myocardial infarction, as indicated by increasingly frequent and prolonged attacks at rest. In all patients with the severe forms of heart disease activity should be kept below the symptomatic threshold; i.e., should be less than that amount which induces dyspnea or pain.

From Dr. Nicholson J. Eastman's (Baltimore):

Particularly appropriate to consider are, first, the abuse of rest as it affects pregnant women in industry and, second, to the abuse of rest of the female reproductive organs as it pertains to "child spacing."

It is certain that most women are better at ordinary work in the home, up to the point of comfort, and it is clearly established that it is just as safe, with certain reservations, for pregnant women to work in industrial plants as it is for them to work at home.

Teaching that babies are less likely to survive if born at intervals of less than two years has had wide circulation and has become both to the physician and to the public almost an axiom of maternity. It is responsible, more than any other doctrine, for the tendency to procrastinate child bearing, and in turn, this procrastination is responsible, more than any other factor perhaps, for the low birth rate among certain very desirable social and economic-income groups.

Recent findings so contradict the old, deep rooted teaching that frequent childbearing is dangerous, as to make them seem on first consideration rather incredible. If these findings are considered in the light of maternal and fetal mortality rates according to the age of the mother they appear altogether logical and, indeed, are exactly what one would expect. Whatever advantage is gained by a rest period of several years between births seems to be offset and in some respects more than counterbalanced by the aging factor, for the most important talisman which a childbearing woman can possess is youth.

From Dr. Ralph H. Gormley's (Mayo Clinic); N. Y.):

Prompt restoration of surgical patients to normal life is an essential feature of convalescent supervison. Early postoperative activity and walking provide manifest modifications in customary convalescent care by which the process of reconditioning may be largely eliminated and early rehabilitation achieved.

From Dr. William Dock's (Los Angeles):

Even prolonged bed rest is rarely followed by serious physical sequelae when young patients are kept in bed without any sedatives, whereas fatal complications are apt to ensue when indolent, obese, elderly patients are confined to bed after prolonged anesthesia, and with enough pain to justify continued use of sedatives and narcotics. The physician must always consider complete bed rest as a highly unphysiologic and definitely hazardous form of therapy, to be ordered only for specific indications and discontinued as early as posible.

From Dr. Ralph H. Gormley's (Mayo Clinic):

The main group of cases in which orthopedic surgeons have to employ rest in bed as a part of the treatment are cases of disease or injury of the spinal column, pelvis, hip or femur. There is scarcely any form of disease or injury of these parts in which efforts to reduce the period of rest in bed have not produced good results. Orthopedic surgeons, realizing the detrimental effects of complete rest in bed, have over the years succeeded in

prescribed treatment for various conditions. Efforts to improve treatment toward this goal continue, and more advances along this line are predicted.

From Dr. Karl Menninger's (Topeka):

The concept of rest as a form of treatment in psychiatry arose in an era characterized by the total neglect of the consideration of psychologic factors in the study of human beings. In the sense of physical inactivity, rest has ceased to be of any importance in psychiatric phenomena. Indeed, the tendency is in precisely the other direction; namely, to utilize, rather than to blockade further, the available energy of the neurotic or psychotic patient.

Successful medicine must envisage the personality as a physiochemopsychologic unit, susceptible of being interpreted and treated from the physical standpoint, the chemical standpoint and the psychologic standpoint, assuming a working knowledge of the instinctual motivations that impel the adjustment patterns of human life.

"The instinctual motivations that impel the adjustment patterns of human life"! In that last line is the key to the whole situation as to our rest needs, our dietary needs—pretty nearly all our needs. For there, expressed in the language of the psychiatrist to be sure, is the statement that our own instincts, our own appetites, our own inclinations, are far more for our weal than for our woe; and plainly intimated it is that our self-regulatory organism's own feeling of need is so much more trustworthy than the food-specialists' tables of calories and vitamins that to forsake the former for the latter would be more than perilous. It would be disastrous. But we will be saved from this disaster. How? Simply enough. By keeping right on eating what our appetite calls for, when it calls for it, and in what quantity it calls for it.

It is encouraging that good doctors are leading the way to a return to the same sanity as to rest—whether real or spurious.

* * * * *

SEROLOGIC REACTIONS IN SYPHILIS

FAR TOO MANY doctors regard a positive blood test as conclusive evidence that a person has syphilis, to the great injury of many an innocent one.

Many a protest against this outrageous error and wrong has been made by Kolmer, of Philadelphia, a scientist and clinician without superior in this field.

A recent such article[1] of his is quoted, in the hope of saving some of those who trustingly put themselves under our care from being done a terrible and inexcusable injury.

1. J. A. Kolmer, in *Amer. Jl. Pub. Health.*

Since no one serologic test is conclusive for the diagnosis of syphilis, two or more approved methods should be used for each serum. In Kolmer's own laboratory all sera are examined routinely by complement fixation, *macro*flocculation and *micro*flocculation tests.

Physicians should not make a diagnosis of syphilis on the basis of a single doubtful or positive reaction, without support of historical or clinical evidence. When the laboratory report is equivocal for patients without knowledge of exposure, treatment should be withheld for at least three to six months, and the tests repeated meanwhile every two to four weeks. If these are repeatedly negative and no physical signs have appeared, syphilis may be excluded. If the reactions are persistently positive, even though weakly so, a *tentative* diagnosis of syphilis is inescapable and the best interest of the patient demands that treatment be instituted. Doubtful reactions sometimes indicate chronic latent syphilis, either congenital or acquired.

Diseases which may cause falsely positive and doubtful reactions include yaws, pinta, leprosy, malaria, vaccinia and vaccinoid, infectious mononucleosis, virus pneumonia, febrile diseases, upper respiratory tract infections, active tuberculosis, septicemia, subacute bacterial endocarditis, acute lupus erythematosus, relapsing fever, ratbite fever, Weil's disease, typhus fever and trypanosomiasis.

REFRESHER COURSES

1. MEDICAL COLLEGE OF THE STATE OF SOUTH CAROLINA

The list of speakers for the course to be held Nov. 1st to 3d. Titles for their papers to be announced later.

Dr. Hilger Perry Jenkins, Surgeon, Associate Professor of Surgery at the University of Chicago.

Dr. Albert David Kaiser, Pediatrician, Associate Professor of Pediatrics at Rochester University and on the Advisory Committee of the Children's Bureau (American Academy of Pediatrics).

Dr. Eugene Markley Landis, Physiologist, former Professor of Internal Medicine at Virginia and now the George Higginson Professor of Physiology at Harvard. In 1942 he was president of the Society for Clinical Investigation. He is co-author of a monograph entitled "Hypertension."

Dr. Bret Ratner, Allergist, Associate Attending Physician of the Children's Division, Bellevue, Attending Allergist, Seaside Hospital, Staten Island and Clinical Professor of Pediatrics at N. Y. U., author of "Allergy, Anaphylaxis and Immunotherapy."

Dr. Harold George Wolff, Internist, formerly Assistant Psychiatrist at Johns Hopkins Medical School, now Associate Professor at Cornell and Associate Attending Physician, New York Hospital. His specialties are neurophysiology and psychosomatic medicine.

Dr. George Edward Pfahler, Radiologist, Philadelphia, author of a monograph on the "Röntgen Treatment of Cervical Adenitis," and "The Diagnosis and Treatment of Tumors of the Bladder."

Dr. Paul Titus, Obstetrician, president of the Executive Council of the American Association of Obstetrics, Gynecology and Abdominal Surgery.

Dr. Henry N. Harkins, Surgeon, Associate Professor of Surgery at Johns Hopkins.

Dr. Julius Lane Wilson, Associate Professor of Medicine

at Tulane, Secretary-Treasurer American Trudeau Society—Charity Hospital Staff.

Registration fee for the course is $5.00.

Requests for hotel reservations should be sent as early as possible to Dr. H. G. Smithy, Medical College of the State of S. C., Lucas St., Charleston, S. C., as Charleston is one of the overcrowded cities.

Special Session on Physical Medicine
November 3d
Stark General Hospital Medical Library
(Transportation furnished)

10:00 a. m. to 10:30 a. m.—Tour of Hospital and Physical Therapy Clinic.

10:30 a. m. to 1:00 p. m.—
1. Address of Welcome—Col. W. W. Vaughan, M.C., Commanding Officer, Stark General Hospital, Charleston.
 Physical Medicine and War Injuries:
 Charles H. Fair, Lt. Col., M.C. Chief Surgical Service.
 John G. Reid, Maj., M.C. Chief, Orthopedic Section
 Arthur M. Pruce, Capt., M.C. Chief Physical Therapy Section.
2. Amputations: Methods and technics in combat zones. Revision, after-care and rehabilitation. Demonstration. Major Reid and Captain Pruce.
3. Peripheral Nerve Injury: The role of splinting and Physical Therapy in pre- and post-operative care. Demonstration.
 (a) Electro diagnosis, Lt. Elizabeth Kelly, P. T. A.
 (b) Presentation of typical nerve injuries and splints. Captain Pruce.

1:00 p. m.—Luncheon. Officers Mess.

2. SOUTH CAROLINA SOCIETY OPHTHALMOLOGY AND OTOLARYNGOLOGY

October 31st
9:00 p. m.—Reception for visiting Speakers and Guests.

November 1st
Speakers

9:00 a. m.—Dr. Henry M. Goodyear, Cincinnati.
11:00 a. m.—Dr. James S. Shipman, Philadelphia.
1:30 p. m.—Luncheon, Medical College Library.
3:00 p. m.—Dr. James Watson White, New York.
4:30 p. m.—Dr. Oscar V. Batson, Philadelphia.
6:00 p. m.—Adjournment.
8:00 p. m.—Smoker by South Carolina Society Ophthalmology and Otolaryngology.

November 2d
9:00 a. m.—Dr. Batson.
10:30 a. m.—Dr. White.
12:00 Noon (Lenses and Their Application)—Mr. Scott Sterling, Bausch and Lomb Scientific Staff.
1:00 p. m.—Luncheon, St. Francis Infirmary.
3:00 p. m.—Dr. Goodyear.
4:30 p. m.—Dr. Shipman.
6:00 p. m.—Adjournment.
8:00 p. m.—Founders Day Banquet.

THIOCYANATE THERAPY IN HYPERTENSION
(T. M. Durant, Philadelphia, in *Penn. Med. Jl.*, Aug.)

The thiocyanates normal range is from 0.51 to 2.55 mg. per 100 c.c. of blood—far in excess of that of any other known depressor substance.

Thiocyanate of sodium's or potassium's upper limit of safety is 12 to 13 mg. per 100 c.c. In many instances satisfactory results will be obtained with as low a level as 4 to 5 mg. per 100 c.c. An initial dosage of 5 to 10 grains continued for four to five days will generally result in a blood level of 4 to 8 mg. If no improvement, the dosage may be continued until a level of 10 to 12 mg. is obtained, after that a maintenance dose, 2½ grains per day average, but the range is wide—2½ grains three times a week for one patient up to 10 grains per day for another.

Thiocyanate therapy has been found to be a valuable therapeutic agent in a considerable number of hypertensive patients. Especially is it likely to be effective in those patients, regardless of age, whose renal function is good and whose retinal vessels demonstrate that slight damage has occurred to the arteriolar system. The benefits to be obtained cannot be had without great risk unless the physician employing the drug is fully cognizant of all the principles involved in its proper administration.

THE EARLY DIAGNOSIS OF ACUTE APPENDICITIS IN CHILDREN
(J. A. Garcia, Corpus Christi, in *Med. Rec.*, Aug.)

The early diagnosis of acute appendicitis in children is extremely difficult. Pain and tenderness are apt to be in the midline and slightly to the left. Pain may never become localized or referred to the right lower quadrant, but progress from pain in this described region to the pain of a general peritonitis.

When a child becomes suddenly but not acutely ill and complains of pain in the midline halfway between the umbilicus and the scymphysis pubis; with no diarrhea, little or no fever, and a fairly normal pulse; with pressure tenderness at the point just mentioned, or tenderness all over the abdomen, and a negative urine, acute appendicitis must be strongly suspected and an exploratory laparotomy is justifiable not later than 18 hours after the onset of the disease.

CRAMP IN THE RECTUM
(M. C. Pruitt, M.D., Atlanta, in *Sou. Med. Jl.*, Aug.)

I have had in the last 16 years, 23 cases of cramp in the rectum. In this group there was a family of three brothers and three sisters. The sisters, in their late fifties and sixties, had attacks of cramp in the rectum at regular intervals over a number of years. These attacks, usually at night, were severe enough to wake the patient from sound sleep.

The relief of the acute attacks is usually spontaneous. Changes of position, walking, rubbing, hot sitz bath, local heat, a warm enema—all have been used and are of value. The giving of opiates is not to be recommended, as the durtion of the attack is short. It is usually over before an apiate could have effect.

It is similar to the unexplained, nocturnal, localized tonic spasm in other parts of the body, coming on during sound sleep, such as cramp in the muscles of the calf of the legs.

Dr. *C. J. Andrews*, Norfolk, Va. (in discussion): The relation between this pain and the cramps during pregnancy are very common and are almost always relieved by calcium. This would suggest that the use of calcium might have some influence in this condition.

A SINGLE DOSE OF EPHEDRINE SULFATE (3/4 gr.) taken by mouth at bedtime has proved extremely helpful in the control of nocturnal enuresis in children. It is well to give it for three weeks continuously. If the habit returns, a second course of three weeks. In favorable cases the child ceases to wet the bed almost immediately, although he may miss one or two nights a week for the first two weeks.

NEWS

MEDICAL COLLEGE OF VIRGINIA

Commencement exercises closing the current session will be held at The Mosque September 23rd, at eight o'clock. Honorable J. Melville Broughton, Governor of North Carolina, will be the speaker. Dr. John Shelton Horsley of Richmond will be the recipient of the honorary degree of Doctor of Science at these exercises. The graduating class will number one hundred and seventy-two.

Dr. Robert W. Ramsey of the University of Rochester faculty will join the staff of the college on September 1st as Associate Professor of Physiology, replacing Dr. Ernest Fischer, who is being transferred to the department of physical medicine with the rank of professor.

Dr. Frances A. Hellebrandt of the University of Wisconsin will join the college staff on October 1st as professor of physical medicine in the department to be set up under the recent Baruch grant.

Dr. W. T. Sanger, Dr. J. P. Gray, Mr. Wortley F. Rudd, Dr. T. D. Rose, Dr. S. S. Arnim and Dr. S. S. Negus attended the workshop at Virginia Polytechnic Institute, August 23rd-30th, as sponsored by the State Board of Education.

UNIVERSITY OF VIRGINIA

Dr. Wendell M. Stanley, of the Rockefeller Institute for Medical Research, Princeton, New Jersey, delivered the annual Phi Beta Pi Medical Fraternity Lecture on July 24th. He spoke on the subject Viruses and Their Relation to the Tumor Problem.

Lieut.-Col. Daniel C. Elkin, Surgeon-in-Chief at the Ashford General Hospital in West Virginia, gave the annual address at the time of the initiation exercises of Alpha Omega Alpha on the night of August 11th. He spoke on the subject of Arteriovenous Aneurysm, Review of Cases Resulting from War Wounds.

Dr. Herbert Silvette, Assistant Professor of Pharmacology, Materia Medica and Toxicology, has received a third grant of $250 from the American Medical Association for continuation of investigations on The Effect of Low Barometic Pressure on Kidneys previously damaged, either surgically or by drugs.

SHACKLEFORD'S HOSPITAL TO CLOSE

Dr. John A. Shackelford, owner and operator of Shackelford's Hospital at Martinsville, Va., which was opened 25 years ago by his father, the late Dr. Jesse M. Shackelford, announces that the institution will be closed upon opening of the new Martinsville General Hospital. A Federal grant and loan, totaling $602,000, has been made to the new project.

Shackelford's Hospital, of 54 beds, is located in the downtown section of the town. When closed, all operational equipment will be moved to the new hospital and the building will be converted into business property.

NEW HOSPITAL AGAIN PLANNED IN PETERSBURG

Efforts are being made by Petersburg hospital authorities to revive plans to build a new hospital, and to obtain a Federal grant for that purpose. The project was started several months ago, and a building was torn down to provide a site. At that time, essential materials were frozen and it was impossible to obtain priorities.

Under the recent grant of the Federal Works Administration for several Virginia hospitals it is believed Petersburg may go ahead with plans.

J. Gordon Bohannan, president of the Hospital Board, is communicating with FWA officials in an effort to determine the status of the project.

DANVILLE HOSPITAL TRUSTEES VOTE TO LIQUIDATE
(From Greensboro News)

The trustees of Danville Community Hospital on August 19th adopted a motion calling for the liquidation of the institution which can no longer function with its present resources. The motion will be passed on by shareholders.

Inability to raise sufficient capital for a new building and the failure of a civic movement to raise funds, together with a large amount representing unpaid bills by patients, were factors in the decision to liquidate. The seriousness of depriving Danville of 70 hospital beds when all hospital facilities are overtaxed was alleviated by a report that the city council at its next meeting might investigate the possibility of a city-owned hospital.

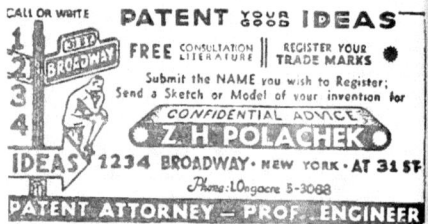

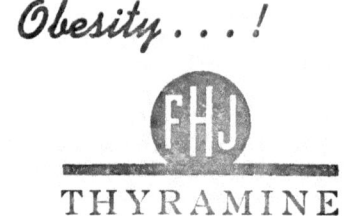

Composition

Thyroid 1 gr. Amphetamine sulphate 5 mgs. Thiamin chloride 1 mg. in suitable combinations with physiological reinforcements.

| No. 1—One Capsule before breakfast |
| No. 2—One Capsule before lunch |
| No. 3—One Capsule at 4 p. m. |

Contraindications
Hypertension .... Hyperthyroidism

Supplied
Capsules: Packages 21 and 42 (one or two weeks supply).

—Professional samples on request—
Available: Any professional pharmacy
F. H. J. PRODUCTS
977 East 176th St., New York 60, N. Y.

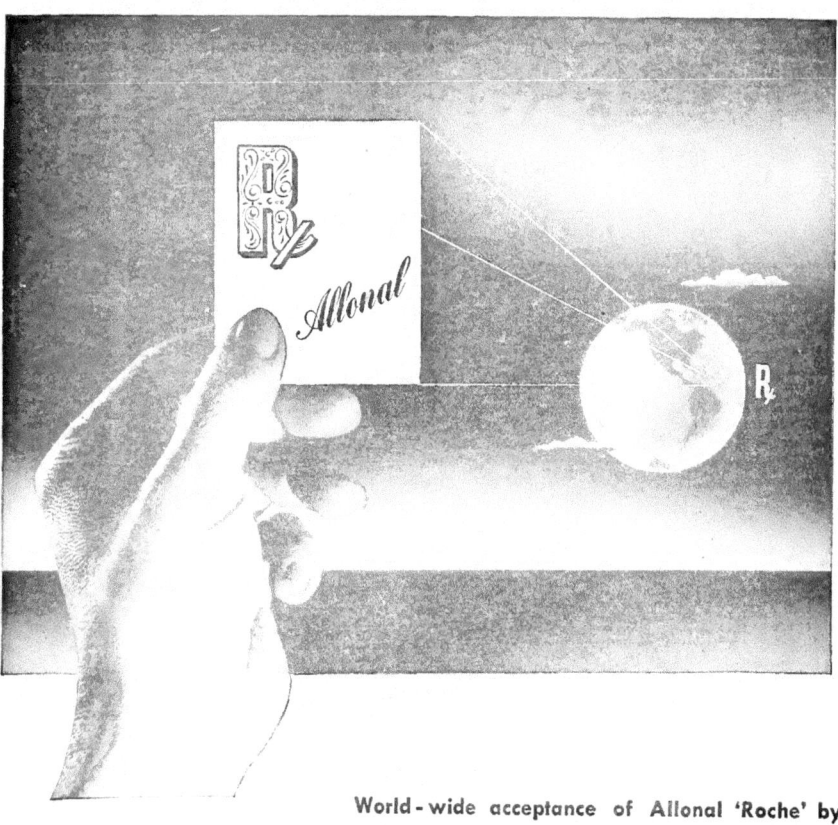

ROCHE PRODUCTS ARE NEVER
ADVERTISED TO THE LAITY

World-wide acceptance of Allonal 'Roche' by the medical profession is a tribute to its efficacy in combating pain and insomnia. Such extensive use is evidence, too, that physicians have found in Allonal their analgesic-hypnotic of choice — one that induces sleep, even in the presence of pain, with very little likelihood of unpleasant reactions following its use. Hoffmann-La Roche, Inc. • Nutley 10 • N. J.

FOR PAIN AND INSOMNIA ALLONAL 'ROCHE'

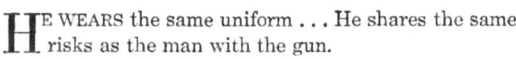

...and Morale

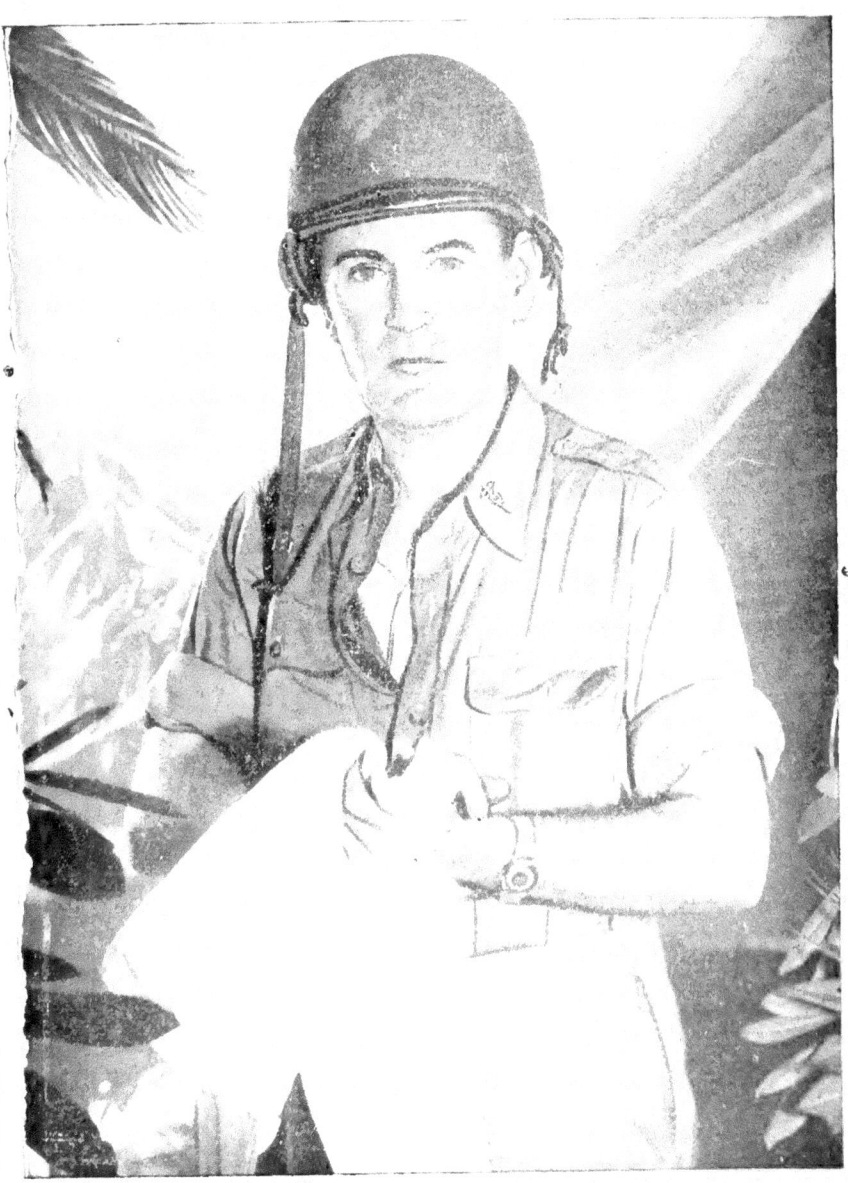

THE AMERICAN COLLEGE OF SURGEONS has cancelled its Annual Clinical Congress because of the great demands upon our transportation systems. From Major General Norman T. Kirk, Surgeon General of the Army, says: "We all like these meetings to be held and to attend them. However, we are needing more and more railroad transportation to move our battle casualties from the ports to our hospitals, and there are still many troops in the United States who require railroad transportation to ports in order to get them overseas. In addition, difficulty is being experienced in obtaining the materials necessary to continue the war. This means transportation for the raw materials and the shipping of the finished munitions to the ports. Each month the need for this material overseas is increasing."

DR. WILLIAM S. CORNELL, now a lieutenant-colonel in the Army, is in charge of an Army hospital on Saipan Island. He left for overseas, after practicing in Charlotte, N. C., for three years, in June, 1942, and was stationed at several points in the Pacific, including Honolulu.

Dr. Chas. N. Wyatt, Greenville, S. C., was promoted to the rank of full Colonel on August 8th. He is now located with the 21st Station Hospital Khouasnshahi in Southern Persia.

Dr. J. S. Gaul, Charlotte, N. C., addressed the Greenville (S. C.) County Medical Society on the evening of August 7th on Shock Treatment for Bulbar Type Poliomyelitis.

MARRIED

Dr. Robert A. McLemore, of Smithfield, North Carolina, and Miss Marjorie Lee Harcourt, of Alliance, Ohio, were married in Philadelphia on August 12th. Dr. McLemore is completing his internship in Jefferson Hospital.

Dr. Robert Payne Beckwith, Jr., of Roanoke Rapids, and Miss Nancy Margaret Kimbrough, of Romney, West Virginia, were married on August 8th. The bride is a graduate of the School of Nursing of the Medical College of Virginia, and is stationed at Valley Forge General Hospital at Phoenixville, Pennsylvania. The bridegroom is completing his internship in the Medical College of Virginia Hospital.

Dr. Matthew Lee Carr and Miss Lilly Belle Rouse, both of LaGrange, North Carolina, were married on August 1st.

DIED

Dr. Alfred A. Kent, 86, former Lenoir, N. C., physician and prominent industrialist, died at his home in Winter Park, Fla., on August 11th, after having been in declining health for several years.

Dr. Kent was graduated from the University of North Carolina and from Jefferson Medical College. In 1905 he entered the industrial field in Lenoir, being one of the pioneer furniture manufacturers of the city. He moved to

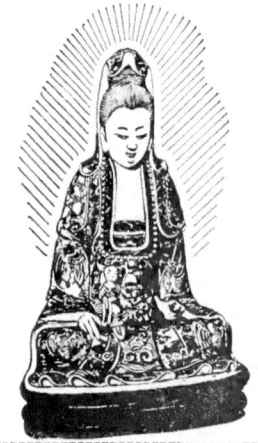

Hotchkiss and Siegler
FERTILITY IN MEN • FERTILITY IN WOMEN

Since the beginning of time, sterility has been a major concern of mankind. Peoples have ransacked apothecary shops, have sought favor with gods and goddesses, that they might beget and multiply. Even today, the treatment of sterility is a maze of pitfalls and indecision. Cutting clearly through this labyrinth, Drs. Hotchkiss and Siegler bring two thoroughly practical books—*Fertility in Men* and *Fertility in Women*—both heralded as real aids to the medical profession.

FERTILITY IN MEN—
Dr. Hotchkiss handles his subject with clarity and perspective. His emphasis on the practical details of treating cases of male sterility makes the volume of great value to the practitioner.

ROBERT S. HOTCHKISS, B. S., M. D., Lt. Com., Medical Corps, U.S.N.R. (now on active duty), is widely known and respected for his work as Assistant Professor of Urology, New York University Medical College, and as Instructor in Surgery, Cornell University Medical College.

FERTILITY IN WOMEN—
Dr. Siegler writes from a functional viewpoint, with structure, function, and disease integrated to present a unified clinical picture. Detailed as to procedure and technic... completely practical... a real, workable guide.

SAMUEL L. SIEGLER, M. O., F. A. C. S., is known for his highly successful work as Attending Obstetrician and Gynecologist, Brooklyn Women's Hospital; Attending Gynecologist, Unity Hospital; and Assistant Obstetrician and Gynecologist, Greenpoint Hospital.

KWAN YIN
Chinese Goddess of Fertility

Fertility • IN MEN $350 • IN WOMEN $450

BOTH BOOKS IN ATTRACTIVE SLIP CASE $800

J. B. LIPPINCOTT COMPANY, Philadelphia 5, Pa.
Enter my order and send me at once—
☐ Fertility in Men—$3.50   ☐ Fertility in Women—$4.50   ☐ Both Books—$8.00
☐ Cash Enclosed   ☐ Charge my account

Send to: NAME_____
STREET ADDRESS_____
CITY & STATE_____

Under your Guarantee, I may return either book in 10 days otherwise I will pay in full in 30 days.

Florida in 1925 after practicing medicine in Caldwell County for 43 years.

Dr. Kent organized Caldwell County Medical Society, was county physician, served on the State Board of Medical Examiners, was president of the Medical Society of the State of North Carolina, a member of the State Board of Health, and served as state legislator.

In 1925 he retired from medical practice and his industrial affairs at Lenoir, and went to Winter Park to assume management of the building and loan association there and he held that position until ill health forced him to retire.

A survivor is a doctor son, Dr. A. A. Kent, Jr., of Granite Falls, N. C.

Maj. Irving I. Shure, Army Medical Corps, who was located at Bethel, N. C., for several years, was killed by accident in Scotland July 27th, memorial services were held at the Temple Israel meeting house in Boston.

Dr. Laurence H. Coffee, Waxhaw, N. C. (Medical College of Va., 1906), died at a Lincolnton, N. C., hospital September 1st, after an illness of one day.

Dr. Benjamin Everett Reeves, 77, one of the most widely knowwn men in northwestern North Carolina, died suddenly at his home at West Jefferson, August 30th.

Graduating from the College of Physicians and Surgeons of Baltimore in 1891, Dr. Reeves immediately entered practice at West Jefferson, and had been active in the practice of medicine for half a century and in public affairs through his life. He had served as a member of the North Carolina legislature in 1899, as county physician and coroner, and as member of the Commission for the State School for the Blind.

Dr. Robert Bennett Bean, 70, for 25 years professor of anatomy at the University of Virginia, died August 27th.

Born at "Pleasant Hill," Galax, Virginia, he was educated at Virginia Polytechnic Institute and Johns Hopkins, and also studied at the Ecole de Medecin, Paris. Before coming to Virginia, he held positions at Johns Hopkins, University of Michigan, University of Philippines, and Tulane.

Dr. Bean was author of several books, including "Racial Anatomy of the Philippine Islander," "The Races of Man," "The Peopling of Virginia."

Former president of New Orleans Academy of Science, and member of American Society of Anatomists, he was first president of University of Virginia Chapter of Sigma Psi, research society.

Dr. Robert Lee Payne, 57, died suddenly at his home at Monroe, N. C., September 7th. Dr. Payne was graduated by Tulane University Medical School in 1911, and had practiced at Monroe and in Union County ever since, with the exception of the period of World War I, when he served in France with the rank of Captain.

RESULTS OF TREATMENT OF THE ACUTE ALCOHOLIC PSYCHOSES BY HYPERTONIC SALINE
(I. J. Silverman, Washington, in *Med. An. D. C.*, Mar.)

The hypertonic saline treatment for the acute alcoholic is seldom contraindicated, but one is hesitant to use it in a case of great renal insufficiency. Occasionally a patient with organic heart disease, just recovering from decompensation, suddenly show psychotic symptoms. Edema might occur in the brain. Giving 100 c.c. or 150 c.c. of 5 per cent saline intravenously has helped many such patients over a stile.

ASAC

15% by volume Alcohol
Each fl. oz. contains:

Sodium Salicylate, U. S. P. Powder........ 40 grains
Sodium Bromide, U. S. P. Granular.......... 20 grains
Caffeine, U. S. P.................................... 4 grains

ANALGESIC, ANTIPYRETIC AND SEDATIVE.

Average Dosage

Two to four teaspoonfuls in one to three ounces of water as prescribed by the physician.

How Supplied

In Pints, Five Pints and Gallons to Physicians and Druggists.

•

Burwell & Dunn Company

Manufacturing 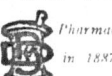 *Pharmacists*
Established *in 1887*

CHARLOTTE, N. C.

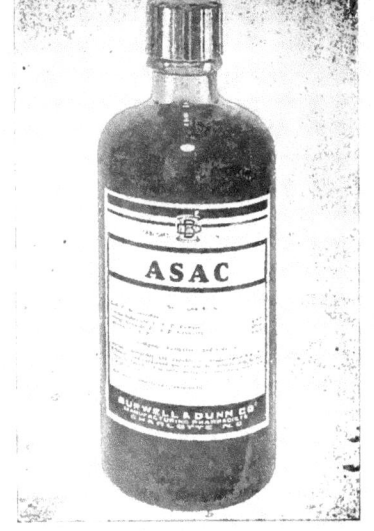

BOOKS

FUNDAMENTALS OF INTERNAL MEDICINE, by WALLACE MASON YATER, A.B., M.D., M.S. (in Med.) F.A.C.P., Professor of Medicine and Director of the Department of Medicine, Georgetown University School of Medicine; Formerly Fellow in Medicine, The Mayo Foundation. Second edition. *D. Appleton Century Co., Inc.*, 35 West 32nd Street, New York City. 1944. $10.00.

In our review of the first edition of this book gratification was expressed at the inclusion of sections on diseases of the skin, diseases of the eyes and diseases of the ears—features not to be found in many books dealing with internal medicine published in the last 50 years. These features are retained in the present edition. Also, it has been kept in mind to exclude all but the essentials in the discussion of any condition. In this way, and in this way only, could the essentials of the subject be embraced in one volume of moderate size.

Considerable attention has been paid to subjects of special interest to internists in the armed forces, who will find the book of great value during the continuation of warfare; and they, along with those of us who did not get into this war, will find this information of great value after the fighting is over.

The author's fine understanding of the practical things of medicine is manifested anew in this edition. He still believes that the most important thing in medicine is to find out what is wrong with the patient and to best help him to get well. The book is excellent in every way.

THE ART OF ANAESTHESIA, by PALUEL J. FLAGG, M.D., Visiting Anaesthetist to Manhattan Eye and Ear Hospital; Consulting Anaesthetist to St. Vincent's, Woman's, Sea View, Jamaica, Mount Vernon, Flushing, Mary Immaculate, St. Mary's and Nassau Hospitals and Chairman of Committee on Asphyxia of the American Medical Association; 7th edition, 166 illustrations. *J. B. Lippincott Co.*, E. Washington Square, Philadelphia 5, Pa. 1944. $6.00.

The author's position in his specialty is well known to all but recent entrants to the profession, and to these the number of hospitals which are glad to avail themselves of his services will be convincing. This conviction will be strengthened on considering that the first edition of this work was published 28 years ago. The final proof will be afforded by study of the book itself and putting its teaching into effect.

A pregnant paragraph is quoted:

"While courses in anaesthesia, arranged for medical officers, stress the importance of cyclopropane, intravenous pentothal sodium, regional block or spinal, etc., little or nothing is said of the most widely used and admittedly the most dependable anaesthetic, ether. Because ether is the most difficult of all anaesthetics to administer, without producing unpleasant after effects, seems to be no reason why its skillful use should not be taught. It is only by such practical experience that the students will learn that its commonly accepted, postoperative ill effects are due to mal-administration. Instead of ignoring ether, therefore, and using it carelessly and inefficiently upon the frequent occasions when it must be used, it is suggested that this agent be stressed and its proper administration intensively taught. The result will be lower morbidity, a better surgical field, and less embarrassment for the anaesthetist."

The newer anaesthetics are not neglected. Nor are they allowed to crowd out the old reliable, the anaesthetic which has been on trial for nearly a hundred years—long enough for physicians and surgeons to learn all its good and all its bad qualities.

Most of those of us who administered anaesthetics when ether was the almost invariable choice retain our belief in, and preference for, ether; and we welcome the author's preference for this old friend in most cases requiring general anaesthesia.

CLINICAL UROLOGY, by OSWALD SWINNEY LOWSLEY, A.B., M.D., F.A.C.S., Director of the Department of Urology (James Buchanan Brady Foundation) of the New York Hospital and THOMAS JOSEPH KIRWIN, M.A., M.S., M.D., F.A.C.S., Attending Surgeon of the Department of Urology (James Buchanan Brady Foundation) of the New York Hospital. Drawings by WILLIAM P. DIDUSCH. Second edition—in two volumes. *The Williams and Wilkins Company*, Mt. Royal & Guilford Aves., Baltimore. 1944. $10.00 for the set.

The plan in this edition is the same as that in the first edition—to supply a text for the medical student, the general practitioner and the general surgeon, and a reference book for the urologist. It represents a survey of diagnosis and treatment of pathological conditions of the urogenital organs according to the present state of knowledge. The urological diseases of women and children are considered in as much detail as are those of men.

Regret is expressed that war conditions have made it impossible to include several hundred illustrations of new operative technics, pathological specimens, and recently designed instruments. New operations and instruments have been described with great particularity in the text, in an attempt to supply information that would have been supplied by the illustrations.

Repetition will be found in various chapters, wherever repetition seemed preferable to cross-reference. The authors endorse the use of anesthetics in urology as preferable in every way to the infliction of any considerable amount of pain. Preference as to treatment of prostatic disease is based on the circumstances of the individual case. Conditions having a large neurologic element and a

(To P. 360)

What happens when your hat comes down?

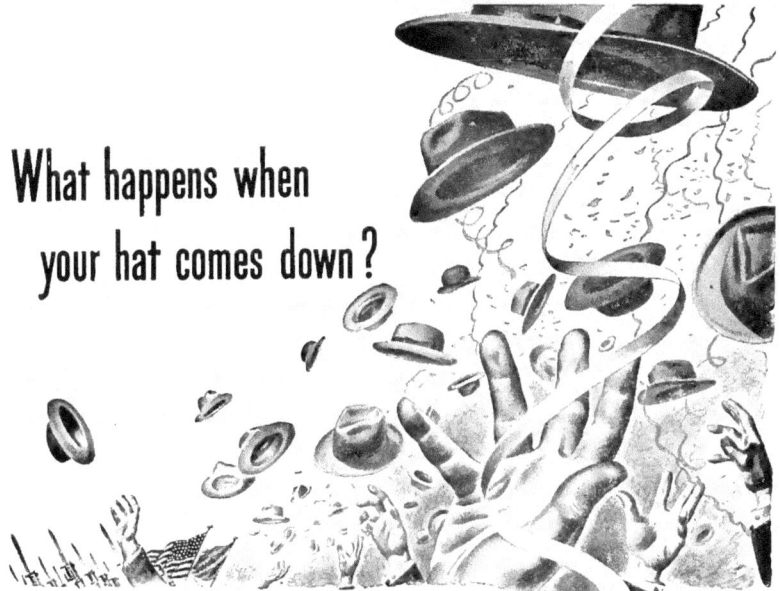

SOMEDAY, the War will be over.

Hats will be tossed into the air all over America on *that* day.

But what about the day after?

No man knows just what's going to happen then. But we know one thing that must *not* happen:

We must *not* have a postwar America fumbling to restore an out-of-gear economy, staggering under a burden of idle factories and idle men, wracked with internal dissension and stricken with poverty and want.

That is why we must buy War Bonds— now.

For every time you buy a Bond, you not only help finance the War. You help to build up a vast reserve of postwar buying power. Buying power that can mean millions of postwar jobs making billions of dollars' worth of postwar goods and a healthy, prosperous, strong America in which there'll be a richer, happier living for every one of us.

To protect your Country, your family, and your job *after* the War—*buy War Bonds now!*

Let's all KEEP BACKING THE ATTACK!

The Treasury Department acknowledges with appreciation the publication of this message by

YOUR NAME HERE

T-3531   5 1-2 x 8 in.   110 screen

NEUROLOGY and PSYCHIATRY

(*Now in the Country's Service*)
*J. FRED MERRITT, M.D.
NERVOUS and MILD MENTAL DISEASES
ALCOHOL and DRUG ADDICTIONS
Glenwood Park Sanitarium   Greensboro

TOM A. WILLIAMS, M.D.
(*Neurologist of Washington, D. C.*)
Consultation by appointment at
Phone 3994-W
77 Kenilworth Ave.   Asheville, N. C.

EYE, EAR, NOSE AND THROAT

H. C. NEBLETT, M.D.
OCULIST
Phone 3-5852
Professional Bldg.   Charlotte

AMZI J. ELLINGTON, M.D.
*DISEASES of the
EYE, EAR, NOSE and THROAT*
Phones: Office 992—Residence 761
Burlington   North Carolina

UROLOGY, DERMATOLOGY and PROCTOLOGY

THE CROWELL CLINIC of UROLOGY and UROLOGICAL SURGERY
Hours—Nine to Five   Telephones—3-7101—3-7102
STAFF
ANDREW J. CROWELL, M.D.
(1911-1938)
*ANGUS M. MCDONALD, M.D.   CLAUDE B. SQUIRES, M.D.
Suite 700-711 Professional Building   Charlotte

RAYMOND THOMPSON, M.D., F.A.C.S.   WALTER E. DANIEL, A.B., M.D.
THE THOMPSON-DANIEL CLINIC
of
UROLOGY & UROLOGICAL SURGERY
Fifth Floor Professional Bldg.   Charlotte

C. C. MASSEY, M.D.
*PRACTICE LIMITED
TO
DISEASES OF THE RECTUM*
Professional Bldg.   Charlotte

WYETT F. SIMPSON, M.D.
GENITO-URINARY DISEASES
Phone 1234
Hot Springs National Park   Arkansas

ORTHOPEDICS

HERBERT F. MUNT, M.D.
*ACCIDENT SURGERY & ORTHOPEDICS
FRACTURES*
Nissen Building   Winston-Salem

GENERAL

Nalle Clinic Building 412 North Church Street, Charlotte
THE NALLE CLINIC
Telephone—C-BVDV (if no answer, call 3-2621)

General Surgery
BRODIE C. NALLE, M.D.
GYNECOLOGY & OBSTETRICS
EDWARD R. HIPP, M.D.
TRAUMATIC SURGERY
*PRESTON NOWLIN, M.D.
UROLOGY

Consulting Staff
R. H. LAFFERTY, M.D.
O. D. BAXTER, M.D.
RADIOLOGY
W. M. SUMMERVILLE, M.D.
PATHOLOGY

General Medicine
LUCIUS G. GAGE, M.D.
DIAGNOSIS

LUTHER W. KELLY, M.D.
CARDIO-RESPIRATORY DISEASES

J. R. ADAMS, M.D.
DISEASES OF INFANTS & CHILDREN

W. B. MAYER, M.D.
DERMATOLOGY & SYPHILOLOGY

(*In Country's Service)

C—H—M MEDICAL OFFICES
DIAGNOSIS—SURGERY
X-RAY—RADIUM
DR. G. CARLYLE COOKE—*Abdominal Surgery & Gynecology*
DR. GEO. W. HOLMES—*Orthopedics*
DR. C. H. MCCANTS—*General Surgery*
222-226 Nissen Bldg. Winston-Salem

WADE CLINIC
Wade Building
Hot Springs National Park, Arkansas

H. KING WADE, M.D.	*Urology*
ERNEST M. MCKENZIE, M.D.	*Medicine*
*FRANK M. ADAMS, M.D.	*Medicine*
*JACK ELLIS, M.D.	*Medicine*
BESSEY H. SHEBESTA, M.D.	*Medicine*
*WM. C. HAYS, M.D.	*Medicine*
N. B. BURCH, M.D.	*Eye, Ear, Nose and Throat*
A. W. SCHEER	*X-ray Technician*
ETTA WADE	*Clinical Laboratory*
MERNA SPRING	*Clinical Pathology*

(*In Military Service)

INTERNAL MEDICINE

ARCHIE A. BARRON, M.D., F.A.C.P.

INTERNAL MEDICINE—NEUROLOGY

Professional Bldg. Charlotte

JOHN DONNELLY, M.D.

DISEASES OF THE LUNGS

Medical Building Charlotte

CLYDE M. GILMORE, A.B., M.D.

CARDIOLOGY—INTERNAL MEDICINE

Dixie Building Greensboro

JAMES M. NORTHINGTON, M.D.

INTERNAL MEDICINE—GERIATRICS

Medical Building Charlotte

SURGERY

(Now in the Country's Service)
R. S. ANDERSON, M. D.

GENERAL SURGERY

144 Coast Line Street   Rocky Mount

R. B. DAVIS, M. D., M. M. S., F. A. C. P.
*GENERAL SURGERY
AND
RADIUM THERAPY*
Hours by Appointment

Piedmont-Memorial Hosp. Greensboro

(Now in the Country's Service)
WILLIAM FRANCIS MARTIN, M.D.

GENERAL SURGERY

Professional Bldg.   Charlotte

OBSTETRICS & GYNECOLOGY

IVAN M. PROCTER, M. D.

OBSTETRICS & GYNECOLOGY

133 Fayetteville Street   Raleigh

SPECIAL NOTICES

TO THE BUSY DOCTOR WHO WANTS TO PASS HIS EXPERIENCE ON TO OTHERS

You have probably been postponing writing that original contribution. You can do it, and save your time and effort by employing an expert literary assistant to prepare the address, article or book under your direction or relieve you of the details of looking up references, translating, indexing, typing, and the complete preparation of your manuscript.

Address: *WRITING AIDE,* care *Southern Medicine & Surgery.*

BOOK REVIEW
(From P. 357)

large urologic element are dealt with in gratifying detail and with proper consideration for each of the two elements.

Modifications and additions to the diagnostic and therapeutic armamentarium of urology are judiciously evaluated. The medical are not subordinated to the surgical aspects. The work has the unreserved endorsement of this reviewer.

THE JOURNAL OF
SOUTHERN MEDICINE AND SURGERY

306 NORTH TRYON STREET, CHARLOTTE, N. C.

The Journal assumes no responsibility for the authenticity of opinion or statements made by authors or in communications submitted to this Journal for publication.

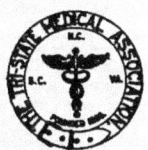

JAMES M. NORTHINGTON, M.D., Editor

| VOL. CVI | OCTOBER, 1944 | No. 10 |

Insulin Resistance: Report of Two Cases*

WILLIAM R. JORDAN, M.D., Richmond

THE CHANGING SEVERITY of diabetes at different times in the same patient makes frequent observations by the patient and by the doctor essential if trouble is to be avoided. Certain conditions, such as inflammation, may produce such a change for the worse, just as control of the diabetes is often followed by lessened severity. At times the severity of the disease changes without detectable cause. In general these changes of either nature are relatively mild. Occasionally they are extreme and constitute the rise and subsidence of insulin resistance. Such resistance may be acute in onset and very severe, or the onset may be gradual and the course prolonged. The first is dramatic and impressive and, if acidosis is present or develops, death is apt to occur. The second gives more warning and greater time for us to realize what is taking place and should give much better results unless it is progressive and persistent, as was true in the case of hemochromatosis reported by Root.[1]

In 1941 Martin et al.[2] reported a fatal case of insulin resistance and summarized the records of 26 cases they collected from the literature. Since then there have been reports[3] of a few other cases. In some it appears that bolder treatment might have given better results as is indicated by the successful use of larger doses of insulin in the case reported by Glass et al. ([3]b) The enormous amount of insulin given in 24 hours by Wiener[4] (3,250 units) was not required while the patient was in clinical acidosis and it did produce hypoglycemia. However, this dosage may well have prevented acidosis which Wiener apparently feared.

The two cases I am reporting represent the acute type which comes without warning and the more gradual kind that persists for many months.

Case No. 207.—A 44-year-old woman with diabetes of 12-years duration was brought to the Stuart Circle Hospital in a semicomatose condition. During the preceding 12 years, dietary treatment was used for control of the sugar, insulin having been employed for one month only of this time. Six days before admission one wrist had become acutely inflamed and other joints had gradually become involved. She had become feverish and had developed a sore throat. Her blood sugar was found to be 536 mg. at the hospital, and I was asked to see her several hours after treatment with insulin and intravenous fluid had been started. At this time the blood CO_2 combining power was found to be 23 vol. per cent.

The physical examination showed a very drowsy, fat woman with slight hyperpnea and considerable dehydration. The involved joints of the arms and legs were acutely inflamed. The tendon jerks were absent. The throat was diffusely red resembling a streptococcal pharyngitis. The blood pressure was 175/102. Otherwise nothing of consequence was noted.

The acidosis and stupor were relieved in 13 hours by 160 units of insulin. During the next few days, under treatment with sulfanilamide, there was a little improvement in the joints but a phlebitis arose in the right thigh. Anemia developed, so the sulfonamide drug was discontinued. The daily insulin dosage rose from 100 units to 151 units of regular insulin. Eight days after admission there was evidence of improvement. The joints were much better and the urine was free of sugar with less insulin which was gradually reduced to 64 units 10 days later. This had to be increased to 97 units 35 days after admission.

At this time protamine insulin was begun in addition to regular insulin. However, there was an exacerbation of the joint condition which increased the insulin need considerably. Fifty-one days after admission the patient was getting 215 units of insulin and from then until discharge at

---
*Presented to Tri-State Medical Association of the Carolinas and Virginia, meeting at Charlotte, Feb. 28th-29th, 1944.

least 200 units were needed daily. The right hip showed marked bone erosion and a cast was applied. On discharge from the hospital 83 days after admission the patient was given a total of 310 units of insulin daily (240 P + 70 R). During the next month only 20 units of regular insulin could be omitted, and it was 6½ months before the insulin requirement fell below 200 units daily. At this time the cast was removed and the hip joint was firmly ankylosed. During the next four months ending one year after admission to the hospital, the dose was gradually reduced to 100 units, at which level it remained for three years, but in the past two years she has taken no insulin. She has made no test for sugar but has remained in good health and done all of her housework.

Case No. 515.—A colored woman, aged 65, was brought to the Retreat for the Sick September 6th, 1941, on account of a sore foot and diabetes. The diabetes of 8-years' duration, had been treated recently at home with a neglected diet and 5 units of regular insulin twice daily, with fairly good urine tests. The sore foot was of 2-months' duration and a discharge from the sore had existed for the three weeks preceding admission. Examination disclosed a drowsy, toxic-appearing woman with obvious weight loss and definite arteriosclerosis. The temperature was moderately elevated. The heart and the blood pressure were normal. There was left footdrop, and the left ankle jerk and pulsation in the dorsalis pedis artery were absent. There was a large abscess of the sole of the left foot originating in a callus. Redness extended up to the ankle. Four ounces of foul pus escaped when the abscess was opened.

The blood sugar on admission was 312 mg. and the urine contained acetone, sugar and albumin, but no diacetic acid. Treatment consisted of diet, fluids, **an immediate dosage** of 20 units each of crystalline and protamine insulin by separate injections, and sulfathiazole by mouth. Continuous wet, boric-acid dressings were used on the foot. The following day the urine showed no acetone and only 24 grams of sugar in 24 hours with an insulin dosage of 57 units, which was continued the third day during which the infection was subsiding.

The morning of the fourth day the patient was vomiting and slightly drowsy but the breathing was normal. Acetone was present in the urine and the blood sugar was 420 mg. The usual morning dose of 47 units of insulin was given, plus an additional 40 units when the blood sugar was reported. In spite of the 87 units of insulin and a rather trivial and subsiding infection, the patient became steadily worse, so that by early afternoon hyperpnea was obvious and the CO_2 combining power of the blood was only 18 vol. per cent. The usual treatment for diabetic coma was given with some caution in view of the unusual occurrence of acidosis in circumstances which should have contributed to improvement of the patient; such as a suitable diet, controlled infection, and a considerable increase in insulin dosage. Improvement in the acidosis was obvious by 7 P. M. Nevertheless, the blood sugar remained over 400 mg. and insulin was continued through the night at frequent intervals. By 4 A. M. clinical acidosis was barely perceptible but the sugar continued high, and the blood sugar at 8 A. M. was 400 mg. in spite of an insulin dosage of 627 units in the preceding 24 hours. The succeeding day brought no particular change, insulin being given at the rate of 60 units every hour with no reduction in the blood sugar, although the CO_2 combining power gradually rose to 33 vol. per cent and by 10 P. M. the urine contained no acetone. At this time the first reduction in blood sugar was noted (to a level of 340 mg.) and the urine became free of sugar. A total of 1,297 units of insulin was given during this 48-hour period and the blood sugar at the end of this period was still 440 mg., although acidosis was not now evident. The third day of this experience passed without incident, only 205 units of insulin being given. At this time amputation through the thigh was done on account of grossly inadequate circulation in the infected foot, and on this day 290 units of insulin were given. After this the insulin dosage was reduced gradually to 135 units daily at the time of discharge 18 days after admission to the hospital. Three weeks later I was called again to see the patient who had been unconscious and taken no food for three days. I found her in typical insulin shock with a blood sugar of 33 mg. A dose of 135 units of insulin had been given daily. No check of the blood sugar or reduction in insulin was made in spite of a very high renal threshold and one definite insulin reaction with unconsciousness. In spite of a return of the blood sugar to normal, the patient never regained consciousness and died with a terminal pneumonia within 24 hours. Autopsy showed no abnormality of the brain or pituitary gland. The liver was normal save for a moderate parenchymatous degeneration. Generalized arteriosclerosis was marked.

In the first case the resistance to insulin is partially understandable on the basis of severe infection and muscle wasting, although it does seem strange that 160 units of insulin will resuscitate a patient with severe acidosis and infection and be totally ineffective later without the acidosis. In the second case the cause of the resistance to insulin is perplexing indeed. Infection would seem to be excluded, since it was not severe on admission and was subsiding at the time of the flare-up in the severity of the diabetes. There was no evidence of pituitary disorder or other glandular upset save the usual mild diabetes of the elderly person until the time of the acute upset. Sections of the pancreas showed only slight hyaline degeneration and fibrosis in a few islets.

One thing these two cases had in common was the transfer from regular insulin to protamine insulin. In each case insulin was used from several bottles, and the protamine was supplemented by injections of clear insulin. The second case was treated during the acidosis purely by clear insulin, two bottles of which were tested on other patients and found to be potent.

The reports[2,6] in the literature and clinical study of my own cases give no real indication of the cause of such insulin resistance. Poor absorption[6] and infection could hardly account for the effectiveness of such huge doses as have been used. I am less concerned at present with the cause than I am with the treatment. The important point seems to be to give insulin according to needs as disclosed by frequent observations rather than by any rules save that alone. Three things seem to stand out.

1. Early recognition made possible by frequent tests and an alert mind probably will prevent the severe acidosis and the associated poor resistance which lead to death.

2. If very large doses of insulin prove ineffective, the timely use of still larger doses seems to work.

3. All insulin resistance seems to be relative and the prolonged use of sufficiently large doses may produce hypoglycemia which in turn may prove disastrous.

REFERENCES
1. ROOT, H. F.: Insulin Resistance and Bronze Diabetes. *New Eng. J. Med.*, 201:201, 1929.
2. MARTIN, W. P., MARTIN, H. E., LYSTER, R. W., and STROUSE, S.: Insulin Resistance. *J. Clin. Endocrin*, 1:387, 1941.
3.
   a. HART, J. F., and VICENS, C. A.: Insulin Resistance. *J. Clin. Endocrin.*, 1:399, 1941
   b. GLASS, W. I., SPINGARN, C. L., and POLLACK, H.: Unusually High Insulin Requirements in Diabetes Mellitus. *Arch. Int. Med.*, 70:221, 1942.
   c. WAYBURN, E., and BECH, W.: Insulin Resistance in Diabetes Mellitus. *J. Clin. Endocrin.*, 2:511, 1942.
   d. SCHRE.ER, H: Insulin Resistance. *N. Y. State J. Med.*, 43:1341, 1943.
4. WIENER, H. J.: Diabetic Coma Requiring an Unprecedented Amount of Insulin. *Am. J. Med. Sc.*, 196:211, 1938.
5.
   a. JOSLIN, E. P., ROOT, H. F., WHITE, P., and MARBLE, A.: The Treatment of Diabetes Mellitus. Ed. 7. Phil. Lea & Febiger, 1940.
   b. MARBLE, A.: Insulin Resistance. *Arch. Int. Med.*, 62:432, 1938.
   c. TAUBENHAUS, M., and SOSKIN, M.: Mechanism of Insulin Resistance in Toxemic State. *J. Clin. Endocrin.*, 2:171, 1942.
6. ROOT, H. F., EVANS, R. D., REINER, L., and CARPENTER, T. N.: Absorption of Insulin Labeled with Radio-active Iodine in Human Diabetes. *J. A. M. A.*, 124:84, 1944.

First two Articles discussed together.

Functional Hypoglycemia*

GRANT L. DONNELLY, M.D., and YATES S. PALMER, M.D., Valdese, North Carolina
Valdese General Hospital

SPONTANEOUS HYPOGLYCEMIA assumed a place of interest in clinical medicine in 1924. At that time Seale Harris noted a close similarity between insulin reactions and symptoms of weakness, nervousness, hunger and sweating occurring three to four hours after meals in non-diabetic patients. This condition was given the name Hyperinsulinism by Harris. It was presumed to be caused by hyperactivity of the pancreas. In 1927 Wilder showed that this hyperactivity was caused by pancreatic adenomata from which he was able to recover insulin. It was further shown that the successful removal of such adenomata resulted in recovery.

The full symptom-complex is related to the central nervous system with flushing, sweating, nervousness, restlessness, weakness, trembles, dizziness, nausea, epigastric pain, hunger, cardiac palpitation, muscle spasm, diplopia, convulsions, and at times aphasia, disorientation and mania.

The diagnosis is based on the following points:
(1) Low fasting blood sugar—below 50
(2) Relief with intravenous glucose
(3) Onset following delayed meals or vigorous exercise
(4) Relentless progress difficult to correct
(5) High carbohydrate intake increases the severity of symptoms.

This is explained by the fact that carbohydrates act as a stimulus to increased insulin production and that the insulin excess outlasts the carbohydrates.

The clinical entity of hyperinsulinism caused by pancreatic adenomata is rare. A more common condition with the same symptoms and most of the same diagnostic points has been recognized. This condition is a *functional* disturbance and is not based on any demonstrable changes in the pancreas. During the past year we have studied nine such patients in the Valdese General Hospital.

Case 1.—A 20-year-old girl, a hosiery machine operator, had complained of weakness and nervousness for one year. She was especially weak before meals, had a poor appetite but felt better after eating. She noted a fine tremor ("trembles") of her hands especially toward the end of the day.

Glucose Tolerance:
  Fasting ½   1   2   3   4   Hours
    37   83   76   71   40   38   Mg. %

On a high-protein diet with frequent feedings this girl gained weight and strength. She now feels well and has no symptoms.

Case 2.—A 36-year-old man for eight months had felt weak and tired. In late morning and late afternoon while at work he had attacks of "trembles" and weakness so severe he could not stand. He gradually became worse and had to quit work for six months but was not much better after the vacation. This patient was not able to say whether or not food gave relief.

Glucose Tolerance:
  Fasting ½   1   2   3   4   Hours
    45   107   75   71   53   50   Mg. %

On a high-protein diet with frequent feedings there was some improvement. This improvement was sharply accelerated by weekly injections of androgenic substance. The patient is now working full time and feels well.

*Presented to Tri-State Medical Association of the Carolinas and Virginia, meeting at Charlotte, Feb. 28th-29th, 1944.

Case 3.—A 16-year-old hosiery inspector had worked one year. She had attacks of unconsciousness following menstrual periods. Sometimes she did not become unconscious. She did not bite her tongue. She ate very poorly and worried a great deal.

Glucose Tolerance:
Fasting ½ 1 2 3 4 Hours
62 100 75 71 71 70 Mg.%

On a high-protein diet, frequent feedings, with iron and brewer's yeast, this patient has shown little or no improvement.

Case 4.—A 16-year-old hosiery worker who complained of attacks of weakness usually following meals and around 10:30-11:30 P. M. These attacks gradually became worse. They lasted for about an hour during which time the patient was not able to stand but did not lose consciousness. She ate very poorly, never taking meat or milk.

Glucose Tolerance:
Fasting ½ 1 2 2½ Hours
26 150 137 120 111 Mg.%

On a high-protein diet with frequent feedings supplemented with brewer's yeast and iron, this patient has gained 15 pounds in two months. She feels well and no longer has attacks of weakness.

Case 5.—A 33-year-old man, a furniture worker, began to have attacks of weakness three years ago, towards the end of the work day. At times he had attacks of palpitation and at times did not sleep well. Food did not relieve his condition. This patient was very unstable.

Glucose Tolerance:

Fasting ½ 1 2 3 4 Hours
48 94 60 60 58 58 Mg.%

With a high-protein diet and frequent feedings and with injections of androgenic substance, he felt well enough to return to work.

Case 6.—A 19-year-old girl for the past year had been operating a full-fashion machine from 4:15 P. M. to 1:15 A. M. She had frequent attacks of weakness around 11:00 P.. M At times she was not able to stand and became semiconscious. Weakness was relieved by coca-cola and prevented by candy eaten around 10:30 P. M.

Glucose Tolerance:
Fasting ½ 1 2 2½ Hours
30 111 69 60 61 Mg.%

A high-protein diet with frequent feedings resulted in complete relief.

Case 7.—A 17-year-old high-school girl, who also works four hours daily, two years ago began to have frequent attacks of weakness and unconsciousness. Fasting blood sugar in hospital was as low as 34 with the weakness.

Glucose Tolerance:
Fasting ½ 1 2 3 4 5 Hours
50 240 120 80 80 75 60 Mg.%

Complete relief from all symptoms was obtained with high-protein diet and frequent feedings.

Case 8.—A 40-year-old business man three years ago began to have weakness and unconsciousness with missed meals and strenuous physical effort. He was thin and under-weight. Attacks were relieved with intravenous glucose.

Glucose Tolerance:
Fasting ½ 1 2 3 4 6
70 70 85 69 69 69 99

A high-protein diet and frequent feedings have given complete relief. This patient has gained 30 pounds.

Case 9.—A 38-year-old hosiery worker began to note a weak, tired feeling toward the end of the day. He felt worse over a period of six months and finally came to the clinic where he was hospitalized.

Glucose Tolerance:
Fasting 1 2 3 3½ Hours
48 49 72 61 66 Mg.%

This patient has gained weight on a high-protein diet and frequent feedings and feels his best in 10 years.

Two factors common to most of the cases were: 1) All were working under conditions of increased stress and strain; 2) With one or two exceptions they were nervous, unstable individuals. In this connection it has already been noted that the symptom-complex is related to the central nervous system.

In conclusion it may be said that with laboratory facilities and adequate history the diagnosis is easy. With reasonable care the treatment is simple and highly satisfactory.

Discussion

DR. GEO. R. WILKINSON, Greenville, S. C.:

The problem of functional hypoglycemia appears to be forever with us. At least the sort of thing that happens between meals when people become irritable and hungry and the blood sugar is found to be below 70.

Some time ago we were content to feed these people some carbohydrates between meals. This more or less quieted them down. More recently it has been shown that a large carbohydrate meal will shoot the blood sugar up, thereby stimulating all the body functions that tend to lower the blood sugar. The blood sugar falls and the symptoms we speak of as hypoglycemia recur. Feeding these people more protein with a small amount of fat and very little carbohydrate seems to level out the curve and the blood sugar has neither its peak nor its depression. The mood continues more or less unchanged from meal to meal. Lately, the discusser has been interested in liver function tests with people who have gastrointestinal complaints, many of which sound like spontaneous hypoglycemia. Many of these people have markedly reduced liver function. In these cases, the protein is stepped up and the carbohydrates kept relatively low and the symptoms frequently disappear. A good many of these people have shown a marked depression in the blood sugar level. We have also found that many of these people have a high blood cholesterol anl low BMR and if put on a high-protein diet will get past the mid-meal point without symptoms. Thyroid extract is useful here. Perhaps our routine dietary which provides a very starchy breakfast starts our people off to work with what is going to preduce the symptoms of hypoglycemia and tends to make them over-eat, when a smaller diet with more proteins would do away with the symptoms and keep the body weight stationary.

DR. WILLIAM R. JORDAN: I'd like to discuss Dr. Donnelly's interesting paper. He made a sharp differentiation

To Page 390

Rehabilitating Those Who Are Psychiatrically Handicapped*

LUTHER E. WOODWARD, Ph.D., Washington
Field Consultant, Division of Rehabilitation

THE WAR has revealed that one-and-a-quarter million men, 13 per cent of all those 18 to 38 years of age coming up for induction board examinations, have some mental or emotional handicap which is believed to make them unfit for military service. Many who were inducted are proving unable, for similar reasons, to serve in the military forces. Forty-five per cent of medical discharges from the armed forces are for some neuropsychiatric condition. Already 300,000 men have been discharged, and 30,000 are being discharged each month, for psychiatric reasons. Sizeable numbers of men and women civilians have suffered mental breakdown or other forms of pronounced nervous instability. Fortunately in some instances mental health has improved with more adequate employment or relief from undue domestic burdens—conditions brought about more or less by the war; but all in all the war has convinced us that our mental health is poorer than we had assumed. A much higher proportion of our fellow citizens than we had thought live rather strained and unhappy lives with varied forms of mental or emotional handicaps.

The degrees of illness and maladjustment range from complete psychoses to very minor maladjustments. A study made in Illinois by Dr. Sommer indicated that 6 per cent of men discharged from the armed forces on psychiatric grounds were so ill as to need hospital care. Veterans' Administration hospitals admit 1,500 to 2,000 veterans each month because of psychiatric disabilities. Fortunately the turnover is rather rapid, 48 per cent of them recovering sufficiently to be discharged from the hospital by the end of the second month.

Others, while not needing hospital care, are unable to work. Many of them attempt one job after another and develop an increasing sense of failure. Others are able to find employment and to say at it although they work under strain and are far from happy in their adjustment. The work itself and the wages received have therapeutic value, and some of these men become more stable after a short period.

The large number of men who have been rejected for military service because of psychiatric conditions is also a matter of concern. Most of them appear able to continue in gainful employment, notwithstanding the fact that an occasional employer has refused to take back men who have been rejected for army duty.

An experiment carried on for one month at the New York City Induction Station revealed that only 15% of the rejections were enough concerned about the causes of rejection to wish to undertake any remedial measures. Fortunately many of the rejected men and a sizeable proportion of those discharged from the armed forces are able to go back into industry and be rather quickly reintegrated into community life. Such recovery and integration must be the goal for all.

Several helpful provisions have been made by the Federal Government but there are also several deficiencies. Veterans' Administration provides hospital care for all who come out of the services in need of it. Because it is army and navy policy to discharge before the completion of treatment tuberculous and psychiatric cases, there is a natural mounting of the numbers of veterans who need hospital care on these two accounts. The Veterans' Administration also provides vocational training and placement in industry for veterans who receive a service-connected rating which entitles them to pension and medical or domiciliary care. The chief gaps as far as the Veterans' Administration services go is for out-patient clinic treatment of men with psychiatric disabilities who do not need to be hospitalized but do require psychiatric treatment, while living at home. The number of veterans' facility neuropsychiatric hospitals is at present limited to thirty and many of them are located outside of large cities; as a result out-patient treatment is rather impracticable for large numbers of these men whose homes are far from the hospital.

The other major provision of the Federal Government is through the establishment of the Vocational Rehabilitation Bureaus of the Federal Security Agency, which pays the administrative costs and 50 per cent of the service and training costs of the State Vocational Bureaus. The Barden-LaFollette Bill removed the restriction which previously limited the service of these bureaus to men with physical handicaps so that the psychiatrically disabled are now eligible for vocational re-training and for medical and psychiatric services if diagnosis indicates a handicap which partially limits the

*Address to a meeting of the Charlotte Mental Hygiene Society, held March 29th, 1944.

man's employability, and if the prognosis indicates likely improvement with vocational training or medical, psychiatric or social services. These bureaus are not expected to establish new clinical facilities but they are clearly authorized to pay for services needed by men who qualify and cannot pay for for such services.

In view of the fact that the Veterans' Administration has thus far granted service-connected ratings to only about 20 per cent of the men with psychiatric handicaps whose claims have been adjudicated, and with only 3 to 5 per cent of discharged men in some states applying to the State Vocational Rehabilitation Bureaus, it is clear that many men who are returning with psychiatric disabilities are not going to get needed service unless communities provide the facilities and see to it that all who want and need such help can get it. There is great need for a broad mental-health program for all—veteran and civilian, male and female, adult and child. Some preliminary planning is being done in the United States Public Health Service which, if implemented by proper legislation, may make more nearly adequate funds available for the development of such programs where needed. This will not, *ipso facto*, provide every community with a clinic. Such programs will call for initiative and organized support in the various localities.

One of the major difficulties in this field is to coördinate the numerous organizations undertaking to serve veterans. In addition to those mentioned there are in many states governors' committees, and in many cities, mayor's committees. The Red Cross plays a major role in advising about claims and giving emergency services of various kinds. State and County Departments of Welfare and Health are interested. There are reëmployment committees of every local board of selective service to insure that veterans get back their jobs if they so desire. U. S. Employment Service is the authorized placement agency for all who wish a different position and there are various groups offering specialized services such as State Tuberculosis Associations, Asociations for the Blind, etc. Army and Navy Relief and the three major veterans' organizations—the American Legion, Veterans of Foreign Wars and Disabled War Veterans—have an active interest in assisting veterans of World War II, but the kinds and amount of service available varies in different places. Mental Hygiene Societies, Councils of Social Agencies, Family Serving Agencies, Young Men's Christian and Hebrew Associations and the churches are all interested. In one state visited recently there are 25 distinct state organizations actively interested in the rehabilitation of veterans.

Obviously no state needs 25 organizations devoted to veterans' interests. Neither is 25 or any other large number of organizations any guarantee that all legitimate needs will be met; in fact, in one state with 25 or more such organizations it is extremely difficult to obtain convalescent care for veterans who very much need it for a few months. In another state equally supplied with organizations virtually no out-patient psychiatric care is available. In this situation certain precautions must be taken and certain needed emphases must be maintained.

We must keep our primary focus on services needed and carefully avoid promoting organizations at the veterans' psychological expense. There is some danger of the mushrooming of new organizations which would only mean more duplication and added confusion. We must avoid the runaround for the veteran. Complaints regarding this have already come from many quarters. It will be unfortunate if not disastrous for morale if large numbers of our service men are permitted to return to civilian life and have an experience of being referred to numerous agencies in succession without getting the particular help needed. Every community is challenged to prevent this.

We need also to ask what specific services the returning service men want and need. It is clear that one of the things most of them want and want promptly is employment. At the far-away battlefronts they have read accounts of soft berths and high wages. Some of them may not be wholly realistic in their employment ambitions but we owe them an opportunity to obtain remunerative employment that uses as fully as possible their various skills. For some who have been wounded and some who have psychiatric disabilities vocational re-training may be necessary. At present, employment opportunities are so plentiful that almost everyone can get work, but it is clear that some men are accepting positions for which they are not fitted and that at a later date they will doubtless need re-training.

Some need convalescent care which in some communities is proving to be a very difficult service to provide. Veterans' facility seems able to provide it for very few because of the constant need for hospital care for those in more serious conditions. Vocational Rehabilitation Bureaus may pay for such care only if the man has been accepted, is engaged in vocational re-training, and cannot pay. Red Cross, Army and Navy Relief, and frequently other veterans' organization services draw the line short of long-term convalescent care.

Some clearly need psychiatric treatment, which in many communities is not available. The acuteness of their need is clear from Dr. Thomas A. C. Rennie's account of the problems of these men.

"The problems facing the men discharged from service are multiple. Perhaps the most common is the mistaken sense of being stigmatized by discharge for a nervous or mental condition. Although employment in the main is now easy to obtain, some employers have refused to take back men diagnosed as psychoneurotic. Socially these men find the adjustment at home difficult. They belong to no recognized group and in many places there are no organized resources for appropriate recreation. Companionship is denied them because their contemporaries are in service. Unable to work or too embarrassed to seek for work, many of them stay at home, occasionally wandering out in the evening alone to a movie—ashamed to telephone former friends, uncertain as to how to explain their reappearance into civilian life, fabricating some physical symptom to explain their discharge. Many of these men know their diagnoses. Their attempts to read up on the subject of psychoneurosis confuse them. Parents are equally baffled and their apprehension, fear and over-solicitude make the problem worse. Well-meaning friends sometimes add the final damage by suggesting that the soldier is entitled to compensation and should become a ward of the government. The man flounders for months while the Veterans' Administration adjudicates his case. He sometimes feels neglected; he believes that his own government has lost interest in him. Fortunately at this moment relatively few of these men are primarily concerned with issues of pension. Not over ten per cent of the men we have seen at the New York Hospital have been involved in government litigations or blame the army experience primarily for their condition, or dwell on dissatisfaction with the treatment that they received in army hospitals. This picture may change radically five years from now but in the main these men are ready now to assume their own responsibility for obtaining help without having their treatment complicated by neurotic compensation patterns.

"When these men finally begin to look around for help, they have little knowledge as to where to go and are apt to be confused by the well-intentioned activities of diverse groups, all of whom are interested in the same problem. Vocational floundering is common. Too many jobs too poorly chosen for their needs are apt to be offered them with the result that they quickly shift from one vocational placement to another. No interpretation of their conditions is available for the many placement agents who want to serve them. Oftentimes they are too sick to work and are doomed to failure. These men are in need of psychiatric help and interpretation. Unless this is first available, floundering is inevitable."

A sound and economical referral system must be established. Two methods are being used by different communities. One is to provide every returning soldier with an informational guide that acknowledges the various types of problems which may confront him and lists the agency or agencies that give the type of service needed in the light of his problem. The Rehabilitation Division of the National Committee for Mental Hygiene, recognizing extensive need for such information, is preparing a sample leaflet which will contain simply stated sound psychological principles that may help to develop proper attitudes toward the veteran on the part of his family and neighbors and at the same time offer some helpful suggestions to the veteran himself. The information regarding agencies and their services would of course have to be compiled by each community, in view of the wide variation in the resources available.

The second method is the establishment of a center to which all veterans are invited to go no matter what particular problems they face. Boston recently established such a center and New York City is in the process of establishing one. Another example is Peoria, Illinois, whose plan has received rather wide publicity. The plan differs somewhat in such centers but in every instance effort is made to use competent interviewers, selected on the basis of skill in making quick diagnoses of difficulties and on the basis of thorough knowledge of the resources. In Peoria the group responsible for the center has insisted that the interviewer who first sees the veteran should be a veteran skilled in interviewing. In Boston the first person to interview him is a veteran who sees that the returning soldier receives information concerning the veterans' organizations and has access to their services. Psychologists are available for testing and social workers for case work interviewing. A doctor is present certain hours and psychiatrists are on call. An unofficial report from Boston indicates that the demand for service has been less than anticipated.

An adaptation of this which is recommended by some thoughtful professional workers is to place, either on a loaned or employed basis, top-notch interviewers in the organizations which have a natural access to the returning soldier, namely, American Red Cross, Veterans' Administration, U. S. Employment Service, State Vocational Rehabilitation Bureaus, and whatever other organizations have contacts with appreciable numbers of veterans. There is a grave question whether the best way to get a job done that is not being done is merely to set up a new agency, when one of the chief causes of confusion is the already existing multiplicity of agencies.

The pattern for bringing about sound and economical referrals may well vary in different communities but the need for this must constantly be kept in mind and effective measures taken to establish it. A runaround with ineffective referrals would quickly add to the confusion and cause justifiable resentment among the men and women returning from the service. Agencies could muff their opportunity quite completely by failing to get men to the agencies that can effectively serve them.

In many communities it will be necessary to establish new facilities for some of the unmet needs. Among those most commonly needed are adult psychiatric clinics and convalescent care. Opportunities for vocational retraining and for occupational replacement are much more adequate than for the services just mentioned. As would be expected, these two services most needed for the returning veteran are also two of the services most commonly needed by sizeable numbers of civilians.

Again the organizational pattern for providing such needed services may well vary. Insofar as trained personnel are available, it will be smart for communities to establish their adult psychiatric clinic services on a permanent basis and make the service available to both men and women, civilians and veterans. Many communities for many years have needed adult out-patient clinics, particularly for people who are employed and can visit such clinics only on evening time.

The problem of finances is sure to arise in this connection. Community chests in some instances may quickly accept the challenge and provide the necessary funds. In view of the needs of veterans and of civilians whose disabilities are more or less war connected, war chests might rightly come forward with the funds. Service clubs and some of the veterans' organizations and their auxiliaries might well assist in such projects.

In other communities, because of lack of funds or personnel, it may not be possible to add to the permanent psychiatric resources, but it may be possible to set up special rehabilitation clinics, drawing in psychiatrists, social workers, and psychologists largely on a voluntary part-time basis. The three rehabilitation clinics in New York City have been set up on that basis. The New York Hospital Rehabilitation Clinic, for example, uses volunteer time of 11 psychiatrists, 7 social workers, 2 clinical psychologists, 2 occupational therapists, and 1 librarian. The only paid staff members are one full-time social worker and one secretary. The clinics at the American Red Cross Headquarters and at Lenox Hill Hospital are similarly on a volunteer basis.

There is marked interest in many parts of the country in establishing such rehabilitation clinics, to meet some of the current needs. Some men need only short treatment, some longer. Others scarcely need therapeutic interviews with a psychiatrist but do need the listening ear and personal guidance of trained social workers, or vocational guidance by the clinical psychologist. Frequently the members of the man's family need to be worked with in the interest of better understanding of the man as he returns, and the man himself may need help in finding appropriate employment, recreation, and opportunities to participate normally in the group life of the community. One of the things he very much needs is to be quickly assimilated into the civilian life of the community and to find avenues of satisfaction.

As evidence of the practicability of such rehabilitation clinics, may I again quote Dr. Rennie.

"After six months of experimentation with a rehabilitation clinic, it becomes perfectly clear that psychiatric rehabilitation is feasible and gratifying. The New York Hospital Rehabilitation Clinic has treated over 175 discharged men. These men were considered not in need of hospitalization at the time of dismissal from the Army. Some of them, however, were psychotic. The majority were psychoneurotic. The results of treatment are gratifying in that over one-half show a favorable response.

"The specific feature of genuine interest is the surprising results that can be achieved by very brief psychotherapeutic methods. It is evident that many of these men are achieving their own rehabilitation spontaneously. A very small group can be oriented towards recovery in a single consultation with guidance as to planning. In about one-fourth of the cases, brief psychotherapy aimed at the discussion of resentment, ventilation of traumatic emotional experiences, together with active social service help in making social contacts and finding appropriate employment brings about speedy improvement. The third group, about one-fifth in all, consisting of depressions, hysterical and hypochondriacal reactions need repeated therapeutic interviews. For groups 2 and 3, group therapy methods can be adopted. In others where the problem is deep-seated and was well established prior to induction, intensive and prolonged individual psychotherapy is necessary. The largest number of the disorders are of a chronic type and are not well suited to treatment in a rehabilitation clinic. They are in need either of hospitalization or protracted psychotherapy in established out-patient departments."

State Mental Hygiene Societies and Mental Hygiene Divisions of State Departments may be expected to take leadership at the state level in efforts to organize such clinics. In many cities the Council of Social Agencies by virtue of being an inclusive planning and coördinating body is perhaps in the most strategic position to give local leadership.

In all communities there is pronounced need for an educational program that will increase the public's understanding of psychiatric disabilities. There has been a marked tendency to regard as generally unfit the men rejected as unfitted for military service. This, of course, is not really true of many of them. One man discharged from the service after a few weeks because of marked depression was treated for a very short interval in a psychiatric clinic and arrangement was made with an aviation company to employ him as a machinist, in which type of work he had had a lot of experience. The manager of the firm, which employs about 15,000 men, reported that this man who was sent to them by the psychiatric clinic proved to be positively the most accurate and productive machinist in the entire employ of the company. It is unfortunate that some employers have questioned whether they should take back into their employ men rejected or discharged on the ground of psychiatric conditions. It merely proves the point of need for an educational program to bring about fuller understanding of such conditions. There needs to be more awareness that many men who would not likely adjust in the Army may nonetheless continue to be productive and get along tolerably well while still living at home and having opportunity to get satisfactions through their usual channels.

The National Committee for Mental Hygiene accepts some responsibility for such education and a joint committee, the Emergency Committee of Psychiatric Societies, which has representation from all the psychiatric and mental hygiene agencies around New York is also promoting such a program. The article by Dr. Binger, appearing in the *Saturday Evening Post* a few weeks ago, was the first in a series that is planned. It will be necessary, however, for each local community to add to this understanding. As communities establish facilities for psychiatric rehabilitation, there will be opportunity for getting information and proper interpretation to the readers of the local papers. Pamphlet material and series of meetings with various lay groups should also be helpful.

To plan, coördinate and maintain these various services effectively, a central planning and coördinating committee will be needed in every community. The make-up of such a committee will vary in different places but certainly in a community such as this the health and family divisions of the Council of Social Agencies would be represented; the various Federal, state and local government bodies interested in rehabilitation would be represented, such as U. S. Employment Service, Veterans' Administration, Red Cross, Veterans' organizations, Vocational Rehabilitation Bureaus, etc.; Mental Hygiene Societies and related clinical groups, no matter whether set up under hospitals as community clinics or in social agencies, should come forward with leadership to provide clinical treatment and mental hygiene interpretation; and industrial, religious, recreational, and arts and craft groups should be included—as professional people we probably need their counsel quite as much as they need ours.

SOME COMMONLY USED LAXATIVES

(H. A. McGuigan et al., Chicago, in *Amer. Jl. Dig. Dis.*, Sept.)

Only when the dose of phenophthalein was raised to 0.1 or 0.12 Gm. did a laxative effect occur in two-thirds of the normal individuals. In constipated cases, the laxative effect passed the 50% mark only after doses of 0.2 Gm., while in some of this group 0.3 Gm. were necessary. It is well to keep the dose near the established optimum. We may assume that the reason larger doses of phenolphthalein are necessary is the insolubility of this substance. When 0.10 Gm. phenolphthalein was given, dissolved in an alcoholic elixir, an 80% laxative effect was obtained in normal subjects and in patients.

The toxicity of phenolphthalein is negligible. Children and the aged up to 12 years of age also need comparatively larger doses than the average adult.

We believe that 0.2 Gm. phenolphthalein represents the optimal dose for laxative and also for minimal side effects.

Habitual constipation is a common disorder, which in many instances requires laxative drugs for its most satisfactory treatment. 0.20 Gm. of phenolphthalein and 4 c.c. of aromatic fluidextract of cascara sagrada are the optimal doses.

BROMIDE INTOXICATION

(Willis Sensenbach, Winston-Salem, in *Jl. A. M. A.*, July 15th)

The degree of intoxication paralleled the height of the blood bromide. In all of the severe cases the blood level was as much as 200 mg. per hundred c.c.

The coexistence of heart failure and bromide poisoning presents a problem for in the treatment of one Na Cl is withheld, while in the other the ingestion of sodium chloride is forced. No patient with heart failure who is being treated with a salt-free or salt-poor diet should be given bromides, and all such patients should be warned of the danger of using the various "patented" bromide-containing remedies. When bromide poisoning exists in a patient with heart failure one may substitute ammonium chloride for sodium chloride, thus supplying the chloride need in the treatment of bromism and eliminating the sodium.

The treatment of bromism is simple and effective—the administration of sodium chloride and the forcing of fluids —and response to therapy often dramatic. Six to 8 Gm. of sodium chloride daily would appear to be the optimum dosage, by mouth or parenterally.

More than 50 per cent of the cases in this series were referrable to the injudicious use of bromides by physicians and their failure to recognize the toxic effects. Other causes were the result of uncontrolled sale of "patented" remedies containing bromide.

Mental symptoms due to bromide poisoning often respond much more slowly to treatment than does the level of bromide in the blood.

CALCIUM CHLORIDE—75 grains of this salt daily will supply 1 Gm. of calcium, the amount in 30 oz. of milk, the daily requirement for a growing child. 50% more is recommended for a pregnant woman, who cannot take milk.

A Concept of Hysteria
With Report of An Instructive Case

SAMUEL P. HUNT, M.D., LT COMDR., M.C., U.S.N.R.
(Home Address), Denmark, South Carolina

MOST OF US know, in a general way, what hysteria is and have seen its manifestations many times in practice. Each doctor formulates his own working idea about it and often suspects its presence when the physical findings in a case do not suggest a medical or surgical diagnosis. Yet the general idea about hysteria varies considerably—anywhere from the belief that it is synonymous with malingering to the conviction that a hysterical patient is crazy or feeble-minded, and that nothing can be done about him. This paper will review briefly an accepted psychiatric concept of this illness. This concept is a hypothesis that can always be tested by the physician in individual cases. The doctor can see for himself whether or not the concept is valid. If it is, then it is reasonable to assume that hysteria is just as clear-cut an entity as malaria or pneumonia. As such it naturally requires certain definite clinical findings for diagnosis. Conversely, it is also logical that hysteria, like any other disease, need not be a diagnosis of exclusion. The practice of good medicine requires an understanding of any illness so general and so incapacitating as hysteria.

The classical symptoms of hysteria are commonly known. They are usually disturbances of motor or sensory function: anesthesias, paralyses of a part of the body, blindness, loss of speech or memory, and tremors and other abnormal movements; pain, headache, post-operative urinary retention, and arthralgia may also be symptoms of hysteria. The symptoms of this neurosis are often subtle and may closely simulate organic disease, and the differential diagnosis is sometimes very difficult. Occasionally it will follow an organic illness, often during convalescence. The hysterical symptoms may develop where the initial organic symptoms leave off, following in their footsteps, so to speak, so that it is doubly hard to tell where the organic ends and the functional begins. It is of vital importance to the patient for the physician to recognize the development of the neurosis because the treatment of a functional disturbance is very different from that of an organic illness.

What are the mechanisms in the development of hysteria? Why should a person develop such striking symptoms for no discernible reason? Here is the generally accepted theory: In any neurotic reaction, certain psychological conditions are in operation *before* the patient develops the symptoms. These conditions are as follows: Two antagonistic sets of ideas exist in the patient's mind. Both sets of these opposing ideas are supported by powerful emotions, and both sets demand expression. It is thought that one of these sets of ideas is conscious, and has the approval of the patient and the people around him. The other sets of ideas is unacceptable, contrary, and out of harmony with what the patient considers he ought to be. This latter set of ideas, which are in conflict with the patient's conscience, have to be dealt with by the patient somehow. As is true of any other manifestations of energy, they cannot be made simply to disappear. The ideas are suppressed (or repressed),* which means that the patient tries to forget them, evade them, put them out of his mind; i.e., one laughs-off a painful experience. In doing this what he actually achieves is not their annihilation; instead he only splits off, so to speak, and buries these ideas in the subconscious part of his mind. But this maneuver does not adequately dispose of the ideas. The conflict between the two opposing sets of ideas still goes on, the suppressed ideas still have energy and demand expression. The attempt at suppression is never completely successful in the neurotic patient, and it is simply the way in which the suppressed ideas manifest themselves that determines the type of neurosis the patient develops. In hysteria, these ideas manifest themselves as physical symptoms: the patient is forced, by the intensity of the emotions involved, to allow at least an indirect or disguised expression of these subconscious ideas. The symptom is therefore a symbol of the suppressed ideas, and the real meaning of the symbol is conveniently hidden from the patient and from others around him. It is because emotions are thus converted into physical symptoms that this disease is often called conversion hysteria. In hysteria, the symptoms sometimes follow in the path of the patient's own experience with his former organic illnesses: if a patient has at one time had appendicitis, for example, his hysterical symptom may be abdominal pain around McBurney's point, even though the appendix has

---
*Suppression is a conscious act of will.
Repression is a similar, but unconscious process.

been removed. If he once had a head injury, he may develop a hysterical headache. An injury or an illness often provides a "catalytic" focus at the site of which the hysterical symptom will "crystallize" out. It is possible that hysteria might be a more accurate diagnosis in the cases of some patients who are thought to have chronic sinusitis, weakness during convalescence from an organic illness, or post-operative abdominal adhesions. Fortunately for making the diagnosis, monosymptomatic hysteria is very rare, and it is usual to discover in the past of the hysterical patient a history of other clearly neurotic symptoms, such as sleep-walking, nervousness, fears, and nightmares.

In hysteria, it is thought that the patient not only has converted a mental conflict into physical symptoms, but that, secondarily, the symptoms provide him with a certain satisfaction or gain as well. This has been spoken of as secondary gain from illness. Unusual attention from the family and from the doctor may constitute this gain. In military service, the two sets of opposing ideas are occasionally simply the conscious desire to carry on at duty and meet with general approval, and the subconscious desire to escape a grim or fearful reality and gain the protection of hospital and home. In many the desire to get home from a combat area is perfectly conscious. In hysteria, the tremendous emotional force motivating a need like this is not conscious, and it is this emotion that is responsible for the hysterical symptom. In service personnel and among civilians, the suppressed ideas are usually more complicated. They lie in the general category of powerful passive and dependent desires for love and protection as well as in needs to escape from a disagreeable or unhappy situation. That this is so provides the attending physician with a clue in establishing a motive for the symptom. In order to make the diagnosis, such a motive should be established. This knowledge can also provide the lead for therapy, since one has simply to discover what is distressing the patient to begin intelligent treatment based on reality.

To illustrate and test this concept of hysteria the following case history is presented.

Case Report

Robert Frazer,[**] a 24-year-old private in an MP Battalion, was admitted to the surgical service of a Naval Hospital in the South Pacific in January, 1944, with the chief complaint of repeated attacks of disabling back pain. Frazer had volunteered for military service in 1940. According to the history, in the spring of 1941 he was struck by a passing truck while standing guard duty. He was not run over or knocked out, and he could walk, but he claimed to feel pain and numbness in the left side of his back. He was taken to a military hospital where examinations were negative and he was treated in the orthodox manner for back strain. Within four months the pain disappeared and he returned to duty. Six months later, the pain reappeared when he lifted a heavy weight. Because of this, he was readmitted to the hospital for one month. When he was again returned to duty he had no complaints. Since that time, however, Frazer has been in various military hospitals *on eight additional occasions*. Each time there was the same sequence of events, as described. He has spent one full year in hospitals since his accident three years ago.

The past history is essentially negative from a surgical viewpoint. Careful examination at the present time reveals no apparent cause for the patient's complaints. X-ray pictures are entirely normal. The conclusion then reached by the surgical and orthopedic consultants was that Frazer was a malingerer. Yet the question arose, why should a soldier, apparently in good health, repeat this unpleasant and time-consuming cycle of hospitalization again and again? In an attempt to answer this question, it was decided to give this patient careful psychiatric study.

Psychiatric History.—On interview it was first found that the patient's father was a chronic alcoholic who abused and threatened the patient and finally deserted the family when Frazer was ten years old. Just before that time, three of his sisters died, one after the other. The atmosphere of the home was continually disturbed. His mother was anxious and solicitous. She was over-concerned and worried that the patient would become like his father or die of illness like his sisters. It is not hard to imagine what was going on in the mind of a ten-year-old boy under these circumstances. After three deaths in the immediate family there remained the problem of a mentally-ill father. He recalled having had many fears about himself. He suffered greatly from feelings of insecurity. When his father deserted the family, Frazer quit school and went to work at the age of ten to help support his mother. He assumed the responsibility of helping her run the farm. When he was 14, his mother remarried, and Frazer left home. He bummed around the West on freight trains, living the life of a tramp. Then he went to California, made a little money, bought a car and got married. He began to help his mother financially, and showed an independent and energetic spirit. But he never really settled down. He never found work that satisfied him. He shifted from job to job. In 1940, he left his wife to join the army,

---
[**]Pseudonym.

and volunteered for foreign duty. He thought he would like combat duty. He said he enjoyed "soldiering" and at that time planned to remain in the regular army. He seemed to feel more protected in military life, and to like the security it provided him. For a while he felt better than he had in civilian life.

His present illness started one year after he had joined the service, when a truck struck him during a black-out at night. It was running without lights and hit him before he saw it. He thinks it spun him around and knocked him to the side of the road. Then it disappeared. (When Frazer told about this his manner was that of a hurt and frightened child. He was shaking and there were tears in his eyes.) He sent a nearby guard to find a doctor. He remembers that he walked over and sat down on a log to wait for help. Many terrifying thoughts were going through his mind. He did not know whether he was badly hurt or not. He was aware that it was painful to move his neck, and he thought it might be broken. He thought of the time when he himself had carried to the hospital a man who was badly injured in a truck accident. He had the idea that his back might be "out of place," or that his ribs were "torn loose." He saw himself an invalid for life, unable to support his wife and his mother. After waiting for what he thought was a long time, he was taken to the hospital in an ambulance. For one month he was allowed to lie flat on his back with nothing to occupy his mind. He began to have nightmares of trucks coming at him. He would awaken from these with a yell of terror. When he recovered, he says he was told two different things by the doctors: first, he was told there was nothing the matter with him and that he was to return to duty. However, at the same time, he claims, he was brought into an office and was urged to accept a certificate of disability discharge from the service. Since that time, he says he has been offered a discharge repeatedly.*** His own situation was not clear to him. He did not understand why he was offered a discharge. To him, this seemed like a contradiction of the recommendation to return to duty and a confirmation of his worst fears that he had a serious physical disability. He became more and more disturbed. He developed the idea that the doctors were trying to get rid of him. He refused to sign any documents. He said he thought the Government at least owed him hospital treatment if there were something wrong with him, because the accident had occurred while in the military service. Although he was physically healthy and able to work in the intervals between hospital admissions, he continued to fret and worry. He phantasied himself eventually paralyzed or impotent, thought at times that he "might not last more than a few years." In a naive way, he became preoccupied with the fear that his children—if he were to have any—might be deformed or blind at birth, because of the effects he imagined his spinal injury would have on his genitalia. He became more and more determined that the Government would have to take care of him in any event. Although he was reassured many times that he was physically well, the repeated suggestions that he accept a discharge convinced him that he must have sustained serious injury, and made him chronically pessimistic and anxious. It is not surprising that in this frame of mind his back hurt him again and again.

In addition, an extremely important point in his thinking was the fact that his father in the last war had received a disability discharge from the army and was still a partial invalid. The patient was afraid that the same fate was in store for him. Another extremely important fact which came out during a psychiatric interview was this: one year ago, in 1943, his wife was struck by an army truck and so injured that her arm had to be amputated. These facts disturbed him extremely, although he rarely mentioned them to anyone. They increased his anxiety and aggravated his hostility toward the service. As a result of these attitudes, his sojourns in the hospitals developed into battles between him and the doctors who "did not understand" him and thought he was a "gold-brick." As time went on Frazer's hostility toward the medical corps mounted with his failure to gain the care he wanted. He became increasingly over-aggressive and bitter, and these attitudes further increased the doctors' inability to understand him. But even under these conditions, he was compelled by his fears for his security to keep on seeking medical care. While on foreign duty, although a conscientious worker, he continued to hurt his back and was finally sent to the naval hospital for reappraisal.

DISCUSSION

Now it is possible to consider the hypothesis proposed at the beginning of this paper and test it against the facts of this case. First, this patient has symptoms for which no organic basis can be found. Second, there is a strongly positive psychiatric family history of mental illness, and an emotionally disturbed family background. In addition, the patient gives a history of neurotic behavior and of a poor work adjustment long before the onset of the present illness. This indicates the kind of emotional instability usually found to be a part of the life of the hysterical individual. Third, there is a logical and intelligible explanation for the development of his symptoms, as outlined

---
***Patient's history is not complete or entirely clear at this point. Social service check-up has been suggested.

above. This mechanism is consistent with the hypothesis that has been stated. Consciously Frazer wants to be an independent man, and he is known to be a good worker. He is aware of his personal responsibilities. He is sensitive and proud, and makes an effort to show how capable and self-sufficient he has been. Yet, subconsciously, in the back of his mind, Frazer retains fears that he will become a chronic invalid as a result of the accident that frightened him so badly. Supporting these fears are powerful, child-like desires to be cared for and protected. He is afraid of a discharge from the service because that might mean he would be thrown out into an indifferent and unfriendly world. He would prefer, unconsciously, to remain in the service and have the protection of the government hospitals. His old fears provide the emotional energy that supports these desires and have driven him to repeated attempts to obtain attention and protection through illness. He is completely unaware of all of this, and in no way realizes that these psychological forces had been operative in his case. He was like a frightened child who wants to climb into his mother's bed. In fact, his mother's extreme solicitude during his childhood, as well as the behavior of his alcoholic father and the death of his sisters, contributed much to the psychological pattern which formed the foundation for his later neurotic reaction. The accident brought out fully his childhood fears and the need for security that accompanied them. In acquiring a pain in his back he was able to obtain protective hospitalization and attention from nurses and doctors, even though this attention did not satisfy him. That is why the symptoms of the hysterical individual are described as being symbolic; they symbolize or represent something the patient unconsciously needs and wants.

In this particular case the theory fits reasonably well with the facts. It can therefore safely be said that hysteria is a definite entity, in certain cases responsible for symptoms. Certainly large numbers of the returned veterans of this war being treated over extended periods of time for what is thought to be organic disease, are suffering from a neurotic personality disturbance, such as Frazer's. Many sick people with chronic symptoms the nature of which is baffling to the physician really have hysteria. It is obvious that hysteria is a disorder to be reckoned with. If it is ignored, patients with this type of reaction will waste much of the time and energy of the physicians who attend them.

Frazer was given eight hourly sessions of simple psychotherapy. The apparent causes of his illness, as outlined above, were gradually explained to him as he himself brought them out in discussion. Much of his fear was relieved by reassurance and suggestion. His understanding of his own condition was increased and his wish to get well was strengthened. Although he was not cured, he improved enough for a trial at duty. Some of his hostility toward doctors and hospitals was reduced by patient and sympathetic handling.

The practice of medicine requires that physicians make a sympathetic and patient effort to understand and treat neurotic patients. Psychotherapy is the form of treatment which gives the best result in cases of hysteria.

The views expressed in the foregoing article are not to be taken as those of the Navy Department, but of the author, individually.

SOME ORIENTAL DISEASES WE ARE TO ENCOUNTER
(G. J. Guldseth, Duluth, in *Minn. Med.*, Aug.)

We may expect a number of our soldiers and sailors to return to their homes in apparent health only to break down, generally after prolonged chilling or fatigue, with malaria or dysentery in bizarre and atypical clinical manifestations as well as in the typical forms.

The great difficulty of finding the specific organisms of malaria and dysentery (especially the latter) in some cases renders a trial of specific therapy justifiable.

Caution is expressed in the interpretation of a positive Wassermann, Kline or Kahn test in patients who may have some oriental disease.

There exists a danger of transmission of malaria in blood or plasma transfusions.

Prophylactic or suppressive treatment may mask a deep-seated insidious malarial process which may later prove very difficult to control.

TRANSFUSION REACTIONS STILL OCCUR
(O .E. Turner, Pittsburgh, in *Pa. Med. Jl.*, Aug.)

Despite all standard precautions for establishing compatibility, blood transfusion reactions are prone to occur. This fact is not well impressed upon some physicians, who believe that every transfusion reaction is one of gross incompatibility.

The Rh factor and technic of eliciting subgroup incompatibility needs development for more practical application.

The occurrence of blood transfusion reactions in patients with malignant disease merits further investigation.

Reactions due to whole-blood transfusions were six times as frequent as reactions from plasma transfusions.

If blood transfusions are to continue in scientific popularity, and to compete with the safety of pooled plasma, improved methods of determining blood compatibility must be forthcoming.

IN CASES OF BLEEDING NIPPLE aspiration biopsy is of little value. It is a warning sign of a malignant lesion or one which frequently terminates in cancer. Over half the bleeding nipple cases may be cured by the simplest type of surgery. Local surgery of this sort is *an important prophylaxis against cancer of the breast*. Every benign tumor demonstrated by palpation or tranillumination should be removed lest it become malignant. Not a radical mastectomy or even a mastectomy unless there are multiple lesions or other conditions which would be of themselves indicate mastectomy even though bleeding were not present.

In a bleeding breast having no demonstrable tumor, prove the nature of the process and proceed with local or general surgery as indicated. If no tumors can be demonstrated the safest procedure is local mastectomy.—*Norman Treves.*

CASE REPORT

SEPTAL ABSCESS
George R. Laub, M.D., Columbia

A 17-year-old colored boy was sent to the office because of an enormous enlargement of his nose. He gave a history of having always been in good health until four weeks previous to his present illness, at which time he contracted a severe influenza. He stayed in bed with high temperature and was dismissed from the care of his doctor after more than two weeks.

Two days before coming to the office he noticed a slight swelling of his nose, which increased continuously so that he was unable to breathe through his nose. The dorsum of the nose was an inch wide and both nostrils were dilated to a maximum, each filled by a reddish mass with a

Septal abscesses are not common. They may be postoperative, caused from injuries, by putrefaction of hematomas, and also as a complication of infectious diseases, such as typhoid, smallpox, influenza (Ballenger). The writer was not able to find any information in the literature to which he had access regarding the frequency of such abscesses. O. Chiari made the statement in his book that he himself saw two or three out of 10,000 cases a year. His observations were mostly of children with injuries of the nose where putrefaction of hematomas occurred. In his opinion the perforation of the septum was due to the original trauma. The description he gave of a typhoid case is very much like the above-quoted case. In the literature nothing is mentioned about the bacteriology. The pus of this patient was cultured and found to be sterile.

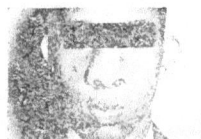
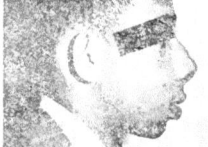
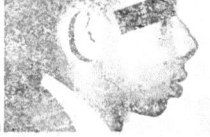
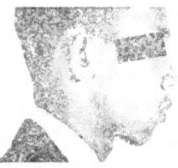

Fig. 1   Fig. 2   Fig. 3   Fig. 4

smooth surface and indolent to touch. (Figs. 1 and 2.) The mass was slightly fluctuating and it was not possible to get a view of the inside of the nose. Physical examination was entirely negative otherwise. He had no fever. Hemoglobin 80%; RBC 5,750,000; WBC 8,200 — polys. 80%, lymphs. 14%, monos. 5%, eos. 1%. Wassermann negative. Urine—1.018, yellow, alkaline, albumin 1-plus, glucose negative.

This patient was admitted to the Good Samaritan-Waverly Hospital for operation. Under pentothal-sodium intravenous anesthesia an incision of the bulging mucous membrane in his left nostril was made. Immediately afterwards greenish, fetid pus came out under pressure. A total of 1½ ounces of pus was drained. A careful examination showed that the cartilaginous septum was perforated. A small drain of iodoform gauze was inserted, just big enough to keep the incision open.

The postoperative course was uneventful. The drain was exchanged daily after syringing the abscess cavity with hydrogen peroxide. Five days after the operation the secretion of pus practically stopped, and two or three days later the nose was completely healed. (Figs. 3 and 4.)

Regarding the treatment, all authors agree on incision and drainage. A. W. Proetz warns that irrigation of the abscess may result in further elevation of the membrane and extension of this process and, therefore, should not be done. Others, among them F. Lederer, recommend irrigation. F. L. Weille and E. DeBlois published a new method with a rubber drain. Due to the rarity of such cases, it is very hard for any one person to evaluate the different methods.

Summary: A case of an unusually large septal abscess as complication of influenza is reported and this rare disease, as well as its treatment, discussed.

BIBLIOGRAPHY
W. L. Ballenger and H. C. Ballenger: Diseases of the Nose, Throat and Ear. Eighth edition. Lea & Febiger, Philadelphia, 1943, 62.
O. Chiari: die Krankheiten Der Oberen Luftwege, Part I: Leipzig und Wien. Franz Deuticke, 1902, 174.
F. L. Lederer: Diseases of Ear, Nose and Throat, F. A. Davis Co., Philadelphia, fourth edition, 1943, 410.
A. W. Proetz, in F. Christopher Textbook of Surgery, second edition. W. B. Saunders Co., Philadelphia and London, 1941, 777.
F. L. Weille and E. DeBlois: "Use of a T-Tube for Drainage of a Septal Abscess." Arch. of Otolaryngology, Vol. 39, Jan., 1944, 85.

DEPARTMENTS

HUMAN BEHAVIOUR

JAMES K. HALL, M.D., *Editor*, Richmond, Va.

ON PSYCHIATRIC BEGINNINGS

THE YEAR 1944 is historic in mental medicine in the United States.

On the tenth of May I attended in Providence, Rhode Island, the centennial exercises in commemoration of the completion of the first hundred years of service of Butler Hospital. It has been said that beginnings are seldom recorded. It would be more accurately stated by saying that the beginning is often not recognized as a beginning. Rhode Island is a small, but not an inconsequential state. Civilization in that state is old, as we count age in our still youthful country. The state is historic. Early in its life it began its contributions to education and to religious freedom and to industry. In war and in peace, the little state has always measured up to the stature of full statehood.

But until 1844 there were no provisions anywhere in Rhode Island for the treatment and the proper care of a mentally sick person. If the mental sickness caused the person's behaviour to be disturbing to the peace of mind and the comfort of others, the person was legally committed to jail. If the mental disorder was less aggravated, the afflicted person was sent to the almshouse. But such care as might be given the patient was altogether custodial, and not at all medical. Fate decreed that Nicholas Brown should die in 1841, and Destiny caused him to provide in his will a bequest of $30,000, a heap of money for a tight-fisted New Englander to give away, "towards the erection or endowment of a retreat for the insane." An "incorporating committee" requested the Legislature of Rhode Island early in 1844 to charter the Rhode Island Asylum for the Insane. And about the same time the spirit moved Cyrus Butler, who had merchandised cumulatively in Providence, to give $40,000 toward the establishment of the asylum, provided an equal amount be contributed by the public. All the conditions were promptly complied with, and a fund of $110,000 was in hand. Almost half the amount was set aside as an endowment fund. With the remaining $60,000 a hospital for the mentally sick was brought into being. Before the year 1844 had passed into history the Legislature had designated the new hospital the Butler Hospital for the Insane.

The Centennial program of today's Butler Hospital occupied the afternoon and the evening of last May the tenth. It was a solemn and also an inspiring occasion. Friends of the hospital and distinguished psychiatrists paid tribute to the fruitful generosity of the Founders and to the memory and the skill and the devotion of those who have exercised administrative directorship of the hospital throughout the hundred years of its life. Amongst the superintendents have been Dr. Isaac Ray, a pioneer in psychiatry; Dr. G. Alder Blumer, an erudite contributor to our profession lent us by England, and Dr. Arthur H. Ruggles, who has been directing the activities of Butler for several years. Each of the three has served as President of the American Psychiatric Association.

In the program of the Centennial there were spoken contributions by Dr. Edward A. Strecker, President of the American Psychiatric Association; by Dr. Gregory Zilboorg, editor of *One Hundred Years of American Psychiatry*, a monumental contribution to American history; by Dr. Karl A. Menninger, of the Menninger Sanitarium, of Topeka; by Elizabeth S. Bixler, R.N., of the School of Nursing of Yale University; and by Dr. Alan Gregg, of the Rockefeller Foundation. I listened with what comprehending intelligence had been granted me to the speakers, and I was impressed most by their modesty and by their recognition of the number of problems that await attention rather than by laudatory references to the achievements of psychiatry. I moved amongst them and communed with them, and I came from the Centennial impressed by the limitations of the knowledge of mental medicine and by the brave stories of high courage and unceasing labour and immortal hope of those of our predecessors who have made it possible for the mentally sick in our country to be treated as sick people and not to be punished as demons.

I would commune with you briefly about the talk of Karl Menninger on: The War Against Fear and Hate. Dr. Karl Menninger is not unacquainted with warfare. As a young medical graduate he participated in the First World War. His brother, Dr. William C. Menninger, a Colonel in the United States Army, is stationed in the office of the Surgeon General as the head of neuropsychiatric medicine. The two brothers, with their father, have brought into being at Topeka, in the midst of what was spoken of almost within my memory as the Great American Desert, a hospital for the understanding and the restoration of the mentally sick that constitutes pioneering in the domain of medical science comparable to that of the Mayo Clinic in Minnesota. The achievement of the human being should be contemplated always in terms of the individual, of his capacity and personality, of his time, and with reference to the place in which he functions. The Menningers think of mental life in terms of spaciousness as vast as that of the boundless plains of Kansas. And in such attitudes they come to their patients who are experiencing difficulty and often distress in living in their various environments and with their numerable selves; and to many mortals, of course, who are the constant recipients of the conflicts that rage within them because they are out of tune with their environment and with themselves. Out of such turmoil within the individual, out of sight of the world, usually a silent, wordless war, come unhappiness, despair, sorrow, doubt, inadequacy, jealousy, envy, hatred, alcoholism, drug addiction, mental disorder, insanity. Such conflict, such warfare, deep within all mortals, is constant, unceasing, often hidden, usually unsuspected, and its existence would generally be denied if it were inquired about. Such conflict tends to make life intolerable. It nullifies the purposeful and helpful utilization of energy. It causes a frittering away of one's hopes and labours. It prevents the synthesizing of activities and the direction of effort.

The function of the psychiatrist is to try to prevent such unhappy maladjustment and to enable the individual to live wholesomely and purposefully by knowing his inner self as well as his environment, so that he may learn to live harmoniously with himself and with the world close about him. Dr. Menninger looks upon man's mightiest conflicts on the field of battle as mere temporary, inconsequential skirmishes in comparison with all the conflicts that are taking place within all of us all the time, whoever we may be and wherever we may be. Those who are bowled over in the combat become patients in mental hospitals, and they are said in legal language to be insane. But communion with such individuals reveals them to be more like than unlike the rest of us, humans. With the help that is brought to them by an understanding of themselves and of what bowled them over, they may step forth, better enabled to run the race of life again.

Dr. Menninger knows that there can be neither peace nor happiness in the world until man banishes envy and jealousy and vengeance and prejudice and covetousness and hatred and cruelty.

Dorothea Dix obtained permission to teach Sunday School in a jail in Boston in 1841. She had probably never before been inside a jail. It was a cold winter day, the jail was unheated, some of those in the jail were insane and were chained to the floor. Dorothea Dix was shocked by the inhumanity with which they were considered. They were cruelly treated; the sane and the insane. Although she was scarcely grown, she moved instantly, in an effort to make possible for the mentally sick medical and nursing and hospital care. She it was who brought into being most of the first hospitals for the mentally sick in our country. She came in 1843 from Boston into Rhode Island to expedite the establishment of Butler Hospital. She moved throughout our spacious country, everywhere, by train, by stagecoach, on horseback and on foot. In North Carolina, by an appeal to the Legislature, she evoked from the civic heart and purse what is now known as the State Hospital on Dix Hill.

Dorothea Dix was one of the most remarkable women of all time. Unhappy in childhood, shielded in girlhood from the roughness of life, frail and probably tuberculous, she reached the age of 85— and in her long life she had spared neither her body nor her emotions. During the Civil War she headed what nursing there was in the Union Army. Every mentally sick person in the United States is indebted to her chiefly for all that mental medicine offers today. Karl Menninger offers a powerful appraisal of her.

If you would, and you should, wish to read Karl Menninger's: The War Against Fear and Hate, ask for a copy of the *Bulletin* of the Menninger Clinic for July, 1944. And if you would know about the psychiatry of today, in contrast with that of the childhood of Dorothea Dix during those next decades after 1800, lay hold of a copy of: One Hundred Years of American Psychiatry, edited by Dr. Gregory Zilboorg, and issued by Columbia University Press. And no nurse, no physician, no citizen proud of his country's marvelous history can be willing to be without a copy of Dorothea Dix, Forgotten Samaritan, by Helen E. Marshall. The volume is highly creditable to the University of North Carolina Press at Chapel Hill.

TUBERCULOSIS

J. DONNELLY, M.D., *Editor*, Charlotte, N. C.

SOME EARLY BRITISH PHTHISIOLOGISTS

ALTHOUGH many of the refinements in the diagnosis of pulmonary tuberculosis have been the result of modern research, the symptoms and pathological changes in the tissues, as visualized by post-mortem specimens alone, were familiar to some of the older British physicians.

Although the disease was at first considered hereditary and not necessarily acquired after birth, it was also considered an air-borne disease by earlier writers and possibly transmissible from parents to children. The disease, however, was not then recognizable until far advanced, and consequently treatment was generally unavailing. Absolute rest was not considered necessary in the treatment and moderate exercise was usually recommended. Earlier diagnosis was urged 250 years ago: "in the beginning it may be cured as other diseases."

In a recent article by Professor Cummins,[1] of

the Royal Society of Medicine (London) several valuable—some remarkable—contributions on tuberculosis by the earlier physicians are discussed.

Richard Morton (1637-1698) was, as far as I can discover, one of the first British physicians to appreciate phthisis pulmonalis as a disease to be closely studied. He was not content to accept anything that he could not see, or at least that he could not explain in terms of what he had been taught. He did not confine himself to the study of the living: *he also followed up fatal cases by autopsy.*

Among the first signs he gives are:

"Being born of consumptive parents; for this Distemper (so far as I have been able to observe) is more Hereditary and *oftener propagated from the parents than any other.*"

It was natural for him to call the disease "hereditary" and we may well pardon him that error, and we must all agree as to the propagation from father and from mother.

"Spitting of blood *though it be accidental."* ....

"But, alas," he adds, "Physicians have very seldom an occasion to give their advice about preventing this Distemper (when at the beginning it may be cured as well as other diseases although, by neglect, it proves fatal) the sick persons seldom imploring Aesculapius' help before the Distemper has run so far as to be a fatal case, and then they expect mircles from the art of Physic when it is more convenient for them to have a good council of a Minister about the future Salvation of their Souls and the advice of a Lawyer about making their last Will."

Benjamin Marten wrote in 1725 on *A New Theory of Consumptions; more especially of a Phthisis of the Lungs.*

After a very good opening on the causation, symptoms and signs of a consumption of the lungs, an opening full of his own experiences and with many quotations, Marten proceeds to enunciate a theory of phthisis so thoroughly explanatory of the phenomena of the disease as to appear to us, nowadays, as almost inspired, though passed unnoticed by the Profession at the time; a theory which goes so far as to anticipate the subsequent discoveries of Villemin and Robert Koch that it should excite our interest and kindle our imagination.

"Some authors who would account for all Diseases by the doctrine of Acid and Alkali think it sufficient to assert that the Blood, abounding with one or other of these, is the cause of the Consumptions and most other Distempers that affect Mankind.

1. Prof. S. L. Cummins, in *Proc. Royal Soc. of Med.* (Lond.), July.

"The original and essential Cause then .... may be some certain species of Animalcula or wonderfully minute living creature that, by their peculiar shape or disagreeable parts are inimicable to our nature, capable of existing in our Juices and Vessels and which, being drove to the Lungs by the circulation of the Blood, or else generated there from their proper ova or Eggs, with which the Juices may abound or which, possibly being carried about in the Air, may be immediately conveyed to the Lungs by that we draw in and, being there deposited, as in a proper Nidus, and being produced into Life, coming to Perfection or increasing in bigness may, by their spontaneous Motion and Injurious Parts, stimulating and perhaps gnawing the tender Vessels of the Lungs, cause all the Disorders." "The Curious, who have turned their thoughts upon the new World of Wonders that microscopical Observations have opened to our View, will easily conceive the Possibility of very minute organisms being not only the original and Essential Cause of this but of many other Diseases hitherto inexplicable."

"How Distempers are apparently communicated from one person to another .... and how they are spread by Degrees and from one County to another may, perhaps, by this Theory, be more easily explained than by any other."

"It seems probable that the minute Animals or their Seed are for the most part either conveyed from the Parents to their Offspring or communicated immediately from the distempered Persons to sound ones. .... The last way, which is properly called infection, we may conceive to be the more reasonable."

William Stark (1741-1770): William Bulloch, in his Horace Dobell Lecture (1910), referred to "a young Physician of St. George's Hospital, whose untimely death at the age of 29, brought about by experiments on his own body, robbed English pathology of one of its earliest and most accurate observers."

It is sad to see so much learning and so much endeavour now quite forgotten amongst the very scenes where it was required.

"His *Experiments on Diet,* or rather the imprudent zeal with which he prosecuted them, proved in the end fatal to himself; at least such was the general opinion of his friends at the time." "He was ill prepared for the cold prudence, the timeserving meanness or the base duplicity which he met with in others."

Others had seen tubercles in the lungs and had noted the presence of "apostemes" and "ulcers" as part of the disease complex, but Stark was the first to examine minutely the growth and development of these little tumors and to show how they might gradually lead to advanced disease and death.

"In the cellular substance of the lungs are found roundish firm bodies, of different sizes, from the smallest granule to half an inch in diameter, the latter often in clusters. The tubercles of a small size are always, those of a larger frequently, of a whitish colour and of a consistency approaching to the hardness of cartilage; when cut through, the surface appears smooth, shining and uniform. No vesicles, cells or vessels are to be seen in them, even when examined with a microscope. On the cut surface of some tubercles one or more cavities containing a thick white fluid-like pus. The cavities are of different sizes, from the smallest perceptible to half an inch in diameter. . . . The cavities of less than half an inch in diameter are always quite shut up; those which are a little larger have, as constantly, a round opening made by a branch of the trachea [producing a] vomica."

"Where ever there is a vomica there is always a broad and firm adhesion of that part of the lungs to the parietes or pleura so as to preclude all communication between the cavity of the parietes or pleura so as to preclude all communication between the cavity of the vomica and that of the chest; even tubercles are seldom without adhesion."

"Those parts of the lungs which are contiguous to tubercles are red, sometimes soft, but more frequently firm and hard; and, while other parts of the lungs unaffected by disease are readily distended by blowing into the trachea, those parts which are contiguous to tubercles or vomicae remain depressed and impervious to air, either blown into the lungs in this manner or forced, by a blow pipe, into incisions made on the surface. So that the function of the lungs, so far as respects the admission of air, seems in those parts, entirely destroyed."

George Bodington (1799-1882), qualified as a medical practitioner in 1825. His pamphlet on *The Treatment and Cure of Pulmonary Consumption* was published in 1840.

He was the first to treat patients suffering from phthisis by giving good, fresh air, a sufficiency of wholesome food and a definite quantity of wine, with a sedative, opium, to ensure sleep and calm apprehension as necessary. And, above all, he asked that they should be taken into a house specially prepared for them and kept under the eye of a specialist in the management of tuberculosis.

"The most important remedial agent in the cure of consumption is the free use of a pure atmosphere . . . . out of doors early in the morning either by riding or walking . . . . with intervals of walking as much as the strength will allow of. . . . The abode of the patient should be in an airy house in the country; if on an eminence so much the better, comparatively free from fog and dampness. . . . . There should be a certain class of practitioners who should pursue this practice as a distinct branch to whom those in large towns should confide their consumptive patients instead of sending them as many do now, to probably fall into the hands of mercenaries at some distant sea port where they commonly die, far away from friends and home."

William Budd wrote a *Memorandum on the Nature and the Mode of Propagation of Phthisis* in 1867.

Budd had been for a long time in practice at Clifton and Bristol to which places many phthisics, among them negroes employed on our ships, came for treatment when they were unable to continue work. "The idea that phthisis is a self-propagating zymotic disease and that all the leading phenomena may be explained by supposing that it is disseminated through specific germs contained in the tuberculous matter cast off by persons suffering from the disease *first came into my mind unbidden* (1856)." With this idea came the sequel: "The Geographical distribution of phthisis in past and present times and especially its great fatality in countries which, when first discovered (by Europeans) were absolutely free from it." . . . . "When the South Sea Islands were first discovered, phthisis did not exist there," and it was now very prevalent. . . . . "Now, everywhere along the African sea-board, where the blacks have come into contact and intimate relations with the whites, phthisis causes a large mortality among them. In the interior, where intercourse with them has been limited to casual contact . . . . there is reason to believe that phthisis does not exist."

PEDIATRICS

DIONNE QUINTUPLETS OUTCLASSED

A GOOD many doctors observed with pain the great to-do about the "miraculous" saving of the five Dionne babies. Data concerning Argentine quintuplets presented in the August 12th issue of *The Journal of the A. M. A.* by its regular Buenos Aires correspondent seem to show that the showmanship and lionizing of the Dionnes' doctor was uncalled-for.

Some months ago the daily papers announced the birth of quintuplets to a couple in Buenos Aires. The parents of the quintuplets wished to keep the information on the matter private. A professor of the obstetric clinic of the Faculty of Medicine of the University of Buenos Aires investigated the case.

"During pregnancy and delivery of the quintuplets the mother was under the care of a midwife. The pregnancy was normal at the beginning. Edema of the legs and the abdomen and severe visual disturbances occurred from the fourth month of pregnancy on. The mother did not stop her daily work as a housewife. The midwife made a diagnosis of twins in the seventh month of pregnancy. In the course of the last month of pregnancy the mother made two excursions of 12 hours each by railroad. According to the midwife, by the end of pregnancy, which went to full term, the abdomen was large; fetal heart beats were heard in several parts of the abdomen. The first symptoms of parturition began on July 14th, 1943, when the patient was transferred from her home to the midwife's house. The infants were delivered at intervals of 10, 20, 20 and 55 minutes. . . . . All the infants breathed normally and cried loudly immediately after birth except the fifth one. . . . . She was treated successfully. . . . . There were two boys and three girls. A second subcutaneous administration of posterior pituitary injection was made before delivery of the fifth baby. Total duration of delivery was 19¾ hrs. The weights of the infants 24 hours after birth were, in order of delivery, 1300, 1200, 1150, 1500, 1250 gm. (300 gm. more for the whole group than for the Dionne sisters). The mother never permitted the midwife to call a physician. The puerperium was normal."

The children were not premature. They showed great vitality. On the second day they began to have a mixture of colostrum from the mother, cow's milk and water. The infants were not put in incubators. Oxygen and carbon dioxide were not administered. The infants were not put in a bath for the first three months of life. The weights at the age of 8 months and 10 days were 8800, 8800, 7500, 8400 and 7500 gm. They were healthy and beginning to cut teeth.

UROLOGY
RAYMOND THOMPSON, M.D., *Editor*, Charlotte, N. C.

INFECTIONS OF THE URINARY TRACT WITHOUT DEMONSTRABLE ORGANISMS

When a doctor is unable to find bacteria in the urine he is apt to conclude that no infection of the genitourinary tract exists, and to think he must look elsewhere for the explanation of symptoms pointing in this direction.

Cook[1] calls attention to this important matter.

Bacteriologic studies, he reminds us, in a small but very interesting group of cases of infection of the urinary tract, fail to demonstrate the causative organism; although the infectious character of the disease cannot be doubted, since there is pyuria, with the characteristic cystoscopic and urographic picture of infection. All of us are familiar with the usual case in which Gram's stain and cultures

1. E. N. Cook, in *Proc. Staff Meet. Mayo Clinic*, July 26th.

of the urinary sediment reveal bacilli or a coccus as the agent responsible for the infection; but there is a group of cases in which pus in the urine contains no microbes. Such a condition must be distinguished from tuberculosis and in many cases this is no easy matter.

It is a serious thing to diagnose tuberculosis where there is no tuberculosis; and in case no acid-fast bacilli are found in the urinary sediment, or inoculations of guinea pigs with urine from the bladder and kidneys produces tuberculosis, *the diagnosis of tuberculosis should not be made.*

Careful physical examination in the male particularly may give important evidence. Bumpus and Thompson state conservatively that in 80 per cent of the cases of renal tuberculosis of males, lesions of tuberculosis will be present in the genitalia also—nodular and thickened epdidymis, beaded or pipestem vas deferens, or nodular prostate gland.

Our experience agrees with the following statement:

"A filterable virus has been suggested as the causative agent. It has been suggested that the reaction in the urinary tract is attributable to toxins liberated elsewhere in the body by some focus of infection which, when excreted in the urine, provokes this inflammatory reaction. Another theory suggests the firm entrenchment of a coccal infection in the renal paranchyma with the resulting inflammatory process producing exudation of pus into the pelvis of the kidney. In the light of our present knowledge, we feel that the second theory is perhaps of more importance than the other two."

The condition is more frequent in the young. Some patients have had their trouble for only a few weeks, others for months or even years when they are seen. Burning on urination, frequent urination, tenesmus and even strangury are commonly complained of. Acute diffuse cystitis, in many cases with ulceration of the bladder, is seen through the cystoscope. The urographic findings are not always characteristic. Enlarged pelves, calices and ureters generally mean an inflammatory process of long standing and tend to arouse suspicion of a tuberculous lesion.

After tuberculosis of the urinary tract has been excluded and stains and cultures of the urine repeatedly fail to provide the explanation, thorough search for foci of infection is in order. In case active foci of infection are found, the extreme bladder distress may contraindicate their removal at once.

Lavage of the bladder with potassium permanganate, 1 in 8,000, alternating with acetic acid, 1 in 3,000; this followed with instillation of silver iodide, are recommended. More recently solutions of silver nitrate have been used for instillation, a weak concentration of 1 in 10,000 first, increased until the solution of 1 in 100 can be tolerated.

Mandelic acid and sulfonamides by mouth have proved of little benefit. Neoarsphenamine started immediately, two or three doses of 0.2 to 0.3 gm. intravenously, five days apart, and eradication of foci have been most valuable weapons in Cook's hands.

Our own management of these cases does not differ essentially. Our main object is to call our readers' attention to this not extremely unusual condition, and to urge that it not be mistakenly diagnosed as tuberculous.

TREATMENT OF SULFONAMIDE-RESISTANT GONORRHEA WITH PENICILLIN SODIUM

IN 15 ARMY HOSPITALS a total of 1,686 patients refractory to at least two courses of a sulfonamide, and in some cases to artificially-induced fever, were treated with total dosages varying from 40,000 to 160,000 Oxford units per case, the individual dose being 10,000 or 20,000 units intramuscularly every three hours.[1]

One course of treatment with a dosage of 160,000 units per case effected cures in 98 per cent; 80,000 to 120,000 units in 96 per cent, and 50,000 units in 86 per cent. No significant differences in the final results were noted when a given total dose was administered in individual injections of either 10,000 or 20,000 units. Little advantage was gained by prolonging the time of treatment schedules beyond 12 hours.

During of infection, previous fever therapy and race appeared to have no effect on the results of therapy.

Of the total of 126 failures to one course of penicillin, 85 were re-treated, using a 100,000 unit dosage. Of these, 78 (91.8%) were cured. Thus, by re-treatment of failures with a second course, 99% of cures were obtained.

Complications of gonorrhea responded well to penicillin, although the more serious forms of complications required prolonged treatment with higher dosage.

Reactions to penicillin were inconsequential, and in no instance was it necessary to discontinue treatment for this reason.

Because of the known effects of penicillin on Treponema pallidum, the possibility of masking or delaying the development of early syphilis must be considered.

One-hundred-and-nine chemoresistant women patients received courses of penicillin;[2] of these, 84 were white women and 25 were Negroes. Failures numbered only five, and in these five cases a favorable response was obtained by giving a second course of the therapy.

It is recommended that 150,000 units be used, although good results may be obtained with as little as 60,000 units. A warning note is sounded that asymptomatic carriers may develop and that penicillin-resistant strains of gonococci may appear.

CLINICAL CHEMISTRY and MICROSCOPY

J. M. FEDER, M.D., and EVELYN TRIBBLE, M.T., *Editors*,
Anderson, S. C.

BLOOD PLASMA
APPLICATION—AVAILABILITY—POTENTIAL HAZARD

THE NEED for blood plasma on the home front should be obvious when the fatality rate of highway accidents in the United States annually surpasses that of our troops in the war in which we are engaged. That blood plasma is a therapeutic success is beyond question, yet its availability on the home front is spotty. A number of years ago when the use of this substance was first suggested and developed by Elliott,* it was his hope, as well as that of this writer and others, to establish in the Tri-State area several central processing depots. How miserably this contemplated program has failed requires no elaboration. Around the larger hospital centers more or less processed plasma is available; in the rural communities and smaller cities little or none. It is commercially available at around $25 per pint, which of course is prohibitive to the average patient.

Although plasma therapy originated in the Southern states, it remained for some of our neighbors in the North to put into effect a program whereby it would be made available to each physician in the state. We have just received a resumé of the procedure as carried out in the State of Michigan under the jurisdiction of the Health Department. From that literature I quote the four essential points necessary for mechanizing this program. All of the sovereign states in the Tri-State Medical Association, with little effort, could meet these specifications:

*Blood plasma has been credited with being one of the trinity that has most reduced mortality on the battlefront. Lest we forget, the original research aimed towards the general avilability of plasma was carried out by Dr. John Elliott, of Salisbury, North Carolina; and unfortunately, it is apparent from the current literature that but scant notation has been made of this fact. Blood plasma was developed here in the Tri-State area, and we believe that the first publication work covering it appeared in the Journal of the Tri-State (*Southern Medicine & Surgery*).

---
1. Lt. Col. T. H. Sternberg & Col. T. B. Turner, M.C., Army of the U. S., in *Jl. A. M. A.*, Sept. 16th.
2. R. B. Greenblatt, Savannah, in *Jl. A. M. A.*, Sept. 16th.

1. A statute providing for free distribution of biologic products of the control of communicable disease.
2. A strong and well organized state public health laboratory with well trained chemists and bacteriologists.
3. The enthusiastic coöperation of the Local, State and National Red Cross.
4. The bleeding unit should be sent into the field from the central headquarters. One cannot depend on local bleeding.

To those engaged in processing plasma, we feel it desirable at this time to raise a red flag to warn of possible disaster which can easily follow the administration of Rh-positive plasma to a Rh-negative sensitized individual. We believe that to eliminate this hazard a much larger pooling volume must be instituted. *Until we reach a stage whereby Rh-negative pools can be established, blood plasma should not be given the pregnant or postpartum patient until she has been proven to be Rh-positive.* In the event that she is Rh-negative, blood plasma should not be administered. It is to be remembered that plasma retains the factor and fatality can result from its use, even in high dilutions. The pregnant and the recently delivered woman must have an Rh determination before a transfusion is given; and if found to be Rh-negative, a Rh-negative donor must be procured.

Blood plasma is the agent of choice in combating shock, but it is of little value if the nearest plasma supply is 80 miles away. This is a proposal that we exert ourselves to the utmost to the end that every drug store in the Tri-State should have on hand for free distribution a supply of blood plasma adequate to meet the need of the immediate district.

It can be done!

THERAPEUTICS

J. F. NASH, M.D., *Editor*, Saint Pauls, N. C.

THE TREATMENT OF SEVERE BURNS

A PHYSIOLOGIST who takes up a clinical problem may be counted on to work out something of value. Harvard's Professor of Physiology[1] tells us how to manage certain burns, and he tells us why.

Our first fear arises from a conviction that the close-fitting, inelastic dressing will cut off the blood supply. Our experiments all showed the circulation in an extremity cast in plaster or enclosed in the usual plaster bandage is unrestricted and wholly adequate. If the dressing is applied over a burn at the middle of an extremity *and the lower part is not enclosed* it will swell promptly and may be made gangrenous if the dressing is left in place.

1. C. K. Drinker, Boston, in Jl. Okla. Med. Assn., Aug.

Leakage from the capillaries in a burned area is the major physiological derangement in the lesion. As soon as the dressing sets, although the vessels are leaky, only minimal damage can occur. The plaster covering will always become stained with foul-smelling exudate, but the loss of plasma may be so much lessened by prompt application of plaster dressings as to reduce the seriousness of the burn in terms of the extent of surface affected.

It is the general impression that lymphatics are pressed shut in the presence of swelling. The opposite is true. The walls of the smallest lymphatics are completely permeable to burn exudates and this results in easy filling for eventual delivery to regions outside of the burn.

We think of mysterious pressure effects against the plaster covering which would be excessively painful. But in a very short time after application, pressures under the dressing become equal in all directions and there is no fluctuant stretching of the tissues. The part in a closed-plaster cast cannot swell beyond the state in which it existed when the dressing was applied. It always shrinks somewhat. Another very real reason why the closed-plaster treatment saves the patient from pain resides in the fact that this dressing once in place is let alone for 21 days. It must contain no windows, and every impulse to open the dressing and ascertain the course of events must be resisted. If regional lymph nodes become inflamed and if fever and leucocytosis indicate an extending infection, it may be necessary to remove the cast; but these are not frequent complications, and in the ordinary case the plaster bandage may remain untouched for three weeks when its removal will not cause the slightest pain.

Local bacterial growth is less with closed treatment than when frequent dressings are used. At the outset the burned surfaces were dusted with one of the sulfa drugs, but this was not continued. If medication by these drugs is thought necessary they are much better given in the usual way. Penicillin locally, because of its effect on staphylococci, has proved well worth while.

As a first covering one or two layers of dry gauze are now used. Grease of any kind has proved quite unnecessary to prevent sticking and may interfere with epithelialization. The fingers need not be wrapped separately. The dressing is applied so as to make a snug fit, but without pressure. Obviously the smaller the part when the dressing is applied the better. Consequently when a patient comes in for treatment the part should be elevated at once and kept so until the dressing is in place.

Many patients could not be treated until some hours after the accident. They were more comfortable at once and they were easily cared for if closed-plaster dressings were used immediately.

The use of rigid plaster instead of the popular pressure dressing is still a matter of careful observation. Between the bandage and the skin there is a variable amount of elastic packing which is bound on so as to make some degree of pressure. How much this is or how much it ought to be no one can tell. From the physiological point of view the technique does not possess the clear-cut advantage of the closed-plaster dressing, but with a good deal of clinical experience, the author has learned that this point of view may readily be wrong. Certainly the use of plaster is largely limited to burns of the extremities; and for those about the genitalia, trunk, neck and head the pressure bandage must be employed in the majority of cases.

GENERAL PRACTICE
D. HERBERT SMITH, M.D., *Editor*, Pauline, S. C.

CHANGE IN BOWEL HABIT—THINK OF BOWEL CANCER

CANCER OF THE BOWEL is prone to come on insidiously, and with no distinctive signs. Over many years we have learned the wisdom of suspecting cancer as the cause when a person at or past middle age gives a history of pronounced change from his or her long-established bowel habit.

The two cases to be reported[1] are illustrative. Also, they teach that acute conditions, demanding prompt surgical intervention, may arise in the right iliac fossa in a man or woman whose appendix has been removed.

Within a period of eight weeks two patients with identical conditions came to Sibley Hospital. Mrs. J., aged 54; Mr. J., aged 65. Both stated that of recent months they had been having difficulty in getting their bowels to move and that there was a sense of fullness in their abdomens and some gas. For some indefinite time they had been resorting to physics. Just previous to the illnesses both patients had taken strong cathartics, which probably had acted as effectively as usually had been the case; but, within 12 to 18 hours each began to suffer severe abdominal pains followed by nausea, vomiting and severe pains in the right lower quadrant. Mr. J.'s temperature 103.8, Mrs. J.'s 100. Ruptured appendix was diagnosed in both cases. Each was operated on during the second day of illness.

Mrs. J. was given ether. In the abdomen there was an excess fluid, brown and foul-smelling, entire cecum and a part of the ascending colon were distended and black, that is, entirely gangrenous. The appendix was retrocecal, adherent, but not involved. The mesentery of the cecum and the ascending colon looked all right but were thought to be thrombosed and it was so mentioned in the

---
1. O. C. Cox, Washington, in *Med. An. D. C.*, Sept.

operative description, but this was not true. There was a carcinoma of the hepatic flexure causing partial obstruction. The terminal ileum, appendix, cecum and one-third of the transverse colon were resected. The incision was closed without drainage and without the use of a sulfonamide.

Mr. J., because of his age, very high temperature and the gravity of his general condition, was operated on under local 2% novocaine. Penicillin was begun before operation without a culture being taken. The same brown fluid was found in the abdomen; the cecum was much distended, entirely black to its mesenteric edge. The appendix was small and fibrous but was not involved. The ascending colon was not gangrenous but was distended and there was a carcinoma at the hepatic flexure. The cecum was exteriorized and a tube was inserted. Iodoform gauze pack about the gut was used to protect the peritoneal cavity. After 12 days of drainage, the temperature was normal and the patient's general condition was better. Under spinal anesthesia the gridiron incision about the opened gut was enlarged and a resection of the gut, including a few inches of the terminal ileum to one-third of the transverse colon with open end-to-end anastomosis, was done. The cecum was entirely sloughed away. The peritoneum was closed and the incision was packed with iodoform gauze, not removed until the ninth day. No sulfonamide was used. There was considerable pus present but no sloughing of the tissue and no bowel leakage.

Mrs. J. was discharged on the 17th day, Mr. J. on the 25th day after the first operation and on the 15th day after the resection.

Cox believes the explanation for the phenomena in these two cases is as follows: Strong physics entered the cecum and became pocketed between the ileocecal valve and the carcinomatous stricture causing the gut to distend, the blood supply to be scanty, the intestinal contents to be irritating, and gangrene to result.

HISTORIC MEDICINE

THE BREVIARY AND DYETARY OF ANDREW BOORDE (1490-1549), PRIEST, PHYSICIAN AND TRAVELLER
In Abstract
DOUGLAS GUTHRIE, in *Proc. Royal Soc. of Med.* (Lond.), July.

ANDREW BOORDE was born about 1490 at Boord's Hill, in Sussex. His name is sometimes written Borde or Boarde, and the fact that he called himself *Andreas Perforatus* suggests that it was pronounced "bored." His career as a Carthusian monk was not long; within a few years he found himself "nott able to byde the rigourosite of your religion," as he wrote his Superior. He went to study medicine at Montpellier, "the nobilist universite of the world for physicians and surgions." On his third continental journey he acted as ambassador for Thomas Cromwell to ascertain the attitude towards King Henry VIII, which he found far from favourable. Next we find Boorde in Scotland, where he spent a year "in a lityl universite namyd Glasco," where he studied and "did practyce physik for the sustentacion of my lyving."

Eventually, Andrew Boorde settled in practice at Winchester, where he was esteemed as "a noted poet, a witty and ingenious person, and an excellent physician." Trouble clouded his later years, when he was accused of keeping at Winchester three women of questionable morals. At all events, he found himself imprisoned in the Fleet in London, and there he died in 1549.

From the medical point of view, Andrew Boorde's most important work is his *Breviary of Health*, 1547, a sort of handbook of domestic medicine, the first medical book, by a medical man, originally written and printed in the English language. From the preface: "The physician must have Grammar to understand what he doth read, Logic to discuss and define truth from falsehood, Geometry to weigh and measure his drugs and potions, and an eloquent tongue to convince his patients." The material is arranged alphabetically from A to Z, from "Abstinence to Zirbus." Abstinence is "the most perfectest medicine that can bee, after repletion or surfet." Virbus (the omentum) is "a pannicle or caule that doth cover the guts; it doth keep the heate of them and d h defend the cold." Of subjects there is an infinite variety; Black Melancholy, King's Evill, Dulness of Wit, Sleep, Memory, Megrim, Warts, Fleas, Pestilence, to mention a few at random. "Musicke" is defined as "one of the liberal sciences comfortable to man in sickness and in health." Gonorrhoea "is named so because Gomorra and Sodom did sinke for such like matter."

Some curious remedies are mentioned. For "Defnes," we are to "take the gall of a hare and mix it with the grece of a Fox and with black woll instill it into the ears"; for "Dronkenness", "drink in the morning a dish of milk"; for "Squint or goggle eye", "put nothing into the eye but the blood of a dove." To counteract fear, "use mery company and feare nothing but God." Treatment of Quinsy: "The 21 Chapter doth shew of the Squincy. Angina is the Latin word, Sinachi the Greek word. It is an impostum in the throat which doth stop up a man's wind or breath. Take a little piece of Pork or Bacon and tie about it a strong thred and let the patient swallow it and by and by pull it out again. Be sure to hold fast the thred and pull it out quickly." Sleeplessness comes of "studying or musyng too much on some matter in the which some persons doth wade too farre, bringing themselves into fantasies." The remedy is leaves of lettuce laid on the temples.

No less than 20 kinds of fevers are described, with curious names—erratic fever, tetrach fever, and putrefied fever, besides the more familiar quartan and tertian. The second book of the *Breviary*, or *Extravagantes*, contains several chapters on examination of the urine, or water casting, as it was called. Boorde wisely remarks that "the best doctour of Physicke may bee deceived in an urine."

The companion volume to the *Breviary* is the *Compendyous Regyment* or *Dyetary of Health*. Commencing with directions on the choosing of a site for one's house, where there is plenty of wood and water and "elbow-rome", he notes that there must be no stinking ponds, nor corrupt dunghills in the vicinity. "As dust doth putrefy the ayre, the swepynge of howses ought nat to be done as long as any honest man is within the precynct." The head of the house must always punish swearers, "for in all the world there is not such odious swearing as is used in Englande, especially among youth and children." Seven hours sleep is enough for most men, and healthy men should not sleep by day, but if they must do so, let them "leanyne and slepe agunst a cupborde, or else syttng upryght in a chayre." "Slepe on your ryght syde . . . with your heed hygh; have a good thycke quylt . . . and let your nyght-cap be of skarlet. When you ryse in the morning, ryse with myrth and remember God."

After eight chapters of such counsel, we come to the main subject of the work, a discussion of diet, first, that for a healthy man, and then the diet advised for the sick. Repletion shortens a man's life, we are told, and two meals a day should suffice, except for a labourer. Water should never be drunk by itself, but may be used to dilute wine. Ale is the natural drink for an Englishman. As for bread, this should be of pure wheat, and not of mixed grains. Despite his dislike of Scotland, the author regards oatcake as "a lordly dish." Milk is good for old men, melancholy men, children, and consumptives. Sea fish are more wholesome than river fish, which may taste of mud. There seems to have been great variety of game in Boorde's day. A bustard is nutritious meat, and a bittern is not so hard to digest as a heron. Plovers and lapwings are not so nourishing as turtle-doves. Of small birds, the lark is best; thrushes are also good, but "not titmonses or wrens, because they eat spiders."

The latter half of the *Dyetary* is devoted to diet in sickness. "A good coke is halfe a physycyon. The chief physick doth come from the kytchen wherefore the physician and the coke for sycke men must consult togyther." It is interesting to note that the sufferer from asthma should avoid nuts, cheese, milk and fish, and should beware of dust and smoke. Lunatics should have hot meals three times a day, but no wine or strong ale. Their heads should be shaven once a month, and they should be kept in a close dark room with a keeper whom they fear.

Boorde pursues his subject to the end, for his last chapter deals with the proper ordering of a deathbed, which should have good nurses, sweet odours, and no babbling women. He was a happy and good-natured man who appears to have taken as his motto his oft-quoted remark that "Myrth is one of the chiefest thynges in Physicke," and who surely deserves to hold a more honoured place in the history of medicine than has hitherto been accorded to him.

GENERAL PRACTICE
JAMES L. HAMNER, M.D., *Editor*, Mannboro, Va.

THE CONSERVATIVE MANAGEMENT OF ACUTE PANCREATITIS

WE HAVE been taught that acute inflammation of the pancreas is a rare, violent disease demanding immediate surgical operation. Now comes an article[1] presenting the picture in a different light.

Acute pancreatitis has been considered to be of extreme rarity, difficult diagnosis, and high mortality. It is a disease of middle and late life in the majority of cases, occurring about equally in both sexes and rarely in the colored race, is more frequent than commonly supposed. In a five-year period in the St. Louis City Hospital the incidence of acute pancreatitis was one-half that of perforated peptic ulcer and *one-tenth that of acute appendicitis*. Not very rare, certainly.

In all patients with severe epigastric or upper abdominal pain, acute pancreatitis should be included as a diagnostic possibility. Diagnosis by clinical methods alone is usually impossible during the acute phase of the disease. The serum-amylase test is practically specific for the lesion, and it seldom if ever presents a false positive.

Delay in operating, with conservative measures directed toward combatting toxicity and altered blood chemistry, has led to a decreased mortality in acute pancreatitis. From 33% treated by operation in the acute stage, to 5% operated on late or not at all. We must be sure the condition is not one demanding immediate surgical intervention.

Since this form of therapy depends on accurate diagnosis for its employment, it is essential that a serum-amylase test be performed in all cases of acute upper abdominal pain in which the diagnosis

1. T. A. Shallow *et al.*, Philadelphia, in *Penn. Med. Jl.*, Sept.

is questionable, because its reliability in diagnosis during the acute phase of pancreatitis has become firmly established.

We must continue to bear this condition in mind. We must make use of this special test on occasion. The diagnosis made, we will use supportive treatment, anodynes, fluids parentally, plasma, blood, oxygen and sulfa drugs or penicillin.

SICK HEADACHES POORLY TREATED

MIGRAINE is little understood and even in high places it is being poorly diagnosed and poorly treated. Thus a master clinician[1] begins an illuminating discussion of this prevalent and disabling affliction.

The cause is a hereditary predisposition, and the attack is a sort of storm which takes place in an overly sensitive brain.

It distresses me that always when a migrainous woman comes in to consult me my assistant's first thought is to put her through the mill. I see no need in these cases for röntgenographing the head or the gallbladder or for sending the patient for a neurologic study. I'd much rather use the time in talking over her life problems and in showing her how to live more calmly and happily, than in making useless examinations.

There is rarely anything organically wrong with the digestive tract, and what the woman needs is not a diet or an operation, but rather information on how to live so calmly that her brain will not get so on edge that the little explosion will take place.

These women are tense, quick in thought and movement; hypersensitive to sounds and lights and smells. They fatigue quickly under any strain or excitement. From girlhood on they tire easily. In the worst cases there is often a combination of migrainous inheritance derived from one ancestor, with a psychopathic inheritance derived from another.

Sensitiveness to chocolate or some other food is often a trigger which can "spring the trap" and bring on a spell. Many a woman will say that, after she discovered all the foods that could give her migraine, she went on having attacks whenever she worried, or menstruated, or took a journey or gave a dinner party, or had a bad night's sleep.

Atypical forms are aches in both sides of the head, or in the back of the head and neck, or headaches so mild that the patient does not complain about them. Similarly, there may be but little nausea and no vomiting. Theye may be only abdominal pain with vomiting.

Often a physician will be puzzled unless he draws out the fact that the woman has two or three different types of headache.

1. W. C. Alvarez, Rochester, Minn., in *R. I. Med. Jl.*, Sept.

Another diagnostic point is that when the woman was a girl in school, she used sometimes to be sent home with an attack of "bilious vomiting." A fact that can almost clinch the diagnosis is that during the woman's pregnancies she was well. Clinching, also, is the fact that an intramuscular injection of gynergen will block or put a stop to an attack.

I know of only one drug that is likely to cut down on the frequency of the spells and that is sodium or potassium thiocyanate. This substance can injure the blood, and it has caused venous thrombosis. I use it only when the patient is having many attacks a month and will not or cannot control the situation by living more calmly and sensibly.

Phenobarbital and dilantin do not affect the triggers which start attacks; no good results seen from treatment with ovarian or pituitary hormones or vitamins.

If she is lucky and if she lives sensibly the headaches should grow less severe with advancing age. They may disappear after the menopause, but she cannot count on that.

The best way in which to get rid of migraine is to solve life's problems and to learn to live free from conflict with self and others.

Often it helps a bit to combat constipation, perhaps with enemas of physiologic saline solution. *Rarely* it helps to get good glasses and to correct any imbalance in the external muscles of the eyes.

Gynergen or ergotamine should not be taken daily to prevent attacks.

In trying to abort an attack an essential point is to begin quickly. Once a patient is nauseated and badly depressed it is useless to put medicine into the stomach. The best drug with which to abort an attack of migraine is ergotamine tartrate or gynergen. In 25 years I have never seen it do any serious harm, even when taken as often as three times a week. In some cases the breathing of pure oxygen for an hour or two works perfectly.

A 3-grain (0.2 gm.) rectal suppository of pentobarbital sodium (nembutal) will often bring rest and sleep and the end of the attack. Sedatives of any type can be given per rectum with the help of a small rectal bulb syringe such as is used for babies.

In all cases it helps greatly if the woman can lie down in a darkened room as soon as an attack threatens. Oftentimes, then, the taking of aspirin with a half grain of codein or two cups of black coffee, or two tablets of bromural will help.

THE CARE OF CLEFT LIP AND PALATE IN BABIES

WHEN I attended on deliveries, I made it a point to get away before a deformed baby was shown to the mother. Arrangements for special care of such babies could be discussed the next day.

The advice of Schultz[1] is conservative and authoritative:

It is preferable that the baby stay in the hospital till the lip has been constructed. Relatives and friends will want to see the baby; if so, show a perfect baby with similar features, because they will gossip, hurt the parents' feelings and later injure those of the child. Instruct the nurse to exhibit the most beautiful blond or brunette baby, and the comment will be favorable.

The child will gain weight rapidly if it expends no energy and all the food is ingested. The best method is to pass a small catheter, put on a glass funnel and pour in the milk. The babies become so lazy they awake only to swallow the tube and then go to sleep again as soon as their stomachs are filled. The first week the baby loses weight, the second week it regains its birth weight and the third week it keeps on gaining weight, showing that the diet is sufficient and agrees with it.

In the first few days of life it can't be known whether all the systems are functioning properly. The ideal time for lip construction is at three or four weeks of age, and for palate construction, three to six months, depending on the width of cleft, the weight of the child and skill of the operator.

1. L. W. Schultz, Chicago, in *Ill. Med. Jl.*, Sept.

DENTISTRY

J. H. GUION, D.D.S., *Editor*, Charlotte, N. C.

THE PATHOLOGY AND TREATMENT OF THE EXPOSED VITAL PULP

IT WILL be of interest to our readers to learn what is high-class English procedure in the treatment of exposed vital pulp. Ross' account before the Royal Medical Society[1] may be taken as affording this information, so it is passed on, considerably abridged:

Many pulpless teeth treated by ordinary routine methods are subsequently found to develop periapical infection. In the case of anterior teeth such infection can be treated by root resection, but in the more inaccessible posterior teeth this often involves the loss of the tooth.

When the pulp is exposed as a result of caries it is always infected. The organisms, however, are usually confined in the first instance to a small corner of the pulp chamber opposite the exposure.

When the crown of a normal healthy tooth is fractured, exposing the pulp, it may be uninfected, but if the pulp remains open to mouth fluids, organisms soon become implanted in the pulp chamber.

1. W. S. Ross, in *Proceedings Royal Soc. of Med.* (Lond.), June.

But for the fact that the area of infection is surrounded by patent dentinal tubules into which the organisms can grow, there is little doubt but that the leucocytes would succeed in destroying the invaders, once the carious cavity is cleaned and filled. As it is, the organisms persist, and a chronic abscess is formed opposite the exposure, but usually the lesion does not remain in this condition for long. Much more often the inflammatory condition of the pulp leads to stasis and death of the pulp. The dentinal tubules then become filled with blood which gives the tooth the familiar blue shade which changes to brown as the haemosiderin crystals coalesce. The organisms are able to grow at will amongst the dead tissue and it is only a matter of time before they reach the peri-apical tissues.

If the cavity is situated on the biting surface, pieces of food debris are likely to be bitten into the carious cavity, and organisms are pushed further into the pulp, with the formation of an acute abscess. This interval may vary from a day to several months or even years, but at its commencement the patient is usually made conscious of the fact that there is a pulp exposure by the exquisite pain which such a condition usually engenders. It is not surprising, then, that the patient at this stage seeks the aid of a dental surgeon. Bearing in mind that the pulp canal is as yet uninfected, the whole aim of root canal treatment must be to see that organisms are not accidentally implanted there during a root-canal instrumentation. Any infection of the peri-apical tissues after removal of a vital pulp must be due to contamination during the operation, unless there is a leak in the crown filling.

There are four principal methods of treatment on teeth with exposed pulps: 1) Pulp capping. 2) Devitalizing the pulp by applying an escharotic sush as arsenic. 3) Removing the pulp under pressure anesthesia. 4) Removing the pulp under a local anesthetic.

1) As it is unlikely that the tissues remain uninfected when the pulp is exposed, no matter from what cause, it is obviously unwise to cover the pulp with a cap without first sterilizing the tissues underneath. The use of a powerful antiseptic causes destruction of tissues, whilst the drug can hardly be expected to destroy every organism present.

Perhaps the only justification of using a pulp cap over an exposure is when it occurs in a young tooth in which the apex is still open. Later the pulp can be extirpated, the root apex having closed in the meantime. Usually the pulp is found to have a chronic ulcer under the pulp cap, although the infection is often limited and gives no discomfort to the patient.

2) A commonly used method is to devitalize the exposed pulp by the application of arsenic. It can be applied simply and quickly and the arsenic can usually be relied upon to kill the pulp without undue pain. The arsenic cannot be depended on to destroy all the organisms present. In a series of experiments in every case a heavy growth of Streptococcus viridans was grown after two-days' incubation.

3) In view of the histological findings that the exposed pulp shows a concentration of organisms in the pulp chamber opposite the exposure, the method of removing the pulp after pressure anesthesia with cocaine pellets need only be mentioned to be condemned.

4) Extirpation of the pulp under local anesthesia is in common use amongst many dental surgeons, but it is at once obvious that the entry of a root-canal instrument such as a barbed broach into the pulp canal, with a view to extirpating the pulp, must first pass through the infected mass, and so contaminate the rest of the pulp tissue.

The method to be described makes use of two electrically heated instruments, which it is believed are capable of destroying bacteria in the carious cavity and in the pulp—the electric cautery and the root desiccator. The latter is an instrument on the lines of the ordinary root-canal drier. A heavy current is needed in order to heat the metal point to a temperature which will burn the contents of the pulp and so destroy the bacteria present. A heavy foot-switch operated by a spring which cuts off the current on being released has been found preferable to the type which is incorporated in the handle of the instrument. After inducing local anesthesia, preferably by intra-osseous injection, the tooth to be operated on is isolated from mouth fluids by means of cotton-wool pads or rubber dam. All burs and instruments are boiled immediately before use and laid in spirit. A few drops of an antiseptic such as one of the formalin-cresol preparations are poured into a dappened glass and placed close to the operator. Every instrument before being introduced into the mouth should be dipped into the formalin solution first in order to eliminate the risk of chance infection.

Enamel edges are chiselled away, and gross caries carefully removed with a large rosehead bur. No pressure is made on the exposed pulp which would introduce fresh organism into the pulp vessels. At this stage the cavity is cauterized with the ordinary electric cautery, and is opened up further to allow of easy access to the pulp chamber, the exposure is widened, and the area cauterized again. The cavity is well soaked with formalin and the electric heated pulp desiccator then introduced into the pulp chamber slowly along the root canal toward the apex. The operator should be able to feel the external surface of the crown of the tooth becoming hot to the finger, and may see the contents of the pulp boiling during the procedure. Formalin is now introduced into the canal by means of a smooth broach and cotton-wool dipped in the antiseptic. When the canal is thoroughly saturated with the solution, the root desiccator is passed into the canal for a second time, and kept there until the formalin boils off. The canal is again filled with formalin, enlarged by suitable root reamers, and immediately filled with an adequate impermeable filling.

OPHTHALMOLOGY
Herbert C. Neblett, M.D., *Editor*, Charlotte, N. C.

A SIMPLE METHOD FOR EARLY DETECTION OF ABNORMALITIES OF PUPILLARY REACTION

Complicated apparatuses with cinematographic registration—only available in a few large research departments—are required to establish early disturbances of the pupillary reaction; the neurologist has usually to content himself with vague expressions as "pupillary reaction perhaps somewhat sluggish." A disturbance of the normal mechanism of the pupillary reaction is in many cases one of the earliest symptoms of a disease of the central nervous system, and of great importance for the diagnosis.

An accidental observation made during slit-lamp examinations demonstrated a way to detect these early disturbances.[1] If a pin-point light is projected on the eye with the slit-lamp in such a way that it just enters the pupil near the margin of the iris, the pupil contracts, the iris margin moves towards the center of the pupil and prevents the light pencil from entering the pupil. As no light now reaches the retina the stimulus for the contraction of the pupil is no longer present, the pupil dilates—and thus again allows the light pencil to reach the retina. This artificial "hippus" continues regularly in a normal eye so long as the light pencil enters the pupil. Physiological differences such as age, colour of the iris, errors of refraction, etc., have no influence on the reaction.

Elderly persons and those with dark irises show less extensive movements; but in every normal person the reaction is easy to produce; the pupil contracts and dilates 10 times in seven to eight seconds, which can easily be measured by the stop watch. The time of 0.7 to 0.8 seconds for one cycle of the "hippus" corresponds with the physiological figure for the pupillary "reflex"; The "reflex time," i.e., the latent period plus contraction time, is in the region of 0.8 seconds. In the method described the contraction does not reach its maximum because the stimulus disappears before it is reached, and the contraction time is therefore shortened. This means that the time of 0.7 to 0.8 seconds consists of 1) the latent period, 2) the shortened contraction time, and 3) the re-dilation time. A disturbance of any one of these three periods would be expected to slow down the "hippus"; this, however, did not occur in the pathological cases so far examined.

In the cases of latent syphilis, early tabes, etc., with clinically normal pupillary reaction the artificial hippus could never be produced by the slit-lamp. Usually a good if not extensive contraction followed the first stimulus; but then, either the pupil did not dilate sufficiently to let the light pencil enter the eye, or a few irregular, sluggish contractions followed, after which the pupil finally remained immobile. In no case could the regular play of the normal pupil be produced.

A large number of cases of, for example, early tabes, with apparently normal pupillary reaction, should be examined with this method. If the results of these investigations are found to agree with these observations, this method might then become a useful diagnostic aid for the physician.

The *method* described by Major Stern for detecting abnormal pupillary reactions should invite the interest particularly of oculists, neurologists and neuro-surgeons, and provoke further investigation by them in this field of eye signs as to their clinical value. The procedure used, however, is available to only a few, unless in large clinics, because the slit-lamp is rarely available except in such clinics. The writer estimates the number in North Carolina not to exceed six which would represent the average number for all states in the union except in those states having large cities. Further, the slit-lamp is an expensive piece of equipment, and its use would necessitate more than casual training by any one who would attempt to use it for the purpose under discussion. It has been suggested (the editor of this Journal) that some simple, less expensive, readily available method, within the reach of all, might be utilized to elicit and correctly interpret these signs.

After some time and thought spent in his office in investigating the matter the writer has been unable to evolve any simple, practicable, inexpensive method which would elicit the pupillary findings in question other than by the use of his own slit-lamp. Since by the use of this instrument at present may be the only feasible method by which these pupillary signs may be correctly determined, other than in large clinics, the procedure would not be practicable except in the hands of the few oculists who own a slit-lamp and are trained in its use.

---
[1]. Maj. H. J. Stern, R.A.M.C. (England), in *Proc. R. of Ophthal.*, June.

HOSPITALS

R. B. Davis, M.D., *Editor*, Greensboro, N. C.

POST-WAR HOSPITALIZATION

A HORDE of people are writing and speaking about post-war conditions; certainly there must be few who have worked out a practical solution for the operation of a post-war world. Since I have not seen or heard any discussion of the post-war hospitalization question, I am venturing to offer for the reader's consideration some thoughts which seem to me to be based on common sense.

That there will be need for hospital services will not be denied by any. How are they to be furnished?

By the Federal Government for all citizens—rich and poor, black and white?

By State, County and City taxpayers?

By the present hospitalization plan which includes the former and private hospitalization service?

Which one of these will be best suited for the post-war world? Whether we be doctors, lawyers or Indian chiefs, we will have to acknowledge the fact that hospitalization is needed more than it is accepted. The cause of this, however, is not due entirely to finances, as some philanthropic politicians would have us to believe. However, this does govern a large percentage of decisions upon the part of the patients whether they will or will not enter the hospitals.

An element that enters largely into the problem is ignorance on the part of the patient. We have professors, lawyers, doctors, preachers, and what not, who are perfectly able to pay the hospital bill but who refuse to go to the hospital. Their argument is that they can get along just as well at home; and that they do not like the odor in the hospital; or that they do not like the food in the hospital; or the noise bothers them; and, sometimes, a timid male objects to nurses waiting on him.

Let us investigate what the Federal hospitalization plan would mean. The first and the biggest problem would be handling the personnel who render the services after the patient is admitted—the doctors, nurses, dietitians, secretaries, engineers. The doctors would have to be on the Federal payroll—at so much per month, with or without maintenance. It would be very hard to convience a patient who was not getting well as fast as he felt that he should that the doctors were doing everything possible to speed up his recovery, if the doctors' checks would be the same whether or not he treated Patient No. 591. Therefore, there would be very little love lost between the patient and the hired doctor. This in itself would defeat one of the most beneficial relationships between the doctor and the patient.

Doctors on the payroll would demand an eight-hour system with double pay for all overtime just as labor-unionists have demanded and obtained. Further, where are the doctors coming from? Under the present system, most doctors are on call twenty-four hours of the day and most doctors actually work more than twelve hours out of the twenty-four. If a system of hired doctors is established, with their certain demands of eight hours with double pay for overtime, we should need at least twice as many doctors in order to see the same number of patients as we are now serving, because vacations would have to be arranged and sick-leave would have to be taken care of in the physician personnel.

We have been continually told for the last three or four years that there are not near enough doctors to carry on as things are. It is evident, therefore, that there must be a number of new medical schools or there must be a doubling of the capacity of the present schools. In this connection, it is an unsolvable problem as to why our medical educators persist in turning down four out of five applicants to study medicine. The American medical colleges are discouraging the enlargement of medical schools and the opening of new medical schools. This truth brings us jam up to the problem of more doctors having to be educated by the Federal medical schools.

It is not an easy prophecy to make that progressive medicine will grow out of Federal control. If progressive medicine is not practiced in the Federal hospitals, the lay people will lose confidence in the Federal hospitals. If a patient does not go to the hospital for that reason, it is safe to say that he will not send for a Federal doctor to see him. And so the latter condition of the man is worse than the first; he could go if he would to the hospital and the worse that could happen to him now is that he can't go on account of finances, but more about that later.

The next great problem with the Federal hospitalization is the nurse personnel. At the present time it takes three years to graduate a nurse. It takes four years to graduate a doctor. But one busy doctor could take care of enough patients to keep ten nurses busy on a twelve-hour shift. Now the nurses, like the doctors, would demand an eight-hour shift, with double pay for all overtime and sick-leave and vacations thrown in. Therefore, it is safe to say that every busy hospital practicing physician will require fifteen nurses under the Federal plan. Where are these nurses coming from? And again, the same professional relationship will exist between the dissatisfied patient and the nurse. If the leaders in the medical profession—i.e., the doctors and the nurses—are going to complicate the policy of the Federal control, what can we expect of the non-professional group? The switch-board operators and elevator operators, the engineers, the cooks and maids, the orderlies—all these would have to be put on a Civil Service basis. The mere bookkeeping required on the personal relationship between government and employees would be a problem that could only be handled by a certified public accountant with ample office assistants. One has very little difficulty in believing this if he has been familiar with the red tape in connection with getting a job under the so-called Emergency Civil Service set-up.

The second way in which hospitalization may be furnished, little different from the first, is through the State, County and City taxpayers; and there are difficulties that might arise to even further complicate the picture. For instance, the State, County and City would hardly be interested in building a medical school which is the only way they could possibly get enough doctors. How would enough beds to take care of all local politician's friends be provided? It would take at least three times as many beds as it takes now with the present system. This would hardly be denied by any of the city hospitals now in operation if the question were asked. The writer has just finished a long-distance conversation with the hospital director of one of the largest city hospitals operated in North Carolina. He was told by that director that their reservations were all filled up until the 15th of September, today being September 5th. The nursing situation might possibly be a bit easier for the reason that the State, County and City hospitals could, if by any chance they could satisfactorily or otherwise control the nursing Council of the State, operate enough Training Schools to supply sufficient nurses.

Some patients who have strong political friends might enjoy a hospital home. At the present time it is not unusual for this type of hospital to carry patients along from three to twelve months, and even up into the years, without being able to discharge them.

If one happens to live in a city where there are both private and city hospitals, it would not be hard for him to determine which hospital comes nearest to satisfying the patients. A satisfied patient will more readily become a well citizen. This should be the function of the hospitals.

The third and final type of hospitalization would be somewhat similar to the present set-up. The writer does not wish to be classified as afraid to adopt anything new that offers a reasonable chance of success. Those who know him best know that he is very far from that type of individual. It would seem, however, to completely disregard all the experiences that we have had in hospitalization of the sick and start out upon an entirely new Political Control System, which would lead us into a lot of pitfalls. These pitfalls would not only involved the pain of kidney colic and the abdominal cramps from ruptured appendix, but would be rooted more deeply than the period of illness would indicate. It would have considerable to do with the initiative and the responsibility of the private citizen. The necessities of life must come as a result of one's labors or be furnished gratis. The citizen with the proper inward feeling is he who by his own efforts builds a financial and a moral relationship by taking care of his own obligations and furnishing himself and those dependent upon him with enough for the necessities of life and a reasonable amount beyond this. When a citizen loses a desire to do this for any reason whatsoever, he becomes a parasite. A lot of people who get something for nothing will abuse that privilege and lose self-respect and regard for their obligations and, therefore, they would not become better citizens but, on the contrary, would increase in shiftlessness. The present system of hospitalization has many faults, but none that cannot be remedied if sound thinking and practical efforts were made to correct it.

One of these that is particularly in need of correcting is the financial side of a hospital stay of many sick citizens. I am proud to state that the medical and hospital authorities have come a long way in this direction, for they have put into effect a plan known as Hospitalization Insurance. There are few who cannot afford to carry this insurance, and those who are not able can be cared for through the Fraternal Orders, Civic Clubs and Religious Organizations, if they would pay the small premium required to take Hospitalization Insurance. The very few remaining could be cared for by the welfare departments of the city, county or state. If this method of taking care of the sick were universally adopted just as the system of furnishing water and electric lights is satisfactory to all citizens, so would be Hospitalization Insurance. It would seem to the author of this article that the responsibility lays fairly and squarely upon the shoulders of the medical profession and its allies, such as the hospital administrators and the nurses.

Have we any other simple way out, but for those of us who are responsible to purge ourselves of this dangerous complacency which is now eating at the very heart of the professions who have to do with the repairing and the maintaining of the human body?

With the State Medical Society, the State Nurses Association and the State Hospital Association the answer rests.

RHINO-OTO-LARYNGOLOGY

CLAY W. EVATT, M.D., *Editor*, Charleston, S. C.

A THERAPEUTIC REGIMEN FOR OTITIS MEDIA

"A Suggested Method of Treatment for Acute and Chronic Infection of the Middle Ear" as published by Dr. R. W. Hanckel in the September *Journal of the South Carolina Medical Association* is a clear-cut, direct method of attack.

In those cases so mild that myringotomy was not indicated sulfadiazine and soda bicarbonate were given in appropriate dosage, with plenty of liquids to eliminate the sulfa. A glycerine compound is dropped into the ear q. 2 to 4 h. to lessen drum congestion by osmosis. A pledget of cotton keeps this solution in the aural canal. Since middle-ear infection starts as nasal and pharyngeal congestion and infection, treatment of this area is of prime importance. In my experience a combination of vasoconstriction and bacteriostatic agent is more efficacious and less troublesome than administering two separate medicaments—mild nose drops of neosynephrine, adrenalin—anyone of the plentiful constricting agents. I have used all the sulfa drugs in the various combinations advocated, but after a few weeks have again come back to glucofedrine or very mild adrenalin in silver for the infants, and adrenalin 1-1000, 20 drops in an ounce of 15% argyrol for the older children. Privine (Ciba) gives the most prolonged constriction—sometimes for six or more hours. A very few drops of privine are as effective as greater amounts of less potent constrictors. These nose drops should be used *correctly* every two four waking hours, to keep the eustachian tube open and aerate the middle ear. With the head hanging upside down over the edge of the bed, the nose drops are to be instilled, the head tilted toward the side involved and this position maintained five minutes. Many myringotomies are prevented by this routine, started early.

Patients are told to return to the office 24 to 48 hours after myringotomy, at which time the canal is wiped clean with 3% hydrogen peroxide on a cotton-tipped applicator. Then the canal is filled with desoxyephedronium sulfathiazole solution (Sulfomone—Park Davis) warmed to body temperature. A Seigle otoscope is now fitted into the ear canal and the attached rubber bulb is compressed and allowed to expand three or four times. Ten per cent argyrol, 5% sodium sulfathiazole have been used. Desoxyephedronium sulfathiazole is non-irritating, vasoconstricting, and antiseptic. This forces the solution through the perforated drum into the middle ear and eustachian canal.

This method of treatment has been used in:

1. Acute purulent infections of the middle ear with an opening in the drum, spontaneous or otherwise.

2. As a postoperative adjunct in cases of simple or modified radical mastoidectomy with remaining purulent otorrhea.

In postoperative radical mastoidectomies a combination of sulfanilamide, sulfapyridine and sulfathiazole powder in equal parts is sprayed through the canal into the operative area at intervals as indicated, until the area becomes completely epithelialized.

3. Chronic purulent infections of the middle ear with no evidence of intracranial or blood stream extension.

After the discharge has ceased the drum membrane may close spontaneously. If not, Stinson's procedure is indicated: *i.e.*, the edges of the perforation are touched with deliquefied trichloracetic acid crystals on a very fine cotton-tipped applicator. If the reaction doesn't initiate closure of the perforation (and it will not do so in medium or large perforations) a patch of Cargyle's membrane one-fourth larger than the perforation is picked up on a moistened cotton-tipped applicator and placed over the perforation. If the patch becomes displaced it is replaced by another and another. If the patch stays in place the perforation may epithelialize across in from a few days to several months. The membrane merely acts as a scaffold to guide the growth of the epithelium. In those cases where a dry ear does not result after six or eight months of weekly treatments, cholesteatoma is suspected. Careful x-ray treatment and radical mastoidectomy are to be considered.

The author reported a total of cured and improved 88.5% in a carefully studied series of 34 patients, a series large enough to suggest value, in that the percentage improved is higher than any reported elsewhere.

DISCUSSION
From P. 364

between the organic hypoglycemia and the functional, which I think is perfectly proper. Hyperinsulinism in patients treated with insulin is another type. Some of the instances he mentioned are most striking. All of them were cases with vague symptoms showing a lowering of blood sugar after glucose, and as Dr. Wilkinson mentioned, need have no relationship to the hypoglycemia. We recently had two cases of organic hyperinsulinism, one nine years in duration and the other eight. One was sent to Williamsburg for insanity. The disease was diagnosed epilepsy in one of the larger hospitals, although hypoglycemia had been found. It seems to me that hypoglycemia is significant only when the patient is obviously disabled. His description of his symptoms may be indefinite but the presence of a definite disabling condition is clear to the family and the doctor. If the blood sugar is low and continues to fall with persistent fasting, I think we should think of a tumor of the pancreas as the cause of it; that is, if the blood sugar falls as low as 50 mgs. One of my patients recently operated on had a fasting blood sugar of 85, but with prolonged fasting it fell to 39 mgm. 20 hours after food. Each had a pancreatic adenoma, and in one case malignancy had begun. I think for that reason reasonably early diagnosis is worth while because removal of the adenoma may cure the patient and, if it stays until it is malignant, cure is not likely.

I think it is a most interesting group of cases and I enjoyed the paper a great deal.

DR. DONNELLY: I think it is possible that two of the patients I mentioned may be of the adenomatous type, that is, the 40-year-old business man and the school-girl who spent four hours in the hosiery mill. The girl has had very definite reactions to missed meals and of course she gets also loss of consciousness if she doesn't eat properly. The business man had an episode three weeks ago when he went to a Lion's Club banquet where he ate the wrong food and on the following day he had to have intravenous glucose. When he goes out in the garden to work, he frequently falls out in a state of semiconsciousness.

Surgical removal of pancreatic adenomata has not proved highly successful in effecting cures and in some instances have left the patients in worse condition than before operation.

SURGERY

GEO. H. BUNCH, M.D., *Editor*, Columbia, S. C.

ERYSIPELOID CANCER OF THE BREAST

EARLY diagnosis is difficult in cases of cancer of the breast that begin with diffuse symmetrical enlargement of the gland. Painless enlargement, without fever, tenderness or discoloration in most cases is indicative of cancer. Fever and redness, when present, are strongly suggestive that the lesion is of inflammatory origin. Erysipeloid cancer, carcinomatous mastitis, lactation cancer are three names for one deceptive and a rapidly fatal type of cancer that manifests itself by symmetrical enlargement with diffuse red discoloration of the skin. It so well simulates inflammatory mastitis that the physician may be lulled into a sense of false security.

Particularly in cases in which a discrete mass has been noted in the breast preceding diffuse enlargement should it be remembered that the apparently benign condition may be malignant. In a case of acute carcinomatous mastitis with painless enlargement there may be fever and leucocytosis with a diffuse purplish red blush over the breast and the contiguous skin. There may or may not be palpable axillary nodes; there may or may not be retraction of the nipple. Such findings in the lactating breast of a young mother will confuse the most astute clinician, if he is not careful. It was DaCosta's rule that, in any case of supposed mastitis persisting for more than two weeks, biopsy be done to rule out inflammatory cancer.

The progressively enlarging, purplish area of skin that has undergone the pig-skin change of lenticular dermatitis is of grave prognostic significance, for it is produced by retrograde invasion of the superficial lymphatics and blood vessels. Duration of life following the appearance of inflammatory signs is about one year. Visceral and skeletal metastases occur early and are widespread.

Geschickter says involvement of the liver, lungs or bone is manifest at the time of initial examination in one-third of the cases; and that in his experience all varieties of therapy were equally unsuccessful in the treatment of erysipeloid cancer. "The majority were treated by radical surgery which by modern standards is contraindicated. This apparently shortened the life of the patient if we compare the duration of life in our series which averaged one year with that of twenty-one months reported by Taylor and Meltzer. In their cases the majority were treated by irradiation. Operation with the cautery or soldering iron had no advantage over the knife. Apparently the response to irradiation is insufficient to affect the rapid spread of the disease. The induction of artificial menopause as reported by Taylor and Meltzer is without benefit."

We have recently had a case of inflammatory cancer in a woman of twenty-five which ran a rapidly fatal postoperative course, in spite of irradiation in maximum dosage over the chest and over the lower abdomen to produce an artificial menopause. The patient lived only six months.

We make this brief presentation of erysipeloid cancer that our readers may recognize the hopelessly fatal condition should it appear.

HOARSENESS—THINK OF CARCINOMA OF THE LARYNX (F. E. LeJeune, New Orleans, in Jl. Med. Assn. Ala., Sept.)

Five per cent of all cancers of the human occur in the larynx; 95% of these in men; 85% of cases occur within the larynx—*intrinsic*—respond favorably to surgery; whereas in *extrinsic* cancer of the larynx the prognosis is bad.

The practitioner could more fully realize that life or death in cases of carcinoma of the larynx depends upon an early diagnosis it cannot be too often repeated that *persistent hoarseness is the one and only unfailing indication of early carcinoma of the larynx.*

IN ALL OUR PATIENTS WITH PEPTIC ULCER who have died and come to autopsy or who, through operative interference, have had the ulcer exposed, the ulcer, if duodenal, has been located on the posterior duodenal wall, has involved the pancreas, and has given rise to hemorrhage through the erosion of the pancreaticoduodenal artery or one of its major branches.

If the ulcer has been gastric, it has been on the lesser curvature and has implicated the right or left gastric artery or their major branches.—G. J. Heuer.

A CASE OF AGRANULOCYTOSIS occurring in an adult male who was receiving sulfamerazine appeared after 22 days of daily administration of the drug. A total dose of 42 Gm. was given. Recovery followed the termination of sulfonamide therapy and treatment with large doses of pentnucleotide and liver extract.

SOUTHERN MEDICINE & SURGERY

Official Organ

JAMES M. NORTHINGTON, M.D., *Editor*

Department Editors

Human Behavior
JAMES K. HALL, M.D.................................Richmond, Va.

Orthopedic Surgery
JOHN T. SAUNDERS, M.D. ....Asheville, N. C.

Urology
RAYMOND THOMPSON, M.D.........................Charlotte, N. C.

Surgery
GEO. H. BUNCH, M.D.................................Columbia, S. C.

Obstetrics
HENRY J. LANGSTON, M.D............................Danville, Va.

Gynecology
CHAS. R. ROBINS, M.D.................................Richmond, Va.
ROBERT T. FERGUSON, M.D. ....Charlotte, N. C.

General Practice
J. L. HAMNER, M.D.................................Mannboro, Va.
J. HERBERT SMITH, M.D. ....Pauline, S. C.

Clinical Chemistry and Microscopy
J. M. FEDER, M.D.,
EVELYN TRIBBLE, M. T. } ....Anderson, S. C.

Hospitals
R. B. DAVIS, M.D.................................Greensboro, N. C.

Cardiology
CLYDE M. GILMORE, A.B., M.D.............Greensboro, N. C.

Public Health
N. THOS. ENNETT, M.D............................Greenville, N. C.

Radiology
R. H. LAFFERTY, M.D., and Associates......Charlotte, N. C.

Therapeutics
J. F. NASH, M.D.................................Saint Pauls, N. C.

Tuberculosis
JOHN DONNELLY, M.D...............................Charlotte, N. C.

Dentistry
J. H. GUION, D.D.S.................................Charlotte, N. C.

Internal Medicine
GEORGE R. WILKINSON, M.D....................Greenville, S. C.

Ophthalmology
HERBERT C. NEBLETT, M.D.........................Charlotte, N. C.

Rhino-Oto-Laryngology
CLAY W. EVATT, M.D.............................Charleston, S. C.

Proctology
RUSSELL L. BUXTON, M.D......................Newport News, Va.

Insurance Medicine
H. F. STARR, M.D.................................Greensboro, N. C.

Dermatology
J. LAMAR CALLAWAY, M.D. ....Durham, N. C.

Pediatrics

Offerings for the pages of this Journal are requested and given careful consideration in each case..... Manuscripts not found suitable for our use will not be returned unless author encloses postage.

As is true of most Medical Journals, all costs of cuts, etc., for illustrating an article must be borne by the author.

THE DIAGNOSIS AND TREATMENT OF MEDICINE'S ILLS

TEN YEARS OR SO AGO a professor in the Medical School of the University of Indiana wrote an article in which he said if his wife ever started computing calories and vitamines in planning his meals he was going to leave home.

A little later a hospital in Indiana, having taken cognizance of the fact that all hospitals have a composite, disagreeable odor, rid itself of that odor and published the means adopted.

Now the dean of Indiana's medical school comes out with the best diagnosis of the *status quo* of Medicine, and the most intelligently conceived plan of treatment, that have come to this desk.[1]

There must be something special in the air, water or soil of the biggest city in the world, not on water.

Dean Gatch's clear-cut ideas, in essentials, are:

Medical science has made spectacular advances which have fascinated the people. Medical education has tried to keep abreast of medical science. The medical curriculum has been overloaded till it now contains more than any mind can master. The people, at great expense and by every possible means of instruction, have been told, chiefly under guidance by lay agencies, all that anybody knows and in most instances a great deal more, about all the mysteries of the human body and the ills which may afflict it.

The investment of money in hospitals is tremendous. Their maintenance is a major industry. It is no longer customary to be born, to be sick, or to die at home. These great events of life now take place in a hospital.

Great numbers of people now carry sickness insurance. Insurance companies are a great power in medicine.

Public health departments are great and opulent. An army of social and welfare workers has moved in between us and the sick poor, and is claiming recognition as a distinct profession.

We no longer have undisputed control of medical care; multitudes of laymen now make a living out of it, and threaten to subjugate us.

We are in an ugly situation which many doctors think is hopeless. It is not! We still have a good fighting chance to save ourselves. It may still be possible to convince the people that we are worthy of the privileges they have granted us, and that lay domination of medical practice is not for their good. The fundamental causes of our troubles are partly the result of social change, partly the result of our own fault, and partly (I think chiefly) the result of lay interference in medical practice.

---
1. W. D. Gatch, Indianapolis, in *Jl. Indiana State Med. Assn.*, Aug.

Lay control of medical practice has increased insidiously. Most physicians are unaware of its extent and sinister characteristics. Much of this work has been beneficial. Most laymen who really want to help medical progress are amenable to guidance by physicians.

Some schemes already in effect, others in prospect, if successful, will greatly limit or even take away entirely our control of medical care. These are being sponsored, for the most part, by individuals who view medical care as a rich prize for commercial and political exploitation—rich in money, in votes, in patronage. They are also sponsored by a large group of social theorists, and by some physicians.

The American Hospital Association and its constituent members possess immense power which is a menace to the medical profession. The American Medical Association and the American College of Surgeons have little power to enforce the recommendations of their hospital inspectors. They have inflicted upon us hospitals too expensive to build and too expensive to operate. They make hospital costs needlessly great. In most cases the hospital bill of the patient is greater than the physician's. The hospital organizations, working in close cooperaton with companies which sell sickness and hospital insurance, promote needless hospitalizations. The natural inclination is to get the value of your money and go to the hospital for illnesses which could safely be treated in the home; also to stay in the hospital much longer than is necessary.

A scheme for a great extension of hospital insurance proposes to lump the cost of the pathologist's services with other hospital expenses. Pathology is perhaps the most important branch of medicine. The need for well-trained pathologists is urgent. What incentive is there to a bright medical student to become a pathologist if he must surrender his status as a physician? So also for the student who thinks of becoming a röntgenologist or anesthetist.

The insurance companies sooner or later, if present forms of insurance persist, are certain to buy the services of all varieties of medical men at the lowest possible cost.

Schemes to socialize medical care are not an immediate danger to us. The cost would be prohibitive; the administration next to impossible. There is no general demand for them outside very limited regions. This demand may come in the future if the forces we have been considering, and others we have but mentioned, are not checked. The practice of medicine as a learned profession cannot exist if it passes under lay control.

We have been widely criticized. We still possess, to an astonishing degree, the confidence of the public. The present shortage of doctors has demonstrated the great love of people for the family doctor. They are not against us. We can show them that our enemies are their enemies. The record of our colleagues in the armed services has been splendid, and is certain to enhance the standing of our profession. Our duty is to preserve its ancient privileges till they come home.

Medicine gives an indispensable service to society. Civilization cannot exist without it. It has survived through the ages under every condition of society and under every form of government. The members of no other calling have the professional pride that physicians have. They will not as a group endure outside control for long. What can we do? I offer, for your consideration, the following ideas:

To drive from medicine the powerful lay groups which are exploiting us will be no easy job, but it can be done.

Our cause is just and in the public interest. Medical care is supporting a great growth of lay parasites. The people should know that this is what makes it expensive.

We are all-powerful as a learned profession which does an indispensable service for society. The people will support us if we act as physicians; not if we act as politicians. We need unity, professional discipline, and the will to fight. A chief danger is that laymen who profit from medical care will disrupt or control or professional organizations.

We must regain control of our hospitals. That the professional affairs of a hospital be made subordinate to its business management is intolerable. even contrary to good business principles. We must oppose, with all our power, the evils of current forms of hospital insurance. The only proper form of insurance is one which pays the patient a lump sum for a given illness, to be used as the insured sees fit, and which also makes the total amount of insurance well below the estimated cost of the illness. To insure a house for its total value or more would be to invite arson.

What is for the general good is for our good. We must be ready and willing to adapt our practice to changing social conditions. We must admit and correct our mistakes. The greatest mistake of our leaders has been to allow an unhealthy growth of specialism at the expense of general practice. A third or more of all physicians are now specialists. They greatly increase the cost of medical care. Diagnosis is now supposed to require a complete study of the entire patient by a group of specialists—a process generally represented to be entirely beyond the ability of a general practitioner.

Very few specialists know enough to do good general practice. The general practitioner and no one else can save the medical profession. No other form of medical care care can compete with that given by a good family doctor. Theorists who would socialize medical care have a very slight conception of what good medical care is.

The Indiana University School of Medicine and the Indianapolis City Hospital have tried out an experimental basis for the training of men for general practice. More than 10 years ago four fellowships were established for this purpose at the Indianapolis City Hospital. These are filled by men who have completed a year of internship. They work for three years in all departments of the dispensary, and review the basic sciences. They learn what we think a man in general practice should know about all human complaints. This plan has been very successful.

We have been remiss as a profession in doing little to refute the teaching that good medical care requires a complete laboratory study of every patient who seeks the advice of a physician. This belief has been fostered by lay influence, and by the over-development of specialism. It can be corrected by the improvement of general practice, and by giving proper information to the people. A good practitioner knows which patients require complete laboratory study, and which ones do not.

We must at all costs rid ourselves of lay domination. We can do this if we stick together. The people are still our friends.

Southern Medicine & Surgery has consistently maintained: that, contrary to the widely proclaimed and accepted belief that the place for a sick person is in a hospital, the place for the vast majority of sick persons is in their own beds; that, instead of the present provision of hospital services on the Cadillac and Rolls-Royce plan, these services should be provided on the Ford and Chevrolet plan (A recent estimate by a hospital "authority" of the need for new hospital beds all over this country places the cost at nearly $7,000.00 per bed!); that public health doctors and nurses should be firmly estopped from encroaching on the field of private practice; that the general practitioner is fully capable of taking care of 80 to 90 per cent of medical practice, yet he has been so belittled and talked down, and the specialist so exalted, as to make the seeking of specialists' and hospitals' services the chief cause for dissatisfaction with the cost of health care; that the function of the specialists is to render service in cases of unusual rarity and severity, not according to sex, age, or the anatomical part affected; that to destroy the general practitioner is to destroy the private practice of medicine, for he is the broad foundation which supports the pyramid of specialism; that for hospitals to control doctors is for the tail to wag the dog.

Southern Medicine & Surgery has maintained all along that we can fight our way out of our present difficulties, if we have the will to fight and not continue the policy of appeasement.

"The general practitioner and no one else can save the medical profession," says this wise and clear-seeing dean. True; but only if the high-priced—and therefore the best in the opinion of the ninety-and-nine whose sole criterion of value is price—members of the profession will awake to the fact that a superstructure must fall when its foundation is completely undermined; and, in self-defense if for no more worthy motive, give the general practitioner his due. In this connection, it is to be borne in mind that medical school faculties are made up wholly of specialists; and that, just as a lawyer on the bench is three-fourths lawyer and one-fourth judge, so a specialist member of the faculty of a medical school is three-fourths specialist and one-fourth teacher of what to do for sick folks.

An article which came to this desk within the past ten days condemns the general practitioner who removes *any* foreign body from the conjunctiva! It may well be doubted whether private medical practice can survive unless it soon comes about that as many patients are referred from specialist to general practitioner as from general practitioner to specialist. And it would help everybody if every dean of a medical school were a genuine family doctor, in active practice.

* * * * *

HEALTH THROUGH MUSIC

THE GREEK TERM from which the word music is derived comprehended all the arts of the nine muses. Anciently, the singing and setting of lyric poetry constituted but a small part of a "musical education," which included reading and writing, all the arts of literature, and even mathematics and astronomy; and was valued chiefly as an important element in character formation.

It is said that magnificent organs were built in a number of the earliest hospitals of Europe—those in Italy.

Towards the end of the 16th century Sir Thomas Gresham established a professorship of Music at Oxford. The first five men to hold this chair were all physicians.[1]

A musician[2] who for three years conducted an orchestra in regular appearances at an Orthopedic Hospital and at a State Hospital for the Insane gives his impressions of music as a therapeutic agent.

Solemn music is out of the question; brightness, gaiety and inspiration, with an occasional note of restfulness—that's the prescription. One who is flat on his back for months does not need restful music; he wants something with life—marches,

---
1. Edward Podolsky, Brooklyn, in *Ohio State Med. Jl.*, Feb., 1940.
2. W. A. Wiant, Charleston, in *W. Va. Med. Jl.*, Nov., 1941

overtures and the like, with a liberal supply of comedy. For the patients at the State Hospital he used an abundance of dance music, hilly-billy and modern jive, with seasoning of comedy numbers and marches.

"At both institutions eyes lit up; faces that had been set with pain looked with interest at the orchestra; lips that had not smiled for weeks were now lifted at the funny songs of our comedians and the comic numbers. The feeble-minded could imagine they were at a formal ball, or else envison themselves as part of a grand cortege for the marches. They went back to their rooms with minds that had been brightened and lifted out of themselves by the power of the music."

"Music can arouse, soothe, anger, quiet, inspire, and if we are to believe rumor, even incite to murder and suicide, we are letting an opportunity slip when we fail to make music available to our sick."

A learned teacher of music[3] says the emotional connotations of music are highly complex, and more powerful than is generally realized. He hesitates to think of what the effect of music upon the next generation will be if the present school of "hot jazz" continues to develop unabated. "It should provide an increasing number of patients for your hospitals and it is, therefore, only poetic justice that musical therapeutics should develop at least to the point where music serves as an antidote for itself!"

Dr. Hanson goes on to tell us: There is first the study of the music as an expression of the individual who creates it, second the study of music in relation to the age from which it springs, third the scientific analysis of musical technics and their relationships to emotional expression, and fourth the study of the effects of these various types of music upon the listener. A combination of the third and fourth categories which would enlist the aid both of skilled musical theorists and psychiatrists should throw much light upon the influence of music, both benevolent and malevolent, in the lives of people. For in this day when through the radio the country is flooded with sound it seems logical to assume that music is destined to play an important part in helping to preserve mental sanity on the one hand or, if misused, to add to the emotional strain of an age already overtaxed by disruptive forces.

An observer[4] of music's effects on patients in hospitals for several different classes of the diseased gives testimony: Most musical instruments can be used for the rehabilitation of movements of fingers, wrist and elbow. For patients with rheumatic fever orchestras have been welcomed by the medical and nursing staff of a research hospital for the study of this disease. For the development of healthful emotional habits and active intellectual life, school is placed next to medical treatment in importance. Musical activity is beneficial to them in developing morale and in providing a practical program of activity with a maximum of rest for the heart. It builds cultural elements into the child's makeup which enrich his whole life.

During the period of rest in bed, the activities of creating music—except those which place demands on the lungs—would give the patient with pulmonary tuberculosis a practical avocation and cultural development and would cultivate a small degree of muscular tonicity. All of the percussion devices permit known and controlled muscular exertion and produce satisfying musical results.

Patients suffering from injuries to nerves are considered from the viewpoint of recoördinating muscular function and movements of joints.

The musician's approach to a psychiatric patient is with a view to having him realize:

"Here is one who is equally aware of intimate subtleties—one who understands—one in whom I can repose confidences." For many such patients music is a means of emotional reëducation and of regaining self control.

In general the aim is to satisfy the cravings of the patient for musical experience and to change the emphasis of the patient's attention to his own disabilities. Musical activity can be participated in by large groups and affords a high degree of personal satisfaction. It is contagious in its spirit and draws the timid person into its numerical anonymity as readily as it encourages others into enthusiastic expression.

The vivid or the subtle protrayal of mood and the revitalizing rhythmic dynamics of music combine to relieve the monotony of disease, dysfunction and depression. Many of the hospitals for patients with mental disease employ directors of music to organize orchestras, glee clubs and other ensemble groups. Often the most disturbed patients are included as orchestra members, playing for dances, dramatic performances and other public functions.

Those aerial vibrations known as music, arranged in certain sequences and produced in certain ways and combinations do something of great importance to the human listener.

Animals other than human do not make music. Birds are said to sing and grouse to drum—but that is not music. Points specially emphasized are the humanity and dignity of music; its tremendous potency; its complexity and variety, from the simple to the sublimely broad and majestic; its unifying effect on listener and performer.

Few will disagree with the author[5] that the world has great need of a feeling for human dignity and

---
3. Howard Hanson, Mus. Doc., Rochester, N. Y., in *Amer Jl. Psychiatry*, Nov., 1942.
4. A. F. Fultz, Brookline, Mass., in *War. Med.*, Mar.
5. J. A. Kindwall, Milwaukee, in *Milwaukee Med. Times*, Sept.

beauty, and that music is one of the purest expressions of what is characteristically human. "The need for emphasis on human dignity is especially great now, when those human inventions—justice and mercy—are temporarily in eclipse. The human element in the present struggle between what is human and what is antihuman, has taken as its symbol the opening notes of a noble Beethoven symphony, notes which it happens, express in their rhythm the telegraphic form of the letter V—for Victory. A more fortunate coincidence could hardly be imagined. Beethoven stands among the giants of the human spirit."

The emphasis now placed on the fact that we are all animals draws the comment we *are* animals, but a great deal more, and it behooves us not to play the moral pauper when we are in truth the princely inheritors of spiritual riches, with a brain which has certain capacities entirely lacking in the lower animals. One of these, perhaps the greatest, is the faculty of imagination—of feeling, or seeing, or hearing something which does not exist.

This doctor-musician goes on to clarify his subject:

Music is one of the purest and finest expressions of the human brain, also one of the most potent influences upon that brain. One of the striking examples is the effect of stirring music upon tired marching men; another is the enticing stimulus one feels from a highly rhythmic dance tune. Certain rhythmic music can also be soothing, sedative; Ravel's "Bolero" was found to have this effect on overly tense, restless patients. The simple, persistent rhythm caught and held their attention, and the increasing and decreasing volume carried them along toward a resting state.

Ancient drawings show musicians playing while workmen are laboring. Heaving up the anchor with the capstan was a heavy job; so was a pull on the halyard or clew-line; and the strength and speed of the seamen were mobilized by the chanty. In a 60-day bicycle race the average speed during the period when music was played was 19.6 miles per hour, while without music the speed was 17.9.

The effect of music on moods can be tremendous. Music is a potent drug in widespread use by many who enjoy it but who do not understand its power. It is doubtful that music, even when poor, inappropriate and excessive, can ever have such bad effects as the improper use of alcohol; but loud, broken rhythms—a certain style of jazz—can have a very unhealthy effect upon the human nervous system.

Rhythm is a basic, constant element in all music, and of all musical elements it seems to have the simplest, most direct appeal. Rhythm may be said to attract and to mobilize the attention. If the attention can be caught and held a change may be produced in the focus of one's mental processes. If this focus has been an unhealthy one, as in a disturbance of mood or in a morbid preoccupation, a shift of the attention can be in the direction of health. This has been found to be the case even in such serious disturbances as those occurring in hospitals for nervous diseases. When a man's mind is disturbed and inaccessible to words and ideas, a short-cut to his attention can be a great help. A more advanced element in music is *melody*—an orderly succession of differences in pitch. If a man is sad, sad music fits his mood as a key does a lock. Having captured his attention, one may gradually shift his mood to a brighter one. Suiting the music to the mood is essentially tact and courtesy, musically expressed.

Still higher in point of development is *harmony*, the simultaneous sounding of several tones and the response to a highly conditioned state both for the group and for the individual. All of these harmonic styles have subtle and powerful effects on those sensitive to them. They are rooted in tradition, or in the revolt against tradition and cannot be ignored as factors in the relation of music to health.

Music may be only a noise to some persons, or to those in certain moods. Addiction can be established to potent drugs which are destructively stimulating. Certain types of music may be considered a drug of this character, the violence of the dose being constantly stepped up as a jaded and irritable nervous system calls out for more and more. A tune normally gay, may, if it was at some time heard under distressing circumstances, give rise to unhappy feelings and considerable tension and discomfort.

Participating in performing music in a group group offers an inspiring opportunity to be a part of a coöperative enterprise, something greater than the individual. Thus diverse moods and temperaments are welded together for one common purpose. Music can "send you out of this world," either in the direction of a screaming, shuddering, jungle world of feverish excitement; or into a higher world of strength, repose and perspective. All this is sorely needed in the world of today. We need to feel, to encourage, and to direct:

"*The desire of the moth for the star, of the night for the morrow,*
The devotion to something afar from the sphere of our sorrow."

"Music is the most potent influence we have to accomplish this purpose. Let us hope that, both in civilian life and in the life of the armed forces, it may be used powerfully and effectively, and not haphazardly or ignorantly. Music is strong medicine. If by health is meant the highest possible functioning of all one's powers, then music is an important element in human health; for it is a peculiarly human phenomenon, and is capable of expressing the most sublime feelings and also of profoundly affecting the mood and thought of us all. Like humor, music removes the sting from the slings and arrows of outrageous fortune, and helps to make brothers of us all."

* * * * *

DOCTOR JAMES H. McINTOSH

DR. JAMES HIGGINS MCINTOSH, widely beloved citzen and highly skilled physician and surgeon in Columbia the last 44 years, died at his home, 1501 Lady street, at 1:15 o'clock yesterday afternoon. He had been ill the last three months and on next October 3rd would have celebrated his 78th anniversary.

Thus *The State* (of Sept. 3d) begins a tribute to our departed friend and brother.

Born at Newberry, S. C., in 1866, the son of a Confederate surgeon whose name he bore, Dr. McIntosh was educated at Newberry Academy, Johns Hopkins and Columbia. He remained in New York City two years, on the staff at Bellevue Hospital. He then returned to Newberry where he practiced until 1900.

In Columbia Dr. McIntosh quickly took a place of leadership in the medical and civic life of his state's capital city. In World War I he gave unstinted service to draft board duties. From 1903 to 1937 he was state referee for the Mutual Life Insurance Company of New York. For a number of years he was chief-of-staff at the Baptist Hospital.

Many honors came to him in organizations of his profession. He had served as president of the Columbia Medical Society, the Seventh District Medical Association, the South Carolina Medical Association and the Tri-State Medical Association of the Carolinas and Virginia. He was a member of the Beta Theta Pi Fraternity at Johns Hopkins.

Two years ago the Columbia Medical Society presented him with a handsome silver service bearing the inscription:

"In appreciation of the long life spent unselfishly in the service of humanity and as an expression of our friendship and esteem, this token is presented to Dr. James H. McIntosh by his medical colleagues of Columbia, May 20, 1942."

Another token of the high esteem in which he was held generally was the gift by his patients of a fine portrait of Dr. McIntosh, which portrait hangs in the lobby of the Columbia Hospital.

Dr. McIntosh was one of the organizers of the Tri-State Medical Association, and was ever one of its most loyal and energetic supporters. Up until the last two or three years he attended every meeting and took an active part in the proceedings.

We have missed him much; we shall miss him more.

NEWS

NORTH CAROLINA EYE, EAR, NOSE AND THROAT SOCIETY

The annual meeting, held at Greensboro, Sept. 27th and 28th, was addressed by Dr. Grady Clay, of Emory University, Atlanta; Dr. Ralph Ellis, of Greensboro; Dr. Kenneth L. Pickrell, of Duke University; Dr. J. A. Harrell, of Winston-Salem; and Dr. V. K. Hart, of Charlotte.

In a report to the afternoon session on the current infantile paralysis epidemic in the state, Dr. Hart said that at the Hickory Poliomyelitis Hospital, 39 out of 200 cases analyzed were of the bulbar type. Two of the patients at Hickory had undergone tonsil operations within 12 days before contracting polio and one had had a tooth extracted four days before.

Although these figures do not warrant stopping all tonsil and adenoid operations during the summer months, Dr. Hart said he recommended that doctors consider that in epidemics or in times of high incidence of polio cases, such operations might add "grave hazards" in lowering the resistance of a child.

Dr. M. E. Bizzell, Goldsboro, was chosen president; Dr. H. C. Neblett, Charlotte, vice-president, and Dr. A. J. Ellington, Burlington, was re-elected secretary-treasurer.

SOUTHSIDE AND FOURTH DISTRICT MEDICAL ASSOCIATION, September 26th, Petersburg, Virginia.

Program

1. Report of Cases: Dr. A. A. Burke, Norfolk, Va.
2. Endocrine Disorders: Dr. Joseph D. Hough, Franklin Va.
3. Surgical Exploration of the Hilum as a Means of Preserving the Function of Inadequate Ovaries: Dr Phillip Jacobson, Petersburg, Va.
4. Some Points in the Differential Diagnosis of Rheumatic and Syphilitic Heart Disease: Dr. Paul D Camp, Richmond, Va.
5. Factors Favoring the Formation of Edema and Its Management: Dr. Douglas G. Chapman, Richmond. Va.
6. Dinner.
7. Brief Business Session.

INSTITUTE OF ALCOHOLISM

On September 14th a meeting was held at Baltimore at which were discussed:

The Effects of Alcohol on the Individual
New Approaches to Understanding the Alcoholic
Alcoholism and Crime
The Problem of the Alcoholic as seen by the Social Worker
The Church and the Alcoholic
The Problem of the Alcoholic as seen by the Probation Department
Alcoholics are Sick People
Alcoholism as Viewed by the U. S. Public Health Service
Alcoholism and Public Health.

This Journal is promised a copy of the Proceedings as soon as they are available.

A Federal grant of $89,000 has been made to aid in the construction of a three-story and basement addition to the RIVERSIDE HOSPITAL at Newport News, Va. The project will be completed at an estimated cost of $180,000. The proposed addition will be a fireproof structure containing living quarters and class-room facilities for 36 student nurses and space for 16 beds which will be used for Negro patients.

DR. K. M. LYNCH—DR. W. R. WALLACE
(Recorder Richland County Med. Soc., October)

At the last meeting of the South Carolina State Board of Health, the chairman, Dr. K. M. Lynch, tendered his resignation from the chairmanship due to his many duties as Professor of Pathology and as Dean of the Medical College.

Dr. W. R. Wallace, President of the South Carolina Medical Association, was elevated to the chairmanship of the Board from the vice-chairmanship and thus brings considerable experience to the office. The South Carolina medical profession should view the future with confidence in these uncertain times with such tried and true men in control of medical affairs in this all-powerful Board of Health.

DR. FRED J. WAMPLER has resigned as Professor of Preventive and Industrial Medicine at the Medical College of Virginia, to take a position as head of the medical department of a large industry in another state. He is an authority on industrial medicine, the author of a textbook on the subject.

He came with the Medical College in 1928, but spent the years of 1930 and 1931 in India and Burma in mission and government hospitals studying public health. He was also for some time in Japan. Dr. Wampler was a medical missionary in China from 1915 to 1926.

DR. WILBURT C. DAVISON, Dean of Duke University's Medical School, heads a group of U. S. medical educators who will give a series of four-week postgraduate medical courses in Dutch universities after Holland's liberation.

Because of German looting of Dutch equipment during four years, the teachers will take with them all material and instruments needed for laboratory and demonstration purposes.

DR. EDWIN LAWRENCE KENDIG, JR., announces the location of his office at 828 West Franklin Street, Richmond 20, Virginia. Practice limited to diseases of infants and children with special interest in diseases of the chest.

DR. WILLIAM P. RICHARDSON has resigned as of September 1st from his position as Orange-Person-Chatham District Health Officer, a position he had held since January, 1936, to go with the State Board of Health as Director of District I, Division of Local Administration, vice Dr. J. C. Knox, who resigned to go into private practice at Wilmington.

MARRIED

Dr. William G. Leary, Jr., of Alexandria, Virginia, and Miss Margaret Conley, of Cincinnati, were married on September 21st.

Dr. Gale Denning Johnson, of Dunn, North Carolina, and Miss Mildred Mariah May, of Roanoke Rapids, were married on September 18th.

Dr. Carroll Thomas Iden II, Lieutenant (jg) USNR, and Miss Mabel Oglesby Tench, of Pulaski, Virginia, were married on September 26th.

Dr. James Given Snead and Miss Frances Maxwell Neal, both of Charlottesville, were married on September 14th. Dr. Snead is serving an internship in the Harper Hospital, Detroit.

Dr. E. J. Pope and Miss Jessie Ellis, of Waverly, Virginia, were married on September 23rd.

Dr. Thomas B. Daniel, of Oxford, North Carolina, and Miss Bette Mazgelis, of Worcester, Massachusetts, were married on September 13th.

Dr. Alexander Webb, Jr., and Miss Mary Louise Hall, both of Raleigh, were married on September 9th.

Dr. Leonard Edward Meisels, of Brooklyn, and Miss Muryal Groh, of Gloucester, Virginia, were married on September 3rd. They will live in Baltimore.

Dr. Geoffrey H. Binneveld and Miss Ellen May Whitt were married at Charlottesville on September 15th. Dr. Binneveld will serve his internship at the Post Graduate Hospital in New York.

Miss Ruth Anne Reed and Dr. Randolph Chitwood, son of Dr. and Mrs. E. M. Whitwood, of Wytheville, Virginia, were married September 18th in the University Chapel, Charlottesville. Dr. Chitwood had as his best man his father, Dr. E. M. Chitwood. The ushers were Dr. Ned Wysor, of Clifton Forge; Dr. Darius Flicham, of Willis, and E. M. Chitwood, Jr., of Wytheville. After October 1st Dr. and Mrs. Chitwood will be at home in Charlottesville, where Dr. Chitwood will have an internship at the University Hospital.

Dr. John Davis Lindner, of Ocala, Florida, and Miss Billie Wyatt Morris, of Roanoke, Virginia, were married on September 24th.

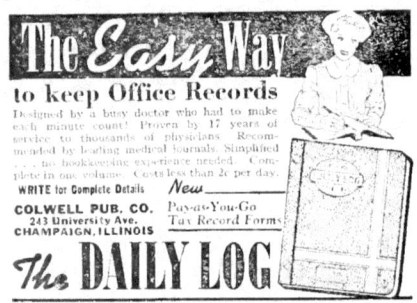

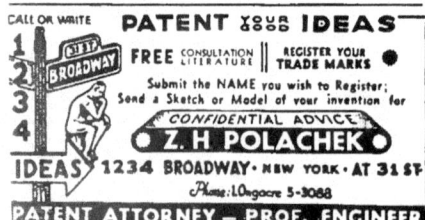

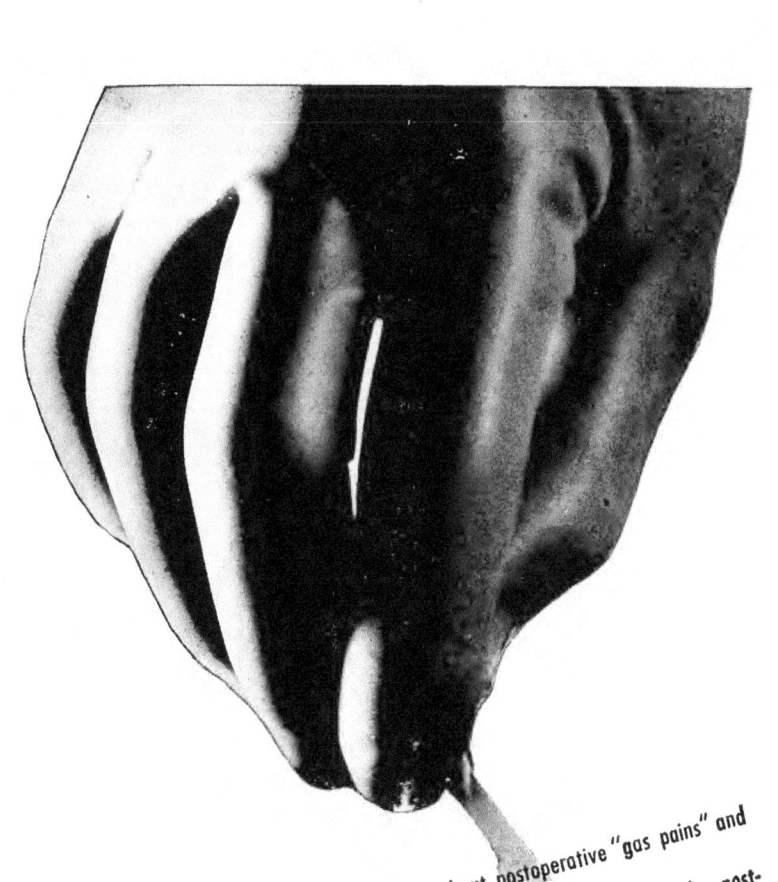

SKILLFUL SURGERY—BUT—how about postoperative "gas pains" and catheterization? Even the most skillful surgery can be followed by the postoperative complications of abdominal distention and urinary retention. The routine use of Prostigmin Methylsulfate* 1:4000, however, provides a convenient and effective means of preventing these distressing and painful disorders, affording the patient a faster, more pleasant recovery ... HOFFMANN-LA ROCHE, INC., NUTLEY 10, N. J.

*Neostigmine Methylsulfate.

Prostigmin Methylsulfate 'Roche'

Dr. Edgar Winslow Lane, Jr., of Bloomsbury, New Jersey, and Miss Gardner Garrou, of Valdese, North Carolina, were married on September 27th.

Dr. Thomas S. Royster, of Henderson, North Carolina, and Miss Caroline Merck Henry, of Philadelphia, were married on September 23rd.

DIED

Dr. Michael Hoke, 70, retired orthopedic surgeon, died Sept. 23rd at the Beaufort (S. C.) Hospital where he had been a patient for several days.

He was the son of Gen. Robert Frederick Hoke, of Lincolnton, N. C. He attended private schools in Raleigh, where he was born and reared. He continued his education at the University of North Carolina, the medical school of the University of Virginia and Johns Hopkins. Later he studied orthopedic surgery in Boston.

Dr. Hoke spent most of his years of practice in Atlanta, where he made a national reputation in his specialty of orthopedic surgery. He went from there to Warm Springs, Ga., where he was chief surgeon of the infantile paralysis foundation. After four years in that post, he retired because of ill health and removed to Beaufort to live in 1937.

Dr. Archibald Alexander McFadyen, 67, for 36 years a Presbyterian medical missionary in China, died suddenly Sept. 23rd from a heart attack at his home at Morganton, N. C.

Dr. McFadyen, who had long suffered from a heart ailment, had worked as usual the day before his death, at the State Hospital, where he had been serving as member of the medical staff for the past two years.

Dr. Walter Hughson, 53, a national authority on deafness, died Sept. 13th in Abington (Pa.) Memorial Hospital six hours after he was discovered—dazed, drenched and his coat and one shoe missing—in a pit at a tree nursery three miles from the hospital from which he disappeared the night of the 11th. Hospital authorities attributed the death to spinal meningitis, but declined to speculate whether he had contracted the illness while lying exposed for hours in a heavy rainstorm or whether it was the cause of his disappearance.

Dr. Hughson was a son of the late Dr. and Mrs. Walter Hughson, who founded Grace Hospital, Morganton, N. C., while his father was rector of Grace Episcopal Church. He resided there as a boy.

Formerly associate professor of otology at Johns Hopkins Medical School, he went to the Abington Hospital in 1935. He was an instructor in otology at the University of Pennsylvania Medical School and a consultant in the Bureau of Child Hygiene of the U. S. Public Health Service. Recently he had been engaged in important studies connected with work on aural casualties at the Philadelphia Naval Hospital.

Dr. Minor Carson Lile, 55, died at his home at Seattle, Wash., on Sunday, September 3rd. Dr. Lile was born at Lynchburg and was brought up at the University of Virginia, where his father was Dean of the Law School. He was graduated from the University of Virginia in both the college and the medical department, served as captain in the Medical Corps of the Army in World War I, as a member of the University of Virginia Base Hospital 41. After the war, he moved to Seattle, where he was a member of the staff of the Virginia Mason Clinic as orthopedic surgeon.

BIPEPSONATE

Calcium Phenolsulphonate	2 grains
Sodium Phenolsulphonate	2 grains
Zinc Phenolsulphonate, N. F.	1 grain
Salol, U. S. P.	2 grains
Bismuth Subsalicylate, U. S. P.	8 grains
Pepsin U. S. P.	4 grains

Average Dosage

For Children—Half drachm every fifteen minutes for six doses, then every hour until relieved.
For Adults—Double the above dose.

How Supplied

In Pints, Five-Pints and Gallons to Physicians and Druggists only.

Burwell & Dunn Company

Manufacturing *Pharmacists*
Established in 1887

CHARLOTTE, N. C.

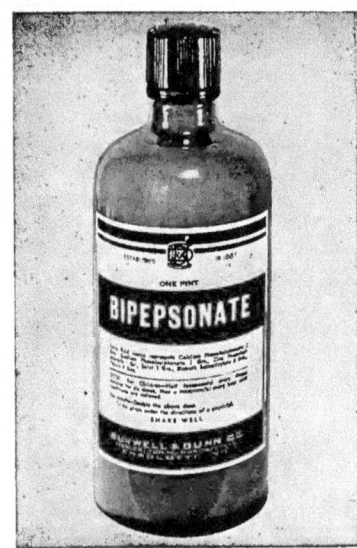

Sample sent to any physician in the U. S. on request

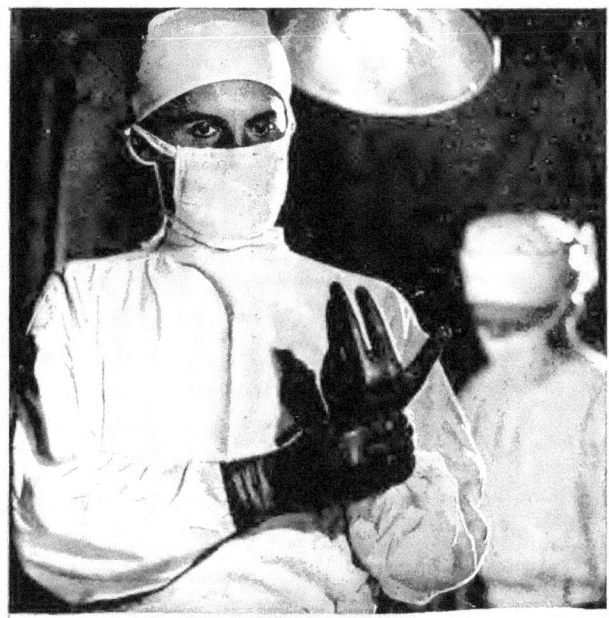

HEROES.. Behind Masks

Bombs screaming down...shells crashing...the crazy chatter of strafing planes' machine guns...they're the "background music" of the drama that's played on every fighting front every day by the surgeons of the field clearing-stations.

"Soldiers in white"...heroes—behind masks.

Naturally we are proud that their choice of a cigarette—in those moments when there's a brief respite for a heartening smoke—is likely to be Camel. The milder, rich, full-flavored brand favored in the Armed Forces all over the world.

Camel is truly "the soldier's cigarette"!

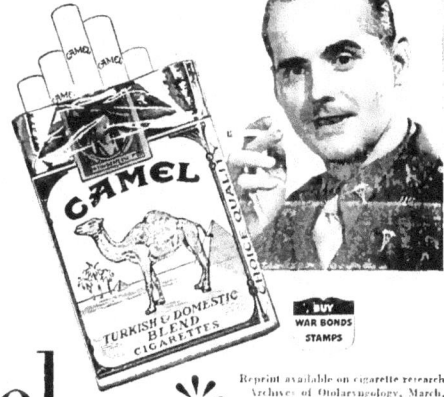

COSTLIER TOBACCOS — Camel

Reprint available on cigarette research Archives of Otolaryngology, March, 1943, pp. 404-410. Camel Cigarettes, Medical Relations Division, One Pershing Square, New York 17, N. Y.

BUY WAR BONDS STAMPS

Dr. Bedford E. Love, 71, Roxboro, N. C., died June 15th of a cerebral hemorrhage. Dr. Love was a graduate of the University of Maryland School of Medicine, 1904, an honorary member of this Association and of the Medical Society of the State of North Carolina, a past president of the Person County Medical Society and physician for the Norfolk and Western Railway. He also served as State Highway and Public Works physician and County physician.

Dr. James Reginald Bailey died at his home at Keysville, Virginia, September 15th. Dr. Bailey was only 43 years of age and was graduated by the Medical College of Virginia in 1926.

DERMATITIS FROM CARROTS
(S. M. Peck et al., in *Arch. Derma. & Syph.*, 49:266, 1944, via *Jl. Mo. Med. Assn.*, Aug.)

The dermatitis occurred in women who were engaged in trimming carrots by hand, working along-side a conveyor belt carrying the carrots and resting their arms on a metal shelf wet with juice coming from cut carrots.

It was determined that carrots contain a skin-sensitizing principle which is found in the raw carrot, in the dried carrot residue, in the carrot juice and in the heated carrot (240° F., 2½ hours).

Since it requires daily contact for seven or more days for carrots to induce dermatitis in the susceptible person, it will not be a frequent factor in the dermatitis of the hands, forearms and face in food handlers.

One has seen isolated cases of occupational eczema due to contact with string beans, parsnips, asparagus, strawberries, uncooked beef, wheat flour and carrots.

HUMAN DANDER AS A CAUSE OF ECZEMA
(F. A. Simon, Louisville, Ky., in *Jl. A. M. A.*, June 3rd)

Evidence demonstrating the etiologic significance of human dander in the genesis of infantile eczema consists of: 1) Positive skin reactions to patch test with human dander in 15 of 20 infants and young children with eczema, whereas in 23 noneczematous infants and young children there was only one positive reaction to the patch test. 2) The fact that all children are exposed to human dander, either from their own scalps or from those of parents and others with whom they come in contact. 3) The prompt clinical improvement in three of four cases following the institution of measures directed at the avoidance of contact with human dander. 4) The reproduction of the lesions at will in four cases (out of four attempts) on a previously uninvolved skin area by exposure of this area to contact with human dander.

COLLODION FOR CHIGGER BITES

A good coating of collodion forms a thin film over the affected area which cuts off the supply of air and causes the death of the parasite. At the same time it prevents clothing and other articles from touching the lesion and this decreases itching. Scratching causes the itching to begin again.

HOME CANNING MAY KILL.—The necessity for *thoroughly* sterilizing all food, and *containers*, is shown by two deaths from eating of beets, twice boiled, but put in cans which had been only "washed." Prolonged boiling is required to kill botulinus spores.

WILLIAM WITHERING reintroduced digitalis into medicine in 1785. It had been known to physicians for perhaps 500 years prior to that time.—*Nelson*.

BOOKS

A TEXTBOOK OF PATHOLOGY, by ROBERT ALLAN MOORE, Edward Mallinckrodt Professor of Pathology, Washington University School of Medicine, St. Louis, Mo. 1338 pages with 513 illustrations, 34 in colors. *W. B. Saunders Company*, Philadelphia and London, 1944. $10.00.

The arrangement of this book is as attractive as it is unique. The approach by disturbances of metabolism rather than by anatomic type of degeneration is a natural and useful departure from the rule, giving more emphasis to the physiologic and chemical aspects of pathology. The same is to be said of grouping diseases by similarity of cause.

The author expresses confidence that preventive medicine will play a more important part in the future of medical science and gives this as a reason for arranging bacterial diseases by the portal through which the bacterium enters the body, and by the source of the bacteria.

His notes on the history of pathology, while giving the usual credit to the Austrians and Germans for their tremendous contributions in this field, point out that they built on a solid foundation of French and English construction, physicians of these nationalities having brought pathology from the realm of speculation to that of objective observation of diseased tissue.

The illustrations strike the eye as quite different from those to be found in the common run of textbooks of pathology. On closer scrutiny it is seen that they are conceived and executed on a different plan. In addition to the usual gross and microscopic photographs there are radiographs, photographs of patients, pictures of great medical men of the past, photographs illustrating paleopathology, and maps showing disease distribution.

It used to be said that one of the very best books on pathology was Osler's "Practice of Medicine." Here we have a textbook of pathology which is one of the best treatises on clinical medicine and surgery.

SIMPLIFIED DIABETIC MANAGEMENT, by JOSEPH T. BEARDWOOD, JR., A.B., M.D., F.A.C.P., Associate Professor of Medicine, and HERBERT T. KELLY, M.D., F.A.C.P., Associate in Medicine, Graduate School of Medicine, University of Pennsylvania. Fourth edition. *J. B. Lippincott Company*, E. Washington Square, Philadelphia 5, Penn. 1944. $1.50.

The methods here outlined will be found helpful in clinic and private practice. The presentation is suitable for physician, nurse, dietitian and the intelligent patient.

OPERATIONS OF GENERAL SURGERY, by THOMAS G. ORR, M.D., Professor of Surgery, University of Kansas School of Medicine, Kansas City, Kansas. 723 pages with 1396 step-by-step illustrations on 570 figures. *W. B. Saunders Company*, Philadelphia & London. 1944. $10.00.

The author is convinced of the need for a book which sets forth the essentials of technic in the field of general surgery. He recognizes that general surgeons are frequently called on to perform operations ordinarily done by one in some surgical specialty, so the technics of many such operations are described. Each operation is described step-by-step.

The indications for operations are summarized. In many instances dangers are pointed out and safeguards described.

The illustrations are superb.

The author is no faddist. In general, as to different methods of performing important operations, each of them the choices of good surgeons, the author is of the opinion that one technic is best at the hands of one surgeon, another at the hands of the other.

For the general surgeon only a short time out on his own, this book will prove a great comfort and aid; and those older in the guild who undertake to keep right in the van will find themselves amply repaid for its study.

MANUAL OF MILITARY NEUROPSYCHIATRY, edited by HARRY C. SOLOMON, M.D., Professor of Psychiatry, Harvard Medical School; and PAUL I. YAKOVLEV, M.D., Instructor in Neurology at the Harvard Medical School. With the Collaboration of 11 Doctors. 764 pages with 15 illustrations. *W. B. Saunders Company*, Philadelphia and London. 1944. $6.00.

This Manual is intended as a reference text of clinical neurology and psychiatry. The neuropsychiatric experiences of the first World War are reviewed, and this review is followed immediately by a description of the organization of this branch of the medical service in the army during the current war.

Induction, administration and disposition details are described. Then we have a section devoted to the different entities in this field—all the way from psychoneuroses to post-traumatic syndromes. It is gratifying to find some hundred-and-fifty pages devoted to preventive and curative therapy.

Among the special topics considered are: Neuropsychiatric Disorders in the Tropics; Physiology of Flying, Hazards and Remedies; Neuropsychiatric Aspects and Treatments of Convoy and Torpedo Casualties; and Electro-Encephalography, Diagnosis Evaluation.

There is hardly a physician among us who will not have to do intimately with neuropsychiatric problems of the discharged soldier. Here is authoritative information on which to proceed.

ELIMINATION DIETS AND THE PATIENT'S ALLERGIES: A Handbook of Allergy, by ALBERT H. ROWE, M.D., Lecturer in Medicine, University of California Medical School, San Francisco, California; Consultant in Allergic Diseases, Alameda County Hospital, Oakland, California. Second edition, thoroughly revised. Octavo, 256 pages. *Lea & Febiger*, Philadelphia 6. 1944. Cloth, $3.50.

The new edition of this valuable work aims to stress the importance of foods in the production of allergic manifestations and the value of elimination diets for the determination of this condition. It discusses the other causes of clinical allergy and the latest methods for their diagnosis and control. The many revisions and additions have required resetting. To make room for this new material, without increasing the number of pages, the type page has been enlarged. The restricted range of usefulness of the skin test and the failure to use trial diet as a routine procedure are given as the chief reasons for the frequent failure to diagnose and control clinical food allergy. The cereal-free elimination diet is used most often because of the frequency of group sensitizations to cereal grains. The indications for the use of the important fruit-free elimination diets are discussed for the first time. A special elimination diet for the control of colitis is presented. Various supplemental diets are advised for the study of unusual types of food allergy—diets to be eaten away from home, diets for obese and diabetic patients and for infants and children. Such menus and recipes have been thoroughly revised, especially because of the war restriction of foods.

The author stresses the frequency of each type of allergy in the production of clinical manifestations, especially of bronchial and nasal allergy and of atopic dermatitis. Cutaneous, gastro-intestinal, neurological, joint, urological and ocular symptoms due to allergy—each receives due attention. This emphasis on the susceptibility of the tissues of the body to allergic reactions indicates the value of this work to all physicians as well as to allergists.

CHUCKLES

A lady on the Madison Avenue bus took the only empty seat—next to a harmless-looking little drunk—and opened a map. It was, a friend of ours discovered by craning his neck a bit, a detailed map of Manchuria. The drunk studied the map for a time, too, and finally addressed the lady in diffident tones. "Sure you're on the right bus?" he asked.—*The New Yorker*.

Selectee: "They can't make me fight."
Draft Board Chairman: "Maybe not, but they can take you where the fighting is, and you can use your own judgment."

BEN TABON, DEAN OF ORDERLIES
(Chapel Hill Weekly)

One of the elder lights of the Durham bar had a period of prostration in Ben's hospital. He was served by Ben as orderly through the whole period. When he had recovered and was leaving the place he was so grateful to Ben for his skilful services that he was impelled to leave with him a substantial reward along with his thanks. The gift was well-earned; but Ben hadn't been working with a view to tips. Therefore he must pay a compliment in turn. So he said: "Thanks, Mr. Will, and I would like to say that you sho' does take a good enema."

NEUROLOGY and PSYCHIATRY

(*Now in the Country's Service*)
*J. FRED MERRITT, M.D.
NERVOUS and MILD MENTAL DISEASES
ALCOHOL and DRUG ADDICTIONS
Glenwood Park Sanitarium   Greensboro

TOM A. WILLIAMS, M.D.
(*Neurologist of Washington, D. C.*)
Consultation by appointment at
Phone 3994-W
77 Kenilworth Ave.   Asheville, N. C.

EYE, EAR, NOSE AND THROAT

H. C. NEBLETT, M.D.
OCULIST
Phone 3-5852
Professional Bldg.   Charlotte

AMZI J. ELLINGTON, M.D.
DISEASES of the
EYE, EAR, NOSE and THROAT
Phones: Office 992—Residence 761
Burlington   North Carolina

UROLOGY, DERMATOLOGY and PROCTOLOGY

THE CROWELL CLINIC of UROLOGY and UROLOGICAL SURGERY
Hours—Nine to Five   Telephones—3-7101—3-7102
STAFF
ANDREW J. CROWELL, M.D.
(1911-1938)
*ANGUS M. McDONALD, M.D.   CLAUDE B. SQUIRES, M.D.
Suite 700-711 Professional Building   Charlotte

RAYMOND THOMPSON, M.D., F.A.C.S.   WALTER E. DANIEL, A.B., M.D.
THE THOMPSON-DANIEL CLINIC
of
UROLOGY & UROLOGICAL SURGERY
Fifth Floor Professional Bldg.   Charlotte

C. C. MASSEY, M.D.
PRACTICE LIMITED
TO
DISEASES OF THE RECTUM
Professional Bldg.   Charlotte

WYETT F. SIMPSON, M.D.
GENITO-URINARY DISEASES
Phone 1234
Hot Springs National Park   Arkansas

ORTHOPEDICS

HERBERT F. MUNT, M.D.
ACCIDENT SURGERY & ORTHOPEDICS
FRACTURES
Nissen Building   Winston-Salem

GENERAL

Nalle Clinic Building 412 North Church Street, Charlotte
THE NALLE CLINIC
Telephone—C-BVDV (*if no answer, call* 3-2621)

General Surgery

BRODIE C. NALLE, M.D.
GYNECOLOGY & OBSTETRICS

EDWARD R. HIPP, M.D.
TRAUMATIC SURGERY

*PRESTON NOWLIN, M.D.
UROLOGY

Consulting Staff

R. H. LAFFERTY, M.D.
O. D. BAXTER, M.D.
RADIOLOGY

W. M. SUMMERVILLE, M.D.
PATHOLOGY

General Medicine

LUCIUS G. GAGE, M.D.
DIAGNOSIS

LUTHER W. KELLY, M.D.
CARDIO-RESPIRATORY DISEASES

J. R. ADAMS, M.D.
DISEASES OF INFANTS & CHILDREN

W. B. MAYER, M.D.
DERMATOLOGY & SYPHILOLOGY

(*In Country's Service)

C—H—M MEDICAL OFFICES
DIAGNOSIS—SURGERY
X-RAY—RADIUM

DR. G. CARLYLE COOKE—*Abdominal Surgery & Gynecology*
DR. GEO. W. HOLMES—*Orthopedics*
DR. C. H. MCCANTS—*General Surgery*
222-226 Nissen Bldg.   Winston-Salem

WADE CLINIC
Wade Building
Hot Springs National Park, Arkansas

H. KING WADE, M.D.	*Urology*
ERNEST M. MCKENZIE, M.D.	*Medicine*
*FRANK M. ADAMS, M.D.	*Medicine*
*JACK ELLIS, M.D.	*Medicine*
BESSEY H. SHEBESTA, M.D.	*Medicine*
*WM. C. HAYS, M.D.	*Medicine*
N. B. BURCH, M.D.	
	Eye, Ear, Nose and Throat
A. W. SCHEER	*X-ray Technician*
ETTA WADE	*Clinical Laboratory*
MERNA SPRING	*Clinical Pathology*

(*In Military Service)

INTERNAL MEDICINE

ARCHIE A. BARRON, M.D., F.A.C.P.

INTERNAL MEDICINE—NEUROLOGY

Professional Bldg.   Charlotte

JOHN DONNELLY, M.D.

DISEASES OF THE LUNGS

Medical Building   Charlotte

CLYDE M. GILMORE, A.B., M.D.

CARDIOLOGY—INTERNAL MEDICINE

Dixie Building   Greensboro

JAMES M. NORTHINGTON, M.D.

INTERNAL MEDICINE—GERIATRICS

Medical Building   Charlotte

SURGERY

(Now in the Country's Service)
R. S. ANDERSON, M. D.

GENERAL SURGERY

144 Coast Line Street   Rocky Mount

R. B. DAVIS, M. D., M. M. S., F. A. C. P.
*GENERAL SURGERY
AND
RADIUM THERAPY*
Hours by Appointment

Piedmont-Memorial Hosp.   Greensboro

(Now in the Country's Service)
WILLIAM FRANCIS MARTIN, M D

GENERAL SURGERY

Professional Bldg.   Charlotte

OBSTETRICS & GYNECOLOGY

IVAN M. PROCTER, M. D.

OBSTETRICS & GYNECOLOGY

133 Fayetteville Street   Raleigh

SPECIAL NOTICES

TO THE BUSY DOCTOR WHO WANTS TO PASS HIS EXPERIENCE ON TO OTHERS

You have probably been postponing writing that original contribution. You can do it, and save your time and effort by employing an expert literary assistant to prepare the address, article or book under your direction or relieve you of the details of looking up references, translating, indexing, typing, and the complete preparation of your manuscript.

Address: *WRITING AIDE*, care *Southern Medicine & Surgery*.

THE JOURNAL OF
SOUTHERN MEDICINE AND SURGERY

306 North Tryon Street, Charlotte, N. C.

The Journal assumes no responsibility for the authenticity of opinion or statements made by authors or in communications submitted to this Journal for publication.

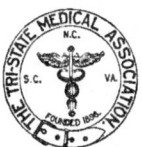

JAMES M. NORTHINGTON, M.D., Editor

Pudendal Block in Obstetrics*

M. Pierce Rucker, M.D., Richmond

OBSTETRICAL ANESTHESIA must be considered not only from the standpoint of both the mother and the baby, but also from the standpoint of hospital and home delivery. It goes without saying that a technic that is hazardous for either mother or baby is fit for neither hospital nor home delivery. There are, however, a number of anesthetics that are useful in the hospital which, for one reason or another, cannot be recommended for home use. Usually an anesthetist is not available for home deliveries. Rarely is more than one nurse to be had, and sometimes you are lucky to have one. Complicated apparatus cannot be carted about from home to home and a complicated technic requires more enthusiasm than the average man has for home deliveries. I wish to direct your attention today to a simple technic that can be used just as readily in the home as in the hospital. It carries practically no danger for either mother or baby, and it can be used either alone or in conjunction with any other analgesia or anesthesia. It is especially useful in poor risks where a general anesthetic is contraindicated.

Denys J. Neal Smith calls attention to a situation that must arise frequently in domiciliary obstetrics. The patient has been delivered without an anesthetic or under the self-administered anesthesia that seems to be so popular in England. She has a laceration of the perineum. To repair the laceration properly you need an anesthetic; which means that you must send for an anesthetist, and that takes time, even if one be available. Pudendal block meets such a situation completely. You can give it yourself and it does not predispose to postpartum bleeding.

The subject has been discussed before this society by W. Z. Bradford, who recommended it for major obstetric procedures. A second discussion seems to be in order because the technic has not had the general consideration that it merits. Recent reviews of obstetric anesthesia by Eastman and by Hellman make no mention of either local infiltration or perineal nerve block. On the other hand, Montgomery in a discussion of analgesia and anesthesia based on a study of the maternal deaths in Philadelphia says that local anesthesia should occupy a more extensive place in obstetrics.

My interest in the use of novocaine in obstetrics dates back several decades. In fact, my probation essay before the American Gynecological Society in 1925 bore that title. That paper dealt chiefly with vaginal delivery under sacral anesthesia, but included one so-called vaginal cesarean section under local infiltration. King in 1916 and Gellhorn in 1913 and 1927 called attention to the possibilities of pudendal nerve blocks and local infiltration of the perineum. King recommended that 1 or 1½ c.c. of 2 per cent solution of novocaine in 1:20,000 adrenalin solution be injected into the anterior triangle of the perineum above Colles' fascia on either side. He gave an excellent picture of the distribution of the perineal and pudendal nerves, but I was unable to get the results with this amount of novocaine that the author reported. Gellhorn's technic of injecting the nerves along the sides of

---
*Presented to Tri-State Medical Association of the Carolinas and Virginia, meeting at Charlotte, Feb. 28th-29th, 1944.

the uterus (Frankenhauser's ganglion) answered very well for curettage, but did not seem to be adapted to full-term deliveries. And so my efforts to make use of novocaine were diverted to the more complicated technics of sacral anesthesia, spinal anesthesia and epidural anesthesia.

There have been several changes in technic of local infiltration and perineal nerve block as I have used it. At first I simply infiltrated the perineum and especially the line of the episiotomy incision. When Walker's article appeared in 1936, I began to inject 10 c.c. of the procaine solution at the ischial spine on either side, in addition to infiltrating the perineum. When Bunim's paper on cervical dystocia appeared last year, I adopted the technic that he described, a technic that had been described previously by Urnes and Timmerman except that the guiding finger is not inserted in the rectum. It consists of injecting 20 c.c. of the solution just below the spine of the ischium, 10 c.c. just inside the tuberosity and 8 to 10 c.c. above the pubes and along the descending ramus. This can be done with a single puncture of the skin on either side. If the patient is not already partially anesthetized a wheal is raised in the skin with a fine needle at the point of injection. The apparatus needed is a hypodermic needle, a 20-gauge needle 10 cms. long, a 10 c.c. luer-lok syringe with ring handles, and an enamel cup that holds 100 c.c.

The only other change, and I think it an important one, is the solvent for the procaine. Stoeckel, a pioneer in sacral anesthesia, carried out a series of experiments to determine the most suitable drug and solution. The solution that gave him the best results was:

novocaine	0.45
suprarenin	0.000325
aqua destil.	3.0
normal salt solution	30.0

For local infiltration and nerve blocking the majority of writers have been content with a solution in either distilled water or sterile tap water, to which is added a few drops of adrenalin solution. DeTakats emphasizes the importance of using an isotonic solution. He says a solution of novocaine in distilled water or tap water hemolyses the red cells, ruptures the connective tissue and fat cells and produces tissue necrosis. Rosenfeld and Greenhill are among the few who mention the use of isotonic solutions.

Sterilization of novocaine presents somewhat of a problem. Boiling or autoclaving a solution of novocaine destroys to some extent its anesthetic properties. Greenhill recommends the use of ampules of concentrated solution. With these and sterile normal salt solution, the desired strength of novocaine-normal salt solution can be made up as needed. The adrenalin solution can then be added with a sterile medicine dropper. Bickers recommends using tablets which can be dropped into sterile normal salt solution with sterile forceps. I use solutions that are made up in the hospital and autoclaved. It is simpler and easier and I use it so constantly that the solution does not get a chance to get old. Some of the efficiency of the novocaine may be lost, but when you start with a 1-per cent solution there is enough margin of safety to more than make up for what deterioration the heat may cause. At first I used distilled water for the solvent. Not infrequently a hematoma would form at the site of injection. Since changing to normal salt solution, I have seen no hematomas.

ANALYSIS OF RESULTS

Since November, 1932, 1693 patients—1064 primiparae and 629 multiparae—have been treated by this method by various members of the staff at the Johnston-Willis Hospital and by me personally at other hospitals. Pudendal block was used either alone or in combination with other analgesics and anesthetics. Tables I and II show these various combinations. It was used without an anesthetic, or when spinal or caudal anesthesia failed, 218 times. Ether was used, along with various analgesics 852 times; sodium pentothal, 515 times; chloroform, 6 times; and ethylene, twice. When an anesthetic was used it was stopped when the head began to crown or the presenting part came into sight, and the rest of the delivery, the episiotomy and the repair were completed under the pudendal nerve block. The following is a list of the operations: Spontaneous delivery, 130; mid-forceps, 269; low-forceps, 1043; version and extraction, 139; breech delivery, 87; Willet forceps, 1; craniotomy, 1; delivery of placenta, 1; curettage, 24; repair of perineum, 2; vaginal salpingectomy, 3; vaginal hysterectomy, 2; Lefort colpocleisis, 1. The discrepancy between the number of patients and the number of operations is due to the fact that there were a number of cases of twins and one case of triplets in the series. The fetal results were as follows: 1639 live babies; 41 neonatal deaths and one baby who died after the two-weeks period of esophageal malformation; 10 non-macerated stillbirths and 6 macerated stillbirths—a total of 1697. In addition there were 18 abortions. The neonatal death rate was 2.47 per cent, and the stillbirth rate was .94 per cent. These results compare favorably with those of Minnitt, who recently reported 1025 labors conducted under self-administered nitrous-oxide-air anesthesia with a stillbirth rate of 1.8 per cent.

The maternal complications include: Febrile puerperium, 116 (including phlebitis, 7; mastitis, 28; cystitis, 9; pyelitis, 40; and cholecystitis, 4); eclampsia, 10; toxemia, 22; ablatio placentae, 7; placenta praevia, 19; detachment of retina, 2; inversion of uterus, 1; inertia, 10; shock, 2; prolapsed arm, 8; prolapsed cord, 5; constriction ring, 39; hour-glass contraction (postpartum), 1; postpartum hemorrhage, 11; and hydramnios, 8. Ten perineorrhaphies broke down. All occurred when I was using novocaine dissolved in distilled water.

There were two maternal deaths. The first was a 35-year-old gravida-VI who gave a history of edema in every pregnancy. She was sent into the hospital in the eighth month of pregnancy because of increasing albuminuria and a rising blood pressure, in spite of treatment at home by her doctor. There was jaundice, and she had marked edema of the sclerae, the abdominal striae, and the hands and feet. The blood pressure was 185/120; hgbn., 43%; red cells, 2,390,000. The urine boiled solid, and contained hyaline and granular casts. Fifteen to 20 red blood cells and 30 to 40 pus cells were found in each highpower field. The patient was semi-comatose. Labor was induced by rupturing the membranes. There was a latent period of 2 hours and 40 minutes, and a labor of 18 hours, terminated by low-forceps operation. The analgesia consisted of 12 grs. of sodium amytal, 1/100 gr. of hyoscine and perineal infiltration with ½-per cent novocaine. The baby cried at once. He weighed 7 lbs. 2¼ oz. and left the hospital in good condition. The mother never regained consciousness. The second maternal death followed symptoms of multiple emboli of the lungs as described by Steiner and Lushbaugh. The patient was an 18-year-old primipara. Labor was induced by rupturing the membranes at term. After a latent period of 5 hours and 12 minutes, and a labor of 17 hours and 39 minutes. The cervix was fully dilated and the head in ROP position. An easy version and extraction was done. The anesthetic agents consisted of sodium amytal grs. VI, hyoscine grs. 5/200, paraldehyde oz. II, rectal ether, sodium pentothal (625 mgm.) and local block. One c.c. of ergotrate was given intravenously and the placenta was delivered intact. It was followed by a little trickle of blood. The cervix was inspected and was intact. The bleeding was easily controlled by manual elevation of the fundus through the abdominal wall and the episiotomy was repaired. The patient regained consciousness during the operation. She was put to bed with a respiration of 60, pulse 200, blood pressure 90/60. The mother died two hours after delivery. A few minutes before she died there was a moderate vaginal hemorrhage.

It has been difficult to estimate the efficiency of pudendal block with any degree of accuracy. Abrams reports failure of the anesthesia in 4 per cent of of his cases and a one-sided failure in 9 per cent. Most of my patients were asleep with some form of analgesia or anesthesia when they came to the delivery room. No more anesthetic was given after the nerve blocking was done, but of course there is often enough hang-over to mask any failure of the local anesthesia. However, the great majority have had some form of perineal repair, and none has complained either of the delivery or of the repair. Twice I have infiltrated the tissues with novocaine to either side of the episiotomy before completing the repair because the patient flinched with each needle-prick. This relieved the situation completely.

SUMMARY

The technic of pudendal block is described and a series of 1693 cases is analyzed to show that pudendal block and/or perineal infiltration has a definite place in obstetrics. It can be used either alone or in conjunction with other analgesia and anesthesia. When used with other anesthesia, that anesthesia can be stopped before the birth of the baby so that the baby is spared most of the effect of a general anesthetic. When used alone pudendal block is adequate for pelvic operations, low and mid-forceps operations, breech extractions, episiotomies and perineal repairs. It is suitable for either hospital or home deliveries and it carries practically no risk to either mother or baby. A series of 1671 deliveries is reported with 2 maternal deaths and an uncorrected fetal mortality of 3.41 per cent. Theoretically an isotonic solution of novocaine should be used and clinical evidence is advanced to support this idea.

TABLE I
Analgesia and Anesthesia with Pudendal Block
Total Cases 1375

Sodium amytal, hyoscine, rectal ether—ether	255	
Sodium amytal, hyoscine—ether	514	
Sodium amytal, hyoscine, paraldehyde, rectal ether—ether	19	
Sodium amytal, hyoscine, paraldehyde—ether	18	
Rectal ether—ether	12	
Morphine—ether	10	
Paraldehyde, hyoscine—ether	1	
Morphine sodium amytal, paraldehyde—ether	1	
Ether	22	852
Sodium amytal, hyoscine, rectal ether—ethylene	1	
Ethylene	1	2
Sodium amytal, hyoscine, rectal ether—sodium pentothal	163	
Sodium amytal, hyoscine—sodium pentothal	297	
Sodium amytal, hyoscine, paraldehyde, rectal ether—sodium pentothal	21	
Sodium amytal, paraldehyde—sodium pentothal	5	
Morphine, hyoscine—sodium pentothal	9	
Sodium amytal, hyoscine—sodium pentothal	19	
Morphine, sodium amytal, paraldehyde—sodium pentothal	1	515
Paraldehyde, hyoscine—chloroform	2	
Paraldehyde—chloroform	1	
Chloroform	3	6

TABLE II
Analgesia with Pudendal Block

Total Cases	318
Morphine, hyoscine	17
Sodium amytal, hyoscine	109
Sodium amytal, hyoscine, rectal ether	3
Sodium amytal, avertin	1
Sodium amytal, caudal	10
Sodium amytal, paraldehyde	4
Sodium amytal, rectal ether	109
Rectal ether	10
Rectal ether, paraldehyde	1
Paraldehyde	28
Paraldehyde, spinal	1
Avertin	6
Caudal	6
Nothing	13
	318

Bibliography

ABRAMS, S. F.: *J. Missouri M. A.*, 35:81, 1938.
BECK, M. C.: *New Orleans M. & S. J.*, 95:278, 1942.
BANSSILLON, E., & BUCKER, P.: *Rev. franc. d. gynéc et d'obst.*, 31:858, 1936. Abst. *Year Book for Obst. & Gynec.*, 1937, p. 167.
BICKERS, W.: *Southern Med. J.*, 35:17, 1942.
BRADFORD, W. Z.: *South. Med. & Surg.*, 98:19, 1936.
BUNIM, L. A.: *Am. J. Obst. & Gynec.*, 45:805, 1943.
BULLAG, K.: *Munchen. med. Wchnschr.*, 62:256, 1915.
DE TAKATS, G.: *Bull. Am. Coll. Surgeons*, 17:40, 1933.
DITTER, F. J. A.: *Northwest. Med.*, 35:150, 1936.
EASTMAN: *Proc. Am. Cong. Obst. & Gynec.* (1939), 1:191, 1941.
FALLS, F. H.: *Mississippi Doctor*, 18:7, 1940.
GELLHORN, G.: *J. A. M. A.*, 61:1354, 1913; *Surg., Gynec. & Obst.*, 45:105, 1927; *Surg., Gynec. & Obst.*, 51:484, 1930.
GREENHILL, J. P.: *West. J. Surg.*, 50:579, 1942; *S. Clin. North America*, 23:143, 1943; *South. M. J.*, 26:37, 1933.
KING, R. W.: *Northwest. Med*, Apr., 1915.
GRIFFIN, E. L., & BENSON, R. C.: *Am. J. Obs. & Gynec.*, 42:862, 1941.
HELLMAN, L. M.: *International Clin.*, 3:300, 1940.
MINNITT, R. J.: *Proc. Roy. Soc. Med.*, 37:45, 1943.
MONTGOMERY, T. L.: *J. A. M. A.*, 108:1679, 1937.
O'CONNOR, C. T.: *New England J. Med.*, 210:758, 1934.
O'HEARN, E., & KNAUER, C. H.: *Am. J. Obst. & Gynec.*, 26:444, 1933.
PHILPOTT, N. W.: *Canad. M. A. J.*, 45:539, 1941.
ROSENFELD, S. S.: *Am. J. Surg.*, 58:207, 1942.
RUCKER, M. P.: *Am. J. Obst. & Gynec.*, 9:35, 1925.
SHELDON, C. P.: *New England J. Med.*, 224:404, 1941.
STOECKEL, W.: *Zentralbl. f. Gynäk.*, 33:1, 1909.
SMITH, D. J. N.: *J. Obst. & Gynaec. Brit. Emp.*, 48:610, 1941.
TORLAND, T.: *Northwest. Med.*, 29:312, 1930.
TRIP, H. D.: *J. Indiana M. A.*, 26:553, 1933.
URNES, M. P., & TIMMERMAN, H. J.: *J. A. M. A.*, 109:1616, 1937.
WALKER, A. T.: *Am. J. Obst. & Gynec.*, 32:60, 1936.

Discussion

DR. C. S. NANCE, Charlotte: I am sure every one of us has enjoyed Dr. Rucker's excellent paper. I had intended asking him some questions. I believe he has already answered most of them.

Two points on which I would like further information are: (1) at what stage he uses his pudendal block; and (2) whether or not pudendal block usually takes the place of a general anesthetic.

DR. RUCKER, closing: The pudendal block is given when you are ready to deliver the patient, or when she is ready to deliver herself. It can take the place of a general anesthetic. In influenza epidemics when there is respiratory infection or toxemia, you can manage the whole thing without a general anesthetic. Most of my patients like to be asleep when the baby is born. For that reason, I combine pentothal sodium or ether or rectal ether with the pudendal block. You can get along with very much less anesthesia with that sort of combination. I have delivered patients with nothing in the world but pudendal block, patients who are brought to the hospital in an ambulance, and they can be managed. They don't blame you for not having them asleep if they get to the hospital just at the time they are right for delivery.

THE ACUTELY CONGESTED EYE
(G. J. Epstein, New York, in *N. Y. Physician*, Oct.

Temporizing with an iritis or a glaucoma may result in irreparable damage to vision, and it would be ridiculous to rush every, even full-blown, conjunctivitis to the ophthalmologist. The patient with an acute keratitis or iritis demands relief from his suffering, and frequently shows his distress by blepharospasm. While lacrimation is not as consistently present as is discharge in conjunctivitis, it is a frequent sign, and sometimes the eye will stream tears.

In general, congestion in conjunctivitis is away from the cornea, while in deeper inflammations it directly surrounds the cornea. But a well-developed pink eye, or acute catarrhal conjunctivitis, will leave very little of the sclera white, and an acute iridocyclitis will evoked such congestion that there is no line of demarcation.

If the physician feels that conjunctivitis is not present, and a more serious lesion is likely to be in progress, it is his duty to dispatch the patient with all promptness to the ophthalmologist.

The diagnosis of acute glaucoma is not difficult and should be familiar to all. The entire globe is affected by a violent congestive lesion; there is intense redness, severe pain and profound loss of vision; a steamy cornea, an extremely hard eye. A combination of these two symptoms and two signs is conclusive evidence of acute glaucoma, and calls for *immediate* intervention by the ophthalmologist.

THE ABUSE OF VASOCONSTRICTORS IN HAY FEVER AND VASOMOTOR RHINITIS
(Louis Sternberg, New York City, in *N. Y. State Jl. of Med.*, July 15th)

A number of patients appear whose nasal discharge and obstruction are more the result of the abuse of various vasoconstrictors than of the underlying vasomotor rhinitis or seasonal hayfever. It seems that the allergic mucous membrane becomes refractory when in frequent and prolonged contact with these drugs for a variable period of time (three to five days), and then remains waterlogged no matter how often the vasoconstrictor is reapplied. At other times those membranes become irritated and inflamed from the same cause.

These drugs may have their place in acute sinusitis or acute rhinitis, when used for a day or two only. They should be used as a spray in an atomizer, never applied as drops into the nasal chambers, into the nose before retiring or during the early morning hours, because symptoms in these patients are usually most distressing then. If drops are applied into a waterlogged nose while the patient is reclining, the drug will keep on its irritating effects for hours while the patient is in that position. In the spray very little of the drug is used up with each application, and it is also dispersed over a bigger surface.

Penetrating Wounds of the Heart*

DANIEL L. MAGUIRE, JR., M. D., Charleston, South Carolina
From the Department of Surgery of the Medical College of the State of South Carolina
and Roper Hospital

FOR MANY CENTURIES, both the layman and the doctor regarded wounds of the heart as being of necessity fatal, so that it was not until the latter part of the nineteenth century that any attempt at surgical treatment was instituted. Three such wounds were sutured in 1896, but only one patient, the one operated upon by Rehn, survived. This is generally conceded to be the first successful cardiorrhaphy. Since this time, more and more cases have been diagnosed and operated upon with increasingly better results. According to Elkin's review of the literature,[3] in 1909 Peck collected 161 cases with a 63 per cent mortality; in 1912, Poole quoted 79 cases with a mortality rate of 49 per cent; in 1923 Smith reported 25 cases with a 36 per cent mortality, and in 1932, Bigger showed a 30 per cent mortality figure in a series of 70 cases. No doubt the percentage of recoveries as gleaned from the literature is too high, since accounts of many single successful cases appear in the journals. It is only in a large number of cases with a recording of the failures as well as the recoveries, that a fairly accurate estimate of the mortality rate can be evaluated. However, it is the best opinion today that in the hands of the average competent surgeon, the mortality rate is about 50 per cent. Obviously, this figure includes only those who reach the operating table, since a large percentage die *en route* to the hospital or in the emergency room.

It has been estimated by observers in large city hospitals that about 2 per cent of all penetrating thoracic wounds involve the heart or pericardium.[1] Undoubtedly the percentage of heart wounds would be greater were included the large number of chest injuries which prove promptly fatal.

The majority of penetrating wounds of the heart are inflicted with homicidal intent with a knife, ice pick or pistol. In the South, a favorite instrument is a long bladed pocket-knife with a push spring on the handle which releases the blade instantly, ready for immediate use. This weapon is known as a "switch blade," and almost every adult Negro has one on his person, and knows how to wield it proficiently. A smaller number of cases are suicidal, a pistol being used in most of these instances. The prognosis is much poorer than in stab wounds, and few gun-shot wounds of the heart ever reach the hospital.

Penetrating wounds of the heart may produce death either by exsanguinating hemorrhage or cardiac tamponade. Those who die of hemorrhage may bleed externally, or may lose vast amounts of blood into the mediastinum or a pleural cavity opened by the stab. However, it is far more common for cardiac tamponade to be the predominant feature. The wound may involve the intrapericardial portion of the great vessels, the coronaries, or any of the chambers of the heart. Not infrequently, the myocardium is lacerated, without extension through the endocardium into the auricles or ventricles. Since the right ventricle occupies most of the anterior surface of the heart, this chamber is most often injured. After that, in order of frequency, come the left ventricle, right auricle, left auricle, coronary vessels and, lastly, the intrapericardial portions of the aorta and pulmonary artery.[3]

The abnormal physiologic changes obtaining in cardiac tamponade are easily comprehended, as blood pours out into and fills the pericardial sac, there results an acute compression of the heart, since the pericardium cannot distend sufficiently to compensate for the added space occupied by the blood. If as little as 200 c.c. of blood passes out into the pericardial sac rapidly, fatal tamponade may ensue. As the intrapericardial pressure rises and the heart becomes more compressed, the inflow of blood from the venae cavae is backed up, and a consequent increase in venous pressure occurs. Because of the tamponade, a proportionately smaller amount of blood is taken into the auricles with each diastole, and a decreased cardiac output from the ventricles in systole results. Thus the blood pressure falls, and the systolic and the diastolic readings approach each other. When the increasing venous pressure can no longer overcome the marked intrapericardial pressure, circulatory arrest occurs with resulting cerebral anoxemia and death. If there is a large rent in the pericardium and the pleura the hemorrhage may decompress itself into the mediastinum and the pleural cavity, in which case tamponade will not ensue, but the patient die of exsanguination. Infrequently, bleeding from the heart is not profuse and it may cease spontaneously. In such cases recovery is apt to come about without surgical intervention.

The diagnosis of cardiac tamponade is not difficult. First of all, it is important for the resident

*Presented to Tri-State Medical Association of the Carolinas and Virginia, meeting at Charlotte, Feb. 28th-29th, 1944.

trauma in all chest wounds, and to be alert to recognize the signs of tamponade. Alcoholism often confuses the clinical picture, but cardiac involvement should be suspected when the degree of circulatory collapse is out of proportion to the visible wound or to the estimated loss of blood.

The history is more or less characteristic. The individual sustains a stab or gunshot wound of the chest, soon followed by collapse and unconsciousness. During the interval of consciousness the person may continue to fight or may walk several blocks. When sufficient time has elapsed for tamponade to be established, cerebral anoxemia is manifested by unconsciousness. If the individual survives the early period of circulatory collapse, there is usually a circulatory adjustment with distinct improvement of the general condition[1] and the blood pressure may rise and consciousness return. The wound may bleed profusely for a few moments at first, then gradually cease to bleed as tamponade progresses.

The physical examination of the patient reveals a stab wound of the chest, most commonly a few inches to the left of the sternum in the second, third, fourth or fifth intercostal space. The direction of the wound is often misleading. The individual is usually stuporous, apathetic and somnolent. The skin is cold and covered with perspiration, and there is cyanosis of the lips, tongue and conjunctivae. The blood pressure is low or unobtainable, the pulse weak or imperceptible, though the rate is not usually as rapid as one would expect with severe hemorrhage. The heart sounds are muffled and distant, but arrhythmia is not necessarily present. One can detect the increased venous pressure clinically by noting the abnormal distention of the cervical veins, and manometric venous pressure recordings in the cubital veins will substantiate this observation. Fluoroscopy of the chest will show the heart shadow not enlarged; but, instead of the normal pulsation, there is almost complete immobility of its outlines.

The treatment of penetrating wounds of the heart obviously depends entirely on the severity of the bleeding and on the degree of tamponade produced. Bigger[1] has classified heart wounds into four groups:

(a) Moderate bleeding without tamponade—This situation usually obtains where there has been a superficial nick of the myocardium or one of the smaller coronary branches. These patients usually recover spontaneously.

(b) Cardiac tamponade responding to conservative measures—In this class of patients, a small laceration of the myocardium seals itself off. Aspirations of the pericardium are performed to relieve the tamponade, and if repeated blood pressure and venous pressure readings fail to reveal evidence of reäccumulating intrapericardial blood, it is safe to continue conservative treatment:[8] If, however, signs of tamponade reäppear, and the patient's general condition does not improve after two or three aspirations, open pericardiotomy is in order to suture the source of hemorrhage.

(c) Severe tamponade—There is no response to conservative measures. Signs of tamponade reöccur immediately after aspiration with no marked improvement in the general condition of the patient. In these cases there is usually a comparatively extensive laceration into one of the chambers of the heart and operation is indicated. Life may be prolonged and the condition of the patient temporarily improved by aspiration of the pericardium while the operating room is prepared.

(d) Severe continued bleeding into a pleural cavity or externally, with or without tamponade. Here the element of marked blood loss further complicates the picture, and usually nothing short of heroic radical measures offer this type of patient a chance of survival. Even though the case appears hopeless, operation should be performed, since occasionally one of these patients will live.

If operation is decided upon, it seems to us wise, if the patient is in deep shock, to begin a continuous slow drip of plasma or compatible whole blood. The infusion can be kept running during the entire operation and the flow speeded up after the tamponade has been relieved. Though no time should be lost getting the patient on the operating table, one should not sacrifice strict asepsis in all details. It would be most disheartening to have the patient survive the cardiorrhaphy to die subsequently of a purulent pericarditis or empyema.

Because of the grave condition of these patients, one would certainly prefer to operate with only local anesthesia if possible. The high degree of anoxemia militates against any type of general anesthesia. Frequently, however, the patient's cerebral state, or often an associated acute alcoholism, makes him either unable or unwilling to coöperate sufficiently, and general anesthesia must be added to keep the patient on the table. When local anesthesia is used, one usually infiltrates the operative site liberally with novocaine ($\frac{1}{2}$-1%), and may also inject the third to the sixth intercostal nerves in the anterior axillary line on that side. During the procedure, it is well to have the patient breathing oxygen. The general anesthetic agents commonly employed include ethylene, cyclopropane, drop ether, or sodium pentothal, since a relatively high oxygen concentration can be maintained. Nitrous oxide is inadvisable because of its tendency to increase the preëxisting the anoxemia. If local infiltration with novocaine is also employed, it definitely decreases the amount of inhalation anesthetic necessary to keep the patient in a satis-

staff to keep in mind the possibility of cardiac factory state for the required surgery.

Unless the wound is well to the right one usually incises to the left of the sternum. If the pleura is obviously torn and a pneumothorax is present, a transverse intercostal, transpleural approach is fast and gives good exposure, but should not be employed if one cannot be sure whether or not the pleura has been injured. A median sternotomy affords excellent exposure of the heart and great vessels, but requires a great deal of time to open and close, and is more shocking than the other approaches. The two most commonly used incisions are the parasternal and the transverse intercostal. The pectoralis fascia and pectoralis muscles are divided and retracted to expose the costal cartilages adjacent to the sternum. Usually the third, fourth and fifth cartilages are resected subchondrally for three inches laterally, taking care to avoid injuring the underlying pleural reflection. The pleura is then gently pushed laterally with a sponge, and a portion of the sternum rongeured away if necessary for a better view. It is essential that the necessary exposure be made before the pericardium is opened. The internal mammary vessels are ligated. The pericardium will appear tense, bulging and blue, and no pulsations of the heart will be seen. The pericardium is opened and all clots and fluid blood evacuated with suction. Upon relief of the tamponade, the heart's action becomes full and vigorous. The wound in the heart can usually be readily discovered by the jet of blood spurting out with each systole. A traction suture is then passed through the apex and, while this is gently held between the third and fourth finger of the left hand, the index finger of the same hand is placed over the heart wound to slow the hemorrhage. Sutures, preferably of silk, are then placed along the wound margins down to, but not into the endocardium and tied just snugly enough to approximate the edges of the laceration. Should there be another opening on the right or posterior aspect of the heart, another traction suture can be utilized to rotate the heart and make the injury accessible. If the coronaries are immediately adjacent to the wound margin, a mattress suture can be passed under the vessels without including them in the tie. If the coronaries are lacerated they will have to be ligated. In such cases, postoperative electrocardiograms show typical changes of coronary infarction, but such ligations are not necessarily fatal. Should fibrillation or asystole develop, satisfactory response will often follow gentle cardiac massage and intramyocardial injections of 3 c.c. of 1:1000 adrenalin.

After the wound is sutured and all active hemorrhage has ceased, the pericardium should be irrigated with normal saline to remove any blood and clots. The pericardium and the wound are sprinkled lightly with sulfathiazole powder, and the wound closed in layers with interrupted silk. We believe that it is best to place a small piece of soft-rubber tissue down to, but not into, the pericardium in order to allow the pericardial fluid to exude through the lower angle of the wound. This drain is removed in 48 hours.

Postoperatively, the patient is placed in an oxygen tent with a back rest. Transfusions of blood or plasma are given as necessary until the blood pressure is stabilized above the shock level. Morphine and barbiturates are employed freely to allay pain and apprehension. Sulfathiazole is begun, and a prophylactic dose of tetanus and gas-gangrene antitoxin is administered. The patient is kept on liquids for the first two or three days, and then the diet is increased as the condition improves. If pleural injury has been sustained, one should be on the alert for the development of a tension pneumothorax (Case I), in which case removal of the air from the pleural cavity by aspiration or by closed thoracotomy with underwater drainage is necessary. Serial electrocardiograms are of interest, and usually present evidence of satisfactory resolution of the sterile pericarditis which invariably follows the trauma of the operation. If then all goes well, these patients can usually be allowed up in three to four weeks and discharged in good condition soon thereafter.

The prognosis depends on the time elapsing from the injury to the operation, the character and the extent of the injury, and whether there exists other intrathoracic involvement such as hemothorax or pneumothorax. These with only temponade usually survive at least one hour. Patients who survive cardiorrhaphy show no evidence later of impaired cardiac reserve, and abnormalities on the electrocardiogram usually disappear within a few months.[5] The most common complications are, in order of frequency: tension pneumothorax, purulent pericarditis, pneumonia, empyema and embolism from endocardial clots.

At the Roper Hospital in Charleston penetrating wounds of the heart are not infrequent, but most of the victims are either dead on admission or die before any surgical measures can be instituted. Only a few reach the operating table, and those that do are often miserable operative risks (Table I). In the last year, however, we had two such patients to be operated upon and survive. Their cases will be reported briefly.

Case 1.—(20049)—A 20-year-old colored man was admitted June 20th, 1943, with a stab wound of the left chest. The clinical findings suggested cardiac tamponade. Fluoroscopy confirmed the diagnosis. There was no evidence of intrapleural involvement. He was taken to the operating room immediately and the heart exposed through a left parasternal incision. A laceration one inch long in

TABLE I

Case No.	Year	Sex	Age	Weapon	Time from injury to operation	Location	Result	Comment
33516	1924	M	19	Knife	2 hrs.	Right Auricle	Recovered	Essentially uneventful postoperative course. Right pleural and pericardial effusions, sterile, absorbed.*
95376	1937	M	30	Knife	90 min.	Left Ventricle and coronary artery	Died	Complicating hemopneumothorax, left. Died on operating table. Hemorrhage and tamponade.
95429	1937	M	25	Bullet	90 min.	Left Ventricle	Died	Laceration of myocardium over, but not into ventricle. Laceration of left lung with massive hemothorax. Death 12 hours after operation—bronchopneumonia, bilateral.
4382	1941	M	18	Knife	90 min.	Right Auricle	Died	Died while heart being sutured. Death apparently due mainly to interference with conduction system, since laceration severed main bundle.
21425	1943	F	49	Knife	50 min.	Left Ventricle and coronary artery	Died	Died on operating table. Also open pneumothorax, left, and massive hemothorax, right. Miserable risk, but operation was only chance.
20049	1943	M	20	Knife	2 hrs.	Right Ventricle	Recovered	See case report. Case No. I.
21840	1943	M	22	Knife	2 hrs.	Right Ventricle	Recovered	See case report. Case No. II.

the wall of the right ventricle was closed with interrupted sutures of chromic catgut. During the operation, the left pleural reflection was nicked and some pneumothorax produced. The pleura was sutured and the free air aspirated from the pleural cavity. Ethylene was used throughout the operation for anesthesia. Five hundred c.c. plasma were given during the operation and 500 c.c. of compatible blood immediately postoperatively. Thirty-six hours after operation, a tension pneumothorax developed on the left, which responded satisfactorily to closed thoracotomy maintained for 48 hours. The wound healed per primam. Discharged in good condition on July 16th. Followed for four months, when last seen he was at work on his farm, felt well, had no complaints, and his electrocardiograms were negative.

Case 2.—(21840)—A 22-year-old colored man was brought to the emergency room of Roper Hospital on August 17th, 1943. He had sustained a stab wound of the left chest and was in deep shock. His appearance suggested cardiac tamponade and the diagnosis was confirmed by fluoroscopy. There was no hemothorax or pneumothorax. Plasma was begun and he was operated on within an hour. The heart was exposed through a left parasternal incision, and a 1-inch laceration in the right ventricle (Fig. 2) was sutured with interrupted silk. The pleural cavity was not entered. Novocaine (3-4%) was used throughout, except for five minutes during the suture of the heart when ethylene was employed to supplement. The postoperative course was uneventful. The blood pressure soon became stabilized above the shock level, and the pulse remained regular and of good quality. No respiratory complications developed. Serial electrocardiograms revealed changes characteristic of healing pericarditis. The wound healed satisfactorily, and the patient was discharged in good condition Sept. 14th, 28 days after admission. He was seen for the last time on December 15th. The wound was healed, he felt well and had no complaints referable to his heart. He had been arrested in November and been sentenced to six months at hard labor.

SUMMARY AND CONCLUSIONS

1. There are now a large number of surgically treated heart wounds recorded in the literature with an average mortality of 50 per cent.

2. Death in these cases is usually due to massive hemorrhage or cardiac tamponade.

3. Cases with cardiac tamponade usually survive long enough for surgical measures to be instituted if the diagnosis is made soon after admission.

4. The cardinal findings in cardiac tamponade are a chest wound with a low arterial pressure, increased venous pressure and a small quiet heart. Fluoroscopy will confirm the clinical diagnosis.

5. If the patient's condition does not improve with aspiration of the hemopericardium, open pericardiotomy with suture of the heart wound is imperative.

6. In cases in which the lung has been injured, tension pneumothorax is a frequent and dangerous complication.

7. Successfully sutured hearts, without involvement of the coronary vessels, show no evidence of decreased cardiac reserve.

Bibliography

1. BIGGER, I. A.: The diagnosis and treatment of heart wounds. Southern Med. Jour., 33:6-11, 1940.

2. CARTER, R. E.: Stab wound of the heart. *Amer. Jour. of Surgery*, 55:143-147, 1942.
3. ELKIN, D. E.: The diagnosis and treatment of cardiac trauma. *Annals of Surgery*, 114:169-185, 1941.
4. GLASSER, S. T., MERSHEIMER, W., & SHINER, I.: Bullet wound of left cardiac auricle with suture and recovery. *Am. Jour. of Surgery*, 53:131-144, 1941.
5. GRISWOLD, A. R., & MAGUIRE, C. H.: Penetrating wounds of the heart and pericardium. *S., G. & O.*, 74: 406-418, 1942.
6. SCHIEBEL, M. H.: Stab wound of pulmonary artery with suture and recovery. *Arch. of Surgery*, 45:957-963, 1942.
7. WARD, T. P., & PARKER, W. G.: Penetrating wounds of the heart. *Am. Jour. of Surgery*, 50:712-714, 1940.
8. BLALOCK, A., & ROVITCH, M. M.: Nonoperative treatment of cardiac tamponade. *Surgery*, 14:157-162, August, 1943.

Discussion

DR. PAUL D. CAMP, Richmond: I don't know surgical technic, however, I have seen several of these cases of wounds of the heart in the cardiac clinic. Some of those Dr. Bigger operated on. I was particularly interested in the cardiographic changes mentioned. Some of the cases gave electrocardiographic evidences of damage within a very few hours after the stab wound.

It is important to note what happens in acute tamponade of the pericardium as contrasted with gradual accumulation of pericardial fluid. Often we get a large amount of fluid without distress of any kind. As the collection of fluid is gradual and the pericardium is being extended gradually, there are no ill effects from it.

DR. H. G. LANGSTON, Danville: To those of us interested in surgical technic in thoracic cases in general, the amount of drainage of the pericardium is quite a point. We all know that the pleura, when drained, is exposed to the rubber catheter, whether under water or open drainage, and produces a degree of susceptibility to infection which could be and should be avoided if it is possible to do so.

In the case of transpleural aspiration of any kind, a sterile effusion generally is a result, which cannot be avoided, but as you know, the pleura can take care of much more accumulation of fluid than can the pericardium. For that reason, it is frequently safe to close the pleura snugly and close the entire wound and make no outlet whatever for drainage. The situation is different from what happens when the pleura produces a large amount of fluid, because as we learned awhile ago, the pericardium is not capable of expanding rapidly. In cases of rheumatic fever the effusion, of course, is slow of onset and slow in development and the progress of such nature as to give the pericardium time to accommodate the fluid, but in case of any pericardial effusion taking place suddenly cardiac tamponade is a probability. Dr. Maguire pointed out very accurately that drainage of the pericardium is necessary in these to obviate a pericardial effusion suddenly and rapidly developing tamponade.

DR. WM. H. PRIOLEAU, Charleston: I have only to say that the degree to which the resident staff are on their toes will determine to a great extent the results in a large series of cases, and it is just to point out that two of the good results in our series occurred during the period Dr. Maguire was in service at the Roper Hospital.

DR. MAGUIRE, closing: Thank you, Dr. Prioleau, but I, in turn, must modestly say that the diagnosis was made for me by the interne who was in the emergency room before I got there.

As to drainage, I feel hesitant in offering an opinion from the small series covered by my observations. Dr. Bigger and Dr. Griswold, I believe, feel that drainage is not necessary; but some of the New York observers have had trouble with marked passive congestion and cyanosis postoperative.

The only other point that might come up for discussion on which some observers are not agreed is giving fluid to these patients preoperatively. You already have an embarrassed circulation, but in both of our cases when plasma was begun dripping slowly, the blood pressure picked up and consciousness returned and they did very well. After we got the heart sewed up, we sped up the plasma and the heart kept going along.

APPENDICITIS COMPLICATED BY RUPTURE OF THE INFERIOR EPIGASTRIC ARTERY

(G. O. Bassett, Prescott, in *Arizona Med.*, Sept.)

Spontaneous hemorrhage from the inferior epigastric artery is not rare. It may be due to trauma or may occur spontaneously, postoperative, or following a severe coughing attack.

A case is reported associated with definite inflammation of the appendix: April 30th, patient stated that he thought he was having an attack of appendicitis. At 10 a. m. a robust male, age 56, seemed in great pain, had awakened at 3 a. m. with sharp pain in the right lower abdomen, was nauseated and vomited shortly afterwards. The pain caused him to draw his right leg up. He had had previous attacks, a severe cold for the past 10 days, and paroxysmal cough. T. 99.2, p. 94, r. 20, b. p. 154/90. Fluoroscopy of the chest and heart was negative. Urine showed albumin 2 plus, pus cells 1 plus, and a few granular casts; negative Wassermann.

Increased fullness tenderness over McBurney's point, muscle spasm. Very light percussion elicited pain and spasm, and nausea, w.b.c. 9,750—poly 65; six hours later white 11,750—Polys 71%. Swelling and muscle spasm increased, less pain, observe for 24 hours. Then w.b.c. 12,400 —polys 74, t. 99, p. 84, r. 18.

A right rectus incision, fascia bluish and very tense, friable, and as it separated a blood clot found extending from the umbilicus downward surrounding the rectus muscle. When the clot was removed the deep epigastric at a point $\frac{1}{2}$ inch within the sheath was found spurting briskly. The peritoneum was opened and the clot was observed to extend under the peritoneal reflection on the bladder. There was a moderate amount of cloudy fluid in the fossa; the appendix was retrocecal, injected and swollen.

Convalescence was uneventful. On the third postoperative day the urine was entirely clear.

CANCER OF THE STOMACH kills more persons than any other malignant disease—125,000 yearly in the United States. It is curable if diagnosed early and in most instances early diagnosis by the x-ray is possible; today we are saving, even with our best surgical technique only 6% of the diagnosed cases. We must insist, and render it possible, that every patient who commits himself to our care and who has any of the symptoms of indigestion get an x-ray examination of his stomach and duodenum.—*T. Grier Miller*.

A WHEEZE appearing for the first time in a patient of cancer age should immediately make one suspect an intrabronchial tumor. While x-ray examination is helpful in diagnosis, inspection of the tracheo-bronchial tree with the bronchoscope is essential.—*E. L. Van Loon*.

EVERY CASE OF HEMATURIA should be subjected to a comprehensive examination to determine, first, the origin of the blood and, second, the cause of the bleeding.—*Alex. Randall*.

Pellagra Sine Pellagra*

ERNEST L. COPLEY, M.D., Richmond

NO MORE DRAMATIC disease than pellagra has ever come to the attention of the medical profession. The tracing of its history through the records that have come down to us reveals many things to be wondered at.

Eberle's two-volume book on "Practice," perhaps the most popular work in the U. S. on this subject 100 years ago, makes no mention of it.

Hughes Bennett, of Edinburgh (1867), in perhaps the most popular book on "Practice of Medicine" in the English language at that time, says nothing on the subject.

Johannes Hermann Baas wrote his scholarly "History of Medicine" in 1885 and made no mention of pellagra.

The "Reference Handbook of the Medical Sciences," 10 large tomes edited by Buck of New York and published in 1887, devotes two pages to the subject and defines it thus: "A complex disease characterized by (1) a squamous erythematous condition confined to those portions of the skin which are exposed to the action of heat and light; (2) a chronic inflammatory condition of the digestive tract; (3) a condition of the nervous system leading in time to mental alienation and paralysis." The Handbook says that the condition has been known as a distinct disease for more than a century.

Surgeon General Billings' "National Medical Dictionary" (1890) defines pellagra as "an endemic disease of Italy characterized by chronic erythematous, desquamative inflammation of the skin, with digestive derangement and neuroses."

The edition of Austin Flint's "Practice" of 1894 has nothing to say on the subject.

The "System of Medicine," edited by Sir Clifford Allbutt, published in 1900, in its five pages on pellagra, says there is no doubt but that the disease is due to bad maize; that in countries where pellagra is known there can be little difficulty in detecting the malady even in its early stage; and that the main pathological changes are to be found in the spinal cord and brain. It is in this "System" that we first encounter the use of the term, *pellagra sine pellagra*.

Yet in Osler's seven-volume "Modern Medicine," published in 1907, only two inches of type are used in the discussion of pellagra and that discussion is in the section on Food poisons, contributed by Novy, a Professor of Bacteriology.

Osler's single volume "Practice," in the edition published in 1912, recorded the reported deaths from the disease in the United States in 1908 as 23, in 1909 as 116, in 1910 as 368, and states that the cause is unknown.

In the official journal of this Association, Dr. James K. Hall, of Richmond, wrote in 1932 what will interest you who have not read it more than anything else I shall say on the subject. He is advising all medical men to read frequently the autobiography of Dr. J. Marion Sims. I can do no better than quote Dr. Hall's own words:

Dr. Sims gives a detailed account of a diarrhea from which he suffered almost continuously from 1848 in Montgomery, until 1855, some time after he had removed to New York. . . . . . I have no doubt that he was suffering from pellagra. Hear Sims' account of his symptoms.

"On Christmas Day (1852) we went to Mount Meigs (near Montgomery), five days after my return from Philadelphia, to dine with our friends the Lucases. There I had a chill. The next day we returned home (to Montgomery). The diarrhea returned and could not be controlled . . . . . within a week I was confined to my house, and within one month . . . . to my bed. By that time my throat and tongue were so ulcerated that I could hardly speak, and any nourishment that I took passed through me like water and almost unchanged.

"Early in February (1853) I had given up all hope, and one day the bell tolled. . . . . . I called to my wife from an adjoining room and wanted to know who was dead. She said it was Mr. Bob Gilmer. . . . . . I . . . . . counted up the numbers. I said 'Bob Gilmer is the eleventh or twelfth important person in this community that has died of this disease that I have since I was taken with it.' I said, 'They have all died, and I have had a hard struggle for my life, and now I must die, too.'
. . . .

'I ought to sell everything, take my wife and children and go to New York, because whenever I have gone to New York I have been better. A few months ago I thought that I was cured. If I could change my climate entirely I believe that

---

*Presented to Tri-State Medical Association of the Carolinas and Virginia, meeting at Charlotte, Feb. 28th-29th, 1944.

even yet I might be cured and restored to health.'"

. . . . .

Dr. Hall comments:

"The wife made the final decision. Montgomery lost the world's great-to-be surgeon. Diarrhea continued to harass him for two or three years, but he finally recovered. Is there any reason to doubt that he had pellagra, and that many of his neighbors were dying of it? Yet the first cases of pellagra in the United States were reported in 1864, by Dr. Gray, in Utica, New York; and by Dr. Tyler, in Somerville, Massachusetts; and Dr. George H. Searcy startled the country by his brief report of an epidemic of the disease in the State Hospital for the colored insane in Alabama in 1907."

The last edition of Osler's "Practice" as revised by Christian in 1942 says that, although the diet plays a very important part, finality has not yet been reached as to the causation. Dr. Christian credits Dr. Searcy with having first described a case in the United States and says that sporadic cases have probably occurred in this country for the last 100 years, and he gives the deaths in 1930 as 6333, in 1940 as 2123.

As is inevitable in the case of a disease dependent on its symptomatology for its diagnosis, most writings on pellagra describe the severe, full-blown cases. While there is such a thing as acute, fulminating pellagra, the vast majority of cases develop gradually with mild manifestations, with remissions or intermissions, and perhaps more cases than any of us realize remain mild throughout.

The purpose of this paper is to present a group of cases, of varying degrees of severity, none of which had the skin changes called typical. For want of a better term, I have accepted the designation *pellagra sine pellagra*.

Reliable information is obtainable of the incidence of the usual forms of pellagra because it is a reportable disease in many states; but I believe that many of the mild cases are never recognized and that most of the cases of usual severity might well be diagnosed earlier. Harris[1] thought the number of such cases to exceed those of full development—whatever the triad of skin, alimentary canal and nervous system symptoms be called, while they are still mild. The important fact is that for these conditions the therapy for pellagra is effective.

Goldberger[2] declared twenty-five years ago the fully developed disease presents such a picture that, once seen, one who is not a physician would not fail to recognize it thereafter. The early manifestations are not easily recognized unless one is alert to their existence.

The full-blown case of pellagra is too familiar to need description here.

It may be well to call attention to the fact that the patient will usually give a history of dyspepsia and anorexia, or gas with bloating or burning in the epigastrium.

Some cases of *pellagra sine pellagra* differ from the classical only in the absence of the characteristic erythema. The most distinctive feature in all cases is the chronicity; the symptoms may extend over a period of several years, with remissions. The symptoms of the earlier stages are not necessarily prodromal to the dermatitis stage—for in the vast majority of instances they continue in various degrees of mildness. The diagnosis of many of these moderately advanced cases is fairly easy. When not recognized as pellagrous, and attributed to some form of avitaminoses, they may still receive the needed therapy.

It must be that many of the milder cases are overlooked, not implying a lack of skill or care, since early pellagra presents a confusing picture. The disease is so insidious the patient cannot date its onset; the symptoms are often multiple and varied, often simulating or existing along with those of other disease conditions. First to attract attention may be an atypical skin lesion, or some vague digestive or nervous manifestation—one or more of which may have recurred in several summers, with winter lapses, before the condition became chronic and disturbing enough for the patient to seek medical advice.

But there is in most cases uniformity enough to give a clue to their diagnosis. Most other organic diseases may be excluded by the use of means at our command, and then anti-pellagra therapy should be instituted. It is generally agreed that the gastrointestinal and mental symptoms antedate the characteristic dermatitis. Dermatitis is apt to be a late development, a part of a stage having a considerable mortality.

I have not included in my series of cases any that did not promptly respond to the use of nicotinamide.

I shall describe briefly some of the features which I regard as diagnostic. Hyperkeratoses occurred frequently in my series, accompanied by an *increase* in the gastrointestinal and mental symptoms. The skin over the knees and insteps became thickened, dry, with some portions pigmented.

In one of my cases, the skin over the dorsal aspects of the forearms and hands was leathery, and covered lightly with dandruff-like scales. It was fissured and cracked over the joints of the fingers. The hyperkeratoses about the insteps were on horizontal lines, as if a tight bandage had been applied. A patient with admittedly poor dietary habits had patches of scaly pigmented areas over the dorsa of the feet. Other symptoms in this case were loss of appetite and insomnia.

In another case the backs of the hands looked and felt hidebound, the skin over the legs was distinctly dry, with many fine scales. There was interference with flexion of the fingers. It was not feasible to expose any of these patients to sunlight.

Ruffin and Smith[3] report hyperkeratoses with pigmentation over the bony prominences of the body. However, they attribute them to rubbing or pressure, and do not think they are otherwise significant. They believe it hazardous to make a diagnosis of pellagra in the absence of typical dermatitis.

Fields et al.[4] describe in much detail the appearance of chronic skin conditions, which they regard as characteristic of the lesser deficiencies. They caution, however, that their significance should be interpreted in the light of other causative factors that may produce like changes.

No doubt, many hyperkeratoses are due to pressure. However, if they are accompanied by other symptoms suspicious of pellagra they are highly suggestive. I have found that small daily doses of nicotinamide markedly improve the majority of such cases, but the matter of diagnosis has been left open.

In two of my cases, in both of which cure was effected, the lesions were far advanced when first seen. The mouth and tongue were of typically pellagrous appearance. In the case of an alcoholic of long standing, desquamation of the epithelium of the entire tongue had left that organ beefy-red and smooth. The mucous membranes of the oral cavity were denuded. There were deeply penetrating ulcers in the buccal mucosa, and the entire fossa was ulcerated so that food intake had become increasingly painful and consequently almost nil.

Only the tongue and lips were involved in the other instance. The tongue was denuded and red in the center, with crusts around the edges in front, alternating with small raw areas. The lips were red, macerated in certain areas, and there were fissures at the angles of the mouth—suggesting an ariboflavinosis. Improvement followed promptly upon institution of therapy in both cases, and continued rapidly thereafter.

Milder forms of glossitis such as the swollen and fissured tongue, with beefy redness at the end, if accompanied by gastric symptoms, should suggest pellagra. Stomatic ulcers are also suggestive, in the absence of other ascertainable causative factors. If the glossitis and stomatitis are accompanied by appropriate gastrointestinal symptoms, treatment should be instituted without waiting for the development of dermatitis, or to expose to sunshine.

The more chronic and recurring the intestinal tract symptoms, the more suggestive they are of pellagra. Severe bouts of diarrhea alternating with constipation, otherwise unexplainable, are common in pellagra. Lesser symptoms which should arouse suspicion are epigastric burning, abdominal discomfort, gas or bloating, and sometimes sick stomach. A history of an inadequate diet lends these symptoms particular significance.

In one of my cases stupor developed, despite energetic treatment, in less than a week after it came under my care. Incontinence of bladder and bowels, dementia and extreme psychosis, disorientation and violence persisted for weeks, so that restraint was necessary and commitment was considered. Another patient remained ambulatory, but developed a food psychosis, delusions of wealth and great personality changes.

Though pellagra is not the explanation of anything like all the complaints of neurotics and psychoneurotics, it should be kept in mind as a likely cause of irritability and fatigability, loss of energy and weakness, mental depression and the lack of zest of living. One of my patients complained of numbness and burning of the extremities and painful joints. X-ray examination revealed no evidence of arthritis. Field et al.[4] state: "Removal of patients from the classification of psychoneurosis and the giving of specific treatment promises to be one of the major accomplishments of medicine."

The following cases were observed in the past two years:

Case No. 1.—A 51-year-old colored woman, with mild diabetes, requiring 15 to 20 units of insulin daily. When first seen, in November, 1942, she had reduced her diet not only in carbohydrate intake, but also in milk products, eggs, meats and liver, and was still taking six units of insulin daily. She had lost fifty pounds in two years, and complained of headache and a burning sensation of the tongue, and had had one bout of diarrhea.

The tongue was smooth and dry, and she had discarded her dentures. Cheilosis was present with maceration of the lips near the angles of the mouth and scabs about the nose. The heart was enlarged to percussion and rapid in rate. The skin was dry, that over the forearms and hands hyperkeratotic, that over the joints of the fingers fissured and cracked.

The hgbn. was 90%, r.b.c. 4,530,000, whites 6,100—neut. 63, lymph. 37. The blood Wassermann was negative for syphilis. The urine was negative for sugar and showed a slight trace of albumin. Fasting, the sugar was 83 mgs. per 100 c.c. of blood. The basal metabolic rate was plus 48. An ECG showed sinus rhythm, and auricular and ventricular rate of 120 and moderate left axis deviation.

Treatment consisted of 200 mgs. of nicotinic acid, and 15 units of protamin zinc insulin daily, a dram of brewer's yeast and 5 m. of Lugol's solution t.i.d., and a diet liberal in carbohydrates and unlimited in proteins and fats.

The headache disappeared promptly, the glossitis and stomatitis cleared and the skin assumed a normal texture. There was a gain of twelve pounds in four weeks, and the pulse slowed to 80 to 90. The nicotinic acid was reduced to 100 mgs., brewer's yeast to a dram daily. Four months later she reported a steady increase in weight and good health.

Case No. 2.—A 40-year-old white woman was first seen August, 1942. For several years she had consumed from a pint to a quart of whiskey daily. The food intake was almost nil. She complained of sore tongue and mouth and pain on deglutition, and gave the "textbook" picture of glossitis and stomatitis found in pellagrins. She complained of a burning sensation of the legs and feet, had tremor of the outstretched fingers, a peculiar stare and reluctance to give the history of her case. She was emaciated and weighed only 80 pounds. Hyperkeratosis was marked about the elbows and knees. There was no abdominal tenderness nor evidence of cirrhosis of the liver.

Treatment consisted of 50 mgs. of nicotinic acid, a dram of brewer's yeast, and capsules containing vitamins A, B and D, t.i.d.

Recovery was dramatic. The oral lesions healed promptly, hyperkeratoses cleared and the appetite became enormous. After the first month, small daily doses of nicotinic acid and brewer's yeast were prescribed. Twelve months after treatment was instituted, she reported excellent health and a gain in weight of 40 pounds.

Case No. 3.—A 75-year-old white woman, first seen September, 1943, with symptoms thought at first to be due to infirmities of age. She was weak and dyspneic on slight exertion, heart fibrillating.

Examination revealed the syndrome of *pellagra sine pellagra*. The present illness had been insidious in onset, the chief symptoms of which were an increasing anorexia, insomnia and nervousness. The history indicated she had been treated for a similar condition, two years before, in a North Carolina hospital.

The diet had consisted chiefly of milk, bread and cereals. She had lost weight and had had several bouts of diarrhea. She had glossitis and stomatitis characteristic of typical pellagra. While there was no florid dermatitis, the skin was hyperkeratotic about the joints, although she had only recently been confined to bed. She was mentally hazy and irritable. All laboratory findings were essentially negatitve. An ECG showed auricular fibrillation and moderate left axis deviation.

Immediate treatment consisted of digitalization and 50 mgs. of nicotinic acid and a dram of brewer's yeast t.i.d. Stupor developed rapidly and hospitalization was necessary.

In the hospital, the nicotinic acid dosage was increased to 500 mgs. daily, given as nicotinamide. Brewer's yeast was supplemented by liver extract, given parenterally, and dilute hydrochloric acid.

Her illness ran a long and stormy course. While the glossitis and stomatitis cleared promptly, and there was a return of appetite, she continued irrational, requiring a constant attendant and some restraint the entire hospital stay of 47 days. Commitment was also considered. As a last measure, she was placed in the care and home of a relative. Whether it was coincidental, or the effect of a change of environment, improvement in her mental condition was immediate and marked. Two months later, she was mentally alert and in good physical condition for her age.

Case No. 4.—A 42-year-old white woman could not date the onset of her illness. For at least a year she had had insomnia, anorexia, weakness and weight loss. Relatives stated she had developed a food psychosis, and that her diet was altogether inadequate. She had delusions of wealth, which members of her family said did not exist, and there were personality changes.

She was emaciated, the tongue was red and the lips parched. The skin was dry. The hgbn. was 75% and the r.b.c. 3,700,000. The blood Wassermann was negative for syphilis, and the urine contained a slight trace of albumin.

Treatment consisted of 50 mgs. of nicotinamide and six brewer's yeast tablets t.i.d., and liver extract parenterally each day.

Improvement in both physical and mental condition ensued promptly on treatment, and persisted. She gained four pounds the first month. In three months, she reported excellent health.

Case No. 5.—A 42-year-old farmer complained of arthritic pains in the extremities, more especially in the right foot and ankle. He had also had indigestion and epigastric burning after eating certain foods for an indefinite time, and was generally unhappy in his work.

The tongue and mouth were normal in appearance. There was thickening of the skin over the hands, interfering with flexion of the fingers, and an ichthyosis-like condition over the calves of the legs, with an abundance of fine scaling.

An x-ray picture of the right foot and ankle showed no evidence of arthritis. The blood Wassermann and urine tests were negative.

He was given 50 mgs. of nicotinamide t.i.d., and thiamin hydrochloride. Two weeks later, marked improvement was noted in the texture of the skin over the hands and about the legs; his attitude and outlook had greatly improved, and the pain in the ankle had almost completely disappeared.

Case No. 6.—A 61-year-old white woman has been seen over a period of a dozen years. Her chief symptom during that time has been nervousness. She has had several bouts of symptoms resembling chorea, and has had to take sedatives of varying strengths almost continuously. In November, 1943, she complained of a thickening of the skin about the ankles, and the perineum, an inflamed area about the anus and dryness of the mouth.

She appeared well developed and nourished. She was nervous, talkative repetitious, with a characteristic use of many "buts" and "ands" while stating her complaint. The tongue was only slightly red around the border, but had furrows. The skin about the ankles was thick, and presented horizontal lines as if a bandage had been about them. The perineum was hyperkeratotic, and there was an area of redness around the anus.

Given 100 mgs. of nicotinamide daily and thiamin hydrochloride, the skin about the ankles was within a week soft and normal in texture, while improvement was felt in the perineal and anal region. Marked improvement was also reported in physical well being.

Strangely enough, during the second week the skin about the perineum and anus became angry red, and had a burning sensation. She was thereupon referred to a dermatologist who gave several doses of x-rays with satisfactory result.

Comment

Three of these six cases, I think, were unquestionably pellagrous. The diagnosis in Case No. 3 was concurred in by a psychiatrist. Case No. 4 was that of the daughter of the patient whose case is No. 3, and the diet had been the same in both instances. Complaints were numerous in Case No. 5. While such factors as fatigue from overwork may have played a part in producing his symptoms, it seems plain that a deficiency state was the chief factor. Case No. 6 was complicated by a mixed skin infection. However, it seems reasonable that the extreme and continuous nervous condition consumed so much of her vitamin intake that there was a definite deficiency which, when replenished gave prompt improvement in her condition.

The treatment of pellagra is simple and reasonably effective for both the severe and mild forms. The diet must be well balanced, of high caloric value and consist of foods containing the water-soluble, heat-stable, (P-P) pellagra-preventing vitamin G *whenever pellagra* is suspected. Especially recommended for their vitamin G value are: sweet and buttermilk; fresh and canned beef; chicken; canned salmon; smoked lean pork; rabbit; fresh or canned collards and kale; and green peas.

There seems to be considerable variation in the individual vitamin requirements. In certain conditions, such as hyperthyroidism, pregnancy and illnesses that may require dietary restrictions, the utilization of vitamins may be either increased or the food intake decreased, so that a vitamin deficiency may result. In all such instances, the vitamin intake must be supplemented.

The generally accepted therapeutic agents are dried yeast powder, liver extract and nicotinic acid. Seventy-five to one hundred grams of yeast daily, recommended by many, has the disadvantage of inducing vomiting and diarrhea in some cases and is very objectionable to the taste of a great number. It is best given in tomato juice. Seventy-five to 100 grams of liver extract orally is also recommended. An equivalent amount of liver in the form of liver extract may also be given parenterally. In severe cases, obviously, large amounts of either or both yeast and liver extract will be required to supply sufficient vitamin G to be effective. As Fields et al.[4] point out, for economic reasons as well as therapeutic, synthetic nicotinic acid is preferable.

The dosage of nicotinic acid required in my experience has varied from 50 to 100 mgs. daily in mild cases, to 150 mgs. in the well advanced; and in one case 500 mgs. was given daily over a considerable period. I think it advisable to supplement the nicotinic acid with dried yeast powder or liver extract or both, and I have done this in the majority of my cases. In two cases, not reported here, I reduced the dosage because headache and epigastric distress were reported, which were thought to be due to the size of the dose. Patients should be watched carefully for any untoward effects of treatment.

Summary

Attention has been called to the lesser vitamin deficiencies under the name *pellagra sine pellagra*.

The features thought to be characteristic of this disease condition have been described, and six cases presented in brief outline.

Nicotinic acid is recommended as the treatment of choice, supplemented by dried yeast powder and liver extract, these in addition to a well balanced diet in as great quantity as the patient can be induced to take.

References

1. Harris, H. F.: *Am. J. M. Sc.*, 141:714-724, 1911.
2. Goldberger, J.: *Pub. Health Rep.*, 33:481-488, 1918.
3. Ruffin, J. M., & Smith, D. T.: *Clinical Pellagra*, p. 210.
4. Field, H., Jr., Parnall, C., Jr., & Robinson, W. D.: *New Eng. J. Med.*, 233: Aug. 29th, 1940.

This paper and the next discussed together.

The Effect of Agricultural Practices on Health and Disease*

James Asa Shield, M.D., Richmond

Assistant Professor of Neuropsychiatry, Medical College of Virginia
Neuropsychiatrist, Tucker Hospital

IT IS THE PURPOSE of this paper to correlate some recorded observations, and interpret them, in terms of possible etiology, of the health and some of the ills of man. Minot[1] states: "It has been proved that certain diseases reflect the character of the social and economic as well as the geographic environment." Snapper[2] indicates that every phase of clinical medicine in Peiping is influenced by the peculiar food situation. One might add that health, too, reflects the character of the social, economic, and geographic environment.

The correct diagnosis and therapy in deficiency diseases has been one of the advances of medicine. However, our desire is the prevention of these deficiency diseases. Although much has been accomplished, there are still many unknown factors in the field of nutrition and its relation to sickness and health.

The medical journals have many papers telling of recently acquired knowledge on almost every variety of deficiency—avitaminosis, hypoproteinemia, and mineral imbalance, with therapeutic response when therapy is based on the proper rationale. There are perhaps no doctors more aware of the value of rational vitamin, mineral, and food concentrate therapy than we in neuropsychiatry. However, the absence of the progressive degenerative disease of the blood vessels—arteriosclerosis;

*Presented to Tri-State Medical Association of the Carolinas and Virginia, meeting at Charlotte, Feb. 28th-29th, 1944.

or the progressive degenerative disease of the nervous system—multiple sclerosis—among the Northern Chinese, whose diet is inadequate in those things we can determine by laboratory analysis; namely, calcium, vitamins, calories, suggests that limited vitamin, mineral, and caloric value is not etiological of these diseases. They have their avitaminoses, their hypocalcemia even to the extent of osteomalacia, but not arteriosclerosis and multiple sclerosis as do their better-fed friends in Continental Europe, England and America. When their food is biologically assayed, who are better off—the Orientals or the Occidentals?

Are the agricultural practices of the Orient and those of Germany, for instance, the reason that multiple sclerosis is unseen in the Orient and so common in Germany? Natural manures have been used in the Orient for centuries, while chemical fertilizers have been championed by the German school of agriculture since 1840. Is this type of soil fertility a factor in giving a food to the population, which, in turn, tends to give them an immunity to arteriosclerosis, thrombophlebitis, multiple sclerosis, Gaucher's disease, renal calculi and gallstones—an immunity which the Chinese seem to have. Does the Oriental agricultural practice give an x value to food that makes its biological assay high in spite of the Chinese diet being low in chemical assay?

Does it follow that people who have an adequate diet will not have deficiency diseases, and, furthermore, may have better natural immunity to disease? The question that presents itself is—what is an adequate diet? Until the present the emphasis has been on the quantities of vitamins, minerals, proteins, fats, carbohydrates, and not on the quality of foods. We may be instructing our patients to ask the questions—how fresh is this food? From where did this food come? What was the nature of the soil fertility that grew this produce? Were natural manures or commercial fertilizers used on the land? What was the fungus and bacteria growth in the soil that grew this food? Was this vegetable grown on a mycorrhizal or non-mycorrhizal soil? What was the quality of the food fed this veal or that beef?

This question of food quality was brought to my attention by Colonel Henry W. Anderson, a lawyer by profession, a scholar by nature, and an agronomist by avocation, when he told me of his observations and presented me with a recent book, *An Agricultural Testament*, by Sir Albert Howard, C.I.E., M.A., formerly Director of the Institute of Plant Industry, Indore, and Agricultural Advisor in Central India and Rajputana. Sir Albert's discussion of the agricultural practices of the Orient caused me to recall that multiple (or disseminated) sclerosis is practically unknown in Japan and China (Miura, Pfister);[3] that there is some question whether one sees genuine pernicious anemia with its severe neurological complications in Northern China;[2] that, although syphilis is as frequent as the common cold in Korea, tabes was not once diagnosed by Wilson, who practiced there thirty years;[4] that there is a remarkable scarcity in China of arteriosclerosis, Gaucher's disease, kidney stones, gallstones and perhaps even thrombophlebitis.[2] (Snapper)

Is it not possible that Nature has presented us with a great many more pertinent facts in the geographic distribution of disease and health? The reasons for the presence and absence of certain diseases among the population of various parts of the world present a complicated and involved question. These natural experiments that are being made all over the world, due to a multiplicity of local circumstances, customs and habits, or changes forced on a people by war or poverty, make available a wealth of material for study and investigation.

What are some of the natural experiments that present material which we may use as indices of health and disease found here and there? And what are the agricultural practices of these respective locations, which may affect the quality of their food?

Heard[5] states: "Dental caries is rare in the town of Hereford and the County of Deaf Smith, Texas. . . . . . After twenty-eight years of interrogating my patients, together with my experience and observation, I am of the opinion that this phenomenon is due to our soil's richness in minerals and vitamins. The growing of plant foods has depleted the soil in most areas of the world of essential mineral elements; and our system of fertilization has failed to restore these elements in adequate quantities." He also comments: "Both physically and mentally this area furnishes superior zoölogical specimens."

McCarrison[6] records an observation: "My own experience provides an example of a race, unsurpassed in perfection of physique and in freedom from disease in general. . . . I refer to the people of the State of Hunza, situated in the extreme northernmost point of India. Amongst these people the span of life is extraördinarily long; and such service as I was able to render them during some seven years spent in their midst was confined chiefly to the treatment of accidental lesions, the removal of senile cataracts, plastic operations for granular eyelids, or the treatment of maladies wholly unconnected with food supply. Appendicitis, so common in Europe, was unknown. . . . It becomes obvious that the enforced restriction to the unsophisticated foodstuffs of nature is compatible with long life, continued vigor and perfect physique."

McCarrison[7] carried out in India some experiments on rats. He mentions first the many different native races of which the population, 350 million, is composed. After describing the experiments he concluded: "What I found in this experiment was that when young growing rats of healthy stock were fed on diets similar to those of people whose physique was good, the physique and health of the rats were good; when they were fed on diets similar to those of people whose physique was bad, the physique and health of the rats were bad; and when they were fed on diets similar to those of people whose physique was middling, the physique and health of the rats were middling."

I would like to mention two observations during World War No. 1—first, Hindhede[8] states: "In Denmark the people received a sufficiency of potatoes, whole-rye bread (containing wheat bran and 24 per cent of barley-meal), barley porridge, grains, milk, abundance of green vegetables and some butter. In consequence of this enforced alteration in the dietetic habits of the Danish people, the death rate dropped as much as 34 per cent, being as low as 10.4 per cent when the regimen had been in force for one year." Hindhede concludes that "the principal cause of death lies in food and drink." The second observation was by Demoor and Slosse,[9] who noted: "Despite the food restrictions imposed upon the people of Belgium during the late war, the infant mortality and infantile diarrhea have decreased greatly;" a circumstance, according to this article, which was "due to organized propaganda encouraging mothers to nurse their infants and to the establishment of national canteens which provided prospective mothers, from the fifth month of pregnancy onward, with eggs, milk, meat, and vegetables."

The Local Medical and Panel Committee of Cheshire, England,[7] representing 600 doctors, reviewed their 25-years experiences, stating: "There has been a fall in fatalities and this was all the more noticeable in view of the rise in sickness. . . . . This illness results from a lifetime of wrong nutrition." They point to the high incidence of bad teeth among English children in the British Isles, but this condition does not exist among their cousins on Tristan da Cunha; also, rickets is still common in England, while in Holland it is relatively rare; there butter, milk and cheese are plentiful. They further point to nutritional anemia and defective diet constipation." They go on to say: "It is far from the purpose of this paper to advocate a particular diet." They remark on the health and the diet of the Eskimos and the Hunzans and the English on Tristan de Cunha and say: "There is some principle or quality in these diets which is absent from, or deficient in, the food of our people today . . . . to decry some factors common to all of these diets is difficult, and an attempt to do so may be misleading since our knowledge of what those factors are is still far from complete; but this at least may be said—that the food is, for the most part, fresh from its source, little altered by preparation, and complete; and that, in the case of those based on agriculture, the natural cycle:

Animal and)   (Animal—)
Vegetable) — Soil — Plant — Food(Man
Waste   )   (———)

is complete: no chemicals or substitution stage intervenes."

This committee refers to the work of Sir Albert Howard, stating: "He has shown that the ancient Chinese method of returning to the soil, after treatment, the whole of animal and vegetable refuse which is produced in the activities of a community, results in the health and productivity of crops and of the animals and men who feed thereon."

In this article it is indicated, not only how bad teeth, rickets, anemia and constipation may be helped, but the observations of the family doctors revealed that the nutrition of expectant mothers was closely supervised in a Cheshire village, the diet being raw milk, butter, Cheshire cheese, oatmeal, eggs, broth, salad in abundance, green leaf vegetables, liver and fish weekly, fruit in abundance, meat and whole-meal bread made of two parts of locally grown wheat and one part of raw wheat-germ, the bread being baked within 36 hours after the milling of the flour. It was noted that mothers were usually able to feed their infants. The nursing mother's food continued as in pregnancy. The children were described as splendid, with perfect sets of teeth common; pulmonary diseases were almost unknown; they slept well, and one of their most striking features was their happy personality. The opinion was expressed: "The human material was entirely unselected, the food was not specially grown but that in spite of these imperfections, the practical application of McCarrison's work should yield recognizable results shows that in a single generation improvement of the race can be achieved."

Sir Albert Howard[10] points out: "Soil fertility is the condition which results from the operation of nature's round, from the orderly revolution of the wheel of life, from the adoption and faithful execution of the first principle of agriculture—there must always be a perfect balance between the processes of growth and the processes of decay. The consequences of this condition are a living soil, abundant crops of good quality, and livestock which possess the bloom of health. The key to a fertile soil and a prosperous agriculture is humus. Humus in the soil affects the plant directly by means of a middle man—fungus—producing the mycorrhizal relationship. Nature has provided an interesting piece of living machinery for joining up fertile soil with the plant."

Does it follow that the agricultural practices of the Orient account for the seeming absence of some of the degenerative diseases that we are more prone to have in America and Europe? Is the produce of our farmers using artificial fertilizer lacking in quality because the chemicals are not sufficient to give food quality? Is there a relationship between food produced on a soil rich in fungus and the absence of susceptibility to diseases of those who live on this food?

In agricultural literature the importance of these fungi in promoting growth and aiding nutrition has been emphasized.[11] Dubois (Rockefeller Foundation) cultured from the soil his gramicidin-producing fungus. Would there be anywhere near as much need for gramicidin and penicillin if our food were derived from a humus-rich soil prolific in its fungus growth? Has the Occidental agricultural practice of using commercial fertilizers been inadequate and destroyed the bacteria and fungus in the soil and, in turn, given us an inferior produce that has reduced our natural immunity to infections?

This paper is presented as a preliminary discussion, and the thoughts are merely suggestive. The scientific investigation of the sources of food supply in this country and the after effect upon health and disease, especially, as we have pointed out, degenerative diseases, has not gone far enough to justify definite conclusions. The observations are certainly indicative of possible fact, and stimulate us in our studies of this x quality factor in food. The studies and results of experiments already made by distinguished scientists, some of which have been mentioned, strongly indicate that efforts toward the prevention of diseases, especially of deficiency diseases and diseases of a degenerative character, and the consequent improvement of the health and happiness of the human race, demand a more thorough study of the sources of food supply, the methods of production, and the soils from which foods are produced. Nutrition is not a question of quantity only but of quality also.

Bibliography

1. MINOT, G. R.: Foreword to *Chinese Lessons to Western Medicine*, Snapper.
2. SNAPPER, I.: *Chinese Lessons to Western Medicine*. Interscience Publishers, Inc., N. Y., 1941.
3. BING and HAYMAKER: *Textbook of Nervous Diseases*. Mosby, 1939.
4. WILSON, R. M.: Impressions of Diet and Disease in Korea. *Virginia Medical Monthly*, Vol. 70, March, 1943.
5. HEARD, G. W., D.D.S.: Low Incidence of Dental Decay in a Texas County. *Southern Medicine & Surgery*, Dec., 1943.
6. MCCARRISON, R.: Studies in Deficiency Disease. *Oxford Medical Publications*, 1921.
7. MCCARRISON, R.: Nutrition, Soil Fertility and the National Health. *British Medical Journal*, 1939.
8. HINDHEDE: *Jour. A. M. A.*, Vol. 74, No. 6, Feb. 7, 1920.
9. DEMOOR and SLOSSE: *Bulletin l'Acad. Roy. de Med. de Belgique*, 1930.
10. HOWARD, SIR ALBERT: *An Agricultural Testament*. Oxford University Press, London, New York, Toronto, 1930.
11. MCCOMB, A. L.: Iowa State College of Agriculture and Mechanic Arts, *Research Bulletin*, Ames, Iowa, 1943.

Discussion

THE SECRETARY: I especially desired to have Dr. J. Adam Hayne talk about this subject. He did the finest job in the saving of life from a condition which is curable and preventable, to wit, pellagra, than any man in the whole world. He bought brewer's yeast, not by the pound, not by the ton, but by the carload, and distributed it in South Carolina, and he has saved more lives than any man that I know of.

DR. J. ADAMS HAYNE, Columbia: Gentlemen of the Tri-State Medical Association: I looked around among you and the young faces that I see before me and I think that 45 years ago I read a paper before this Association on "The Medicinal Treatment of Gall Stones." I remember with a good deal of shame having read such a paper, but that is what I thought at the time. I was nearly thrown out of the organization for saying the internist cleverly untied the Gordian knot while the surgeon deftly tied it

Pellagra is one of the things we have made a profound study of. We started in 1910 in Columbia with a Pellagra Conference, the first one held in this country. We had men from Romania, Egypt and Italy and all over the world to come there and discuss pellagra. There were just about as many theories as there were people present and no one had any solution. All the theories that you hear, from calcium up and down, were presented at this particular meeting. Goldberger was laughed at. Noguchi said it was the most unscientific study of a disease that was ever made by anyone who was supposed to be a scientist. The experiments in Mississippi were not based on any control of any sort. They took people out of the penitentiary that were there for crime and it was agreed if they developed any symptoms of pellagra they were to be turned loose. About the only thing that they did develop was a condition of the scrotum that was not then recognized as pellagra. Yet, Goldberger was on the right track and later on we had to agree that he had something that he made available as pellagra preventive or p.p.

We had in 1929 in South Carolina 950 deaths from that disease and 40,000 or 50,000 cases. Our asylum was full of people. It was no question of pellagra sine pellagra. It was all pellagra cum pellagra. We didn't have trouble finding pellagrins. They were everywhere. They went insane. They died. The veriest tyro in medicine could diagnose a case of pellagra, because there was nothing in the world like it. Nothing had ever been seen like it. There was a lot of discussion, as you heard in some of these papers, about it being here in 1850 and long before that, and all that, but until a surgeon in Alabama discovered it and wrote about it in 1908 nobody else ever thought of pellagra in this country. Manson, a great man on tropical diseases, said there was no pellagra in the United States. As mentioned by the essayist, many other men said the same thing. You can go back over the records and seem to think you see pellagra among the very poor people who ate corn bread, molasses and fatback. That was the diet of the South and that was said to be the occasion of pellagra, but they ate cornbread, molasses and fatback when I practiced medicine and they did not have pellagra.

The second paper gave some possible clue as to why pellagra occurred in the period from 1908 to 1930 in the South. It was at that time that it was first mentioned to us that nitrate of soda was a good preparation for fertilizer for grain and for other vegetables and other foods. Now the nitrate of soda as sold by the Chilean Government for the last five years has had the iodine taken out of it. For years it was sold with the iodine content and you may remember that South Carolina was known as the Iodine State and we had quite a lot of money spent on advertising that point. The reason why we had the iodine in South Carolina was because South Carolina used more nitrate of soda with iodine in it than any other state in the Union, and consequently the plants absorbed the iodine and analyses were made by scientific tests show more iodine than other parts of the United States.

DR. R. C. MILLER, Gastonia: I read a paper before the Gaston County Medical Society in 1936 on Pellagra. Dr. Copley mentioned that Dr. Sims improved with change of locality. My theory is that it is not vitamin deficiency at all. We have overlooked some element of the soil. The most important element of the soil is calcium. Sims went to New York where there is lime in the water. He got well of pellagra. If we check the calcium content of the blood, we may have something, because calcium is in the blood in two forms, available and non-available. It is like having a mortgage that you can't cash in when you want to pay off some of your debts.

In his third case there where his patient improved, he will probably find that she had some calcium in the water. I have cured numerous ones with one nickel's worth of lime water. I didn't change the diet, let them eat what they had been eating. It is cheap treatment, and it does not taste or smell nearly as bad as yeast and liver. There is little pellagra in hard-water sections.

DR. R. B. DAVIS, Greensboro: Last year a doctor friend of mine's baby showed allergy to eggs. I said, "Durham, I never heard of a baby who couldn't eat eggs when I was small." I believe they use fish mash to make hens lay. I get as many as 333 eggs a day and I haven't bought and don't intend to buy any fish mash. I have a 50-acre lot and the hens have all the vitamins and minerals they want. I said, "Let me feed your baby from my farm where no artificial food is used." The baby began eating those eggs and immediately recovered from the allergic condition and has had no more trouble that I know of. I don't know whether it can take city eggs or not because when the baby got well, Durham come for no more eggs.

DR. CLAY EVATT, Charleston: It is delightful to be here among this learned company where so many things of import are being definitely settled, and the last word has been said on pellagra. One of our doctors has some beautiful charts illustrating the Catamenic Age. During that period of life it seems four women die to one man. I would ask the learned ones whether or not that is due to endocrine deficiency, or is it that these women got to eat only what the men left?

DR. C. M. GILMORE, Greensboro: Dr. Shield opened up to medical men a vast new field of thought, of possible research and development. His work is, as yet, incomplete. As he goes on, I think he will uncover many other important data. Five or six thousand years of history confirm some of his speculations. It takes about 200 years of use without replenishing to exhaust the minerals and other native elements of soil. If you will check the civilization for the last 6000 years, with the exception of those soils locked by freezing six months of the year, the average climate in 200 years or 300, will show decline of a new civilization. There must be some connection between the properties of the soil and the characteristics of a people. We particularly need to study this problem here in our portion of the South because the hot weather, sunshine and frequent floods speed up the natural erosion and depletion of our soil. If we are to survive agriculturally and continue as a virile, hard-hitting, working, fighting people, then we must pay much more attention in the future, to the conservation, to the retaining of minerals and humus elements in our soil. I think that one factor, its absence or its presence in our soil has, we will find in the years to come, a far greater influence on our health, our virility, our daily life than any one has heretofore suspected.

DR. G. G. DIXON, Ayden, N. C.: Concerning pellagra, I saw my first case of it when I was an interne in the city of Detroit. The patient had been in the hospital for six weeks. All kinds of men in the city had undertaken to diagnose the condition. The A. M. A. met there at that particular time and a skin clinic was held and some of the Southern men said, "What a wonderful case of pellagra!"

Concerning the paper on modern trends of agriculture— I was reared in eastern North Carolina. The dairymen say they cannot raise milk to advantage in the east for the manufacture of cheese because we do not have sufficient lime in our soil. I know the eastern part of North Carolina and South Carolina are great pellagra centers and it only came after the South had risen from its destruction during the Civil War and gotten back to the place where we could buy commercial fertilizers, which by then had replaced the natural guano—sea-bird manure—formerly brought by dozens of shiploads from the coast and islands of Peru. Before the Civil War North Carolina, South Carolina and Georgia were considered the very best in the nation and the most of the meat consumed by the whole nation was grown in the South, so was bread—wheat and other grain. After the Civil War, the meat production center moved west. We produced some grain, further depleting our soil, but we had to use home-grown fertilizer. We were using mostly commercial fertilizer by 1900, and just a few years later we began to develop pellagra. Whether that has anything to do with it or not, I do not know.

DR. E. L. COPLEY, closing: I want to thank these gentlemen for their discussion of my paper. My father was a farmer and he used to send us out in pairs, a good worker and one not so good. I have the feeling that Dr. Northington, in arranging this program, was kind enough to place my paper along with the stimulating and provocative paper of Dr. Shield. I am glad that I have had the support of his excellent paper to help me with mine.

I want to say, in the matter of calcium, that I am very happy to know about it. I ran into Dr. Morrison Hutcheson some time back when I had a very ill patient and had tried nearly all the remedies on the patient, and I asked Dr. Hutcheson what he thought I'd better do about it. He said, "Suppose you leave off treatment. Maybe the patient will get well." Some fifteen years ago everybody apparently was using urotropin for urinary infections. We may find something better than nicotinamide for pellagra. At the present time I do feel that in preventing pellagra, it is a most effective agent and also in the treatment of these deficiencies.

DR. JAMES ASA SHIELD, closing: I want to thank the gentlemen for their discussion. This subject interested me immensely after it was brought to my attention, and as it was brought out by one of the discussers, there is a possi-

COPLEY & SHIELD—To P. 428

Meningococcemia*

ROY S. BIGHAM, JR., A.B., M.D., Baltimore, Maryland
Instructor in Medicine, Johns Hopkins Hospital

From the University of Virginia Hospital, Department of Internal Medicine

THE PRESENT tendency is to avoid distinctions in naming meningococcic diseases specifically. We speak of meningococcic infection and define the stage of the invasion present in the individual. The idea of infection of the meninges through the cribriform plate has been discarded, except in rare cases of fracture followed by clinical meningitis. We now visualize the meningococcus as a fairly common inhabitant of the upper respiratory tract, present in some 4 to 5 per cent of normal individuals and, under certain conditions of weather, environment, and associated respiratory diseases, found with increasing frequency up to a level of about 30 per cent, at which point clinical epidemics of infection seem to appear.

At any point during the stage of endemic or epidemic presence of the organism, under conditions which are not understood as yet, clinical manifestations of meningococcic infection may appear in the individual. In the simplest form, this infection appears as a nasopharyngitis distinguished from an ordinary sore throat or tonsillitis only by culture. This may progress to an invasion of the blood stream and the organisms, finally, may localize in the joints, lungs, meninges, skin, or even in several of these locations. The infection may stop its spread at any stage and may even regress spontaneously. Localization in the meninges has been by far the most common manifestation and is the usual picture brought to mind when we speak of "meningococcic infection." The Waterhouse-Friedrichson syndrome, however, is a meningococcic septicemia frequently unaccompanied by meningitis and such localizations as meningococcic arthritis and sinusitis are described unaccompanied by meningitis.

Since the advent of the sulfonamide drugs, earlier treatment of meningococcic infections has become feasible and, by the same token, earlier recognition of the stages and types of infection has become necessary and desirable.

We are concerned primarily in this report with the stage of infection consisting of invasion of the blood stream, and more particularly with that group of infections consisting of septicemia (1) without demonstrable focus and (2) of long duration. In this respect we avoid those cases which are acute when first seen and in which ordinarily death or progress to clinical meningitis is a matter of a few hours or a day or so at most. We also exclude the occasional case of meningococcic endocarditis which may extend over some weeks or months before death, because a definite localization of infection and thus a focus of recurring bacteremia is present. A dividing line cannot be drawn sharply, but we would not feel justified in calling a case true chronic meningococcemia with a history of less than two to three weeks' duration.

The following case is, we believe, a typical example:

A 29-year-old white man employed in highway maintenance, first seen as an out-patient in the University of Virginia Hospital on June 7th, 1943, complained of episodes of chills, fever and pains in the calves of both legs. Attacks had occurred 14 and 3 days previously, on each occasion with the appearance of pink spots on the arms and legs. Each attack lasted three days. He was asymptomatic and afebrile and was advised to return at the time of the next attack. The impression, because of the history of associating the symptoms with unusual food intake, was a possible allergic reaction.

The following day he was seen in the emergency room with t. of 102° and a maculopapular rash over the thorax, arms and legs. These lesions differed from urticaria in having fairly sharp margins. They were pale pink and 0.5 to 1.0 cm. in diameter. No central red spots were noted. Because of the history, a test dose of adrenalin was administered—without effect. He was unable to enter the hospital at the time, but returned for admission 12 hours later. Temperature then was 98.6°; he was asymptomatic except for residual soreness in the legs; skin lesions were not recorded. The examiner advised him, again, to return during an attack.

On July 3rd, he was admitted during an attack, the seventh in a period of less than six weeks. The first two attacks were ushered in by a chill, but in the succeeding spells, a prodromal stage of several hours, during which he was drowsy and irritable, preceded the chill, according to the patient's wife. The chills were always severe and lasted for as long as 30 minutes, following which an eruption described as "pink spots the size of a bean" would appear on the trunk, arms and legs. These areas were not painful or pruritic and, as we recorded, were attributed during the two initial attacks to eating tomatoes. Fever persisted for 12 hours after the chill and was followed by cramping in the calf muscles. The whole course of events would last 12-24 hours and he usually resumed work on the following day, not being hampered by the residual soreness in the legs.

The patient was well developed but slightly undernourished, mentally alert and in no obvious discomfort. Temperature was 101.8°, p. 80, r. 20, b. p. 130/68. The skin was hot and dry. A moderate number of scattered erythematous maculopapular lesions, from 0.5 to 1.0 cm. in

---

*Presented to Tri-State Medical Association of the Carolinas and Virginia, meeting at Charlotte, Feb. 28th-29th, 1944.

diameter, were present over the trunk, arms and legs, most prominent on the abdomen, flexor surfaces of the forearms and upper legs. The rash faded on pressure, but a red central spot, which did not fade, was present in several of the lesions. The conjunctivae were slightly injected. An old herniorrhaphy scar was present in the right lower quadrant. Physical examination was otherwise negative.

Erythrocytes were normal, leukocyte count 16,400 with a shift to the left in the neutrophile series. Urine, stool, and serological test for syphilis were negative. No malaria parasites were found in smears. Agglutinations for Brucella abortus and suis, Eberthella typhosa (H antigen), Salmonella paratyphosi A and B, Pasteurella tularense, and the O strains of Proteus X-19, X-2 and X-K were negative. Brucellergen intradermal test was negative, as were blood cultures for Brucella abortus.

The leukocyte count fell to normal and the patient became afebrile and asymptomatic on the second hospital day. He was kept under observation in the hope of observing a complete attack, but another episode did not materialize and he was discharged after six days.

A blood culture taken on July 3rd, and kept under observation for Brucella abortus, was reported as positive for Neisseria meningitidis on July 16th, four days after the patient was discharged. A culture taken from the nasopharynx on July 8th also showed a colony of N. meningitidis at this time.

The patient was communicated with and he was readmitted to the hospital on July 19th, having had no further attacks in the preceding week. Examination and routine laboratory procedures were negative. He was given sulfadiazine, 6 gm. daily, for six days, at the end of which time 4 nasopharyngeal and 3 blood cultures were negative. Röntgenological examinations of the teeth and sinuses, as well as clinical examination of the teeth, sinuses, nasopharynx, and throat were negative.

The patient had been asymptomatic for more than three months and had had three further negative blood and nasopharyngeal cultures for N. meningitidis when last seen.

Chronic meningococcemia was first described as a syndrome by Solomon in 1902,[1] the acute phase of meningococcic septicemia having been recognized several years earlier. Most of the early reports are in the foreign literature, and in 1934 the ratio of foreign to American reports was stated to be 6:1.[2] Carbonell and Campbell reviewed the American literature in 1938 and presented 33 cases, including three of their own.[3] Several new series appeared, including those of Applebaum[5] and Heinle,[6] together with many individual case reports,[7,8,9,10,11] so that in 1942 Ney, Semisch and Merves were able to collect about 70 cases.[4]

In the past one and one-half years, meningococcic infections have increased in frequency, particularly in Army establishments, and there has apparently been a concomitant rise in the frequency of meningococcemia.[16] This rise may be due, in part, to better recognition of the disease and earlier observation of patients, since relatively few cases were reported following similar outbreaks of infection due to N. meningitidis in 1918.

However, in November of 1943 Campbell was able to add three new cases of his own and enough reports from the literature to bring his series of American cases to 88.[20] I have presented one case and have a second unreported case from University of Virginia Hospital records, treated with serum in the pre-sulfonamide days and terminating fatally from septicemia some nine months after the initial symptoms. This patient was a 56-year-old white housewife who had the clinical syndrome and who in addition passed through an attack of meningitis during the fourth month of her illness. Her death occurred after the development of serum sensitivity and cessation of treatment. Her blood cultures were repeatedly positive for N. meningitidis and she presented intermittant chills and fever, headache, myalgia, nausea and vomiting, a palpable spleen and a skin rash, symptoms occurring at intervals of about three weeks and lasting for periods of from 3 to 30 days.

In addition to these, I have personal knowledge of two other unreported cases which fit our criteria of prolonged septicemia without demonstrable focus, both in the past year. Two large series concerning meningococcic infections from Army installations[16,17] and one from a metropolitan hospital[15] in the last six months have presented, respectively, 32, 13 and 8 cases of meningococcemia, some of which are certainly chronic. The syndrome is mentioned, but no cases quoted specifically, in still another recent paper.[18] We may assume that the number of American cases reported has, in the past five years, been at least three times the number reported in the previous thirty years. Clinical recognition of this syndrome, then, is proceeding rapidly and cases are no longer as rare as they once appeared to be.

The epidemiology of meningococcemia is no better understood than that of meningococcic infections in general. Meningococcemia seems to be more prevalent in the present exacerbation of meningococcic infections, but the majority of the case reports of chronic meningococcemia have concerned sporadic and endemic cases. One case has been reported following the occurrence of meningitis in two other members of the same family.[12] The only reported multiple cases in one family occurred several years apart, in mother and son.[13]

Contact cases for meningitis itself are rare and no studies have been carried out with meningococcemia. Cross-infection, however, is suggested in the fact that two visitors in the home of our recent patient, his sister-in-law and a nephew, were found to have nasopharyngeal cultures positive for N. meningitidis. Aside from one report of a meningococcic sinus infection associated with meningococcemia,[14] there is no evidence to support the association of foci with meningococcemia. A careful focal hunt in our case failed to show any localized infection other than the presence of the organism in the nasopharynx.

The syndrome has been found predominantly in males (69%) and the average age is about 29.[20] The course may run from two weeks upward, averaging about twelve weeks. One case has been reported as presenting attacks over a period of 14 years.[6]

The symptoms of intermittent chills and fever, arthritis or arthralgia, and a rash constitute the outstanding clinical manifestations. Campbell[04] gives the following percentages in his 88 cases:

		%
1.	Fever	93.4
2.	Rash	88.8
3.	Arthralgia	62.5
4.	Chills	54.5
5.	Headache	45
6.	Myalgia	25
7.	Arthritis	13.6
8.	Vomiting	11.4
9.	Palpable spleen	11.4
10.	Sore throat	10.3
11.	Sweating	10.3
12.	Weakness	8
13.	Herpes	5.7
14.	Epistaxis	4.5

The fever is characteristically intermittent. It may follow a tertian, quartan, or quotidian curve, but is different from some gonococcic septicemias in, apparently, never showing a double quotidian type of curve. The curves may reach 102-105°.

The rash may vary from a frankly hemorrhagic area to small erythematous macules. A central hemorrhagic spot is not invariable. Not infrequently, as in our case, the lesions resemble those of erythema nodosum, but are far more transient.

Pains in the back and legs are usually present and pain in the joints may occur. These are usually unaccompanied by any objective changes, such as redness and swelling, however.

The headache, when present, is generalized and severe, but is not as severe or incapacitating as the headache of meningococcic meningitis. Nausea and vomiting may accompany the more severe headaches.

A palpable spleen can usually be found in the cases of long duration of the infection.

The disease may be suspected from the clinical picture presented, but absolute diagnosis cannot be made unless the organism is identified in the blood stream. The cultural characteristics of Neisseria meningitidis present certain difficulties which are not insuperable providing care is taken in suspected cases. The blood is more likely to yield a positive culture if taken at the height of a febrile reaction, but will also give a high percentage of positives at any stage. We grew the organism from dextrose carbonate broth, with added paraäminobenzoic acid. A more rapid growth, however, is to be expected from a blood medium under decreased oxygen tension. A culture on a plain broth medium should not be considered negative in a period of less than two weeks.

A more rapid diagnostic aid suitable for bedside use has been described.[19] This depends entirely on the presence of petechial lesions, and when such small hemorrhagic areas can be found in the skin lesions, intracellular diplococci may sometimes be identified by staining tissue juice obtained from the center of the area.

Prior to the development of the sulfonamide series of drugs, treatment of this condition was limited to serum or vaccine, or to no treatment at all. The death rate was 12.3 per cent in these cases. Since the introduction of sulfanilamide and the later drugs of this group and their use in the management of meningococcemia, only two deaths have been reported,[4,6] both in the early days of the sulfonamides and neither in a case treated with a sulfonamide alone. The cautious statement made by Heinle in 1938, that "sulfanilamide seems to be the treatment of choice" would seem to be adequately confirmed.

Endocarditis has been observed in meningococcemia, and while the continued bacteremia may be secondary in these cases to an original implantation on a valve, the possibility of endocarditis occurring as a complication of prolonged meningococcemia from an unknown focus cannot be ignored. The fatality rate of meningococcic endocarditis is very high.

Meningococcic meningitis is occasionally followed by a chronic meningococcemia as a complication; but the reverse, the development of clinical meningitis in a case of meningococcemia, is far more likely to occur. If early recognition and treatment of the meningococcemia is obtained, there are no complications. However, if the case progresses to meningitis, the sequelae of the meningitis, regardless of treatment, are frequent enough to be of concern to both the physician and the patient.

Summary

1. An increased incidence of chronic meningococcemia might have been expected and is to be found at the present time, accompanying the general rise in the incidence of meningococcic infections.

2. The disease can be recognized clinically and the diagnosis confirmed with relative ease by the practitioner.

3. While management of the complications is difficult or unsatisfactory, chemotherapy of chronic meningococcemia is highly satisfactory both as regards survival and absence of disability.

Bibliography

1. SALOMON, H.: Uber Meningokokkenseptikamie. Berl. klin. wchnschr., 39:1045, 1902.
2. RICHTER, A. B.: Meningococcemia. J. A. M. A., 102:2012, 1934.
3. CARBONELL, A., & CAMPBELL, E.: Prolonged meningococcemia. Arch. Int. Med., 61:646, 1938.
4. NYE, R., SEMISCH, C., & MERVES, L.: Chronic meningococcemia complicated by acute endocarditis. Ann. Int. Med., 16:1245, 1939.
5. APPLEBAUM, E.: Chronic meningococcus septicemia. Am. J. Med. Sci., 193:96, 1937.
6. HEINLE, R. W.: Meningococcic septicemia. Arch. Int. Med., 63:575, 1939.
7. CRAVEN, E. B., JR.: Chronic meningococcic septicemia. South. Med. & Surg., 101:367, 1939.
8. FRIEDMAN, J. J., & BUCHANAN, J. A.: Chronic meningococcemia. New York State J. Med., 39:1662, 1939.
9. KATTWINKEL, E. E.: Meningococcemia. New England J. Med., 224:685, 1941.
10. HAYES, M. G.: Meningococcic septicemia. Northwest. Med., 40:284, 1941.
11. WATSON, L. D.: Meningococcemia without meningitis. New England J. Med., 225:685, 1941.
12. LEMANN, I. I., & TEASLEY, H. E.: Meningococcemia following meningitis. New Orleans M. & S. J., 83:448, 1931.
13. CLARKE, F. B.: Chronic meningococcemia. California & West. Med., 34:361, 1931.
14. HERRICK, W. W.: Extrameningeal meningococcus infections. Arch. Int. Med., 23:409, 1919.
15. SMITH, H. W., THOMAS, L., DINGLE, J. H., & FINLAND, M.: Meningococcic infections. Ann. Int. Med., 20:12, 1944.
16. DANIELS, W. B., SOLOMON, S., & JAQUETTE, W. H.: Meningococcic infections in soldiers. J. A. M. A., 123:1, 1943.
17. HILL, L. W., & LEVER, H. S.: Meningococcic infection in an army camp. J. A. M. A., 123:9, 1943.
18. ADAMS, F. D.: Clinical aspects of meningococcic infection. Ann. Int. Med., 20:33, 1944.
19. TOMPKINS, V. N.: Diagnostic value of smears from purpuric lesions of the skin in meningococcic disease. J. A. M. A., 123:31, 1943.
20. CAMPBELL, E. P., Meningococcemia. Am. J. Med. Sci., 206:566, 1943.

Discussion

DR. K. B. PACE, Greenville, N. C.: Dr. Bigham covered the subject thoroughly. Chronic cases keep us busy keeping up with them. For us in general practice diagnosis is even more important, than for those of you who are expected to require more time.

I have recently seen two cases of meningitis, one that of a man 40 years old, which began with unconsciousness. His wife weighed 250 pounds, and she shook him for an hour and failed to wake him. Since that didn't wake him, I realized that he was really unconscious. Some of these cases are not nearly as rapid as others. That gives a much better chance to get the drug in time.

As brought out, sulfadiazine is the drug of choice. I have seen recently an acute case in a girl of 17. She came home from school at 4 o'clock and at 5 had a terrific headache and in an hour was unconscious. She had vomiting and high fever and she was started within two hours' time on large doses of sulfadiazine and within four days was well on the way to recovery.

I have seen a great many of these cases treated by baby specialists and to us, it is almost unbelievable the large doses of sulfadiazine they use in children of six weeks to four months. Evidently, if they can stand the dose, that is what they need.

DEATHS FROM ASTHMA
(F. M. Rackeman, in Jl. Allergy, 15:249-258)

Suffocation from complete occlusion of smaller bronchi by mucus plugs is the immediate cause of deaths which occur during a severe paroxysm of asthma.

The duration of asthma and mode of death in each of 50 patients who died with asthma and were examined postmortem are shown. The pathologic conditions described were found in 27 of these.

Among the younger patients seven who had asthma of the extrinsic (probably allergic) type, which began early in life, died from complicating conditions, such as pneumonia. Other younger patients had had asthma since about the age of 20, with progression until death in the early 30s; in none was a specific allergen demonstrable and death occurred from pneumonia, acute cor pulmonale or coronary disease.

Twenty-eight individuals with asthma beginning between the ages of 40 and 50 died suddenly in an asthmatic seizure. The disease in several of these patients was of short duration and probably not of allergic origin. Drug sensitivity, especially to aspirin, may have been a precipitating factor in some instances. Several of the older patients died in the emergency ward after receiving morphine, a warning that this drug should not be used for patients with severe asthma. Bacterial allergy, perverted reflexes from the nose and throat, endocrine disturbances, vitamin deficiencies, degenerative pulmonary fibrosis and pulmonary fibrosis and arteriosclerosis are other possible etiologic considerations.

Bronchial obstruction in younger individuals, particularly those in whom the asthma is primarily allergic, is generally due to bronchial spasm with edema, but little or no exudate. Death in such a case is similar to that from anaphylactic shock induced in guinea pigs.

In older patients bronchial obstruction results primarily from plugs of tenacious, viscid mucus in the small bronchioles; bronchial spasm is associated in some cases.

IT IS PROBABLE that, if laymen were educated to consult a physician within one month after the onset of symptoms and the physician utilized only digital rectal examination, proctosigmoidoscopy, and barium enema, the curability rate of carcinoma of the rectum and colon would be doubled.—*H. L. Bockus.*

ABNORMAL UTERINE BLEEDING, not only at the time of the menopause but at any period in a woman's life, demands prompt and thorough pelvic examination, adequate investigation and appropriate treatment.—*L. C. Scheffey.*

COPLEY & SHIELD—From P. 424

bility of a lot of explanations, a lot of things we may learn by studying the geography of disease.

I can't tell you anything about the death ratio of women to men, but I have been very much impressed with the fact that the capacity to reproduce seems to be associated with agricultural practices. In some observations made and recorded by Mace in New Zealand, he found there in a study of deficiency diseases that they have had a lot of trouble with their sheep. There was a paralysis among their sheep for several years and they thought it was due to cobalt deficiency. However, they continued to have trouble with their cattle's low fertility and high death rate, and Mace reports that by changing the practice of agriculture over a four-year period and discontinuing use of commercial fertilizers and using a natural manure and following that applying humus to the soil, the sterility of cattle was reduced from 28 per cent to 2 per cent.

The Interpretation and Treatment of the Discharging Breast*

J. D. GILLAND, M.D., Charlotte

THIS SUBJECT is chosen for the reason that too often this clinico-pathological syndrome is very perplexing. To intelligently interpret, evaluate and lay out a plan of therapy, its clinical significance must be clearly understood. Discharge is well recognized as indicative of morbid changes within the ductile and secretory systems of the breast, but it affords in itself scant information concerning the provocative factor. The heads of clinics, who see large numbers of breast cases and are able to draw statistical conclusions, vary so in their statistics and express opinions so diverse as to be matched by few other clinical problems. A discharge from the nipple of a non-lactating breast is frequently the initial sign which impels the patient to seek medical advice. No one has claimed, except in the rare cases of true vicarious menstruation, that bleeding can come from a healthy breast.

Incidence: In 8 per cent of all mammary lesions, some type of discharge occurs from the nipple—a sanguinous discharge in 6 per cent. Of early signs of cancer of the breast discharge from the nipple is second only to the presence of a lump. It is the first sign in 1 per cent of all breast cancers, and 4 per cent of breast cancers discharge. Bleeding from the nipple occurs with equal frequency in malignant and benign conditions. One-half of benign tumors, having a discharge, are papillomatous; 47 per cent of duct papillomata discharge blood. There is a discharge in 7 to 15 per cent of cases of chronic cystic mastitis. The incidence of mammary cancer is only 9 per cent in cases of discharge from the nipple, *without* a palpable mass; 75 per cent of discharges are due to three lesions—cancer, chronic cystic mastitis and ductal papilloma. The papilloma and chronic cystic mastitis with epithelial hyperplasia is regarded as precancerous. The age at which bleeding occurs in the malignant cases is about that of the usual appearance of cancer. As far as can be determined, there is no indication that having nursed predisposes to bleeding breasts, malignant or benign.

Types of Discharge: The amount, color, consistency and odor of the discharge depend on the nature of the causative lesion and the degree to which the secretion is altered before reaching the surface of the nipple. If bleeding arises near the orifice of a duct, the escaping fluid is frankly hemorrhagic; but if the site is deep within the matrix, the fluid may assume a serosanguinous or a serous character or even a brownish chocolate color, due to the degeneration of the retained blood and its admixture with other secretions from the duct. The character of the discharge may also be altered by infection or necrosis.

Blood is discharged in such a variety of pathologic conditions in the breast as to possess little diagnostic value. In the absence of trauma or a palpable tumor, it is most likely to be caused by a papilloma of the duct. It is imperative that the primary cause be determined. The bloody discharge may be of traumatic origin, and if so, is easily recognized by the history and on examination there may be evidence of ecchymoses. Carcinoma cannot be excluded because the discharge is free of blood. In only half such cases is the discharge bloody.

A *serous* discharge from the nipple is, in too many cases, regarded as inconsequential. A thin, clear, straw-colored fluid escapes from the breast in 10 per cent of all cases of sarcoma; in many cases of carcinoma. Early the discharge may be serous, and as degenerative changes occur it become hemorrhagic. A mammary cancer may produce a serohemorrhagic discharge from one duct and a serous discharge from an adjacent duct. A serous discharge is seldom a feature of papilloma. Serous fluid comprises 22 per cent of all discharges.

A thick, *greenish-yellow* discharge from the nipple, usually bilateral, does not discharge itself spontaneously, and is caused by the retention of secretion in dilated ducts following lactation. A mild secondary infection combined with the degenerative products of desquamation may account for the color of the discharge.

Occasionally a *whitish* discharge will seep from the nipples of the newborn, in which instance both breasts are hypertrophied, tense and tender. All symptoms subside spontaneously within two or three days. Sometimes a milky fluid escapes from virginal breasts during pregnancy. Retarded post-lactation involution may cause a spontaneous leakage of milk for several months after active nursing has been discontinued. The discharge may contain pus, or in rare cases, masses of desquamated epithelial cells.

---
*Presented to Tri-State Medical Association of the Carolinas and Virginia, meeting at Charlotte, Feb. 28th-29th, 1944.

Etiology of Discharge: The three most common causes of discharge from the breast are duct papilloma, carcinoma and chronic cystic mastitis, in that order of frequency. Other causative factors: non-specific infection of dilated ducts, endocrine factors (as yet unconfirmed), trauma, sarcoma, fibroadenoma, luetic mastitis, tuberculous mastitis, Paget's disease of the nipple, inflammatory cysts and fibrous mastitis.

Examination of the Breast: Inspect and *palpate* in the upright and the supine position; palpate between the hand and chest wall, between the two hands, and between the thumb and fingers. In spite of the accessibility of the mammary gland, few small infiltrating carcinomata, papillomata, dilated lactiferous ducts or compressible cysts can be palpated. The presence of a small lesion, such as a papilloma, is occasionally demonstrated by the positive pressure test, whereby pressure over a constant segment within or near the areolar border or in the periphery of the breast causes a discharge to emit from the nipple.

Transillumination will distinguish between a solid tumor and a cyst containing clear fluid, and will often reveal impalpable papilloma which may be multiple. The character of the opacity does not diefferentiate between benign and malignant tumors. Blood is intensely opaque. The most striking feature of transillumination of the normal breast is the prominence of the blood vessels. If the papilloma has not bled it may escape detection, as opacity is usually due to the collection of blood about it. It is important to emphasize that minute papillomata may fail to cast shadows, even when the intensity of the light is reduced to a minimum.

Soft-tissue *röntgenography* has failed to clearly depict the identifying characteristics of mammary neoplasms. All pathologic conditions with a discharge from the breast must originate within or secondarily involve the ductile system. Any procedure, therefore, which visualizes the lactiferous ducts should possess diagnostic value. A technic of contrast röntgenograms has been developed. A radiopaque material, such as stabilized thorium dioxide, is introduced into the milk ducts by cannulating their orifices with a blunt 26-gauge needle. By use of stereoscopic röntgenograms an alteration in the size, shape or conformation of these ducts can be detected readily and the causative agent identified. The possibility of serious tissue reactions to the radiopaque material, plus the possibilities of diagnostic error, minimize the value of mammographic studies.

Microscopic examination of the discharge is often necessary in order to demonstrate the presence of blood, but is of no help in revealing the presence of malignant cells. The attempt to diagnose a carcinoma under these circumstances requires a special knowledge of the differentiation of morphological appearances of benign, inflamed and atypical epithelial cells, from those definitely malignant. The absence of malignant epithelial cells does not negative the diagnosis.

Frozen-section diagnosis of lesions manifesting a nipple discharge is sometimes difficult, because early or uncommon types of cancer may be encountered for the diagnosis of which permanent sections may be necessary. Upon the microscopic study of the cells of the lesion the final diagnosis is obtained. It is on this diagnosis that additional surgery may be done, radiation therapy instituted, and the prognosis given.

Interpretation: Unless there are contraindications, every benign tumor should be removed, lest it become malignant. In any case of tumor with bleeding, surgery should be adopted to reach a diagnosis, and a local or radical excision carried out accordingly. It is important to realize that bleeding from such a tumor is not even presumptive evidence that it is malignant. Bleeding should not stampede one into a radical operation; a complete mastectomy, even, is not indicated unless there are multiple lesions or other conditions which would, without discharge, indicate mastectomy. Any woman who has had a local operation for a condition presenting a discharge should be watched with extra care at more frequent intervals than usual; for we know that multiple lesions may and do exist and the lesion previously excised may not be the one responsible for the discharge. Repetition of the discharge demands careful consideration of more extensive removal. In discharging breasts with no demonstrable tumor, it is exceedingly difficult to determine the best procedure. The unnecessary removal of a breast is a calamity. Some students of this question, however, hold the opinion that bleeding from the breast is an exceedingly grave symptom, often demanding operative interference. To await the clinical detection of a gross lesion may spell the difference between a prevented or cured malignant growth, and the palliative removal of a malignant breast. When a tumor cannot be demonstrated by any method, the proper safeguard will usually be removal of the entire breast. Papilloma may be single, or multiple (30% of cases); and, when multiple, they may be found in separate ducts. A papilloma may become malignant: the majority of papillary carcinomata are thought to represent a late development in pre-existing benign papillomata. The carcinomata associated with nipple discharge are often the more localized, slowly-growing papillary or comedo types. One never knows from a clinical examination whether there is only one papilloma or many papillomata, or whether there is or is not a carcinoma. These matters cannot be decided by anything else than a careful examination with many microscopic sections of the whole breast.

Therapy: The method of treatment in cases of discharging breast must be influenced by the number of cases of cancer of the breast in which a discharge occurs, and upon the incidence of malignancy which ultimately follows such a sign. Individualization in therapy is one of the secrets of success in the handling of breast cases. The case in which both tumor and discharge are present arouses no controversy. The presence of the mass is an indication for surgery, independent of discharge. The troublesome and dangerous problem is the discharging breast which, on examination, contains no mass. The surgeon should offer no apology for performing many biopsies and, finally, simple mastectomy rather than local excision in borderline cases, where the picture suggests the possibility of carcinoma. However, the psychic and cosmetic arguments against mastectomy are prominent in the minds of patients, and demand consideration. There are both operative and non-operative forms of therapy, each adequate in specific cases.

Operative—1. When transillumination demonstrates an area of opacity in one of the large ducts near the nipple, the diagnosis of probable papilloma may be made. Local excision of the offending duct is indicated. A technic that is satisfactory for identifying the diseased duct is that of canalizing with a blunt needle or probe the duct orifice from which the discharge may be expressed. An incision is then made at the areolar border and the duct is distinguished by tilting the inserted needle. The offending duct is thus removed.

2. In those cases exhibiting a positive pressure sign, a local excision of the duct or a block excision of a segment should be done.

3. Breasts exhibiting a localized nodularity should have quadrant excision or a simple mastectomy.

4. Breasts manifesting a generalized nodularity should have a simple mastectomy. Localized or diffuse "shottiness" is apt to present a picture of epithelial overgrowth—potentially malignant.

5. In case of discharge after the menopause, the psychic and cosmetic arguments against mastectomy are so weakened, and the threat of cancer so real, it is safer to do a simple mastectomy, unless some definite local lesion can be identified.

6. One should not hesitate to advise and perform a simple mastectomy for continued bleeding of undetermined origin of one month or more.

Non-operative: It must be borne in mind that all cases treated medically are done so empirically, without a definite diagnosis.

1. Radiation of the discharging breast will stop the discharge in half the cases; but in some, cessation is only temporary.

2. Dilatation of the duct with the injection of sclerosing solutions has been tried, and, while the discharge may cease, such a procedure is not recommended.

3. Good results have been obtained after estrogen therapy in some women in whose breast bleeding occurred at the time of the menopause. This postulates a lobular proliferation of epithelium due to a deranged hormonal physiology, and has clinical and experimental evidence in support. The therapy rests upon the clinical diagnosis, and the clinical diagnosis in this age-group is not to be relied upon to this extent.

4. If trauma is established beyond all doubt to be the etiological factor, leave the breast alone and the hemorrhage will stop.

5. Observation may be the treatment of choice —the facts in each case to be carefully analyzed.

Further aids in individualizing patients with a breast discharge as to surgery may be had from a consideration of the following facts: (1) the age of the patient; (2) the duration of the discharge; (3) the type of discharge; (4) a family history of cancer; (5) the size of the breast; (6) the psychology of the patient, and (7) the question of an adequate follow-up, essential to a program of observation. Errors in treatment may be avoided if exploration be instituted, and the most suspicious zone excised and examined microscopically. A discharge from the nipple with or without a palpable tumor is a surgical condition.

SUMMARY

1. A discharge from the nipple of a non-lacting breast is a warning sign of exceedingly grave significance.

2. A discharge occurs from the breast in equal proportions in benign and malignant conditions.

3. Seventy-five per cent of such discharges are due to three lesions: cancer, chronic cystic mastitis and ductal papilloma. The papilloma and chronic cystic mastitis, with epithelial hyperplasia, are regarded as precancerous.

4. The character of the discharge cannot be relied upon to identify the underlying etiologic factor.

5. Given a case of a discharging breast, every effort should be made to arrive at a definite diagnosis, using any or all of our means of physical examination.

6. Interpretation of this important sign revolves about the presence or absence of a demonstrable mass.

7. In discharging breasts in which a mass is detected, the treatment is of the mass and not the

discharge, and should be the removal of the tumefaction for histological study. The differential diagnosis must be made with a microscope. Excised tissue is always sent to a pathologist. Should malignancy be encountered, radical treatment is instituted at once.

8. Various forms of therapy are presented for the handling of those cases in which no tumefaction is detected.

Conclusions

In the light of all that has been said, I feel that it is imperative in protracted discharge from the nipple, either continuous or intermittent, regardless of its character and regardless of whether a tumor is demonstrable, be given serious consideration; and that, in most instances, the bleeding tissue be removed, in order that the exact nature of the lesion may be determined. If a palpable tumor is present, a local excision may suffice. If several tumors or diffuse thickening can be felt, or if no tumor can be demonstrated, the entire breast should be removed. All cases, no matter how treated, should be watched with unusual care. Important cancer-preventive surgery can and should be performed and the surgeon will occasionally be rewarded by the discovery of an early, impalpable cancer.

Case History

A 40-year-old colored woman, admitted to Good Samaritan Hospital, Charlotte, on October 19th, 1943.

C. C. Bleeding from the left breast.

P. I. On October 17th, two days prior to admission, patient first noticed a soreness in the left breast, and on that date blood was expressed from the nipple. The patient attributes her present illness to the lid of a victrola falling on her left breast last summer (1943), after which the breast was sore for two weeks.

Patient has had 12 pregnancies, has 12 children, the baby being 18 months of age. One menstruation has occurred since last delivery.

T. P. R.—Normal. B. P. 130/82, middle-aged, very obese, seemingly in good health and free of distress.

Both breasts are very large, pendulous, symmetrical. Right: Non-tender, normal to palpation, no masses. Left: No definite mass palpated, though there is a sense or feel of increased nodularity throughout. An area of tenderness is present mesial to the nipple and pressure on this area causes a small amount of dark reddish-brown fluid to be extruded from the nipple. No glands palpable beyond the breast.

No specific diagnosis but this onset of bleeding considered a warning sign of grave significance.

I had the choice of three courses—

1. *Observation*— considered unwise.

2. *Local excision*—of the segment mesial to the nipple—considered inadequate, because of inability to obtain a frozen section at this hospital and to follow through with a more radical operation, if malignancy were reported.

3. *Mastectomy*—which was done. A left simple mastectomy was performed on October 20th. A simple, rather than a radical, operation because of hesitancy to do a radical without a positive pathological report of a malignancy and if it was malignant, it was an early malignancy.

It was about a foot away from the chest wall and a simple mastectomy should thus suffice. Mastectomy was decided on because:

1. I considered the percentage incidence in favor of malignancy.

2. If it was malignant, it was an early lesion and I could probably effect a cure.

3. If it was benign, the patient had lost little compared to what she would gain if it was malignant.

4. The breast would probably never be used again functionally.

5. If I had done some other procedure, and the lesion had been malignant, the patient may have succumbed to a cancer death in a few years, and there would then be 12 little motherless Negro children.

Pathological Report: "Involuting breast with atypical glandular and ductal epithelium with hemorrhage at nipple. The case is to be looked upon as a border-line case. The epithelial hyperplasia is intraductal."—Dr. Paul Kimmelstiel.

The patient left the hospital on the 9th day, post-operative, in good general condition. The incision had healed by primary union.

Bibliography

1. Adair, F. E.: Sanguineous Discharge from the Nipple, Relation to Cancer of the Breast. *Ann. Surg.*, 91:197, 1930.
2. Babcock, W. W.: A Simple Operation for the Discharging Nipple. *Surgery*, 4:914, 1938.
3. Cheatle, G. L., & Cutler, Max: *Tumors of the Breast*. J. B. Lippincott Co., Philadelphia, 1931.
4. Cutler, Max: Transillumination as an Aid in the Diagnosis of Breast Lesions. *S., G. & O.*, 48:721, 1929.
5. Davidoff, R. B., & Friedman, H. F.: The Treatment of Discharge from the Nipple. *New Eng. J. of M.*, 216:1072, 1937.
6. Geschichter, C. F.: *Diseases of the Breast*. J. B. Lippincott Co., Philadelphia, 1943.
7. Gray, H. K., & Wood, G. A.: Significance of Mammary Discharge in Cases of Papilloma of the Breast. *Arch. Surg.*, 42:203, 1941.
8. Hicken, N. F., Best, R. R., & Hunt, H. B.: Discharges from the Nipple. *Arch. Surg.*, 35:1079, 1937.
9. Hichly, P. R.: Nipple Discharge. *Ann. Surg.*, 113:341, 1941.
10. Miller, E. M., & Lewis, D.: The Significance of a Scrobemorrhagic Discharge from the Nipple. *J. A. M. A.*, 8:1651, 1923.
11. Petersen, H. A.: Benign Tumors of the Breast. *J. Nat. Med. Assn.*, 33:4:113.
12. Stowers, J. E.: The Significance of Bleeding or Discharge from the Nipple. *S., G. & O.*, 61:537, 1935.
13. Wainwright, J. M.: The Treatment of the Bleeding Breast. *Amer. J. Cancer*, 19:339, 1933.

Discussion

Dr. A. E. Baker, Charleston: Discharges from the nipple are associated with a variety of breast conditions. Some are serous or milky discharges, others bloody or sanguinous. The milky secretions are caused by an irregularity or impairment in the endocrine system of which the pituitary gland and the ovaries play the leading part, as they do in the function of the normal breast from time of birth. One-tenth of the newborn babies develop enlarged secreting breasts because of maternal hormones born in them. Shortly these breasts subside and remain dormant until puberty, when the gonads mature and their own endocrine secretions are established. The breasts then enlarge and remain so until menopause when the gonads atrophy, and so do the breasts. This is nature's plan.

GILLAND—To P. 442

CLINIC
Conducted by
FREDERICK R. TAYLOR, B.S., M.D., F.A.C.P.,
High Point, N. C.

A 34-YEAR-OLD LOOPER complained of soreness in the right lower quadrant of the abdomen and nausea, on Aug. 8th, 1942. She stated she had had trouble with pus in her kidneys for about 9 years, for which a physician had treated her off and on. At the onset of this trouble she began having pelvic pains on both sides, no worse on voiding. Though they kept up for 2 weeks, she paid no attention to them, though for the last 3 or 4 days of this 2-weeks period she had fever and vomited every time she ate. She did not have a doctor at this time. At the end of this 2-weeks period she went to bed one night and her husband said she raved all night, though she remembers little about it. A physician, called at 3:00 a. m., told her she had "poisoned kidneys." He gave her medicine, but she remembers nothing of the next 4 days. She stayed in bed at home for 6 to 8 weeks. Then she seemed to get all right for awhile, but later her trouble kept recurring. After going to the same physician off and on for about 8 years, she developed gross hematuria for the first time, and having heard that Dr. E. A. Sumner was especially good at urology, just about this time she consulted Dr. Sumner, who made pyelograms, gave her cystoscopic treatments, etc., and she improved the most she had done since the onset of her trouble. She last saw him 3 or 4 weeks before consulting me, just before he left to go into military service. He told her she was doing well then, and she was feeling pretty well, but the week she came to me her old symptoms of bilateral pelvic pain, right-sided lumbar pain and nausea returned. She has not vomited this time. At times she has noted pitting edema of her feet and swelling of her face. No headache. There is discomfort on voiding, though it is hard for her to say whether it hurts or burns. She has no frequency now, but some urgency. It is very difficult at times for her to void at all. She had a surgical menopause in 1937 because of continuous menstruation. Her appendix, right ovary and uterus were removed.

She had typhoid fever in childhood, pneumonia at 15. Because of the latter she had been examined several times at the Guilford County Sanatorium for tuberculosis, the last time a year ago, and her lungs had always been pronounced normal. Her habits were not contributory.

Her mother died of asthma at 52; one sister has pus in her kidneys; 2 brothers are well; husband is well. She has never been pregnant. During the taking of this history, the patient became faint and the Trendelenburg position relieved her at once.

Height 5 ft. 6¾ in., wt. 103¼ lbs. (standard wt. 143 lbs.), T. 98.6, P. 68—weak, but regular, R. 18, B. P. 130 84. She had had an attempt at tonsillectomy by a general practitioner years before, but a large amount of the left tonsil remains, and a small shred of the right one. There is a very slight symmetrical, smooth enlargement of the thyroid, without exophthalmos or tremor. Her thorax is long and narrow, heart and lungs seem normal, and spine negative. She is very tender over both kidneys, especially the right. Abdomen shows exquisite tenderness in right hypochondrium, presumably due to right kidney rather than to gallbladder trouble. There is marked tenderness in both iliac fossae, but not in the pelvis, and marked tenderness over the left kidney. Pelvic examination not made, as 3 weeks ago Dr. Sumner made one and told her everything was all right in that region. Extremities negative—no edema now. No edema of face. Urine negative, both chemically and microscopically. Weight light, but more now than ever before. She states that Dr. Sumner told her he found no ureteral kinks or strictures after a 3-day study. Despite all this, I suspected an extreme type of floating kidney, and referred her to another urologist, Dr. Sumner being in the army. He had her admitted to a hospital in another city and, after finding marked nephroptosis, decided it was severe enough to warrant a nephropexy, and did this.

One week after an apparently successful nephropexy, soreness and pain developed in her right lower chest and rapidly progressing dyspnea. A medical man on the staff of the hospital was asked to see her and found evidence of consolidation of the lower lobe of her right lung and right pleural effusion. Tapping obtained 300 c.c. of serosanguinous fluid. Her dyspnea was not relieved by this. A diagnosis of pulmonary infarction was made. She was sent home with a poor prognosis by the medical man. I saw her very shortly after this (Sept. 21st) and found her very dyspneic and too sick to be at home with no one to care for her. Sent back to the hospital more fluid was removed from her chest. This fluid failed to infect guinea pigs. Extensive laboratory studies were negative. She was afebrile at this time. However, one internist strongly suspected a tuberculous pleurisy. She came home later much improved. Since that time she has been examined clinically and röntgenologically at the Guilford County Sanatorium on 3 occasions, and no evidence of active tuberculosis has been found. We agreed with the man who made the diagnosis of pulmonary infarction, but could not understand his poor prognosis. We felt that if pulmonary infarction did not kill promptly, or set up an abscess in the lung or cause a severe acute cor pulmonale, the prognosis was reasonably good.

My last notes on her case, dated Aug. 24th, 1943, show no evidence of further trouble in her chest.

Diagnosis: Pulmonary infarction due to postoperative embolism.

ON DECEMBER 9th, 1941, I was called to see a 28-year-old doctor whom I had known from his early childhood. He had come home on vacation from a New York hospital, where he was a resident in obstetrics and gynecology. He had hunted all day, and then danced most of the night. The next day he played golf, took cold and, 2 days later, called me. He was aching all over and had an intractable, rather productive cough. The sputum was tenacious and purulent, but contained no blood. Two days after I first saw him, his t. reached its maximum of 105° F. and then gradually declined with an irregular curve. Large doses of codeine, intravenous iodide, etc., had little effect on the cough. Insomnia, too, was obstinate, despite rather heavy sedation. Sulfadiazine was given when his t. was very high, for 10 doses, without benefit. Dr. M. B. Leath examined his sinuses and said they were normal. Early in the course of his disease I could find no signs of pulmonary consolidation. Another internist, in consultation, transilluminated his sinuses and said the left antrum was cloudy, so Dr. Leath punched a hole and washed it out—washings entirely clear. He had about as extreme sweating as any patient I ever saw, for which frequent intravenous injections of 1000 c.c. glucose-saline were given. All this was done at home, as he did not care to go into the local hospital. For 10 days his respiratory rate was slightly elevated, running from 20 to 26 per minute; on the 9th day, for the first time, there were definite chest signs of bronchopneumonia. He was put back on sulfadiazine, 2 Gm. the first dose, then 1 Gm. q. 4 hrs. On the 11th day his r. rate rose to 40 and and his breathing was shallow, p. rate 96. The physical signs in his chest seemed rather better, but he was greatly prostrated and his cough would not stop. *Throughout his entire illness he had a definite feeling that it would be fatal,* and this was one reason he did not want to go to the hospital. At this time Dr. Tinsley R. Harrison, then Professor of Medicine in the Bowman Gray School of Medicine, called in consultation, made a remarkable diagnosis, on clinical grounds only, of probable staphylococcus bronchopneumonia. A smear of the sputum showed few but varied organisms with many neutrophiles. His sputum was taken for culture. To provide every facility for study, he was sent to the Baptist Hospital at Winston-Salem, and Dr. George T. Harrell took charge of him, as it was impossible for me to be in Winston-Salem every day. While he was at home, blood culture for E. typhosus was negative. His white cell count on the 5th day of his disease was 10,700 with 79% neutrophiles. At the hospital, x-ray films of his chest showed involvement of both lungs, especially the left, far out of proportion to the physical signs, suggesting to Dr. J. P. Rousseau a virus influenza plus a secondary invasion of the lungs by Pfeiffer's bacilli. The sputum was negative for tuberculosis. The serum chlorides were 3.5 mg. per 100 c.c. He was given glucose and hypertonic (3%) sodium chloride intravenously, sulfathiazole (sputum culture showed a non-hemolytic staphylococcus), and x-ray treatments of his lungs. By December 23rd, he had improved remarkably, both clinically and röntgenologically. His t. had come down to normal. He had laughed and joked with his friends and members of his family. He stated that when he left his home in the ambulance for the hospital, it was a sore trial to him, for *he had firmly believed that he would never see his home again.* He seemed, however, to have recovered completely from this foreboding. Indeed, he had talked only a short time before with Dr. Harrison, who dropped in to see him, about going to Florida to convalesce, after leaving the hospital. At 9 o'clock that evening he complained of pain in his right groin. Dr. Harrell examined him an hour later, and gave special attention to the veins in that region, but could find no evidence of thrombophlebitis. The patient suggested that his prolonged and violent coughing (by that time happily well-controlled) might have stretched his right inguinal ring, and that he might be developing a hernia. Dr. Harrell found that the ring was rather large and there was an impulse on coughing. The next morning Dr. Harrell phoned me that at 4 a. m., while talking to his nurse, the patient suddenly became speechless and died almost instantly, without a sound.

Necropsy showed an extensive bilateral resolving bronchopneumonia, worse in left lung, the right thigh 4 cm. more in circumference than the left at the same level (Dr. Harrell had made these measurements the night before and they were equal then), without edema of the right foot. There was thrombosis of the right common iliac vein, and a huge embolus practically occluding the left main branch of the pulmonary artery, which was obviously the cause of death. There was marked dilatation of the right heart. The skull was not opened. Artificial respiration at the time the embolism occurred, and intracardiac injection of adrenalin and coramine were all given.

Diagnosis: Resolving extensive bilateral non-hemolytic staphylococcic bronchopneumonia, thrombosis of right common iliac vein, massive embolism of left main branch of pulmonary artery, dilatation of right heart (acute cor pulmonale).

DEPARTMENTS

HUMAN BEHAVIOUR

James K. Hall, M.D., *Editor*, Richmond, Va.

AN AWFUL RESPONSIBILITY

THE RETIREMENT of Alfred E. Smith from public life came at the most inopportune time. His cheery speech and his uncanny administrative capacity were badly needed by the American people during the period of the long economic depression, and they are needed even more throughout the present war. He must have possessed genius as a public official. Few citizens in the history of our country have been so blessed as he with the linguistic gift that enabled him to translate for the people into their own every-day language just how their government takes their financial contributions in the form of taxes, imposed and collected, and transmutes those contributions into services rendered to all the people. Governor Smith was able to make the complex simple; the obscure lucid; the ambiguous no longer doubtful. He was the gifted and unselfish public servant who made it possible often for the citizen to do by the state's help what he could not do without that help. As a citizen and as an official Governor Smith could help the people to understand that one of their very own was sincere, honest, capable, unselfish, incorruptible and courageous. And in the time of need he was both able and willing to stand up either for the under dog or for the upper dog. He was religious and reverent, but his kind of reverence did not cause him to have too much respect for man-made fabrications. He seemed to feel certain that few things had reached a state of perfection and to believe that many things might be improved, even by man.

And one of those things was criminal procedure. I think I can remember with a degree of tolerable accuracy that in addressing the Bar Association, perhaps of New York State, that Governor Smith advocated radical changes in the customary method of trying the individual charged with violating the criminal law. He suggested that, as soon as the jury pronounced the defendant guilty the procedure be stopped there, and that the convicted defendant then be placed in the care of a board. And the board, carefully selected by the Governor, would be empowered to place the criminal—in a penitentiary, in a mental hospital, in a reformatory, in an institution for the feeble-minded, or in a hospital for the criminal insane, or, perhaps, under probation out in the world.

The board would be guided in dealing with the prisoner by its conception of his condition obtained from the history and from the examination of the prisoner. Governor Smith advocated the exercise by the board of all authority over the convicted individual—in placing him, in having him cared for and treated; and the board, by the knowledge it would eventually acquire of the prisoner, would be in position to measure properly the period of control to be exercised by the state over the convicted person. And the board would possess the authority to keep the person under restraint for life, if advisable; or to discharge the person out into society, when the person would become fit for such a change.

But unless some such change in the criminal procedure were brought about, Governor Smith thought the power to pardon the prisoner sentenced to death should not be taken from the Governor. Even though the pleas of loved ones that a criminal be saved from electrocution might cause the Governor to suffer anguish and to lose sleep, Governor Smith thought it better that one man, the Governor, rather than a board, should hear such pleas, and should exercise the pardoning power. I believe he was of the opinion that such awful responsibility should not be diluted through a board, but that it should be borne by one, and that one should be the Governor.

The General Assembly of New York did not adopt the suggestion of Governor Smith by creating a board to take over the defendant found guilty by the jury. And in not yielding to the suggestion of Governor Smith the State of New York was prevented from taking a forward step in the treatment of so-called criminals. A well-selected board, vested with the contemplated authority, would have come upon some understanding of criminal behaviour and of the criminal by its investigations and examinations of prisoners.

At present there is little understanding of either. In the criminal court room only a cross-section of the defendant's life is dealt with, the violation of law with which he is charged; and usually little effort is made to find out what manner of individual the defendant is. A brief trial affords no opportunity for such investigation, even if there were any inclination to make it. The so-called criminal trial is generally characterized by lack of interest in truth, by unilateral unfairness and by apparent relative unconcern about justice. There is seldom any evidence of judiciousness except that afforded by the presence of the trial judge.

Not long ago I heard a studious and philosophic judge remark that within fifty years our descendants would be speaking altogether truthfully of the barbarity of the criminal procedures of today. It would be difficult to conceive of the behaviour of any individual as more criminal than that of many criminal trials. In our lack of understanding and in our care of those who are aberrant in conduct because of mental deprivation, because of mental disease, or because of so-called criminalistic urges, we are still uncivilized. Warfare between groups—modern war—and warfare between society and the so-called criminal, is in each instance unintelligent and therefore senseless and in consequence destructive.

At the approaching election on November 7th, already held when you shall have read this, I shall vote against both of the proposed amendments to the Constitution of Virginia. But the amendment to which I object most vigorously is that one which would "authorize the General Assembly to provide for a board to be appointed by the Governor and to vest in such board the power to commute capital punishment and to grant reprieves and pardons." Yet I doubt not that the amendment will be adopted. There has been little discussion of it in the press or elsewhere; and that little has been concerned more about the distress experienced by the Governor than about the agony suffered by the prisoner. The pardoning power should not be divided amongst three or five members of a board; it should remain one of the Governor's responsibilities. If the Governor is unable to hear the pleas for commutation of sentences and to act upon them because they tear his heart-strings, his suffering could be prevented by the abolition of capital punishment. Civilized people do not kill each other.

Not too much concern is devoted to the prisoner after his incarceration, but there is too little investigation of the defendant before and during the trial. What does criminal behaviour mean? Why and under what circumstances does it occur? Little dispassionate concern is ever devoted to those interrogatories. No individual should be marked by conviction of a crime, if such conviction can be justly avoided. Conviction stigmatizes generally, brands ineradicably, and often degrades. The attitude and the activities and the hope of society should be constructive, not destructive.

Lately a man whom competent psychiatrists had pronounced insane was electrocuted by the State of Virginia. The Governor of Virginia had been given their diagnosis of the prisoner's mental condition. The prisoner had been declared to be sane by the jury that convicted him. The inference is unavoidable that the Governor of Virginia had more respect for the medical opinion of the lay trial jury than for the opinions reported to him of the several psychiatrists who repeatedly examined the prisoner in the penitentiary and concluded that he was insane.

But in spite of a Governor's willingness in a tragic instance to accept the diagnostic opinion of a lay jury, rather than the opinions of examining physicians, I continue to believe that the pardoning power should remain the Governor's responsibility.

The tendency of the day is to create too many governmental boards. Eventually they cannot be numbered for their multitude. The group cannot think. The group cannot reason. The group cannot exercise judgment. The group can feel; or it may not be emotionally stirred. Thinking and reasoning and reaching conclusions and formulating opinions and exercising judgment are functions of the individual only; never of the group.

Intelligent human beings insist upon having God, not gods. The Governor of the state goes into office of his own volition. He seeks and secures from the people all the pleasures and all the responsibilities, including the agonies, that go with the governorship. Let him hold fast to those responsibilities that are awful because of their necessity. No Governor in office can possibly suffer, qualitatively or quantitatively, as the prisoner suffers who awaits at the break of day his legal electrocution by the state of which he is a constituent. Let the Governor continue to suffer; no board can so suffer. The people unschooled in formal psychological pedantry instinctively know such things. And because they know that no board can take the place of a human being they object to the performances of so many governmental functions by the myriad governmental boards. No board can intellectualize any problem. A board may exhibit emotion but not intelligence. There is valid basis for the objection of the people to so-called bureaucratic government. No bureau drawer ever contains what one is looking for and what one needs.

OPHTHALMOLOGY

Herbert C. Neblett, M.D., *Editor*, Charlotte, N. C.

SOME LATE COMPLICATIONS AND SEQUELAE FOLLOWING BLUNT TRAUMA TO THE EYE AND ORBITAL WALL

Following any injury to the globe or the anterior orbital wall or both, however trivial, by any blunt instrument it is well for the physician to be guarded in his prognosis. Even in the absence of any demonstrable injury to the eyeball, externally or internally, serious complications and sequelae may ensue. An early report of negative findings and normal function of the allegedly injured eye may later result in embarrassment to the reporting physician, and to his colleague who may later be asked to review the case and report his findings because something has occurred in the interim to the eye that was injured. Should the case come under the Workman's Compensation Act further complications of a legal nature are sure to arise which are time-consuming, annoying and unprofitable in every respect to the physicians concerned.

In industrial accident cases pressure is brought to bear upon all physicians doing that work through the medium of the Industrial Courts, the employer and the insurance carrier to expedite the return of the injured workman to duty and the report that must follow. This for the purpose to conserve man hours and to lessen the cost of medical care. The main point, the conservation of vision, is often submerged in the effort to expedite the case, rather than to promote proper medical care; and a hurried, rather than an adequate, appraisal of the case is made. This in turn resolves itself into a greater cost for medical care in the treatment of delayed complications. To illustrate some of these problems the following cases are submitted which came to the writer recently for review, diagnosis, treatment and for final status of disability. In all of these cases a period of from 2 to 6 months had elapsed since occurrence of an an alleged injury.

1—Man, aged 50, 2 months prior to being seen by me, while unloading 2-by-4 timbers was struck over the left brow by a piece of the timber. The report of the findings by the physician who first saw him and who treated him for 3 days said of the eye only that there was an abrasion of the upper lid and a moderate contusion over the supraorbital wall. When seen by me the patient stated the eye had felt uneasy since the injury and 10 days ago had become very painful with decreasing vision, all of which had become progressively worse. At my examination there was no evidence of injury to the globe or to the orbital wall but the entire eyeball was highly injected and painful, and vision was light perception only. Tension by tonometer was 90 plus. No details of the interior of the eye could be seen.

Diagnosis: Glaucoma, acute, probably secondary to trauma. The following day a broad basal iridectomy was done and a few moments after its completion it was seen that the crystalline lens was dislocated upward and nasalward. Operation gave prompt relief of the glaucoma and convalescence was uneventful. Three or four weeks later, as was to be expected from the presence of the dislocated lens, there began a slow rise of intraocular pressure. A complete extraction of the lens was accomplished without complications, and an uneventful convalescence. Following this a study of the fundus showed many gray-black opacities in the vitreous which suggested an intraocular hemorrhage the result of the initial trauma. Vision with correction 20/40 plus.

2—Man, aged 47, 6 months previously had been struck over the left eye by a heavy rope breaking loose from a pulley, causing a severe contusion of the globe and intraocular hemorrhage. This case was thoroughly and properly handled and discharged with a minor degree of disability as cured. Subsequently the vision gradually deteriorated and when seen by me was less than 20/200, due to delayed changes in the vitreous, optic nerve and macula.

3—This man 4 months ago was struck over the left brow by the end of a cable breaking under tension. He was unconscious for 24 hours and treated in a hospital for 3 days and discharged as recovered without any visual disability. Patient stated when seen by me that 3 days following the injury he became aware of disturbance of vision of left eye, but upon examinations he was told that the eye was uninvolved. My examination showed a dilated and faintly mobile pupil and vision of hand movements, due to a large hole in the macula the result of the accident described.

4—A boy, aged 12, was struck in the left eye by a chinaberry shot from a sling. The history given by the examining physician was that there was no evidence of injury, pain or altered function in the eye. Four days later a massive intraocular hemorrhage occurred, partly cleared up, then a second, and later a third, hemorrhage occurred and when seen by me secondary glaucoma was present and vision was reduced to light perception. Under treatment over a period of three weeks convalescence was well established with the final result normal vision and no sequelae.

Resumé—Patients 1 to 3 inclusive had been examined prior to employment and had normal vision each eye. Patients 2 and 3 employed legal counsel to present their cases before the Industrial Commission for compensation. Under the industrial law patients 1 to 3 inclusive are industrially blind in the eye involved and therefore entitled to and will receive full compensation for their visual disability. These four cases show the delayed complications and sequelae of two slight and two severe injuries: in one directly to the globe without any demonstrable injury thereto, in one a definite injury to the globe, and in the remaining two to the orbital wall, without any appreciable external trauma to the eyeball.

SURGERY

GEO. H. BUNCH, M.D., *Editor*, Columbia, S. C.

UROGENITAL RETROPERITONEAL CYSTS

LARGELY because of their rarity, retroperitoneal cysts present an interesting problem in differential diagnosis. Cysts of the kidney and of the pancreas are not true retroperitoneal cysts, as defined by Handfield-Jones: "those cysts lying in the retroperitoneal fatty tissues which have no apparent connection with any adult structures save by areolar tissue." Under this classification there are:

A—Chylous cysts from lymphatic obstruction
B—Parasitic cysts usually caused by echinococcus infection
C—Dermoid cysts from imperfect closure of the abdominal plates. These may contain bone and cartilage. They include the enteric cysts which form from the remains of isolated segments of intestine that for some reason have not developed and have not become connected with the alimentary tract.
D—Urogenital cysts which develop from the remains of the Wolffian duct.

Evolution in man is shown admirably in the embryology of the kidney and of the ureter. Their origin is associated with the development of two fetal structures, the pronephros, which becomes the kidney of amphibians, and the mesonephros which becomes the kidney of fishes. In man the former never functions and soon completely disappears: the latter excretes urine prior to the development of the permanent kidney from the metanephros. The mesonephros, which at first extends from the 6th cervical to the 3rd lumbar segment, also disappears except the 3 caudal segments. The Wolffian duct, which is the excretory duct of both the pronephros and the mesonephros, becomes the tubular portion of the genital system in the male. The Mullerian duct, except for the ovaries, becomes the internal genital organs in the female. Both ducts discharge into the cloaca. The gonads in both sexes develop from the Wolffian body. Wolffian cysts occur only in women, for in them the Wolffian duct remain unutilized.

Urogenital retroperitoneal cyst, Wolffian cyst, manifests itself as a painless, progressive enlargement of the abdomen, which in the beginning may be unilateral but becomes general with increase in size. Although the kidneys and the intestine may be mechanically displaced there are no obstructive symptoms.

Diagnosis is largely made by elimination. Intravenous pyelograms and x-ray study of the colon after the giving of barium enemas are helpful in identifying the site of the cyst in relation to the kidney and to the bowel.

The treatment is exclusively surgical. At operation transperitoneal removal is the procedure of choice. When the posterior peritoneum has been incised and the cyst is exposed its eneucleation is readily accomplished by blunt dissection with the gloved hand. There is no pedicle. The wall is thin and fibrous and presents a line of cleavage that is easily followed. The tissues are so avascular that no bloodvessels may have to be tied. Cysts that are too adherent may be cured by marsupialization.

Wolffian cysts are rare. Lahey in 1934 had had only two cases in the clinic. We have recently had a case in a fat woman of 45 years in whom the preöperative diagnosis of retroperitoneal cyst was made with the help of the urologist and the röntgenologist.

DENTISTRY

J. H. GUION, D.D.S., *Editor*, Charlotte, N. C.

INFECTION IN FILLED, VITAL, ROENTGENOGRAPHICALLY NEGATIVE TEETH

PULPLESS TEETH, irrespective of whether they gave röntgenographic evidence of changes, have been proved to harbor streptococci which on injection into animals tend to produce disease resembling that of the patient from whom the teeth were removed. The removal of pulpless teeth often results in improvement of patients ill with systemic diseases due to streptococci. Some patients, not so benefited, have improved after removal of röntgenographically negative teeth that contained large restorations and that responded to vitality tests.

The results obtained from a recent bacteriologic and histologic study of seven vital teeth with fillings and of diseased bone in which some of the teeth were embedded are so striking it was felt that a report[1] be made.

Substance of the report:

A physician, 68, had had repeated attacks of neuromyositis, bursitis and mild arthritis at widely separated intervals for many years, but otherwise had remained in excellent health. After removal of one or two pulpless teeth from which streptococci were isolated, these recurring attacks disappeared promptly and remained absent for years. In the past two years there was a mild recurrence of symptoms with a lack of endurance, increasing tremor of one hand and dull aching pain in the mandible, especially surrounding teeth containing large restorations, to which bridges were attached. There were no pulpless teeth. All upper teeth had been removed some years before and a well-fitting dnture supplied. The tonsils had been cleanly removed many years before. There was no evidence of sinusitis or prostatitis.

Röntgenograms of the upper jaw showed no residual areas of infection. The mucous membrane over the alveolar process appeared normal and there was no tenderness on palpation. Five of the lower teeth had been removed, four of these six years before. The right lower second bicuspid which had contained a deep gold inlay and supported one end of a bridge contained three teeth, was removed seven months before, 12 hours after several sharp twinges of pain suggestive of acute pulpitis had occurred during an attack of neuromuscular pain.

---
1. E. C. Rosenow, Rochester, Minn., in *Cincinnati Jl. of Med.*, Oct.

After its aseptic removal, the tooth was split in a rigid vise with sterile technic, and the apex and the pulp were found severely congested. From this tooth a pure culture of streptococci was isolated in dextrose-brain broth and dextrose-brain agar. Two rabbits were inoculated, one intracerebrally with 0.1 c.c. of a 1:10,000 dilution of the culture from the pulp and the other intravenously with 10 c.c. of the undiluted primary dextrose-brain broth culture from the apex. Lesions of muscles, fascia and periarticular structures developed in both animals.

Following extraction an exacerbation of neuromuscular pain occurred, but, except for a second mild attack two weeks later, there was relative freedom from symptoms for several months. Then similar attacks, with undue fatigability, again occurred.

Of the 11 remaining teeth in the lower jaw six contained small to large gold fillings. Two, the left lower second bicuspid and the second molar, harbored deep gold inlays to which a contact bridge containing two teeth was attached. The left third molar was capped with a large, shallow gold inlay. The left lower cuspid contained a small gold filling near the margin of the gum. All 11 teeth responded to vitality tests and in consequence were considered normal by the best dentists and exodontists as having nothing to do with symptoms.

The episodes of neuromuscular pains and fatigability increased in severity. Sensitiveness to cold developed in several teeth with twinges of sharp pain.

The six filled teeth and surrounding diseased bone were removed at one sitting under local block anesthesia. Two abscesses containing foul pus were found under the bridge and one was found at the lingual side of the roots of the third right molar, so situated that röntgenograms could not reveal its presence. The bone surrounding these abscesses was badly and deeply infected. This bone and the alveolar processes surrounding the remaining teeth were removed surgically. The recurring attacks of dull pain in the lower jaw, all other pains and the undue fatigability have disappeared.

Apices and pulps of filled, x-ray negative, vital teeth were found to be infected by streptococci. The bone in which the infected teeth were embedded showed condensing osteitis, cystic degeneration, localized regions of necrosis and leukocytic infiltration in which large numbers of streptococci and fusiform bacilli were found. Since the streptococci that grew in the brain-containing mediums had specific localizing power and they did not grow on blood agar, and since they were agglutinated specifically by the patient's convalescent serum, it may be concluded that the streptococci isolated were not contaminants.

GENERAL PRACTICE

D. HERBERT SMITH, M.D., *Editor*, Pauline, S. C.

THE TREATMENT OF MULTIPLE FURUNCULOSIS WITH PENICILLIN

A RECENT REPORT[1] of the treatment of crops of boils with penicillin is gratifying to all of us who have to do with this common condition.

An initial dose of 20,000 units intramuscularly followed by 10,000 additional units every three hours—a total of 440,000 units, within 24 hours after treatment was begun produced distinct improvement. Without the aid of any local therapy all of the lesions were healed in four days except for a large abscess on the left thigh, which drained spontaneously and healed two days later.

In another case 5,000 units was administered intramuscularly q. 3 h. to a total of 200,000 units of penicillin. Within 48 hours the furuncles began to regress, and hard papular swellings as well as the small fluctuant furuncles became absorbed and completely disappeared after four days. Discharged after six days.

In the third case an initial intramuscular injection of 10,000 units of penicillin was given followed by an additional 5,000 units every three hours to a total of 230,000 units. The furuncles began to regress in 24 hours and completely disappeared in 2 hours except for two large fluctuant abscesses of the scalp, which were incised and drained and completely healed two days later.

The rapid cure of multiple furunculosis observed in six children under penicillin treatment indicates a result far superior to any previously known therapy for this condition.

Urticarial reactions to penicillin have been described as occurring[2] in 12 of 209 cases treated in army hospitals. None of the patients included in the report quoted showed precipitins or positive skin reactions to penicillin. Present evidence indicates, however, that the sensitivity is to penicillin itself.

1. Rose Coleman & Wallace Sako, New Orleans, in Jl. A. M. A., Oct. 14th.
2. Leo H. Criep, Pittsburgh, in Jl. A. M. A., Oct. 14th.

* * * * *

TREATMENT OF SCARLET FEVER

SCARLET FEVER is not a common disease in this section, and with us it is apt to pursue a mild course. Nevertheless, it is in order that we keep posted on the most improved method of treatment, such as that herewith outlined from an authoritative contribution.[1]

During the past 20 years the treatment of scarlet fever has been radically changed. Three types of therapy are now possible. Sulfonamide com-

1. M. J. Fox & N. F. Gordon, in Arch. Int. Med., July.

pounds find their chief value in the treatment of certain complications. They are of no value in the management of the toxic phase or type. Commercial antitoxin, prepared with horse serum, combats the toxic phase of the disease but introduces the danger of foreign-protein reactions.

Pooled human convalescent serum offers the best means of therapy—prompt subsidence of fever, alleviation of signs and symptoms, avoidance or improvement of most complications, shortened period of hospitalization and lower mortality rate.

A series of 1,000 patients of 1937 to 1943 contained a far higher percentage of seriously ill persons than did the 1,000 patients of 1923. The average duration of fever for the serum-treated patients was 2.1 days, in the control 5.5 days; average duration 24.5 days for serum-treated, 43.5 days for the control series. Although the patients receiving the serum were more seriously ill, only 17 deaths occurred, whereas there were 20 fatalities in the control group.

Dosage—

	Present Doses c.c.
Infants:	
Moderate	10-20
Severe	20-40
Children:	
Moderate	20-30
Severe	30-60
Adults:	
Moderate	20-40
Severe	40-80

It was found that smaller doses proved to be as effective as the former larger doses and were especially efficacious if the patient received the serum early in the course of the disease.

LABORATORY MEDICINE AND IMMUNOLOGY

J. M. Flore, M.D., and Evelyn Tribble, M.T., *Editors*,
Anderson, S. C.

FORENSIC LABORATORY MEDICINE

Forensic Medicine has a large element of laboratory medicine and perhaps in no field of scientific endeavor does one find more cases bungled. Example: A machinist working at a lathe fell dead. The coroner promptly signed a death certificate bearing the trite term, Heart Failure. Several hours later at the request of the man's family, the senior editor of this column performed an autopsy. There was a tiny bluish wound just to the left of the sternum in the third interspace. It was found that a spicule of steel propelled at great velocity had nicked the aorta. Result: $5,000 collected by the family on a double-indemnity insurance policy, and precautions taken against repetition of the accident.

Some pertinent medicolegal facts are presented in tabulated form:

I. *Blood*—Blood stains found at the scene of a crime or upon the clothing or person of the deceased or suspect can reveal the following information:

a. The simple benzidine test will determine at once if the substance is blood or some other reddish matter.

b. By extracting the blood with a few drops of warm saline solution, and using this as typing serum against known type-2 and type-3 red blood cells, the blood group of the individual can be determined. This can be of great value in freeing, but is of very little service in convicting. Example: Blood is found at the scene of a crime. A suspect has a cut hand; the blood spot is type-2 and the suspect is type-2. The examiner is exactly where he started as there are many type-2 individuals. On the other hand if the blood spot is type-2 and the suspect's blood type-3, the two bloods did not come from the same individual.

c. By a rather complicated procedure, it is possible to determine whether the blood is human or from some other animal. This technique is outside the scope of the average chemical laboratory being performed by a few hematologists at established medicolegal laboratories.

d. There is no test available to prove that a given specimen of blood came from any certain individual.

II. *Spermatozoa*—Seminal stains may be obtainable from the person of the alleged victim of rape, from her underclothing, or from material at the scene of the attack. Spermatozoa correspond to the blood group of the individual from whom they were derived. This should make a very important diagnostic link.

III. *Poisoning*—In all autopsy cases in which death has occurred under suspicious circumstances, exhaustive examination for poison should be made.

a. In ordinary screw-top fruit jars, place the stomach, tied at either end to prevent leakage, sections of kidney, liver and intestine. Label these properly and seal with wax to be sent to a chemical laboratory in the custody of a duly authorized officer. These must not be mailed or shipped by express. If the journey is a lengthy one, the containers should be packed in ice to prevent decomposition. A specimen of urine obtained from the bladder and 10 c.c. of blood drawn from the ventricle of the heart should also be sent. *The routine clinical laboratory worker, whether director or technician, who attempts forensic toxicology heads for disaster or at least embarrassment.* It is a job for a laboratory properly equipped and staffed by workers having specialized training.

The nearest the senior editor of this column ever approached homicide was a time in another location when a son of Hippocrates handed him a pill with a blunt, "What's in that?" Upon being informed that the laboratory director was not a medicolegal chemist, the ill-informed purveyor of physic replied, "Hell, ye're a pathologist, ain't chu? Finding out what's in things is your job, ain't it?"

IV. *Drowning*—The question will frequently arise: Was this person drowned or was he killed in some other manner and the body then thrown into the water? Blood is drawn from the right ventricle and from the left ventricle of the heart. Then a chloride estimation is performed on both specimens. If the amount present in both chambers corresponds, death was not due to drowning. If the chloride content of the left ventricle blood is found much lower than that of the right, and assuming that fresh water was the medium, death was probably due to submersion. If the suspected drowning took place in salt water, the chloride content of the left ventricle blood will be much greater than that of the right.

V. *Marking of Bullets*—When a doctor removes a bullet in a case of gun-shot wound, he will be wise to mark the bullet in some way whereby he can later identify it. *Be sure to place this marking on the nose or butt: do not mark the sides, and parenthetically, care should be exercised in extracting the missle to avoid forcep marks.* These precautions are necessary in aiding the ballistic expert in his search for rifling marks.

This is not by any means a comprehensive review of the medicolegal field. The final word of admonition is—don't do it. A man's life or liberty may depend upon the findings. Medicolegal toxicology has no place in the ordinary hospital laboratory. On the other hand, every doctor and technical worker will want to properly prepare and forward specimens to State Chemists and others qualified and legally empowered to make such examinations.

GENERAL PRACTICE

JAMES L. HAMNER, M.D., *Editor*, Mannboro, Va.

THE DIFFERENTIAL DIAGNOSIS OF GLYCOSURIA

A POSITIVE TEST for sugar in the urine does not mean that the patient has diabetes. It does mean that the doctor should proceed to find out what is wrong.

John[1] plainly directs what should be done:

Have the patient eat a heavy carbohydrate lunch and note the exact time he *started* eating. Then

---
1. H. J. John, Lt. Col. M. C., U.S.A., in *Am. Jl. Digestive Diseases*, Oct.

$2\frac{1}{2}$ hours later obtain 2 c.c. of blood with the syringe found in any doctor's bag. A pinch of sodium or potassium oxalate in the tube will prevent coagulation if the tube is inverted a few times. A laboratory will have the answer in less than one hour.

If the blood sugar is below 120 mg. per cent, the patient is *non*-diabetic.

If the blood sugar is above 120 mg. per cent, he is *probably* a diabetic.

If it is well above 120, say 200 or more, a *frank diabetes* exists.

If it is 126 or 136, one needs to go into the problem further and do a glucose tolerance test the following morning.

One hundred gm. of glucose is given orally after a night's fasting and blood and urine are obtained before and one half, one, two, and three hours after the administration of the glucose.

If the curve descends in $2\frac{1}{2}$ hours to 120 mg. per cent or below, the patient is *not* diabetic.

If it is 200 or more at two and a half hours, the patient is a *frank* diabetic.

If it is 126 to 136, then we are dealing with a *potential or pre-diabetic* state. A real chance for the practice of preventive medicine.

All that is necessary is slight restriction of diet which eliminates the excessive use of carbohydrates or overeating, and annual examination.

There is no indication for doing a glucose tolerance test if the $2\frac{1}{2}$ hours post-prandial blood sugar is 200 mg. per cent or more, for the glucose tolerance test will give no more information. It is already known that the patient is a diabetic. The extreme height and prolongation of the curve, if it starts with a normal blood sugar or a near normal, is not an index to the severity of the patient's diabetes. *Some patients with the most abnormal glucose tolerance curves turn out to be the mildest diabetics.*

Symptoms or lack of symptoms alone prove nothing. It is the laboratory evidence which is of diagnostic value, regardless of the presence or absence of symptoms. One can be easily misled if he finds classical symptoms and a glycosuria.

A patient with a non-diabetic glycosuria does not drift into diabetes. In our population one to two per cent are diabetic. A case of non-diabetic glycosuria is not exempt from this incidence. If the patient with proven non-diabetic glycosuria is shown to have diabetes in later years, this is probably fortuitous, and will occur in one to two per cent of such patients. If non-diabetic glycosuria were a precursor of diabetes, a high percentage of these patients would develop diabetes. That is not the case, for several hundred such cases have been followed over a period of 23 years, and not more than three of these patients have developed diabetes in later life.

The differential diagnosis between a diabetic and a non-diabetic glycosuria can be made only by a glucose tolerance test or by a blood sugar estimation 2½ hours following a heavy carbohydrate meal.

Numerous urine estimations for sugar for diagnostic purposes settle nothing and waste time.

Non-diabetic glycosuria is not a precursor of diabetes.

Upon a finding of glycosuria, a diagnosis should be arrived at without delay (within 24 hours). This will eliminate the possibility of self-imposed dietary restrictions which distort the glucose tolerance curve (toward the diabetic side) and thus give false information.

There is no treatment for non-diabetic glycosuria, and none is needed.

* * * * *

MASKED HYPOGLYCEMIA

IN ANY GENERAL practice there is a large group of patients who are tentatively classified as psychoneurotics or neurasthenics and who later turn out to have organic disease. This percentage varies greatly with the diagnostic curiosity and thoroughness of the physician and with his threshold of suspicion in the matter of spontaneous hypoglycemia.

Dyer[1] writes helpfully on this subject:

The symptomatology is varied and often bizarre, but usually remains constant in a particular patient. In the mild cases there may simply be a feeling of weakness, slight dizziness, perhaps a sense of hunger, or excessive perspiration. In the more severe cases the patient will often complain of diplopia, headache, occasionally nausea, extreme weakness ataxia, and loss of mental equilibrium. In the severe case the symptoms are much more dramatic where the patient suddenly becomes unconscious, has convulsions, breaks out into cold, clammy perspiration, and is revived best by the use of glucose intravenously.

Where spontaneous hypoglycemia is suspected, all of my patients have this test: A fasting blood sugar is taken; 1.5 Gm. of glucose per kilogram of body weight is given and specimens of blood taken at hourly intervals up to and including the five-hour specimen. No previous dietary regimen or limitation of activity is required.

Most cases of functional hypoglycemia have fasting blood sugars above 50 mg. per 100 c.c.

Of factors in the evaluation of spontaneous hypoglycemia among the most important are: 1) the level of blood sugar at the time of the reaction; 2) the rapidity of fall of the blood sugar; and 3) the previous level of blood sugar. It is just as possible to have hypoglycemic reactions when, in the course of one to three hours, a blood sugar is brought from a level of 300 to 100 as when a blood sugar is brought from a level of 150 to 50.

An isolated laboratory finding must be taken with a grain of salt, and if a patient fails to respond to the therapy, one must continue investigation.

In our experience the greatest benefit has arisen from a regimen of low carbohydrate, moderately high fat, and high protein at the three usual meals with interval and bedtime feedings.

There are probably many cases of spontaneous hypoglycemia masquerading as epilepsy, psychoneurosis, neurasthenia, menopausal neurosis, etc. The diagnosis in these patients can be established by a simple and common laboratory procedure if care is taken to insist upon a normal diet preceding the tolerance test and to insist upon a five-hour examination rather than the conventional three-hour test. Complete medical study of a patient must be done as well as the glucose-tolerance test. After the diagnosis is established, many of these patients respond to a simple dietary regimen and appropriate treatment of the attendant disease, if any.

The prevalence and the gravity of hypoglycemia are matters of wide differences of opinion. There are enough cases in which great relief can be afforded by very simple measures to make it worthy of our attention.

GILLAND—From P. 432

Pathological conditions also cause milky discharges from the breasts, such as the forms of chronic mastitis which are due to endocrine disturbance. It is estimated that milky discharges occur in 5 per cent of cystic mastitis, 4 per cent of cases of mastodynia (very soft painful breasts) and 2 per cent of cases of adenosis (hard, painful, thick, knotty breasts). It also occurs in residual lactation from one to several years after pregnancy. All these conditions usually respond to estrogen or testosterone propionate.

The bloody discharges from the nipple are due to carcinoma, benign intracystic, papilloma or a proliferative type of cystic mastitis (adenosis). Tissue for microscopic study should determine the type of treatment indicated in these cases.

It was a pleasure to have heard Dr. Gilland's excellent paper.

DR. GILLAND, closing: Endocrinology we know is one of our youngest of the fields of medicine. There is no other part of the body where you see endocrines in action more than in the breast. As we learn more of the physiology of the breast and endocrine association, the more will we use endocrines in the treatment of our breast conditions.

CAUSE OF CANCER.—We do not believe that a single injury is the direct or exciting cause, but it is impressive to note the frequency with which a single trauma may appear to bring to light a pre-existing bone tumor lesion.—*P. C. Colonia.*

---

1. W. W. Dyer, Philadelphia, in *Penn. Med. Jl.*, Sept.

PROCTOLOGY

Russell Buxton, M.D., F.A.C.S., *Editor*
Newport News, Va.

INTERNAL HEMORRHOIDS

Internal hemorrhoids are those masses of enlarged veins which lie above the mucocutaneous junction just above the anorectal line. The mass is usually divisible into four quadrants and is of a bluish color. Internal hemorrhoids are usually seen above the age of 20, and by far the most constant cause is constipation with straining at stool. Uncomplicated internal hemorrhoids ordinarily are seen first after bleeding, as bleeding occurs after bowel movement or during it and is without pain. It is usually bright red blood. If the hemorrhoids are not treated, sooner or later fibrosis takes place and protrusion occurs. Pain is remarkable only by its absence, however, backache and a feeling of fulness in the rectum is often present. Diagnosis is made by history and by rectal examination. With the patient in the Sims' or in the knee-chest position, a request to bear down will usually show the piles. If these are not seen by this method, an anoscope may be used.

The treatment divides itself into three stages. The early treatment of this disease is palliative, with mild laxatives such as mineral oil or petrolagar, antispasmodics, rectal lubrication at night using one or two ounces of warm olive oil or cottonseed oil. Many types of suppositories are of value. Bland anesthetic ointment also will help. Rest, particularly bed rest, will often give relief.

The second stage of treatment is at that time before protrusion of the hemorrhoids take place and consists of injection. The injection treatment is quite simple, but the following precautions must be observed: The treatment must be used early in the course of the disease before any complications such as protrusion, necrosis, or strangulation have occurred. It must not be used when external hemorrhoids are present.

The patient is placed in the knee-chest position and a Brinkerhoff anoscope is used to isolate the hemorrhoids. Any one of a number of solutions may be injected—quinine, urethene, carbolic acid solutions, synlasol. After the anoscope is introduced, the slide is removed and the pile prolapses in the slide. The tuberculin syringe equipped with a long offset needle is the best type. For small hemorrhoids .2 to .3 c.c. and for larger hemorrhoids .5 c.c. of the chosen solution is injected. Not more than two hemorrhoids are treated at any one sitting and the patient is instructed to use a rectal ointment and to take mineral oil for 10 days following injection, at which time he returns for further treatment. The results of the injection treatment are usually good but the patient should be instructed that the hemorrhoids may recur in the course of time, particularly if constipation is allowed to develop.

The final stage in the treatment of internal hemorrhoids is surgical. Surgical treatment should be used in cases of long-standing prolapsed internal hemorrhoids. No matter what type of operation is used, the patient should be seen three times a week for three weeks following operation and once a week for an additional three weeks, and at each of these visits rectal dilatation should be carried out to insure a competent anal opening at the time the patient is finally discharged.

UROLOGY

Raymond Thompson, M.D., *Editor*, Charlotte, N. C.

TRANSURETHRAL DRAINAGE OF THE SEMINAL VESICLES IN SEMINAL VESICULITIS

In a paper which considered involvement of the seminal vesicles along with obstructive vesiculitis, prostatic calculi, hemospermia, and obstructive sterility, the present status of catheterization of the ejaculatory is presented by Herbst and Merricks.[1]

Their clinical experience now consists of the transurethral dilatation and catheterization of 730 ejaculatory ducts. Obstructive vesiculitis they have found to result from the obstruction of the ejaculatory ducts chiefly by stricture, the aftermath of gonorrhea. Prostatitis is frequently associated. These patients had been treated by prostatic massage, urethral sounds, irrigations and other procedures for more than three years.

The chief complaints were of pains in the genitals and perineum and repeated attacks of epididymitis. Backache and pains, malaise with chills and fever were worse when tension of infected vesicular contents reached its height. Pain on ejaculation and hemospermia were features of some of the cases.

Massage of a seminal vesicle full of infected material or straining, compresses the vesicles and by forcing the infection back up the vas deferens often produces epididymitis.

In the cases reported, relief was best afforded by repeated transurethral dilatation of the obstructed ejaculatory ducts, vasotomy offering nothing in the way of removing these obstructions.

Visualization of the vesicles was accomplished by the retrograde injection of full strength diodrast through the indwelling catheter, one side after the other. Caudal anesthesia, using 25-30 c.c. of freshly

---
1. R. H. Herbst & J. W. Merricks, Chicago, in *Ill. Med. Jl.*, Oct.

prepared 1 per cent novocaine, gave adequate relaxation. Failures were less than one per cent and were mostly due to distortion of the posterior urethra, acquired or congenital. Only one or two dilatations were needed in some, many in others.

Attention is called to the fact that prostatic calculi have been found in half of the prostate glands removed at routine postmortem examinations in a hospital in which these urologists do a great deal of work. In such cases dilatation of the ejaculatory ducts may provide adequate drainage of the infected vesicles, yet transurethral prostatomy with removal of the stones may be required.

Hemospermia they have found to mean tuberculosis, malignant lesions at the bladder neck; or polyps, calculi, or benign prostatic hyperplasia; or occurring with no demonstrable cause. They have had a huge vesicle filled with blood respond well to nitrate of silver instillations into the vesicle.

Sterility is a subject of perennial interest. Obstructive sterility results more frequently from obstruction in the terminal portion of the seminal system than the proximal, near the epididymis. We are cautioned to not neglect investigation of the ejaculatory ducts in case bladder-neck disorder is suspected.

In a case reported in some detail, manifested by pain on ejaculation, hemospermia, stones in the prostate and sterility, stones were removed by transurethral prostototomy; and the ejaculatory ducts, which were extremely distorted and difficult to catheterize, were straightened out. The wife conceived six months later.

When routine treatment by massage and instillations, with removal of distant foci of infection, fails to relieve infection involving the prostate and seminal vesicles, often satisfactory results have been obtained by providing adequate drainage of obstructed infected seminal vesicles. Transurethral dilatation of the ejaculatory ducts alone, or at times combined with transurethral prostatotomy for removal of prostatic calculi, are considered the methods of choice.

Some years ago a good many urologists grew quite enthusiastic about the possibilities of transurethral catheterizaton of the seminal vesicles. Then, for some reason, apparently this enthusiasm waned.

This favorable experience in a large series of cases of so eminent a urologist as Herbst can not fail to stimulate many of us to make use of catheterization of the seminal vesicles and the other means of treatment recommended by him and his coworker.

HOSPITALS

R. B. DAVIS, M.D., *Editor*, Greensboro, N. C.

SAY WHAT YOU THINK

MUCH CRITICISM would be avoided and many hospital mistakes would never have been made if the owners and operators of the hospitals would say what they think about matters pertaining to hospitalization for the citizens of the community.

The Honorable Governor of North Carolina has appointed a Medical Advisory Committee to investigate the practicability of building a large central hospital, out of the taxpayers' money, and a group of smaller hospitals scattered throughout the state, all to be maintained with the taxpayers' money. The responsibility of operating these institutions would be placed upon the politicians, a long step in the direction of State Medicine, which some choose to call Socialized Medicine.

If one caters to a certain class of citizens, it would seem very plausible that we should socialize everything. Whole countries have set up governments on this principle. Those in favor of socialized medicine use the argument that, with the present system of hospitalization and medical services, the poor man does not obtain adequate services when they are most needed. Does the poor man always get adequate meat and bread, adequate clothing, or adequate housing? Does the poor man get adequate legal advice? Does the poor man get a college education?

In fact, the poor man can and does get medical and hospital services more adequately than he gets any other necessity or decent comfort of life.

In North Carolina there are 100 hospitals which maintain a free medical service for those unable to pay. Each of these hospitals maintains a ward with many beds, at a charge of less than cost or no charge. Under the present system, at least 25 per cent of the medical services rendered by the doctors in the state are either rendered below cost or out-and-out charity.

I know of no free grocery store in the state of North Carolina where the poor can go and get a week's ration; no clothing store advertising that those needing clothes may come and receive, gratis, first-class clothing outfits; no college where the poor and needy student may attend without money; no real estate office furnishing rent-free quarters to those unable to pay for housing. But 100 hospitals and 2000 doctors over the State maintain a 24-hour medical service free to the indigent.

In the face of all that has been done and is being done, the population at large is of the opinion that more should be done, and quickly. And if not, the politicians of our state and other states are willing to turn to state and socialized medicine unless we medical and hospital people grasp the opportunity to satisfy them without delay.

Services rendered by state, county and city health departments of the country are closely connected with state medicine or socialized medicine. However, the services rendered by these organizations are less valued by the poor than are the services rendered by the hospitals and medical profession on an individual basis. It is also a fact that funds for medical and hospital services rendered by the state, county or city have never come anywhere near being adequate. It is nothing unusual for a "public health" or "contract" doctor to have 25 patients in his office in one afternoon. No doctor can render efficient service under these circumstances. Politicians have never yet been educated to the fact that time is essential for efficient medical services. The same lawyer who requires a week to try a beggar for murder would expect the doctor to save that same person's life by an examination and treating him 5 or 10 minutes. As hinted before, the charity patient is seldom cooperative and as helpful as he or she could be in regard to carrying out instructions.

As a medical man and hospital administrator, I say that it is largely our fault that this matter has not been worked out to a more satisfactory end. However, the politicians and the lay people generally would do well to give us some praise for what we have done.

The Governor's Plan can be measured by the same rule applied in this discussion. It is true that we have provided more colleges for young men to study medicine. The medical profession is at fault, particularly those few so-called leaders who think they represent the combined medical profession, who serve as directors of medical education and promote the forming of many medical schools so that, for every new school opened, there have been two or more old schools closed in the last 20 years. Even in North Carolina, we have had two medical schools to die and only one new one to open since 1915.

A great effort was made not many years ago to drop two medical schools in the state which were at that time only giving two years of medicine. A sad situation it is in any country when *dictators* assume the roll of *saviors*. If every doctor and every hospital administrator would take the pains to investigate, they would find that if we are to clean our own house in regard to these matters, a way would open up that would be plain and broad and satisfactory to the people of our country.

The people must think constructively, and then say what they think before any progress can be made. The writer of this paper pleads with those who read it to make it known to their politicians, lay and professional, that we will take care of the poor if only given a legitimate chance. And that we do not propose to practice under dictatorship—whether by doctors, hospital administrators, or who nots?—who demand and put before all else artificial and absurd "standards" according to their rules and regulations.

No two medical students are alike. No two nurses are alike. No two doctors are alike. Therefore, it is criminal to demand that every hospital and every medical school have its applicants dragged through the same keyhole before they are admitted to the profession.

TREATMENT OF AMEBIC DYSENTERY
(C. C. Wu, in *Chinese Med. Jl.*, 61:337-341, 1943)

Ya Tan Tzu, the seed of *Brucea javanica* used for 25 patients by C. C. Wu, M.B., effected cures in 19, improved 3.

The following six-day treatment was used routinely: On the first, third and fifth days, 20 seeds, with shells removed but seeds not broken, were given in capsule form, t.i.d., p.c.; on the second, fourth and sixth days, 20 seeds with shells removed, were soaked in 200 c.c. of 1% $NaHCO_3$ solution for two hours, and given as a retention enema, following a cleansing enema, b.i.d. In addition, two patients required 20 seeds in capsules t.i.d., p.c.; for three days, and four needed a similar dosage for six days. *Entamoeba hystolytica* disappeared in two to five days from stools of patients treated successfully, and the lesions healed in five to 16 days.

One patient whose condition was improved but who was not cured refused further treatment, another's case was complicated by syphilis and anemia, and a third had both amebic infection and bacillary dysentery. In one case of failure, complicated with malaria and polyp of the colon, five days' medication did not influence the bowel symptoms, although amebae disappeared on the third day. Another patient received no symptomatic relief from six days' medication and motile amoebae were found in the stools daily. In the third case of failure, the patient had a slightly enlarged liver and a t. 38-39° C. Ya Tan Tzu relieved the symptoms, but the fever persisted. A diagnosis of liver abscess was established. Emetine was immediately used.

Among the 19 patients who responded satisfactorily, two had relapses—one at three weeks and the other six weeks after discharge. One was again controlled with Ya Tan Tzu and the other with emetine injections.

EPHEDRINE SULFATE IN THE TREATMENT OF NOCTURNAL ENURESIS
(W. E. Kittredge & H. G. Brown, New Orleans, in *New Orleans Med. & Surg. Jl.*, June)

A dose of ephedrine sulfate (1/4th gr.) taken by mouth at bedtime has proved extremely helpful in the control of nocturnal enuresis in children.

It is well to give it for three weeks continuously. If the habit returns, a second course of three weeks. In favorable cases the child ceases to wet the bed almost immediately, although he may miss one or two nights a week for the first two weeks.

SOUTHERN MEDICINE & SURGERY

Official Organ

JAMES M. NORTHINGTON, M.D., *Editor*

Department Editors

Human Behavior
JAMES K. HALL, M.D.................................Richmond, Va.

Orthopedic Surgery
JOHN T. SAUNDERS, M.D. ....Asheville, N. C.

Urology
RAYMOND THOMPSON, M.D..........................Charlotte, N. C.

Surgery
GEO. H. BUNCH, M.D..................................Columbia, S. C.

Obstetrics
HENRY J. LANGSTON, M.D.............................Danville, Va

Gynecology
CHAS. R. ROBINS, M.D.................................Richmond, Va.
ROBERT T. FERGUSON, M.D. ....Charlotte, N. C.

General Practice
J. L. HAMNER, M.D......................................Mannboro, Va.
J. HERBERT SMITH, M.D..............................Pauline, S. C.

Clinical Chemistry and Microscopy
J. M. FEDER, M.D.,
EVELYN TRIBBLE, M. T. } ....Anderson, S. C.

Hospitals
R. B. DAVIS, M.D..Greensboro, N. C.

Cardiology
CLYDE M. GILMORE, A.B., M.D..................Greensboro, N. C.

Public Health
N. THOS. ENNETT, M.D.................................Greenville, N. C.

Radiology
R. H. LAFFERTY, M.D., and Associates.......Charlotte, N. C.

Therapeutics
J. F. NASH, M.D..Saint Pauls, N. C.

Tuberculosis
JOHN DONNELLY, M.D..................................Charlotte, N. C.

Dentistry
J. H. GUION, D.D.S.......................................Charlotte, N. C.

Internal Medicine
GEORGE R. WILKINSON, M.D.......................Greenville, S. C.

Ophthalmology
HERBERT C. NEBLETT, M.D..........................Charlotte, N. C.

Rhino-Oto-Laryngology
CLAY W. EVATT, M.D...................................Charleston, S. C.

Proctology
RUSSELL L. BUXTON, M.D..........................Newport News, Va.

Insurance Medicine
H. F. STARR, M.D..Greensboro, N. C

Dermatology
J. LAMAR CALLAWAY, M.D. ....Durham, N. C.

Pediatrics

Offerings for the pages of this Journal are requested and given careful consideration in each case.... Manuscripts not found suitable for our use will not be returned unless author encloses postage.

As is true of most Medical Journals, all costs of cuts, etc., for illustrating an article must be borne by the author.

HOW TO GET DOCTORS TO PRACTICE IN THE COUNTRY

IT IS PROFOUNDLY GRATIFYING to learn from the current issue of the *North Carolina Medical Journal* that the mind of Dr. Isaac Manning goes right along with my own, a good part of the way, as to ways and means of improving the amount and the quality of the medical care rendered our country people.

He accepts it as a fact that the rural population as a whole is not receiving adequate medical care. Agreed, but *only* that this medical care is not far from adequate. In his common-sense way he points out that the good roads and automobiles have made a doctor 20 miles away nearer in point of availability than was one five miles away 40 years ago. "If, therefore (in rural counties having hospitals), the rural population is not receiving adequate medical service the explanation is not the scarcity of doctors, but is largely, if not wholly, economic."

In counties having neither adequate hospital facilities nor a sufficient number of doctors, the problem is again an economic one. "Doctors cannot be expected to locate in any section in which they cannot make a living. For this situation the only remedy is the subsidy. There are, however, other factors."

Recognizing as we all do that doctors being graduated now, thoroughly instructed and trained in scientific medicine, will not be content to practice "without laboratory and hospital facilities, although not necessarily hospital accommodations"; we should consider the feasibility of making these facilities available in the villages and rural sections remote from the towns.

The Duke Foundation's aid in building and helping support hospitals in various counties of North Carolina had for one of its purposes attracting doctors to the rural sections. However, as Dr. Manning says, generous and helpful as this aid is, the main burden is still on the community, and the economic condition of the community may not and does not in many counties justify the erection of a hospital as a solution of the problem.

Then he suggests as a less costly alternative the establishment of a diagnostic laboratory, a means which has been successfully tried out in Michigan. "The laboratories are equipped to furnish at low cost such laboratory information as the doctor may desire." Such a laboratory has become self-supporting within 18 months. It may become the nucleus of a clinic or hospital. Another alternative is to set up such a laboratory in connection with the County Health Department.

The clinic seems to this thoughtful doctor to offer the most promising solution of the problem of making the rural sections more attractive to the doctors. He cites a number of such clinics already operating successfully in North Carolina—all provided by doctors in private practice; all equipped for doing essential laboratory work, also minor surgical operations and obstetrics.

Dr. Manning thinks the young doctor, fresh from a hospital training and perhaps in debt for his education, may not be able to establish such a clinic; but, where such clinics are made available recent graduates who prefer an independent practice and the opportunity offered by provision of such a clinic by others, to get on promptly with the job of making a living, will accept the chance of a rural practice, and later may take over the clinic as a private enterprise.

The suggestion is made that revolving funds should finance these ventures and that some foundation might be willing to render such a real service to the rural population.

To provide for major surgical operations the rural population "must depend upon hospitals in nearby towns or cities, or upon a state-supported general hospital as suggested by the Governor." For major health hazards insurance is regarded as the only solution, and this can be brought within reach of the rural population through voluntary health insurance associations, which are designed for the protection of the low-income groups and furnish the service at the lowest possible cost.

Still further, those called leaders in the profession by newspapers and medical journals must cease to "damn with faint praise" the general practitioner.

Propagandists in the field of cancer have been great offenders in this matter. How many and many a time have you heard one of these proclaim: "It's just a matter of education." "Cancer taken in time is curable." And along with it a statement or a strong implication that, since the general practitioner sees the patient first (which is by no means always true), his is the responsibility for every death from cancer.

Repeatedly this editor has pointed to the high death rate from cancer among the leaders in the warfare on cancer. Dr. Wm. H. Welch died of cancer. So did Dr. Charles Lucas, the only cancer specialist Charlotte ever had. It is noted as a change of attitude, that the August issue of the *Bulletin of The American Cancer Society*, in an article, "The Family Doctor and Cancer," has this to say:

"Curability rates for early and late lesions are difficult to reduce to terms of statistics. It is generally agreed that *if it were possible* to bring to bear on every cancer patient the sum total of our present knowledge as soon as the patient is able to discover a deviation from normality, the cancer death rate could be reduced by *from 1-3 to 1-2* of its present 160,000 annual deaths. Specifically, the following claims are made for the curability of early cancer compared with the curability of late lesions:

	Early %	Late %
Skin	95	30
Mouth	80	20
Uterus	80	10
Breast	75	20
Rectum	50	0

It will be noted that no claim whatever is made as to cancer of the stomach, the cancer causing more deaths than cancer of any other organ.

That's a lot better. And we dare predict it will be appreciated by the scapegoats of the profession, the general practitioners, and will spur them to even better efforts since it does not hold them responsible for the attainment of the extravagantly impossible.

It so haps that the ex-president of the Tri-State Medical Association who died last month, chose as the subject of his presidential address, "The Effects of Present-day Medical Education on the Rural Physician"; and 20 years ago come next January, recommended some of the practical measures now being put forward, for meeting the situation.

Your attention is invited to these words of his: "Could it be that those of us who are privileged to deal with referred cases have forgotten the rights of the doctors at home? This is easy to do, in view of the fact that many patients have exaggerated the worth of the specialist and already may have mistrust of the home physician."

Masterly understatement that, for which the Scots are famous and Dr. McLeod went on:

It is the part of "those of us who are privileged to deal with referred cases" to *remember* the rights and the competency of the doctor at home. Suitable action following on this remembering rehabilitate the home doctor in the estimate of his people, will remove the mistrust, and go far in influencing recent graduates in medicine and surgery to adopt country practice as a lifetime vocation.

With Dr. McLeod I would urge, that specialists and teachers can make rural practice attractive by giving the general practitioner his just credit for being competent to take care of 80 to 85 per cent of the health problems of his community.

There was never a time when it was so easy to hire money, and at so cheap a rate. At 3½ or 4 per cent, any doctor could obtain money for establishing a clinic. Further, instead of a big hospital at Chapel Hill, if the State would provide half the funds, the other half to be provided by the county, in each county not having adequate hospital facilities, the country doctor could put his patient in the local hospital and see after him or her, himself.

thereby building up his prestige, his pride and his income in such a way as can never be done so long as he must refer to a specialist everything but the trivialities of practice.

* * * * *

DOCTOR FRANK HILTON McLEOD

After many years of semi-invalidism Dr. Frank McLeod is dead. He was born in Robeson County, N. C., in 1868, won his medical degree at the University of Tennessee Medical School, Memphis, in 1888, and soon thereafter opened an office across the border in the town of Florence, S. C., for the practice of medicine and surgery.

Soon his skill in office and home surgery won recognition and stimulated him to provide a small hospital for the better care of those who make up his large practice. Always he kept abreast of the progress of his art, and not a few contributions he made thereto. He made frequent visits to the great medical centers. From time to time he enlarged his hospital and improved its facilities, until from the little wooden building with accommodations for a dozen or so patients, evolved the magnificent temple to Hygieia in which his son, Dr. James McLeod, and his associates, will carry on the great work.

Dr. McLeod early took, and maintained to the end, the commanding place in the medicine of his state and section to which his talents and his energy entitled him. He was a Founding Fellow of the American College of Surgeons. All the high offices of the South Carolina Medical Association were his. As president of the Tri-State Medical Association in 1925, it is of special interest to observe, he addressed the association on "The Effects of Present-day Medical Education on the Rural Physician." Ideas expressed by him in 1925 are pertinent to the great problem of rendering medical care to our country people today.

"Could it be," he asked, "that those of us who are privileged to deal with referred cases have forgotten the rights of the doctor at home?" And he went on to say this is easy to do, in view of the fact that many patients have exaggerated the worth of the specialist and already may have mistrust for the home physician."

Medical education he said was now beyond the means of poor boys. He declared our rural districts must not be depleted of doctors and thought the State should lend aid to those who would undertake the study of medicine and would "agree to locate for periods of five to 10 years in rural districts." His closing sentence was:

"While one does not desire state medicine, yet state aid for the poor boy who would undertake the study of medicine may be his only chance, and certainly a very commendable way to aid suffering humanity."

Dr. McLeod foresaw much of what we are undergoing today. He was wise and resourceful and energetic in the prosecution of his professional duties, but he did not, while cultivating his special talent, neglect to improve his whole capital as a man. He was a power for all kinds of good over a large area for more than half a century; indeed, he still is, and always will be a great power, for those great influences he brought to bear will be continually exerted by those he stimulated and taught by precept and example. He ceased from his labors on the 24th of October, but his works do follow him.

* * * * *

DOCTOR JOHN McCAMPBELL

At the ripe age of 76, at the Davis Hospital of Statesville, N. C., on the fifth of November, died John McCampbell, Ph.G., M.D. Although he had been in ill health for many months, death came suddenly, of a heart attack.

It was in 1894 that he came to the State Hospital at Morganton. His first services to the patients in this hospital was as pharmacist, although he was a graduate in both pharmacy and medicine when he came. After three or four years he was made assistant physician. He was superintendent from 1907 until his resignation in 1939—only a little short of a third of a century. About all his medical life was given to the mentally sick there. His patients were devoted to him and he to them. His earliest and his best medical years were lived there in obscurity — unknown to the world — as druggist and as assistant physician.

Dr. McCampbell had a powerful intellect. He did his own thinking in his own way. He had a good command of language. He had a profound understanding of what we call human nature in all its mutations. With a few intimates he was genial and lively and entertaining; with a crowd he was withdrawn, reserved, almost mute. He was too modest to be assertive, even in his own defense.

A distinguished psychiatrist who knew him well writes: "He would not let himself become known. At a national medical meeting, when I would try to introduce him to my friends and to some of the big ones he would slip away. Pedestalization was painful to him; some such reasons as these kept him from becoming widely known. I know some psychiatrists of wide fame who lacked such intelligence as his, and such understanding of the human heart as his. He was a too-little-known great man."

Dr. McCampbell had served as chairman of the District Medical Board during the first World War and as president of the North Carolina Neuropsychiatric Society; he was a member of the State and Tri-State Medical Associations, and the American Association of Psychiatrists.

His wife, Miss Margaret Thompson, of Morganton, was Superintendent of Nurses at the hospital when they were married. Their only child they named for the great editor of the *Charlotte Observer*, Joseph P. Caldwell. Mr. Caldwell was at that time president of the Hospital Board. This son, a geologist, was teaching at his alma mater, the University of North Carolina, when he was called a few months ago to the Chair of Geology at Rutgers.

From 1939 to the time of his death Dr. McCampbell had done private practice in psychiatry, first at Wilmington, Delaware, later at Morganton

---

RENAL FAILURE DUE TO LOSS OF SALT AND WATER
(G. W. Thorn *et al.*, in *New Eng. Jl. of Med.*, 231:76-85, 1944)

The clinical picture is that of a shock-like state produced by excessive loss of sodium chloride and water and, as a consequence, dehydration, hemoconcentration, hypertension and collapse, which suggests Addison's disease. However, at autopsy the adrenal glands and the kidneys are found to be intact. Sodium chloride and water were lost because of the damage to the absorbing epithelium of the tubules.

Two patients representative of this form of nephritis were a man and a woman, each aged 21, who apparently had had no previous kidney disease. When first seen neither protein nor formed elements were noted in the urine of either. The initial state of collapse was successfully treated by administration of sodium chloride, glucose and adrenocortical hormone. However, the elevated blood urea nitrogen did not return to normal with such treatment and kidney-function tests indicated renal insufficiency.

Both patients were able to tolerate large quantities of sodium chloride (10 to 15 Gm. daily) and sodium bicarbonate (4 to 6 Gm. daily) without the development of edema and hypertension, in spite of renal insufficiency. This phenomenon persisted for two years in one case and for four years in the other, until one to two months prior to death in each instance. The ability of the kidneys to reabsorb sodium chloride in excess of water was greatly impaired in both patients, and large doses of sodium chloride were therefore necessary for the maintenance of an adequate plasma volume. Neither individual could maintain a sodium chloride level that would prevent rise in the blood urea nitrogen, hypertension or edema. Definite changes eventually appeared in the retinal vessels, hypertension developed, and death occurred in the same manner as from chronic nephritis.

The syndrome of "salt-losing nephritis" is probably not due to a particular lesion in the kidney, but rather to conditions which occur late in the course of slowly progressive renal disease. A small excess loss of sodium chloride daily results ultimately in severe depletion of extracellular fluid volume, hemoconcentration and terminally, from impaired function of the few remaining nephrons, in edema, hypertension and cardiac failure. Impending heart failure and excessive hypertension contraindicate the use of sodium chloride even in uremia.

"COURAGE AND DEVOTION BEYOND THE CALL OF DUTY"

Through the coöperation of Mead Johnson & Company, $40,000 in War Bonds are being offered to physician-artists (both in civilian and in military service) for art works best illustrating the above title.

This contest is open to members of the American Physicians Art Association. For full details, write *Dr. F. H. Redewill, Secretary, Flood Building, San Fransico.*

NEWS

MATHESON LECTURE FOUNDATION

The Opening Series of Annual Medical Lectures under the Matheson Lecture Foundation established by the will of Dr. J. P. Matheson, who died in 1937, were given at Central High School Auditorium, Charlotte, October 26th and 27th.

Speakers and Subjects:

Dr. Watson S. Rankin, born Mooresville, N. C., is now Trustee and Director of Hospital and Orphan Section, Duke Foundation.

Brigadier General James S. Simmons, USA, born Newton, N. C., is now Chief of Preventive Medicine, Army Service Forces.

Dr. John W. Moore, born McConnellsville, S. C., is now Dean and Professor of Medicine, University of Louisville School of Medicine.

Dr. John de J. Pemberton, born Wadesboro, N. C., is now Professor of Surgery, University of Minnesota Graduate School, Mayo Clinic.

Dr. William S. Tillett, born Charlotte, N. C., is now Professor of Medicine, New York University College of Medicine.

Dr. Joseph T. Wearn, born Charlotte, N. C., is now Professor of Medicine, Western Reserve University School of Medicine.

Dr. T. Grier Miller, born Statesville, N. C., is now Professor of Clinical Medicine, University of Pennsylvania School of Medicine.

Dr. Algernon B. Reese, born Charlotte, N. C., is now Associate Professor of Clinical Ophthalmology, College of Physicians and Surgeons, Columbia University.

> The Matheson Foundation
> Health, the Number-One Freedom
> Some Studies in Hemodynamics in Man
> Carcinoma of the Colon and Rectum
> A Survey of the Current Uses of Chemotherapy
> Some of the Contributions of the Committee on Medical Research to Medicine
> Management of the Medical Complications of Peptic Ulcer
> Participation of the Eye in General Diseases

The Matheson Lecture Foundation was established in 1937 as an annual lectureship under the will of Dr. James Pleasant Matheson, physician and long-time member of the Mecklenburg County Medical Society. Dr. Matheson was born at Taylorsville, North Carolina, graduated from Davidson College in the class of 1899 and in Medicine from the University of Maryland, class of 1905. He spent the greater part of his active life as an Ear, Nose and Throat Specialist in Charlotte and was one of North Carolina's most widely known and beloved physicians. His death on August 5th, 1937, resulted from an automobile accident. The influence of his life and character will be long perpetuated in the Medical Lecture Foundation which he established. Heretofore unavoidably deferred on account of the world conflict, the opening series of lectures is now presented.

STATESVILLE HOSPITAL FUND GROWS

The fund for the proposed new hospital for the Negroes of Statesville, N. C., and vicinity has reached $21,000. Latest contributions included $5,000 from Statesville Flour Mills and $700 from Belk Stores. The money is being raised through the efforts of the Negro Hospital Association which was organized a year ago. The goal of the association is $50,000.

Urology Award

The American Urological Association offers an annual award not to exceed $500 for an essay (or essays) on the result of some specific clinical or laboratory research in Urology. The amount of the prize is based on the merits of the work presented, and if the Committee on Scientific Research deem none of the offerings worthy, no award will be made. Competitors shall be limited to residents in urology in recognized hospitals and to urologists who have been in such specific practice for not more than five years. All interested should write the Secretary, for full particulars.

The selected essay (or essays) will appear on the program of the forthcoming June meeting of the American Urological Association.

Essays must be in the hands of the Secretary, Dr. Thomas D. Moore, 899 Madison Avenue, Memphis, Tenn., on or before March 15th, 1945.

SIXTH DISTRICT SOCIETY, Chapel Hill, Nov. 4th.—Dr. W. R. Berryhill welcomed the visitors. Dr. Paul Whitaker, president of the Medical Society of the State of North Carolina, spoke on "The Proposal for the Extension of Medical and Hospital Care in North Carolina."

Papers were read by Dr. Samuel A. Vest and Dr. Bruno Barclare, Jr., of the University of Virginia; Dr. F. T. Harper, of Graham; Dr. J. D. Fitzgerald, of Roxboro; Dr. Raney Stanford of Durham, and Dr. Verne S. Caviness, of Raleigh.

Dr. R. E. Brooks, Burlington, is president of the District Society, Dr. Carl Liles of Raleigh is vice-president, and Dr. Sidney Smith of Raleigh is secretary-treasurer.

The North Carolina Section of the AMERICAN COLLEGE OF PHYSICIANS held a meeting at Chapel Hill on the 3rd. Papers read by Dr. Edward S. Orgain of the Duke University Medical School, Dr. J. P. Rousseau of the Bowman Gray Medical School in Winston-Salem, Dr. William deB. MacNider of the University of North Carolina Medical School, Dr. P. P. McCain of the State Tuberculosis Sanatorium, Dr. Donnell B. Cobb, of Goldsboro, and Dr. C. T. Smith of Rocky Mount.

NEGRO PHYSICIAN NAMED AS AIDE AT PINE CAMP

Dr. Jack B. Porterfield, Director of the Richmond Health Department, announces the appointment of Dr. Felix J. Brown, as part-time physician at Pine Camp Hospital. He is the first Negro doctor to be employed at the hospital for tuberculous patients, and will treat the Negro patients at the hospital. The employment of Negro physicians for Negro patients had been advocated by Governor Darden, and by Dr. Riggin, of the State Health Department.

Dr. Brown is a native of Richmond and a graduate of Armstrong High School. He was graduated from Virginia Union University in 1926, and received his M.D. from Howard University. He interned at Freedner's Sanitarium for tuberculous patients in Washington.

A Unique Palatable Calcium Wafer

Hoffman-La Roche announces to the medical profession a new pleasant-tasting wafer for oral calcium therapy called Larocal Wafers with Vitamins C and D. Larocal Wafers contain a generous amount of calcium in the form of calcium arabonate—a readily-soluble, well-tolerated, and promptly-absorbed salt which is free from chalky taste. In addition, Larocal Wafers supply vitamins C and D in generous quantities—the latter for its important role in the absorption and utilization of calcium and the former for its part in the formation of dentine and bone matrix.

JOHN P. KENNEDY, M.D., F.A.C.S., Charlotte, N. C., announces to the members of the profession that he has discontinued cystoscopic examinations and treatments in order to devote his entire time to general surgery.

DR. E. S. KING, Professor of Bacteriology in the Bowman Gray School of Medicine, Winston-Salem, spent July and August in Washington at the Army Medical School taking the special course in Tropical Diseases. This was their 20th class since war began. After eight weeks there he was sent to Central America for five weeks, spending most of the time in Costa Rica and Guatemala visiting institutions having specially to do with preventive practices.

DR. ARNOLD J. LEHMAN is the new head of the Pharmacology Department in the University of North Carolina Medical School, DR. WILLIAM DEB. MACNIDER having retired from active teaching last year in order to devote himself entirely to research.

Dr. Lehman had his academic education at the University of Washington; took his M.D. degree at Leland Stan-

---

PRIMER OF SCLEROTHERAPY

by

H. I. Biegeleisen, M.D.

The first simplified explanation of Injection Therapy in any language. A clear presentation, with illustration and tables, of the essentials of the subject. Based on the author's original work which for the past twelve years has been published in the leading medical and surgical Journals.

Cloth, $2.00 postpaid.

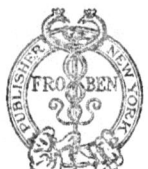

FROBEN PRESS PUBLISHERS

4 St. Luke's Place
New York 14, N. Y.

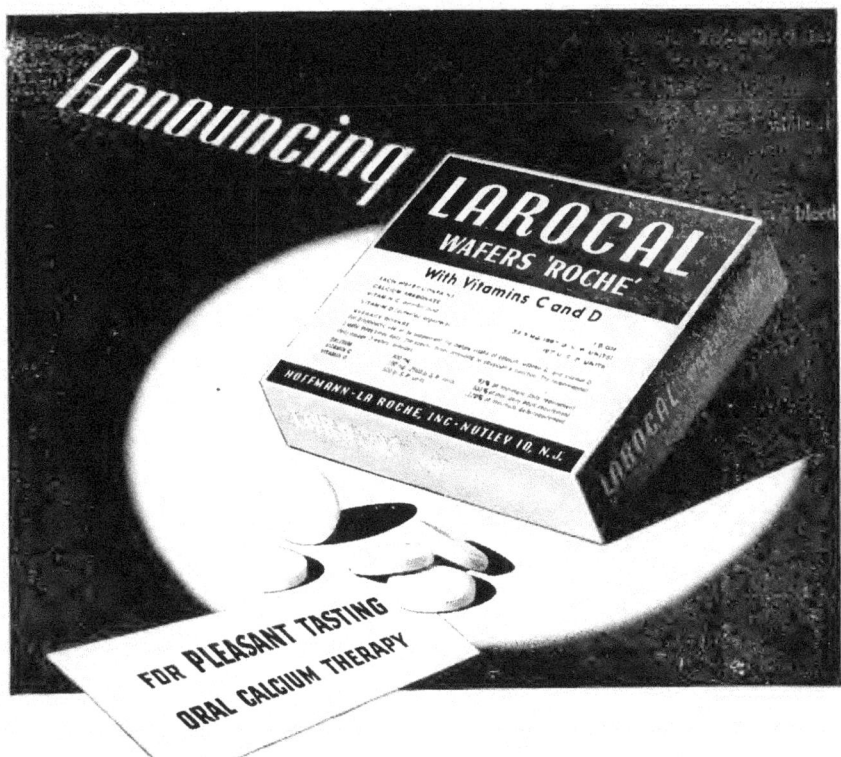

Roche now makes available to the medical profession Larocal Wafers 'Roche' with Vitamins C and D. These exceptionally pleasant-tasting wafers contain calcium arabonate which is promptly absorbed, non-irritating, and well-tolerated by the digestive tract; in addition, Larocal Wafers supply generous quantities of vitamins C and D.

INDICATIONS: During the period of growth, for proper tooth, bone and tissue development; to meet the highly increased calcium demands during pregnancy and lactation; as an adjunct to vitamin D therapy in the treatment of rickets; to supplement parenteral therapy in other calcium deficiencies. Supplied in boxes of 30 and 100 wafers.

HOFFMANN-LA ROCHE, INC.
ROCHE PARK · NUTLEY 10 · N. J.

LAROCAL WAFERS 'ROCHE' · CALCIUM WITH VITAMINS C and D

ford, Jr., University in California, and was in the Pharmacology Department at Stanford under the celebrated Dr. John Paul Hanzlik. In the last few years he has been at Wayne University in Detroit.

DIED

Dr. Charles B. Wilkerson died at his home at Raleigh September 20th, after a year's illness of cancer of the pancreas. He was a member of the staffs of Rex Hospital, and Saint Agnes Hospital, Raleigh. He was Wake County physician from 1921 to 1931.

Dr. Wilkerson began the practice of medicine at Apex in 1906 immediately after receiving his medical degree from the University of North Carolina, where he had transferred after attending Trinity College, now Duke University.

Dr. Frank H. McLeod, 76, founder of the McLeod Infirmary, Florence, S. C., died October 24th at his home after a long period of ill health.

Dr. McLeod established the McLeod Infirmary in 1906 in a small frame building. It is now a modern seven-story building with 200 hospital beds. He was a past president of the South Carolina Medical Association, also of the Tri-State Medical Association. He was a charter member of the American College of Surgeons, a recipient of the Sullivan award and of the LL.D. degree from the University of South Carolina.

One son, Major James McLeod, U. S. Army Medical Corps, stationed at Fort Dix, N. J., is a survivor.

Dr. Brown Carpenter, Major in the Medical Corps of the Army, was found in the wreckage of an army plane near Allentown, Pa., October 12th. Burial was at Danville, Va., where Dr. Carpenter had been in practice until he volunteered his services two years ago.

Dr. James R. Parker, 69, died suddenly at his home at Norfolk, Va., October 5th, of a heart attack. Dr. Parker was a former resident and practitioner of Clinton, N. C., moving to Norfolk 15 years ago.

FOR SALE—X-RAY EQUIPMENT

One G.E. Model B Victor 30 MA 85 KV. P. shockproof X-ray unit complete with curved movable table, built-in Bucky diaphragm, fluoroscopic screen for upright and horizontal fluoroscopy, dark-room fixtures, lead apron and gloves. Machine in excellent condition, has had minimum of use and is suitable for large office or small hospital. Owner is in service and will sacrifice all for $1,200. Terms arranged if desired. See at *Morrison Clinic*, Lancaster, S. C.

PATHOLOGIST (CLINICAL & GENERAL), widely known in Piedmont Carolina, with complete technical staff —wants location on straight commission basis with guarantee. Would equip laboratory under favorable circumstances. Address *Pathologist*, care S. M. & S.

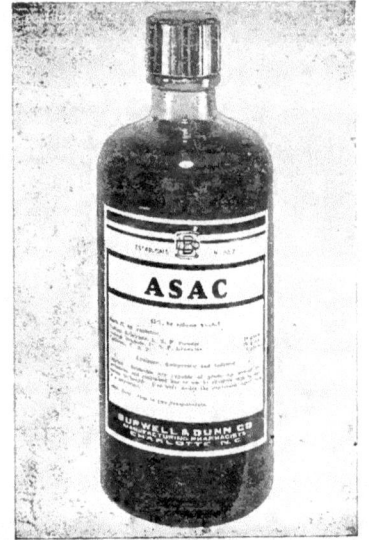

ASAC

15%, by volume Alcohol
Each fl. oz. contains:
Sodium Salicylate, U. S. P. Powder..........40 grains
Sodium Bromide, U. S. P. Granular..........20 grains
Caffeine, U. S. P.................................... 4 grains

ANALGESIC, ANTIPYRETIC AND SEDATIVE.

Average Dosage

Two to four teaspoonfuls in one to three ounces of water as prescribed by the physician.

How Supplied

In Pints, Five Pints and Gallons to Physicians and Druggists.

Burwell & Dunn Company

Manufacturing Pharmacists
Established in 1887

CHARLOTTE, N. C.

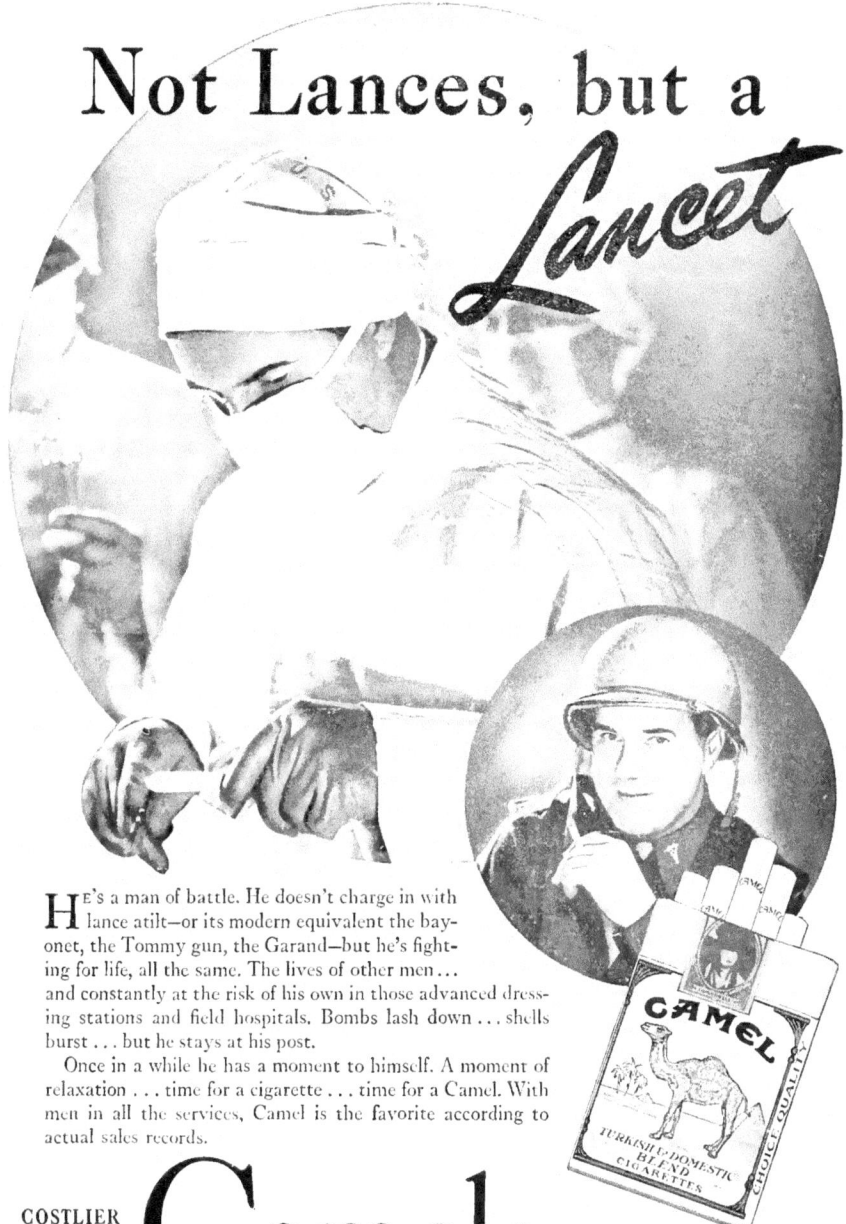

Vaughan Memorial Clinic

On September 1st, Dr. John W. Thomas joined Dr. W. Randolph Graham in the establishment of the Vaughan Memorial Clinic in Richmond, so that the splendid work of the late Dr. Warren T. Vaughan and of Dr. Graham can be continued. Dr. Thomas gives up the headship of the Department of Allergy of the Cleveland Clinic, where he has been for some time, in order to come to Richmond. In Cleveland he was President of the Cleveland Allergy Society; he edited *Allergy in Clinical Practice*, and he was assistant editor of the *Annals of Allergy*.

But in coming to Richmond he is coming again home, for he was associated for some time with Dr. Vaughan a few years ago.

And Dr. Thomas had his origin in the South and he is a graduate in medicine of the University of Georgia, and his internship was served in the University Hospital in Augusta. Dr. Thomas is assured a cordial return to Richmond and a busy professional life.

Danville Hospital Will Be Opened

A survey of Danville's (Va.) hospital needs made by representatives of a Federal body has been followed by a report that the city cannot expect to obtain funds under the Lanham Act. Steps were taken to reorganize Community Hospital, which closed its doors recently, and the city council agreed to give the stock company $4,000 to permit reopening until ways can be found for reorganizing the company.

The council, acting in executive session, took this action after the medical profession of Danville had endorsed the position that Danville needs two hospitals and cannot provide adequate service with one.

Dr. S. V. Lewis has been appointed Health Officer of Burke and Caldwell Counties to serve during the leave of Dr. L. D. Hagaman, now a Lieutenant in the United States Naval Reserve.

Dr. Lewis is a native of Nash County and a graduate of the Medical College of Virginia. He has had graduate work in the School of Public Health of the University of North Carolina and he has been in public health work for several years. He will live at Lenoir.

Dr. Hudnall Ware, Jr., of Richmond, has been elected president of the Virginia League for Planned Parenthood.

Why Treat Latent Syphilis?

(C. W. Barnett, in *Stanford Med. Bul.*, 2:51-54, 1944)

About the only justification for treating persons with latent, asymptomatic syphilis is the demonstration of positive evidence in the spinal fluid. Sixty-four per cent of persons with syphilitic infection of 15 to 40 years' duration will never have any symptoms, and 22% will die of other causes; benign conditions may occur late in 15%, neurosyphilis will develop in 10% and lesions of the cardiovascular system in 13%.

Women in the childbearing period should be treated because of the possibility of infection in the offspring. Negroes are more prone to syphilitic cardiovascular disease, and consequently should probably be treated. The obligation to treat asymptomatic, latent syphilis weakens as the age of the patient and the duration of the infection increases.

As It Came to the Registrar

Woman, age 35. Cause of death: Mr. and Mrs. Johnson were out driving. They had an argument. Mrs. Johnson jumped out. Mr. Johnson drove on home.

BOOKS

HISTORY OF GYNECOLOGY, by Richard A. Leonardo, M.D., Ch.M., F.I.C.S., Fellow Royal Society of Medicine (London); Fellow American Medical Association; Member American Association of the History of Medicine; Member American Medical Association of Vienna (Austria). Forewords by Prof. J. P. Greenhill (Loyola University) and Prof. Victor Robinson (Temple University). *Froben Press*, 4 St. Luke's Place, New York 14, N. Y. 1944. $5.00.

This informative book tells us that the ancient Hebrews practiced Caeserean section, and their midwives used the vaginal speculum and performed version; that Soranus (2nd century) inserted an astringent solution on soft linen by means of a sound for checking hemorrhage, and vaginal plugs of sponge to prevent conception, and enlarged a tight cervix for the cure of dysmenorrhea; that as Christianity became powerful science was stifled; that excision of the clitoris was a common practice among the Egyptians; that while Christian Europe wallowed in ignorance and filth, Mohammedan Spain had public schools, libraries, a high order of architecture, famous hospitals and baths.

John Hunter is credited with having been the first to advocate removal of diseased ovaries. Due credit is given Charles White (1728-1813) for his teaching of careful cleanliness in obstetrics. John P. Mettauer is given honorable mention for his repairs of fistulae. Marion Sims' statue is shown on the cover and his title of Father of Gynecology amply justified.

There is an account of the introduction by Battey, of Augusta, Ga., of the removal of the ovaries for the cure of dysmenorrhea and neuroses.

Improvements in instruments and techniques are recorded all the way down to 1942.

A unique contribution to the history of this large department of medicine and surgery. Every doctor of medicine will find it instructive and stimulating.

DERMATOLOGIC THERAPY IN GENERAL PRACTICE, by Marion B. Sulzberger, M.D., Commander (M.C.) U. S. N. R., Assistant Clinical Professor of Dermatology and Syphilology, Skin and Cancer Unit of the New York Post-Graduate Medical School and Hospital of Columbia University; and Jack Wolf, M.D., Attending Dermatologist and Syphilologist, Skin and Cancer Unit of the New York Post Graduate Medical School and Hospital of Columbia University. *The Year Book Publishers, Inc.*, 304 South Dearborn Street, Chicago 4, Ill. 1943. $5.00.

This book is written in response to a need long felt by medical officers of the Navy for a hand book which would make available for all practitioners of medicine the essentials of skin diseases and syphilis. The first edition proved of such high quality as to be commended by the Surgeon General of the Navy to all students and practitioners.

The principal changes made in this, the second edition, have been in a general condensation, a more useful indexing, and the addition of advances made in the interval.

We are under obligation to the authors for taking cognizance of the fact that the vast majority of cases of skin disease should be treated by the general practitioner, and for making available a book supplying the necessary information. Every doctor in general practice should have a copy and make daily use of it.

NEUROLOGY OF THE EYE, EAR, NOSE AND THROAT, by E. A. Spiegel, M.D., Professor of Experimental and Applied Neurology and Head of Department of Experimental Neurology, Temple University School of Medicine: and I. Sommer, M.D., Lecturer in Ophthalmology, Long Island College of Medicine; Consultant Ophthalmologist and Otolaryngologist, Chicago Eye and Ear Hospital. *Grune and Stratton, Inc.*, 443 Fourth Ave., New York. 1944. $7.50.

It is recognized that many have been the recent developments in what might be called the borderland between neurology and diseases of the eye, ear, nose and throat. This book is made up largely of postgraduate lectures in this field given in the past quarter-century at the University of Vienna, at Temple University and to various groups in this country. Many students have expressed a desire for the essence of these lectures in book form, so it was decided to make this provision.

So many of the symptoms, so many of the disease processes, in this field, have to do mainly with the nerve elements, as to make Neurology of the Eye, Ear, Nose and Throat a fairly comprehensive text on diseases of this specialty. Careful reading of the book will add greatly to the understanding of these diseases and of the rationale of a good many of the commonly used tests used by these specialists.

PRINCIPLES AND PRACTICE OF SURGERY, by Wayne Babcock, M.D., F.A.C.S., Emeritus Professor of Surgery, Temple University; Acting Consultant, Philadelphia General Hospital; with the collaboration of 37 members of the Faculty of Temple University. Illustrated with 1141 engravings and 8 colored plates. *Lea & Febiger*, Washington Square, Philadelphia 6, Pa. 1944. $12.00.

For a third of a century Babcock has pursued with great energy the practice of clinical surgery and research in the fundamentals of the surgical art. Now he has interested twoscore of his associates in working with him to produce a text covering the best in surgical practice of today. The surgery of trauma, the surgery of infections, thoracic surgery, orthopedic surgery, neurosurgery—all surgery is covered as to diagnosis, preöperative treatment, operative treatment, postoperative treatment, and in cases as needed, follow-up treatment.

The section on anesthesiology is quite complete, also that dealing with sutures, drains and dressings. A reliable textbook covering the whole of the art and science of modern surgery.

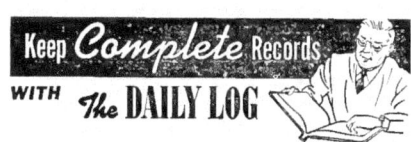

Dr. Colwell's DAILY LOG: A Brief, Simple, Accurate Financial Record for the Physician's Desk. *Colwell Publishing Company*, Champaign, Ill. $6.00.

This account book continues to meet the needs of the physician in a remarkably efficient way. If it has a defect, this examiner has not discovered it in making personal use of it over a number of years. No doctor of medicine could spend the price to better advantage, nor could he serve a doctor-friend better than by presenting him a copy as a Christmas present.

METHOD OF ANATOMY: Descriptive and Deductive. by J. C. Boileau Grant, M.C., M.B., Ch.B., F.R.C.S. (Edin.), Professor of Anatomy in the University of Toronto. Third edition. *The Williams and Wilkins Company*, Mt. Royal and Guilford Aves., Baltimore. 1944. $6.00.

This great teacher of anatomy has original ideas of how a subject should be taught. He realizes the need for presenting the subject by correlating facts and studying them in their mutual relationships. The human body is studied by regions, the parts considered according to the functions they serve. The illustrations consist entirely of line drawings, simple and accurate and conveying a definite idea.

The book represents the greatest advance in textbook teaching of anatomy since Gray.

MEDICAL WRITING: The Technic and the Art, by Morris Fishbein, M.D., Editor, *The Journal of the American Medical Association*; with the assistance of Jewel F. Whelan, Assistant to the Editor. *Press of American Medical Association*, 535 N. Dearborn St., Chicago.

It is generally said that the *Journal of the American Medical Association* is the best edited medical publication in the world. This book is written to teach the methods developed over many years by the editors of that journal.

TABER'S DICTIONARY OF GYNECOLOGY AND OBSTETRICS, by Clarence Wilbur Taber, Medical Editor, and Author of Taber's Cyclopedic Medical Dictionary, etc.; with the collaboration of Mario A. Castallo, M.D., F.A.C.S., Assistant Professor of Obstetrics, Jefferson Medical College. Illustrated. *F. A. Davis Company*, 1914-16 Cherry St., Philadelphia 3, Pa. 1944. $3.50.

An unusual kind of medical dictionary, reminiscent of the Century Dictionary and Cyclopedia, provided for every one concerned professionally with obstetrics and gynecology: in addition to doctors of medicine, the obstetrical supervisor, the medical student, and the nurse devoting special attention to these subjects.

The Century has well met a special need among the literate generally; Taber's Dictionary will well meet a special need among those having to do with Obstetrics and Gynecology.

OFFICE TREATMENT OF THE NOSE, THROAT AND EAR, by ABRAHAM R. HOLLENDER, M.Sc., M.D., F.A.C.S. Associate Professor of Laryngology, Rhinology and Otology, University of Illinois College of Medicine. *The Year Book Publishers, Inc.,* 304 S. Dearborn St., Chicago. 1943. $5.00.

As the author sees it, neither college curriculum nor training in special hospitals properly stresses the details of office management of otolaryngologic diseases; and there is a lack of this information in textbooks and monographs. To meet these needs he has written a book which will serve well the specialist in this field and the general practitioner who sees no reason why he should not treat the greater part of these ills among his patients.

With the idea that more patients could be adequately treated in offices and homes than is now the general practice, this reviewer is in strong agreement. This could be done with no detriment to the patient, and to the great advantage of patient and doctor.

Hollender's book is a conservative, sound dealing with this important field of medicine and surgery, which will be welcomed by doctors generally.

SEXUAL ANOMALIES. The Origins, Nature and Treatment of Sexual Disorders, by MAGNUS HIRSCHFELD, M.D., Former President, World League for Sexual Reform; Director, Institute of Sexual Science. Authorized Translation. *Emerson Books, Inc.,* 251 West 19th Street, New York 11, N. Y. 1944. $4.95.

This book is written for students, criminologists, educators, doctors and lawyers. It may be considered an addendum to the writings of Krafft-Ebing and Havelock Ellis. The publication's preface states "The essence of Hirschfeld's teaching was that he traced the development of sexuality to the action of the hormones on the germinal glands" ..... "formulated it with a greater precision and gave it a firm basis."

The arrangement is logical, sequential.

Book 1. The normal development of sexuality from conception to death.

Book 2. The quantitative irregularities of sexual development—under- or over-development of sexual impulse.

Book 3. Anomalies due to deflection of the sexual impulse—a deviation from the normal direction.

Books 4 and 5. Anomalies arising from independent development of component impulses which under normal circumstances merge with the sexual impulse.

The subjects dealt with in this book are those with which every physician should be familiar. Everybody dabbles in these subjects nowadays, and every physician should have authoritative information for passing on to his patient, somewhat for instruction, more for correction of what the patient already assumes that he or she knows.

HOMICIDE INVESTIGATION — LEMOYNE SNYDER, Medicolegal Director, Michigan State Police. *Charles C. Thomas,* Publisher, Springfield, Illinois. $5.00.

This is more than a textbook; it is a scathing indictment of the laxness of the average medicolegal investigation. Doctor Snyder, well trained both in law and medicine and with years of experience, is in an enviable position to make a contribution to criminal investigation.

Any serious act of violence upon the person can best be unraveled by a doctor, well trained in medicolegal methods, working in close coöperation with the police; preferably holding a commission in the department which places him upon an equal official plane with the investigating officials. It would not seem too much to expect that each state should have on the staff of its State Police such a specially qualified doctor, whose services could be placed at the disposal of any legal agency within the State at a moment's notice. Many are roaming the streets today who would have graced the electric chair, gallows, or gas chamber had an investigation been made by a medical man with proper experience and training.

Doctor Snyder well says: "Dead men tell no tales. Too often this is true. How much they tell may be in direct proportion to the care, diligence and conscientious effort that the investigators and laboratory technicians apply to the investigation. Sometimes the dead man becomes eloquent. As the science of homicide investigation advances, dead men will tell more and more." In most cases, medicolegal examinations should be made by an expert. Thousands of dollars are involved in many cases that come to post mortem study, so why should a hundred or two dollars autopsy physician's fee be a quibbling point? This book implies that 20 per cent of all persons die under circumstances that require an official probe into the cause of death. In the experience of the Michigan State Police, no serious crime has ever been committed by a person who was under the influence of marihuana.

"Homicide Investigation" is a succinct presentation of what to do and how to do it, and—of perhaps more importance—what-not-to-do is emphasized. Usually, when evidence has been destroyed or distorted by bungling, many links in the chain have been lost.

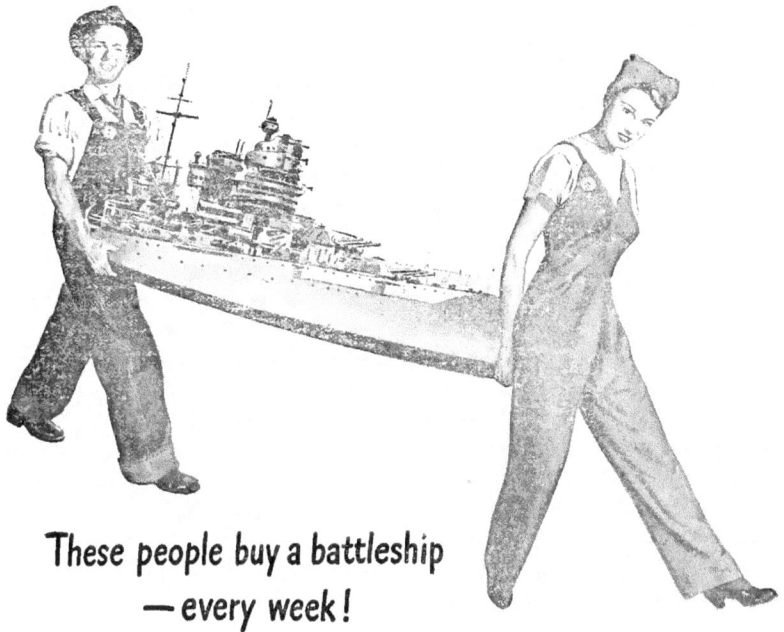

These people buy a battleship
— every week!

Meet John S. . . . . and Mary D. . . . . ,

John works at an electronics plant on Long Island, and makes $85 a week. Almost 16% of it goes into War Bonds.

Mary has been driving rivets into bombers at an airplane plant on the West Coast. She makes $55 a week, and puts 14% of it into War Bonds.

John and Mary are typical of more than 27 million Americans on the Payroll Savings Plan who, every single month, put half a BILLION dollars into War Bonds. That's enough to buy one of those hundred-million-dollar battleships every week, with enough money for an aircraft carrier and three or four cruisers left over.

In addition, John and Mary and the other people on the Payroll Plan have been among the biggest buyers of *extra* Bonds in every War Loan Drive.

They've financed a good share of our war effort all by themselves, and they've tucked away billions of dollars in savings that are going to come in mighty handy for both them and their country later on.

When this war is won, and we start giving credit where credit is due, don't forget John and Mary. After the fighting men, they deserve a place at the top. They've earned it.

You've backed the attack—now speed the victory!

YOUR NAME GOES HERE

This is an official U. S. Treasury advertisement—prepared under auspices of Treasury Department and War Advertising Council

T-126   5 1-2 x 8 in.   100 Screen   General Magazine Ad   Final Proof, 9-15-44

It is only logical for physicians to play a major role in the field of crime detection when one reflects that all modern criminal investigation is based upon a character who was the figment of a doctor's imagination — Sir Conan Doyle's "Sherlock Holmes."

It is to be hoped that Doctor Snyder will give us a "Medicolegal Pathology" at some time in the near future, as most books on general pathology miss this field by a wide margin.

—J. M. FEDER, M.D.

THERAPEUTICS

J. F. NASH, M.D., *Editor*, Saint Pauls, N. C.

THE PROBLEM OF THE RUPTURED INTERVERTEBRAL DISK

THE IMPORTANCE of rupture and extrusion of the intervertebral disk as a cause of disability and low-back pain is variously estimated. Some surgeons have gone so far as to predict that, with better recognition of the condition, soon more surgical operations would be done because of this than because of any other ailment.

Doughty's[1] presentation of the subject, with the discussion, provides a conservative guide.

Somewhat nearer the posterior edge of the intervertebral disk is a soft mass of fibro-cartilage with irregular connective tissue bands called the nucleus pulposus. The entire disk is held between the vertebrae by a capsule which is weakest on each side of the midline posteriorly. Flexion of the spine puts the joint surfaces of the vertebrae in a V shaped position. If a compression force is then applied the soft nucleus pulposus is forced backward, away from the point of the V and against the wall of the capsule. Rupture of the capsule frequently occurs to one side or the other of the midline. Through this tear a portion of the soft nucleus pulposus extrudes into the bony canal, and presses upon the nervous tissues.

A sudden fall to a sitting posture is often the exciting cause, in many cases so slight as to be forgotten. Pain in the back usually follows immediately often mild at first. This is the local backache due to joint trauma, relieved by rest and made worse by movement.

The immediate protrusion of a large cartilaginous mass does not occur in most instances. Should this happen, however, the pressure upon the cord, cauda equina or, as is most usual, upon the emerging nerve, gives rise at once to symptoms in more distant parts of the body. The picture is from that of a complete section of the cord to that of a mild irritation of a spinal nerve.

1. R. G. Doughty, Columbia, in *Jl. S. C. Med. Assn.*, Sept.

The amount of cartilage extruded is usually small, or there is simply a bulge of the capsule. In this event pressure on the emerging nerve, or other nerve elements, develops only at a later date as the mass slowly increases by further extrusion. As a result of the narrowing of the intevertebral space edema of the facet joints begins, further increasing the pressure upon the nerve root.

While any vertebral joint may be involved, 95% of all ruptured disks are in the 4th and 5th lumbar joints. The usual history is of a low-back injury or strain followed by low-back pain, relieved by simple measures but recurring on exercise. Sooner or later it is followed by sciatica, usually in one leg, but again not continuous. The pain may be severe during the acute phase; it is made worse by coughing, sneezing and straining at stool.

If the patient lies on his back with the edge of the table somewhat above the knees so that the legs hang free pain is so severe the position cannot be maintained.

The Achilles reflex is abolished in half the cases. Pain in the thigh and a disturbance of sensation in that location point to L 3. Lumbar puncture usually yields nothing worth while.

The frequency with which ruptured disks occurs and the percentage of spontaneous cures are both as yet unknown. It is only in instances where the attacks are so mild that they do not interfere with the normal life of the patient that operation is deferred. Complete curetage of the joint removes pathological tissue and produces an almost ideal type of fusion.

In discussing Dr. Doughty's paper:

Dr. J. W. White (Greenville):

This disc operation has been too frequently condemned because of the extravagant claims by overenthusiastic surgeons who follow their cases only a few months, barely beyond their acute convalescence. The insurance companies are still far from being satisfied with the results in their series of cases. Many cases, showing typical disc symptoms get well with conservative treatment, regulation of activity, general supportive treatment and proper mechanical use of the back.

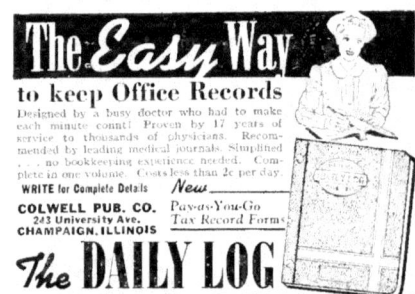

How a Dane Saved 4 Million Americans!

ONE of the world's greatest benefactors was Einar Holboell, Danish postal clerk.

As he worked long hours sorting Christmas mail, he thought of a way to put it to work for humanity ... and in 1904 started the sale of Christmas Seals to combat tuberculosis. Introduced in America in 1907, the Seals have helped cut the T.B. death rate 75%, have helped save 4,000,000 lives!

But T.B. still kills more people between 15 and 45 than any other disease. Your dollars are urgently needed now. Send in your contribution *today* — please.

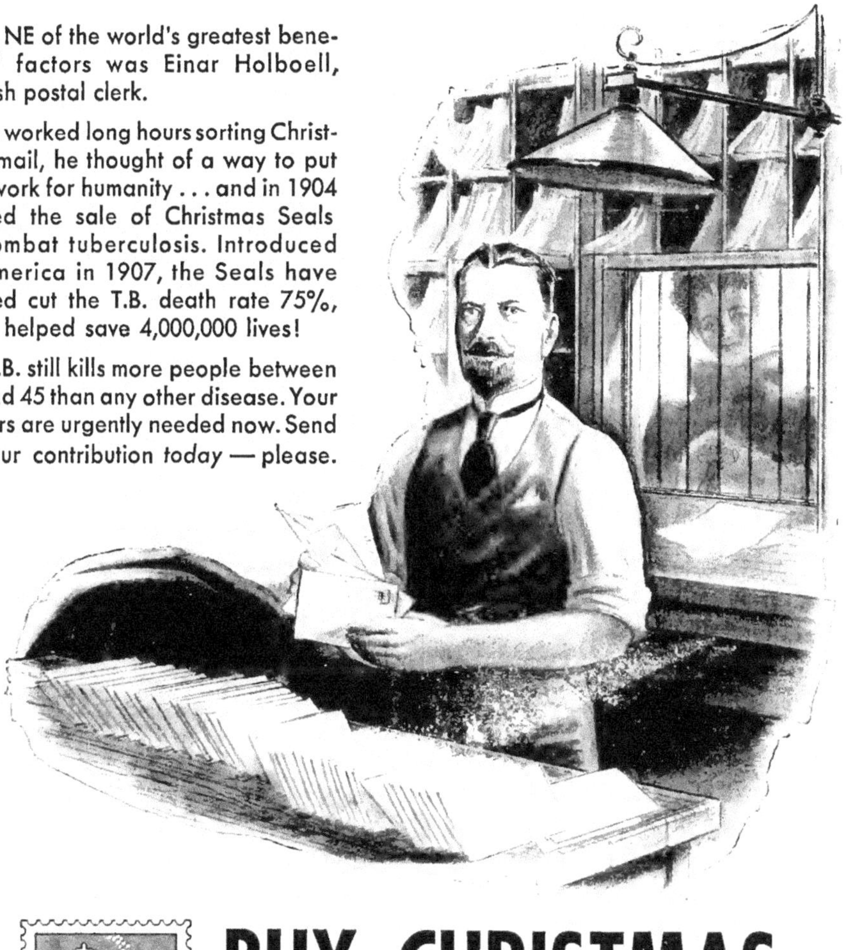

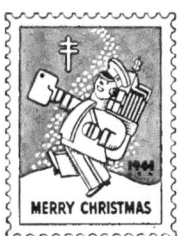

BUY CHRISTMAS SEALS!

The National, State and Local Tuberculosis Associations in the United States

NEUROLOGY and PSYCHIATRY

(*Now in the Country's Service*)
*J. FRED MERRITT, M.D.
NERVOUS and MILD MENTAL DISEASES
ALCOHOL and DRUG ADDICTIONS
Glenwood Park Sanitarium   Greensboro

TOM A. WILLIAMS, M.D.
(*Neurologist of Washington, D. C.*)
Consultation by appointment at
Phone 3994-W
77 Kenilworth Ave.   Asheville, N. C.

EYE, EAR, NOSE AND THROAT

H. C. NEBLETT, M.D.
OCULIST
Phone 3-5852
Professional Bldg.   Charlotte

AMZI J. ELLINGTON, M.D.
DISEASES of the EYE, EAR, NOSE and THROAT
Phones: Office 992—Residence 761
Burlington   North Carolina

UROLOGY, DERMATOLOGY and PROCTOLOGY

THE CROWELL CLINIC of UROLOGY and UROLOGICAL SURGERY
Hours—Nine to Five   Telephones—3-7101—3-7102
STAFF
ANDREW J. CROWELL, M.D.
(1911-1938)
*ANGUS M. MCDONALD, M.D.   CLAUDE B. SQUIRES, M.D.
Suite 700-711 Professional Building   Charlotte

RAYMOND THOMPSON, M.D., F.A.C.S.   WALTER E. DANIEL, A.B., M.D.
THE THOMPSON-DANIEL CLINIC
of
UROLOGY & UROLOGICAL SURGERY
Fifth Floor Professional Bldg.   Charlotte

C. C. MASSEY, M.D.
PRACTICE LIMITED TO DISEASES OF THE RECTUM
Professional Bldg.   Charlotte

WYETT F. SIMPSON, M.D.
GENITO-URINARY DISEASES
Phone 1234
Hot Springs National Park   Arkansas

ORTHOPEDICS

HERBERT F. MUNT, M.D.
ACCIDENT SURGERY & ORTHOPEDICS
FRACTURES
Nissen Building   Winston-Salem

GENERAL

Nalle Clinic Building 412 North Church Street, Charlotte
THE NALLE CLINIC
Telephone—C-BVDV (*if no answer, call 3-2621*)

General Surgery

BRODIE C. NALLE, M.D.
GYNECOLOGY & OBSTETRICS

EDWARD R. HIPP, M.D.
TRAUMATIC SURGERY

*PRESTON NOWLIN, M.D.
UROLOGY

Consulting Staff

R. H. LAFFERTY, M.D.
O. D. BAXTER, M.D.
RADIOLOGY

W. M. SUMMERVILLE, M.D.
PATHOLOGY

General Medicine

LUCIUS G. GAGE, M.D.
DIAGNOSIS

LUTHER W. KELLY, M.D.
CARDIO-RESPIRATORY DISEASES

J. R. ADAMS, M.D.
DISEASES OF INFANTS & CHILDREN

W. B. MAYER, M.D.
DERMATOLOGY & SYPHILOLOGY

(*In Country's Service)

C—H—M MEDICAL OFFICES
DIAGNOSIS—SURGERY
X-RAY—RADIUM

DR. G. CARLYLE COOKE—*Abdominal Surgery & Gynecology*
DR. GEO. W. HOLMES—*Orthopedics*
DR. C. H. McCANTS—*General Surgery*
222-226 Nissen Bldg.   Winston-Salem

WADE CLINIC
Wade Building
Hot Springs National Park, Arkansas

H. KING WADE, M.D.	*Urology*
ERNEST M. MCKENZIE, M.D.	*Medicine*
*FRANK M. ADAMS, M.D.	*Medicine*
*JACK ELLIS, M.D.	*Medicine*
BESSEY H. SHEBESTA, M.D.	*Medicine*
*WM. C. HAYS, M.D.	*Medicine*
N. B. BURCH, M.D.	
	Eye, Ear, Nose and Throat
A. W. SCHEER	*X-ray Technician*
ETTA WADE	*Clinical Laboratory*
MERNA SPRING	*Clinical Pathology*

(*In Military Service)

INTERNAL MEDICINE

ARCHIE A. BARRON, M.D., F.A.C.P.

INTERNAL MEDICINE—NEUROLOGY

Professional Bldg.   Charlotte

JOHN DONNELLY, M.D.

DISEASES OF THE LUNGS

Medical Building   Charlotte

CLYDE M. GILMORE, A.B., M.D.

CARDIOLOGY—INTERNAL MEDICINE

Dixie Building   Greensboro

JAMES M. NORTHINGTON, M.D.

INTERNAL MEDICINE—GERIATRICS

Medical Building   Charlotte

SURGERY

(*Now in the Country's Service*)
R. S. ANDERSON, M. D.

GENERAL SURGERY

144 Coast Line Street   Rocky Mount

R. B. DAVIS, M. D., M. M. S., F. A. C. P.
*GENERAL SURGERY
AND
RADIUM THERAPY*
Hours by Appointment

Piedmont-Memorial Hosp.   Greensboro

(*Now in the Country's Service*)
WILLIAM FRANCIS MARTIN, M.D.

GENERAL SURGERY

Professional Bldg.   Charlotte

OBSTETRICS & GYNECOLOGY

IVAN M. PROCTER, M. D.

OBSTETRICS & GYNECOLOGY

133 Fayetteville Street   Raleigh

SPECIAL NOTICES

TO THE BUSY DOCTOR WHO WANTS TO PASS HIS EXPERIENCE ON TO OTHERS

You have probably been postponing writing that original contribution. You can do it, and save your time and effort by employing an expert literary assistant to prepare the address, article or book under your direction or relieve you of the details of looking up references, translating, indexing, typing, and the complete preparation of your manuscript.

Address: *WRITING AIDE*, care *Southern Medicine & Surgery*.

THE JOURNAL OF SOUTHERN MEDICINE AND SURGERY

306 North Tryon Street, Charlotte, N. C.

The Journal assumes no responsibility for the authenticity of opinion or statements made by authors or in communications submitted to this Journal for publication.

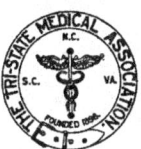

JAMES M. NORTHINGTON, M.D., Editor

Present-Day Concepts of the Rapid Treatment of Syphilis*

J. Lamar Callaway, M.D., and Ray O. Noojin, M.D., Durham

From the Division of Dermatology and Syphilology of the Department of Medicine, Duke University School of Medicine, Durham, North Carolina

SINCE Ehrlich's discovery of arsphenamine, syphilologists have been searching for a drug or treatment regimen that will effect an immediate biologic cure in which all spirocheta pallida are eliminated from the organism. Various saturation methods with the arsenicals alone or in conjunction with fever therapy or bismuth are being used in an attempt to effect a complete biologic cure. Recently penicillin has been introduced.

We shall attempt to survey critically several of the representative treatment schedules now in use, but we do not wish to imply that any treatment regimen omitted in this summary is not deserving of special comment.

All of the many rapid-treatment methods have as yet been in use too short a time to determine their eventual value. What will a 10- or 20-year evaluation reveal? Will the incidence of cardiovascular syphilis be greater in those treated by rapid-treatment methods than in those treated by the regimen as advocated by the Clinical Coöperative Group? Will the incidence of syphilis of the central nervous system be greater in the rapid-treatment group? Until these and similar questions are answered one will not be able to evaluate the newer forms of treatment. The importance, however, of investigation toward a solution of the syphilis-control problem can hardly be overemphasized.

It appears certain that out of the extensive and careful investigations now under way, there will come a form of short-course therapy for syphilis which will produce better results and, because of the short time involved, will enable us to hold our patients more easily.

Fleming[1] reviewed the subject of intensive therapy in early syphilis in May, 1943. The major contribution since that time has been the work initiated by Mahoney and his co-workers[2] with penicillin.

Five-Day Intravenous-Drip Therapy

It has long been recognized that the major difficulties in treating syphilis arise from the fact that, although trivalent arsenicals are spirocheticidal *in vitro* and *in vivo*, unfortunately they cannot be administered in doses sufficiently large to effect immediate cure.

In 1931 the syndrome of speed shock was described by Hirshfeld, Hyman and Wanger[3], who demonstrated that large doses of substances ordinarily highly toxic might be introduced safely into the blood stream by a slow intravenous-drip technique. Dr. Louis Chargin in 1932 suggested that a rapid antisyphilitic regimen might be evolved from the use of slow intravenous-drip therapy with trivalent arsenicals.[4] In 1933 Chargin, Leifer and Hyman[5] began treatment with this new regimen administering 4 to 4.5 grams of neoarsphenamine over a period of five days. To 50 c.c. of a 5 per cent dextrose solution 0.1 gram neoarsphenamine was added and this was administered intravenously at the rate of 100 c.c. per hour. After each 0.1 gram of neoarsphenamine had been received, the patient was then given 100 c.c. of 5 per cent dex-

*Presented to Tri-State Medical Association of the Carolinas and Virginia, meeting at Charlotte, Feb. 28th-29th, 1944.

trose solution without addition of the drug. Ordinarily during the average day the patient received 1,500 c.c. of 5 per cent dextrose solution and 1 gram of neoarsphenamine. Twenty-five patients were treated in this manner in the first series. Five years later 15 of the original 25 patients were available for reëxamination. Thirteen of 15 patients were felt to have been cured, with persistent negative blood and spinal-fluid serologic tests at the end of the period. Only two patients of the group were regarded as possibly having failed of cure. Although febrile reactions, toxicodermas, mild gastrointestinal symptoms, and polyneuritis frequently occurred during or following this rapid form of therapy, it was felt that the clinical results warranted further investigation. Dr. John L. Rice, Commissioner of Health of the City of New York, accordingly appointed a large committee to study the problem of rapid antisyphilitic therapy and they in turn agreed that the question should have additional investigation.[6] Further studies were continued by Chargin, Leifer and Hyman, and in 1941 they reported a recapitulation of all of their data accumulated from 1933 to 1941.[7] After treating a total of 111 patients with neoarsphenamine, it was discontinued because of a fatal case of hemorrhagic encephalitis and the frequent occurrence of peripheral neuritis. Mapharsen was substituted and at first was given in a total dosage of 400 mgm. in five days. Because of the frequent occurrence of infectious relapse, plus the infrequency of toxic reaction with mapharsen, it was gradually increased until a total dosage of 1,200 mgm. was administered. By 1941 they had treated 382 cases of early syphilis with either neoarsphenamine or mapharsen. Treatment with neoarsphenamine produced one death. There were no deaths due to mapharsen. Toxic symptoms in general due to mapharsen were many times less common than when neoarsphenamine was used. The authors felt that at least 81 per cent of their cases, whether treated with neoarsphenamine or mapharsen, had a completely satisfactory course (as regards serologic studies and mucocutaneous relapse), and that the figure might rise to 88 per cent, since the developments in several cases were still indeterminate. They felt that irrevocable failures approximated 5 per cent in the series, and pointed out that 41 patients were treated in the seronegative primary state with uniformly satisfactory results. This fact should be emphasized again and again. It is of course worthwhile to recognize that only a small number of these patients have been observed for a follow-up period for as long a period as five years. This New York group is deserving of high commendation for the impetus they have given to the study of rapid-treatment methods of syphilis.

The status of massive therapy with the intravenous-drip technique or a modification of it was reviewed by Elliott et al.[8] The results in 968 patients with early syphilis treated in 13 hospitals, indicate that the failures were only 5 to 15 per cent within 12 months when 1,200 mgm. of arsenoxide was used. There were five deaths due to toxic encephalitis in so treating 1,600 patients—a fatality rate of 0.3 per cent or 1:320. It was pointed out that the public-health value of controlling infection in at least 85 per cent of the cases of early syphilis by five successive days of treatment was of considerable significance.

MULTIPLE-SYRINGE THERAPY

In 1939 Thomas and Wexler[9] decided to modify the five-day intravenous-drip technique to the extent of giving 1,200 mgm. of mapharsen by the usual syringe technique in divided dosages. Sixty mgm. of mapharsen, dissolved in 10 c.c. of sterile distilled water, was given twice daily for ten days. After treating 38 patients in this manner, they decided to shorten the treatment period to six days because of the frequency of acute arsenical erythemas toward the end of the treatment period. The total dosage was maintained at 1,200 mgm., 0.1 gm. being given twice daily for six days. The 111th patient developed hemorrhagic encephalitis and died. Following this the daily dosages were decreased from 0.1 to .08, or .09 gm. in males, and .06 or .07 in females. Even with this reduction in dosages, two additional cases of hemorrhagic encephalitis occurred, neither, however, terminating fatally. Altogether they administered 280 treatment courses with mapharsen alone, before turning to the administration of smaller doses of mapharsen plus fever therapy in an attempt to reduce the incidence of hemorrhagic encephalitis.[10] Six to 29 months following treatment with 0.9 to 1.2 gm. of mapharsen in 151 patients, approximately 83 per cent had probable favorable results. There were three cases of toxic encephalitis in 280 patients, only one of which terminated fatally.

Schoch and Alexander[11,12] independently published in 1941 and 1942 reports of treatment of over 350 patients. Two-hundred and eight of this group were given a total of 1,200 mgm. of mapharsen in 10 days, 120 mgm. being given each day by the usual syringe technique. One-hundred and forty-two were given smaller individual doses over a longer period of time. In this group of 350 patients, hemorrhagic encephalitis occurred in three cases, one of which proved fatal. One-hundred and three of the patients treated by the 10-day regimen and observed for 6-18 months resulted in 77 per cent satisfactory results with an additional 11 per cent of the cases pending at the time of the report.

CHEMOTHERAPY COMBINED WITH FEVER

Boak, Carpenter and Warren reported in 1942[13] upon the combined use of neoarsphenamine and fever in experimental rabbit syphilis. Ten milligrams of neoarsphenamine per Kg. of body weight were administered in a single injection followed by 3 to 4 hours of fever at 40.5 C. This cured 98 per cent of 43 test animals. If the fever was induced before the arsenical, however, the percentage of cure was reduced. If only the drug was used and even with slightly larger doses, the percentage of cures was decidedly reduced.

At about the same time Boak and her colloborators[14] treated eight cases of primary and secondary syphilis with a single prolonged fever treatment for from 10 to 15 hours at 41 C. or above. The local lesions healed promptly and were usually dark-field negative before the treatment period had ended; however, four out of five patients who received no subsequent chemotherapy within four months, had a mucocutaneous relapse. Serologic tests for syphilis were not significantly altered.

Thomas and Wexler in 1941[9,10] combined fever therapy with mapharsen to avoid using more than .84 gms. of mapharsen in their rapid-treatment course. They hoped to get the same therapeutic results obtained with total dosages of 1,200 mgm., and at the same time to avoid the too-frequent occurrence of toxic encephalitis of large dosages. One of their treatment schemes was the administration of 0.54 gms. mapharsen in divided doses and four bouts of fever in nine days. They obtained 86 per cent probably favorable results in 299 cases followed six months or longer after treatment. Seven cerebral reactions and one death occurred among the 549 patients that were treated.

Simpson, Rose and Kendell,[15] after treating eight patients with early syphilis with 10 weekly five-hour fever treatments (40.6 to 41.1) without combined chemotherapy, abandoned its use because of the frequent occurrence of clinical relapses. The same authors[16] followed 27 patients with early syphilis for four to eight years after treatment with 10 to 12 fever sessions at weekly or semiweekly intervals, plus in most cases 30 weeks of concurrent neoarsphenamine 0.3 gm. or mapharsen .04 gm., and a compound containing 0.2 gm. of metallic bismuth. All patients had a satisfactory result, none showing clinical or serological relapse during the follow-up period.

Interestingly enough the same group[17] combined fever with chemotherapy, both given within a single day. Twenty-three patients with early syphilis were given one fever treatment lasting 10 hours at 41.1 C., plus administration of 0.25 gms. of bismuth subsalicylate just prior to starting fever. During the fever episode most patients received 120 to 240 mgm. mapharsen in divided dosages. No further treatment was given and all patients were followed at least six months after treatment. In all cases there was a progressive decline in titre in the Kahn quantitative procedure to negativity, as well as apparently satisfactory clinical results during the short interval followed. The authors recognized that the series was small and the observation period short, yet they felt that the method seemed sufficiently satisfactory to warrant further trial. There were apparently no fatal reactions.

PENICILLIN THERAPY

In a recent preliminary report Mahoney, Arnold and Harris[2] described the treatment of four cases of primary syphilis with the intramuscular injection of 25,000 units of penicillin at four-hour intervals until 48 injections or 1,200,000 units were given over a period of eight days. Evidence of clinical reactions during the period included malaise, headache, slight fever, and pain at the sites of the chancre and regional lymph-nodes. All lesions were dark-field negative 16 hours after initiating treatment. Frequent and varied serologic studies were carried out on each of the four patients. The decline in titre in each case was more or less rapid, indicating very favorable spirocheticidal effect of penicillin *in vivo*. This may well represent the most revolutionary contribution in antisyphilitic therapy since Ehrlich presented the arsphenamines. The results of further studies now under way will be eagerly awaited. A new era in syphilology may be in the making.

EXPERIMENTAL INTENSIVE EARLY SYPHILITIC THERAPY

Eagle and Hogan[18] recently pointed out the too-frequent occurrence of fatalities and serious central nervous system injuries in over 2,000 patients treated with intravenous-drip technique. One of every 250 patients treated in that manner has died as a result of the therapy. These investigators set out to establish certain criteria in the rapid treatment of experimentally-produced syphilis in rabbits which might also be applicable to man. The total duration of treatment in these animals varied from 10 seconds to six weeks.

It was learned that the maximum tolerated dose of mapharsen in rabbits with a single injection was 10 mgm. per Kg. More than 65 per cent of this dosage was excreted in one week. If injections were given three times weekly only 8 mgm. per Kg. could be tolerated over a four-week period. If four daily injections were given at two-hour intervals over a four-day period the amount tolerated per injection decreased to 2.4 mgm. per Kg. By administering a single intravenous drip for six hours daily over a period of four days, 50 per cent more drug could be tolerated than by four consecutive daily injections by syringe. In brief, these results reveal essentially the fact that by prolongation of the treatment period and by increasing the frequency of injections the total tolerated dose is significantly increased.

The same authors released additional interesting figures in a second publication[19] in which they stated that the total curative dose of mapharsen in syphilitic rabbits was 6.3 mgm. per Kg. for a single injection, 8.1 mgm. per Kg. divided into six weekly injections, 7.7 mgm. per Kg. divided into 12 tri-weekly injections, and 6.4 mgm. per Kg. divided into 12 daily injections. It is interesting to note that a single dose of 6.3 mgm. per Kg. accomplished no more than a total dosage of practically the same figure, 6.4 mgm. given in divided daily doses over a period of 12 days. Thus the size of the curative dose was affected to a minor degree only by varying the number of injections or duration of treatment. The suggested safety measure present with the smaller doses given over a longer period of time are obvious. The multiple-syringe technique was considerably more effective than the intravenous-drip method using smilar dosages over the same period and the margin of safety with the multiple-syringe injections was greater. All their experiments definitely indicated that tri-weekly injections represent the method with the maximum efficiently as regards the shortest interval between injections, and at the same time using therapeutically-effective doses with a large safety margin.

In summarizing the clinical implications[20] it was pointed out that the optimum intensive treatment schedule covers the shortest period within which a curative dose can be given with safety. It is revealed that the curative dose in man is 20-30 mgm. per Kg.—1,500 mgm. for a man of average size. The administration of 1,200 mgm. in five days by intravenous drip results in one death in each 200 patients treated, as compared with less than one in 3,000 in present schedules utilizingly weekly injections. They indicated that no regimen completed in less than 20 days can be curative and produce less than one fatality in each 1,000 cases, utilizing arsenicals, bismuth or fever. These same authors have interested 80 clinics in carrying out treatment using that regimen which to them seems from animal experimentation to be most logical, viz: tri-weekly injections, each injection approximately 1 mgm./Kg., with duration of treatment six to 12 weeks. The necessity of concomitant bismuth therapy is also under study. The results of the aforementioned investigations should prove of great value.

Resume

In brief several methods of rapid treatment for early syphilis are described, viz.: (1) five-day intravenous-drip, (2) multiple-syringe injections, (3) chemotherapy combined with fever, (4) Eagle's triweekly regimen, and (5) penicillin.

Hahn[21] reviewed the deaths occurring over a 27-year period in the syphilis clinic of Johns Hopkins Hospital. With routine therapy one death occurred in 1,250 patients treated with trivalent arsenicals, whereas in early syphilitics the mortality rate was one to 2,800 treated patients. It was felt that the lower fatality rate was due to their younger age and relative lack of concurrent disease. Hemorrhagic encephalitis occurred only twice among 27,400 patients given 270,000 injections. He points out that massive dose therapy may produce seven times as many fatalities as routine therapy, whereas hemorrhagic encephalitis may occur 60 to 70 times as often.

There are many pros and cons to the question of hospitalizing patients for rapid-treatment methods. Whether isolating a patient during treatment to make certain of complete therapy and to avoid contacts justified the expense, loss of time, and lowered morale will perhaps be eventually decided only when a definite satisfactory routine has been worked out.

The effects of the therapeutic measures discussed are as yet insufficiently tried in late syphilis and its variable complications.

Mapharsen has established itself as a very definitely active drug therapeutically and as having a greater safety margin than neoarsphenamine as regards untoward reactions.

It would appear that sufficient evidence has accumulated to sustain the fact that the use of 1,200 mgm. of mapharsen in 10 days or less is not justifiable because of the too-frequent occurrence of toxic encephalitis. Unless the combination of fever or other concurrent medication considerably enhances the curative effect of smaller doses of mapharsen, a therapeutic period longer than 10 days will be required. These considerations would seem to eliminate five-day intravenous-drip therapy as well as the 10-day (or less) multiple-syringe methods. The results of fever therapy combined with mapharsen are perhaps as yet insufficiently tested.

Turner and Sternberg[24] recently revealed that the U. S. Army had adopted a method of treating early and latent syphilis which is considerably more intensified and shortened than the usual alternating regimen. Forty injections of arsenoxide are administered in 26 weeks, injections being given twice weekly during the first and last ten-week periods. Bismuth subsalicylate is given weekly during the first to the sixth week, the eleventh to the seventeenth week, and the twenty-second through the twenty-sixth week. Thus from the eleventh to the seventeenth week only bismuth therapy is administered. This method has been in effect only a year.

Additional rapid-treatment centers are scattered throughout the country under the direction of the

United States Public Health Service and are doing an excellent job in this respect. The Army and Navy are also using modified short-course therapy.

The combination of 10 weekly or semiweekly fever treatments, plus an additional 30 weeks of concomitant arsenical and bismuth therapy, gave good results in a small series. There are, however, several obvious disadvantages to this method, particularly because it involves hospitalization, special equipment, specially trained personnel, etc.

Verbal reports on some 2,000 cases of syphilis now under treatment with penicillin indicate a most promising outcome. Detailed written reports and analyses will testify to the enthusiasm now rampant. Time alone will settle the validity of all treatment procedures.

Reinfection following intensive rapid treatment has been discussed thoroughly by Schoch and Alexander[22], Moore[23] and others. Many patients who have been classed as relapsed, and thus failures, in the newer systems are in all probability examples of reinfection.

Conclusions

1. There is at this writing no reported completely safe, adequately tested, and clinically satisfactory rapid treatment method for curing syphilis.

2. Although therapeutic results in many of the various rapid-massive-treatment regimens are good, the incidence of serious reactions including fatalities as a result of therapy is too great.

3. The average physician must for the present continue to consider the conventional system of alternating courses of trivalent arsenicals and bismuth advocated by the Clinical Coöperative Group as the treatment of choice.

4. Penicillin therapy appears to be the most promising method of treatment advocated. The triweekly treatment advocated by Eagle and his coworkers, with minor modifications, seems one of the next best methods in the light of present reports. However, there are definite objections to the triweekly treatment because of high morbidity rates, morbidity being not so great in the 26-week treatment regimen advocated by the Army and this less intensive method appears to offer a middle course.

Addendum.—Since these conclusions were drawn, additional experience with penicillin has been reported in papers by Moore, Sternberg *et al.*,[25] and Stokes and his co-workers,[26] on the use of penicillin in the treatment of early and late syphilis. From their published results it appears that penicillin bids fair to replace in a large degree the use of arsenicals, and or bismuth. At least penicillin. with various combinations of hyperpyrexia, arsenicals, and or bismuth, appears to bring the cure of syphilis nearer than ever before. In preliminary studies which we are conducting in the treatment of early and central nervous system syphilis under a contract with the Office of Scientific Research and Development of the National Research Council we concur in the enthusiasm they have expressed.

Results to be published by those coöperating in the studies now under way under the auspices of the National Research Council, together with the experience of the Army, Navy and United States Public Health Service, will demonstrate the eventual effectiveness of penicillin.

Bibliography

1. Fleming, W. L.: Intensive Treatment of Early Syphilis. *North Carolina Med. J.*, 5:6-12 (Jan.), 1944.
2. Mahoney, J. F., Arnold, R. C., and Harris, A.: Penicillin Treatment of Early Syphilis: A Preliminary Report. *Ven. Ds. Inform.*, 24-355-357 (Dec.), 1943.
3. Hirshfeld, S., Hyman, H. R., and Wanger, J. J.: Influence of Velocity on the Response to Intravenous Injections. II *Arch. Int. Med.*, 47:259 (Feb.), 1931.
4. Baehr, F.: Massive Arsenotherapy in Early Syphilis by the Continuous Intravenous Drip Method; the Preliminary Work with Neoarsphenamine. *Arch. Dermat. & Syph.*, 42:239-244 (Aug.), 1940.
5. Chargin, L., Leifer, W., and Hyman, H. T.: The Application of the Intravenous Drip Method to Chemotherapy as Illustrated by Massive Doses of Arsphenamine in the Treatment of Early Syphilis. *J. A. M. A.*, 104:878 (March 16th), 1935.
6. Hyman, H. T., Chargin, L., Rice, J. L., and Leifer, W.: Massive Dose Chemotherapy of Early Syphilis by the Intravenous Drip Method. *J. A. M. A.*, 113:1208-1215 (Sept. 23rd), 1939.
7. Leifer, W., Chargin, L., and Hyman, H. T.: Massive Dose Arsenotherapy of Early Syphilis by Intravenous Drip Method: Recapitulation of the Data (1933 to 1941). *J. A. M. A.*, 117:1154-1160 (Oct. 4th), 1941.
8. Elliott, D. C., Baehr, G., Shaffer, L. W., Usher, G. S., and Lough, S. A.: An Evaluation of the Massive Dose Therapy of Early Syphilis. *J. A. M. A.*, 117:1160-1164 (Oct.), 1941.
9. Thomas, E. W., and Wexler, G.: Rapid Treatment of Early Syphilis with Multiple Injections of Mapharsen-Preliminary Report of 275 Cases Treated with Mapharsen Alone and 141 Cases Treated with Mapharsen and Fever. *Am. J. of Publ. Health*, 31:545-556 (June), 1941.
10. Thomas, E. W., and Wexler, G.: Rapid Treatment of Early Syphilis. Report of Two Hundred and Eighty Treatment Courses with Mapharsen Alone and Five Hundred and Forty-nine Treatment Courses with Mapharsen Combined with Fever. *Arch. Dermat. & Syph.*, 47:553-568 (April), 1943.
11. Schoch, A., and Alexander, L. J.: Short Term Intensive Arsenotherapy of Early Syphilis. *Am. J. Syph., Gonor. & Ven. Dis.*, 25:607-609 (Sept.), 1941.
12. Schoch, A., and Alexander, L. J.: Intensive Arsenotherapy of Early Syphilis: Follow-up Report on the Ten-day Method. *Arch. Dermat. & Syph.*, 46:128-129 (July), 1942.
13. Boak, R. A., Carpenter, C. M. and Warren, S. L.: The Concurrent Treatment with Fever and Neoarsphenamine of Experimental Syphilis in Rabbits. *Am. J. Syph., Gonor. & Ven. Dis.*, 26:282-290 (May), 1942.

14. BOAK, R. A., CARPENTER, C. M., JONES, N., KAMP-MEIER, R. H., McCANN, W. S., WARREN, S. L., and WILLIAMS, JR., J. R.: The Inadequacy of a Single Prolonged Fever for the Treatment of Early Acute Syphilis. *Am. J. Syph., Gonor. & Ven. Dis.*, 26:291-298 (May), 1942.
15. SIMPSON, W. M., ROSE, D. L., and KENDELL, H. W.: Quantitative Serologic Studies in Early Syphilis. I Treatment with Artificial Fever Alone. *Ven. Dis. Inform*, 23:403-407 (Nov.), 1942.
16. KENDELL, H. W., ROSE, D. L., and SIMPSON, W. M.: Quantitative Serologic Studies in Early Syphilis. II Treatment with Artificial Fever Combined with Chemotherapy. *Ven. Dis. Inform.*, 23:408-411 (Nov.), 1942.
17. ROSE, D. L., SIMPSON, W. M., and KENDELL, H. W.: Quantitative Serologic Studies in Early Syphilis. III Treatment with a Single Intensive Session of Combined Fever-Chemotherapy. *Ven. Dis. Inform.*, 23:411-415 (Nov.), 1942.
18. EAGLE, H., and HOGAN, R. B.: An Experimental Evaluation of Intensive Methods for the Treatment of Early Syphilis. I. Toxicity and Excretion. *Ven. Dis. Inform.*, Vol. 24:33-44 (Feb.), 1943.
19. EAGLE, H., and HOGAN, R. B.: An Experimental Evaluation of Intensive Methods for the Treatment of Early Syphilis. II. Therapeutic Efficacy and Margin of Safety. *Ven. Dis. Inform.*, Vol. 24:69-79 (March), 1943.
20. EAGLE, H., and HOGAN, R. B.:: An Experimental Evaluation of Intensive Methods for the Treatment of Early Syphilis. III. Clinical Implications. *Ven. Dis. Inform.*, Vol. 24:159-170 (June), 1943.
21. HAHN, R. D.: Antisyphilitic Treatment: Mortality Studies. *Am. J. Syph., Gonor. & Ven. Dis.*, Vol. 25: 659-686.
22. SCHOCH, A. G., and ALEXANDER, L. J.: Reinfection in Syphilis: Newer Concept of Reinfection Encountered with Ten-day Arsenotherapy of Early Syphilis. *Am. J. Syph., Gonor. & Ven. Dis.*, 27:15 (Jan.), 1943.
23. MOORE, J. E., Editorial: Intensive Arsenotherapy and the Curability of Early Syphilis as Measured by the Criterion of Reinfection. *Am. J. Syph., Gonor. & Ven. Dis.*, 27:108 (Jan.), 1943.
24. TURNER, T. B., and STERNBERG, T. H.: Management of the Venereal Diseases in the Army. *J. A. M. A.*, 124: 133 (Jan. 15th), 1944.
25. MOORE, J. E., MAHONEY, J. F., SCHWARTZ, COMDR. W. H. (MC) USN, STERNBERG, LT. COL. T. H. (MC) AUS, WOOD, W. B.: The Treatment of Early Syphilis With Penicillin. *J. A. M. A.*, 126-67 (Sept. 9th), 1944.
26. STOKES, J. H., STERNBERG, LT. COL. T. H. (MC) AUS, SCHWARTZ, COMDR. W. H. (MC) USN, MAHONEY, J. F., MOORE, J. E., and WOOD, W. B.: The Action of Penicillin in Late Syphilis. *J. A. M. A.*, 126:73 (Sept. 9th), 1944.

DISCUSSION

DR. R. L. RAIFORD, Franklin, Va.: During my years of practice, I have seen some pretty severe cases of dermatitis from giving the arsenicals. The last case that I had—somebody had advised me to give mapharsen for shingles or herpes, and I gave it just because so very distinguished a man gave me this advice. I gave two minimum doses of mapharsen and the patient developed the most aggravating arsenical dermatitis that one ever saw. I came up particularly to ask the question—what would happen in this intensive syphilis treatment if you happened to strike a person susceptible to arsenicals to the extent this was as indicated by response to two treatments of mapharsen at intervals for some other disease? Would it cause such an intense dermatitis? It seems to me unless there is some way to rule that type of person out, it would give a lot of trouble. I'd like to have Dr. Callaway express himself on that line.

DR. T. C. BRITT, Mount Airy, N. C.: Gentlemen, a few years ago I had an experience with neoarsphenamine which I have been asked to report after ten years out of Public Health work.

The nearest approximation to giving a lethal dose of neoarsphenamine in my experience happened in Durham in 1928. I was ill. It was just after Christmas and we had a large clinic and I had invited two young fellows from Watts Hospital who had little experience in giving mass treatment. I crawled from the bedside and asked the two young men to come down for me. On this afternoon I went over the size of ampules that I had in the office. The first five patients were given 4.5 grams of neoarsphenamine. They fell out on the way down from the office. There were two colored people, one man and one woman, and one white woman and two men. It was a very sad experience. I learned about the thing on Saturday morning and we visited all those patients. They were all hospitalized save one. Three died and two survived—one a Negro boy 18 or 20 years old, and when we went back to look for him, he was standing behind the door. We asked for him and he said, "Here I is," and apparently it didn't affect him at all. The other patient who survived was a woman who had neuritis and partial paralysis, with atrophy of muscles and lower extremities. I had occasion to pass through Durham some time after that and I was interested to look her up. At that time she was going to a chiropractor and she was getting well. Three patients died of multiple small hemorrhages over the body. Two of them developed severe jaundice. The entire report I can't give, but I thought at thi stime I would mention that. The Public Health Service told me after that that it was the approximated maximum dose a man might take and live.

DR. HOWARD P. STEIGER, Charlotte: I agree with Dr. Calloway that in new procedures, treatment schemes, etc., conservative reasoning and caution must be used. When the sulfonamides first came into use we followed conservative methods. I'm sure that most of you now agree that all patients receiving sulfonamides do not have to be admitted to the hospital and receive daily complete blood counts and all the other laboratory data that these patients received six or seven years ago.

Dr. Ca'loway in quoting Hahn states that encephalopathy occurred in two of 27,400 cases treated by routine methods whereas it occurs in one of 320 cases treated intensively. This appears to be a great difference and certainly speaks against intensive therapy. There are a few loopholes in that statement, however. First—what percentage of that 27,400 patients completed treatment?, and second—how many reactions occurred in patients who left the clinic or in patients who later died from "other causes," or simply lapsed from treatment.

It is estimated that less than one-third of all patients started on antiluetic therapy ever complete, say, 20 arsenical and 20 bismuth injections, with enough regularity to prevent relapse or late complications of the disease. The average clinic patient in North Carolina receives only 16 injections in a period of 12 months. The greatest difficulty, however, is that the clandestine, the transient and even the truck-driver, who is more likely to disseminate the disease, is less likely to take treatment regularly than the less promiscuous individual. In other words, when we talk about conservative treatment, that is, 18-months treatment, for the greatest disseminators of this disease, we are talking about a treatment that doesn't exist. What have we ac-

To Page 475

Utilization (at Suprapubic Hysterectomy) of the Round Ligaments of the Uterus to Insure Better Bladder Support*

GEORGE H. BUNCH, M.D., Columbia

CYSTOCELE, or herniation of the urinary bladder into the vagina, is a steadily progressive disabling condition which, if unrelieved, inevitably leads to chronic invalidism. This results from the dragging weight of the prolapsed bladder and from ascending urinary infection caused by inability of the atonic bladder to completely empty itself. Although cystocele may be of congenital origin most cases result from weakening or disruption of supportive tissues in the anterior vaginal wall at childbirth. That the condition may also be caused by loss of bladder support incident to suprapubic hysterectomy, whether total or subtotal, is not generally appreciated. Though the rate of occurrence is relatively small, after such a common operation as hysterectomy, the total number of cases is considerable. The complication is found more frequently in elderly multiparae in many of whom a relaxed perineum and moderate loss of bladder support are already present before hysterectomy is done. After hysterectomy, as after childbirth, failing support may remain symptomless and unsuspected until made manifest in old age by loss of muscle tone.

In the lacerations of childbirth the posterior perineal muscles almost always give way first and rectocele of some degree is practically a universal complication of torn perineum. It is the usual finding in cystocele. In our experience rectocele, uncomplicated by cystocele, uterine prolapse or bowel incontinence from a completely torn sphincter ani muscle, causes but few symptoms and is readily cured by perineal repair. However, a wide-open vaginal outlet affords no support and invites herniation. For this reason perineorrhaphy is an essential procedure in the prevention and in the cure of cystocele.

In women the bladder is supported from below by a strong plane of fascia which, forming an integral part of the anterior vaginal wall, is attached anteriorly to the symphysis pubis, laterally to the pubic rami and posteriorly to the anterior wall of the internal os up to the peritoneal reflexion. It is longer antero-posteriorly than it is laterally and the only opening in it is for the urethral meatus. Firm bony attachment in front and on the sides makes the posterior or cervical attachment the more vulnerable to injury from either childbirth or hysterectomy. The fascia forms a supportive floor under the bladder which, as it fills, extends into the pelvis rather than into the vagina. In large cystoceles the fascia becomes thin and attenuated from stretching. The cervix is dependent upon the uterine ligaments for support and when this fails, whether from childbirth or from operation, the posterior anchorage of the fascia becomes insecure. From this the fascia sags under the weight of the full bladder and a vicious cycle begins: the greater the weight of the progressively enlarging cystocele the greater the sag, and the greater the sag the greater the distention and the weight. The supportive power of the fascia depends primarily upon the security of its posterior mooring, which, as has been shown, may be lost after suprapubic hysterectomy if care is not taken at operation to prevent it.

The cure of cystocele from any cause once it has developed is a problem in mechanics and in anatomy that severely taxes the judgment and the skill of the gynecologist. There are but two operative procedures that have proven to be generally effective: first, the Watkins interposition operation; and second, vaginal hysterectomy. In the Watkins operation the bladder is made to lie upon the posterior surface of the fundus of the uterus which is held permanently in acute antefiexion by being sutured to the periosteum of the pubic rami and to the anterior vaginal fascia. At the operation the fallopian tubes should be resected. The possibility of pregnancy is a contraindication. Vaginal hysterectomy should be done when there is the suspicion of uterine or of cervical malignancy. In this procedure, after the uterus has been removed, the ligatured ends of the ligaments are sutured to those of the opposite side under the bladder across the midline and also to the periosteum of the pubic rami so as to form a supportive sling for the bladder.

Both operations are done vaginally. It is a surgical axiom that cystocele cannot be cured by laparotomy alone. In the Watkins operation the fundus, and in vaginal hysterectomy the ligaments of the uterus, are used to restore the bladder to its normal position and to maintain it there by

---

*Presented to Tri-State Medical Association of the Carolinas and Virginia, meeting at Charlotte, Feb. 28th-29th, 1944.

adequate support. Because neither the uterus nor the ligaments are available for this purpose, the treatment of cystocele developing after suprapubic hysterectomy is unsatisfactory. In these cases, at subsequent laparotomy the retracted atrophic uterine ligaments may be identified and sutured to the vaginal vault, and at colporrhaphy a longitudinal strip may be removed from the anterior vaginal fascia and the defect closed by suture to give better support to the bladder by reducing the width of the fascia. After both procedures have been done, however, many cases recur and the patient then faces the alternative of wearing a pessary for bladder support, which is ineffective, or of being denied marital relationship by having total ablation of the vagina done. These cases are not rare. We all see them. Disappointed and unrelieved they become derelicts going the rounds. They are the victims of surgery who suffer more from the effects of operation than many of them would have suffered from their disease.

As postoperative cystocele has been found to be intractable to surgical treatment the writer has sought a way at suprapubic hysterectomy of utilizing available anatomic structures to suspend the vaginal vault after total or subtotal removal of the uterus, and to provide lasting support to the bladder postoperatively. He has not seen the method described in operative gynecologies but has made no complete study of the literature. As details in technique have been perfected in about a hundred cases done over a period of nearly five years, neither the operative time nor the hazard is appreciably greater in his hands than in hysterectomy done in the ordinary way. When routine work is resumed after operation the patients have a feeling of support and of security. Those who have returned for examination months after operation have, without exception, had satisfactory support.

The Method: Through a midline incision the uterus and the cervix are removed after both the round and the broad ligaments have been severed flush with the uterus, so they remain uninjured throughout their full length. The vaginal vault is closed with an interlocking catgut suture. The ligatured stumps of the uterine vessels are securely sutured to the vault at the line of closure. When traction is made upon the vault an avascular line of cleavage in uncomplicated cases may be demonstrated between the bladder and the vault anteriorly, so that the bladder, by blunt dissection, may be readily separated as far as may be desired from the white anterior vaginal fascia lying under it. The round ligaments are sutured under the retracted bladder to the fascia an inch or more anterior to its line of closure instead of being sutured to this line as in ordinary hysterectomy. If each ligament is first sutured at a suitable point, near its origin from the internal inguinal ring, to the edge of the fascia on the same side, the distal end of the ligament reaches across the fascia to the opposite edge and may be sutured there without undue tension. Ordinarily for this purpose a running mattress suture of chromic catgut is used, each stitch passing through the center of the ligament. The suture line should extend along the middle of the ligament so as not to impair its blood supply. The round ligament from the other side, when sutured in a similar way to the fascia, should lie beside the first without overlapping, so as to afford maximum surface contact of the ligaments with the fascia. To maintain the length of the vagina, whether the adnexae have been removed or not, the ligatured ends of the broad and the sacro-uterine ligaments are sutured to the vaginal vault at its line of closure. Finally, the operative field is peritonealized in the usual way. If subtotal hysterectomy is done the round ligaments are sutured under the retracted bladder to the anterior vaginal fascia just as in the total operation.

It is surprising how the elastic round ligaments may be made to stretch so that they may be sutured to the fascia under the bladder almost to the region of the trigone without undue tension. In this operation this quality enables us to use them to reinforce and to strengthen the fascia where it is weakest and to support the bladder in much the same way as in vaginal hysterectomy. The development of cystocele after suprapubic hysterectomy should be prevented at the time of operation. That the round ligaments when sutured to the fascia under it give better support to the bladder than when sutured to the vaginal vault above is a sound mechanical principle.

DISCUSSION

DR. W. M. SCRUGGS, Charlotte: Gentlemen, I am sure we appreciate Dr. Bunch's presentation of this subject, as we recognize him not only as an able surgeon, but an ingenious technician.

There probably isn't anything that presents itself to those of us who do much gynecology so embarrassing as one of those postoperative cystoceles following a suprapubic hysterectomy. For a good many years I have tried to obviate the possibility of the development of the cystocele in those cases in which it seemed most likely to develop by resorting to vaginal hysterectomy in all cases in which this was possible. As Dr. Bunch says, a vaginal hysterectomy properly done and the refastening of the bladder resorted to at the same time provides against the development of cystocele. His experience with this operation is going to be of great benefit to a great many of us, and to our patients. For a good many years in a patient who has had children, I have resorted in practically 90 per cent of the cases to clamp hysterectomy, for the reason that so many of these patients come back with a troublesome cervix and the number of malignant growths that develop. I feel that the additional hazard does not justify leaving in a cervix in most of these cases and it is probably in that type of case that we are most likely to get a cystocele. For a long time I have recognized that the

To Page 472

Hemorrhagic Encephalitis Following Neoarsphenamine in Late Pregnancy*

JOHN Z. PRESTON, M.D., Tryon, North Carolina

AN ARMY PILOT recently returned from the Mediterranean theatre with the Purple Heart decoration was asked at Kiwanis to tell about the time his plane was shot down. He slowly got to his feet and smiled. "I'd rather tell about the time I shot down the Hun, not the time he got me." Ordinarily I'd prefer to talk about the patients I think I cure, rather than the ones that die.

These cases are reported to remind you that hemorrhagic encephalitis can easily happen.

Case I.—A colored girl, 18, was first seen as a maternity case on February 15th, 1938. She was then 7½ months pregnant. Her general physical examination was negative. A Wassermann was taken and reported 4+. On March 1st, she was given neoarsphenamine 0.45 gm. She had no symptoms, and therefore was given the same dose intravenously on March 8th.

On the night of March 10th, I was called to the Cotton Club, where she lived. It was a large rooming house, and when I arrived, was filled with boisterous, drinking Negroes. The patient was dressed, but disheveled. My immediate, although false, impression was that she, too, was intoxicated. I asked her questions, which she attempted to answer, but her words were jumbled and confused. She tried to walk, but was unsteady on her feet. She had low blood pressure, was not having uterine contractions, and there was no edema. I left her in disgust, but asked that I be notified of her condition on the following day. I was called, and was told that she was worse. I went by, and found her in much the same condition. This time, I thought she was hyterical or malingering. But I ordered her by taxi to the hospital. She was admitted by wheelchair.

On admission, she could swallow and talk, and could use her hands. This condition rapidly changed to stupor, coma and death. She had glucose intravenously. The record states that a spinal puncture was attempted and failed. That may mean that bloody spinal fluid was confused with poor technique. She died with axillary temperature of 108, on March 12th, four days after the neoarsphenamine.

Case II.—Colored woman, aged 25, married, first seen on April 3d, 1941, when a positive Wassermann was found on a routine health-certificate examination. A second positive Wassermann was reported on September 10th, 1941. Treatment was begun on September 15th, with bismuth. On October 30th, she had a severe reaction to neoarsphenamine, at the 6th dose; but she tolerated mapharsen fairly well except for occasional nausea. She was given 59 weekly treatments: 6 of neoarsphenamine, 27 of bismuth in oil 2 c.c.; and 26 treatments of mapharsen, either 0.04 or 0.06 gm. Her blood Wassermann was reported negative on May 5th and November 12th of 1942; and on February 11th, August 31st and December 28th of 1943. She had a negative spinal Wassermann on November 30th, 1942.

Her husband had a negative Wassermann on September 17th, 1941, when the wife was started on treatment, but he later developed typical secondaries, with the result that he still is under treatment with a persistently positive Wassermann.

On January 18th, 1944, the nurse in the prenatal clinic asked if the wife shouldn't have some more treatment. She was answered that under no circumstances would we give her any more treatment. She understood, and so instructed the clinic secretary. But the husband had been told to bring his wife to the syphilis clinic. He did, and the following note was made: "Patient is 6½ to 7 months pregnant. Will give weekly injections of neo, in interest of baby, until confined." She was given neoarsphenamine 0.45 gm. on January 20th, 1944. She was dead on January 27th. She developed "a terrible feeling all over" on the fourth day. She couldn't describe this specifically, except that she was terrified. She then lost the ability to hold food or water in her mouth, or to swallow. Then her speech became muffled and disconnected.

On January 25th, her blood pressure was 86/60, with T. P. & R. normal. She was hard to examine because she was constantly trying to get up and walk. She answered questions, but the answers were not often applicable to the questions. She stared, but apparently did not see what she was looking at. She could not swallow.

She was taken to the hospital and given glucose and saline intravenously; vitamin C intravenously; phenobarbital; and adrenalin subcutaneously. A spinal puncture was done, removing 30 c.c. of bloody fluid, but apparently without increased pressure. She rapidly sank into stupor, coma and then death.

Here are two unnecessary deaths in healthy young primiparas in the third trimester, due to hemorrhagic encephalitis following neoarsphenamine intravenously. The first patient died after being given the second dose, with a positive Wassermann, as a result of inexperience. The second patient died after the first dose, following a year's rest, with a negative Wassermann for 21 months, as the result of a misapprehension.

As a result of these cases, there are the following DON'TS to guide my future treatment of syphilis, especially in late pregnancy.

1. DON'T start off with neoarsphenamine.

2. DON'T give neoarsphenamine to a pregnant woman in the third trimester, unless she has been treated in the second.

3. DON'T give neoarsphenamine to a pregnant woman who has a history of arsenical reaction.

4. DON'T expect recovery unless heroic treatment of hemorrhagic encephalitis is begun early.

DISCUSSION

DR. B. C. NALLE, Charlotte: Dr. Preston's paper presents a subject of great interest. Since we are going to have syphilis and pregnancy we are obliged to use treatment we think best. I don't see a great deal of syphilis in obstetrical patients, but in the few that I have seen, I am glad to say, I haven't had a death, but I have had a few very severe reactions in the way of dermatitis, which have scared me to death. But I continue to give neoarsphenamine in pregnancy before the fourth month, before the baby has a chance to get syphius from the mother, and arsenicals have helped in the fourth month. After 7½ months, it seems very dangerous, even as the doctor said after six months. In the latter part of pregnancy if she is without symptoms and getting along well, I don't dare give arsenicals. And if there is the slightest sign of toxemia, especially from the kidneys, I do not give it in any stage of pregnancy. Certainly, as the doctor has already suggested, no woman who gives a history of any sensitivity to arsenicals, should be given these drugs.

These cases bring to our attention that in late pregnancy it must be quite dangerous, very much more so than in early pregnancy. We should certainly get it in before four months, starting with small doses and go up to 7 or 7½ months if they are without symptoms.

DR. M. PIERCE RUCKER, Richmond: Dr. Preston's communication is very important because it is so diametrically opposed to the committee on 100, or whatever the number is, that was supposed to outline treatment necessary for women who have any suspicion of syphilis. We are told from above (Washington, I think) that every woman who has a positive Wassermann should be treated and you should plan your treatment so as to finish the arsenicals just before delivery. We are also told that a woman who has had a positive Wassermann previously should be treated through every subsequent pregnancy, regardless of Wassermann. For that reason, I think Dr. Preston's communication is a very pertinent one.

DR. G. G. DIXON, Ayden, N. C.: In the early 20s Dr. Pace and myself had a small obstetric clinic in Greenville which we operated for ten years with one fatality. That was in a colored girl. She had an acute nephritis. She had complete suppression of urine after the first dose of neoarsphenamine and died six days later from acute uremia.

For the past 2½ years, I have been operating one of the State Board of Health clinics in Pitt County, treating from 50 to 100 patients a week. About 50 per cent of them are women, about 20 per cent of the women are pregnant some time during the course of the treatment. We begin to treat them when we get them, whether first, third, fifth or seventh month. In some of them we have had untoward reactions. I am of the opinion that people do have encephalitis or meningitis that do not get neoarsphenamine. There is great probability that a good many of these women die of some infection, a condition we do not discover, and not from neoarsphenamine. When I have a death, I take that attitude because I hate to think that I killed one.

DR. H. J. LANGSTON, Danville: I am very much obliged to Dr. Preston for bringing these two stories to us, for the same reason that Dr. Rucker mentioned about this information or direction we are getting from Washington. I have been irritated by the instructions, and by the attitude the Army and the Navy with regard to syphilis.

I am very sure I know three or four competent fliers that you can turn loose in Buffalo and without chart or maps they can get in at Buffalo to come to Charlotte and hit Charlotte right on the nose—and yet the Army and Navy take the same attitude about treatment of fliers as they do a pregnant woman—treat her, treat her, treat her and keep on treating her. Some syphilologists call attention to the fact that if you didn't even treat the syphilis, some of these women would get well. The same thing is true of a flier. If you don't treat him, but give him plenty of food, he seems to get well. I think we should be scientific and when we get them free from syphilis and reports keep coming and coming and coming negative and a woman is well, we should discard treatment. Give it when it is necessary and when it is not necessary, don't give it.

Dr. Dixon says maybe something else is wrong with those patients. I don't know about that. I have seen two or three fatalities, not in pregnant women, but in other persons, who have been given over and over neoarsphenamine and bismuth. I would like to suggest that these cases, when we have treated them and they go along—Dr. Rucker may say this is all right and he may not—we can't do them any harm—give them a grain or a half-grain of iodide of mercury t.i.d., over six or eight months. I have seen some terrible reactions in these patients and they have to go to the hospital and stay six or eight weeks from skin irritations and developing kidney and pulmonary edema, almost went out, but they didn't die.

DR. PRESTON, closing: Thank you, all of you, and I am quite pleased at so much discussion. I came down here to learn. I believe these deaths were due to neoarsphenamine. At the time, one of the men in the hospital, when I had the first case, said, "Oh, John, that is an alcoholic and the death was not due to arsenic." The girl hadn't had anything to drink. So far as I know, they were killed by neoarsphenamine. I feel that I will know a little more about how to deal with such cases in the future.

Better Bladder Support—From P. 470

simple standardized operation of anchoring the ligaments into the vaginal stump was very ineffective in preventing the cystocele.

I was not familiar with Dr. Bunch's technic, but for a long time I have done a somewhat similar operation. It was called to my attention a good many years ago by Floyd Dean, who had practiced plicating round ligaments anterior to the stump after he had pushed the bladder back and fixed it to the fascia with silk, and that has been my practice. I usually anchor it with very fine silk.

This is a very able presentation and well worthy of our consideration, and a credit to our Association.

DR. OREN MOORE, Charlotte: Mr. President and Gentlemen: I am very happy to have learned that little trick. There is no question of the gravity of the situation, for the patient and for the surgeon, when a woman returns in the condition Dr. Bunch has described. You spend practically the rest of your life trying to make her life livable. I shall make use of the technic Dr. Bunch has worked out. I want to agree, along with Dr. Scruggs, that the possibilities of this happening are greater in total hysterectomy, but the operative difficulty in total hysterectomy is not much greater than in subtotal. Certain clinics have no greater mortality or morbidity rate when total hysterectomy is done at the hands of competent operators. Occasionally an operator should and will stick to the subtotal as being less likely to end in diaster of one kind and another, with regard to bladder and with regard to uterus. Again I say I like the trick Dr. Bunch brought out. It is good common sense. It affords the support needed, and it affords it at the right place. Like most inventions, with my superior mind, I am wondering why I hadn't thought of it myself. I think it was becauses I was so busy with so many other things I hadn't got around to it.

I will take up the rest of my time singing loud hymns of praise to the Manchester operation, in which the bladder pillars are used below in a splendid and efficient fashion and the cardinal ligaments are employed to the full extent of their splendid capability forever holding the uterus up and the bladder up thereafter. The old objection of shortening the vagina and interfering with marital relations, which was the end result of the interposition operation, is completely done away with.

The Aid That May Be Had From the Electrocardiogram*

PAUL D. CAMP, M.D., Richmond

AT THE END of the Eighteenth Century, Luigi Galvani (1737-1798), Professor of Anatomy at the University of Bologna, discovered by accident that stimulating the nerves of a frog's leg with electricity caused the leg to contract vigorously. Albert von Kolliker and Müller, in 1856, discovered that an exposed frog's heart produced an electrical current each time it beat. In 1878 in England, John B. Sanderson and F. M. J. Page were the first to record this electrical current, using a capillary electrometer.

Augustus D. Waller, in 1887, published a paper entitled "A Demonstration on Man of the Electromotive Changes Accompanying the Heart's Beat," describing the first successful electrocardiogram obtained from man and animals using electrodes placed on the body and without opening the thorax. His method was not practicable since, due to the inherent inertia of the mercury used, each curve had to be plotted again in a corrected form.

William Einthoven, in 1903, introduced the string galvanometer, the invention of Johannes S. C. Schweigger (1779-1857), for the measurement of electrical current produced by the human heart, and thus was begun a practical method of electrocardiography. Einthoven did most of the pioneer work in this field.

Sir Thomas Lewis soon began to use the electrocardiogram in London, correlating the clinical data with observations arising from the use of the new instrument. Most of his observations have stood the test of time. However, he later lost interest in electrocardiographic research. When I was working with him in London in 1931-1932, it was my opinion that he felt that the electrocardiograph would not offer in the future much that was new and of aid to cardiology. However, the contributions of Barker et al., through their studies made from the exposed human heart and the introduction of the chest leads, have certainly been a definite advance.

The electrocardiogram is an indispensable aid to modern cardiologists, but its scope and limitations must be recognized. I feel sure that the pioneers in this field, if they were here, would emphatically agree to this statement. Marvin has rather recently published an excellent article deploring the abuse of electrocardiography and stating that: "one of the principal reasons why the electrocardiographic method is doing widespread harm today is that many physicians over-emphasize its value and underestimate its limitations. They confidently expect it to accomplish much the same thing that a surgeon expects of an exploratory laparotomy; that it will disclose the nature of the pathologic process, reveal its exact location and extent, and tell a great deal about the immediate treatment and prognosis."

Quite frequently physicians who refer patients to me for an electrocardiogram seem rather puzzled when I try to explain to them the limitations of electrodardiography. At times patients will come in and ask for an electrocardiogram and—judging from their expressed expectations—it would seem that some doctor, or some of the patient's friends, had been telling the patient that the electrocardiogram always diagnoses types of heart disease present and that a normal record ruled out the possibility of heart disease. That such is not the case is an established fact. In angina pectoris one-third of the cases will present a normal electrocardiogram; and diseases other than heart disease may cause an abnormal ecgm. Further, the ecgm. may be normal in a patient with congestive heart failure.

It must be emphasized again and again that the electrocardiogram is a part—a very important one, it is true, but still only a part—of the complete cardiological examination. The findings must be correlated with the history, the physical examination, the x-ray examination, and other laboratory procedures.

Willius writes very interestingly of the "so-called electrocardiographer . . . . who fails to conform to the requisites of the physician and perilously exceeds the limitations of a good technician," who acquires an electrocardiograph and thinks that by doing so he acquires the experience and knowledge necessary to correctly interpret all records. Such a person, unfortunately, goes farther and renders a complete diagnosis from the electrocardiogram alone. Many patients have been wrongly diagnosed as having heart disease and forced to live very limited lives, while others have developed serious neurocirculatory asthenia, because ignorant electrocardiographers have put great stress on low voltage

*Presented to Tri-State Medical Association of the Carolinas and Virginia, meeting at Charlotte, Feb. 28th-29th, 1944.

of the Q-R-S complex in one lead, or minimal slurring of the Q-R-S in one lead, or an inverted T-3 or large Q-3.

There are, of course, certain instances in which the ecgm. gives invaluable aid, and in some cases it only will supply the essential information.

The most exact and, at times, most enlightening information we get from the ecgm. is that concerning the arrhythmias. The ecgm. very rarely fails to record the exact nature of an arrhythmia. It is not always possible to diagnose the arrhythmias by other means. Certain cases of rapid premature contractions resemble auricular fibrillation, and in auricular fibrillation ectopic ventricular contractions cannot be detected without the aid of the ecgm. In some cases in which the rhythm is apparently regular by clinical examination, we may find by electrocardiographic study auricular flutter with a normal ventricular rate, or a partial first-degree heart block, or a complete A-V dissociation with a normal ventricular rate. The exact diagnosis of the mechanism of an abnormal rhythm is of importance in treatment and prognosis.

Perhaps the greatest value of the ecgm. is the aid it renders in the recognition of acute myocardial infarction. The picture presented by the ecgm. in cases of acute anterior and posterior infarction is well known. Likewise, the progressive changes occurring in the ecgm. in different phases after the infarction have been described again and again. I would call special attention to the fact that the initial positive deflection of the Q-R-S complex in the chest lead is often absent soon after the infarction and this absence may persist for a long time. This is often of help in the proper evaluation as to whether or not an existing left-bundle-branch block is due to a quite recent or not distant acute coronary thrombosis. Despite certain opinions to the contrary, coronary occlusion is not always the cause of intraventricular block or bundle-branch block. Serial ecgms. are of a distinct value in following a case of coronary thrombosis, yet it must be realized that a patient may show marked improvement from the electrocardiographic viewpoint and yet may fail to show other improvement and even die suddenly. Likewise, if the injury happen to be in a point of great electrical activity, a small scar may cause a markedly abnormal ecgm. as long as the patient lives, although the patient may return to a normal, useful life.

The help of the ecgm. in the more chronic types of coronary-artery disease is not so clear-cut. We know that coronary arteriosclerosis and its resultant myocardial ischemia do cause certain changes in the ecgm., if properly correlated with the other clinical findings, are of great help. However, I feel sure that a great deal is read into ecgms. that should not be. Low voltage of the Q-R-S complex in all leads has been adjudged by some to indicate definite and widespread coronary disease; but it must be remembered that other types of heart involvement, as well as extracardiac factors, cause low voltage. Large Q waves in lead-3, without other changes, are often interpreted as indicative of coronary disease. This is not necessarily the case. Likewise a large Q-3 and inverted T3 do not necessarily indicate a past or present disturbance in the posterior myocardial circulation. Perhaps the greatest difficulty of all is that of attaching the proper significance to changes in the S-T segment and T waves. These changes from the accepted normal are too frequently interpreted as indicating coronary disease or myocardial damage. Howard Sprague lists forty-one conditions other than coronary arteriosclerosis causing changes in the S-T segment and T waves, and thirty-three of these do not imply heart disease. It thus behooves us to be very careful in using the term coronary disease in the interpretation of electrocardiograms. I am inclined to agree with Frank Wilson, who states: "It would be better if this term (coronary disease) were never used under any circumstances in connection with the interpretation of the electrocardiogram."

The ecgm. is sometimes of help in the detection of transitory coronary insufficiency; for example, during an attack of angina pectoris or paroxysmal tachycardia.

We are all familiar with the picture of right and left electrical axis deviation suggesting shift of the heart muscle mass to the left or the right. These records may or may not present abnormal S-T and T wave changes. Even if abnormal S-T and T wave changes are present, these may or may not be associated with coronary artery disease. Rather recently attempts have been made to differentiate the two types of S-T and T changes. Probably one should be able to differentiate the ecgm. of simple anatomical shift of preponderant centricular hypertrophy and strain, and of preponderant hypertrophy with definite coronary-artery disease. The type of ventricular strain is of help in confirming a valvular lesion, at times. Mitral stenosis, and especially pulmonary valve stenosis, tend to show right ventricular strain. Aortic valve lesions and coarctation of the aorta are likely to present left ventricular strain.

In addition to showing which ventricle is undergoing the most strain in congenital heart disease, the ecgm. presents a rather characteristic Q-R-S in certain cases; namely, diphasic Q-R-S complexes of great amplitude in the limb leads, with a deep Q or S in more than one of these leads. The ecgm. of dextrocardia is of course diagnostic.

The ecgm. may be of value in various acute illnesses, especially in diphtheria and rheumatic fever. As is well known, involvement of the heart during diphtheria to such an extent as to cause any type of heart block is of extremely grave prognostic significance. Most cases of rheumatic fever have some degree of myocarditis at some phase of the illness. We have found in our Rheumatic Fever Program that the ecgm. is often of help in the diagnosis and handling of such cases, and we do routine ecgms. in these cases. The prolonged *P-R* interval is the most definite abnormality. Serial ecgms. will often be of infinitely greater value than single ones.

In certain chronic diseases the electrocardiogram findings often prove helpful. Chronic rheumatic heart disease often shows right ventricular preponderance and abnormal *P* waves. Syphilitic heart disease may show marked left ventricular hypertrophy and strain and evidence of coronary artery involvement. Recently, prolongation of the *O-R-S-T* interval (normal .22 to .44) has been noted in the hypocalcemia of parathyroid disease. Hypertension may cause the changes discussed under ventricular strain. Arteriosclerosis and diabetes mellitus are usually associated and hence abnormal ecg. findings are common.

Drugs may affect the heart either by direct action, e.g., digitalis; or by indirect action, e.g., ephedrine or iodine. It is wise to learn if the patient is taking, or has recently taken, any drugs before arriving at the final interpretation. Digitalis, the most widely used drug in the treatment of cardiac disease, reflects the most marked changes in the ecgm., causing the characteristic *S-T* and *T* wave changes. In certain cases the ecgm. is the only means of making an accurate diagnosis and of guiding us as to the advisability of increasing or decreasing the dose of digitalis. However, it is not wise to rely upon the electrocardiographic findings alone as a guide to the degree of digitalization.

An ecgm. should be made in each case of suspected neurocirculatory asthenia before arriving at a definite diagnosis. By doing this, we may find certain things pointing toward organic heart disease. If the ecgm. is normal, then the doctor can with greater confidence reassure the patient that he or she does not have organic heart disease. A graphic record is oftentimes of more psychological value to a nervous, apprehensive patient, than a learned clinical opinion. This is true among doctor patients as well as others. The knowledge of a normal ecgm. often takes a great burden off their minds.

Again, however, the physician must remember that a normal ecgm. does not always rule out heart disease, and that it must be correlated with all the other clinical and laboratory findings.

DISCUSSION

DR. S. H. SHIPPEY, Rock Hill, S. C.: I don't come as a cardiologist, but one who tries to use the electrocardiograph in my work, and I am glad to have an opportunity to hear this very fine paper. Really, there isn't anything to discuss about the case. The essayist has covered it so well that I can't take issue with anything that he has said. The only thing I do want to do is to lay emphasis on what he has said.

The electrocardiogram is becoming so prominently before the people that everyone is wanting to have one made. It is a very valuable aid when used in conjunction with all other aids in the diagnosis of heart disease, but certainly the most important thing is proper interpretation of the symptoms.

DR. CAMP, closing: First, I want to thank Dr. Shippey for his discussion. I appreciated it very much. I shall take just a minute of your time to show you a graphic representation of certain things that we talked about. (Shows slides.)

SYPHILIS—From P. 468

complished if we treat 27,400 people conservatively and, during the course of their treatment, we have 27,400 additional cases of syphilis as contacts of these individuals?

During the last six months we have treated 748 cases of infectious syphilis at the Charlotte Rapid-Treatment Center—572 by the 12-day multiple-syringe method, and 176 by the drip method. Technique of the "12-day" method: 1.2 mapharsen and 1.0 Gm. bismuth subsalicylate are given a patient of average weight in a period of 10 to 14 days by multiple injections.

We have had two fatalities. One of these was a 15-year-old the multiple-syringe method. The other was an 18-year-additional cases of encephalopathy with recovery.

Our average syphilis patient stays in the hospital 16 days. He is followed at monthly intervals for a year upon his return home and if his physical and serological findings are not considered satisfactory he is given some additional therapy. The number of patients requiring this additional therapy to date have been negligible, which may be a fault of our follow-up, rather than an argument for the type of therapy they have received.

I think we will have the answer to this question in a few years. I predict that in the future the more progressive health departments and private hospitals will have beds available for the isolation and intensive therapy of all infectious cases. Whether the method of treatment will be arsenical, arsenical and fever, penicillin, or some other method remains to be seen.

I do not think that the intensive therapy of syphilis has reached the point where individuals not familiar with the reactions or who do not have the necessary physical equipment can use it. Any form of therapy more intensive than the triweekly regimen of Eagle is a hospital procedure.

Addendum (Dec. 10th).—Since giving the foregoing discussion we have treated 495 additional cases by the multiple-syringe method, and 367 additional cases by the drip method, without a fatality.

DR. CALLAWAY, closing: I think Dr. Steiger has pointed out the main reason for using the rapid treatment in that it affords one an opportunity to complete treatment in the majority of patients. Even though rapid treatment did not result in a greater number of cures than the conventional type of therapy in the percentage of patients completing treatment, an infinitely greater number will complete the short-course treatment. The infectious patient, who is the

To Page 482

Some Common Diseases of the Rectum*

R. B. DAVIS, M.D., F.A.C.S., Greensboro

TO UNDERSTAND the pathology of any organ one must have a clear insight of its physiology and anatomy. The functions of the rectum are storage and transportation, for the most part transportation. Let us call it, if you please, the low highway to good health.

In some cases the symptoms come on so insidiously that the patient cannot give you the date of onset, and it may be difficult to locate the origin of the discomfort. The result is that we frequently miss making a diagnosis because we do not examine the rectum.

Almost 10 years ago I read a paper before the Medical Society of North Carolina entitled "The Uses and Abuses of the Rectum"; in this paper I reported 700 rectal examinations. Since that time we have added 800 more cases. The testimonies of grateful patients have prompted me to further urge attention to the rectum.

Anatomy.—The rectum begins at the 3rd sacral vertebra and extends downward in a curve conforming to the curve of the sacrum and coccyx, terminating in the perineum at the anus. It is 6 to 7 inches long, narrow above and below, and contains circular and longitudinal muscle in its walls. Within its lumen are contained three halfmoon valves. At its lower end are two strong circular bands of muscle, between which is a superabundance of lymphatic and blood vessels.

Physiology.—As the rectum becomes filled with fecal matter the half-moon valves knead the mass into a formed stool. As pressure is brought to bear upon these valves the first sensation for defecation is felt. As this pressure increases on the valves, stimulation is increased until the sphincter muscle is automatically urged to relax. Then follows the contraction of the levator ani muscle, which has a tendency to straighten and fix the rectal canal, so that intraäbdominal and pelvic pressure, plus that of the peristaltic wave from above, presses the fecal matter through the anus.

We shall attempt to discuss only four or five of the most common of the non-malignant rectal diseases.

Hemorrhoids.—Hemorrhoids are one of the most common ailments for which surgical treatment is sought. There are internal and eternal hemorrhoids, bleeding and protruding hemorrhoids; accordingly as they arise from the internal or external hemorrhoidal veins, or whether the strangulation is severe enough to produce ulceration, or whether the dilated veins are large enough and long enough to protrude.

Obstruction to the return flow of blood in the veins is the immediate cause, this obstruction in 90 per cent of the cases being a bolus of fecal matter within the rectum. The extrarectal causes, such as tumors in the pelvis, pregnancies and abdominal ascites, are less frequently the cause, mainly for the reason that the pressure is exerted first upon some msculature, before it reaches the vein walls. With a mass within the rectum the converse is true.

The most common and distressing complication of hemorrhoids is muscular spasm due to irritation of the sphincter muscle, which creates a vicious circle—irritation from hemorrhoids causes spasm of the sphincter; spasm of the sphincter muscle produces more obstruction, thereby more hemorrhoids.

It follows that treatment should aim at removal of the hemorrhoidal veins and relief of muscular spasm and so prevention of a recurrence. This means dilation of the constricting muscle and good elimination following operation.

Fissure.—A fissure can be likened unto a military guard at the gate with a nervous trigger finger. The pain and discomfort is of little significance until a passage is attempted. The pathologic changes here begin with a break in the mucous membrane, then infection, then an inflammatory reaction exerted upon the sphincter muscle. Here again a vicious circle is created as the fecal mass stretches the inflammatory area. Stretching the fissure causes pain, pain causes spasm of the sphincter, spasm of the sphincter prevents normal passage of the fecal mass. The passage of a large fecal mass is the primary cause of a fissure.

The treatment of fissure is directed not only to the healing of the ulcer, but also to preventing pain and spasm and thereby a recurrence.

Fistula in Ano.—Most fistulas begin as fissures, therefore the exciting factors are the same. However, the infection here burrows deeply and passes through the rectal wall, spreading into the perirectal fatty tissue and muscle. This creates a blind

---

*Presented to Tri-State Medical Association of the Carolinas and Virginia, meeting at Charlotte, Feb. 28th-29th, 1944.

pocket of pus which travels in the line of least resistance and eventually produces an abscess.

The symptoms are both local and systemic. The pain in the rectum is continuous until the pus is evacuated. Here, as formerly, pain is due to inflammation and spasm.

The treatment then should consist of relief of the systemic condition by relieving the pressure in the abscess cavity, with complete drainage, the healing of the fistulous tract, dilating the muscle to prevent spasm, and providing adequate elimination postoperatively.

Pruritis Ani.—I can think of no minor disease which creates more disturbance in the peace of mind and disposition of a patient than pruritis ani. Every member of the household suffers as a result of the patient's bad disposition and restless nights.

The causes of this condition are many. Most common, however, are dietary disturbance, notably too much carbohydrate, avitaminoses, lack of proper hygiene, the sitting position embarrassing the circulation of the mucocutaneous area, and senile debility. It has been the writer's experience, however, that whatever the predisposing cause, in any severe case of pruritis ani, the immediate cause is constipation. It would seem that embarrassed circulation here affects the lymph channels rather than the venous channels.

It is generally said that the retention of lymph in the tissues creates the terible itching. This must be true because in the beginning neither the mucous membrane nor the skin is broken.

Treatment should be directed toward cure of the disease, relief of pain and prevention of recurrence. Topical applications will relieve the itching as a rule. Nature will repair the surface damage done by the scratching. The irritable sphincter muscle should be dilated; and free elimination provided forever afterwards will help to prevent a recurrence.

In conclusion let us consider that all rectal diseases mentioned in this article produce an abnormal function of the rectum. The abnormal function expresses itself in the spasm of the sphincter muscle and retention of the feces. The one causes the other, and the other causes the one.

DISCUSSION

Dr. Wm. H. Prioleau, Charleston: I enjoyed Dr. Davis' presentation no little. I'd like to comment on one or two remarks. He referred to the rectum as having a function of storage. I think that is very, very limited. The normal rectum is an empty rectum. The constant taking of mineral oil prevents the rectum from being properly emptied. Anybody who does proctologic work knows as soon as he sees a patient who has been taking mineral oil that he cannot empty his rectum. If so, not for very long. There is constant seepage downward. Only by having normal stools is the anal region going to be kept healthful.

These conditions, of course, cause some trouble to correct. They are as difficult to readjust as bad constipation and lead to just as much trouble.

Dr. Thomas Brockman, Greenville, S. C.: Mr. Chairman and Friends: I appreciate Dr. Davis' paper. I want to agree with Dr. Prioleau that the normal individual's stool should stay in the lower sigmoid and unless he takes laxatives and mineral oil, it will not accumulate in the rectum. We all know the physiology of the sigmoid is to straighten much like the neck of a choked goose in trying to swallow some bigger dose of food than he should have taken, and this sigmoid colon is supposed to have enough of, say redundancy, to squeeze that stool on down into the rectum and out the anal outlet.

I will have to disagree with Dr. Davis on the cause of fissure—that it is due to over-stretching the anal outlet. If that is true, then a lot of little boys and girls that many of us see ought to have a fissure early in life because we see in these little bellows the largest stools we will ever see any more. As we grow older, we all pass smaller-sized stools. I believe a fissure in a great majority of cases is due to infection in the anal crypt. In the large majority, hemorrhoids are associated with fissure. This fissure has brought the patient in. It is true they all come in complaining of hemorrhoids; but close examination or close history-taking before we take that patient in will tell us that we are dealing with a fissure. Patients will come, as Dr. Davis said, complaining of lots of pain from stools, pain that lasts several hours. There are very few things that will do that other than a fissure and if we will use an angle probe—after that pain has been eased entirely, but not before—we will find a sinus extending back from the crypt, on the posterior margin, and the undermining of this crypt has caused the fissure. The fissure broke because the tissue had been undermined by infection.

Dr. Wm. W. Rixey, Richmond: I want to say that there is a lot of truth in Dr. Davis' paper. Perhaps it is all true. I am going to disagree with some of it, but I can be wrong. He said something about rectal valves as not very important structures. In any proctological examination, you can see one valve, two valves and in the majority of cases three valves. We find a patient with some incontinence and we can't get in to the colon to repair the pelvic floor because that is where the trouble is. I don't believe it is from fissures ordinarily, certainly not the majority from fissures.

Dr. Davis, closing: I want to say, gentlemen, that I appreciate the discussion that the paper doesn't merit; and I want to make a correction. Speaking of the physiology of the rectum, I should have said, if I didn't say, it is in my paper, "the functions of the rectum are storage and transportation, but for the most part transportation." I might not have read it, and I certainly didn't make it clear, and appreciate that the men brought it out.

Amazing DDT

In 1939 Paul Muller, scientist of J. R. Geigy, of Basle, Switzerland, determined that this drug was an effective insecticide as protection for the potato crop.

Geigy produced it in large quantities for the Swiss farmers to use against agricultural insects, and it was imported to the United States for the same purpose. Geigy, having discovered that it was effective against the typhus louse, so informed the American military attache in Berne in August, 1942.

Spraying of cattle will protect them from the pest of flies. Fly-transmitted diseases, like diarrhea and dysentery which plague armies in the field, will thus be prevented. Likewise it can be applied to civilian life as a protection against typhoid and other diseases transmitted by flies. The number of garden pests which it is believed may be eliminated is astounding. Most of the fruit and vegetable pests are included in this enumeration.—*Northwest Medicine*, July, 1944.

Splenic Rupture With Case Report*

WILLIAM A. JOHNS, M.D., Richmond
Lieutenant Medical Corps, U. S. Naval Reserve

ABOUT five hundred cases of rupture of the spleen have been recorded in the medical literature. The vast majority of these are traumatic in origin, resulting from severe trauma and present the usual signs and symptoms of severe intra-abdominal hemorrhage. About sixty cases fall into the classification of delayed hemorrhage following traumatic rupture of the spleen. In this group a certain period of time elapsed between the injury and the time the hemorrhage occurred which is called the period of symptomatic silence or the latent period. The time element of this period has varied from a few hours to several months. Non-traumatic rupture of an enlarged chronically pathologic spleen as seen in leukemias and malaria is not infrequent. Such mild trauma as straining at stool or dressing has been associated with these cases. Non-traumatic rupture of a previously normal spleen was described in 1696 by Vanselow and since this date some twenty-five cases have been recorded in the medical literature. It has been designated as a spontaneous rupture of the normal spleen. Grossman points out correctly that spontaneous rupture of the normal spleen does not occur and suggests the following classification:

1. Traumatic rupture of the spleen.
2. Non-traumatic rupture of the spleen in (a) Chronically pathologic spleen. (b) Acutely pathologic spleen.

Once the diagnosis of a ruptured spleen is made the treatment is surgical removal. Conservative treatment results in 100 per cent mortality. Surgical procedures other than removal, such as some form of repair or tamponment, have been tried and found to be unsuccessful. Immediate surgery is urgent as about fifty per cent die within one hour of the injury.

In the classical traumatic cases, except when complicated by severe injury to other organs, the diagnosis is not too difficult. It is in the cases of delayed rupture and non-traumatic rupture of a previously normal spleen that the diagnosis is obscured. McIndoe, in speaking of delayed hemorrhage following traumatic rupture of the spleen, states "the diagnosis may be made from a knowledge of the injury and the site of the primary injury; from the presence of a persistent dull ache in the left side with slight left upper-abdominal rigidity during the latent period; from the later sudden onset of signs of severe internal hemorrhage, and in conjunction with the appearance of Ballance's sign, elevation of the left diaphragmatic dome, or pain in the left shoulder referred from the splenic region." Pain in the left shoulder as a symptom of this condition, referred to as Kehr's sign, has been described by many writers, most graphically by Dr. A. Murat Willis in 1919. Some have described it as almost diagnostic, others have noted it only by its absence. It is certainly suggestive, and at least should make one suspect the diagnosis of rupture of the spleen, with blood or blood clots causing an irritation to the diaphragm and phrenic nerve, thus producing the pain in the shoulder. Its presence was very obvious in my case. It is seen more frequently in cases of delayed hemorrhage than in the acute traumatic rupture.

Case Report

A white man, aged 18, was admitted to a United States Naval Hospital on November 8th, 1943, on the neurological service. His history was that of difficulty with his right side of five-years duration, and of several momentary attacks when his right side would become useless. Immediate recovery would occur after a short period of rest. His past history was essentially negative except for an appendectomy in 1938. In March, 1943, his ship was torpedoed and sunk and he was rescued after several hours in the water. Physical examination on admission, which included a neurological examination, was negative. The Kahn test was negative; urine and stool findings were within normal limits; r.b.c. 5,180,000; hemoglobin 95%; w.b.c. 12,500 with 59% segmented cells; 35% lymphocytes, 4% eosinophiles, and 2% basophiles.

On December 12th he was granted liberty from the hospital and left at 11 a. m. with no complaints. At 2:50 p. m. he developed a gnawing pain in the left side of his abdomen which he attributed to gas on his stomach. He remained on liberty and called for his girl at 6 p. m. He did not feel like eating dinner. At 9:45 p. m. he was seized with a sudden severe pain in his epigastrium which radiated to his left shoulder. He stated his shoulder pain was very severe. He was brought to the hospital at once. His entire abdomen was rigid, blood pressure 110/80, pulse 100, respirations 24, w.b.c. 25,000 with 80% segmented cells, urine findings within normal limits.

A preöperative diagnosis of perforated peptic ulcer was made and under spinal anesthesia the abdomen was opened through a right rectus incision. To my surprise the peritoneal cavity was found full of blood. The stomach, duodenum and liver appeared normal. A large blood clot was felt around the spleen and the capsule of the spleen was felt to be torn. The incision was enlarged transversely to

*Presented to Tri-State Medical Association of the Carolinas and Virginia, meeting at Charlotte, Feb. 28th-29th, 1944.

the left. The large blood clot between the spleen and diaphragm was removed. The pedicle of the spleen was clamped, the spleen was removed and the pedicle ligated with chromic catgut. The abdominal wall was closed quickly with through-and-through sutures of braided silk. The operative procedure lasted 45 minutes. A few minutes after the peritoneal cavity was opened the patient showed signs of profound shock. Plasma was started intravenously immediately and a total of 1500 c.c. given, this followed by 1750 c.c. of whole blood from universal donors. These procedures proved life-saving.

His postoperative course was satisfactory except for some consolidation at the left base. A type-32 pneumococcus was isolated from his sputum and he was treated with sulfadiazine. His temperature returned to normal on the sixth postoperative day and convalescence was uneventful.

On December 21st, his r.b.c. was 5,160,000, hemoglobin 100%, w.b.c. 14,000 with 67% segmented cells, platelet count 577,600, bleeding time 2 minutes and 55 seconds, clotting time 2 minutes and 30 seconds. On January 10th, 1944, r.b.c. was 4,450,000, w.b.c. 8,300 with 51% segmented cells, hemoglobin 90%.

The spleen was of normal size and weighed 155 grams. No definite tear into splenic pulp could be demonstrated. The capsule on the lateral surface was torn and this surface of the spleen was covered with a partially organized blood clot. On cutting the spleen a blood clot was found in the lower half beginning in the center of the organ and gradually making its way to the periphery.

Blocks of tissue for microscopic examination taken from an area of the spleen not involved in the hemorrhage showed normal appearing spleen tissue including a moderated amount of phagocytized hemosiderin. Blocks taken from the hemorrhagic area showed a fresh, irregular, linear, unorganized area of hemorrhage which had separated the splenic tissue. The general appearance of the tissue between the Malpighian bodies indicated dilatation of the blood spaces, although they did not contain blood. There was a small area where the normal living cells were replaced by degenerating cells showing only residual nuclei. Between them was homogeneous red material. This was consistent with an infarct.

The Pathologist, Commander R. H. Goodale, commented: "The infarct and focal area of dilated blood spaces suggest that a thrombus or other process has obstructed a venous branch causing congestion in part of the spleen. With increasing pressure from the arterial side the spleen finally ruptured. The underlying pathology may be a sequel of a previous injury."

The only history of injury that can be obtained was the fact the patient was skylarking with a shipmate about 10 a. m. on the same date. On investigation this proved most trivial in nature. When his ship was torpedoed seven months previously he received a severe blow to his left flank. He complained of pain in his left side, nausea and vomiting, for a week following this experience.

It is thought that this is a case of delayed hemorrhage from a ruptured spleen, the original injury having occurred seven months previously. This is a longer latent period than has been reported, but the pathology was certainly that of a delayed hemorrhage.

CONCLUSION

Splenic rupture with delayed hemorrhage is not a rare condition. It has been and will continue to be seen more frequently as a result of war injuries.

Its diagnosis is somewhat difficult. Generalized abdominal tenderness and rigidity with pain in the left shoulder should make one suspicious of the condition.

The treatment is immediate splenectomy.

The life-saving value of plasma and whole blood in the treatment of shock due to hemorrhage is again emphasized.

Bibliography

BUERMANN: *U. S. Nav. M. Bull.*, 51:73-93, Jan., 1943.
COLEMAN, A. H.: *Brit. J. Surg.*, 27:173-175, July, 1939.
CURTIS, G. M.: *Am. J. Surg.*, 59:292-317, Feb., 1943.
GROSSMAN, L. L.: *Wisconsin M. J.*, 41:477-482, June, 1942.
HARKINS, H. N.: *Am. J. Surg.*, 57:159-161, July, 1942.
MCLOCHLIN, A. D.: *Am. J. Surg.*, 1117:476-479, March, 1943.
MCINDOE, A. H.: *Brit. J. Surg.*, 20:249, 1932.
PEMBERTON, J.: *South. Med. & Surg.*, 102:46-52, Feb., 1940.
WILLIS, A. M.: *Surg., Gyn. & Obst.*, 29:33-39, 1919.

DISCUSSION

DR. WM. H. PRIOLEAU, Charleston: I enjoyed this timely presentation, and I say timely, particularly because this is the age not only of war, but also of an over-activated civilian industry. Lieutenant Johns has covered the subject thoroughly. There is little I can add; however, I would like to emphasize one or two features.

One is, and I am not sure it is always present, increase of white count as an indication of hemorrhage. That is an almost invariably present feature of a rapidly progressing hemorrhage. The other point is of approach. If the diagnosis can be made, that is in regard to the spleen or slit in the abdomen, I wish to make a plea for the use of a transverse incision. In a father limited experience with such cases in which I failed to make a diagnosis, I have had subsequent trouble with herniation following the use of the combined incision, first straight and having to go transversely to make a proper approach. If the diagnosis can be made, transverse incision will give better approach and is more likely to heal and give no subsequent trouble, even in the presence of infection.

DR. R. B. MCKNIGHT, Charlotte: I have seen three ruptured spleens in my life, the last years ago. Dr. Johns has ably presented this subject and Dr. Prioleau followed up just as splendidly.

It opens up a larger field for discussion of non-penetrating injuries of the abdomen. The liver being so large and so friable is much more subject to rupture. Following ruptures in the abdomen in ordinary industrial life, the particular sign I want to point out is the almost constant bradycardia which occurs in cases of ruptured liver. I wish some other physicians would talk on injuries following non-penetrating wounds.

Two or three years ago, a young man of 18, working on a scaffold, fell and landed on his abdomen on a board lying on the floor transversely. I made a diagnosis of ruptured spleen. He did not have ruptured spleen, but did have ruptured transverse colon and duodenum. Thanks to the sulfa drugs, plus transfusion, he was pulled through. The only mark on the abdomen was the slightest redness where he struck the board in falling.

LT. JOHNS, closing: I'd like to say, in conclusion, the Navy Military surgeons frequently see what are called near-misses or water explosions, and that frequently non-penetrating wounds of the abdomen are seen following these mass injuries.

ruptured spleen because in the Navy alone within the past
I'd like to reëmphasize delayed hemorrhage following

To Page 481

The Treatment of Intertrochanteric Fractures of the Neck of the Femur*

JAMES W. DAVIS, M.D., Statesville

INTERTROCHANTERIC FRACTURES of the neck of the femur occur principally in the aged. Every patient with a fracture of this kind presents a multitude of problems, all of which are important. A fracture of the neck of the femur with involvement of the intertrochanteric portion of the bone can be treated best by internal fixation. For obvious reasons treatment by other means is either impossible or very unsatisfactory. The skin will not stand traction from adhesive plaster. Skeletal traction is not advisable usually. Reduction and fixation with a plaster spica is not satisfactory because these patients do not stand plaster well and, besides, to keep an aged person in one position too long may be fatal. In addition, the mental effect of a plaster spica upon a patient is not good.

We see each year a large number of intertrochanteric fractures of the neck of the femur, most of them in patients beyond seventy years of age. These fractures usually occur at a time in life when the patient is in poor physical condition. There is usually some cardiorenal trouble present. The nervous system is not any too stable. The victim of the accident is susceptible to many complications, the majority of them at least potentially serious. A fracture of the neck of the femur in an aged person causes severe shock, both mental and physical. The pain from a fracture of the hip is distressing. In addition, most patients have heard of others who, following this accident, have had to spend their remaining days in bed or in a wheel-chair and are fearful of the possibility of a life of invalidism and helplessness.

The treatment of a patient with an intertrochanteric fracture of the neck of the femur should be prompt. It is true that many apparently are extremely bad risks for any form of surgery, but it is my opinion that where there is the least possible chance the patient should be given the benefit of the doubt. Years ago we had numbers of patients who were extremely poor risks but wanted to take the chance and, since most of them not only stood the operation well but made a good recovery, we have been greatly encouraged to do a reduction and internal fixation on practically all of these patients. The good results have more than justified this method.

The excellent results obtained and the low mortality, considering everything, have been due to the fact that the proper anesthetic was given and proper pre- and post-operative treatment were followed out in detail. The internal fixation can usually be done within twenty-four hours after the injury. The patient can move about in bed freely, can be up in a wheel-chair within twenty-four hours after the operation, and can sit up without pain—all of which gives confidence and hope.

The method of internal fixation which we use in a majority of cases is that of the insertion of a Smith-Petersen nail in the neck of the femur and attaching an angle bar to this. The angle bar is attached to the upper end of the femur by screws. This arrangement holds the fragments in proper position until union takes place and, meantime, the patient can move about freely in bed and can be up in a wheel-chair in a day or two after the operation. Occasionally Parham bands are used. Screws or nails to hold fragments in position may be necessary in addition to the angle bar. We usually allow these patients to return home at the end of a week to ten days, depending upon the general condition.

After having two patients, both of whom were ninety-five years of age, treated by this method and recover, we have felt more encouraged than ever about this method of treating intertrochanteric fractures.

In addition to the reduction and internal fixation of the fracture, there are, of course, a great many things that must be done for these patients. Every possible thing that can be done for them in the way of medical attention and nursing is necessary and should not be overlooked.

Except in patients who are actually moribund and obviously about to perish, almost all cases of intertrochanteric fracture should be treated by internal fixation. The immediate relief from pain and the fact that the patient can be up in a wheel-chair the next day will turn the tide in many cases in favor of the patient, because by this method we have given the patient not only relief from pain but hope as well.

*Presented to Tri-State Medical Association of the Carolinas and Virginia, meeting at Charlotte, Feb. 28th-29th, 1944.

DISCUSSION

Dr. O. L. Miller, Charlotte: Mr. President and Members of the Tri-State: I want to commend the essayist for calling to our attention this very modern treatment of intertrochanteric fracture, and to invite your attention to the difference between intertrochanteric fracture and fracure of the surgical neck. Interference with the blood supply to the head of the femur is not very likely in intertrochanteric fracture, but it is likely in fracture of the surgical neck of the femur. If you have to select another fracture of the lower extremity or an intertrochanteric fracture of the femur, you'd better select the intertrochanteric, because it is the one in which you can be most assured of union. Even without reduction, you will get union. It is difficult to get non-union in intertrochanteric fracture of the femur. I have treated them in the beginning days with Buck's extension. They will unite in Buck's extension. I have used spica casts. They unite nicely in spica casts. Naturally, we try to get away from nursing them in spica casts if we can because of the patient's inactivity. If the well leg and the fractured leg are both tied up, the patient is able to be up. That will reduce them. In most of these patients the fracture will unite in 12 to 14 weeks. The patients usually end up with a good walking leg.

Dr. Davis showed us an interesting case of an old person with good reduction. More recently we have been doing reduction of intertrochanteric fractures with that technic. It doesn't tie up either leg.

I want to show a slide or two. The first is a well-leg traction apparatus, which I am sure some of you have used with good results. It ties up both legs. You have to get both legs back into action again.

The second is an intertrochanteric fracture cared for with a well-leg traction splint. That was an advance over the use of spica.

The third shows the technic of Dr. Davis, an advance over either, in which the patient gets some active reduction. It is a question of whether it was not put on the well leg.

Something was said about anesthetics. Dr. Davis referred to the fact that he used low, light spinal. That is the same technic we use and its disturbs the patients very little.

More recently this apparatus is succeeding the Smith-Petersen nail. It is the Brown plate or the Moore plate. Dr. Moore, of Columbia, has done an interesting open reduction fracture and provided a plate similar to this. It is one instrument that can be bent to fit. Anyway the effect is the reverse of the old Thomas splint, the Buck traction or the well-leg splint. Incidentally, the operation causes very little shock. There is no blood supply to be concerned about. You can put this type of apparatus on, or one similar to it, and the result is excellent.

Dr. Davis, closing: As I came in this morning, I saw my good friend Banks, who has helped us a great deal in getting special apparatus for fractures, so if you have to do this work, I suggest that you see him. He is a good man.

A life depends sometimes on the anesthetic and the low spinal anesthesia apparently gives no shock. We have found the older they are, the better they stand it, and the point is to give very little, just enough, and it has no effect on the blood pressure. High spinal anesthesia in an elderly person is not a good thing.

This plate is one of the newest helps in such cases, and I believe it was devised by Dr. Austin Moore of Columbia. It is very fine. We are using these, but not very much. We use mostly a combination of Smith-Petersen nail and angle bar. The blade gives good reduction and yet the surface exposed is not quite so great and the three blades of Smith-Petersen give a large surface and obtain fixation. This may suit the others of you here. I understand Dr. Moore will be here this afternoon and may talk on this particular subject. I hope you hear him because he is the man that devised this instrument and I am sure he will have a lo tof new light to give us on the subject of intertrochanteric fractures.

NO SEX IN MEDICINE
(Norfolk District Medical News, Boston, Mass.)

Gradually women have found their way into the study of medicine and been licensed to practice. By 1941 all medical schools but five in the United States admitted women; but most of them still strictly limited their numbers, and today only 5 per cent of all physicians in the country are women as compared to 17 per cent in England and 85 per cent in Russia.

With World War II came a tremendous demand for doctors for the armed forces. Almost immediately women physicians, particularly those recently graduated, became popular on the home front. Hospitals that had previously refused to consider women interns are now glad to accept them. Medical schools, finding themselves faced with a 23 per cent reduction in student enrollment because of curtailment of the Army and Navy medical training program, have decided to increase the enrollment of women! Harvard Medical School, after 163 years, has decided women and medicine are not antipathetic and may become candidates for the M.D. degree. Only Georgetown, St. Louis, Dartmouth (which gives only a two-year course) and Jefferson Medical Schools still stand pat, hugging the antiquated precept that women have no place in medicine.

May we suggest that since women are now on their way to sharing equal rights with men in medical institutions, women's medical schools and hospitals should accept men as students, interns and staff members, thus further demonstrating that there is no sex in medicine.

SYPHILIS—From P. 475.

public health problem, can be held until treatment is finished. Dr. Steiger is to be complimented on having treated more patients with rapid therapy than any other individual in the country.

In answer to Dr. Raiford, I feel that the patient he described would have reacted to massive therapy. No one can predict these idiosyncratic reactions. A good feature of rapid treatment is that one sees the patients daily instead of weekly and reactions can be recognized and treated early. Careful questioning, examination of the skin, white blood cell counts with differential study enable one to pick up reactions immediately.

I was interested in hearing Dr. Britt's description of the fatal reactions to a single dose of 4.5 grams of neoarsphenamine. This represents roughly ten times the normal dosage and is disastrous. The reason neoarsphenamine was dicontinued as an agent in massive rapid treatment was because of the high incidence of reactions.

SPLENIC RUPTURE—From 479

year four such cases have occurred following torpedo accident, which have been reported. No doubt there are many others which have not been reported, and since in these cases symptoms develop sometimes several months after the original injury, I think it is important that we all keep this fact in mind.

Wassermann reaction was negative in a mother just prior to giving birth to a child that, at the age of 10 months, was found to have a 3+ Wassermann reaction.

CLINIC
Conducted by
FREDERICK R. TAYLOR, B.S., M.D., F.A.C.P.,
High Point, N. C.

ON AUGUST 22nd, 1930, I was asked to see a public health officer who had been admitted to the Burrus Memorial Hospital.

Case taking.—He complains of pain in his left leg. He has had varicose veins in that leg for 35 years. They are also present in slight degree in his right leg. He has worn elastic bandages, stockings, etc., and has never had a varicose ulcer. He had typhoid fever 34 years ago and thinks it may have left him with chronic infection in his gallbladder, though he did not suspect this until 11 years ago, when he had an attack of what he believed and gave himself a hypodermic. This was the only attack he has ever had severe enough to require a hypodermic, though he can always tell when 6 p. m. comes from soreness in his right hypochondrium. Eleven years ago he consulted Dr. John B. Deaver in Philadelphia, who thought he had cholecystitis and possibly cholelithiasis, but advised him to let it alone. He has had duodenal tube drainage on several occasions with slight benefit. Never had jaundice and never had renal colic. He had lobar pneumonia in Camp Greenleaf in 1918 and nearly died, but recovered without sequelae. One and one-half to 2 years ago he thought he noticed a painless terminal hematuria only on the 1st urination in the morning. He has never had any venereal disease, and has no nocturia, and never had any prostatic trouble. Dr. C. B. Squires at the Crowell Clinic found an infected verumontanum, treated it with silver nitrate, and it cleared up. Cystoscopy 2 weeks after treatment was begun showed everything normal. Four months ago his car ran off a 30-foot embankment and he suffered unbearable pain in the coccyx, but could not stop working. Dr. H. H. Bass sent him to Dr. McCrae, Philadelphia, who studied him and Dr. Manges x-rayed him thoroughly, and the final diagnosis was shock from an automobile accident plus overwork and a near-neurasthenia. Dr. McCrae was rather non-committal about the gallbladder, and would not advise for or against operation. Surgical consultants thought him in no condition for operation. Then Dr. John Deaver came in one day and told him he ought to forget his gallbladder.

A month ago, he was on a train going from Raleigh to Washington, D. C. For 3 weeks before, due to overwork and worry, he had not averaged 4 hours' sleep a night. Sometimes he would drive all night long. He had had to let 23 of his employes go because of a state economy program, and he was trying to find them work, and did find work for every one of them. While on the train he woke up with severe pain in his right lower and posterior chest. Another public health officer was on the train, but had nothing with him to use in treatment, so he arranged for a doctor to meet the train. This doctor diagnosed pleurisy and gave him a hypodermic. Later an official on the train gave him a drink of liquor. His temperature was 103. His medical friend took him to a hotel in Washington and strapped his chest, and he attended a drought conference all day. The next day he returned to Raleigh and went to bed. At this time he had typical pleural friction. He stayed in bed 2 days and then went back to work with a t. of 100° F., but finally recovered. A week after that, the Executive Committee of the State Board of Health went to Montreat to check a budget, and while there, the patient climbed a mountain to see a water supply, and got a phlebitis in his left leg. Then another special meeting came on 3 weeks ago, and this patient went to that with a severe cellulitis in his leg. He suffered much after that, but kept on working. Then he went to a big pellagra meeting at Raeford, and later to a tuberculosis meeting in Salisbury, where his suffering became intense.

Day before yesterday he tried to get up and couldn't, so came to High Point from Raleigh in an ambulance, to be under the care of his friend Dr. John T. Burrus. Night before last he was given a hypodermic, and he said he "went crazy from it" and vomited the next morning. Otherwise he had no nausea or vomiting. His back aches from lying in bed, he says. There is some soreness in his head and aching in his finger joints. Otherwise his history is essentially negative. His past history is unimportant except for tertian and quotidian malaria 14 years ago, and very severe influenza in 1891.

As is obvious, the patient overworks excessively. Usually his appetite is good, but it has been poor for the past 2 weeks. He smokes 50 to 60 cigarettes a day. Otherwise his habits are moderate. He has had insufficient sleep for the past 5 or 6 months— less than 6 hrs. a night. Before that, he averaged only about 6 hours.

His father died of apoplexy at 80, his mother suddenly of unknown cause while patient was in France in World War I. One sister has had arthritis, psoriasis, and a nervous breakdown due to her husband's death. One sister died of tuberculous enteritis, the patient always thought, though no less a person than Dr. Osler thought not, though he said he did not know what it was. One sister died of a typhoid perforation of the intestine. One brother died of apoplexy, aged 36, precipitated by a very severe fit of influenzal coughing. Wife and 3 children well.

A large, well-developed man, of a peculiar yellowish clay-like complexion. Head otherwise negative. Neck negative. Heart seems normal, though some rales are heard at left base which disappear after a deep breath. Back of his chest incompletely examined because too painful to his leg to turn over. Abdomen negative except for some tenderness on ulnar percussion just below right costal margin. Genitals negative. B. P. 132/92. The whole left lower extremity is swollen and inflamed, an obvious phlebitis. Rectal examination not made —it was imperative that he should not move much. Urine shows a light cloud of albumin and 5 to 6 granular casts per h. p. f. Blood normal.

Diagnosis: Thrombophlebitis of left lower extremity. Probable chronic gallbladder disease. Chronic renal irritation.

August 23rd (next day): Not feeling so well. Tired out.

Aug. 24th: Feels better, though leg looks bad—very red—better around knee, worse in Scarpa's triangle. Phthalein total output 40%; blood urea nitrogen 72 mg. per 100 c.c.

Aug. 25th: Improving greatly. Enjoyed breakfast. Looks like himself.

Aug. 26th: No special change in morning. At 5 p. m. complained of weakness and wanted his bed lowered. This was done. He seemed in critical condition. The only physician in the hospital at that hour was an eye-ear-nose-throat man, and he was called and came at once. The patient was given caffeine, ammonia and amyl nitrite, but died at 5:10 p. m.

Diagnosis: Pulmonary embolism secondary to thrombophlebitis of femoral vein.

ON MAY 24th, 1922, a 56-year-old executive complained of pain in his right chest, which began 3 days ago from sitting in a draft with his right chest pressing against the arm of a chair. The pain came on suddenly. Yesterday morning he had a slight fever, and his pain was so severe he wanted me to come at once to see him. Being unable to respond, I sent another physician who thought he had an intercostal neuralgia and gave him a mixture of codeine, atophan and caffeine without much relief. The pain is about in the midaxillary line, just above the liver. It prevents him from taking a deep breath. Appetite rather poor. Constipated despite a dose of castor oil.

Respiration rapid and shallow, voluntarily limited because of pain. He says he can't rest in bed. Given a mixture of Dover's powder and acetphenetidine, also solution of magnesium citrate for his constipation. At this time he made no mention of pain in his leg, but on my next visit did so, and a thrombus was found in his right leg. The diagnosis now is pretty obviously pulmonary embolism. Patient now states that at times within the past day or so he has had blood-streaked sputum. On June 3rd, 10 days after I first saw him, he consented to go to the hospital. He was there only a few days, but while there developed a thrombus in his left leg, then another embolus in his other (left) lung. Dr. Frederic M. Hanes, then of Winston-Salem, saw him in consultation and agreed on the diagnosis. While the patient was in the hospital, I reported his case to the Guilford County Medical Society and noted the remarkable multiplicity of thrombi and emboli, and expressed a wonder as to the probable outcome. When I got back from the meeting, which was held in Greensboro, the patient was dead. The nurse was just outside his door and heard him beating on the wall with his fist, went in, and, before she had time to call anyone, he was dead. A few days before his death the patient asked me to tell him what his outlook was, saying that if his life were in danger, he wanted to make some important business arrangements. I told him he might make an uninterrupted recovery, might have more thrombi and emboli, and then recover, or a big embolus might hit him like a bullet in the chest and kill him. He thanked me. His brother came down from Baltimore to attend his funeral and expressed his gratitude at my frankness, saying that it had enabled the patient to save his family from severe financial loss.

Discussions These 4 cases (2 reported in November) illustrate various etiologic factors. The first one was postoperative; the second came in convalescence from a severe infection; the third was associated with varicose veins in addition to respiratory infection; the fourth seemed to develop the thrombus spontaneously. Case 4 teaches the lesson that in any case of pain in the chest, pulmonary embolism should be considered and possible sources for such investigated carefully.

NEW HOSPITAL CAR

On November 13th, the first of a new type hospital car for use in the United States was opened for inspection at Washington. These new unit-type cars are designed and built as hospital cars. They are ten feet longer than pullmans, are air-conditioned, accommodate 38 patients and attendant personnel. Each includes two rows of triple-tiered beds, two compartments with three beds each, a stainless-steel kitchen equipped with refrigeration, ice-cream cabinet and coal range; a receiving room with four-foot side doors for loading and unloading litter patients; two roomettes, each with toilet and shower, for the medical staff or seriously ill patients; and a baggage compartment. The car also carries a modern pharmacy unit and sterilizing equipment and in case of emergency either the receiving room or one of the roomettes can be converted quickly into an operating room.

The Glennon-type, steel-frame beds are adjustable, and unoccupied center bunks can be dropped to provide seating accommodations for ambulatory patients.

Six more of these cars were put in operation in November; 18 are due in December and 75 during January, February and March of next year—bringing the total to 100, in addition to the 120 converted hospital cars now in use.

DEPARTMENTS

HUMAN BEHAVIOUR

JAMES K. HALL, M.D., *Editor*, Richmond, Va.

POLITICAL ALCOHOLISM

I DO NOT BURDEN my memory with the statistical statements I read from time to time of the number of arrests made in Richmond and throughout Virginia of individuals charged with being drunk, or drunk and disorderly. I should be unwilling to attempt to record the total number of such arrests for any one month, lest I might make a mistake. Yet it lies upon my mind that I read not long ago the statement that seemed to be authoritative that of all the arrests made within this ancient commonwealth within the span of a year, at least 80 per cent of them were attributed by the apprehending officers to disorders of behaviour caused by alcoholic intoxication.

The alcoholic beverages of the best quality are supposed to be dispensed to the thirsty citizens through agencies maintained by the state and approved by the local community, rural or urban, and by the all-embracing United States government. The Federal government is constantly protruding some one of its many digits into so many pies that were once thought to be reserved to the citizens that it must now be almost impossible to declare that the national government either does or does not participate at all in a specific activity. But I know of no other poison except alcohol that the various units of government offer openly for sale for the purpose of making money. I think I know that I shall be told that no department of government, local or Federal, actually sells alcoholic potables for the purpose of making money. I shall be told, to be sure, that the government does, in spite of its wishes, make money out of its whiskey business, but that the so-called A B C stores were set up, not for the purpose of causing people to drink, but to induce them not to drink. Lying is an almost invariable accompaniment of alcoholism, whether the alcoholic be an individual or the government—represented by the rural area, the village, the city, the state, or the United States.

Once I heard a great man, who was not infrequently embarrassed by his periodic indulgence in alcohol, remark that no one could have anything to do with whiskey without being tarnished by it. The truth is, perhaps, axiomatic. I am offered frequent entertainment by the expressed opinion of some citizen that even over-indulgence in whiskey legally obtained cannot be biologically or psychologically hurtful. Alcohol got from such a source must be free from all deleterious substances, one must infer, because the citizen's own government proffers it to him for his own good. But alcohol is alcohol, a toxic chemical substance, whether it comes into being in an elaborate distillery licensed and supervised by the Federal government, or whether it be concocted in crude crockery and in home-made tubs in a crypt on a branch-bank remote from human habitation. The cell of the human body neither knows nor cares where the alcohol molecule comes from that at first stimulates and later narcotize the cell. The epigram reputed to the Scot, traditionally fond of his toddy, comprehends the truth about alcohol's pharmacology: It preserves what is put into it and destroys what it is put into.

The earth is spheroidal. The universe may be a vast globe. There are those who believe that straightness exists nowhere except in fragmentary fashion; and that the straight line is not straight, but is only a portion of a circle whose diameter is endlessly long. And there are those who believe that the present state of things may continue; but that if it does not, it will be succeeded by a former way—that what has been is that which shall be. So, I surmise that, at some day not distant, there may be a bioscopic study of the governmental adventure into alcoholic merchandising. And such a biopsy would eventually be followed by an autopsy. Then prohibition will come again. And those same legislators and those numerous other office-holders who gave us state liquor stores may again be addressing Sunday School picnics as they did in the first flower of prohibition in denunciation of the sale of rum by the individual and by the state.

Were it possible to charge the A B C stores as associates of most of those citizens who are tried for the commission of crimes, then the government whiskey stores would be convicted by the **very** government that maintains them, and they would each be sentenced to incarceration for a thousand years. The one problem in our own national life that is larger, more complex, more difficult, more destructive to life, to health, to efficiency, to happiness; and that is farther away from understanding than any other problem, is alcoholism. The alcoholic is robbed by the manufacturer and by the seller of whiskey; he is denounced and punished by others. The alcoholic is the victim of his pathologic thirst and of his sadistic fellow-man. Nothing is done for him; many things are done to him. The government that sells him beverage alcohol is his enemy. It should be possible for the citizen to bring his enemy to the bar of public and of scientific opinion for trial, for conviction and for punishment.

OPHTHALMOLOGY

Herbert C. Neblett, M.D., *Editor*, Charlotte, N. C.

THE SURGICAL REMOVAL OF THE CHALAZION

The surgical removal of this small cystic tumor of the lid is not difficult but requires a special technique for prevention of pain and hemorrhage and for postoperative results. The operation is usually an office procedure safely carried out under sterile precautions with the patient in the prone position. Only on rare occasions when the tumor has perforated the skin surface of the lid or is seen as a hard mass on the upper surface of the tarsal plate is it necessary to remove it through a (horizontal) skin incision and close with sutures. If removal of the tumor is done via a vertical incision over its site on the under surface of the tarsal plate, sutures and a dressing are dispensed with to the gratification of the patient, and if properly done no or very slight reaction follows.

Technique: Instill into the eye sac a few drops of ½ of 1% solution of pontocain for surface anesthesia. Cocaine is contraindicated because of its mydriatic effect. Installation of any amount of anesthetic will not make the operation painless, but by the additional injection of novocain-adrenalin chloride 1% solution will make the operation painless. With the proper ring clamp holding the everted lid with the tumor presenting through the ring, 0.5 c.c. of the solution injected in the mucous membrane fold just behind the upper border of the tarsal plate in the area behind the site of the chalazion, will give full anesthesia at the operative site in the tarsal plate but not to the skin and muscle on the outer surface of the lid. In order to do this the chalazion clamp is removed and reversed so that the site of the tumor presents through the ring in the clamp on the skin surface of the lid. In this area inject 0.5 c.c. of the anesthetic, carrying it down to the lid margin. Remove the clamp and for a moment or two massage over the area of the injection with the index finger to dessiminate the anesthetic and promote its absorption. A drop or two of pontocain and one of adrenalin 1 to 1000 are now instilled in the eye sac, the clamp firmly applied with its ring inclosing the chalazion on the upper or under surface of the lid as the case may be and the operation begun by incising the cyst and curetting its cavity with a sharp serrated curette. The incision in the tarsal plate should extend from below upward to within 2 mm. of the lid margin and in the channel of the gland involved if possible, so that it is incised to its orifice and all inspissated material may be removed therefrom. In addition the lid margin should be firmly compressed at the site of the cyst to bring away any residue from the mouth of the gland. Some of these cysts are lobulated or have very small cystic areas adjacent to the sides of the main cyst. After this, a tight-wound wet cotton applicator is introduced with a twisting motion to the depth of the cyst to clear out any remaining detritus and dry out the pockets for inspection and for the next step, cauterization of the entire cavity with a cotton-wound applicator saturated with 3% tincture of iodine and neutralization with alcohol. Wash out the sac, remove the clamp and apply a cold, wet cotton pack over the lid for 5 minutes to control hemorrhage which after removal of the clamp is slight and brief.

If the cyst is removed through an incision in the skin surface of the lid the technique as outlined may suffice, or in addition the cyst may have to be dissected out.

Little or no discoloration of the skin surface of the lid or of its mucous membrane surface should result following this operation whether done on the outer or inner surface of the lid. A considerable discoloration of the lid will occur if a vessel in the skin is punctured by the injecting needle. This should not occur if some care is used to avoid puncturing the vessels which can be clearly seen through the taut skin within the ring of the lid clamp. Those in the mucous membrane are easily seen when the lid is everted.

UROLOGY

Raymond Thompson, M.D., *Editor*, Charlotte, N. C.

MEATOTOMY A VALUABLE AND NEGLECTED THERAPEUTIC MEASURE

Of all the parts of the human body, Ballenger[1] says none is more neglected by doctors than the urethra; although here there is little difficulty of diagnosis, and no unusual skill is required. The trouble is that "the symptoms frequently do not suggest the obstructions of the anterior urethra and hyperemia and lesions of the prostatic urethra."

Some symptoms pointing to such lesions are:
1. Enuresis
2. Itching of the urethra and non-specific urethritis in men
3. Cystitis or symptoms suggesting cystitis in women
4. Pain and discomfort in the pelvic and postpubic region
5. Backache
6. Pain in the perineal region.

Children complaining of these symptoms should be examined for a small meatus, urethral stricture or vesical-neck obstruction. In women these same

1. E. G. Ballenger, Atlanta, in *Clin. Med.*, Nov.

lesions may be found, also urethral caruncle infected glands or polypoid growths at the vesical neck.

In men, the posterior urethra may require special investigation. Hyperemia and hypersensitive conditions, common deep urethral disorders, are readily detected by the passage of urethral sounds.

It is suggested that the main reason for the neglect of the urethra when obstructions or hyperemia of the urethra remain, is that it does not seem rational to dilate a urethra already irritated or chronically inflamed. For the major part of urologic problems, this concept of dilation in the presence of chronic infection or persisting irritation now seems to this urologist to be the most important fact learned in many years of work in urology.

To diagnose and to treat disorders of the urethra, he regards as an art and a science, both easily acquired if the value of urethral dilation is recognized and the procedure gently carried out. Realization of the obstructive problem will greatly assist in the management of many common conditions in everyday practice in men, women and children.

In the majority of cases relief of urethral disorders has been afforded by meatotomy, and/or other means of correcting obstructions. In the cases requiring further measures urethroscopic studies may be carried out far more satisfactorily than if the dilation had not been employed as a preliminary.

Non-specific urethritis is one of man's commonest affections and we agree that its usual cause is a small meatus or urethral strictures, and that meatotomy and dilation of strictures afford prompter and more beneficial results than do urinary antiseptics, astringent injections, irrigations and dietary changes. When gonorrhea is not responding to appropriate treatment by local measures and sulfa drugs, likely hindering factors are a small meatus, urethral strictures, poor drainage from the glands of Littre or the prostate.

Obstructions or other lesions should not be sought or treated until acute inflammatory symptoms have been subdued by milder measures.

Patients with no urethral discharge or infection but who have pelvic or perineal pain or discomfort, those who have premature ejaculation, are sexually weak, or children who have enuresis usually respond to the same plan of treatment; that is—meatotomy when needed, urethral dilation and instillation of 1 or 2 per cent solution nitrate of silver into the deep urethra or later to endoscopic applications of stronger solutions to the verumontanum.

The mere introduction of sounds is not sufficient. They should be left in place for about 10 minutes, if the maximum good is to be derived from their use in dilating strictures or in correcting deep urethral irritation. In case these mild measures are not effective, careful endoscopic studies should be made to determine the presence or absence of retarding lesions.

Many of the perineal pains and the various symptoms of the sexual neurasthenic will respond well to this plan of treatment, though no urethral lesion exists; and many disturbing pelvic, perineal, urinary and sexual disturbances may be cured by correcting anterior urethral obstructions and posterior urethral disorders.

DENTISTRY

J. H. GUION, D.D.S., *Editor*, Charlotte, N. C.

THE CASE AGAINST THE IMPACTED TOOTH

MANY hold that the impacted tooth should be left alone so long as there are no subjective or objective symptoms attributable to the impaction. In many cases dental surgery and orthodontia in combination can achieve the successful eruption of a tooth in cases in which orthodontia alone would be unsuccessful.

A New England dental surgeon[1] discusses this problem from what is probably the general viewpoint. He exposes as much of the crown of the tooth as possible and removes any bony impediment to its eruption; then instructs the patient in inhibiting the regrowth of soft tissues over the tooth by the daily use of a sterile orange woodstick. If the tooth does not erupt of its own accord, orthodontia treatment is instituted to bring the tooth to its proper place in the arch.

While any of the permanent dentition may be impacted, the teeth most often aected are the third molars and cuspids. The rare fourth molars are more often impacted than not.

An impacted tooth may remain for years and may never give rise to symptoms or it may give rise to confusing symptoms—pain in various parts of the head, often pain seeming to originate in areas not immediately surrounding the impaction area, local swelling and diffuse cellulitis of the face. Pericoronal infection in this area most commonly brings the patient to seek treatment. An impacted tooth can cause a multiplicity of systemic disturbances because it is generally found to be cystic and as such a potential primary focus of infection. By its intermittent activity causing pressure it can damage nervous tissue and give rise to symptoms that often defy our best efforts at detection of cause. In the search for focus of infection causing pain in the head, a full dental radiographic examination should be made.

1. H. A. McGuirl, Providence, in *R. I. Med. Jl.*, Nov.

An impacted tooth should be removed while the tooth is quiescent and there is no evidence of any acute inflammation in the area. Some believe that with the proper anesthesia it is permissible to remove the offender in the acute condition.

One patient seen several years ago had an onset of violent head pains at 70 years of age and had been wearing full upper and lower dentures for 30 years. There was a suspicion of brain tumor and a radiographic examination showed a deeply impacted cuspid, the removal of which gave prompt and permanent relief from pain.

SURGERY

Geo. H. Bunch, M.D., *Editor*, Columbia, S. C.

GASTROJEJUNOCOLIC FISTULA

Only after thousands of patients had had posterior gastroenterostomy done as an almost routine treatment of peptic ulcer did the medical profession awake to the fact that, except for its complications, the treatment of ulcer should be medical; that when surgery is indicated subtotal gastrectomy is the procedure of choice, and that anastomosis of the stomach to the jejunum after gastric resection should be antecolic. The antecolic site is preferable because the field at any subsequent operation is accessible, and because of the very real hazard to the patient from gastrojejunocolic fistula after postcolic operations. In America the popularity of posterior gastroenterostomy as an effective treatment for ulcer followed its advocacy by the Mayos. It is interesting to note that after many years it has been found in the Mayo Clinic that 11 per cent of the patients undergoing posterior gastroenterostomy developed jejunal ulcer; and that of these developing jejunal ulcer, 11 per cent developed gastrojejunocolic fistula.

The symptoms of gastrojejunocolic fistula are progressive loss of weight, persistant diarrhea and in some cases regurgitation from the stomach of material having the odor of feces. When suspected the fistulous passage between the stomach and the transverse colon may be readily recognized by fluoroscopic study after the ingestion of barium. The prognosis is grave. All those treated medically die, and the mortality rate from the operative closure of the fistula approaches 50 per cent.

Our experience with the condition is confined to a single case, that of a man of 50 years, who eight years ago had subtotal gastric resection done by us for a large indurated ulcer that had penetrated into the pancreas. A postcolic anastomosis of the end of the stomach to the side of the jejunum had been made. His convalescence had been uneventful. For two years he has had a return of ulcer symptoms.

In the last three months he has lost 40 pounds from intractable diarrhea caused by the escape through the fistula of fluids from the stomach to the colon. The diagnosis of gastrocolic fistula was confirmed by x-ray examination. After avitaminosis and hypoproteinemia had been overcome he was operated upon.

We had planned at the first stage to do an end-to-end anastomosis of the terminal ileum and the sigmoid colon, closing the distal end of the ileum and bringing the proximal end of the sigmoid through the abdominal wall as a colostomy. Jejunostomy in a loop distal to the gastrojejunal union was to be done. This would permit adequate feeding through the jejunostomy tube and keep the stomach at rest until healing had been complete, after the proximal colon had been removed and the fistulous opening closed at a subsequent operation.

Fortunately, however, at operation we were able to close the fistulous opening into the colon and to restore the gastrojejunal anastomosis, after having completely separated the three structures—stomach, jejunum and colon. Sulfathiazole powder was dusted over the operative field and the wound closed without drainage. Convalescence was uneventful and the patient was dismissed on the 21st postoperative day again free from symptoms.

In this case it would have been possible to restore the stomach to its antecolic position and to make the anastomosis to the jejunum antecolic, but because of the extra hazard it was not attempted. We feel that without the use of sulfathiazole we might have lost this patient from peritonitis.

THERAPEUTICS

J. F. Nash, M.D., *Editor*, Saint Pauls, N. C.

INTRAVENOUS ANESTHESIA IN CHILDREN

Frequently do we need to produce anesthesia in a child. Holly[1] presents the advantages of pentothal as the agent.

To make a 2.5 per cent solution, add 20 c.c. of c. p. water to 0.5 gram (7.5 grains) of pentothal. The water is aspirated into a 20-c.c. syringe and injected into an ampoule containing pentothal. The resulting solution should be clear. Should a precipitate occur, do not use but prepare another solution. Each c.c. of the solution will contain 25 mg. of pentothal. Discard the solution if it is not used within four hours, as it deteriorates rapidly.

The equipment consists of one 3-way valve, a piece of rubber tubing 8 inches long; at the end of the tubing, a luer glass tip; to this is attached an

1. J. D. Holly, Miami Beach, in *Sou. Med. Jl.*, Nov.

intravenous needle; also a glass for the mixing solution, a 20-c.c. luer-lok syringe and stand for holding the syringe, and needles 1¼ inches, 22-24 gauge, beveled and sharp-pointed.

The veins in the antecubital fossa, those on the dorsum of the hand, or the great saphenous vein, anterior to the internal malleolus may be used.

Atropine sulphate gr. 1-250th is given by hypo. up to 5 years of age 30 min. before operation; children over 5 years of age are given nembutal 1-1½ 1 hr. before operation and atropine gr. 1 150 30 min. before operation. Atropine prevents laryngeal spasm, salivation, hiccough and respiratory depression.

One or 2 c.c. of the solution is injected slowly, and one waits for it to take effect (15-30 seconds), then prepares the operative site. Anesthesia comes on in a few seconds; respiration becomes quiet and regular. If the child moves his extremities or begins to moan, inject 0.5-1 c.c. additional. At the sign of a "snore," insert an airway. Do not allow the surgeon to begin until anesthesia has become established. As anesthesia deepens, respiration becomes depressed in rate and amplitude, eyeballs are centrally fixed, and then the lid reflex is lost. Phonation and increased rate and depth of respiration are the first indications of awakening, and call for a fraction of a c.c. of the pentothal solution.

If the anticipated operation is to be over 30 minutes, glucose or saline solution is given by attaching the tube from the infusion set to the small rubber tubing on the 3-way valve. In this manner intravenous fluids given to support the circulation, replace fluids lost by hemorrhage, and at the same time keep the intravenous needle from plugging due to clotting of blood. Oxygen is administered throughout the operation.

Pentothal can be used in children for any type of operation except bronchoscopy. The more severe the illness, the greater the indication for its use. Since it produces no irritation of the lungs, it can be used during acute coryza or colds if surgical procedures are indicated.

Pentothal is contraindicated as an anesthetic agent in inflammations that encroach on the trachea, neck, posterior pharyngeal wall, and operations that involve the skin only. It is a useful and safe anesthetic agent for children. The equipment is simple and can easily be carried in a small case. Hazards of inflammability and explosion are eliminated. The action of pentothal is rapid, and its elimination is likewise rapid. Relaxation is comparable to that from inhalation anesthesia.

Pentothal administration is economical. One gram will suffice for an operation lasting one hour or more. Repeated administrations produce no deleterious effects. It is particularly adaptable for use in emergency cases following a full meal; since it does not produce nausea or vomiting, the constant dread of aspirating vomitus is eliminated.

The anesthetist is out of the way of the operating field in operations in the region of the face and throat.

Overaction is combatted by artificial respiration, and stimulation of respiration with picrotoxin, coramine, caffeine-sodium benzoate, carbon dioxide and oxygen.

DERMATOLOGY

For this issue RAY O. NOOJIN, M.D., Durham

ROSACEA

THE ROSACEA COMPLEX is a member of that large dermatological group for which completely satisfactory causes have yet to be clearly demonstrated. This dermatosis is chronic and recognized usually by flushing, seborrhea, papules, pustules, and in some cases tissue hypertrophy. The region involved usually includes an oval area made up of the chin, nose, cheeks and middle forehead. Women are more commonly affected than men, and the patient is usually past the age of thirty at the time of onset.

There continues to be considerable controversy regarding the cause of this disease. Emotional disturbances, a seborrheic diathesis, and a dysfunctioning gastrointestinal tract are perhaps the most significant contributory factors. In certain cases, foci of infection, endocrine imbalance, diet inadequacy, or chronic alcoholism may be significant.

The fact that the Demodex folliculorum may be found microscopically in the sebum expressed from the follicles of the local areas may be of little significance, since the organism is frequently found in the skin of patients without rosacea.

At the time of onset there tends to be a temporary flushing of the face and neck. This flushing mechanism is under a sensitive vasomotor control, and these patients may be seen to flush in the physician's office at the time of examination due to the tension incident to the occasion. Anger, menses, excitement, alcohol, and numerous other factors may produce the flushing episodes. Later the flushing tends to develop into a permanent hyperemia of the involved areas with numerous superficial dilated capillaries becoming visible, probably resulting from the long-standing congestion. The formation of papules usually follows the increased vascularity. The papules may pustulate due to infection or follicular necrosis. These lesions are acneform in appearance. The sebaceous glands eventually become hypertrophied, and it has been suggested that this results from the local increased vascular congestion. The increased activity of the sebaceous glands produces a local seborrhea. Comedones are not a feature of this affection.

Gastroscopic examination in patients with rosacea has revealed gastritis to be present considerably more frequently than in normal controls. Rosacea and gastrointestinal disturbances occur together too frequently to be simply incidental. The significance of the contribution that gastric abnormality makes to the syndrome is not entirely understood.

After the disease has been present for several years there may occur hypertrophy of the tissues of the nose to produce rhinophyma. Lobulated masses of tissue may be formed in this area, and the nose may become greatly increased in size.

Subjectively the patients complain of little in the way of local symptoms, except for occasional burning or stinging during the episodes of flushing.

In 5 per cent or less of the cases of facial rosacea a complicating ocular rosacea occurs—rosacea blepharitis, conjunctivitis, keratitis, or iritis, in this order of frequency. A contributory factor to this complication has been ascribed to riboflavin deficiency by some; however, all investigators are not in agreement on this point.

The diagnosis of rosacea is not difficult in the typical case. The flushing, telangectasia, limitation of the disease to the flush areas, presence of acneform lesions, and the occurrence of the syndrome in middle age tend to make the diagnosis obvious. Acne vulgaris, acneform drug eruptions, lupus erythematosus, seborrheic dermatitis, rosacea-like tuberculid, the nodular syphiloderm, and atopic eczema are to be considered in the differential diagnosis.

Treatment is at times difficult and should always consist of local and constitutional measures. Well organized therapy usually results in improvement even in the more severely involved patients. An attempt should be made to find the factor, or factors, which seem most contributory in the individual.

(1) Search for and eliminate foci of infection.

(2) Psychiatric help is sometimes needed, if emotional conflicts are disturbing.

(3) The diet should be bland. Coffee, tea, alcohol, tobacco, fried, hot and cold foods or drinks, overeating, nuts, iodides, bromides, chocolate, condiments and hurried eating are contra-indicated.

(4) Dilute hydrochloric acid is usually helpful to patients with achlorhydria. One to five cubic centimeters in milk or fruit juice is to be sipped through a glass tube following meals. Patients with hyperacidity should be tried on aluminum hydroxide or magnesium trisilicate.

(5) Chronic constipation should be corrected with mineral oil and sufficient fluid intake rather than by irritating laxatives.

(6) Every effort should be made to improve the physical and mental health of the patient.

(7) Sedation, generalized ultraviolet light, rest and daily naps are indicated for the patient with obvious nervous tension.

The following local measures are suggested:

(1) Lotio alba may be applied to the affected areas one to three times daily.

(2) No cremes or oily lotions should be applied locally.

(3) In bathing the face cool water only should be used. Strong soaps should be avoided. A mild soap may be used one to three times daily.

(4) The patient should not pick at the pustules, because of the possibility of further dissemination of the infection and increased scarring.

(5) The telangectasias may be eliminated by means of local electrodesiccation.

(6) Surgical removal of the redundant nasal tissue may be necessary when rhinophyma develops.

(7) X-ray therapy in fractional doses is advocated locally if the lesions are predominantly acneform. Only one well experienced in roentgen therapy should administer this treatment.

(8) An ophthalmological consultation is indicated if ocular rosacea occurs.

GENERAL PRACTICE

JAMES L. HAMNER, M.D., *Editor*, Mannboro, Va.

FETAL ASPHYXIATION

THERE IS a lot in the public prints about resuscitation, most of it with emphasis on complicated, expensive machinery. From Kansas comes a report of well-nigh perfect results from the use of methods of the utmost simplicity. Many a person has lost his life because the would-be helper ran for an expert or a machine instead of using his hands and breath in a commonsense way.

In 2404 consecutive deliveries, half of them made by interns, only one baby born alive failed to breathe; four babies requiring one-half hour or longer to resuscitate, died subsequently. Two babies were found at autopsy to have large brain hemorrhages and two clinically appeared to have brain injury. The uncorrected stillbirth rate for this series was 1.01%. No complicated apparatus was used for resuscitation; only simple methods, available to everyone.

As soon as the baby's head emerges, mucus squeezed out of the baby's chest should be milked out of its neck and mouth and wiped away. A soft rubber ear syringe can be inserted quickly into its mouth and throat and mucus aspirated before the

1. R. E. Pfuetze, Topeka, in *Jl. Kansas Med. Soc.*, Oct.

first breath. The baby should then be held briefly in the lap of the obstetrician to allow additional blood to flow into the baby from the placenta.

The baby may be stimulated to breathe by rubbing its back, slapping its feet or shaking it gently. If breathing did not begin immediately, the baby was covered with a towel, the mucus removed from its trachea by a catheter and artificial respiration begun. No delay should be allowed in trying less efficient or more shocking methods.

A great many simple and complicated machines have been invented to carry on artificial respiration in the newborn and many of them are good. The Drinker "Iron Lung" is perhaps the most spectacular. But a tracheal catheter may be purchased for $1.00 and is all that is needed in the way of equipment. With it, mucus may be effectively aspirated from the mouth and trachea and respiration established. The baby's head should be extended somewhat and the index finger inserted to a point just behind the epiglottis and the arytenoid cartilage to prevent the catheter going down the esophagus. The catheter may then be inserted along the underside of the finger and its tip pushed into the trachea. After removing the mucus from the throat and trachea, it is reinserted and artificial respiration begun gently. Only the amount of air that can be held in the mouth without distending the cheeks is pushed into the baby's lungs, repeating 15 times or more a minute.

Some skill is required to quickly pass the catheter and it is best learned on babies that are stillborn or die shortly thereafter. It is very difficult to insert a catheter in a baby with all reflexes present.

In the absence of a tracheal catheter, mouth-to-mouth insufflation may be used. This has the disadvantage that mucus or meconium will be blown into the baby's lungs rather than be cleaned out first and air will be frequently forced into the baby's stomach.

THE FALLACY OF MASSAGE IN THE TREATMENT OF OBESITY (S. W. Kalb, Newark, in Jl. Med. Soc. N. J., Nov.)

Since the dawn of civilization, massage, rubbing, or pounding has been used as a means for reducing the overweight individual. Millions of persons have accepted it in the hope of finding an easy way to lose weight.

In order to determine the value of massage as a therapeutic aid in the treatment of obesity, this study was undertaken.

In 40 patients with obesity on low-calory diets, there was a less in total body weight and a decrease in the circumference of the limb which was massaged. There was a similar decrease in the measurements of the opposite limb which was not massaged.

In 20 patients with obesity which no dietary restrictions but who received body massage, there was no loss in total body weight and no decrease in the circumference of the limb which was also massaged with a vibratic machine.

DISEASES OF THE DIGESTIVE SYSTEM, edited by SIDNEY A. PORTIS, B.S., M.D., F.A.C.P., Associate Professor of Medicine, University of Illinois Medical School (Rush). Second Edition, Illustrated with 182 Engravings. Lea & Febiger, Washington Square, Philadelphia 6. 1944. $11.00.

The second edition following so promptly testifies to the popular acceptance of this work. A discussion of the physiology of each organ just before the discussion of its disease conditions is a valuable feature; another is the dealing with complaints thought by patients to be of gastrointestinal origin which turn out to be due to disease outside the abdomen.

The 50 contributors have labored successfully to reduce to essentials of the subjects they discuss to a reasonable volume. In less than 1,000 pages are presented all the essentials for a proper diagnosis and treatment of diseases of the digestive system.

THE ART OF RESUSCITATION, by PALUEL J. FLAGG, M.D., Chairman, Committee on Asphyxia, A. M. A. Reinhold Publishing Corporation, 330 W. 42nd Street, New York City. 1944. $5.00.

In resuscitation as in anesthesia Flagg is an authority second to none. In a foreword Chevalier Jackson says his first thought in reviewing the book is the great number of lives it will save. That, its teachings, put into effect, will certainly do; and certainly that is the chief aim and end of all medical books. A book in a class by itself.

THE MODERN TREATMENT OF SYPHILIS, by JOSEPH EARLE MOORE, M.D., Associate Professor of Medicine and Adjunct Professor of Public Health Administration, The Johns Hopkins University, with the Collaboration of JAROLD E. KEMP, M.D., Late Associate in Venereal Diseases; HARRY EAGLE, M.D., Surgeon U.S.P.H.S., and Lecturer in Medicine; PAUL PADGET, M.D., Associate in Medicine; MARY STEWART GOODWIN, M.D., Instructor in Pediatrics; and FRANK W. REYNOLDS, M.D., Instructor in Medicine. Lt. M.C.-V. (G), U.S.N.R., all of The Johns Hopkins University. Third Printing. Charles C. Thomas, Springfield, Ill 1944. $7.50.

The author's plan for the study of syphilis by himself and his associates, unique in conception and modified as it went on over the years, has produced results which as presented up to date in this printing, are deserving of the highest praise and the widest diffusion. First he discusses the biology of syphilitic infection in relation to treatment, then the prognosis of syphilis, treated and untreated, as to infectiousness and cure. The individualization of treatment according to many various factors are made on all the evidence. Perhaps in no other book is so emphasized the study of syphilis as an entity, in whatever part of the human economy the disease may be making its greatest ravages. The book has no superior for use in the private office, the syphilis clinics, the general or the special hospital.

PRESIDENT'S PAGE

SOLDIERS DISCHARGED ON ACCOUNT OF NERVOUS DISABILITIES

Not only after the war will there be in our states many marines, sailors and other soldiers discharged on account of nervous diseases, but already many have been. In spite of the fact that hundreds of our best psychiatrists have been carefully examining and rejecting applicants for enlistments and draftees who present a nervous background or family history, many still have gotten into the various services whom the psychiatrists were unable to detect at the time of enlistment.

Many more of the above type of disease will come back from the battle fronts whose illness was caused by hardships of warfare. Many of these will be discharged on S. C. D. with disability benefits and rightfully so. The mere payment of dollars in varying amounts to these former soldiers is not sufficient. There is something vastly more important, that is to get these men to work. Occupation is the answer, and the remedy for the great majority of nervous diseases real as well as imaginary. Physical work with little or no mental problems to solve. Eight hours a day is not too much. This does a double-barreled function. First, it gives to the patient a feeling of well-being in that he is a producer paying his way through. Second, it takes away from him eight hours that he would be thinking of his disability were he unemployed.

I know of no more terrible calamity to befall anyone than for these young men (and they are all young, 20 to 30) to have too much time to reflect that at this youthful age their usefulness in filling a place in civil and community enterprise is over. Their entire life insofar as business management and employment is before them. Their past years at this young age cover nothing but schooldays.

Many, many times have I seen from the results of World War I, young men who about all they had to do in the twenty-four hours a day was to sleep eight hours and sixteen hours left to constantly carry over in their minds the thoughts of having no part in world affairs except to remain sick and wait for their next pay check. What can we doctors of Virginia, North Carolina and South Carolina do about it? Quite a great deal, and any doctor of the U. S. A. will have the same opportunity. For in the first place, we will all agree that any nervous patient will most certainly seek a physician for advice and treatment. While talking to these boys, let then run through your mind the thought of what physical work is this man best suited for and help him get a job. Talk with his employer at intervals. Tell him to give the employee plenty of work, often hard work so long as it is mostly physical. I have recently had the opportunity to observe several of these cases discharged from service in the present war. You will be surprised and highly pleased the way these boys change their attitude from one of depending upon the Federal Government to one of filling a place in human affairs which was exactly their object and desire before entering the armed service. This physical work is the best medicine for many nervous disorders that has ever been prescribed. The recovery is remarkable from the beginning and continues until anyone who was not aware of it would never know the individual ever was mentally sick. Of course, for the greatly depressed patient, the neurasthenic and neurocirculatory asthenic, we, as physicians, must help decide the type of work these men should do and help put them at it as early as circumstances in the individual case permit.

In the cases where the patient wants to know and asks you what is his trouble or diagnosis, we should never use the word shell-shock. It is hard for some patients to ever divorce themselves from this word and it is a great detriment to recovery.

If the doctors of the entire nation will help these nervous patients to get on a job, almost regardless of what type of labor it is, they will do the patient and the American people a great service; and the doctors will be wholly paid in satisfaction of a job well done.

Remember that these ex-service men are mere youths willing and ready for advice, and what we do for them will go farther and be much more beneficial than what they get merely through the small pay check for disability.

Thousands of other youths will enter college after the war. These will come largely from another group, those whose nerves stood up under the strain better than the first group. We can advise boys as to what college course they are best fitted for.

This is the last issue of the *Journal of Medicine & Surgery* for 1944. In the closing days, I want to thank all who have contributed to making this a successful year.

To one and all of these doctors, both at home and abroad, a most pleasant Christmas and for those in the armed services, our prayer is that the war may terminate at an early date and all of you may soon return to your family and loved ones.

K. B. Pace.

SOUTHERN MEDICINE & SURGERY

Official Organ

JAMES M. NORTHINGTON, M.D., *Editor*

Department Editors

Human Behavior
JAMES K. HALL, M.D. .... Richmond, Va.

Orthopedic Surgery
JOHN T. SAUNDERS, M.D. .... Asheville, N. C.

Urology
RAYMOND THOMPSON, M.D. .... Charlotte, N. C.

Surgery
GEO. H. BUNCH, M.D. .... Columbia, S. C.

Obstetrics
HENRY J. LANGSTON, M.D. .... Danville, Va.

Gynecology
CHAS. R. ROBINS, M.D. .... Richmond, Va.
ROBERT T. FERGUSON, M.D. .... Charlotte, N. C.

General Practice
I. L. HAMNER, M.D. .... Mannboro, Va.
J. HERBERT SMITH, M.D. .... Pauline, S. C.

Clinical Chemistry and Microscopy
J. M. FEDER, M.D.,
EVELYN TRIBBLE, M. T. } .... Anderson, S. C.

Hospitals
R. B. DAVIS, M.D. .... Greensboro, N. C.

Cardiology
CLYDE M. GILMORE, A.B., M.D. .... Greensboro, N. C.

Public Health
N. THOS. ENNETT, M.D. .... Greenville, N. C.

Radiology
R. H. LAFFERTY, M.D., and Associates .... Charlotte, N. C.

Therapeutics
J. F. NASH, M.D. .... Saint Pauls, N. C.

Tuberculosis
JOHN DONNELLY, M.D. .... Charlotte, N. C.

Dentistry
J. H. GUION, D.D.S. .... Charlotte, N. C.

Internal Medicine
GEORGE R. WILKINSON, M.D. .... Greenville, S. C.

Ophthalmology
HERBERT C. NEBLETT, M.D. .... Charlotte, N. C.

Rhino-Oto-Laryngology
CLAY W. EVATT, M.D. .... Charleston, S. C.

Proctology
RUSSELL L. BUXTON, M.D. .... Newport News, Va.

Insurance Medicine
H. F. STARR, M.D. .... Greensboro, N. C.

Dermatology
J. LAMAR CALLAWAY, M.D. .... Durham, N. C.

Pediatrics

Offerings for the pages of this Journal are requested and given careful consideration in each case. Manuscripts not found suitable for our use will not be returned unless author encloses postage.

It is true of most Medical Journals, all costs of cuts, etc., for illustrating an article must be borne by the author.

DOCTOR DARDEN DIES

This issue was almost off the press when news came of the sudden death of Dr. O. B. Darden, on Sunday, December 10th. There is just time to put in this brief notice to every Tri-State member, that this loyal Fellow will gather with us no more. Our next issue will carry a full account of this distressful happening.

* * * * *

THE COMING TRI-STATE MEETING

PREPARATIONS are well advanced for our meeting in February. Not so many papers will be scheduled as were accepted for our last meeting, when, for the first time in Tri-State history, all those who had been placed on the program showed up. Allowance had been made for at least ten per cent notifying by wire at the last moment that illness in the person of the doctor or of a member of his family, or of patients who could not be left, made it impossible that they attend.

The next meeting is to be held at Columbia, February 26th and 27th; headquarters will be the Wade Hampton Hotel. Our meetings at Columbia have always been well attended and enthusiastic, and all the portents show that the approaching meeting will be another of the same kind.

Every member is charged to be especially careful to extend an invitation to each qualified prospective member with whom he comes into contact. The secretary is greatly hampered in his canvassing by the absorption into Armed Services of the great majority of our new eligibles, and by his lack of knowledge of the distribution of those who, for various reasons, have been rejected by the Services.

Members who desire place on the program should so notify the secretary immediately. Also bear it in mind that a *candidate* with something very special to say is given opportunity to say it in a paper or in discussions.

Write the Manager, Wade Hampton Hotel, Columbia, S. C.; and the Secretary, as soon as you can possibly complete your plans.

* * * * *

ABOUT MEDICAL NEEDS IN NORTH CAROLINA

As TO DIAGNOSIS AND TREATMENT of the medical needs of the people of this state, this journal is in disagreement with the Governor, his Committee, and what appears to be the majority sentiment of those who express themselves on the subject. We have in previous issues pointed out the fact that in states in which there is no medical school, right alongside states which have a medical school and have had it for years on years, the two states as alike as two peas in a pod, the distribution of doctors is to all intents and purposes the same. This by way of comment on the contention that in order to have doctors to care for our people we must educate them within the borders of the State.

Then, when we did not have a school in the State which gave the third and fourth years in medicine, the distribution of doctors in the State was practically the same as in other states of the same per capita wealth, yet having one or more medical schools graduating doctors of medicine every June.

Mr. Clarence Poe is a man held in high esteem for his qualities of head and heart. It is hard to understand just what he means by stating that North Carolina is the fourth State in the Union in the payment of Federal taxes. As a bald statement of fact it is true; but the conclusion seems inescapable that to make the statement in arguing that North Carolina can afford to do this or that, it is meant to say that our State is the fourth wealthiest State in the Union; and everybody knows that such a statement would be absurd. North Carolina pays so much in Federal taxes because within her borders are manufactured most of the cigarettes consumed in this country—in the whole world; and cigarettes are enormously taxed as a luxury—on the good old plan enunciated by Mark Hanna, in order "to get the most feathers with the least squawking." The man, woman or child who smokes a cigarette pays the tax, whether he live in Charlotte, Washington, Paris or Singapore.

The only state in the Union of population comparable to that of North Carolina which has three medical schools is Tennessee, and one of these schools graduates only Negro doctors. Only one medical school would constitute a high average for North Carolina's population and wealth, and, despite statements of enthusiastic citizens to the contrary, North Carolina is away down toward the bottom in per capita wealth.

In no ordinary sense of the words can it be said that we need to graduate more doctors than we are graduating. But if we are determined to give the last two years to the students in medicine at Chapel Hill, within the borders of the State, it can be much better and more cheaply done in Charlotte or in Asheville than at Chapel Hill. I know of no medical educator who does not look upon a large out-patient department as an essential for the instruction of medical students. Charlotte or Asheville could furnish these patients; Chapel Hill cannot. Teachers in all the branches are available in either city; no importation necessary to teach the medicine and surgery of today, and teach it as well as it is taught anywhere. It is claimed by the supporters of this plan that the state badly needs another large hospital to which patients with obscure disease conditions may be sent for expert study. Maybe so, but if so why place it within a dozen miles of Duke University Hospital? It is evident that such a hospital in Charlotte would much better serve a much larger number of the people of the State. Incidentally there seems no reason to believe that, in case this large hospital is built at Chapel Hill, it will provide any better service than is being provided by a number of hospitals in Charlotte and in Asheville. And everybody knows a great number will continue to go out of the State for medical and surgical care.

A good deal is said about University atmosphere. A medical school's third- and fourth-year teaching may be on the campus, but it is not of it. The first two years in medicine are taught in the lecture rooms and the laboratories; the last two in the hospitals—in-patient and out-patient departments.

This journal is steadfastly of the opinion that the surplus which has accumulated in the treasury of the State will be urgently needed in the near future to take care of real needs. It fully expects to see the present hospitals of North Carolina, their bed occupancy no more than 60 per cent, and so large a proportion of the 60 per cent non-pay that great difficulty will be experienced meeting monthly bills. It does not believe that enlargement of the medical school at Chapel Hill is needed. If the powers that be are bent and determined that the medical school of the University of North Carolina give the third and fourth year of medicine, we are firm in the belief that the proper place to give this instruction is either Charlotte or Asheville, that in either of these cities better doctors would be made, and at fraction of the cost.

* * * * *

THE FALLIBILITY OF THE BLOOD TEST FOR SYPHILIS AS ILLUSTRATED BY A PRELIMINARY REPORT OF BLOOD TESTING, AS REQUIRED BY ALABAMA LAW

IN 1943 the Legislature of Alabama passed a law requiring all civilians between the ages of 14 and 50 years residing or living in that State to have their blood examined for syphilis. The law also stipulates that all members of a family under 14 and over 50 years of age, living in the same household in which a positive reactionh as been found, shall be blood tested.

The procedure as carried out is as follows: A modified one-tube Kahn test is used, and a standard Kahn test antigen, the results recorded as positive, doubtful, or negative. In all instances in which a positive or doubtful report was made on an original blood specimen, a second specimen was obtained and examined by the three-tube Kahn

―――――――――
J. W. H. Y. Smith et al., in Venereal Disease Information, Nov.

standard technic. The results of these tests were recorded also as positive, doubtful, or negative.

All persons with positive, doubtful and unsatisfactory tests are notified by letter to appear at a specific clinic or at the health department. All persons with suspected syphilis, as shown by two positive or three doubtful reactions or a combination of these findings after more than three tests, are requested to present themselves to their own physician or to a clinic. An examination is made and if syphilis is diagnosed the patient is admitted and treatment begun.

The experience in two counties is thus reported[1] as to some features:

All clinic patients with *early* syphilis were treated by the 8-, 16-, or 30-week plan (Eagle), the *late latent* by the 40-week alternating course of bismuth and arsenicals.

The percentage of positive tests by race for three counties were: White, 2.2; Negro, 20.5.

In one county, of the 1,544 positive reactions found following a first serologic test, 127 (8.2%) proved by repeated tests not to be syphilitic; 185 have not been found as yet to be syphilitic; and 2,219 have been shown to *probably* have syphilis.

In the second county, where the follow-up work is still in progress, 2,252 were found to have a positive reaction to the first Kahn test. Of these, 197 (8.7%) were found not to be syphilitic; 588 have not yet been completely studied, and 1,367 were shown to *probably* have syphilis.

Note that in the reports for the two counties here reported 8.5 per cent of those persons whose first blood test was positive for syphilis have, as the result of further examination, "found not to be syphilitic;" and in a much larger percentage the examiners remain in doubt; and that the remainder have been shown only "to *probably* have syphilis."

This journal believes that Alabama is wise in taking this forward step, since it is fortunate enough to have its administration in the hands of doctors who do not regard any blood test as meaning that a person certainly has syphilis. We would advocate such a law in North Carolina. But it needs no exceptional foresight to know that putting such a law into effect will give its enforcers many a headache. Labeling a man, woman or child who does not have syphilis, as "syphilitic" involves heavy responsibilities—moral, legal, even physical.

Lispth

The Professor was questioning his class about the constituent parts of a tree. A student answered to his satisfaction, telling of the inner and outer bark and the core or pith. At this point, the instructor, noting an apparently inattentive co-ed, thought to trip her with a "surprise" question. "Miss Robinson," he asked, "do you know what pith is?" Whereupon the young lady disarmingly, but simply replied, "Yethir!"

NEWS

The Seventh District Medical Society Meeting, Nov. 8th.
Program

Meeting called to order at 4 p. m. by Dr. J. A. Elliott, Councilor, Charlotte.

"Pneumoconiosis—With Special Emphasis on Silicosis," Dr. W. Henry Hill, Albemarle.

"Intensive Therapy of Syphilis," Dr. Howard P. Steiger, Charlotte.

"Socialized Medicine or What?", Dr. W. C. Bostic, Sr., Forest City.

"The Effect of Fear on Diagnosis," Dr. J. P. U. McLeod, Marshville.

"Poliomyelitis—An Acute Emergency," Dr. H. C. Whims, Newton, N. C.

Dinner 7:30 p. m., Hotel Albemarle.

Invocation—Dr. George H. Rhodes, Albemarle.

Address of Welcome, Attorney A. C. Huneycutt, Albemarle.

Response, Dr. L. A. Crowell, Sr., Lincolnton.

Dr. John Stuart Gaul, Charlotte, made a detailed, instructive report, in elaboration of Dr. Whims' paper.

Dr. Roscoe McMillan, Secretary-Treasurer of the State Medical Society, spoke in the stead of the President, Dr. Paul F. Whitaker, who was detained at home by illness.

Promotions

Some recent promotions of medical corps officers are from Lieutenant Colonel to Colonel, Dr. John Powell Williams of Richmond; from Major to Lieutenant Colonel, Dr. James P. Baker, Richmond, Dr. G. A. Duncan, Norfolk, Dr. A. DeJ. Hart of Charlottesville, and Dr. J. W. Blanton of Fairmont, W. V.

Lieutenant Colonel William H. L. Westbrook, Jr., M.D., of Franklin, Va., formerly assigned Administrative Branch, Hospital Division, Operations Service, assigned as Executive Officer of McGuire General Hospital, Richmond, Va.

Legion of Merit

Major Saul Greizman, M.C., of Pittsburgh, has recently been awarded the Legion of Merit for "exceptionally meritorious conduct in the performance of distinguished service in the Solomon Islands from July 22nd, 1943, to April 7th, 1944." Born in Romanov, Russia, Captain Greizman graduated from the University of Pittsburgh in 1929 with the degree of B.S., and received his medical degree from the Vanderbilt University School of Medicine in 1934. He entered the Medical Corps as a first lieutenant in 1942, and was promoted to major in July of this year.

Silver Star

Captain Edward I. Lederman, M.C., of Baltimore, has recently been awarded the Silver Star. The citation accompanying the award declares that he was the assistant surgeon of an infantry battalion engaged in combat with a determined group of enemy located in advantageous positions on high ridges on Biak Island, New Guinea, May 28th. Captain Lederman moved forward to advance units to render medical assistance with less delay. Under severe fire, he gave medical assistance to the wounded and expedited their evacuation to the rear. During withdrawal from the position across an open beach, he stopped to aid a severely wounded man. These acts required exceptional courage and initiative, and the results of his work saved the lives of many soldiers.

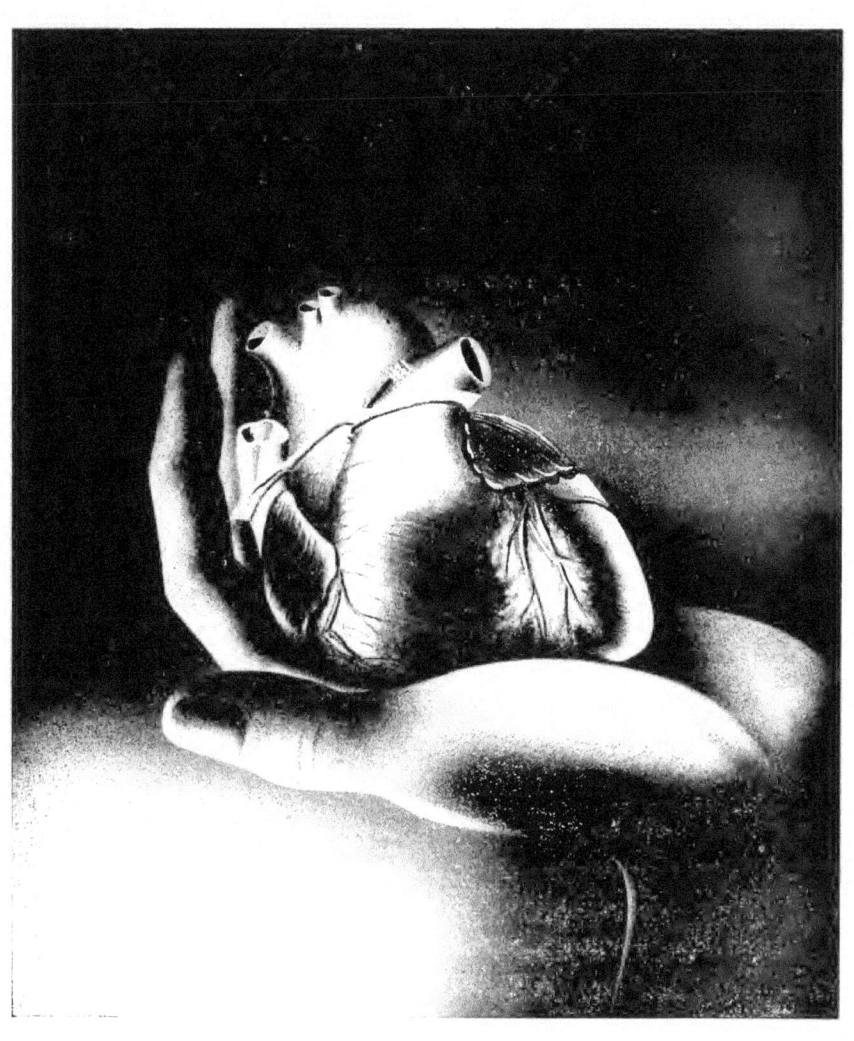

SUPPORT FOR THE FAILING HEART... *Digalen® Roche®*

Dr. Beverley R. Tucker has been elected chairman of the board of the Richmond Public Library.

UNIVERSITY OF VIRGINIA

Dr. Fletcher D. Woodward gave the American Board Fall Examination on Otolaryngology in Chicago on October 4th to 6th. Also he attended the Annual Meeting of the American Academy of Ophthalmology and Otolaryngology in Chicago the week of October 9th through 14th and gave three lectures on "The Management of Recent Fractures of the Face."

Dr. Ralph B. Houlihan received a grant of $2,000 from the John and Mary R. Markle Foundation for a period of one year (November 1st) to aid in his Research Study of Agglutinative Action of Streptococcus Viridans on Blood Platelets.

Dr. Beverly C. Smith, Associate in Surgery at the College of Physicians and Surgeons, Columbia University, spoke at the meeting of the University of Virginia Medical Society on November 10th on "The Use of Radio-Active Sodium as a Tracer Substance in the Study of Peripheral Vascular Disease."

Dr. Dudley C. Smith attended a National Venereal Disease Control Conference in St. Louis November 9th to 11th. This conference was under the auspices of the National Research Council and the U. S. Public Health Service. The theme of the conference was "Problems in Venereal Disease Control After the War." Dr. Smith is a member of the investigating unit of the Penicillin Panel of the Office of Scientific Research and Development.

On final settlement of the estate of the late Dr. William Evelyn Hopkins, noted Ophthalmologist of Los Angeles, Calif., the sum of $29,094.00 became available to the Hopkins Medical Library Fund in addition to an earlier installment of $13,432.00.

Dr. W. W. Waddell, Professor of Pediatrics, attended the meeting of the Southern Medical Association in St. Louis on November 14th and spoke on "Neonatal Mortality Rates in Infants Receiving Prophylactic Doses of Vitamin K."

MEDICAL COLLEGE OF VIRGINIA

Dr. Ernest J. Jaqua, Educational Director, Baruch Committee on Physical Medicine; and Dr. A. R. Mann, Vice-President of the General Education Board, were recent college visitors.

Dr. W. T. Sanger, President, and Dr. J. P. Gray, Dean of the School of Medicine, attended the annual meeting of the Association of American Medical Colleges in Detroit, October 23rd-25th.

Gifts in the amount of $950.00 have been received during the past two months for loan and scholarship funds in the School of Pharmacy. The Office of Scientific Research and Development of the Federal Government has made an allotment of $11,025.00 for the continuation of research on shock and burns under the direction of Dr. E. I. Evans, Associate Professor of Surgery.

Armistice Day exercises were held at Monument Church at noon on November 11th in conjunction with the veterans of Base Hospital 45. Rev. George Ossman, rector of the church, gave the invocation and benediction. President Sanger welcomed the assembly and introduced the speakers. Dr. John Bell Williams represented Dr. Stuart McGuire, commander of Base Hospital 45 in World War I. Lieutenant Mary V. Duncan, who had served in Africa and Italy with the present General Hospital 45, spoke briefly. Dr. A. L. Currie, rector of Second Presbyterian Church, made the principal address.

Dr. J. P. Gray, Dean of the School of Medicine; Dr. Porter P. Vinson, Professor of Bronchoscopy, Esophagoscopy, and Gastroscopy; Dr. Austin I. Dodson, Professor of Urology; Dr. T. Dewey Davis, Associate Professor of Medicine; Dr. E. I. Evans, Associate Professor of Surgery; Dr. Lawther J. Whitehead, Associate Professor of Radiology; and Dr. Bernard Black-Schaffer participated in the program of the Southern Medical Association at Saint Louis, November 13th-16th. Others of the faculty attending the meeting were: Dr. Thomas W. Murrell, Professor of Dermatology; Dr. H. H. Ware, Jr., Professor of Obstetrics; Dr. Lee E. Sutton, Jr., Professor of Pediatrics; and Dr. Frances A. Hellebrandt, Professor of Physical Medicine.

MARRIED

Miss Anna Lee Carner, of Glen Allen, Virginia, and Dr. Edgar Clyde Garber, Jr., of Greensboro, N. C., were married in Richmond, December 9th. The bride was given in marriage by her uncle, Dr. Waverly R. Payne, of Newport News. Among the attendants were Drs. William W. Kersey, Wm. P. Morrison, Thos. L. Howard and Raymond D. Adams.

Dr. Lynwood Earl Williams and Miss Dorothy Dean Wells, of Kinston, were married on November 25th.

Dr. Gus Evans Forbes, of Greenville, North Carolina, and Miss Nancy Burnette Armistead, of South Hill, Virginia, were married on November 25th.

Dr. P. C. Purvis, of Fairmont, North Carolina, and Miss Peggy Joyce Haynie, of Decatur, Georgia, were married on November 11th.

DIED

Dr. John Quincy Myers, prominent Charlotte physician, died at a local hospital December 3d of a heart attack. He had been confined to the hospital for two months under treatment for recurring symptoms of peptic ulcer.

Dr. Myers was born in Wilkes County in 1877, pursued his academic and medical studies at Davidson College, receiving his M.D. degree in 1904. From 1904 to 1909 he practiced his profession in his native county.

Soon after coming to Charlotte in 1909 he became interested in the formation of the North Carolina Medical College and was one of its founders, and a teacher there throughout the life of the college. For many years he was physician-in-chief to Tranquil Park Sanitarium.

He was the first secretary-treasurer of the North Carolina Hospital Association, and had been president of the State Medical Society, of the State Board of Medical Examiners and of the Board of U. S. Pension Examiners. He was a member of the Charlotte draft board in World War I and a Fellow of the Tri-State and the American Medical Associations. A number of times he had been a delegate to the the latter association's meetings.

Captain Charles Walton Purcell, 36, a native of Louisa County, Virginia, Army Air Forces Medical Corps, was instantly killed in an automobile-bus collision near Napa, Calif., Nov. 11th. Captain Purcell had been stationed at the Army Air Base in Fairfield, Calif., for the past year and was en route from his home to the base hospital when the accident occurred.

Dr. Purcell was graduated in 1933 from the University of Virginia Medical School, interned at Orange Memorial Hospital in New Jersey and Post-Graduate Hospital in New York. He returned to the University of Virginia in 1936 and took special training in pediatrics at the Univer-

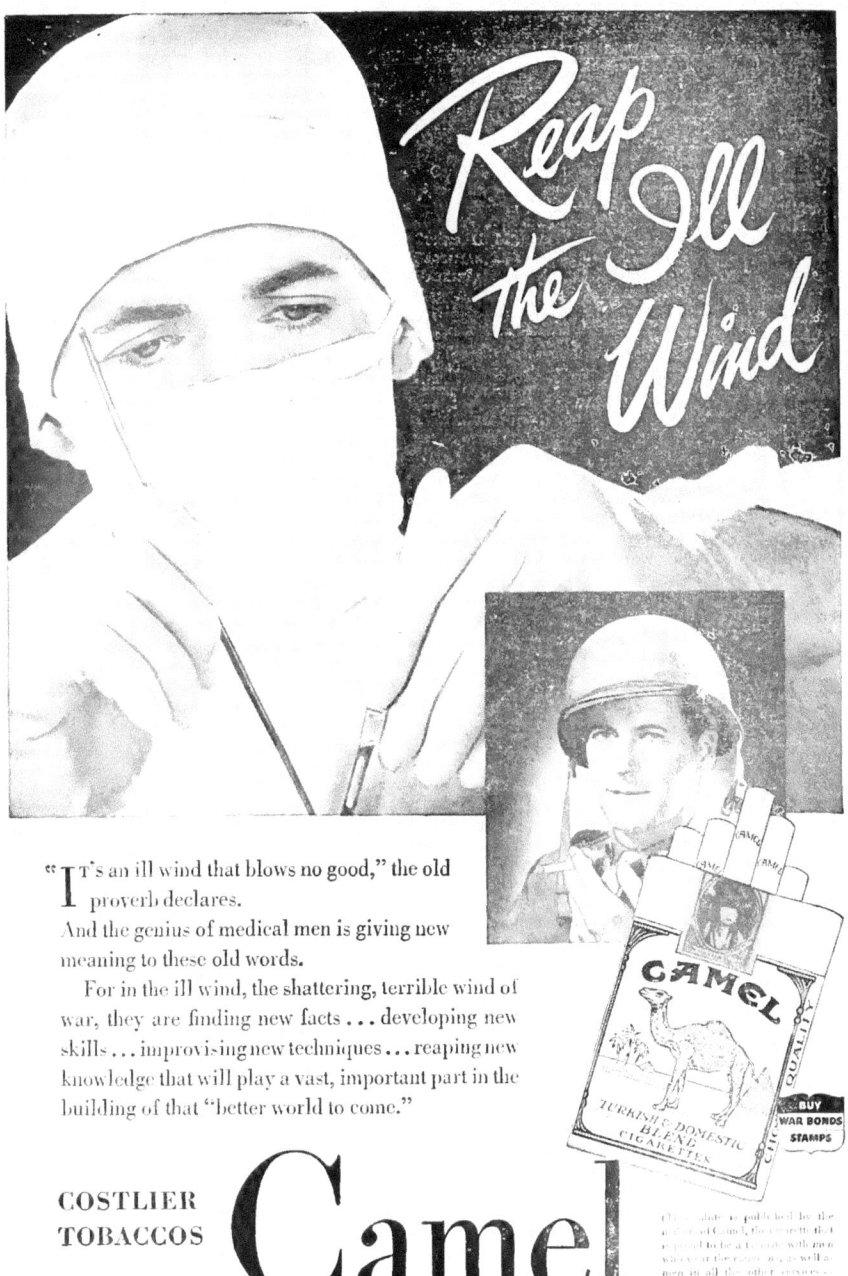

sity Hospital. In 1937 he went to Danville to live and built up a large practice there as a pediatrician. He served as a flight surgeon in the Pacific area for a year, returning to the States in December, 1943.

Dr. John Reeves Gamble, 59, owner and founder of the Reeves Gamble Hospital of Lincolnton, N. C., died Dec. 1st, after an illness of several months. He had been active until his last illness.

Dr. Gamble was educated at the University of Tennessee Medical School and began practice in Lincoln County in 1911. He had lived in Lincolnton since 1915. He founded his hospital in 1930.

Dr. William James Knight, 72, one of Newport News' leading physicians, died Nov. 15th at his home.

Dr. Knight, a pioneer resident of Newport News, was graduated by the Medical College of Virginia in 1897, and had spent 47 years in the practice of medicine and surgery. He established a hospital at his residence in 1905 and was one of five doctors in this section who founded the old St. Francis Hospital and the last surviving member of its staff. He had been a member of Riverside Hospital staff since it was established.

PREVENTION OF BLINDNESS—$500 PRIZE

A prize of $500 for the most valuable original paper on the diagnosis of early glaucoma or the medical treatment of non-congestive glaucoma is being offered by the National Society for the Prevention of Blindness, 1790 Broadway, New York 19, N. Y. This award will take the place of two separate prizes of $250 each announced some time ago.

Papers may be presented by any practicing ophthalmologist of the Western Hemisphere and may be written in English, French, German, Italian, Spanish or Portuguese. Those written in either of the last four languages should be accompanied by a summary in English.

The award will be made by the Society with the guidance of a committee composed of Doctors John N. Evans, Frank C. Keil, Daniel B. Kirby, Arnold Knapp, John M. McLean, R. Townley Paton, Algernon B. Reese, Bernard Samuels, Kaufman Schlivek, Mark J. Schoenberg, Manuel Uribe Troncoso, David H. Webster.

THE USE OF HONEY IN THE TREATMENT OF CHILBLAINS, NON-SPECIFIC ULCERS, AND SMALL WOUNDS
(K. L. Yang, in Chinese Med. Jl., Jan.-Mar.)

In a series of 50 cases, there were 38 complete cures, 10 showing marked improvement or partial cures, and 2 no improvement. Several patients stopped attending after healing had started. Of the 2 unimproved cases, one was a chronic ulcer (4 x 2.5 x 0.3 cm) on the anterior and middle parts of the right leg for half a year; the color was light gray, the surrounding tissue fibrotic and indurated, varicose veins on the back of the leg. The other was a chilblain ulcer of the right index finger. Response to the honey treatment was similar to that in the first case. As the patient did not appear again after three weeks of treatment, there was no way of observing the ultimate result.

Report is made of the use of 80 per cent honey in lard, in the treatment of 50 cases of chilblain, chilblain ulcers, ordinary ulcers and small wounds; its success in hastening the subsidence of passive hyperemia and edematous swelling, and in stimulating epithelization and granulation tissue formation.

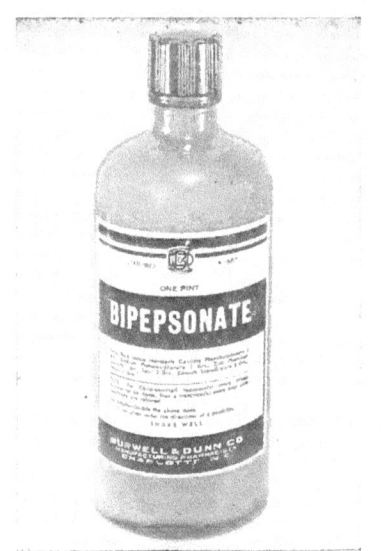

Sample sent to any physician in the U. S. on request

BOOKS

MODERN CLINICAL SYPHILOLOGY, by JOHN H. STOKES, M.D., Professor of Dermatology and Syphilology, School of Medicine and Graduate School of Medicine, University of Pennsylvania; HERMAN BEERMAN, M.D., Sc.D. (Med.), Assistant Professor of Dermatology and Syphilology, School of Medicine and Graduate School of Medicine, University of Pennsylvania; and NORMAN R. INGRAHAM, JR., M.D., Assistant Professor of Dermatology and Syphilology, School of Medicine, University of Pennsylvaria. Third Edition, Reset. 1332 pages with 911 illustrations. *W. B. Saunders Company*, Philadelphia and London. 1944. $10.00.

The fundamental bacteriology, pathology and immunology of syphilis are carefully reviewed; then the clinical approach to syphilis is made, the fundamental diagnostic tests described and the fundamental principles of treatment laid down. There are chapters on the heavy metals and iodides; the arsenicals; technical considerations in diagnosis and treatment; reactions, complications and contraindications of treatment; latent syphilis and special problems; diagnosis of early syphilis; relapse, reinfection and progression; treatment in the various stages; separate chapters for syphilis of the various systems. The final chapter is entitled "The Current Developments—Penicillin."

This is a truly encyclopedic coverage of clinical syphilis. The senior author has devoted his great talents largely to the study of syphilis over a quarter of a century. No one can speak more authoritatively or more helpfully on this subject of the first importance.

DERMATOLOGIC THERAPY IN GENERAL PRACTICE, by MARION B. SULZBERGER, M.D., Commander, M.C., U.S.N.R., Assistant Clinical Professor of Dermatology and Syphilology, Skin and Cancer Unit of the New York Post-Graduate Medical School; and JACK WOLF, M.D., Attending Dermatologist and Syphilologist, Skin and Cancer Unit of the New York Post-Graduate Medical School and Hospital of Columbia University. *The Year Book Publishers, Inc.*, 304 S. Dearborn St., Chicago. 1943. $5.00.

It is generally said that the general practitioner knows less about dermatology than about any other division of medicine. This is largely because of the needless confusion of the presentation of the subject in the average text. The text under review is remarkably clear and covers the subject in a way to meet the need of the nonspecialist and to enable him to successfully diagnose and treat the larger number of dermatologic cases in his practice.

CLINICAL DIAGNOSIS BY LABORATORY EXAMINATIONS, by JOHN A. KOLMER, M.S., M.D., Dr. P.H., Sc.D., LL.D., F.A.C.P., Professor of Medicine in the School of Medicine and the School of Dentistry of Temple University. First Edition, Revised. *D. Appleton-Century Company, Inc.*, 35 West 32nd Street, New York City. 1944. $10.00.

The author came into clinical medicine through the door of pathology, which gives him a very special qualification for writing on this subject. The title is significant. He does not think of "laboratory diagnosis" but of "clinical diagnosis by laboratory examinations."

His long experience as a pathologist and bacteriologist, working in close association with clinical teachers, gives him exceptional capacity as a practitioner and teacher of medicine. As an illustration of the clarity of Dr. Kolmer's thought, and the precision of his diction, the reviewer, in his capacity as editor of a medical journal, once had an address made by the author without the use of notes put into type from the stenographer's notes without submitting them to the speaker for revision.

The very best book in this field.

PROTEINS AND AMINO ACIDS: Physiology, Pathology, Therapeutics, The Arlington Chemical Company, Yonkers 1, New York. 1944. *Complimentary* to any physician applying to publishers.

Proteins: Amino Acids:: Atoms: Electrons— and just as we need to go further than the atom in our study of physics, so we need to go beyond protein in our study of the most important element in nutrition. This booklet supplies this essential information with the needs of the physician in view.

PRIMER OF SCLEROTHERAPY: Injection Treatment, by H. I. BIEGELEISEN, M.D. *Froben Press*, 4 St. Luke's Place, New York 14, N. Y. 1944. $2.00.

The author is credited with being the deviser of the term sclerotherapy. This primer is an introduction to the author's textbook of the subject, soon to be published.

CHUCKLES

Visitor to Church Custodian: "How do you get along with the Women's Society of Christian Service?"
Custodian: "I just get in neutral and let' em push me around."

Clothing Store Proprietor:: "How's that new salesman?"
Manager: "Best in the world. He's just sold a double-breasted suit to the owner of a Phi Beta Kappa key!"

Will: "I told her that each hour I spent with her was like a pearl to me."
Bill: "And did that impress her?"
Will: "No. She told me to quit stringing her."

A little girl went to the grocery store on an errand for her mother, and asked for a roll of bathroom tissue, the purchase to be charged. Remembering the little girl's face but forgetting the name, the grocer asked, "Now who is this for?"
"Oh, we're all going to use it," answered the little girl.

Old Lady (at the zoo): "Is that a man-eating lion?"
Fed-up Keeper: "Yes, lady, but we're short of men this week, so all he gets is beef."

Three managers of chicken farms in Germany were being questioned by a gastapo man. "What do you feed your chickens?" the first was asked.
"Corn."
"You're under arrest! We use corn to feed the people."
The second manager overheard the conversation, and tried to play safe.
"What do you feed your chickens?" came the question.
"Corn husks."
"You're under arrest! We use the husks to make cloth. And you?" he asked, turning to the third man.
"I give my chickens the money and tell them to go and buy their own food."

Member of a Gasoline Rationing Board came across an application from a local doctor for a large amount of gasoline. Having his doubts, the ingenious board member telephoned the doctor:
"Can you come out right away?" he asked. "My daughter is very sick."
"Sorry," said the physician, "I don't make house calls at all."
So—he didn't get the gas!

"She has a very magnetic personality," said one.
"She ought to have," said the other, "everything she has on is charged."

"Mr. Jones, dad wants to borrow your corkscrew."
"All right, sonny. You run along home—I'll bring it over."

How the Southern Voice Was Lost

Mrs. A. C. McIntosh made her screen debut, at the age of seventy-something, on Thursday of last week in the Forest Theatre, in the movie of Tom Wolfe's novel, "Look Homeward, Angel." She sang—along with four hundred other people—the University song, "Hark the Sound." Two or three days earlier, in the lobby of the Carolina Inn, a visitor with whom she had become acquainted said to her: "You don't talk like a Southerner—you don't have the familiar accent." She replied: "Young man, if I talk like a Yankee it is because I have two sets of false teeth, one above and one below."

—*Chapel Hill Weekly.*

When the newlyweds boarded the train, the embarrassed groom tipped the porter liberally, to not disclose that they were just married. Next morning, on the way to breakfast in the diner, they were greeted with many grins, stares and craning necks. The groom upbraided the porter.
"Nassuh, Boss," George replied, "Ah didn't tell 'em. When dey asked me if you was just married, Ah says, 'No suh, dey is just chums.'"

One hears a great deal about the absent-minded professors, but none more absent-minded than the dentist who said soothingly as he applied the pliers to the tack in his tire:
"Now, this is going to hurt just a little."

The Game of "What's My Name?"
(The *New England Townsman*, April, 1944)

Father Begin, who besides being a genealogist, and a first rate French scholar, is a bit of a wag, tells this one for true. Four sons of one father use for surnames Roi, Roy, King, and Ware. Now the Roi-Roy-King combination is well known to the file searchers of the Division, but in the matter of "Ware" something new has been added. Father Begin explains that the boy, being able neither to write nor to spell Roi, his oral, rolling-r rendering of it to his Yankee boss would make like M. G. M.'s movie lion's "Rrrowar," interpreted to Ware by the boss. So Ware became the boy's name for all time.

The young bear woke up happily from hibernation. "I'm a ready Teddy," he cried joyously, looking around for entertainment.
Several days later, he returned, showing big bags under his eyes. "I'm a ruined Bruin," he declared.

PRIMER
OF
SCLEROTHERAPY

by
H. I. Biegeleisen, M.D.

The first simplified explanation of Injection Therapy in any language. A clear presentation, with illustration and tables, of the essentials of the subject. Based on the author's original work which for the past twelve years has been published in the leading medical and surgical Journals.

Cloth, $2.00 postpaid.

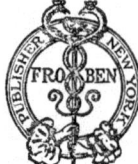

**FROBEN PRESS
PUBLISHERS**

4 St. Luke's Place

New York 14, N. Y.

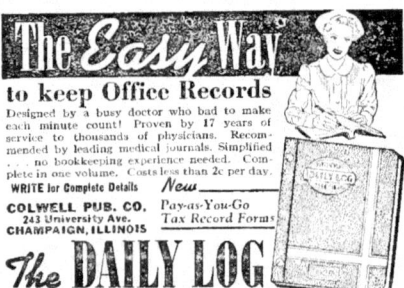

PRODUCTS OF MERIT

FERROSEL "B" ENKOTES

Indicated in the treatment of iron deficiencies.

For use where Vitamin B Complex factors are desirable in addition to iron in the prevention and treatment of Microcytic or secondary anemia, and in the Macrocytic anemias where a deficiency of iron also exists. Recommended for use in anemia following gastrointestinal surgery, and routinely during last months of pregnancy.

COMPOSITION

Thiamin Chloride 1 mg., Riboflavin 0.5 mg., Nicotinamide 1 mg., Ferrous Sulphate gr. 5—in a special enteric coating.

DOSAGE

One tablet three times daily.
Bottles of 100 and 1000 tablets.

Available

At your own Pharmacy or write to Vitamix Corporation

CHLOROID ENKOTES

Indicated in the treatment of Obesity

The rationale of combining Ammonium Chloride with Thyroid in the treatment of obesity:

Thyroid increases the metabolic rate. The lower the rate the better the action.

Urea is known as a powerful diuretic and the ammonium salts which are constituted in the body into Urea acts as a diuretic in a similar manner.

COMPOSITION

Ammonium Chloride 5 gr. and Powdered Thyroid gr. 1/3 in a special enteric coating.

CHLOROID ENKOTES NO. 2

Indicated in the treatment of Obesity

Each tablet contains Amphetamine 5 mg., Pd. Thyroid gr. 1/3, Amm. Chloride gr. 5. Especially indicated where Amphetamine Sulphate is tolerated.

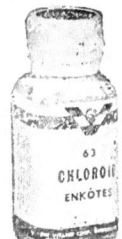

DOSAGE

One tablet three times daily.
Bottles of 63 and 1000.

Available

At your own Pharmacy or write to Vitamix Corporation

GENEROUS SAMPLES ON REQUEST FROM

VITAMIX CORP. 382 Broadway, Brooklyn 11, N. Y.

GENERAL PRACTICE

D. HERBERT SMITH, M.D., *Editor*, Pauline, S. C.

THE CLINICAL VALUE OF LIVER FUNCTION TESTS

Just what may be learned of value to the patient by making "liver function" tests? A teacher of pharmacology[1] gives his opinions:

These tests are not intended to furnish diagnoses.

Such powerful and valuable drugs as diethylstilbestrol and sulfonamides are apparently not causing any significant reduction of liver function.

In many instances clinical recovery advances much faster than restoration of function as determined by such tests as the prothrombin response to vitamin K, and the synthesis of hippuric acid. On the other hand, a slow-subsiding jaundice may erroneously suggest a delayed return of function, wherea sdeterminations of hippuric acid synthesis may clearly indicate satisfactory progress.

The teratment of liver disease has been and is still unsatisfactory and disappointing.

The hippuric acid test is based on the well known chemical reaction which occurs when benzoic acid, taken into the body is conjugated with the simple amino acid, glycine, with the formation of hippuric acid and water.

The synthesis requires two mechanisms: 1) a conjugating force uniting the two substances and 2) a prompt and continuous synthesis of glycine. In the human, both appear to be localized in the liver and any injury of the organ brings about a reduction in the ability to form hippuric acid.

To perform the test ,the sodium benzoate may be given either orally or intravenously; six Gm. dissolved in 30 c.c. of water one hour after a light breakfast. The urine is collected every hour for four hours and analyzed for hippuric acid by the author's method.[2] A normal adult excretes 3 to 3.5 Gm. of zenboic acid as hippuric acid in that period.

The oral test is inexpensive, easy to carry out in the home, office or hospital, and is entirely harmless. Vomiting is infrequent even in patients who complain of nausea. The rate of absorption of sodium benzoate may be delayed due to gastric stasis or other causes, but this is rare.

The intravenous test consists in injecting 1.77 Gm. of sodium benzoate dissolved in 20 c.c. of water. The urine is collected one hour after the injection and the hippuric acid is determined. A normal adult will excrete 1 to 1.4 Gm. of hippuric acid. If given too fast, a transient but severe pain along the course of the vein may result. The influence of body weight is too small to necesitate the introduction of a correcting factor.

The hippuric acid test is not reliable in severe dehydration and other states that interfere with proper renal function. Hippuric acid output is reduced during the end of pregnancy and the beginning of menstruation.

The meaning of high values of hippuric acid excretion is not known. They have been found in cholecystitis and in a mild arsphenamine hypertrophic hepatitis.

One hour before the test (oral or intravenous) the patient should eat a light breakfast, should drink a moderate amount of water to insure urine 50 c.c. or more per hour. If possible the administration of all drugs should be stopped a day or two prior to the test. Repeated or serial tests usually furnish much more valuable and trustworthy information.

Two factors are necessary for maintaining the normal level of prothrombin in the blood: 1) vitamin K and 2) adequate liver function. If the prothrombin is low, and is not significantly increased when excess vitamin K is administered, one can concluded that liver function is impaired.

Inject daily for three days 2 mg. of menadione in oil intramuscularly. The prothrombin level is determined before the menadione is given and thereafter daily for three or four days. If not increased to a level of 75 per cent of normal or more, hepatic damage is indicated.

In many cases of jaundice, particularly catarrhal, the prothrombin is little altered, whereas the marked reduction in the hippuric acid synthesis which is usually found indicates definite liver injury. Moreover hypoprothrombinemia resistant to vitamin & can occur in the absence of demonstrable liver disease. In idiopathic hypoprothrombinemia no signs of hepatic disease can be found.

The chief value of the prothrombin test is in studying the jaundiced patient. If the prothrombin rises promptly after vitamin K is administered, one can conclude that the liver is functionally normal and the prothrombinopenia is primarily the result of lack of vitamin K. If, on the other hand, vitamin K fails to elevate the prothrombin, it appears reasonably certain that the cause of the hypoprothrombinemia is primary hepatitis, or liver injury secondary to the biliary obstruction.

DENTAL REQUIREMENTS MADE SENSIBLE

According to Lieutenant Colonel John C. Brauer, Assistant to the Director of Dental Division, any man who has two jaws can now qualify dentally for the Army. In a paper which was read to the Military Surgeons at their 52nd annual meeting, Colonel Brauer said that over a million men who lacked the teeth to chew their food had been rehabilitated by the Army Dental Corps and made eligible for Army service. In addition, thousands of other men have been made eligible or kept dentally fit for Army service through the insertion of 55,000,000 fillings.

---

1. A. J. Quick, Milwaukee, in *Wisc. Med. Jl.*, April.

NEUROLOGY and PSYCHIATRY

(*Now in the Country's Service*)
*J. FRED MERRITT, M.D.
NERVOUS and MILD MENTAL DISEASES
ALCOHOL and DRUG ADDICTIONS
Glenwood Park Sanitarium   Greensboro

TOM A. WILLIAMS, M.D.
(*Neurologist of Washington, D. C.*)
Consultation by appointment at
Phone 3994-W
77 Kenilworth Ave.   Asheville, N. C.

EYE, EAR, NOSE AND THROAT

H. C. NEBLETT, M.D.
OCULIST
Phone 3-5852
Professional Bldg.   Charlotte

AMZI J. ELLINGTON, M.D.
DISEASES of the EYE, EAR, NOSE and THROAT
Phones: Office 992—Residence 761
Burlington   North Carolina

UROLOGY, DERMATOLOGY and PROCTOLOGY

THE CROWELL CLINIC of UROLOGY and UROLOGICAL SURGERY
Hours—Nine to Five   Telephones—3-7101—3-7102
STAFF
ANDREW J. CROWELL, M.D.
(1911-1938)
*ANGUS M. McDONALD, M.D.   CLAUDE B. SQUIRES, M.D.
Suite 700-711 Professional Building   Charlotte

RAYMOND THOMPSON, M.D., F.A.C.S.   WALTER E. DANIEL, A.B., M.D.
THE THOMPSON-DANIEL CLINIC
of
UROLOGY & UROLOGICAL SURGERY
Fifth Floor Professional Bldg.   Charlotte

C. C. MASSEY, M.D.
PRACTICE LIMITED TO DISEASES OF THE RECTUM
Professional Bldg.   Charlotte

WYETT F. SIMPSON, M.D.
GENITO-URINARY DISEASES
Phone 1234
Hot Springs National Park   Arkansas

ORTHOPEDICS

HERBERT F. MUNT, M.D.
ACCIDENT SURGERY & ORTHOPEDICS FRACTURES
Nissen Building   Winston-Salem

GENERAL

Nalle Clinic Building   412 North Church Street, Charlotte
THE NALLE CLINIC
Telephone—C-BVDY (if no answer, call 3-2621)

General Surgery	*General Medicine*
BRODIE C. NALLE, M.D.	LUCIUS G. GAGE, M.D.
GYNECOLOGY & OBSTETRICS	DIAGNOSIS
EDWARD R. HIPP, M.D.	
TRAUMATIC SURGERY	LUTHER W. KELLY, M.D.
*PRESTON NOWLIN, M.D.	CARDIO-RESPIRATORY DISEASES
UROLOGY	
	J. R. ADAMS, M.D.
Consulting Staff	DISEASES OF INFANTS & CHILDREN
R. H. LAFFERTY, M.D.	
O. D. BAXTER, M.D.	W. B. MAYER, M.D.
RADIOLOGY	DERMATOLOGY & SYPHILOLOGY
W. M. SUMMERVILLE, M.D.	
PATHOLOGY	(*In Country's Service)

C—H—M MEDICAL OFFICES	WADE CLINIC
DIAGNOSIS—SURGERY	Wade Building
X-RAY—RADIUM	Hot Springs National Park, Arkansas
DR. G. CARLYLE COOKE—*Abdominal Surgery & Gynecology*	H. KING WADE, M.D. — *Urology*
DR. GEO. W. HOLMES—*Orthopedics*	ERNEST M. McKENZIE, M.D. — *Medicine*
DR. C. H. McCANTS—*General Surgery*	*FRANK M. ADAMS, M.D. — *Medicine*
222-226 Nissen Bldg. Winston-Salem	*JACK ELLIS, M.D. — *Medicine*
	BESSEY H. SHEBESTA, M.D. — *Medicine*
	*WM. C. HAYS, M.D. — *Medicine*
	N. B. BURCH, M.D.
	Eye, Ear, Nose and Throat
	A. W. SCHEER — *X-ray Technician*
	ETTA WADE — *Clinical Laboratory*
	MERNA SPRING — *Clinical Pathology*
	(*In Military Service)

INTERNAL MEDICINE

ARCHIE A. BARRON, M.D., F.A.C.P.	JOHN DONNELLY, M.D.
INTERNAL MEDICINE—NEUROLOGY	*DISEASES OF THE LUNGS*
Professional Bldg. Charlotte	Medical Building Charlotte

CLYDE M. GILMORE, A.B., M.D.	JAMES M. NORTHINGTON, M.D.
CARDIOLOGY—INTERNAL MEDICINE	*INTERNAL MEDICINE—GERIATRICS*
Dixie Building Greensboro	Medical Building Charlotte

SURGERY

(Now in the Country's Service)
R. S. ANDERSON, M. D.

GENERAL SURGERY

144 Coast Line Street   Rocky Mount

R. B. DAVIS, M. D., M. M. S., F. A. C. P.
GENERAL SURGERY
AND
RADIUM THERAPY
Hours by Appointment
Piedmont-Memorial Hosp.   Greensboro

(Now in the Country's Service)
WILLIAM FRANCIS MARTIN, M.D.
GENERAL SURGERY

Professional Bldg.   Charlotte

OBSTETRICS & GYNECOLOGY

IVAN M. PROCTER, M. D.

OBSTETRICS & GYNECOLOGY

133 Fayetteville Street   Raleigh

SPECIAL NOTICES

TO THE BUSY DOCTOR WHO WANTS TO PASS HIS EXPERIENCE ON TO OTHERS

You have probably been postponing writing that original contribution. You can do it, and save your time and effort by employing an expert literary assistant to prepare the address, article or book under your direction or relieve you of the details of looking up references, translating, indexing, typing, and the complete preparation of your manuscript.

Address: *WRITING AIDE,* care *Southern Medicine & Surgery.*

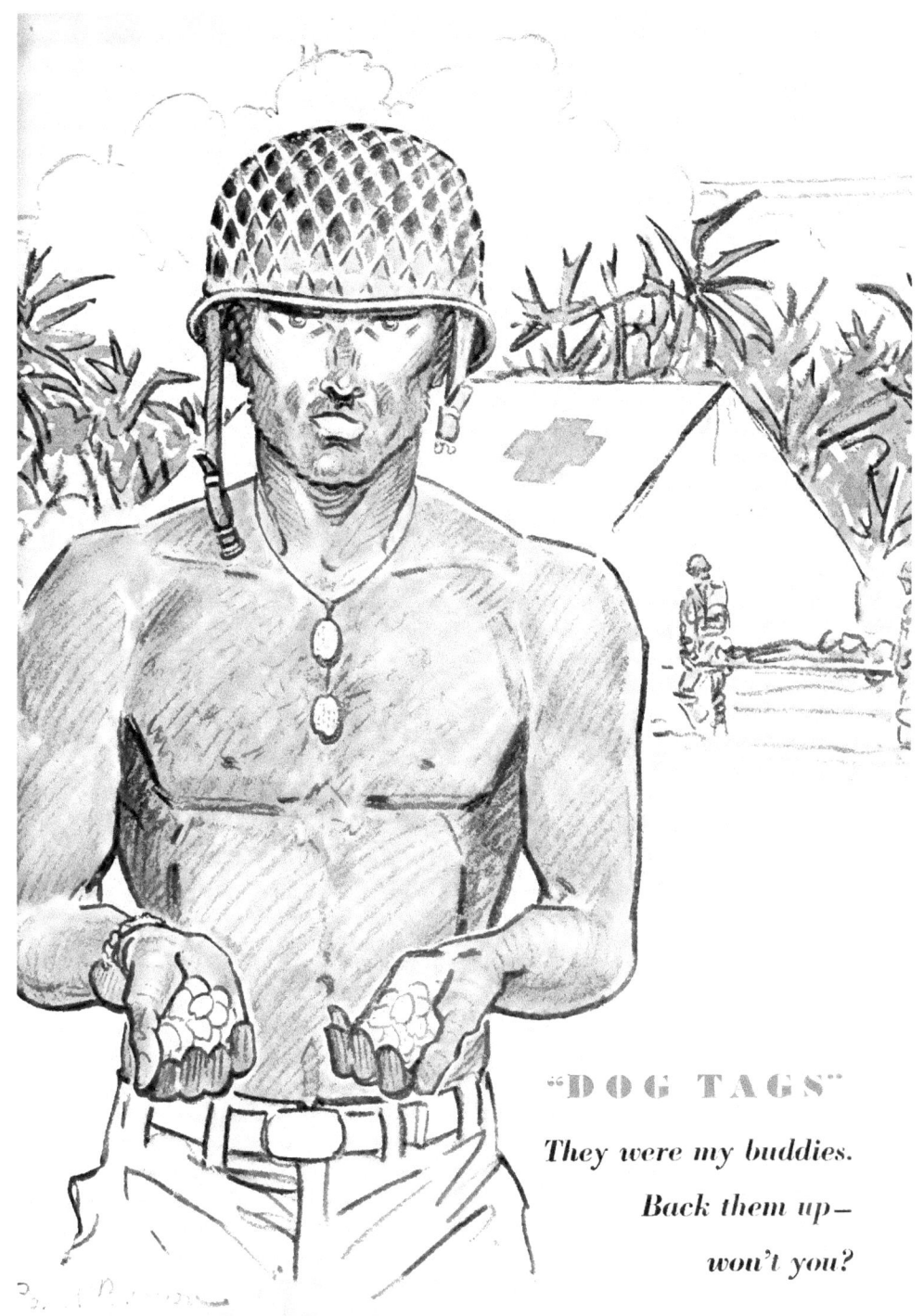

WE TAKE PRIDE

IN SHARING IN THE MAINTENANCE OF THE HIGH STANDARDS OF MEDICAL SCIENCE. TO THIS END WE PLEDGE CONTINUED PARTICIPATION IN ORIGINAL LABORATORY AND CLINICAL RESEARCH WITH THE OBJECT OF DEVELOPING AND MAKING AVAILABLE NEW AND VALUABLE PHARMACEUTICALS FOR DIAGNOSIS AND RELIEF OF HUMAN SUFFERING.

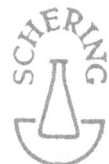

SCHERING CORPORATION
Bloomfield, New Jersey

INDEX

ADDRESSES, ORIGINAL ARTICLES AND CASE REPORTS

Abscess, Septal, Case Report, *G. R. Laub* 374
Address of the President of the Tri-State Medical Association of the Carolinas and Virginia, *F. S. Johns* 75
Adiposo-Genital Dystrophy, The Relationship of Tonsillectomy and, *M. A. Goldzieher* 39
Agricultural Practices on Health and Disease, The Effect of, *J. A. Shield* 420
Aid That May Be Had From the Electrocardiogram, The, *P. D. Camp* 473
Allergic Individual, Some Military Considerations of the, *L. C. Todd* 287
Asthma, The Important Role of Bronchoscopy in the Occasional Case of, *V. K. Hart* 167
Bladder Support, Utilization of Round Ligaments to Insure Better, *G. H. Bunch* 469
Breast, The Interpretation and Treatment of the Discharging, *J. D. Gilland* 429
Bronchoscopy, The Important Role of, in the Occasional Case of Asthma, *V. K. Hart* 167
Burns, The Local Treatment of Surface, *W. H. Prioleau* 201
Cardiovascular Disease, Differential Diagnostic Implications From the Complaints of Patients with, *T. S. Ussery* 3
China, Medicine in, *R. T. Shields* 113
Clinical Laboratory; The, Its Personnel and Some of Their Problems, *J. M. Feder* 247
Differential Diagnostic Implications From the Complaints of Patients With Cardiovascular Disease, *T. S. Ussery* 3
Discharging Breast, The Interpretation and Treatment of the, *J. D. Gilland* 429
Doctors' Responsibility for Expansion of Medical and Hospital Facilities, *K. B. Pace* 329
Electrocardiogram, The Aid That May Be Had From the, *P. D. Camp* 473
Encephalitis Following Neoarsphenamine, *J. Z. Preston* 471
Estrone and Stilbestrol, Clinical Effects of Suspension of, *H. S. Kupperman & R. B. Greenblatt* 1
Fractures in the Insane, Treatment of Hip, *J. R. Saunders & Y. S. Palmer* 203
Fractures of the Neck of the Femur, The Treatment of Intertrochanteric, *J. W. Davis* 480
Functional Hypoglycemia, *G. L. Donnelly & Y. S. Palmer* 363
Gastrointestinal Function: Neurophysiological Aspects of, *F. H. Hesser* 120
General Hospital, The Role of a Neuropsychiatric Service in a, *J. M. Fearing* 164
Grind With Water That is Past," "The Mill Cannot, *C. V. Reynolds* 281
Handicapped, Rehabilitating Those Who Are Psychiatrically, *L. E. Woodward* 365
Health Alone is Victory, *J. K. Hall* 321
Heart, Penetrating Wounds of the, *D. L. Maguire, Jr.* 411
Help, *R. M. Yergason* 37
Hemorrhagic Encephalitis Following Neoarsphenamine in Late Pregnancy, *J. Z. Preston* 471
Hip Fractures of the Insane, Treatment of, *J. R. Saunders & Y. S. Palmer* 203
Hold the Line, *E. J. Williams* 197
Hypoglycemia, Functional, *G. L. Donnelly & Y. S. Palmer* 363
Hysteria, A Concept of, *S. P. Hunt* 370
Insane, Treatment of Hip Fractures of the, *J. R. Saunders & Y. S. Palmer* 203
Insulin Resistance: Report of Two Cases, *W. R. Jordan* 361
Intertrochanteric Fractures, The Treatment of, *J. W. Davis* 480
Involutional Melancholia, Prefrontal Lobotomy With Reference to, *J. G. Lyerly* 124
Johnston, George Ben, Pioneer of Modern Surgery in the South, *F. S. Johns* 75
Laboratory:, The Clinical, Its Personnel and Some of Their Problems, *J. M. Feder* 247
Line, Hold The, *E. J. Williams* 197
Lobotomy, Social Adjustment in Obsessive Tension States Following Prefrontal, *J. W. Watts & Walter Freeman* 233
Lobotomy With Reference to Involutional Melancholia, Prefrontal, *J. G. Lyerly* 124
Local Treatment of Surface Burns, The, *W. H. Prioleau* 201
Medicine in China, *R. T. Shields* 113
Medicine, The Politico-Economic Situation in Reference to, *H. F. Starr* 85
Melancholia, Prefrontal Lobotomy With Reference to Involutional, *J. G. Lyerly* 124
Meningococcemia, *R. S. Bigham, Jr.* 425
Military Considerations of the Allergic Individual, Some, *L. C. Todd* 287
Mill Cannot Grind With the Water That is Past," "The, *C. V. Reynolds* 281
Neoarsphenamine in Late Pregnancy, Hemorrhagic Encephalitis Following, *J. Z. Preston* ... 471
Neurophysiological Aspects of Gastrointestinal Function:, *F. H. Hesser* 120
Neuropsychiatric Service in a General Hospital, The Role of a, *J. M. Fearing* 164
Neuropsychiatry, The Pituitary in Relation to, *B. R. Tucker* 117
Obsessive Tension States Following Prefrontal Lobotomy, *J. W. Watts & Walter Freeman* ... 233
Obstetrics, Pudendal Block in, *M. P. Rucker* 407
Pellagra Sine Pellagra, *E. L. Copley* 416
Penetrating Wounds of the Heart, *D. L. Maguire, Jr.* 411
Penicillin, *E. McG. Hedgpeth* 238

Physician as Teacher, The. *Karl Schaffle* 243
Pituitary in Relation to Neuropsychiatry, The. *B. R. Tucker* 117
Pneumonia, Diagnosis and Treatment of Primary Atypical. *V. D. Offutt* 5
Political-Economic Situation in Reference to Medicine. *H. F. Starr* 83
Prefrontal Lobotomy, Social Adjustment in Obsessive Tension States Following. *J. W. Watts & Walter Freeman* 233
Prefrontal Lobotomy With Reference to Involutional Melancholia. *J. G. Lyerly* 124
Pregnancy, Hemorrhagic Encephalitis Following Neoarsphenamine in Late. *J. Z. Preston* 471
President of the Tri-State Medical Association of the Carolinas and Virginia, Address of the. *F. S. Johns* 75
Proctologic Practices. *W. J. Morris, Jr.* 159
Psychically Handicapped, Rehabilitating Those Who Are. *L. E. Woodward* 365
Pudendal Block in Obstetrics. *M. P. Rucker* 407
Rapid Treatment of Syphilis. *J. L. Callaway & R. O. Noojin* 463
Rectum, Some Common Diseases of the. *R. B. Davis* 476
Rehabilitating Those Who Are Physically Handicapped. *L. E. Woodward* 365
Rorschach Work, A Practical Introduction to. *V. Cranford & R. V. Seliger* 327
Septal Abscess: Case Report, *G. R. Laub* 374
Social Adjustment in Obsessive Tension States Following Prefrontal Lobotomy. *J. W. Watts & Walter Freeman* 233
Splenic Rupture With Case Report. *Wm. A. Johns* 478
Stilbestrol, Clinical Effects of Suspension of Estrone and. *H. S. Kupperman & R. B. Greenblatt* 1
S-T Segment and T Wave Change in Transitory Insufficiency: Case Report. *E. L. Copley* 170
Surface Burns, The Local Treatment of. *W. H. Prioleau* 201
Syphilis, Rapid Treatment of. *J. L. Callaway & R. O. Noojin* 463
Tonsilectomy and Adiposo-Genital Dystrophy, The Relationship of. *M. A. Goldzieher* 39
Transitory Insufficiency, S-T Segment and T Wave Change in, Case Report. *E. L. Copley* 170
Tri-State Medical Association of the Carolinas and Virginia, Address of the President of the. *F. S. Johns* 75
Victory, Health Alone Is. *J. K. Hall* 321
Waters That Is Past," "The Mill Cannot Grind With the. *C. V. Reynolds* 281

EDITORIALS
(Unsigned Editorials are by the Editor)

Alumni, Charles Willis Calls Medical College of Virginia 145
Angioneurotic Edema and Urticaria 26
Armed Services No Reflection on Doctors of Medicine, The Record of Rejections for the 24
Aspirin 186
Beveridge Plan, British Doctors on the 58
Blood Test for Syphilis, The Fallibility of the 493
Country, How to Get Doctors to Practice in the 446
Barden Dies, Burton 492
Department Editors, Two New 24
Diagnosis, More About Relative Importance and Expense in 306
Diagnosis and Treatment of Medicine's Ills, The 392
Editing and Ignoring the G. P. and Doctors Will Locate in the Villages, Stop 268
Doctor John McCampbell 448
Doctor James H. McIntosh 397
Doctor Frank Hilton McLeod 448
Doctors to Practice in the Country, How to Get 446
Dressed Sons, Medical Men Should Be 59
Editors, Two New Department 24
Education of the Medical Student, The 59
Expense in Diagnosis, More About Relative Importance and 306
Farmers' Program to Lead to Health Cost and Need for More Hospitals and More Medical Inspectors in North Carolina 184
Fire Insurance Costs, How You May Save on 25
General Practitioner to be Paid Same as Specialists: A New Thing Under the Sun 25
Gone, Medicine Is Not 221
Head of the Tri-State Medical Association of 144
Hippocratic Oath Made 394
How to Get Doctors to Practice in the Country 446
Insurance Costs, How You May Save on Fire 25
Liaison Medical Committee, Reports to A. M. A. on the 269
Lead Health Cost and Need for More Hospitals and More Medical Inspectors in North Carolina, Farmers' Program to 184
Locate in the Villages, Stop 59
Medical 448
McIntosh, Doctor James H. 397

McLeod, Doctor Frank Hilton 448
Medical College of Virginia Alumni, Charles Willis Calls 145
Medical Needs in North Carolina, About 492
Medicine Is Not Guilty 221
Medicine, The Tri-State Medical Association's Special Place in 101
Medicine's Ills, The Diagnosis and Treatment of 392
Mental Health 102
More Hospitals and More Medical Instruction in North Carolina, Facts vs Fiction as to Lack of Health Care and Need for 184
Music, Health Through 394
New Thing Under the Sun:, A, General Practitioner to be Paid Same as Specialist.......... 25
Penicillin 307
Plan, British Doctors on the Beveridge 58
Poliomyelitis, A Possible Preventive Measure As to 304
Rejections for the Armed Services no Reflection on Doctors of Medicine, The Record of 24
Respiration, The Restoration of Breathing in Emergencies and the Maintenance of 305
Rest Possible Only to the Weary 346
Serologic Reactions in Syphilis Not Infallible 348
Specialization on the Education of the Medical Student, The Effect of 59
Stop Discrediting and Ignoring the G. P. and Doctors Will Locate in the Villages 268
Syphilis, The Fallibility of the Blood Test for 493
Tri-State Medical Association's Special Place in Medicine 101
Tri-State Meeting, The Coming 492
Tri-State Program, The 27
Urticaria and Angioneurotic Edema 26
Weary, Rest Possible Only to the 346
Wilson Resigns, Dr. Robert, *The Recorder* of Columbia (S. C.) Medical Society 23

MEDICAL AND SURGICAL OBSERVATIONS

Anesthesia and the Reduction of Mortality in Surgery, Spinal 22
Armed Forces, Keep Record of Examination and Treatment of Patients Discharged From 23
Cardiovascular Symptoms as Seen in the Military Hospital, Psychosomatic Disorders Manifested Mainly by 263
Fractures of the Neck of the Femur, Treatment of 22
Kidney, Ptosis or Prolapse of the 55
Letter, A 23
Penicillin 141
Penicillin in the Treatment of Syphilis 303
Psychosomatic Disorders Manifested Mainly by Cardiovascular Symptoms 263
Ptosis or Prolapse of the Kidney 55
Spinal Anesthesia and the Reduction of Mortality in Surgery 22
Syphilis, Penicillin in the Treatment of 303
Davis Hospital Staff

CLINICS

Bronchopneumonia, Thrombosis Iliac Vein, Embolism Pulmonary Artery, Acute Cor Pulmonale 434
Constitutional Psychopathic Inadequacy or Mental Deficiency 250
Muscular Atrophy, Progressive Spinal 160
Psoas Abscess 57
Pulmonary Embolism Second to Thrombophlebitis of Femoral Vein 482
Pulmonary Infarction Due to Postoperative Embolism 433
F. R. Taylor

DEPARTMENTS

(Unsigned Department Editorials are by the Editor of the Department; in Departments in which there is more than one Editor, each Editorial is signed)

HUMAN BEHAVIOR

Ageing and Adaptation, On 262
Alcoholism, Political 484
Barbiturates and Bromides As Causes of Mental Disease 332
Death, Fear of 205
History of Medicine, On the 171
Illiteracy and Warfare 54
Medicine, On the History of 171
Medicine in North Carolina 293
Mental Disease, Barbiturates and Bromides as Causes of 332
Political Alcoholism 484
Prohibition Resurgent? 7

Psychiatric Beginnings, On 375
Responsibility, An Awful 435
Rum and War 87
Vaughan, Dr. Warren Taylor 140
War, Rum and 87
Warfare, Illiteracy and 54

DEPARTMENT EDITOR—*J. K. Hall*

ORTHOPEDIC SURGERY

Brachialgia 90
Hip Fractures 48
Low-Back Problem, The 7

DEPARTMENT EDITOR—*J. T. Saunders*

UROLOGY

Army, Venereal Diseases of the 45
Dysuria and Nocturia in the Female 134
Gonococcic Infections, Sulfonamide-Resistant 15
Gonorrhea in General Practice, Management of 344
Gonorrhea With Penicillin Sodium, Treatment of Sulfonamide-Resistant 380
Infections of the Urinary Tract Without Demonstrable Organisms 379
Lower Urinary Tract, Indications for Visual Examination of 257
Meatotomy a Valuable and Neglected Therapeutic Measure 485
Nocturia in the Female, Dysuria and... 134
Penicillin-Sodium, Treatment of Sulfonamide-Resistant Gonorrhea With 380
Prostatic Disease and Seminal Vesiculitis 213
Prostatic Disease: Prevention Suggested 177
Seminal Vesiculitis, Transurethral Drainage of the Seminal Vesicles in 443
Serious Urologic Disease May Be Painless, Even Symptomless 297
Sulfonamide-Resistant Gonococcic Infections 15
Sulfonamide-Resistant Gonorrhea With Penicillin Sodium, Treatment of 380
Transurethral Drainage of the Seminal Vesicles 443
Urologic Disease May Be Painless, Serious, Even Symptomless 297
Venereal Diseases of the Army 45
Vesiculitis: Prostatic and Seminal, Acute and Chronic 213
Visual Examination of the Lower Urinary Tract, Indications for 257

DEPARTMENT EDITOR—*Raymond Thompson*

SURGERY

Anesthesia, Refrigeration 259
Backache From Ruptured Intervertebral Disks 44
Bad-Risk Patient, Preoperative and Postoperative Care for the 294
Cancer of the Breast, Erysipeloid 391
Cancer, Skin 335
Cysts, Urogenital Retroperitoneal 437
Gangrene of the Testicle, Torsion of the Spermatic Cord With 174
Gastrojejunocolic Fistula 487
Intervertebral Disks, Backache From Ruptured 44
Laparotomy, The Right of the Surgeon to be Governed by his Judgment at 184
Linen as a Suture Material 210
Peritoneal Transplants After Traumatic Rupture of the Non-malignant Spleen.............. 87
Preoperative and Postoperative Care for the Bad-Risk Patient 294
Refrigeration Anesthesia 259
Right of the Surgeon to be Governed by his Judgment at Laparotomy, The.................. 134
Skin Cancer 335
Sodium Chloride Poisoning 16
Spermatic Cord With Gangrene of the Testicle, Torsion of the 174
Spleen, Peritoneal Transplants After Traumatic Rupture of the Non-malignant 87
Suture Material, Linen as a 210
Torsion of the Spermatic Cord With Gangrene of the Testicle 174
Traumatic Rupture of the Non-malignant Spleen, Peritoneal Transplants After 87
Urogenital Retroperitoneal Cysts 437

DEPARTMENT EDITOR—*G. H. Bunch*

OBSTETRICS

Anesthesia, Present Status of 211
Bicornate Uterus With Pregnancy in Each Horn 14
Ergot, Induction and Stimulation of Labor With 93
Fetus During Labor, The Care of the 93

Labor With Ergot, Induction and Stimulation of 93
Obstetrical Emergencies From the Standpoint of the General Practitioner 182
Office Delivery in Rural Obstetrics 131
Pregnancy Test, A Two- and Six-Hour 94

DEPARTMENT EDITOR—*H. J. Langston*

GYNECOLOGY

Cancer, Especially Gynecological Cancer, R. T. Ferguson 8
Eczema-Dermatitis of the External Genitalia, E. L. Lowenberg 216
Hormonal Therapy in Gynecologic Disorders, Injudicious, R. T. Ferguson 42
Octofollin in Estrogen Deficiencies and in Gonorrheal Vulvovaginitis, The Use of, R. T. Ferguson 97
Pelvic Examinations, Pertinent Points as to, R .T. Ferguson 298

DEPARTMENT EDITORS—*Chas. R. Robins & R. T. Ferguson*

GENERAL PRACTICE

Anemia in Pregnancy, J. L. Hamner 136
Angina Pectoris, The Prognosis of, J. L. Hamner 10
Appendicitis, Acute Virus Infection With Nerve Root Involvement Simulating, D. H. Smith.... 138
Asphyxiation, Fetal, J. L. Hamner 489
Bowel Habit—Think of Bowel Cancer, Change in, D. H. Smith 382
Cancer, Change in Bowel Habit—Think of Bowel, D. H. Smith 382
Cardiovascular Emergencies in the Home, The Treatment of, J. L. Hamner 9
Cardiovascular Round Table, J. L. Hamner 338
Chronic Heart Disease, Care of the Patient With, J. L. Hamner 337
Clept Lip and Palate in Babies, The Care of, J. L. Hamner 385
Colds, About Immunity to, J. L. Hamner 52
Coronary Disease: Its Recognition and Management, J. L. Hamner 51
Diabetes, Simplification of the Treatment of, J. L. Hamner 97
Endocrine Diagnosis and Therapy, Short Cuts in, J. L. Hamner 179
Endocrine Disease, Peptic Ulcer and, J. L. Hamner 51
Ethyl Chloride Spray for Freezing Donor Area in Skin Grafting, J. L. Hamner 214
Fetal Asphyxiation, J. L. Hamner 489
Fracture Treatment, Simplicity in, J. L. Hamner 181
Furunculosis, The Treatment of Multiple With Penicillin, D. H. Smith 439
Gingivostomatitis (Vincent), The Treatment of Acute, J. L. Hamner 137
Glycosuria, The Differential Diagnosis of, J. L. Hamner 441
Heart Disease, Care of the Patient With Chronic, J. L. Hamner 337
Hypertension, Potassium Thiocyanate in, D. H. Smith 176
Hypertension, Vitamin A in the Treatment of, D. H. Smith 175
Hypoglycemia, Masked, J. L. Hamner 442
Hypothyroidism, The Incidence of, D. H. Smith 254
Intravenous Therapy Technique, Practical Points in, D. H. Smith 92
Ivy Dermatitis, Evaluation of Measures for the Prevention of, D. H. Smith 50
Liver Function Tests, The Clinical Value of, D. H. Smith 502
Malaria, J. L. Hamner 299
Malaria, Encouragement As to, D. H. Smith 139
Ophthalmology in General Practice, D. H. Smith 234
Pancreatitis, The Conservative Management of Acute, J. L. Hamner 384
Paralysis, Sleep, J. L. Hamner 98
Peptic Ulcer, An Endocrine Disease, J. L. Hamner 51
Potassium Thiocyanate in Hypertension, D. H. Smith 176
Pregnancy, Anemia in, J. L. Hamner 136
Scabies, Another Rapid Treatment for, D. H. Smith 343
Scarlet Fever, Treatment of, D. H. Smith 439
Sick Headache Poorly Treated, J. L. Hamner 384
Skin Diseases, Therapy of Common, D. H. Smith 49
Skin Grafting, Ethyl Chloride-Spray for Freezing Donor Area in, J. L. Hamner 214
Sleep Paralysis, J. L. Hamner 98
Syphilis in Practice, Management of Some Common Phases of Late, D. H. Smith 343
Virus Infection With Nerve Root Involvement Simulating Appendicitis, Acute, D. H. Smith 138
Vitamin A in the Treatment of Hypertension, D. H. Smith 175

DEPARTMENT EDITORS—*J. L. Hamner & D. H. Smith*

LABORATORY MEDICINE & IMMUNOLOGY

Allergic?, A New Hope for the 52
Allergy, Leucopenic Index With Reference to Gastrointestinal 253
Blood Plasma 380
Collecting Specimens and Getting Them to the Laboratory, The Art of 334

Darling, Histoplasmosis of 20
False Positive Serologic Reactions, On the Importance of Malaria as a Cause of.................. 53
Forensic Laboratory Medicine 440
Gastrointestinal Allergy, Leucopenic Index With Reference to 253
Gynecology, A Synopsis of Laboratory Diagnosis 208
Histoplasmosis of Darling 20
Leucopenic Index With Reference to Gastrointestinal Allergy 253
Malaria as a Cause of False Positive Serologic Reactions, On the Importance of.................. 53
Plasma, Blood 380
Registered Medical Technologist Get That Way?, How Does a 301
Specimens and Getting Them to the Laboratory, The Art of Collecting 334

DEPARTMENT EDITORS—*J. M. Feder & Evelyn Tribble*

HOSPITALS

Build Additional Rooms Now, Most Hospitals Would Do Well to 47
Carolinas-Virginia Hospital Association, The Annual Meeting of the 252
Days Go By, As the 207
Post-war Hospitalization 388
Say What You Think 444

DEPARTMENT EDITOR—*R. B. Davis*

PUBLIC HEALTH

Step in Advance, A 213
War Manpower Commission Employment Stabilization Program, Health Workers Now Subject to 154

DEPARTMENT EDITOR—*N. T. Ennett*

THERAPEUTICS

Adolescence, Menstrual Problems of 99
Ambulatory Treatment of Cerebral Concussion 100
Anesthesia in Children, Intravenous 487
Anesthesia in Office Practice 341
Arteriosclerotic Heart Disease, Two Cases of Inflammatory and 220
Burns, The Treatment of Severe 381
Cerebral Concussion, Ambulatory Treatment of 100
Children, Intravenous Anesthesia in 487
Cyanide Poisoning, Treatment of 300
Gout, Successful Treatment of 46
Hand Infections 259
Heart Disease Seems Promising, New Treatment of 46
Heart Disease, Two Cases of Inflammatory and Arteriosclerotic 220
Malaria Treatment Today 172
Meningococcic Meningitis, The Treatment of 137
Menstrual Problems of Adolescence 99
Neurological Treatment in General Practice 11
Psychiatric Treatment Methods 193
Ruptured Intervertebral Disk, The 458

DEPARTMENT EDITOR—*J. F. Nash*

TUBERCULOSIS

British Phthisiologists, Some Early 376
Diagnosis and Treatment of Tuberculosis 176
Important Facts About Tuberculosis 128
Pulmonary Tuberculosis in supposedly Screened Selectees 212

DEPARTMENT EDITOR—*John Donnelly*

DENTISTRY

Ageing, The Teeth and 258
Bacteria Sealed in Dental Caries, The Fate of 16
Impacted Tooth, The Case Against 486
Infection in Filled, Vital, X-ray Negative Teeth 438
Oral Surgery by the General Practitioner of Dentistry, The Practice of................................ 91
Pulp, The Pathology and Treatment of the Exposed Vital 385
Sodium Fluoride on Dental Caries, The Effect of Topically Applied..................................... 136

DEPARTMENT EDITOR—*J. H. Guion*

INTERNAL MEDICINE

Dysentery and Its Treatment 18

DEPARTMENT EDITOR—*G. R. Wilkinson*

OPHTHALMOLOGY

Abnormalities of Pupillary Reaction, A Simple Method for Early Detection of 387
Asthenopia—"Eye Strain" 339
Cataract and That of Trauma, The Handling of Myopia of Incipient Senile 215
Cataract From Electrical Shock?, Bilateral, Case Report 12
Blunt Trauma to the Eye and Orbital Wall, Some Late Complications and Sequelae Following .. 436
Chalazion, The Surgical Removal of the 485
Children?, Rheumatic Fever or Syphilis in 50
Enucleation With Ball Implant, Verhoeff's Spectacle As an 251
"Eye Strain"—Asthenopia 339
Myope at the Beginning of Presbyopia, The 174
Myopia of Incipient Senile Cataract and That of Trauma, The Handling of 215
Myopia Sine Myopia (Incipient Myopia) 135
Phorometer *verus* The Trial Frame in Refraction, The 296
Presbyopia, The Myope at the Beginning of 174
Pupillary Reaction, A Simple Method for Early Detection of Abnormalities of 387
Refraction, The Phorometer *versus* the Trial Frame in 296
Rheumatic Fever or Syphilis in Children? 50
Rimless and Half-rimless Spectacle as an Eye Hazard, The 251
Verhoeff's Method of Unucleation With Ball Implant 91

DEPARTMENT EDITOR—*H. C. Neblett*

RHINO-OTO-LARYNGOLOGY

Epistaxis, Orbital 183
Hemorrhage, Control of Nasal 55
Otitis Media, A Therapeutic Regimen for 390
Tonsillitis, etc., Bismuth Salt of Heptadiene-Carboxylic Acid in Suppositories in 257

DEPARTMENT EDITOR—*C. W. Evatt*

PROCTOLOGY

Anal Fissue 209
Examinations, On the Importance of Making Rectal 260
Hemorrhoids 302
Hemorrhoids, Internal 443

DEPARTMENT EDITOR—*Russell Buxton*

INSURANCE MEDICINE

Applicant for Life Insurance, The 13
Heart Murmurs in Life Insurance 255
Mortality Increase Due to War, 1943 48

DEPARTMENT EDITOR—*H. F. Starr*

DERMATOLOGY

Cutaneous Medicine 43
Dermatologic Therapy, Recent Adjuncts to 210
Dermatophytid 21
Lupus Erythematosus, *R. O. Noojin* 88
Rosacea, *R. O. Noojin* 488
Wart, The Common 340

DEPARTMENT EDITOR—*J. L. Callaway*

PEDIATRICS

Acute Infectious Diseases in Childhood, Management of, *A. L. Hoyne* 345
Allergy in Childhood, The American Approach. *Lt. Col. H. N. Pratt* 291
American Paedriatricians, Papers by a Group of (Abs.) 291
Blood in the Stools of Infants and Children, *M. S. Rosenblatt* 133
Breast Milk for Emergency Feeding, *W. Ripley* 89
Convulsions in Childhood, *M. G. Peterman* 17
Deaths, The Lessons to be Learned From a Study of Infant, *E. L. Potter* 132
Dionne Quintuplets Outclassed (Abs. *H. A. M. A.*) 378
Emergency Feeding, Breast Milk for, *W. Ripley* 89
Enteric Diseases of Children, The Significance of the Widal Reaction in, *Morris Greenberg* ... 18

Enuresis, Discussion on, *T. H. Higgins et al.*, ... 292
Fibrosis of the Pancreas in Infants and Children, *Major C. D. May* 291
Hemorrhagic Disease in the Newborn, *L. P. Gray* 44
Herpetic Stomatitis in Infants and Children, *Major T. F. McN. Scott* 291
Immunization of Children, *M. W. Beach & B. O. Ravenel* 299
Infectious Diseases of Childhood, Management of Acute, *A. L. Hoyne* 345
Intravenous Injection in Infants, Technic of, *M. L. Spivek* 17
Lessons to be Learned From a Study of Infant Deaths, The, *E. L. Potter* 132
Pancreas in Infants and Children, Fibrosis of the, *Major C. D. May* 291
Poliomyelitis Prevention, Suggestions From the National Foundation for Infant Paralysis........ 261
Quintuplets Outclassed, Dionne (Abs. *J. A. M. A.*) 378
Stomatitis in Infants and Children, Herpetic, *Major T. F. McN. Scott* 291
Widal Reaction in Enteric Disease of Children, The Significance of the, *Morris Greenberg*........ 18

HISTORIC MEDICINE

Broode (1490-1549), Priest, Physician and Traveller, The Breviary and Dietary of Andrew
 (Abs.), *Douglas Guthrie* 382
Confederate States Hospital, The Great, Richmond *Times-Dispatch* 336
Gunshot Wounds of Three Presidents of the United States, *S. B. Harper* 129
Heberden and the Age of Reason, William, *Sir Walter Langdon-Brown* 94

TRI-STATE MEDICAL ASSOCIATION

Address of the President, *F. S. Johns* 75
Darden Dies, Dr. 492
McCampbell, Dr. John 438
McIntosh, Dr. James H. 397
McLeod, Dr. Frank Hilton 438
President's Page, *K. B. Pace* 143, 267
Program 27, 60
Soldiers Discharged on Account of Nervous Disabilities, *K. B. Pace* 491
Special Place in Medicine 101
Tri-State Meeting, The Coming 492

AUTHORS

Bigham, R. S., Jr. 425	Lyerly, J. G. 124
Bunch, G. H. 469	Maguire, D. L., Jr. 411
Callaway, J. L. 463	Martin, W. J. 159
Camp, P. D. 473	Noojin, R. O. 463
Copley, E. L. 170, 416	Offutt, V. D. 5
Cranford, V. 327	Pace, K. B. 329
Davis, J. W. 480	Palmer, Y. S. 203, 363
Davis, R. B. 476	Preston, J. Z. 471
Donnelly, G. L. 363	Prioleau, W. H. 201
Fearing, J. M. 164	Reynolds, C. V. 281
Feder, J. M. 247	Rucker, M. P. 407
Freeman, W. 233	Saunders, J. R. 203
Gilland, J. D. 420	Schafile, Karl 243
Goldzicher, M. A. 39	Seliger, R. V. 327
Greenblatt, R. B. 1	Shield, J. A. 420
Hall, J. K. 321	Shields, R. T. 113
Hart, V. K. 167	Starr, H. F. 83
Hedgpeth, E. McG. 238	Todd, L. C. 287
Hesser, F. H. 120	Tucker, B. R. 117
Hunt, S. P. 370	Ussery, T. S. 3
Johns, Wm. A. 478	Watts, J. W. 233
Johns, F. S. 75	Williams, E. J. 197
Jordan, W. R. 364	Woodward, L. F. 365
Kupperman, H. L. 1	Yerguson, R. M. 37
Laub, G. R. 374	

Lightning Source UK Ltd.
Milton Keynes UK
UKHW040929180920
370091UK00001BA/62